MANUAL OF CLINICAL ONCOLOGY

Sixth Edition

MANUAL OF CLINICAL ONCOLOGY
Sixth Edition

Editor

Dennis A. Casciato, MD
Clinical Professor of Medicine
David Geffen School of Medicine at UCLA
Los Angeles, California

Associate Editor

Mary C. Territo, MD
Professor of Medicine
David Geffen School of Medicine at UCLA
Hematopoietic Stem Transplantation Program
UCLA Center for the Health Sciences
Los Angeles, California

Wolters Kluwer | Lippincott Williams & Wilkins
Health
Philadelphia · Baltimore · New York · London
Buenos Aires · Hong Kong · Sydney · Tokyo

Senior Executive Editor: Jonathan W. Pine, Jr.
Senior Managing Editor: Anne E. Jacobs
Senior Project Manager: Rosanne Hallowell
Senior Manufacturing Manager: Benjamin Rivera
Marketing Manager: Angela Panetta
Art Director: Risa Clow
Production Services: Aptara, Inc.

Sixth Edition
© 2009 by Lippincott Williams & Wilkins, a Wolters Kluwer business
530 Walnut Street
Philadelphia, PA 19106
LWW.com

© 2000, 2004 by Lippincott Williams & Wilkins. © 1983, 1988, 1995 by Little, Brown & Company.

Printed in the United States

Library of Congress Cataloging-in-Publication Data

Manual of clinical oncology / editor, Dennis A. Casciato; associate editor, Mary C. Territo. — 6th ed.
   p. ; cm.
   Includes bibliographical references and index.
   ISBN-13: 978-0-7817-6884-9
   ISBN-10: 0-7817-6884-5
1. Cancer—Handbooks, manuals, etc.   2. Oncology—Handbooks, manuals, etc.   I. Casciato, Dennis Albert.   II. Territo, Mary C.
   [DNLM: 1. Medical Oncology—methods—Handbooks.   2. Neoplasms—diagnosis—Handbooks.
   3. Neoplasms—therapy—Handbooks.   QZ 39 M2943 2009]
   RC262.5.M36 2009
   616.99′4—dc22

                                                              2008026304

                                        10 9 8 7 6 5 4 3 2 1

CONTENTS

I: GENERAL ASPECTS

II: SOLID TUMORS

III: HEMATOPOIETIC MALIGNANCIES

IV: COMPLICATIONS

APPENDICES

*T*he *Manual of Clinical Oncology,* which has attained major popularity as a reference source for oncology fellows, residents, and medical students, is completely revised for its sixth edition. Like its predecessors, it focuses on information useful for making diagnostic and therapeutic decisions at the bedside of patients with cancer. The goal for the Manual has been to remain comprehensive, current, and concise, without being susceptible to rapid obsolescence. Redundancy is not allowed. Evanescent aspects of oncology, such as chemotherapy "regimens of the month," have been assiduously avoided.

The chapters are grouped into four parts. Part I presents the principles of diagnosis and treatment of cancer. Parts II and III address the specific malignancies in a uniform format. Part IV presents complications of cancer according to end-organ involvement, whether by local invasion, metastasis, paraneoplasia, or therapy. The Appendices present cytogenetic nomenclature (Appendix A); the complications of chemotherapy and toxicity criteria for evaluating patients in clinical trials (Appendix B); tumor identifiers, such as immunohistochemical differential diagnosis, leukocyte differentiation antigens, and the World Health Organization's classifications of hematopoietic malignancies (Appendix C); and the most useful chemotherapeutic regimens for lymphomas (Appendix D).

The first edition was written nearly exclusively by Dr. Barry Lowitz and me. New authors contributing to subsequent editions significantly expanded the expertise and geographic distribution of the faculty. Yet, every line of the entire book has been punctiliously redacted by this editor to ensure consistency in organization, content, style, and philosophy. For the current edition, we gratefully welcome the important contributions of the following "first-time" authors: Dr. Bartosz Chmielowski, Dr. Nancy Klipfel, Dr. Dan Leibovici, Dr. Theodore Moore, Dr. Ron Paquette, Dr. Mark Pegram, Dr. Lauren Pinter-Brown, Dr. Antoni Ribas, Dr. Gary Schiller, Dr. Eric Sherman, and Dr. Przemyslaw Twardowski. I am most pleased to welcome my friend and colleague, Dr. Mary Territo, not only as a new contributor, but also as Associate Editor. Her work in organizing the hematologic malignancies with their enormous changes was greatly appreciated.

Cancer management involves so many clinical and psychosocial parameters that treatment based on any finite number of data points is patently illogical. Each patient is unique and almost never has a clinical course that follows a predictable statistical model. The complex and unpredictable nature of cancer makes treatment decisions a high art, refined by a balance of science, personal experience, common sense, and sound synthesis.

This sixth edition of the *Manual of Clinical Oncology* reaffirms the unique relationship between patient and doctor and continues its commitment to provide the caregiver with the ability to temper today's popular interventions with good judgment and a cautious openmindedness to the promise of tomorrow.

D.A.C.

*T*his sixth edition of the *Manual of Clinical Oncology* is earnestly dedicated to Registered Nurses working oncology units and offices everywhere. Their special calling is highly respected and greatly appreciated by both oncologists and their patients.

Specifically, this edition is dedicated to those RNs with whom I have worked directly and continuously for one to two decades, both in my private clinic and at the Providence Tarzana Medical Center Oncology Unit in Tarzana, California. (To those who are not familiar with the territory: Yes, Tarzana is named for Edgar Rice Burroughs' progeny and is located in the western section of San Fernando Valley in Los Angeles County.) I highly value their sincere sensitivity to patients' needs. I am comforted by their funds of knowledge. I trust their clinical judgments. I rest calmly knowing that they are taking care of my patients when I am not there. These ladies are established role models for their profession.

To:

Denise Rebbie-Galpin
Ellen Madey
Leslie Rosenberg
Lisa Edwards
Felicia Kidd
Elana Farquhason
Marlene Organ
Robin Sartellano
Laurie Haynes
Nida Delarmente
Yunche Smith
Jan Richter
Susie Loomis
Kelly McIntyre

Thank you for being there for my patients and for me,

Dennis A. Casciato, MD

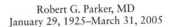
Robert G. Parker, MD
January 29, 1925–March 31, 2005

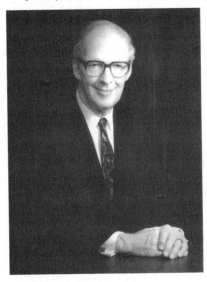

$\mathcal{D}$r. Parker was a pioneer in the field of Radiation Oncology. In fact, he was one of the founding fathers of the discipline that seceded from its cousin, Diagnostic Radiology.

Dr. Parker received his college education at the University of Michigan and earned his Doctor of Medicine degree from the University of Wisconsin in 1948. After internship at the University of Nebraska, he fulfilled residency training in pathology at Western Reserve University and then completed a residency in radiology at the University of Michigan. He subsequently completed postdoctoral work at the Tumor Institute of the Swedish Hospital in Seattle, Washington, and pursued further postgraduate education in nuclear medicine at Columbia University.

From 1958 to 1977, he served as the Director of Therapeutic Radiology at the University of Washington. He was the founding chairman of the Department of Radiation Oncology at the University of California at Los Angeles in 1977, and he served in that capacity until 1994. He remained active clinically until his retirement in January, 2005.

Dr. Parker achieved a long list of academic accomplishments, including publication of more than 155 peer-reviewed articles and 43 book chapters. He was the lead author for Chapters 3 and 7 for this *Manual of Clinical Oncology* since its second edition. He also held visiting professorships at many major universities in the United States and abroad and was invited to deliver numerous prestigious lectureships.

He served as the President of several leading professional organizations, including the American Society of Radiology and Oncology (ASTRO), the Radiological Society of North

America (RSNA), the American Board of Radiology (ABR), and the American Radium Society (ARS), all of which have honored him with either a gold medal or life-achievement recognition.

A true gentleman and scholar, Dr. Parker represents the aggregate epitome of a clinical scientist, an effective educator, and a compassionate physician. His legacy in the field of radiation oncology is perhaps best portrayed by his presidential address for ASTRO in 1976:

> Each of you has made a primary responsibility to humans afflicted by cancer. Such a responsibility requires interests far beyond what is included in a restrictive definition of therapeutic radiology. Indeed, your highest responsibility is to reduce the frequency of or even eliminate cancer, even though radiation therapy is the sustaining base of your current intellectual and economic activities. Thus maintenance of your recognized central position in clinical cancer activities ultimately will not rest on advocacy of a treatment method, but on a myriad of activities which have an underlying common objective of reducing or even eliminating the need for such treatment.

As witnessed by medical students and residents, Dr. Parker spent most of his time with patients in the clinic talking not about cancer, but rather about *living*. In private life, he once scrimmaged with the Detroit Red Wings, played trombone for the Woody Herman Orchestra, led the University of Michigan marching band, and was a gourmet cook and a jazz piano player. His office at UCLA was decorated with magnificent photographs taken from his trips around the world. He made the physicians at UCLA use blue and gold as background colors for presentation slides, but some continue to suspect that it was meant for the Michigan Wolverines rather than for the UCLA Bruins. During the memorial to celebrate his life at UCLA on June 23, 2005, friends and distinguished scholars from all over the country came and paid tribute to this wonderful human being so loved by everyone. We miss you, Professor!

Steve P. Lee, MD
For the Editors

ACKNOWLEDGMENTS

The Editor extends his most sincere gratitude to Eve Perkins and her staff for their continued assistance to the *Manual of Clinical Oncology*. Eve is the medical librarian at Northridge Hospital Medical Center in Northridge, California. Her literature searches for me were indispensable. I also graciously thank Anne E. Jacobs, Senior Managing Editor for Medicine at Lippincott Williams & Wilkins, and Donna Kessler of Aptara, Inc. for their personal support and efforts to make this publication a success.

Dennis A. Casciato, MD

*It is not hard to compose,
but it is wonderfully hard to let the superfluous notes
fall under the table.*

—Johannes Brahms

*No passion in the world is equal to the passion to
alter someone else's draft.*

—H.G. Wells

CONTRIBUTORS

Steven R. Alberts, MD
Associate Professor of Oncology
Mayo Medical School
Rochester, Minnesota

Jonathan S. Berek, MD, MMS
Professor and Chair
Department of Obstetrics and Gynecology
Stanford University School of Medicine
Palo Alto, California

James R. Berenson, MD
Medical and Scientific Director
President and CEO
Institute for Myeloma & Bone Cancer
   Research
Hollywood, California

Russell K. Brynes, MD
Professor of Clinical Pathology
University of Southern California Keck
   School of Medicine
Director of Special Hematology Laboratory
Los Angeles County—USC Medical Center
Los Angeles, California

Harold E. Carlson, MD
Professor of Medicine
Head of Endocrinology Division
Stony Brook University School of Medicine
Stony Brook, New York

Dennis A. Casciato, MD
Clinical Professor of Medicine
David Geffen School of Medicine at UCLA
Attending Physician
Hematology-Oncology Section, VA Greater
   Los Angeles Healthcare System
Los Angeles, California

Howard A. Chansky, MD
Professor and Co-vice Chair,
Department of Orthopaedics and Sports
   Medicine
University of Washington School of
   Medicine
Chief, Section of Orthopaedics,
VA Puget Sound Healthcare System
Seattle, Washington

Bartosz Chmielowski, MD, PhD
Fellow
Division of Hematology-Oncology
David Geffen School of Medicine at UCLA
Los Angeles, California

Lisa M. DeAngelis, MD
Professor of Neurology
Weill Medical College of Cornell University
Chairman, Department of Neurology
Lillian Rojtman Berkman Chair in Honor of
   Jerome B. Posner
Memorial Sloan-Kettering Cancer Center
New York, New York

Chaitanya R. Divgi, MD
Professor of Radiology
University of Pennsylvania
Chief of Nuclear Medicine and Clinical
   Molecular Imaging
University of Pennsylvania
Philadelphia, Pennsylvania

Martin J. Edelman, MD
Professor of Medicine
Division of Medical Thoracic Oncology
University of Maryland Greenebaum
   Cancer Center
Baltimore, Maryland

Lawrence H. Einhorn, MD
Distinguished Professor of Medicine
Indiana University
Indianapolis, Indiana

Robert A. Figlin, MD, FACP
Professor, Beckman Research Institute
City of Hope National Medical Center
Chair, Division of Medical Oncology &
   Experimental Therapeutics
City of Hope National Medical Center
Duarte, California
Emeritus Professor
David Geffen School of Medicine at UCLA
Los Angeles, California

Charles A. Forscher, MD
Assistant Clinical Professor of Medicine
David Geffen School of Medicine at UCLA
Sarcoma Program Director
Cedars-Sinai Outpatient Cancer Center
Los Angeles, California

David R. Gandara, MD
Professor of Medicine
Associate Director of Clinical Research
University of California Davis Medical
Center
Sacramento, California

W. Lance George, MD
Professor of Medicine
David Geffen School of Medicine at UCLA
Associate Chief of Medicine
VA Greater Los Angeles Healthcare System
Los Angeles, California

Richard M. Goldberg, MD
Professor and Chief of Hematology and
Oncology
University of North Carolina at Chapel
Hill
Associate Director, University of North
Carolina Lineberger Comprehensive
Cancer Center
Chapel Hill, North Carolina

Carole G. H. Hurvitz, MD
Clinical Professor of Pediatrics
David Geffen School of Medicine at UCLA
Director of Pediatric Hematology/
Oncology
Cedars-Sinai Medical Center
Los Angeles, California

Nancy Klipfel, MD
Assistant Professor of Clinical Pathology
University of Southern California Keck
School of Medicine
Los Angeles, California

David W. Knutson, MD
Professor of Medicine
The Pennsylvania State University College
of Medicine
Hershey, Pennsylvania

Steve P. Lee, MD
Associate Professor in Clinical Radiation
Oncology
David Geffen School of Medicine at UCLA
Los Angeles, California

Dan Leibovici, MD
The Urology Department
Assaf Harofeh Medical Center
Zerifin, Israel

Alexandra M. Levine, MD
Distinguished Professor of Medicine
University of Southern California Keck
School of Medicine
Los Angeles, California
Chief Medical Officer
City of Hope Medical Center
Duarte, California

Barry B. Lowitz, MD
Emeritus Associate Clinical Professor of
Medicine
David Geffen School of Medicine at UCLA
Los Angeles, California

Sanaz Memarzadeh, MD, PhD
Assistant Professor
David Geffen School of Medicine at UCLA
Department of Obstetrics and Gynecology
Division of Gynecologic Oncology
Los Angeles, California

Theodore B. Moore, MD
Associate Professor of Pediatrics
Director of Pediatric Blood and Marrow
Transplant Program
David Geffen School of Medicine at UCLA
Los Angeles, California

Ronald L. Paquette, MD
Associate Professor Medicine
David Geffen School of Medicine at UCLA
Los Angeles, California

Robert G. Parker, MD
Professor of Radiation Oncology
David Geffen School of Medicine at UCLA
Los Angeles, California

Mark D. Pegram, MD
Professor of Medicine
University of Miami, Miller School of
Medicine
Director of Translational Research
Braman Breast Cancer Research Institute
University of Miami—Sylvester
Comprehensive Cancer Center
Miami, Florida

Lauren C. Pinter-Brown, MD
Clinical Professor of Medicine
Director, Lymphoma Program
David Geffen School of Medicine at UCLA
Los Angeles, California

Eric E. Prommer, MD
Assistant Professor Medicine
Mayo Clinic College of Medicine
Director of Palliative Care
Scottsdale, Arizona

Antoni Ribas, MD
Assistant Professor of Medicine and
    Surgery
David Geffen School of Medicine at UCLA
Los Angeles, California

Dale H. Rice, MD
Tiber/Alpert Professor and Chair
Department of Otolaryngology—Head and
    Neck Surgery
University of Southern California Keck
    School of Medicine
Los Angeles, California

Gary J. Schiller, MD
Professor-in-Residence
David Geffen School of Medicine at UCLA
Director of Hematopoietic Stem Cell
    Transplantation
UCLA Center for the Health Sciences
Los Angeles, California

Eric J. Sherman, MD
Assistant Attending Physician
Memorial Sloan Kettering Cancer Center
New York, New York

Mary C. Territo, MD
Professor of Medicine
David Geffen School of Medicine at UCLA
Hematopoietic Stem Cell Transplantation
    Program
UCLA Center for the Health Sciences
Los Angeles, California

Przemyslaw Twardowski, MD
Assistant Professor of Medicine
Department of Medical Oncology and
    Experimental Therapeutics
City of Hope Medical Center
Duarte, California

Richard F. Wagner, Jr., MD
Professor of Dermatology
University of Texas Medical Branch at
    Galveston
Galveston, Texas

Amnon Zisman, MD
Vice Chairman
Department of Urology
Assaf-Harofeh Medical Center
Tel Aviv University
Tel Aviv, Israel

General Aspects

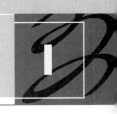

PRINCIPLES, DEFINITIONS, AND STATISTICS

Barry B. Lowitz and Dennis A. Casciato

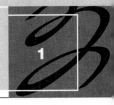

No one can get tomorrow's news before it happens.—BL

I. SOME PRINCIPLES OF CANCER BIOLOGY AND CANCER TREATMENT

A. Normal cell reproduction

1. **The cell cycle** is depicted in Fig. 1.1. Cell replication proceeds through a number of phases that are biochemically initiated by external stimuli and modulated by both external and internal growth controls. Certain oncogenes and cell cycle–specific proteins are activated and deactivated synchronously as the cell progresses through the phases of the cell cycle. Most cells must enter the cell cycle to be killed by chemotherapy or radiation therapy. Many cytotoxic agents act at more than one phase of the cell cycle, including those classified as *phase specific*.

   a. In the **G_0 phase** (gap 0 or resting phase), cells are generally programmed to perform specialized functions. An example of drugs that are active in this phase is glucocorticoids for mature lymphocytes.

   b. In the **G_1 phase** (gap 1 or interphase), proteins and RNA are synthesized for specialized cell functions. In late G_1, a burst of RNA synthesis occurs, and many of the enzymes necessary for DNA synthesis are manufactured. An example of drugs that are active in this phase is L-asparaginase.

   c. In the **S phase** (DNA synthesis), the cellular content of DNA doubles. Examples of drugs that are active in this phase are procarbazine and antimetabolites.

   d. In the **G_2 phase** (gap 2), DNA synthesis ceases, protein and RNA synthesis continues, and the microtubular precursors of the mitotic spindle are produced. Examples of drugs that are active in this phase are bleomycin and plant alkaloids.

   e. In the **M phase** (mitosis), the rates of protein and RNA synthesis diminish abruptly while the genetic material is segregated into daughter cells. After completion of mitosis, the new cells enter either the G_0 or the G_1 phase. Examples of drugs that are active in this phase are plant alkaloids.

2. **Cyclins** activate the various phases of the cell cycle. Most normal cells capable of reproduction proliferate in response to external stimuli, such as growth factors, certain hormones, and antigen–histocompatibility complexes, which affect cell-surface receptors. These receptors then transduce the signal that results in cell division. Tyrosine kinases (TKs) are an essential part of the cascade of proliferative signals, from extracellular growth factors to the nucleus. Cyclins combine with, activate, and direct the action of special TKs, called *cyclin-dependent kinases*.

3. **Cell cycle *checkpoints*.** Cells that are capable of reproducing are normally stopped at specific phases of the cell cycle called *checkpoints*. The most important of these are immediately preceding the initiation of DNA synthesis and immediately preceding the act of mitosis. These histologically quiescent periods are probably mediated by decreased activity of cyclin-associated kinases and tumor-suppressor proteins. In fact, the cells in these phases are biochemically active as they prepare proteins to enter the next phase of the cell cycle and correct any genetic defects before going on to reproduce.

   a. **Normal cells have mechanisms that detect abnormalities in DNA sequences.** When DNA is damaged, a number of repair mechanisms replace

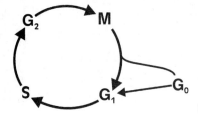

Figure 1.1. Phases of cell growth.

damaged nucleotides with normal molecules. These mechanisms are most important during cellular reproduction to ensure that new genetic material in daughter cells is an exact copy of the parent cell.

b. The first checkpoint occurs in the late G_1 phase, just before cells enter the S phase. Even if the proper extracellular signals are received and all of the machinery is in place for DNA synthesis, the DNA must be in an acceptable state, with no lesions, before the cell can leave G_1. If lesions are detected, they either are repaired or the cell is made to undergo apoptosis. This stopping point is one of the actions of the *p53* protein (see section I.C.3.b).

c. The second checkpoint occurs just before the cell enters the M phase; the cell cycle inhibitors stop the cell until it is determined whether the new progeny are worthy successors with accurate genetic copies of the parent. A cell that has not completely and accurately replicated all of its DNA or that does not have the full complement of proteins, spindle materials, and other substances to complete mitosis is arrested at this checkpoint until everything is in order and before the M phase can begin.

4. Normal populations of cells have a small component of "immortal cells," which, when called on by signals from other parts of the organism, can replenish themselves and also supply daughter cells that mature and differentiate into specialized tissue cells necessary for the function of the whole organism. Although a few types of tissue can dedifferentiate, most cell types lose their vitality as they differentiate, enter senescence, and eventually die. The following four populations of normal cells can be identified in eukaryotes:

a. Germ cells, which are capable of reproducing themselves indefinitely, possibly as a result of going through meiosis. Unlike cancer cells, these cells must undergo a meiotic "event" to produce an immortal cell line.

b. Stem cells, whose only two functions are to reproduce and to produce cells destined to differentiate and perform specialized functions for the host. Unlike cancer cells, these cells have a limited biological number of reproductive cycles.

c. Partially differentiated cells, which have limited capability to reproduce and whose progeny eventually become fully differentiated, nonreproducing cells.

d. Fully mature specialized cells, which cannot reproduce further generations.

5. Differentiation is inversely related to immortality. Unlike cancer cell lines that are immortal by definition, differentiated normal cells have a biological "clock" that counts the number of times the cell can divide, after which no further division is possible. For example, a human fibroblast in culture can divide about 50 times, no matter what it is fed or the conditions of its culture, and then it and its progeny can divide no further.

B. Characteristics of cancer cells. Cancer can be defined as a cellular disorder characterized by progressive accumulation of a mass of cells, as a result of excessive reproduction of cells not compensated by appropriate cell loss; these cells progressively invade and damage the tissues and organs of the host. Although cancer cells are abnormal and die at a faster rate than their normal counterparts, the death rate is not able to keep up with the formation of new cells. This imbalance is the result both of genetic abnormalities in cancer cells and of the inability of the host to detect and destroy such cells. Some of the unique characteristics of cancer cells follow.

1. **Clonal origin.** Most cancer cells appear to originate from a single abnormal cell. Some cancers arise from multiple malignant clones either as a result of a *field defect*, in which multiple cells of a tissue are exposed to a carcinogen (such as the upper airways in smokers), or as a result of inherited defects in certain genes.

2. **Immortality and telomeres.** Most normal cells have limits on the number of reproductive cycles that a cell can have as it matures. Cancer cells, on the other hand, can proliferate indefinitely, providing an inexhaustible pool of precursor cells. One mechanism for immortality involves telomeres, the ends of chromosomes. Telomeres of most types of normal cells progressively shorten as the cells differentiate. In contrast, the telomeres of cancer cells and stem cells are replenished by the enzyme telomerase. This enzyme normally progressively decreases in a programmed manner as cells differentiate; the fully differentiated cell becomes senescent and eventually dies as it loses its ability to reproduce. In contrast, telomerase production is preserved or activated in many types of cancer cells; consequently, the length of the telomeres remains intact, and the cell remains "immortal."

3. **Genetic instability** due to defects in DNA repair and in detection of DNA mismatches leads to heterogeneity of cancer cells. The cancer cells produce clones that become progressively less responsive to control mechanisms of proliferation and have an increased capacity to survive in "foreign environments" as metastases.

4. **Loss of contact inhibition and anchorage-dependent growth.** Normal cells grown in tissue culture do not divide unless they become anchored to a solid substratum to which they can adhere. Normal cells also stop dividing when they attain a confluent monolayer, even if the culture medium contains all the growth factors and nutrients necessary for further division. Cancer cells can grow independently in a semisolid medium without the requirement for substrate adherence; they continue to proliferate beyond a confluent monolayer in cell culture.

5. **Progressive independence of proliferation from growth factors and nutrients** is noted in cancer cell cultures. Cancer cells can actually self-destruct by continuing to divide even after they have consumed the nutritional factors in the culture media necessary for their survival.

6. **Metastasis** is a feature of cancer that is not found in normal tissues or benign tumors. The ability to metastasize results from the loss of or abnormalities of cellular proteins responsible for adhesion to the extracellular matrix, abnormalities in the interaction between cells, abnormal attachment to basement membrane, abnormal production of basement membrane, destruction of basement membrane by enzymes such as the metalloproteases (collagenases), and many other factors.

C. **Causes of overproduction of cancer cells**

1. **Failure of abnormal cells to undergo apoptosis.** Apoptosis is *programmed cell death.* An initial stimulus sets off an extremely complex cascade of events eventually resulting in apoptosis.

    a. **Apoptosis occurs in normal tissue reabsorption;** the classic example is the disappearance of tadpoles' tails. Apoptosis also results in the disappearance during embryogenesis of webs between fingers of primates, allowing the formation of individual digits. Apoptosis results in the elimination of normal senescent cells when they become old and useless and, of thymic T cells that recognize "self" and thereby prevent immune attack by these cells on the host.

    b. **Apoptosis eliminates cells with abnormal DNA** caused by either irreparable DNA damage or by inaccurate, incomplete, or redundant transcription of DNA. This is a major mechanism for maintaining chromosome number in cells of a particular species and in preventing aneuploidy. The process ensures that only cells that have fully and accurately replicated their entire DNA can enter mitosis.

    c. **Apoptotic cells can be recognized microscopically.** Apoptotic cells show clumps of intracellular organelles in the absence of necrosis. The nuclei are condensed and fragmented; intracellular structures are degenerated and compartmentalized. As the cell falls apart, phagocytes take up the fragments. Unlike the process of cell necrosis, apoptosis does not cause an inflammatory response. Apoptosis requires synthesis of specific proteins that have been highly conserved throughout evolution.

d. Apoptosis is genetically regulated and may be perturbed in malignant cells. Cancer cells and some immunologic cells produce substances that promote inappropriate apoptosis in normal tissues (and may contribute to the cachexia of malignancy). For example, the *p53* tumor-suppressor oncogene stimulates apoptosis. The *Bcl-2* oncogene inhibits apoptosis, decreases normal cell death, and increases cell populations. Apoptosis may be the major mechanism by which tumor cell populations are decreased by hormones, cytotoxic chemotherapy, and radiation therapy.

e. Caspases. The final stage of the various death pathways is mediated through activation of the caspases, which represent a family of cysteine proteases. The activation of caspases is determined by the intrinsic and extrinsic pathways of apoptosis.

The intrinsic pathway is a mitochondrial-dependent pathway mediated by the *Bcl-2* family of proteins. Exposure to cytotoxic stress results in disruption of the mitochondrial membrane, which then leads to release of protease activators. Caspase-9 is subsequently activated, setting off a cascade of events that commits the cell to undergo apoptosis.

The extrinsic pathway is mediated by ligand binding to the tumor necrosis factor (TNF) family of receptors, which includes TNF-related apoptosis-inducing ligand (TRAIL) and others, and certain essential adaptor proteins. These adaptor proteins recruit various proteases that cleave the N-terminal domain of caspase-8, which leads to activation of the caspase cascade.

2. Genetic abnormalities that inappropriately stimulate cell proliferation, independent of normal proliferation signals, occur through a variety of mechanisms. Mutations or overproduction of receptors or transducing proteins can cause the cell to become independent of growth factor or other triggers and to initiate cell division independently. These gene abnormalities are usually dominant (i.e., normal cells hybridized with abnormal cells become phenotypically malignant).

3. Abnormalities of tumor-suppressor genes (genes that are responsible for suppressing cell division) probably result in cancer through failure of the host to destroy genetically abnormal cells. These genes are recessive; malignant cells hybridized with normal cells become normal.

a. Hereditary tumors. Retinoblastoma gene (*RB1*) was the first of these abnormal genes to be discovered. Subsequently, a number of other suppressor gene abnormalities have been found, particularly in uncommon or rare hereditary diseases. Examples include Wilms' tumor (*WT1*), familial polyposis (*APC*), familial melanoma (*CDKN20*), and familial breast and ovarian cancers (*BRCA-1* and *BRCA-2*).

b. *p53* Suppressor gene. The most important example of these genes is the *p53* suppressor gene. The *p53* protein is a gene product that suppresses the cell cycle with multiple complex activities. It can detect DNA lesions, such as nucleotide mismatches and DNA strand breaks, including those caused by radiation and chemotherapy. This function of *p53* is thought to be critical in preserving the integrity of the cellular genome.

(1) When DNA lesions are detected, the *p53* protein arrests cells in the quiescent G_1 and G_2 phases of the cell cycle, preventing cells from entering the DNA synthetic (S) phase of the cell cycle. The *p53* protein can then induce repair mechanism proteins or trigger proteins, which cause apoptosis.

(2) In the absence of intact apoptosis, cancer cells can continue through sequential cell divisions and accumulate nucleotide mismatches and progressive DNA mutations.

(3) *In vitro* studies have shown that chemotherapy and radiation kill cancer cells through DNA damage, which triggers *p53* protein–induced apoptosis. In contrast, *p53* protein–deficient mouse thymocytes and resting lymphocytes remain viable after irradiation.

(4) Many human cancers are found to have mutant *p53* suppressor genes. Mutant *p53* is characteristic of Li-Fraumeni syndrome, a hereditary autosomal dominant syndrome of both soft tissue and epithelial cancers at multiple sites starting at an early age.

4. **Tumor angiogenesis.** Cancer colonies are not larger than about 1 mm in diameter unless they have a blood supply. Colonies without adequate blood supply are not resting (not in the G_0 cell cycle phase); they typically have a high rate of proliferation but a fully compensating cellular death rate. After the blood supply is established, the cellular death rate decreases, and the tumor grows rapidly.

   a. **Several substances are required to promote formation of new blood vessels** (angiogenesis) in normal tissues. Almost all measurable cancers, however, are limited to the production of only one of these factors, called *vascular endothelial growth factor* (VEGF), which induces blood vessel formation. VEGF has a number of interesting properties that may be useful for cancer treatment, including the following:

   (1) VEGF induces receptors for itself on mature and nonproliferating blood vessel endothelial cells. These normal, resting endothelial cells do not have the receptor until they are exposed to VEGF.

   (2) VEGF induces the production and activity of multiple other growth factors that contribute to blood vessel formation.

   (3) VEGF can be induced by *c-ras* and by other oncogenes and growth factors, which then induce further production of VEGF.

   (4) Unlike normal blood vessels that require other factors for normal development, blood vessels induced by VEGF are "leaky." VEGF-induced plasma proteins, such as fibrinogen, can leak out of the new vessels, forming a spongy gel around the tumor. This gel contains VEGF, which induces further angiogenesis.

   (5) VEGF appears to prevent apoptosis in induced endothelial cells.

   b. **Tumors also elaborate angiogenesis inhibitors,** which can decrease growth of tumor at distant sites. One form of murine lung cancer gives rise to metastases that elaborate such inhibitors and suppress the growth of the primary site. This mechanism may account for the difficulty in locating primary tumors that present with metastases and for the absence of a detectable primary tumor (metastases of unknown origin).

5. **Population kinetics.** Tumor growth depends on the size of the proliferating pool of cells and the number of cells dying spontaneously. The larger the tumor mass, the greater the percentage of nondividing and dying cells and the longer it takes for the average cell to divide. Fig. 1.2 demonstrates the theoretic tumor growth curve based on the Gompertzian model of tumor growth and regression. Some features of this sigmoid-shaped curve on logarithmic coordinates are as follows:

   a. **The lag phase.** During the earliest phase of tumor development, a small mass of a tumor does not enlarge very much. The working hypotheses about this lag phase are that the "pre-cancer" cells are dividing, but the rate of birth of new cells is offset by cell death. During this phase, the dividing cells are accumulating various mutations. These mutations help the surviving cells improve their adaptivity to the supply of nutrients, increase the rate at which the mutated cells divide, decrease the rate of apoptosis sensitivity (e.g., c-kit factor), provide them with invasive properties, make the mutated cells more responsiveness to host factors, and produce angiogenesis factors. Before the angiogenesis factors are expressed, the small tumor does not have its own blood supply and is dependent on local factors to get all the necessary nutrients. Although not shown on the graph, animal models suggested that these tiny cancers may remain unchanged in size and undetectable for many years before they enter the logarithmic phase and are large enough to be detectable.

   b. **The log phase.** The tumor now shows rapid exponential growth of the tumor mass. Hypothetically, the reasons for this phase are a relatively high proportion of cells are undergoing division, with rapidly declining rates of cell death; the *growth fraction* (ratio of dividing to total cells) is high. This rapid growth also reflects the adaptivity of the cells and the production by the tumor cells of angiogenesis factors which induce the surrounding tissues to form new blood vessels that "feed" the tumor mass. When the tumor's growth fraction is at its

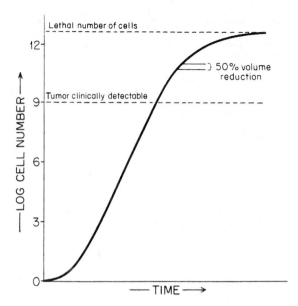

Figure 1.2. Tumor growth in diameter found on chest x-ray film or by breast examination. Tumors with 10^{12} and 10^{13} cells (about 2 to 20 lb of cancer) usually result in damage to vital organs and death of the patient.

highest level, it is still clinically undetectable. Although the reduction in cell number is small, the fractional cell kill from a dose of effective chemotherapy would be significantly higher than later in the course of the tumor.

   c. The plateau phase. Tumor growth slows down as the percentage of dividing cells decreases, and a larger percentage of cells are dying. The hypotheses are that growth rates eventually plateau because of restrictions of space and nutrient availability, of blood supply, and of genetic mutations, which cause a higher death rate of cells. The curve becomes asymptotic with some maximum.

   d. 1 × 10^9 cells represents one gram of tissue and the smallest number of tumor cells required to be clinically detectable (equivalent to a mass of 1 cm). A 50% reduction in tumor mass represents only a one-third log decrease in tumor volume. For example, a tumor mass on x-ray film containing 8×10^{10} cells that is reduced to half its volume by chemotherapy still contains 4×10^{10} cells.

II. PRINCIPLES OF CANCER TREATMENT

A. Categories of chemotherapeutic drugs. Cytotoxic agents can be roughly categorized by their activities relative to the cell generation cycle.

   1. Phase nonspecific

   a. Cycle-nonspecific drugs kill nondividing cells (e.g., steroid hormones, antitumor antibiotics except bleomycin).

   b. Cycle-specific, phase-nonspecific drugs are effective only if the cells proceed through the generation cycle, but they can inflict injury at any point in the cycle (e.g., alkylating agents).

   c. Pharmacokinetics. Cycle-nonspecific and cycle-specific, phase-nonspecific drugs generally have a linear dose–response curve: the greater the amount of drug administered, the greater the fraction of cells killed.

   2. Phase specific

   a. Cycle-specific, phase-specific drugs are effective only if present during a particular phase of the cell cycle.

    b. Pharmacokinetics. Cycle-specific, phase-specific drugs reach a limit in cell-killing ability, but their effect is a function of both time and concentration. Above a certain dosage level, further increases in drug dose do not result in more cell killing. If the drug concentration is maintained over a period of time, however, more cells enter the specific lethal phase of the cycle and are killed.

B. Cancer treatment involves the exploitation of the biological characteristics of cancer cells to make them susceptible to drug therapy. Although malignant cellular proliferation occurs in the absence of normal internal and external growth controls, cancer cells depend on the same mechanisms for cell division that are found in normal cells. Damage to those mechanisms leads to cell death in both normal and malignant tissues.

    1. Therapeutic selectivity. Both radiation therapy and chemotherapy exert their initial effects greater in neoplastic cells than in normal host tissues because normal tissues have intact genetic machinery. Normal cells, for example, in the bone marrow and gut and in contrast to cancer cells, are able to repair DNA damage and to destroy cells with irreparable DNA, rather than allowing damaged cells to progress through the normal cell cycle and potentially replicate their damaged DNA. Loss of normal tissue cells as the result of DNA damage triggers proliferation of normal tissue cells and replacement of the lost cells in a self-limited manner.

    2. Exploitation of apoptosis in cancer. Cancer cells with intact mechanisms for apoptosis can be forced to undergo apoptosis by irreversible damage to their DNA. Radiation therapy and most cytotoxic antineoplastic agents kill cancer cells by damaging the cell and inducing apoptosis. Ideally, when cancer stem cells are destroyed, the cellular "template" for the production of the malignant phenotype is diminished or destroyed; thereby, these cells would not be replaced by more of their kind.

    3. Exploitation of proliferation control factors in cancer

        a. Biological response modifiers have been used primarily to stimulate selected immune system cells, which then demonstrate anticancer activity. These modifiers include interferons, interleukins, and several growth factors.

        b. Activation of epidermal growth factor receptors (EGFR) and its downstream signaling events play a key role in regulating tumor cell growth and proliferation, DNA repair, invasion, metastasis, and angiogenesis. Increased expression of EGFR is observed in a broad range of solid tumors. A number of clinical studies have correlated the expression of EGFR with disease progression, poor treatment outcome, and poor patient survival. Other studies have shown no such relationship with EGFR expression as measured in the laboratory. Several chemotherapeutic agents, such as erlotinib and lapatinib, exert their antitumor effect by inhibiting the tyrosine kinases of EGFR.

    4. Exploitation of maturation abnormalities in cancer cells

        a. Directly acting maturation factors force incompletely differentiated cells to fully mature. This technique is exemplified by transretinoic acid for the treatment of acute promyelocytic leukemia. Other agents, such as vitamin D and cytosine arabinoside, can induce maturation of some types of leukemic stem cells *in vitro*.

        b. Eradication of stem cells can leave behind a population of maturing cells, which then complete their differentiation into mature, nonmalignant tissues. This phenomenon is demonstrated by the finding of residual tumor masses of benign teratoma cells after successful treatment of germ cell tumors.

    5. Angiogenesis inhibition: exploitation of the dependence of cancer cells to induce the formation of their own blood supply to proliferate. Angiogenesis inhibition has potential in controlling tumor growth by limiting tumor blood supply, with only limited effects on normal revascularization. Counteraction of the antiapoptosis effect of VEGF may prevent accumulation of genetic defects that make cancers more aggressive with time. Many inhibitors of angiogenesis are known. Some of these agents are useful in cancer therapy, including pentostatin, interferons, glucocorticoids, and bevacizumab.

C. Mechanisms of drug resistance

1. **Tumor cell heterogeneity.** Spontaneous genetic mutations occur in subpopulations of cancer cells before their exposure to chemotherapy. Some of these subpopulations are drug resistant and grow to become the predominant cell type after chemotherapy has eliminated the sensitive cell lines. The **Goldie-Coldman hypothesis** indicates that the probability of a tumor population containing resistant cells is a function of the total number of cells present and its inherent mutation rate. This hypothesis asserts the high likelihood of the presence of drug-resistant mutants at the time of clinical presentation, even with small tumors. The Goldie-Coldman model also predicts that the maximal chance for cure occurs when all available effective drugs are given simultaneously (an impossibility to execute).

2. **Single-drug resistance**

   a. **Catabolic enzymes.** Exposure to a drug can induce the production of catabolic enzymes that result in drug resistance. The drug is catabolized more rapidly inside the cell by gene amplification of DNA for the specific catabolic enzymes. Examples include increased dihydrofolic reductase, which metabolizes methotrexate; deaminase, which deactivates cytarabine; and glutathione (GSH), which inactivates alkylating agents.

   b. **GSH** is essential for the synthesis of DNA precursors. Increased levels of GSH enzymes have been found in various cancers and not in their surrounding normal tissues. GSH and its enzymes scavenge free radicals and appear to play some role in inactivation of alkylating agents through direct binding, increased metabolism, detoxification, or repairing DNA damage.

   c. **Resistance to topoisomerase inhibitors** may develop with decreased drug access to the enzyme, alteration of the enzyme structure or activity, and increased rate of DNA repair, and as the result of the action of multidrug-resistance protein.

   d. **Transport proteins.** Exposure to a drug can induce the production of transport proteins that lead to drug resistance. As a result, smaller amounts of the drug enter the cell or larger amounts are carried out because of adaptive changes in cell membrane transport. Examples include methotrexate transport and the multidrug-resistance gene.

D. Mechanisms of multidrug resistance. Resistance to many agents, particularly antimetabolites, may result from mutational changes unique to that agent. In other cases, however, a single mutational change after exposure to a single drug may lead to resistance to apparently unrelated chemotherapeutic agents.

1. **P-170 and the *mdr-1* gene.** The process of multidrug resistance appears to occur as a result of induction or amplification of the *mdr-1* gene. The gene product is a 170-dalton membrane glycoprotein (P-170), which functions as a pump and rapidly exports hydrophobic chemicals out of the cell. P-170 is a normal product of cells with inherent resistance to chemotherapy, including kidney, colon, and adrenal cells.

   P-170 membrane glycoprotein can be induced by and mediates the efflux of vinca alkaloids, anthracyclines, dactinomycin, epipodophyllotoxins, and colchicine. When exposed to one of these drugs, the cells become resistant to the others but remain sensitive to drugs of other classes (e.g., alkylating agents or antimetabolites). Calcium-channel blockers (e.g., verapamil), amiodarone, quinidine, cyclosporine, phenothiazines, and other agents have been studied for their ability to reverse or block the effects of P-170.

2. **Loss of apoptosis as a mechanism of drug resistance.** All cells, including cancer cells, must have intact mechanisms for replication and repair to avoid loss of information necessary for survival. Loss of apoptosis is manifested by the increasing aneuploidy often seen as cancers become more aggressive and by the very high frequency of mutations in the *p53* suppressor gene.

   a. ***p53* is a tumor-suppressor protein and is a potent inducer of apoptosis** within a cell in which DNA damage has occurred (see section I.C.3.b). DNA-damaging agents cause increased levels of *p53* in normal cells. Mutations in the *p53* gene are present in >50% of all human tumors.

The wild-type *p53* suppresses the promoter of the *mdr-1* gene, while mutant *p53* protein can stimulate the promoter. Various tumors expressing mutant *p53* or deleted *p53* are resistant to a wide range of anticancer agents. Dysregulation of the *p53* pathway might well be a prominent mechanism of drug resistance due to the overproduction of gene products responsible for entry into S-phase and rapid cell growth. However, loss of *p53* function is not always associated with chemoresistance.

   b. *Bcl-2* is a potent suppressor of apoptotic cell death. Permutations of *Bcl-2* expression (or related genes) can result in either repression or promotion of apoptosis triggered by γ-irradiation or chemotherapeutic agents. *Bcl-x$_L$*, a functional and structural homologue of *Bcl-2*, is also able to confer protection against apoptosis induced by radiation as well as by several anticancer agents, including bleomycin, cisplatin, etoposide, and vincristine.

   c. NF-κB (nuclear factor-kappa B) activation results in potent suppression of the apoptotic potential of a number of external stimuli, including various cytokines, tumor necrosis factor-α (TNF-α), and radiation. Activation of NF-κB expression in response to chemotherapy may represent an important mechanism of inducible tumor chemoresistance.

   d. The relationships among *p53* status, NF-κB, *Bcl-2,* the caspase cascades, and chemotherapy sensitivity and resistance are obviously complex.

III. CLINICAL USES OF CYTOTOXIC AGENTS

   A. Indications. Chemotherapy is used in the following circumstances:
   1. To cure certain malignancies
   2. To palliate symptoms in patients with disseminated cancer when the potential benefits of treatment exceed the side effects of treatment
   3. To treat asymptomatic patients in the following circumstances:
      a. When the cancer is aggressive and treatable (e.g., acute leukemia, small cell lung cancer, lymphoma)
      b. When treatment has been proved to decrease the rate of relapse and increase the disease-free interval or increase the absolute survival (stage III colon carcinoma, stages I or II breast carcinoma, osteogenic sarcoma)
   4. To allow less-mutilating surgery by treating first with chemotherapy alone or in combination with RT (sarcomas and carcinomas of the anus, breast, esophagus, and larynx)

   B. Contraindications. Chemotherapeutic agents are relatively or absolutely contraindicated in the following situations:
   1. When facilities are inadequate to evaluate the patient's response to therapy and to monitor and manage toxic reactions
   2. When the patient is not likely to survive longer even if tumor shrinkage could be accomplished
   3. When the patient is not likely to survive long enough to obtain benefits from the drugs (e.g., severely debilitated patients)
   4. When the patient is asymptomatic with slow-growing, incurable tumors, in which case chemotherapy should be postponed until symptoms require palliation

   C. Adjuvant chemotherapy is given to patients who have no evidence of residual disease but who are at high risk for relapse. The justifications for adjuvant chemotherapy are the high recurrence rate after surgery for apparently localized tumors, the inability to identify cured patients at the time of surgery, and the failure of therapy to cure these patients after recurrence of disease. The disadvantages of this therapy are the immediate patient discomfort and the short- and long-term risks associated with such treatment. To date, the only malignancies for which adjuvant chemotherapy has proved beneficial are breast cancer, colon cancer, and osteogenic sarcoma.

   D. Dose intensification and dose density have received increasing emphasis in recent years as strategies for overcoming resistance to chemotherapy and improving results. Dose intensification has generated the notion that drugs in combination chemotherapy regimens should be given in the highest tolerated dose over the briefest interval, perhaps even with patient rescue maneuvers, such as the intensive use of hematopoietic growth factors, autologous marrow stem cell infusion, or allogeneic bone marrow transplantation. Dose density involves administering chemotherapy using cumbersome protocols on an increased number of days per cycle to increase drug exposure over time. Although these concepts are being tested in certain malignancies, the concept that more chemotherapy is better than regimens using standard doses remains to be proved.

    E. Sequential versus alternating cycles. The Norton-Day model indicates that the sequential use of combinations of chemotherapy is likely to outperform alternating cycles because no two combinations are likely to be strictly non-cross-resistant or have equal killing capacity.

IV. MEDICAL PRACTICE AND ITS TOOLS

    A. The principal goal of medical care is to provide the most beneficial treatment at the lowest risk. Although most patients and physicians consider this as self-evident for medical care, this axiom is no simple matter to implement. Every person is different from every other—even for one of a pair of identical twins. The meaning of "benefit" and "optimal" is a highly personal matter; a very large number of interacting parameters make it impossible to have a preconceived idea of the meaning of benefit for each patient. We tend to think of a benefit as solely a physical result of a medical decision—the benefit may be partial or complete eradication of a disease, optimization of patient's physical ability to function, or the psychological comfort of the patient and significant others in the patient's life. Similarly, acceptable risk is a special idea. The optimal care in each situation requires the experience and judgment of the physician on a very individualized basis.

    B. Medical care is an art; science, technology, and statistics are important tools. Too often, the tools of medicine are mistaken for the art of care. Like all arts, there is no satisfactory "one size fits all" approach to patient care. Attempts to reduce medical practice into a fixed set of algorithms creates "one size fits nobody" programs and damages optimal care for individual patients.

    The tools of art are necessary but alone do not determine the quality of the art. Quality requires experience, thoroughness, attention to detail, good judgment, and, most of all, caring about the quality of the resulting product.

    Most people think of science as a mathematical description of cause and effect— "if you do A, then B will occur." People are so complex that cause-and-effect thinking is all but useless. If we recommend active treatment, the best we can do is to guess what will happen. But, we can often estimate the probabilities of obtaining a result and the probability of the risk and degree of side effects.

    C. Statistics as a tool of medicine. Statistics helps doctors to maximize the benefits and minimize the risks in recommending treatment. Although statistics uses some fancy equations, these are not what medical statistics is about. Statistics is a kind of ruler that measures the probability of what happens to a large number of people who participate in a study but never predicts the future or the positive benefits or harm for any individual patient.

V. STATISTICS IN MEDICAL PRACTICE

    A. The basic idea. Clinical treatment trials are usually based on stochastic hypotheses; this boils down to making our best guess. Initial guesses usually come from personal experience and the experience found in published studies. After an experimental trial of a treatment, we learn how often a treatment was associated with particular effects, what kinds of adverse effects it produces, and most importantly, which patient parameters best correlate with obvious outcomes. These parameters help define subpopulations that can be used to make better hypotheses for future clinical trials.

    B. Statistics is a tool that measures probability of future events. Imagine a universe that has two million inhabitants and every one of them has metastatic colon cancer. Aside from this malady in common, no one of these patients is exactly like another; they are of different ages, genders, races, levels of activity, extent of the tumor, and so on. Now, let us suppose that there is one lonely investigator who wants to try a particular treatment. The researcher cannot physically conduct the study on all two million people. The best the researcher can do is to try to determine how closely the results for the population studied looks like the whole two million. The researcher knows that the measurement will not be completely accurate, but it is possible to measure the probability of inaccuracy, that the error will fall into some range of values. By studying the variation of results in the sample, the researcher can make a more consistent hypothesis of the risks and benefits of a diagnostic study or treatment.

1. **The single most important statistical concept for the clinician.** Many studies that show initial "promising results" ultimately prove the ineffectiveness of such therapy. Most initially exciting "state-of-the-art" therapies provide no improvement. It is essential that the clinician avoid "one-article quotes," early data, and data reported only in abstract form as a basis for making clinical decisions.

2. **Sufficient duration in a clinical study** is essential for determining the effectiveness of treatment. Inadequate duration of a study may result in an effective therapy being considered ineffective. Studies of a treatment for most of the common cancers require at least 5 to 10 years for any meaningful interpretation. Earlier data are characteristically misleading.

   a. In rapidly lethal cancers or in widespread malignancies for which survival expectancy is short, it is usually easy to determine whether a treatment is effective in a relatively short period of time.

   b. Tumors that are likely to be associated with a long survival without treatment require long periods of study to determine whether a treatment is beneficial. An example is prostate cancer, in which most untreated patients survive 15 or more years from the time of diagnosis. Prostate cancer studies are also confounded by the fact that the disease affects older men, who often succumb to unrelated illnesses before reaching the terminal stage of their cancer.

3. **Matched populations.** Treated and untreated patients must be closely matched for particular characteristics. For example, no information can be drawn about the effectiveness of a sarcoma therapy if the treated group consists of otherwise healthy, young Asian women with low-grade localized sarcomas and the untreated group consists of elderly diabetic white men with high-grade metastatic sarcomas.

   a. **Numbers of patients used** to compare treated and untreated groups strongly affect the statistical power and needed duration of a study to determine effectiveness. Inadequate numbers of patients may make it impossible to find a subgroup of treated patients with readily identifiable prognostic factors who significantly benefit from a treatment.

   b. **Risks and benefits of a treatment** are an essential part of statistical study design. For example, a study that conclusively demonstrates that a treatment results in 1% improvement in 5-month survival but increases time in the hospital for therapy of treatment-related complications in 50% of patients and causes death in 15% should probably not be recommended.

C. **Definitions of terms used to describe frequency of cancers**

1. **Incidence** refers to the overall number of people developing cancer in a particular time frame, usually 1 year.

2. **Incidence rate** is the number of people developing cancer per 100,000 population per year.

3. **Mortality rate** refers to the number of people dying from cancer per 100,000 population per year.

4. **Case fatality rate** is the percentage of people with a particular cancer who die from that cancer.

5. **Prevalence** is the number of cases of cancer in a population at a specific point in time.

D. **Definition of terms used in survival analysis**

1. **Cure** is a statistical term that applies to groups of cancer patients rather than to individual patients; it describes those patients who are rendered clinically free of detectable cancer and who have the same survival expectancy as a healthy age-matched control group. A cure does not guarantee that the particular patient meeting these criteria will not eventually die from the original cancer.

2. **Actuarial survival** (or life table survival) is the life expectancy from a specified age of a group of patients with a particular cancer. These data are used to determine the chance that an individual patient will survive for a specified time. This parameter is useful in determining both the natural history of the cancer and the effectiveness of treatment by comparing patient survival with actuarial survival tables of a matched healthy population.

3. **Observed survival rate** is the percentage of patients alive at the end of a specified interval of observation from the time of diagnosis.

4. **Relative survival rate** corrects the survival rate for the "normal mortality expectation" in a matched population.

5. **Adjusted survival rate** corrects the survival rate by discounting deaths from causes other than cancer or cancer treatment in those patients who are free of cancer at the time of death.

6. **Median survival** is the time when 50% of patients are dead and 50% are still alive. Average or mean survival rates are meaningless because survival of patients with similar tumors may range from a few weeks to years. Median survival may be a useful index for comparison of clinical trials but can be misleading. In "mature studies," a significant group of patients may survive for many months or years after the time that 50% of the patients have died.

7. **Disease-free interval** is the time from when the patient is rendered free of clinically detectable cancer until recurrent cancer is diagnosed.

8. **Censored data.** Data for patients who are still living and discontinue the trial therapy or whose fate is unknown are frequently excluded (censored) from statistical analysis. Censoring data can severely skew results and make a study uninterpretable. The larger the number of censored data in relationship to the overall study, the more likely it is that the study is not interpretable. Good reporting carefully defines the reasons for censoring data, what the data would look like if censored data were included, and the percentage of data points that were censored.

9. **Overall 5-year survival rate** is an arbitrary but convenient rate used to provide a short-range assessment of the value of therapy and the adverse effects of therapy. It is used for all cancers and cancer therapies, because most of the frequency and long-term adverse effect of drugs are found within this time frame. Five-year survival does not represent cure or complete eradication of detectable tumor, nor does it predict future tumor recurrence in complete responders. However, the rate of future recurrences for many tumors declines significantly. This is especially true for rapidly growing, aggressive cancers.

   a. **Early detection.** Most of the treatment-related improvement in survival has occurred as the result of early detection of common cancers; it is not yet clear whether some of these early cancers have the same lethal biological potential as cancers discovered in a more advanced state. Early detection and diagnosis of cancers that appear histologically identical but are biologically less lethal can yield misleading survival figures.

   b. **Lead-time bias.** Patients appear to live longer from the time of diagnosis only because the cancer was detected earlier rather than because of treatment.

E. **Definition of terms used for describing types of drug development trials**

   1. **Phase I trials** determine the optimal dose, schedule, and side effects of a new therapy.

   2. **Phase II trials** determine what kinds of cancer respond to a particular treatment.

   3. **Phase III trials** compare a treatment shown to have some effectiveness in a phase II trial with no treatment or with a treatment that has also shown effectiveness.

   4. **Meta-analysis** is a retrospective study in which data from multiple randomized trials are pooled and analyzed. All patients, including those being treated but not entered into each study, must be accounted for. Meta-analysis is most useful for evaluating many small, randomized trials to look for an effect not evident in a single small study and for identifying subsets (by prognostic strata) of patients who benefit from treatment.

F. Definition of terms used in describing the design of a study

1. **Sample space** is the number of patients, tests, treatments, or other data points used to represent the entire "universe" of all such patients, tests, and outcomes.

2. **Stratification** of patients according to known prognostic factors (such as age, ethnicity, sex, performance status, and extent of disease) is essential if a clinical study is to be useful for the clinician making treatment decisions. Randomizing patients between a treated group and an untreated group is a technique used to deal with unknown factors that affect prognosis. Proper stratification helps the clinician to determine whether a particular patient is represented in the population of a published study and whether that therapy has a reasonable chance of being effective.

3. **Randomization** is the assignment of a patient to a particular treatment by random chance. Randomization is done when a treatment is being compared with another treatment or with no treatment. Each of the treatments or nontreatments is called an *arm* of the study.

4. **Blinded studies.** Studies in which patients do not know to what treatment arm of the study they have been assigned. In a double-blinded study, neither the patients nor the investigators know to what arm of the study any patient has been assigned. The data are codified; the study is stopped ("broken") if one arm is significantly providing better or worse results than another study arm.

G. Definition of terms used to describe response to treatment

1. **Complete remission (CR).** No clinically detectable cancer is found after treatment.

2. **Partial response (PR).** Measurable tumor mass decreases by 50% after treatment, no new areas of tumor develop, and no area of tumor shows progression. The approximation of the mass of an individual area of tumor is usually given as the product of two diameters of the lesion; the measurable tumor mass is the sum of the masses of all measurable lesions.

3. **Minimal response (MR)** is the same as partial response, but the response does not meet the criteria of 50% reduction.

4. **Progression.** The mass (product of diameters) of one or more sites of tumor increases >25%, new lesions appear, or the patient dies as a result of the tumor.

5. **Stable disease.** Measurable tumor does not meet the criteria for CR, PR, MR, or progression.

H. Statistical measurements used to assess clinical research results

Figures don't lie, but liars figure.—Old aphorism

1. **Experimental trials: Kaplan-Maier graphs and "acceptable error."** When we try to estimate the effectiveness or ineffectiveness of a treatment based on a clinical trial or meta-analysis, we can estimate the probability that the sample of patients, stratified by various parameters, is representative of the whole universe of patients with the same disease and the same treatment. On the standard survival curve the x-axis is marked off in equal time divisions (usually 1-month intervals) and the number of patients who are alive from the time they started participating in the study is plotted on the y-axis. A stepladder-shaped "curve" called a Kaplan Maier plot results when the dots are connected. This curve can be made smoother by decreasing the time intervals.

Each curve is composed only of samples of the "universe" of all untreated and all treated patients. Consequently, we have the probability of several errors that can be estimated by statistically measuring the differences between curves. One way of determining the differences is to measure how different averages of the populations are between the curves. Another way to look at differences is to use the hazard ratio, which is discussed in the next section.

We must define an "acceptable" percentage error in deciding whether curves are different. We can never be sure that there is or there is not a difference, or even what is the best way to measure the differences. Each of the ways of evaluating experimental data produces quite different results. Do we want to be 95% certain (two standard deviations from the mean) or 99.7% certain (three standard deviations from the mean)? The less error we accept, the fewer the number of patients we would treat. For example, if we are willing to accept a 5% error, we would have a 5% chance of treating patients who would not benefit but who would be exposed to the toxicities of treatment, and we would have a 95% chance to treat and benefit many more patients.

Some investigators design experimental trials with the assumption that there will be no difference (the *null hypothesis* [or "show me it really works"]). Other investigators assume that the result of a step in a study cannot completely predict the next result (so-called *stochastic models*); the best one can do is to make a "best guess" for the next step. Other investigators assume that defined parameters must be included in an experimental plan, while others use nonparametric statistical methods and want the data from the experiment to speak for themselves without imposing preconceived ideas about which parameters might be important. All of these experimental statistical approaches have their own mathematics and applications and can affect the results we read about.

2. **Hazard ratios** are another way of looking at survival. Some types of clinical trials *test* hypotheses made in advance of the study. Hazard ratio analyses generate hypotheses; we get a result and then try to determine what might have caused it.

   The general idea is to determine the number of people who experience a single kind of event (e.g., death in a survival analysis) out of the number of patients during *a specific sequential time frame*. This is called the **hazard rate** for this time frame. This rate identifies those patients who are alive at the beginning of that interval and who die later in that time frame. In a clinical study, the hazard rates for each treatment group are calculated for a large number of time frames. At each time interval, the hazard rate of the treatment group is divided by the hazard rate of the control group (with application of an array of mathematical probability functions), resulting in the *hazard ratio* for the particular time frame.

   One needs to have some sort of average hazard ratio so that the hazard ratio measured is likely to contain this average. As in other forms of survival analysis, one would want to have a two–standard deviation (95%) confidence interval for ratios so that the measured hazard ratio contains this average. Suppose the calculated hazard ratio was 2 over a 3-month period. A patient asks you, "How much better off will I be if I take the treatment?" You can tell the patient that her or his chance of living for the next 3 months is twice as good as patients who don't take the treatment.

3. **Confidence intervals, ratio tests, and statistical significance.** Confidence intervals are used for assessing response rate in single-arm trials and for comparing and assessing the magnitude of differences between treatments in phase III studies. For single-treatment studies, the confidence interval is the **range of values** around a measured result that would be 95% certain to contain that measured result if the entire universe of patients were tested. The more patients included in a trial, the more likely the measured value will be closer to the "true" value; the higher the number of measured responses, the higher the likelihood that the "true" response rate will be higher.

4. **Proportion tests** compare the ratio of positive treatment outcome to the sample size in each study arm.

   a. **Confidence interval comparison of two proportions** gives the range of numbers that will contain the actual numeric difference between the ratios with 95% certainty. The confidence interval comparison is a statistical assessment of the probable magnitude of the difference between the two treatments being compared. These statistical tests are used in both one- and two-tailed clinical trials.

   b. **Statistical significance comparison of two proportions** evaluates whether there is a false-positive result rate <5% in studies showing a difference in the ratios. It does not provide a range for the probable magnitude of the difference. The χ^2 (chi square) test, or the more politically correct Fisher's exact test, is used to determine statistically significant differences that can be correlated with the p value (see next paragraph) for significant differences.

5. **p Value (the false-positive value)** is the probability that a measured difference between results of two arms of a study, or a confidence interval difference, would disappear if the entire universe of identical patients could be tested. When the p value is <0.05, the probability that measured differences occurred by chance is $<5\%$. The choice of a 5% false-positive error is somewhat arbitrary and is used to give a value that is two standard deviations from the average value that test results are "the true value." The p value has no significance in studies of small numbers of patients evaluated over a short time. Interval p values showing a difference in treatment arms reported before the planned number of patients are entered are usually false-positive results and should be ignored, unless the "power" of the study is also reported and has a high value.

6. **β Error (the false-negative value)** is the probability that two treatments that appear to have identical results would be different if the entire universe of patients were tested. This error is not usually reported in clinical research reports because it is a part of study design and is used in advance to determine the number of patients who must be entered into the study to meaningfully interpret a p value.

7. **One- and two-tailed (-sided) tests.** A one-tailed test gives the p value for the hypothesis that the experimental treatment arm of a randomized study is better than the control arm; it provides no statistical information regarding whether the treatment arm is the same or worse than the control arm. A two-tailed test is the same as a one-tailed test but also evaluates whether the experimental treatment is actually worse than the control arm. Two-tailed tests are really answering the question; consequently, they require twice as many patients in each study arm. The first "tail" determines whether a treatment is better than the control. If the first study tail is not statistically different from the control, the second tail tells us whether the control is the same as or better than the treatment group. This is particularly helpful in planning future studies—if the control study is better than the treatment, it can be used again as a control for new treatment studies.

8. **Power of a statistical test.** The power of a test is calculated as "$1-\beta$." Reported studies done with small numbers of patients typically have p values of <0.05 and appear to be positive. The p value tends to increase both as the duration of the study becomes longer and as more patients are accrued into the study. For the p value to be interpretable and to have clinical applicability, statisticians require that a predetermined number of patients be entered into the study and evaluated for a predetermined amount of time. The *power of a statistical test* takes into account the number of patients enrolled; higher powers give increasing confidence that any observed differences between arms are less likely to be by chance, no matter how many patients are enrolled.

I. **Summary of recommendations for the clinical application of the literature to patient care decisions**

> *Medical therapy is like computers and software: The most important reason to know the current state of the art is to be certain that you stay 5 years behind it when you treat most of your patients.—BL*

The status of ongoing clinical trials must be reported before the data are "mature" to allow coordination of trials among different institutions and investigators. Thus, critical evaluation of research reports is essential for clinicians who are deciding whether to recommend a new treatment for a patient. No trial result, however, is a substitute for sound clinical judgment or for individualization of treatment for patients not enrolled in a study. The clinician should ask the following questions when reading the literature:

1. Are patients who benefited from the study treatment substantially like your patient with regard to age, sex, stage of disease, performance status, and other prognostic factors?

2. Does the study exclude certain patients? If so, what were the reasons for exclusion?
3. Did the study treatment produce toxicity that is unacceptable in view of the potential benefits? On the other hand, was improvement in survival so superior that the risk for toxicity and drug-related death is warranted?
4. Did the study stratify and randomize patients in a manner that allows clear interpretation of the data?
5. Was the study large enough to provide sufficient confidence that observed differences were not by random chance? Optimally, the most useful studies are two-tailed tests with p values <0.05 and a power ≥ 80.

2

NUCLEAR MEDICINE

Chaitanya R. Divgi

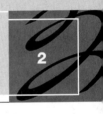

I. DEFINITIONS

A. **Nuclear medicine** is the use of radioactive tracers in the form of unsealed sources for the diagnosis, therapy, and laboratory testing of human diseases. The common radiopharmaceuticals include 25 forms for diagnostic imaging applications and 5 forms for therapy (Table 2.1).

B. **Radioactivity, radioisotopes, and radionuclides.** The nucleus contains a variety of subatomic particles, such as protons and neutrons, which are held together by incredibly strong short-range forces. The **atomic number** (Z) of an atom is the number of protons in the nucleus and is characteristic of a particular element. The **mass number** of an atom is the sum of the protons and the neutrons (A); it is this number that we refer to in this section unless otherwise specified. For most of the common elements in the earth, the nucleus is completely stable and unchanging. Radioactive elements occur when the balance of subatomic particles in the nucleus is inherently unstable. Each radionuclide has specific radioactive decay characteristics in terms of half-life and radioactive emissions.

1. **The half-life** $(t_{1/2})$ is the time required for one half of the atoms to undergo radioactive decay.

   a. The half-life of most of the radioisotopes is short, and they therefore do not exist in nature. Some naturally occurring elements are radioactive; for example, ^{40}K accounts for 0.1% of the potassium found within the human body and has a half-life of 1.26×10^9 years. Other naturally occurring radioactive elements include radium, thorium, lead, and carbon. All elements with atomic weights greater than ^{209}Bi are radioactive. The transuranium elements may also have half-lives of 10,000 years or more.

   b. Most of the radioactivity used in nuclear medicine is artificially produced in a cyclotron or reactor (see sections I.D.5 and 6). ^{131}I, for example, has a half-life of 8 days and emits a gamma ray of 364 keV, along with several beta particles, including one with a maximum energy of 0.606 MeV. These radioactive emissions can be detected externally and permit ^{131}I to be useful as a tracer for the study of thyroid physiology.

2. **Forms of radioactive emissions**

   a. **Gamma rays:** photoelectric energy that is capable of penetrating a meter or more through human tissue.

   b. **Beta rays:** particulate emissions with the mass of an electron and a negative charge that are capable of penetrating from a few millimeters to about a centimeter in tissue.

   c. **Positrons:** particulate emissions with the mass of an electron and a positive charge that travel for a few millimeters in tissue and then interact with an electron, forming annihilation radiation.

   d. **Annihilation radiation:** two gamma photons of 511-keV energy traveling at 180 degrees from each other that are created when a beta ray and a positron combine.

   e. **Alpha particles:** two neutrons and two protons (a helium nucleus) that are capable of traveling for about 10 to 20 cell diameters in tissues.

   f. **X-rays:** result from rearrangement of electrons in orbit around the nucleus.

TABLE 2.1 Some Diagnostic and Therapeutic Radiopharmaceuticals

Nuclide	Pharmaceutical	Pharmacology	Dosage	Patient preparation	Use
^{18}F	FDG	Glycolysis	10 mCi	Fasting	Tumor viability
^{67}Ga	Citrate	Transferrin receptor	10 mCi	Laxatives	Lymphoma, inflammation
^{131}I	MIBG	Catecholamine uptake	0.5 mCi	Off α-, β-blockers	Neuroendocrine tumor
^{131}I	Bexxar	Anti-CD20 MoAb	65–75 cGy WB	Iodide; see text	Refractory lymphoma
^{123}I	Sodium iodide	Thyroid hormone	25 μCi	Off thyroid hormone, iodides	Thyroid dysfunction
^{111}In	Leukocytes	Target inflammation	5 mCi	None	Phelgmon
^{111}In	Pentetreotide	Somatostatin receptors	5 mCi	Off steroids; laxatives	Endocrine malignancy
^{111}In	Prostascint	Anti-PSMA MoAb	6 mCi	Laxatives, enema	Prostate cancer recurrence
^{153}Sm	Quadramet	Hydroxyapatite	1 mCi/kg	Positive bone scan	Bone pain in prostate, breast, lung cancers
^{89}Sr	Metastron	Bone mineralization	4 mCi/70 kg	Positive bone scan	Bone pain in prostate cancer
^{99m}Tc	Phosphonates	Bone mineralization	25 mCi	None	Bone disease
^{99m}Tc	Sulfur colloid	Lymphatic clearance	0.2–0.5 mCi	None	Identify sentinel node
^{99m}Tc	Albumin	Lymphatic clearance	1 mCi	None	Lymphatic drainage
^{99m}Tc	Aggregated albumin	Capillary blockade	5 mCi	None	Pulmonary emboli
^{99m}Tc	Erythrocytes	Vascular markers	30 mCi	Off β-blockers	Measure LVEF
^{99m}Tc	Pertechnetates	Thyroid iodine trap	10 mCi	Off thyroxine, iodide	Thyroid nodule
^{99m}Tc	MIBI	Lipophilicity and intracellular binding	20 mCi	Fasting; stop xanthines	Tumor viability, cardiac perfusion
^{99m}Tc	CEAScan	Anti-CEA MoAb	20–30 mCi	Laxatives	Colorectal cancer
^{201}Tl	Chloride	NA$^+$–K$^+$ pump	5 mCi	None	Tumor viability
^{90}Y	Zevalin	Anti-CD20 MoAb	0.3–0.4 mCi/kg	See text	Refractory lymphoma

Key: CEA, carcinoembryonic antigen; FDG, fluorodeoxyglucose; LVEF, left ventricular ejection fraction; MIBG, metaiodobenzylguanidine; MIBI, methoxyisobutyl isonitrile; MoAb, monoclonal antibody; PSMA, prostate-specific membrane antigen; WB, whole-body dose.

g. **Auger electrons:** low-energy electrons that are emitted from the orbits around the nucleus and travel only a few microns in tissue.

h. **Applications.** Gamma rays and annihilation radiation in particular are useful for various diagnostic imaging applications. The shorter range particles, such as alpha particles, beta rays, and Auger electrons, are used for therapeutic applications.

3. **Quantity of radioactivity**

a. **Becquerel (Bq).** One disintegration per second (dps) is defined as 1 Bq of radioactivity, in honor of the discoverer of radioactivity. Typical doses used for imaging are often 37 MegaBecquerels (MBq), which is 1 milliCurie (mCi).

b. **Curies (Ci).** The curie unit is based on the amount of radioactivity in 1 g of radium or 3.7×10^{10} dps. Typical diagnostic doses range from 1 mCi (37 MBq) to 30 mCi (1,110 MBq).

4. **Quantity of absorbed radiation**

a. **Rads.** When radioactive emissions interact with matter, a fraction of the total energy is absorbed. The rad is equivalent to one erg of energy absorbed per gram of tissue.

b. **Gray** (Gy) is the newer unit replacing the rad. One Gray is 100 rad; 1 centiGray (cGy) is 1 rad.

c. **Rem** (R), or roentgen equivalent man, was introduced as a unit because not all radiation emitted has equivalent potency for the biological effects that it exerts for a given amount of radiation dose absorbed. For gamma photons and x-rays, the rad dose and the rem dose are the same. For larger particles (e.g., the alpha particle), the rem is the rad dose times a "quality factor." For alpha particles, the quality factor is much higher, so that for a given rad dose, the rem for alpha-particle exposure is much greater than that for gamma exposure: the exact value is under debate but is typically assumed to be at least 20-fold higher.

d. **Sieverts** (Sv). One Sv is 100 rem.

C	Carbon (^{11}C)	**P**	Phosphorus (^{32}P)
F	Fluorine (^{18}F)	**S**	Sulfur (^{35}S)
Ga	Gallium (^{67}Ga)	**Sr**	Strontium (^{89}Sr)
I	Iodine (^{123}I, ^{125}I, ^{131}I)	**Tc**	Technetium (^{99m}Tc); *m*
In	Indium (^{111}In)		means *metastable*
Kr	Krypton (^{81}Kr)	**Tl**	Thallium (^{201}Tl)
Lu	Lutetium (^{177}Lu)	**U**	Uranium (^{235}U, ^{238}U)
Mo	Molybdenum (^{99}Mo)	**Xe**	Xenon (^{127}Xe, ^{133}Xe)
N	Nitrogen (^{13}N)	**Y**	Yttrium (^{90}Y)
O	Oxygen (^{15}O)		

C. **How much radiation exposure is safe?** The answer is the ALARA principle, which means "as low as reasonably achievable."

1. **In the workplace,** a maximum of 5,000 milliRem (mRem) per year is permitted; 25% of this dose (1,250 mRem) is sought. Several decades of exposure of large populations of workers to the 5,000 mR/year limit has demonstrated no adverse effects. The U.S. Food and Drug Administration (FDA) has used this definition for what could be considered "safe" levels of total-body radiation exposure. Directives for pregnant workers permit 500 mR per 9-month gestational period.

2. **The general public** in the United States receives an average of 290 mR/year from naturally occurring radiation. Up to 10 times this exposure may occur at high altitudes, again with no discernible adverse effects. The mandated level for the general public is now set at 100 mR/year.

3. **Diagnostic exposure** for the purpose of patient management has no limits because the doses involved are relatively low, and it is generally believed that the benefits outweigh the risks associated with indicated studies.

4. **Therapeutic radioisotopes** sometimes require admission to the hospital. In the United States, the Nuclear Regulatory Commission has established guidelines

such that therapy may be administered on an outpatient basis provided the radiation dose to the general public is within acceptable limits (see above), usually calculated based on the amount and effective residence time of the administered radioactivity; if data are not available for such determination to be made, hospitalization with radiation isolation precautions needs to be carried out until the radiation levels fall to 5–7 mR/hour at 1 m from the treated subject. After that point, the patient is not subjected to special precautions.

Photons can set off radiation detectors, increasingly in use in the United States after September 11, 2001. Thus, the patient needs to be advised about the potential for activation of such detectors—most institutions now provide patients with written directives including amount and type of radioactivity received.

D. Instrumentation

1. **Well counters.** A radiation-sensitive crystal (usually sodium iodide) is fashioned so that a small test tube containing a body fluid can be placed in a well. For each decay, the energy from the emitted radiation is deposited in the crystal, and the crystal is induced to emit a pulse of light. This light pulse is converted to a weak electrical signal by a photoelectric tube. Further amplification results in a signal that can be read as an individual "count." Typical samples have 10,000 to 20,000 counts per minute (cpm). The amount of the radiotracer present is proportional to the total amount (cpm) detected. By reference to standards of known activity, the absolute amount of tracer can be detected.

2. **Gamma camera devices** are the most commonly used imaging device for the widely available radiopharmaceuticals, such as ^{99m}Tc, ^{111}In, and ^{131}I. The gamma camera is designed as a circular sheet of sodium iodide crystal, encased in a lead shield and directly coupled to 90 or more photoelectric tubes. A collimator device in front of the crystal serves to focus the radiation; it is a 1-in. thick lead shield with holes punched in the lead. Every disintegration in the patient that results in a gamma ray travels to the collimator and passes through the holes in the lead to strike the radiation-sensitive crystal. A light pulse is created in the crystal and is detected by several photomultiplier tubes simultaneously. A computer calculates where the photon hit the crystal, with the strongest signal being nearest the site where the photon struck the detector. Resolution is about 1 cm or so for most planar gamma cameras.

3. **Single photon emission computerized tomography (SPECT).** In this form of imaging, radioactivity within the patient is collected at 360 degrees around the patient, and the data are reconstructed into a three-dimensional representation. The data are collected by rotating a specialized gamma camera around a patient who has received an injection of radioactivity that is stable in distribution for the 45- to 60-minute collection times typically required. SPECT is commonly used for the imaging of ^{67}Ga citrate in the mediastinum of patients with lymphoma, ^{201}Tl in myocardial perfusion studies, hemangiomas within the liver, and radiolabeled antitumor antibodies.

The typical in-depth resolution is 16 mm, somewhat more coarse than for planar imaging. Planar gamma camera imaging provides better contrast resolution, whereas SPECT provides better images of small, deep lesions, especially when **attenuation correction** (whereby radioactivity emitted from deeper in the body is corrected based on the amount and type of tissue between the source and the detector) is carried out, using either assumptions or actual measurements of the density of tissue and nature of the attenuation.

4. **Positron emission tomography** (PET) has the highest resolution and is the most sensitive imaging device available for nuclear medicine. For reasons related to the physics of positron emission decay, the image can be converted into an accurate, quantitative three-dimensional distribution of radioactivity with a resolution of about 3 to 5 mm in depth within the body. The radiotracers used with PET are ^{18}F, ^{15}O, ^{13}N, and ^{11}C; these elements are readily incorporated into biological molecules. Most of these radiotracers have half-lives that are too short for

shipping. Thus, they must be produced in a hospital-based cyclotron. Nonetheless, clinical applications are emerging, especially using ^{18}F-labeled tracers (which are now commonly being produced by commercial radiopharmaceutical manufacturers). ^{18}F-fluorodeoxyglucose (^{18}F-FDG) imaging of glycolysis by tumors has become the archetypal molecular imaging agent and is increasingly used to diagnose and stage cancer, as well as to demonstrate tumor viability after treatment with radiation or drugs.

5. **Cyclotron.** The cyclotron accelerates subatomic particles (e.g., protons, deuterons, helium nuclei, alpha particles) to speeds approaching the speed of light. The particle strikes a "target" atom and produces radioactivity. For example, by accelerating protons to about 11 MeV and striking a target that contains an enriched isotope of oxygen (^{18}O), ^{18}F in the form of fluoride ion is produced. These *accelerator systems* produce a large variety of the radiotracers useful in nuclear medicine, including ^{11}C, ^{15}O, ^{13}N, ^{67}Ga, ^{111}In, ^{123}I, and ^{18}F.

6. **Reactors.** The reactor is fueled by heavy elements, such as ^{238}U and ^{235}U, which undergo spontaneous fission. Neutrons are emitted from the nucleus and, when present in sufficient quantities, "split" the uranium atoms, with the consequent release of large amounts of energy. An entire cascade of radioactive elements is produced in this process; these elements, called *fission products,* include ^{99}Mo (from which ^{99m}Tc is derived), ^{131}I, ^{125}I, ^{32}P, and ^{35}S. In some cases, a target element is bombarded with neutrons to produce the radioactive element used in medicine (e.g., ^{89}Sr). In other cases, separation of fission products may produce the radioisotope as a by-product of reactor operation (^{131}I, ^{125}I).

II. TUMOR IMAGING STUDIES

A. Bone scanning

1. **Indications** for bone scanning are to determine the presence and extent of primary and metastatic tumor involving bone and to provide a baseline in early malignancy if the patient has a cancer that notoriously metastasizes to bone (e.g., prostate cancer, stage II or III breast cancer) or has significant bony abnormalities of a benign nature. Some cancers that metastasize to bone do not provoke increased hydroxyapatite turnover, and bone scans are not very useful in these cancers (multiple myeloma, thyroid cancer). Bone scans are frequently used for evaluation (not measurement) of bone metastases, most often in prostate and breast cancer, as well as in lung and colon cancer; bone scans are used less frequently in kidney cancer.

2. **Radiopharmaceutical.** A pyrophosphate or other phosphonate derivative is labeled with ^{99m}Tc.

3. **Principle.** Primary or metastatic tumor provokes a reaction in the adjacent bone that causes the bone crystal to remodel and in the process take up the ^{99m}Tc bone agent. Even small tumors can evoke a considerable response. (See Chapter 33, section I.D.3.)

4. **Procedural notes.** Whole-body scans are ordinarily obtained using gamma cameras with large fields of view. SPECT imaging is performed on suspect regions and is particularly helpful in the spine.

5. **Interpretation.** Against a background of bone turnover, a metastatic site stands out as avid uptake. Bone scans are more sensitive than computed tomography (CT) and magnetic resonance imaging (MRI) for detection of metastases in cortical bone. MRI may detect metastases in the bone marrow before cortical bone is affected.

B. ^{18}F-FDG imaging with PET

1. **Indications**

    a. To distinguish radiation necrosis from recurrent glioblastoma.

    b. To evaluate dedifferentiation of brain tumor from low grade to high grade.

    c. To evaluate the potential for recurrence of meningioma.

    d. To assess tumor viability and monitor treatment response.

    e. To differentiate benign from malignant pulmonary nodules.

f. To evaluate staging, restaging, and response to therapy; local and distant metastasis; and response to treatment in patients with a variety of hematologic and solid cancers, including lymphoma, breast, GI, lung, melanoma, and others (note g and h below).

g. For the diagnosis, staging, and restaging of hormone-refractory prostate cancer.

h. For restaging of recurrent or residual thyroid cancers, of follicular cell origin, that have been previously treated by thyroidectomy and radioiodine ablation with serum thyroglobulin levels >10 ng/mL and negative ^{131}I whole-body scans.

2. Radiopharmaceutical: $[^{18}F]$-2-fluoro-2-deoxy-d-glucose (or FDG) is an analog of glucose.

3. Principle. Tumors have markedly accelerated glycolysis in comparison to the tissues from which they arise. FDG enters the tumor cell through the glucose transporter and is phosphorylated to FDG-6-phosphate (FDG-6P). FDG-6P, however, is not a suitable substrate for other glycolytic enzymes, is "metabolically trapped," and accumulates in the tumor tissue in proportion to the rate of phosphorylation of FDG. Although FDG-6P can be dephosphorylated by glucose-6-phosphatase, this enzyme is not expressed in actively proliferating tumors. Most normal tissues, with the exception of brain and heart, do have glucose-6-phosphatase and rapidly clear the FDG. Thus, a gradient develops between tumor and background over time and can be readily detected by a PET scanner.

4. Procedural notes. ^{18}FDG is injected into a fasting, euglycemic patient 45 to 60 minutes before PET scanning. Patients with blood glucose levels >200 mg/dL are typically not studied; patients who have received insulin immediately prior to study may also have altered biodistribution.

Increasingly, PET is carried out using a PET/CT instrument. The CT under such circumstances is carried out primarily to obtain a measure of tissue density for attenuation correction, and for anatomic localization. Frequently, oral contrast is administered (except when head and neck cancers are being evaluated), and an IV-contrast CT may also be carried out, usually after the PET/CT is completed.

5. Interpretation. ^{18}FDG PET imaging is likely to be of great use in the scanning of many malignancies.

a. For primary brain tumors, a comparison is made to the "contralateral" white matter; a hyperactive tumor has a ratio of 1.4 times the concentration of FDG. Increased uptake is characteristic of high-grade primary and metastatic neoplasms. The more active the uptake, the more rapid the growth pattern. Areas of decreased uptake are seen with low-grade tumors and radiation necrosis.

b. Solitary pulmonary nodules are commonly managed with thoracotomy because of uncertainty about the benign or malignant nature of this finding. If the ratio of ^{18}FDG PET uptake between a nodule and a normal control region is ≥2.5, the lesion is almost certainly malignant. The ratio varies between instruments and methodology; in general, the higher the cutoff value, the greater the specificity and the less the sensitivity.

c. False-negative studies are more common in those cancers that have a low metabolic rate; notably bronchioloalveolar carcinoma, well-differentiated (papillary or follicular) thyroid carcinomas particularly when the patient is on thyroid hormone, and hormone-sensitive, well-differentiated (Gleason ≤7) prostate carcinoma.

d. False-positive studies occur as a result of increased tracer concentration in nonmalignant regions with increased glucose metabolism. Infectious foci are the common false-positive abnormalities (for neoplasia); these may be acute infections, as well as chronic granulomatous diseases, notably tuberculosis and sarcoidosis. In most cases, the intensity of uptake is less than that noted in neoplasia. False-positive uptake has also been noted in muscle caused by tension or movement (especially of the vocalis muscles as a result of the patient talking after tracer injection) and in brown adipose tissue (the former may be decreased by encouraging the patient to relax, or by administration of short-acting benzodiazepines). To the trained interpreter, these latter appearances are usually distinguishable from neoplastic foci.

e. The concept of "metabolic response" is evolving. Most groups have accepted complete metabolic response (CMR) as representative of no viable tumor, and several studies have shown a correlation between CMR and survival in a variety of diseases, particularly lymphoma and breast cancer. Partial responses are being defined but currently utilize numerical criteria analogous to those used in **response evaluation criteria in solid tumors** (RECIST) and other similar response sets.

f. Standardized uptake value (SUV) is a semiquantitative index of glycolytic rate. It is usually calculated based on the patient's body weight, as follows:

$$SUV = \frac{\text{Activity concentration in volume of interest (KBq/mL)}}{\text{Activity injected (KBq)/Weight (g)}}$$

Several studies have suggested that an SUV >2.5 is representative of malignancy. SUVs are rarely >8 in infectious foci. It must be remembered that SUV is dependent on equipment and image reconstruction methodology as well as time after injection, among other factors, and therefore may be more useful for intrapatient comparison rather than group analyses.

C. ^{67}Ga imaging

1. Indications. The use of radiogallium imaging has significantly decreased since the introduction of FDG PET. Positron-emitting isotopes of gallium (^{68}Ga, ^{66}Ga) are available and are currently being evaluated.

a. To evaluate response to treatment of patients with Hodgkin lymphoma and intermediate- or high-grade (but not low-grade) non-Hodgkin lymphoma (NHL). A baseline assessment is performed before therapy and repeated at the time of restaging procedures.

b. To evaluate viability selectively in other tumors (e.g., hepatoma, sarcoma, melanoma). These patients are studied as far from the completion of treatment as possible.

2. Radiopharmaceutical: ^{67}Ga citrate

3. Principle. ^{67}Ga is a transition element that shares a variety of properties with iron, including rapid binding to transferrin (TF) after intravenous injection. Thereafter, the ^{67}Ga-TF is taken up by tumor cells through binding to the TF receptor on the membrane of tumor cells. The expression of the TF receptor is proportional to growth; the more rapidly proliferating the tumor, the more avid the uptake.

4. Procedural notes. The patient is imaged 48 to 72 hours after injection. A purgative may be administered the night before imaging. SPECT is significantly more sensitive than planar imaging for detecting active tumor sites. Anatomic correlation with CT or MRI helps greatly in interpretation. Where available, images from two different imaging modalities can be coregistered ("fused") in the computer. The anatomic image is used as a template on which the ^{67}Ga image is laid to identify the tumor-avid sites.

5. Interpretation

a. ^{67}Ga citrate imaging is not normally used for staging purposes, but a baseline scan is helpful for later comparisons to help determine tumor response, particularly in patients with lymphomatous mediastinal involvement. Tumor sites may take up ^{67}Ga with strong avidity, which is greatly reduced when the tumor has responded to treatment. Persistence of ^{67}Ga is a sign of poor prognosis.

b. ^{67}Ga imaging is nonspecific; the isotope is avidly taken up in inflammatory lesions (e.g., diffusely in the lungs with *Pneumocystis carinii* and other pneumonitides). ^{201}Tl has been found to be useful when the cause of uptake on a ^{67}Ga scan is questioned. ^{201}Tl is normally concentrated in viable tumor and is rarely positive in lymphatic inflammation.

D. Lymphoscintigraphy

1. **Indications:** To determine the direction of lymph node drainage from truncal skin lesions (e.g., for melanoma) or the status of lymph ducts in regions of lymphedema.

2. **Radiopharmaceutical:** ^{99m}Tc-labeled albumin or sulfur colloid.

3. **Procedural notes.** Typically, injections are made into the webbing between the toes or fingers to assess the lower limbs or arms, respectively. Gamma camera imaging is performed to assess the direction of drainage as a guide to determining what lymph node–bearing region should undergo surgical exploration.

4. **Interpretation.** Careful attention to detailed imaging in the early images may show the sites of interruption of draining lymphatic ducts, which in some patients can be used as a basis for correcting the problem.

E. Lymphoscintigraphy: sentinel node detection

1. **Indication:** Detection of the sentinel lymph node in patients scheduled to undergo surgical resection of primary breast carcinoma or melanoma.

2. **Radiopharmaceutical:** ^{99m}Tc sulfur colloid (in many cases, particularly for melanoma, passed through a 0.22-μ filter to decrease particle size). When filtered radiopharmaceutical is used, lymphatic channels are seen more frequently, and sentinel nodes are seen earlier. Several groups in the United States use unfiltered ^{99m}Tc sulfur colloid; this may permit greater flexibility from injection time to intra-operative detection, but may result in a lower proportion of sentinel nodes being visualized by imaging up to 2 hours after injection, though detection at surgery by intra-operative gamma probes remains feasible.

3. **Procedural notes.** After perilesional intradermal injection (or other site optimized for delineation of draining nodes) of the radiocolloid, serial gamma camera imaging (anterior and lateral views) is carried out to determine the lymphatic drainage and identify the first node that concentrates tracer. This is usually supplemented by intra-operative detection of nodal radioactivity using a gamma probe.

4. **Interpretation.** Serial images permit detection of the first node to concentrate radioactivity. It has been proposed that disease status of this node is representative of overall nodal status.

F. Metaiodobenzylguanidine (MIBG) imaging for catecholamines

1. **Indication:** To identify metastatic and primary tumor sites for pheochromocytoma and neuroblastoma.

2. **Radiopharmaceutical:** Iobenguane sulfate, ^{131}I-(MIBG sulfate), or ^{123}I-(MIBG sulfate).

3. **Principle.** MIBG is normally concentrated by adrenergic tissues in cytoplasmic storage granules that also contain other catecholamines. Anything that blocks uptake or promotes release of these storage granules can potentially lead to false-negative results (see section II.F.6).

4. **Procedural notes**

   a. **The typical dose** for an adult is 0.5 mCi of ^{131}I and 10 mCi of ^{123}I. For children under 18 years of age, a body surface area adjustment is made assuming the adult dose is for a 1.7 m^2 individual. Patients are pretreated with stable iodide (for adults, 10 drops daily of a 1g/mL solution starting just before injection and continuing until the last day of imaging).

   b. **Technique:** When ^{131}I is administered, the patient is imaged with the whole-body camera at 24 hours, and at 48 hours if necessary, with special attention to the retroperitoneum and adrenal region. SPECT of regions of interest is possible in most instances the day after ^{123}I-MIBG injection.

   c. **Warning.** Hypertensive crises have occurred after injection of MIBG, especially in patients with pheochromocytoma. Pregnancy is not an absolute contraindication, but the potential risk to the fetus should be carefully assessed.

5. **Interpretation.** MIBG is cleared by glomerular filtration from the plasma and is rapidly taken up in catecholamine storage granules in tissue sites containing sympathetic nerves or adrenergic storage sites. Thus, uptake occurs in the heart, kidneys, liver, and adrenals at most imaging times. Tumors show up as areas of increased uptake.

6. **Drug interactions.** The following drugs have the potential to interfere with the uptake of MIBG by neuroblastoma and pheochromocytoma and should be stopped a few days to weeks before beginning the imaging, depending on the pharmacology of the drug.
   a. Antihypertensives: labetalol, reserpine, calcium-channel blockers
   b. Amytriptyline, imipramine, and derivatives
   c. Doxepin
   d. Sympathetic amines (pseudoephedrine, ephedrine, phenylpropanol-amine, phenylephrine)
   e. Cocaine
7. **MIBG as treatment.** Several groups, notably in Canada and Europe, have used ^{131}I-MIBG as therapy for the neuroendocrine tumors listed above. Typical doses range up to 200 mCi ^{131}I. Dose-limiting toxicity is hematopoietic; most patients recover their blood counts completely and are eligible to be retreated in the absence of disease progression at 3- to 6-month intervals. For therapy studies, saturation with saturated solution of potassium iodide (SSKI) is carried out typically for a week after therapy.

G. **Pentetreotide (octreotide) imaging**
   1. **Indication:** For diagnostic workup of neuroendocrine tumors that bear somatostatin receptors.
   2. **Radiopharmaceutical.** Pentetreotide is a diethylenetriaminepentaacetic acid (DPTA) conjugate of octreotide, which is a long-acting analog of human somatostatin. ^{111}In is bound to the agent.
   3. **Principle.** ^{111}In-pentetreotide binds to somatostatin receptors throughout the body. Neuroendocrine tumors highly express these receptors and thus concentrate sufficient amounts of the radioactive agent to be seen by scintigraphy.
   4. **Procedural notes.** The patient undergoes daily planar and SPECT imaging until it is determined whether the agent is helpful. Typical imaging times are 4, 24, and 48 hours after injection. Because the agent is excreted into the bowel, the patient should be given a mild laxative the evening before the 24- and 48-hour imaging times.
      a. **False-negative results** may occur in patients who are concurrently taking octreotide acetate (Sandostatin®) for control of symptoms related to neuroendocrine tumors. If possible, patients should stop taking this medication 2 weeks before the scan. Also, corticosteroids by prescription should be stopped before scanning, as these and adrenocorticotropic hormone–producing tumors can reduce the expression of somatostatin receptors.
      b. **Warnings and adverse reactions.** Transient symptoms are occasionally seen, including dizziness, hypotension, and headache. Patients with known or suspected insulinomas should have an intravenous line running with 5% dextrose in normal saline before and during administration to avoid possible hypoglycemia.
   5. **Interpretation.** The normal pituitary gland, thyroid gland, and liver are seen. To a lesser extent, the gall bladder, kidney, and bladder are also visible. Uptake in tumors bearing somatostatin receptors is apparent beginning at 4 hours, with the 24- and 48-hour images showing the greatest tissue contrast. The sensitivity for detecting tumor types depends on the frequency of somatostatin receptor. Those patients with strongly positive scans may be most likely to benefit from treatment with octreotide.
      a. **New lesions that were previously occult,** despite extensive workup, were identified in nearly 30% of patients studied with ^{111}In-pentetreotide. Carcinoid tumors, neuroblastomas, pheochromocytoma, paragangliomas, small cell lung cancer, and meningiomas were detected in about 90% of cases. Lymphomas, pituitary tumors, and medullary tumors were detected in high but more variable percentages.
      b. **Granulomatous lesions** and other types of inflammatory lesions were also positive, including tuberculosis, sarcoidosis, rheumatoid arthritis, and Graves' disease ophthalmopathy.

H. Prostascint for prostate tumor imaging

1. **Indications:** Detection of prostate cancer outside the prostatic bed or recurrent prostate cancer in the prostatic bed.

2. **Radiopharmaceutical.** ^{111}In-capromab pendetide (Prostascint) consists of a monoclonal antibody, to which ^{111}In is attached by a chelate, against the prostate-specific membrane antigen (PSMA).

3. **Principle.** The antibody reacts with an antigen specifically found in prostate cancer cells. After intravenous administration, the antibody is gradually cleared from the circulation while localizing in tumor tissue.

4. **Procedural notes.** Anterior and posterior whole-body images are obtained starting about 30 minutes after injection, followed by SPECT of the infrahepatic abdomen and pelvis. Comparable images are obtained typically 4 days after injection. Because the radioactivity may be concentrated in the liver and is usually excreted through the bowel, it is important to prepare the bowel with an oral laxative the night before.

5. **Interpretation.** The whole-body images are searched for areas of increased uptake in the region of the aortic and iliac nodal groups, as well as for recurrence in the prostate bed. The SPECT images are important for the region of the prostate bed and the obturator nodes. Because the antibody remains in circulation and because the increased uptake in diseased areas is sometimes difficult to distinguish from normal vascular activity, it is important to compare the early and delayed image sets to ensure that the area of uptake seen in the delayed imaging is not in a vascular region. Some groups do not carry out the early image sets and instead carry out "dual-isotope" imaging using ^{99m}Tc-labeled red cells to delineate the vascular structures. Increasingly, groups are beginning to use SPECT/CT so that the CT component can provide anatomic localization of radioactivity distribution. It is also important to ensure that the patient voids urine as completely as possible before imaging and to image comparable areas of the body.

I. Tumor viability imaging: ^{201}Tl chloride and ^{99m}Tc sestaMIBI

1. **Indications.** FDG PET/CT is increasingly used in place of these agents, particularly in areas outside the brain.
   a. Differential diagnosis of breast masses
   b. Viability assessment of primary bone tumors after chemotherapy
   c. Monitoring viability of well-differentiated thyroid cancer
   d. Imaging of parathyroid adenomas
   e. Imaging of brain tumors (SPECT)

2. **Radiopharmaceutical**
   a. **^{99m}Tc methoxyisobutyl isonitrile** (MIBI) is a monovalent cationic form of ^{99m}Tc that is highly lipid soluble. The agent is formed as a central ^{99m}Tc atom surrounded by six isobutyl nitrile molecules; for this reason, it is sometimes referred to as *sestaMIBI*.
   b. **^{201}Tl (thallous) chloride** is a radioisotope of thallium, which is in the actinide series of elements and behaves *in vivo* as an analog of potassium.

3. **Principle.** ^{201}Tl chloride is a widely used cardiac perfusion agent that is taken up by most viable cells as a potassium analog and transported by the Na^+–K^+ pump. ^{99m}Tc sestaMIBI is also used to monitor cardiac perfusion. In addition, when taken up into the cell by a different mechanism, it can be used as a marker for cellular viability. After introduction into the bloodstream, both of these agents are rapidly cleared from the circulation in proportion to cardiac output.

4. **Procedural notes.** The tracer is injected intravenously, and imaging is begun over the region of interest within 20 minutes of injection, frequently at an early and a late time after injection (e.g., 5 minutes and 60 minutes after injection). For breast imaging, a special breast apparatus permits planar lateral views of the breast in the prone position. This appears to be a technical advance. For brain and other imaging, SPECT scanning is performed.

5. **Interpretation**
   a. **Breast masses.** About 25% of patients who are subjected to screening mammography have "dense" breasts that obfuscate interpretation. If these patients

also have palpable breast masses, there may be a clinical dilemma in regard to biopsy of these lesions. It has been reported that uptake of ^{201}Tl is negative in fibrocystic disease and positive in 96% of breast cancer nodules. Similar results have been observed in patients with breast masses imaged with MIBI. The negative predictive value for breast cancer with these studies is likely to improve the specificity of breast mammography and is applicable to both dense breasts and normal breasts.

  b. Primary bone tumors are frequently treated with chemotherapy before surgery. ^{201}Tl and ^{99m}Tc sestaMIBI are both taken up with high sensitivity into primary bone tumors and extremity sarcomas. Chondrosarcoma is an exception. MIBI uptake is lost in tumors responding to chemotherapy and has also been shown to correlate well with response to therapy.

  c. Brain tumors. ^{201}Tl chloride appears to be the agent of choice for evaluating supratentorial primary brain tumors when FDG PET is not available. SPECT imaging is accurate for assessing the viability of brain tumors. In our experience, ^{201}Tl is preferred over ^{99m}Tc sestaMIBI because uptake in the choroid plexus is not as marked.

  d. Thyroid cancer imaging. ^{201}Tl whole-body imaging is a good way to monitor the activity of well-differentiated thyroid cancer during the interval when the patient is fully suppressed on thyroid hormone. The total uptake, as a percentage of the total-body uptake, is a monitor of the cellular viability of the tumor and can be used to assess the effectiveness of primary cancer treatment.

  e. Parathyroid imaging. With careful comparisons of ^{201}Tl or ^{99m}Tc sestaMIBI imaging, it is sometimes possible to detect parathyroid adenomas in the neck or upper mediastinum when other modalities are negative. Still, the sensitivity of these techniques is disappointingly low (about 50%) in patients with intact parathyroid glands and considerably higher (about 80%) for the detection of recurrence. FDG PET has not been found to be useful for parathyroid imaging.

III. OTHER IMAGING STUDIES USED IN ONCOLOGY

  A. Cardiac functional studies. Equilibrium (gated) blood pool imaging is used to evaluate possible cardiac failure and to monitor changes after treatment with cardiotoxic drugs.

  1. Radiopharmaceutical. Red blood cells (RBCs) may be labeled *in vivo*. Stannous pyrophosphate (1 mg) is administered 20 minutes before injecting ^{99m}Tc pertechnetate. The stannous pyrophosphate enters and is trapped in the RBCs. The ^{99m}Tc pertechnetate diffuses into the RBCs and is bound to the β chain of hemoglobin. About 75% of the dose is labeled to the RBCs. An electrocardiogram R-wave signal serves as a physiological "gate" for collection of timed "frames" (often called *gated blood pool imaging*).

  2. Interpretation. Images obtained during rest are interpreted qualitatively to determine areas of abnormal wall motion, size of cardiac chambers, presence of intrinsic or extrinsic compression of the cardiac contour, and size and shape of the outflow tracts. Images are interpreted quantitatively for a physiological assessment of the quantity of blood ejected from the left ventricle with each beat (the left ventricular ejection fraction [LVEF]). A normal LVEF is usually >50%. LVEFs <30% are usually but not always associated with clinical congestive heart failure. A decrease of >10% in LVEF is highly significant. Cardiotoxic chemotherapeutic agents should be stopped when ejection fractions fall to below normal.

  B. Vascular flow and bleeding studies can be used to detect the patency of venous access in the upper extremities (e.g., post-subclavian catheter-placement swelling, superior vena cava syndrome), to assess for the presence of hemangioma as a space-occupying lesion, or to determine a site for bleeding. ^{99m}Tc pertechnetate or ^{99m}Tc sulfur colloid can be used as transient labels of the vasculature. *In vivo* labeling of RBCs with ^{99m}Tc may be used as more long-term vascular labels (see section III.A.1).

  C. ^{99m}Tc-macroaggregated albumin for lung perfusion can be used to evaluate patients suspected of having pulmonary embolism and to determine the lung function capacity before pulmonary resection. ^{99m}Tc-labeled to macroaggregates of albumin

(30 to 60 μm in diameter) are injected intravenously and are cleared in the first pass through the pulmonary circulation. The distribution of radioactivity is proportional to blood flow to the lungs.

D. Studies of pulmonary ventilation can be used to determine whether a ventilation-perfusion "mismatch" exists as an aid in the differential diagnosis of pulmonary embolism and to assess the ventilatory capacity of the human lung. ^{133}Xe gas, ^{127}Xe gas, ^{81m}Kr, and ^{99m}Tc-DPTA aerosol are used to label the inspiratory air. As the patient breathes, a gamma camera obtains an image of the distribution of radioactivity. Several minutes of breathing is required to achieve equilibrium with bullae and fistulous tracts.

E. Infection imaging

1. **^{67}Ga citrate appears to be taken up by the cells near the region of the infection.** ^{67}Ga imaging requires several days to complete, and normal physiological uptake (especially in the abdomen) interferes with interpretation. ^{67}Ga citrate imaging is sensitive for making the diagnosis of *P. carinii* pneumonia at a relatively early stage. It is somewhat less sensitive than ^{111}In-labeled white blood cells (WBCs) in the postsurgical setting; the normal excretion of ^{67}Ga into the bowel is a drawback. Nevertheless, by using imaging methods that increase contrast, such as SPECT, satisfactory imaging can be obtained in most cases.

2. **Radiolabeled (^{111}In or ^{99m}Tc) WBCs** progressively accumulate at the site of infection. The labeled WBC method requires external manipulation and labeling of the patient's blood. WBC imaging with ^{111}In shows uptake in the liver, spleen, and bone marrow, but not in other sites within the abdomen. Sensitivity for acute infection approaches 90%.

3. **FDG PET** has a high sensitivity rate for detection of infection. Its utility in patients with cancer is limited by its comparable sensitivity for viable cancer detection, with consequent inability to differentiate infection from recurrent cancer.

4. **New directions for inflammation imaging.** Radiolabeled monoclonal antibodies that label WBC *in vivo*, a variety of leukotropic peptides (that also label WBC *in vivo*), and a radiolabeled nonspecific immunoglobulin (with accuracy rates of close to 90%) are in various stages of development and approval.

IV. THERAPEUTIC RADIOISOTOPES

A. ^{131}I for well-differentiated thyroid cancer

1. **Radiopharmaceutical:** sodium iodide (^{131}I), oral solution

2. **Patient selection** (see Chapter 15, section III). Patients are selected for study after surgery has established the diagnosis of thyroid cancer. Patients considered for radioactive ^{131}I are those at high risk for recurrence of well-differentiated thyroid cancer, either papillary or follicular, or one of the well-known variants to these tumors. Patients are considered at "high risk" if they are older than 40 years of age; if the primary tumor is large (>2 cm), locally invasive, or multicentric in the neck; or if there is metastatic tumor in the neck.

3. **Procedural notes.** There is considerable variation in the study and treatment protocol for thyroid carcinoma.

   a. Some experts simply treat all high-risk patients after surgery with >100 mCi of ^{131}I. A thyroid remnant, if present, is ablated with administered doses sufficient to deliver at least 300 Gy to the normal thyroid.

   b. In most situations, some form of testing is performed for the ability of the tumor to concentrate radioactive iodine, and patients are treated if there is residual ^{131}I-concentrating tissue in the neck. At the time of testing, patients are expected to be hypothyroid (thyroid-stimulating hormone level >30 IU/mL) and to have a low serum iodine concentration (<5 μg/dL). Patients are prepared by being off thyroid hormone (thyroxine for 6 weeks and tri-iodothyronine for 3 weeks) and on a low-iodide diet (for 3 weeks before treatment).

   c. The recent approval of recombinant thyrotropin (rhTSH, Thyrogen) has enabled the evaluation of patients in the euthyroid state. The recommended dose of rhTSH is 0.9 mg IM daily for 2 days. Typically, diagnostic ^{131}I is given on the third day, and imaging and thyroglobulin estimation are carried out on the fifth day.

4. **Dose selection.** Several authorities treat with standard doses after uptake in thyroid cancer is demonstrated. If lymph nodal metastases are demonstrated in the neck only, a dose of 150 mCi is sometimes used. For pulmonary, bone, or central nervous system metastases, a dose of 200 mCi may be used.

At Memorial Sloan Kettering Cancer Center (MSKCC), a higher dose protocol has been developed, which depends on more careful dosimetry and is called the *highest safe dose* approach. Dosimetry testing for 3 to 5 days in the well-prepared patient is used to select a dose that delivers at least 2 Gy (200 cGy) to the blood, not >140 mCi retained in the whole body at 48 hours, and in patients with metastatic lung disease, <80 mCi retained in the lungs at 48 hours. With this set of dosing rules, several hundred patients have been treated with good treatment response and without major complications.

5. **Treatment response.** Patients respond best to treatment when the tumor is small (total tumor burden <200 g) and confined to local or regional areas of the body. The cure rate at MSKCC was >95% for patients younger than 40 years of age and 50% for those older than 40 years of age. Even when cure is not achieved, significant palliation can be obtained with ^{131}I treatment.

6. **Follow-up.** Patients are normally evaluated at yearly intervals. Consideration for retreatment requires taking the patient off thyroid hormone, allowing hypothyroidism to develop, and treating with high-dose ^{131}I until no appreciable ^{131}I tissue is present ("clean slate"). Elevation of thyroglobulin levels indicates a high likelihood of recurrence of thyroid cancer at some time in the next 5 years in patients with well-differentiated thyroid cancer. In patients with unusually aggressive thyroid cancers, retreatment at a shorter interval can be considered (usually at about 6 months). We usually require tumor doses of at least 20 Gy. Ablation of known metastases has occurred with doses as low as 35 Gy, but 100 Gy is usually required for lymph nodes containing tumor.

7. **Treatment complications.** The most common complication of high-dose ^{131}I treatment is sialadenitis, which occurs in about 20% of patients at doses >200 mCi; a few patients develop chronic sialadenitis.

With any exposure to whole-body irradiation, there is always the concern that an increase in malignancies may occur, particularly leukemias. However, no increase in leukemia was seen in a large group of Swedish patients treated with an average dose of 160 mCi. At higher average doses in more than 500 patients at Memorial Sloan-Kettering Cancer Center, no leukemias have occurred in the treatment group. These data suggest that ^{131}I does not significantly increase the risk for leukemia.

B. **Bone pain palliation with radioisotopes**

1. **Radiopharmaceuticals:** [89]Sr chloride (Metastron), 4 mCi; or [153]Sm-EDTMP (Lexidronam), 1 mCi/kg. [153]Sm emits gamma rays and thus can be evaluated for radioactivity distribution.

2. **Principle.** Various human tumors produce a strong osteoblastic reaction that results in the deposition of bone-seeking radionuclides in the hydroxyapatite crystal in the region of the tumor. When given in sufficient quantity, the radionuclide radiates the active bony regions near the metastases sufficiently to relieve pain. It is unclear whether the benefits of treatment are due to the irradiation of the bone or of the tumor itself. The usual dose is thought to be about 7 to 10 Gy.

3. **Procedural notes.** Patients should have platelet counts >60,000/μL and WBC counts >2,400/μL, and painful bone lesions should be demonstrated as being positive on bone scan preferably carried out within 3 weeks of the treatment. Patients should not be treated with ^{89}Sr unless their life expectancy is at least 3 months. Patients with platelet counts >150,000/μL may be treated at the recommended dose; those with lower platelet counts should be treated at lower doses and monitored carefully for hematopoietic toxicity.

    a. Complete blood counts should be repeated every 2 weeks for 4 months. Platelet and WBC counts are typically decreased by about 30%, and the nadir counts occur 12 to 16 weeks after injection.

    b. Because the radioactivity is primarily excreted in the urine, the patient should be continent or catheterized to minimize contamination of clothing and the patient's home environment.

  4. Treatment response. Patients with cancers of the prostate, breast, and lung have been treated with these radiopharmaceuticals, but, in principle, any tumor with an osteoblastic component on bone scan could be treated. The usual onset of pain relief occurs within 7 to 21 days after administration (earlier for Lexidronam). Patients should be counseled about the possibility of a "flare response," in which pain is increased for a period of days to weeks after the treatment. A significant proportion of patients (75% to 80%) do get significant pain relief, and the typical duration of response is 3 to 4 months.

  5. Contraindications and precautions. Pregnancy is an absolute contraindication, and women of childbearing age should have a pregnancy test the day before administration of a radiopharmaceutical. Patients may be considered for retreatment, usually after 90 days, if they have responded well to initial therapy and provided that hematopoietic toxicity was not excessively severe. Most patients tolerate multiple injections without major side effects.

C. ^{32}P for polycythemia vera (PV)

  1. Radiopharmaceutical: buffered sodium ^{32}P-phosphate solution

  2. Dosage. Intravenous doses of 2.3 mCi/m^2 (dose not to exceed 5.0 mCi) are administered at 3-month intervals to induce remission or to control excessive cellular proliferation. The dose may be repeated twice if a remission is not achieved and is increased by 25% each dose (not to exceed 7 mCi as a single dose).

  3. Treatment response. About 80% of patients with PV achieve remission after one injection of ^{32}P. In comparison with phlebotomy alone, patients treated with ^{32}P survive longer and have fewer thrombotic complications but have a significantly increased incidence of acute myelogenous leukemia.

  4. Contraindications. Pregnancy is an absolute contraindication because of the possibility of teratogenic effects. In PV, the drug should not be administered when the WBC count is <5,000/μL or platelets are <150,000/μL.

D. Colloidal ^{32}P for malignant effusions

  1. Radiopharmaceutical: chromic ^{32}P-phosphate colloidal suspension

  2. Dosage. In a 70-kg patient, 6 to 12 mCi is used for intrapleural administration and 10 to 20 mCi for intraperitoneal administration. Great care should be taken to ensure that all radioactivity is deposited in the intended body cavity. Large tumor masses or loculation of fluid is a relative contraindication to treatment.

  3. Treatment response. Most patients receive some benefit from treatment in terms of control of effusions. There is a growing interest in the use of ^{32}P in the treatment of low-volume ovarian cancer.

E. ^{90}Y-labeled anti-CD20 antibody for lymphoma

  1. Radiopharmaceutical: ^{90}Y-labeled ibritumomab tiuxetan (Zevalin)

  2. Indications. Zevalin, as part of the Zevalin therapeutic regimen, is indicated for the treatment of patients with relapsed or refractory low-grade follicular or transformed B-cell non-Hodgkin lymphoma, including patients with rituximab-refractory follicular NHL.

  3. Dosage. Ibritumomab is a murine antibody that reacts with CD20, a cell-surface receptor found on most B-cell lymphomas. Tiuxetan is a proprietary chelate that binds radioactive metals to antibody. The dose of ibritumomab tiuxetan in patients with platelet counts >150,000/μL is 0.4 mCi/kg body weight, and in patients with platelets between 100,000 and 149,000/μL is 0.3 mCi/kg. In both instances, the maximum administered dose should not exceed 32 mCi ^{90}Y. Patients with >25% lymphomatous involvement of marrow should not be treated with this agent.

    a. Assessing biodistribution. The patient initially receives 250 mg/m^2 of rituximab (Rituxan, Mabthera), a chimeric (Fv-grafted human IgG$_1$) monoclonal antibody that recognizes the CD20 receptor (for details on rituximab administration, see Chapter 4, section VII.G4.). The rituximab is followed by 5 mCi ^{111}In-labeled ibritumomab tiuxetan. Whole-body ^{111}In images are then carried out 2 to 24 hours and 48 to 72 hours after injection to assess biodistribution. Visual assessment of favorable biodistribution is defined by tumor uptake of radioactivity; easily detectable uptake in blood pool on the first-day image, decreasing subsequently; and moderate uptake in normal liver and spleen with low uptake in normal kidneys and normal bowel.

   b. Treatment is carried out in an identical manner to the diagnostic infusion. The patient is treated between 7 and 9 days after this first infusion. The patient receives 250 mg/m^2 of rituximab. This is followed by ^{90}Y-labeled ibritumomab tiuxetan at a dose of 0.3 to 0.4 mCi/kg body weight (to a maximum of 32 mCi), usually given over 10 minutes.

4. Toxicity. Acute side effects following Zevalin are rare; nonspecific symptoms following rituximab are more common after the first treatment than after the second. Grade 3 or greater hematologic toxicity occurs in almost half of all treated patients and requires support (G-CSF for neutropenia, transfusions for thrombocytopenia) in about 10% to 30%. Toxicity nadirs occur between 7 and 9 weeks after treatment and last for about 3 weeks. Patients should be monitored closely for hematologic toxicity for at least 8 weeks or until recovery (usually 12 weeks).

5. Efficacy. Ibritumomab tiuxetan in combination with rituximab gives significantly higher overall response rates compared with rituximab alone (80% vs. 56%). The complete response rate with ibritumomab tiuxetan is also higher than with rituximab alone (30% to 34% vs. 16% to 20%). The secondary end points, duration of response and time to progression, are not significantly different between the two treatment arms; however, there is a trend toward longer time to progression in patients with follicular NHL (15 months in the ibritumomab tiuxetan arm vs. 10 months in the rituximab arm) and in patients who have achieved a complete response (25 months vs. 13 months, respectively).

F. ^{131}I-labeled anti-CD20 antibody for lymphoma

   1. Radiopharmaceutical: ^{131}I-labeled tositumomab (Bexxar)

   2. Indications: The Bexxar therapeutic regimen (tositumomab and ^{131}I-tositumomab) is indicated for the treatment of patients with CD20-positive, follicular NHL, with and without transformation, whose disease is refractory to rituximab and has relapsed following chemotherapy. The Bexxar therapeutic regimen, like the Zevalin regimen, is not indicated for the initial treatment of patients with CD20-positive NHL. Patients with >25% lymphomatous involvement of marrow should not be treated with this agent.

   3. Dosage. Tositumomab is a murine antibody that reacts with CD20, a cell-surface receptor found on most B-cell lymphomas. In contrast to Zevalin, which is administered on an activity per unit weight basis, Bexxar is administered on a whole-body radiation absorbed dose calculation. The dose of ^{131}I-tositumomab in patients with platelet counts >150,000/μL is 0.75 Gy to the whole body and 0.65 Gy in patients with platelets between 100,000 and 149,000/μL.

   a. Preparation. A day prior to initiation of therapy, the patient starts oral iodide therapy for thyroid protection (typically 10 drops of SSKI solution daily), which continues until 2 weeks after the therapeutic dose.

   b. Biodistribution and dosimetry. The patient initially receives 450 mg of tositumomab over an hour. Nonspecific symptoms are rare (fatigue, low-grade fever, and chills) and can be controlled if necessary with oral acetaminophen and diphenhydramine. This is followed by 5 mCi ^{131}I-labeled tositumomab (35 mg), given over 20 minutes. Whole-body ^{131}I images (dosimetry scans, carried out at speeds of about 30 cm/minute) are carried out immediately on completion of infusion, and again 2 to 4 days and 6 to 7 days after injection. These images are used to calculate the amount of ^{131}I that will deliver no >0.75 Gy radiation absorbed dose to the whole body. As with Zevalin, visual assessment of favorable biodistribution is defined by easily detectable uptake in the blood pool on the first-day image, decreasing subsequently, and by moderate uptake in normal liver and spleen, with low uptake in normal kidneys and normal bowel.

   c. Treatment. The patient is treated between 7 and 14 days after this first infusion. Treatment is carried out in an identical manner to the diagnostic infusion. The patient receives 450 mg of tositumomab, followed by ^{131}I-labeled tositumomab (mass 35 mg). The amount of ^{131}I administered is calculated based on whole-body clearance of the dosimetric radioactivity.

  4. Toxicity. The most common adverse reaction is hematopoietic, with most patients having grade 3 or 4 toxicity, with a time to nadir of 4 to 7 weeks, lasting for approximately a month. Due to the variable nature in the onset of cytopenias, complete blood counts should be obtained weekly for 10 to 12 weeks. Hematopoietic toxicity follows patterns comparable to those with Zevalin.

  5. Efficacy. Bexxar therapy results in responses and response durations comparable to those with Zevalin. The overall response rates have ranged from 47% to 64% and the median durations of response from 12 to 18 months. These response rates have been comparable in patients refractory to rituximab.

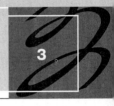

RADIATION ONCOLOGY
Steve P. Lee

3

I. RADIATION ONCOLOGY

A. Radiation oncology is a discipline specializing in the use of radiation for therapeutic purposes. It is synonymous with *therapeutic radiology*, an older name created to distinguish the specialty from *diagnostic radiology*. **Radiation therapy** (RT) is a treatment modality in which ionizing radiation is used for patients with cancers and other diseases.

   The first therapeutic use of radiation dates back to 1896, almost immediately after the discovery of x-rays. For more than a century, RT continues to play a significant role in the fight against cancer, with its progress intimately supported by the advances in modern science and technology. Among the main cancer treatment modalities, RT and surgery aim to provide local-regional tumor control, while chemotherapy addresses systemic metastases in addition to serving frequently as a radiation-sensitizing agent.

B. A **radiation oncologist** is a physician trained in cancer medicine who uses radiation for the treatment of cancer patients. The radiation oncologist discusses the benefits and risks of the proposed treatment, designs and controls the treatment process, cares for the patient's treatment-induced side effects, and continually monitors the patient's disease status. The delivery of RT necessitates the efforts of other health care professionals.

   1. Medical physicists ensure the proper functioning of radiation-producing machines and maintain treatment planning hardware and software.

   2. Dosimetrists and physicists perform treatment planning for individual patients to the specifications of radiation oncologists.

   3. Radiation therapists operate treatment machines to irradiate patients according to specific treatment plans.

   4. Collaborators. To deal with a patient's cancer problem, a radiation oncologist must also collaborate closely with diagnostic radiologists, pathologists, surgeons, and medical oncologists.

II. PHYSICAL, CHEMICAL, AND BIOLOGICAL BASIS OF RADIATION ACTION

A. Ionizing radiations. Radiations in the energy range used for RT can cause the ejection of orbital electrons and result in the *ionization* of atoms or molecules. The amount of energy deposited within a certain amount of tissue is defined as the *absorbed dose* with a unit of **gray** (Gy; 1 Gy = 1 joule/kg). The older unit of **rad** is equivalent to 1 centigray (cGy; 1 rad = 1 cGy). The types of radiation commonly used clinically are:

   1. Photons are identical to *electromagnetic waves*. The energy range used for RT pertains to either **x-rays,** which are commonly produced by a *linear accelerator* (LINAC), or **γ-rays,** which are emitted from radioactive isotopes. Photons of different energies interact with matters differently: from low to high energy, the absorption mechanism ranges from *photoelectric effect*, *Compton effect* to *pair production*. Modern therapeutic machines produce photon beams with energy of *megavoltage* (or *million electron volt*, MeV) range rather than *kilovoltage* (*kilo electron volt*, KeV), as used in diagnostic radiology. In general, the higher the photon energy, the greater the depth of penetration into the body and the more "skin-sparing" effect with less radiation dermatitis.

2. **Electron beams** dissipate their energy rapidly as they enter tissue. Thus, they have a relatively short depth of penetration and generally are used to treat superficial lesions. The effective range in tissue also depends on their energy. Each modern LINAC usually provides one or two energies of photons and several levels of electron energies.

3. **Other radiation particles** used for RT include **protons, neutrons,** and **heavy ions,** such as carbon anions. These particles are characterized by the so-called **linear energy transfer** (LET), a quantity measuring the rate of energy loss per length of path. Heavy ions have high LET and thus are "densely ionizing," compared with the low-LET photons and electrons, which are "sparsely ionizing."

   a. **Relative biologic effectiveness** (RBE) is defined as the ratio of doses needed to produce the same biologic endpoint between a standard low-LET photon beam (by convention 250 KeV x-ray) and another radiation of different LET. The term relates LET to an actual biological effect, such as cell death. In general, higher LET particles have higher RBE up to a certain level ($\sim$100 KeV/μ), beyond which RBE actually declines due to "wastage" of further energy transfer.

   b. Another factor that depends on LET is the efficiency of oxygen molecules to enhance radiation cell killing (mediated by oxygen radical formation). Lower LET radiation, compared with higher LET particles, tends to depend more on the presence of oxygen to effect cellular damage and thus have a higher **oxygen enhancement ratio** (OER, defined as the ratio of doses needed for a particular radiation to produce the same cell survival between anoxic and oxic environments).

   c. **Protons** have a level of LET similar to photons, and thus have no significant biological advantage over high-energy photons or electrons. A proton beam, however, has a special physical property of releasing very little energy as it traverses into tissue until a fixed depth is reached where almost all the dose is deposited (called a "Bragg peak"). The depth of this peak can be manipulated electronically to coincide with the target by varying the incident energy of the protons. Thus, proton radiation has a dosimetric advantage when treating a deep-seated tumor next to a critical normal structure.

   d. **Neutrons** do not possess the dosimetric advantage of protons because they do not have the depth-dose characteristic of a Bragg peak. Nevertheless, neutrons have high LET and low OER. That is, their cell-killing function does not depend on the presence of oxygen. Thus, neutrons have the biological advantage of treating tumors that are relatively resistant to photons due to the presence of significant hypoxia (see III.C.1).

   e. **Heavy ions** have high LET and low OER, as well as the presence of a Bragg peak. Thus, if used properly they possess both the biological and physical advantages seen in neutrons and protons, respectively.

B. **Mechanism of damage to cellular targets.** Where water is abundant, short-lived (10^{-10} to 10^{-12} seconds) hydroxyl radicals can be formed by ionizing radiation (via a process called *radiolysis*) and impact on a nearby ($\sim$100 Å) macromolecule such as DNA to damage its chemical bonds (**indirect action**). Alternatively, such chemical bond damage can result directly from the deposition of radiation energy (**direct action**). Evidence suggests DNA to be the main target of radiation action in cells. The "elementary lesions" include *base damages, cross-links, single-strand breaks,* and *double-strand breaks.* Recent studies show the presence of "complex clustered damages" or "multiply damaged sites," each of which consists of multiple elementary lesions within a few nanometers, or about 20 base pairs of DNA. These damages remain unrepaired and can lead to eventual cell "lethality," which is defined operationally as the *loss of reproductive integrity* (i.e., clonogenicity). Such mode of *mitotic death* is considered a predominant mechanism of radiation killing, but other processes such as *interphase death* and *apoptosis* (programmed cell death) also play important roles.

C. Cellular and tissue response to radiation damage. Some molecular mechanisms have been identified to govern a cell's response to radiation damage, with an intricate network of signal transduction pathways leading to either cell death or survival. The ultimate outcome is a result of complex chain events dictated not only by the biophysical interaction between radiation particles and DNA, but also by molecular and genetic determinants such as oncogenes, tumor-suppressor genes, and cell cycle regulation. In addition, extracellular and tissue conditions such as hypoxia, cell–cell interaction, and extracellular matrix can also modify the final expression of radiation effects to cells and tissues. Despite these complexities, certain clinical-pathologic outcomes can still be predicted due to the simplicity of direct radiation action on critical cellular targets.

III. BIOLOGICAL BASIS OF RADIATION THERAPY

A. Target cell hypothesis. A biophysical interpretation of the radiation mechanism can be made between a given dose, D, and the observed fraction of clonogenic cells surviving (*surviving fraction, SF*). The basic assumption is that critical targets exist within each cell; when ionizing radiation particles hit these targets, loss of cellular clonogenicity may result. This is the essence of the so-called *target-cell hypothesis* or *hit theory*.

B. Cell survival curves. When plotted as a semilog graph of $\log_e SF$ vs. D, almost all mammalian radiation survival curves reveal a very similar shape with a "curvy shoulder" at the low-dose region in contiguity with a relatively linear tail toward the high-dose region. This suggests that at least two biophysical mechanisms seem to be operating simultaneously to produce such a result.

1. The **linear component** signifies that radiation action on the critical target within a cell is a *random* process, resulting in *logarithmic* decrease in survival such that equal dose increments cause a constant logarithmic proportion of cell deaths. It is commonly described as a *single-hit* killing, which results in nonrepairable damage leading to direct cell death.

2. The **curvy shoulder,** however, reflects a much more complex situation whereby interactions of more than one target lesion are at work to result in eventual cell lethality (thus described as *multitarget* killing). Before subsequent interacting events can take place, the initial lesion may be repaired. Thus, the ultimate expression of this mode of cell killing depends on the kinetics and efficiency of the repair process.

3. Quantitative models. The most popular is the **linear-quadratic (LQ) model.** Based on this model, the SF after a single treatment of radiation dose D can be characterized by the following equation:

$$SF = exp(-\alpha D - \beta D^2),$$

where α and β are tissue-specific parameters governing intrinsic radiation sensitivity. The LQ model can be used to explain the differential sensitivities of malignant tumors versus normal tissues to fractionation radiotherapy (i.e., dividing the overall therapy into numerous fractions of small-dose irradiation). The **α/β ratio** is used clinically to characterize how various tissues respond to fractionation treatment.

a. Acute-responding tissues, such as cancers and fast-dividing normal cells, typically have high α/β ($\sim$8 to 10 Gy), and upon irradiation experience **acute effects** (e.g., tumor shrinkage, dermatitis, mucositis, or esophagitis).

b. Late-responding tissues (normal cells that rarely proliferate but can experience **late effects** such as fibrosis, xerostomia, and nerve damage) have low α/β ($\sim$2 to 5 Gy).

c. Upon fractionation, it is seen that acute-responding cells are killed predominantly, while the late-responding tissues are relatively spared due to their higher capacity to repair (see III.C.3).

C. Fractionation radiobiology. The biological processes occurring in between the treatment fractions have been summarized as the **4 Rs of fractionation radiobiology:**

1. **Reoxygenation.** The damage of tissues by radiation depends largely on the formation of hydroxyl radicals, which in turn depend on the availability of oxygen molecules in close proximity. Fractionation allows oxygen to diffuse into the usually hypoxic center of an expanding tumor during the interval between fractions and thus enables more tumor cell killing during the subsequent treatment.

2. **Repopulation.** All living tissues have the potential to repopulate by mitotic (clonogenic) growth. If normal tissue progenitor cells repopulate more adequately than malignant cells during the treatment course, then a therapeutic gain may be obtained by fractionation. Moreover, a phenomenon of **accelerated repopulation,** which is stimulated by cytotoxic intervention such as radiation, has been described for fast-growing malignant and normal cells. Thus, the *overall treatment time* is an important clinical variable affecting the chance of tumor control. As cancer cells quickly repopulate, further protraction of overall treatment time is disadvantageous. Once radiation treatment commences, unnecessary interruption of treatment course is discouraged.

3. **Repair.** Repair machinery within cells can reverse partial damage caused by a small fraction of the radiation dose. The cells would die if such damage fails to be repaired sufficiently and the damage is exacerbated by further radiation insults. One possible contributing mechanism is called **sublethal damage (SLD) repair.** As the dose per fraction decreases and interfractional time interval increases enough to allow for complete SLD repair, the total dose required to achieve a certain level of cell death would be increased. Thus, fractionation spares cells from radiation damage compared with single-dose irradiation. Furthermore, late-responding tissues, which have higher SLD repair capacity, would be spared preferentially over acute-responding malignant cells, which might lack adequate repair mechanisms.

4. **Redistribution.** Cells exhibit differential sensitivities toward radiation at different phases of the cell cycle. Most mammalian cells are more sensitive at the junction between G2 and M phases. After an initial fraction of dose, the cells at a more resistant phase (e.g., late S) may survive but then progress eventually to the sensitive phases in time, allowing more efficient killing during the next fraction. Thus, fast-cycling cells (like skin or mucosal cells and most cancers) are more prone to radiation killing than slow or dormant ones (such as muscle or skeletal cells).

D. Dose rate effect. The biological effect of a given radiation dose also depends on the rate it is delivered. With decreasing dose rate, the cell survival increases due to SLD repair. Cell survival is also enhanced due to repopulation as the treatment course gets further protracted until a limit (characterized by nonrepairable single-hit killing) is reached. Beyond this limit further decrease of dose rate will in fact give rise to more cell death (*inverse dose rate effect*) due to cell cycle arrest at G2 phase where cells are most vulnerable to radiation killing.

1. Once daily fractionated RT typically uses a dose rate of about 1 Gy/minute.

2. For **continuous low-dose rate brachytherapy** (or *implant*), radioactive seeds are typically inserted into a patient's body (either *interstitial* or *intracavitary*) for a long period of time, with radiation dose emitting at a rate of about 1 cGy/minute.

3. **High-dose rate brachytherapy** has gained wide popularity, using a dose rate of about 1 Gy/minute, as is used with external beam *teletherapy*.

E. Altered fractionation. The fractionation scheme used in conventional RT usually utilizes 1.8 to 2 Gy per fraction to a total dose that is required for a particular malignancy (e.g., about 70 Gy for gross epithelial cancers, or much less for radiosensitive tumors such as lymphomas). However, by exploiting the radiobiologic principles as listed earlier, therapeutic benefit can be increased via *altered fractionation* regimens.

1. Because fractionation preferentially spares late-responding normal tissues, a strategy of **hyperfractionation** can be used to enhance tumor cell killing while maintaining the same degree of late normal tissue damage. More fractions are delivered

(usually twice daily) by using a smaller dose per fraction to a higher total dose, while keeping overall treatment time about the same as conventional fractionation.

2. To overcome the potential bottleneck for tumor control due to accelerated repopulation of cancer cells, the strategy of **accelerated fractionation** can be used to deliver a conventional total dose but shorten the overall treatment time with more intensely fractionated patterns. A lower dose per fraction is delivered two or three times daily.

3. Based on the LQ model, a quantity termed **biologically effective dose** (BED) has proved to be convenient in quantifying radiobiological effects and has enabled comparisons among various clinical trials using different fractionation schemes. For late-responding tissues,

$$BED = D \cdot \{1 + [d/(\alpha/\beta)]\}$$

where D is the total dose and d is the dose per fraction. BED is versatile because it is *linearly additive*; that is, one can sum up directly all BED values for partial treatments with various fractionation regimens or special techniques such as brachytherapy, to predict the net biological effect to a tissue characterized by a specific α/β.

F. **Dose response curves.** The terms **tumor control probability** (TCP) and **normal tissue complication probability** (NTCP) can be used to assess clinical consequences of RT quantitatively as functions of dose. As probability curves, they both exhibit rising sigmoid shapes from 0% to 100% when plotted linearly against increasing dose. Only when the NTCP curve is sufficiently to the right (higher dose region) of the TCP is it warranted clinically to irradiate. Many innovations in clinical radiation oncology have been based on attempts to separate these two curves.

1. The **therapeutic ratio** is the relative degree of tumor control (measured as TCP) over normal tissue damage (NTCP). There exists an optimal dose for which this ratio, or the **uncomplicated TCP (UTCP)**, is maximized:

$$UTCP = TCP \cdot (1 - NTCP)$$

2. With a sharply rising sigmoid shape, TCP dictates that once a certain dose is deemed necessary to achieve adequate tumor control, the treatment should not be terminated prematurely because almost no therapeutic gain would be expected until the whole course is near completion (i.e., "all or nothing" response).

3. Both TCP and NTCP depend not only on the dose, but also on the size or volume (i.e., the number of clonogenic cells in a tumor for TCP or the so-called **functional subunits** (FSUs) of a normal tissue for NTCP, respectively). The higher the number of cells to irradiate, the more the dose response curve shifts to the right.

4. For a specific malignancy or normal tissue, factors that may "flatten" (i.e., decrease slope of) the respective sigmoid TCP or NTCP curves include the wide variation of radiation sensitivity in a patient population.

5. For the prophylactic control of subclinical micrometastases by radiation, the dose response curve is flattened due to the heterogeneous distribution of metastatic tumor burdens in the targeted volume. Thus, a small amount of dose can still be beneficial, in contrast to the substantially larger dose required for the control of bulky tumors.

G. **Tissue organization.** The structural organization of the FSUs in a normal tissue may be critical in determining the kinetics of its damage expression, as well as the effect of heterogeneous dose distribution across its volume.

1. Based on physiological and cellular kinetics reasoning, some normal tissues can be separated structurally into **type-H (hierarchical)** or **type-F (flexible)** tissues.

   a. **Type-H tissues** (e.g., bone marrow, skin, and gastrointestinal tract) contain stem cells that are destined to mature into functional cells. As they lose clonogenicity in the process, these cells become radioresistant because only the rapidly proliferating stem cells are likely to be sensitive to radiation killing.

     b. Type-F tissues (e.g., lung, liver, and kidney) contain cells that can simultaneously maintain their proliferation capacity (thus are radiosensitive) and serve their normal physiological function.

     c. Upon irradiation, type-F tissues can exhibit a dose-dependent kinetics of damage expression—the higher the dose, the earlier the time of expression. In contrast, the kinetics of damage for type-H tissues is relatively independent of the dose.

  2. The spatial orientation of normal tissue can be separated into **parallel** and **series** structures. Parallel structures are typified by kidney, liver, lung, and tumors, whereas series structures include the GI tract, spinal cord, and peritoneal sheath. Most normal tissues have mixed characteristics of both parallel and series structures. The concept of *relative seriality* has been proposed, based on the perceived organization of FSUs. This concept is useful when dealing with heterogeneous dose distribution across a structure of interest (see III.H.3 and 4).

H. Heterogeneous dose distribution. The biological effect of radiation on a particular normal **organ at risk** (OAR) can vary significantly with the amount of volume as well as which portion or region of the organ is treated. Clinicians have been trained to be familiar with the overall radiation effect (e.g., NTCP) of an OAR being irradiated with *uniform* dose distribution. However, modern treatment techniques using inverse planning and intensity modulated radiation therapy (IMRT) (see IV.C.2) often involve heterogeneous dose distribution.

  1. The cumulative biological effects of partial volume irradiations that might not amount to the effect predicted based on the same total physical dose assumed to be uniformly deposited for the whole organ is called the **volume effect**.

  2. For a grossly heterogeneous dose distribution across a significant portion of an OAR, the degree of such heterogeneity can be quantified using the **dose volume histogram** (DVH). It takes a shape of a monotonically decreasing sigmoid curve on a fractional volume versus dose plot.

  3. Tissues in parallel have been modeled along the so-called *critical volume* argument. The total volume irradiated has direct impact on NTCP. Irradiating a significant volume of such tissue, even if with moderate doses, would be more detrimental than giving an extremely high dose but to only a small volume of the organ. Thus, the bulk of the volume irradiated does matter significantly.

  4. Tissues in series have *critical elements* arranged in chains upon which irradiating even a small volume of the structure to a sufficiently high dose might incur a complication. The prime example would be spinal cord, which needs only a hot spot at a given segment to manifest transverse myelitis. The *incidence* of a complication increases in proportion to the volume irradiated for series tissues.

  5. Equivalent uniform dose (EUD) has been defined to address heterogeneous dose distribution and is the dose that, when distributed uniformly across the target volume, gives rise to the same biological effect.

IV. CLINICAL PRACTICE OF RT

A. Consultation. Patients are usually referred by surgeons, medical oncologists, primary care physicians, or other specialists for consultation, during which the history and physical examination are done by radiation oncologists. The indications for RT, as well as its associated short- and long-term side effects, are explained to the patient in detail.

  1. Indications. Like surgery and chemotherapy, RT has definite indications and contraindications for clinical application. RT can be used alone or in combination with other methods, as the major component of treatment or as an adjuvant modality. Approximately 50% to 60% of all patients with cancer receive RT during the course of their illness. Properly used, the intent of RT for about 60% of these patients will be curative. For others incurable by any current method of treatment, palliation of symptoms and signs by RT can improve their quality of life.

  a. Treatment with curative intent is often complicated and requires professional skills and facilities that may be distant from the patient's home. Usually the doses are higher and, consequently, the risks of sequelae are greater than for palliative treatment.

  b. Palliative treatment should have a specific objective. Inconvenience, cost, discomfort, risk, and overall treatment time should be minimized. Objectives of palliative RT include: relief of pain, usually from metastases to bone; relief of neurological dysfunction from intracranial metastases; relief of obstruction of the ureter, esophagus, or bronchus; promotion of healing of surface wounds caused by tumor; preservation of the weight-bearing skeleton compromised by metastases; or preservation of vision by controlling metastases to or tumor invasion of the eye or its orbit.

2. Negative side effects. Most normal tissue effects of RT are related to cell killing. Some effects, such as nausea, vomiting, fatigue, and somnolence, remain unexplained, although there may be a relationship to radiation-induced cytokines. Some late effects may be related to radiation-induced proliferative responses such as gliosis or fibrosis.

  Side effects of RT are influenced by other treatments. Acute skin or mucous reactions may be accentuated by the concurrent or even later administration of chemotherapy agents (e.g., doxorubicin). Radiation-induced bowel damage may be accentuated by prior surgery. The appearance of clinical injury after cell killing will depend on factors such as cell turnover time and differentiation kinetics. For convenience, these time-related responses are arbitrarily divided into:

  a. Acute responses that appear usually within 2 to 3 weeks after treatment commences, such as mucositis and diarrhea, are secondary to the depletion of stem cells (especially for type-H tissues, see III.F.1) and are expected to subside gradually once the treatment course is over.

  b. Subacute responses, such as *Lhermitte's syndrome* (electric shock-like sensation down the periphery upon sudden flexion of neck, due to demyelination) or *somnolent syndrome*, occur after several months and are nearly always transient.

  c. Late responses are secondary to the depletion of slowly proliferating cells and are nearly always permanent. These are usually the critical structures that limit the dose prescribed by the radiation oncologists.

B. Treatment preparation. Once the patient agrees and provides the informed consent to proceed with RT, the next step is usually a simulation process and subsequent treatment planning.

  1. Simulation is a procedure when the radiation oncologist tries to determine how to aim the beams of RT according to the patient's anatomy and the locations of the target lesions, as well as the OARs. A conventional *simulator* may be used, which has the geometric construct of the beam source and patient couch movement identical to the actual treatment machine. Such machines are being replaced by CT simulators, where tomographic scans form the basis of subsequent 3-dimensional (3-D)–oriented treatment planning. During simulation, the patient is placed on a treatment couch and certain immobilization measures are often implemented because the positioning must be reproducible for subsequent daily treatments with acceptable precision. Frequently, permanent tattoos are marked on the patient's body surface.

  2. Treatment planning. Other than fairly simple cases, for which old techniques continue to serve well, modern RT requires complex treatment planning. Computerized data are essential to this process to produce a finalized plan that can be transferred seamlessly to computer-controlled therapy equipment. It requires the integrated efforts of radiation oncologists, medical physicists, dosimetrists, and radiation therapists.

  a. The first step of treatment planning is the identification of essential anatomic structures relevant to the goal of the treatment. The 3-D extent of each structure of interest can be traced in contoured forms, section by section, on the tomographic images.

b. Conceptually the treatment volume incorporates the **gross tumor volume** (GTV), which represents the detectable extent of the tumor target, the **clinical target volume** (CTV), which includes microscopic tumor extensions, and the **planning target volume** (PTV), which includes margins around the CTV to allow for positional uncertainty.

c. Normal structures of interest are also identified, contoured, and designated as OARs.

C. Precision-oriented RT. Computerized treatment planning now allows for delivering RT with ultraprecision.

1. **Conformal RT.** Because the structures of interest are often irregular in shape, devices such as metal blocks have been constructed manually and customized for individual patients, and the treatment planning has been rather rudimentary with a 2-D dosimetry plan used as a basis for 3-D extrapolation. When CT-based imaging became available and adapted for simulation, truly 3-D–oriented **conformal radiotherapy** became common practice.

a. Computer technology allows for a very slick 3-D treatment planning approach using a machine-driven beam-shaping device called **multileaf collimators** (MLC). The target structures are basically sliced one beam path at a time with a width measuring from a few millimeters to a centimeter, and the radiation dose within each slice is calculated to precision and spatially conformed to the edge of the desired target. One useful tool is the **beam's eye view**, which simulates looking along the axes of multiple radiation beams to plan the best arrangement.

b. During the treatment, the automated MLCs restrict the delivered dose to tightly conform to the target. Thus, precise dosimetric determination for any 3-D irregularly shaped tumor target or OAR is theoretically feasible. Tools are available to maximize the therapeutic ratio by a process of optimizing various treatment parameters.

2. **IMRT** is a technique that allows photon beams modulated by MLCs to deliver specific doses to irregular-shaped target volumes while sparing nearby OARs.

a. The essence of IMRT is **inverse planning.** The physicist feeds in the anatomic information of tumors and OARs, specifies the desired outcome with dose constraint for each structure of interest, and then lets the computer search for the best solution to achieve such goal. The answer will dictate how the treatment machine might adjust (or "modulate") the radiation beam intensity in an automated fashion by moving the MLCs rapidly across the irradiated target, while constantly avoiding the OARs.

b. The computer-generated IMRT plan allows for a much higher dose within and tighter dose distribution around the irregular target border, while the adjacent normal tissues receive relatively little dose.

c. Higher doses can be given via IMRT as a "boost" to the primary tumor bed *sequentially* after a course of RT aimed at a broader coverage of the head and neck region. This follows the traditional practice of the **shrinking-field technique,** with the dosages of various structures (including the tumor) prescribed to commonly accepted values.

d. IMRT is now often used from the very beginning of the treatment course with the so-called **simultaneous integrated boost** (SIB) technique. For each fraction, the subclinical spread of cancer cells in the broad area is treated to a relatively lower dose, while the primary tumor is irradiated *simultaneously* with a higher dose. Therefore, the total dose received at any structure of interest and its subsequent clinical effect can vary widely depending on the fractionation schemes. It is less meaningful to use total *physical* doses for intercomparison of treatment results using different SIB techniques. Instead, some sort of quantitative *biological* correction is usually needed.

e. IMRT has the potential of introducing dose heterogeneity (see III.H) *within* a specific structure because of intensity modulation. The biological consequence due to such effect is still not very well understood because clinicians have traditionally been trained to be familiar with the consequences of only homogeneous dose distribution across an anatomic object.

3. **Particle therapy.** Particle beams such as protons and heavy ions have dosimetric characteristics of the Bragg peak (see II.A.3), thus can be exploited for ultraprecision treatment. may be done in an inverse manner, with intensity modulation amounting to "dose painting." This may represent the most sophisticated form of precision-oriented RT, although many technical details remain to be worked out. The main disadvantage of praticle beams is their extremely high cost of production and operation.

4. **Brachytherapy (implants)** is another form of precision irradiation. Because the "fall off" of energy is inversely proportional to distance from the radioactive sources, the tissues adjacent to the target receive relatively lower doses. Thus, the main advantage of brachytherapy is its extremely low dose to the rest of the patient's body (termed "integral dose," the sum of the total body dose). Its disadvantages mainly involve the operative risks (anesthesia, bleeding, infection, etc.) and the need to observe radiation precautions for health care personnel and patients.

D. **Stereotactic irradiation.** Precision-oriented treatment planning loses its meaning if the positions of the target and OARs are deviated during actual treatment because of setup uncertainty or motion. Patient immobilization is thus crucial, especially for tumors in the brain and the head and neck.

1. **Stereotactic radiosurgery (SRS).** For relatively few and small tumors, *ablating* each lesion precisely with an exceptionally high level of radiation dose using the so-called SRS technique may be indicated.

   a. Originally developed by neurosurgeons to locate brain lesions with pinpoint accuracy using a 3-D coordinate system in reference to a rigid frame attached to the patient's skull, the stereotactic localization technique is utilized when high-dose radiation is used to substitute invasive surgical resection.

   b. Two different ways of producing the radiation for SRS are commercially available. For systems such as the Gamma Knife, about 200 ^{60}Cobalt radioisotope sources emitting γ-rays are oriented in a hemispherical fashion, or other similar geometrical construct, to focus all the beams on a central point. Alternatively, such focused radiation can be produced via a LINAC, which generates an x-ray beam as a single source and can be rotated or moved around a central focus.

   c. Feasible SRS targets must be small (usually ≤ 3 cm in diameter), and the number of lesions to be treated must be few (usually ≤ 4).

   d. SRS has gained wide popularity to treat central nervous system tumors (both benign and malignant) and, at times, neurophysiological disorders such as trigeminal neuralgia.

   e. The use of SRS for head and neck tumors is usually limited to administering an additional "boost" beyond conventional radiation treatment or as salvage for local recurrence.

   f. Extracranial tumors (such as in the spine, lung, or liver) are also being explored for possible SRS treatment as long as single or few fractions of large-dose irradiation (an approach called **hypofractionation**) is deemed appropriate and the problem of motion uncertainty can be resolved (e.g., with technical innovation to compensate respiratory motion for lesions in the trunk; see IV.F.1).

2. **Stereotactic radiotherapy (SRT).** For many malignancies, the size of primary tumor is typically larger than what SRS can accommodate, and more importantly, its edges are often mingled with normal tissues. In such cases, stereotactic technique can be combined with the biological advantages of fractionation to provide SRT as a treatment option. SRT is done often with removable body-fixation frames for daily treatments.

3. **Selection of SRS versus SRT** (guidelines):

   a. SRT will in general have a theoretical biological advantage over SRS for most malignancies. SRS is often favored for logistic reasons rather than biological considerations per se.

    b. Whenever an aggressive tumor is found located in close proximity to a critical normal tissue, SRT would probably be more beneficial than SRS because the biological advantage of fractionation can be exploited.

    c. If there is not much biological difference between tumor (e.g., a benign or low-grade lesion) and the surrounding normal tissue, it may be legitimate to offer patients SRS treatment, serving just like a surgical tool.

    d. Perhaps due to the wide acceptance of SRS, or because SRT is simply a more tedious procedure, clinicians might develop a lingering desire to minimize the number of fractions for patient treatment. Only with precision treatment is it safe to do so. By spatially segregating tumors from normal tissues, one can treat the former without too much concern of deleterious biologic effect over the latter.

E. Functional image-guided RT. The development of functional imaging studies like *positron emission tomography* or *magnetic resonance spectroscopy* has allowed physicians to contemplate whether dose escalation to metabolically active or radiation-resistant spots within a tumor might help raise the local tumor control rate. These sophisticated imaging techniques may unite modern molecular biology to clinical radiation oncology using IMRT or particle beams for dose-painting purpose. As it stands today, much remains to be researched before their clinical application becomes routine.

F. Image-guided radiation therapy (IGRT). IGRT is preoccupied with precise tracing of the radiation target to compensate for motion uncertainty. An example is to implement *respiratory gating* for tumors in the trunk during each fraction of irradiation by synchronizing the treatment field coverage precisely over a target that moves with respiration. Another frequent application of IGRT is for prostate cancer, because the prostate gland can move (mostly depending on the content of the rectum behind it) from day to day through the long course of radiation therapy.

    1. The internal soft-tissue structures, which ordinarily will escape radiographic detection, can be illuminated. For example, metal seeds could be inserted as "fiducial markers." For relatively fixed tumors, internal bony landmarks can be used for x-ray positioning.

    2. Special imaging devices such as a perpendicular pair of diagnostic x-ray systems or "cone-beam CT" can be added to currently existing LINACs for the purpose of IGRT. Commercially available ultrasound systems (suitable for imaging soft-tissue structures) or traceable radiofrequency/infrared signal–emitting devices can also be used for daily image guidance.

    3. Another option is to acquire a system such as Tomotherapy, which can serve the functional duality of both a rotational (or "axial") RT machine as well as provide frequent tomographic images for IGRT.

G. Adaptive radiation therapy. Initially bulky tumors can often shrink readily during the long course of radiation and chemotherapy treatment. The anatomic uncertainty is thus introduced not because of patient motion or setup error, but because of the significant anatomic deviations of relevant internal structures due to the progressive change of the tumor bulk (or the patient's significant weight loss). Adaptive radiation therapy aims to keep track of this dynamic situation and issue appropriate countermeasures as frequently as possible. The goal is to modify sequentially the treatment plan based on the initial simulation scan and the subsequent daily image verifications, using a sophisticated mathematical algorithm for mitigation of the geometrical incongruities and variations, without actually repeating the laborious simulation and treatment planning.

V. TREATMENT RESPONSE ASSESSMENT

Once RT is finished, or even during the treatment course, assessment of tumor response may be desirable. However, the efficacy of radiation-induced cell killing may not be directly related to the rate of gross tumor regression because of the wide range of cell turnover kinetics. The terms *radioresistance* and *radiosensitivity* are frequently misused because of the misconception that the rate of gross reduction of tumor size is a measure of radiosensitivity and a surrogate for therapeutic effectiveness.

VI. LONG-TERM SIDE EFFECTS OF RT

Every effective therapy may generate undesirable and even dangerous side effects. Despite the nearly instantaneous initiation of the radiation process, its biological effects may be delayed for weeks (skin, mucous reactions), decades (carcinogenesis), or generations (genetic changes in offspring). Although these side effects are inherent in the treatment modality itself, their frequency and severity are influenced by physician competence and philosophy, adequacy of equipment and facilities, operational quality assurance, and attitudes of the patient and his or her family.

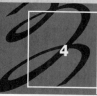

4 CANCER CHEMOTHERAPEUTIC AGENTS
Dennis A. Casciato

CONTENTS

I. ALKYLATING AGENTS

A. General pharmacology of alkylating agents. Alkylating agents target DNA and are cytotoxic, mutagenic, and carcinogenic. All agents produce alkylation through the formation of intermediates.

1. Alkylating agents impair cell function by transferring alkyl groups to amino, carboxyl, sulfhydryl, or phosphate groups of biologically important molecules. Most important, nucleic acids (DNA and RNA) and proteins are alkylated. The number 7 (N-7) position of guanine in DNA and RNA is the most actively alkylated site; the O-6 group of guanine is alkylated by nitrosoureas. Alkylation of guanine results in abnormal nucleotide sequences, miscoding of messenger RNA, cross-linked DNA strands that cannot replicate, breakage of DNA strands, and other damage to the transcription and translation of genetic material.

2. The primary mode of action for most alkylating agents is by means of cross-linking of DNA strands. Cytotoxicity is probably a result of damage to the DNA templates rather than inactivation of DNA polymerase and other enzymes responsible for DNA synthesis. DNA strand breakage also appears to be a minor determinant of cytotoxicity.

3. Alkylating agents are cell cycle–specific but not phase-specific. The drugs kill a fixed percentage of cells at a given dose.

4. Tumor resistance to these drugs appears to be related to the capacity of cells to repair nucleic acid damage and to inactivate the drugs by conjugation with glutathione.

B. Busulfan (Myleran)

1. **Indications.** Chronic myelogenous leukemia (CML), bone marrow transplantation (high doses)

2. **Pharmacology**
   a. **Mechanism.** Alkylation (see section A)
   b. **Metabolism.** Acts directly; catabolized to inactive products that are excreted in the urine.

3. **Toxicity**
   a. **Dose-limiting.** Reversible and irreversible myelosuppression with slow recovery; blood cell counts fall for about 2 weeks after discontinuation of drug.
   b. **Common.** Gastrointestinal (GI) upset (mild), sterility
   c. **Occasional.** Skin hyperpigmentation, alopecia, rash; gynecomastia, cataracts, LFT abnormalities; seizures
   d. **Rare.** Pulmonary fibrosis ("busulfan lung"; see Chapter 29, section IV.A), retroperitoneal fibrosis, endocardial fibrosis; addisonian-like asthenia (without biochemical evidence of adrenal insufficiency); hypotension, impotence, hemorrhagic cystitis, secondary neoplasms

4. **Administration**
   a. **Supplied** as 2-mg tablets
   b. **Dose modification.** Hematologic
   c. **Dose.** Usually 2 to 8 mg/day PO; or 0.05 mg/kg/day for CML
   d. **Drug interactions.** Itraconazole and phenytoin respectively reduce and increase busulfan metabolism.

C. Chlorambucil (Leukeran)

1. **Indications.** Chronic lymphocytic leukemia (CLL), Waldenström macroglobulinemia

2. **Pharmacology**
   a. **Mechanism.** Alkylation (see section I.A)
   b. **Metabolism.** Acts directly; spontaneously hydrolyzed to inactive and active products (e.g., phenylacetic acid mustard); also is extensively metabolized by the hepatic P450 microsomal system. The drug and metabolic products are excreted in urine.

3. **Toxicity.** Least toxic alkylating agent
   a. **Dose-limiting.** Myelosuppression
   b. **Occasional.** GI upset (minimal or absent at usual doses), mild LFT abnormalities, sterility

      c. Rare. Rash, alopecia, fever; cachexia, pulmonary fibrosis, neurological or ocular toxicity, cystitis; acute leukemia

    4. Administration

      a. Supplied as 2-mg tablets

      b. Dose modification. Hematologic

      c. Dose. Various dosage schedules are used. For example, 0.1 to 0.2 mg/kg/day PO for 3 to 6 weeks, then decrease dose for maintenance

      d. Drug interactions. Phenobarbital, phenytoin, and other drugs that stimulate the liver's P450 system may lead to increased production of toxic metabolites.

D. Cyclophosphamide (Cytoxan)

    1. Indications. Used in a wide variety of conditions

    2. Pharmacology

      a. Mechanism. Alkylation (see section I.A); also inhibits DNA synthesis. Cell cycle–nonspecific and active in all phases of the cell cycle.

      b. Metabolism. Native drug is inactive and requires activation by liver P450 microsomal oxidase system to form an aldehyde that decomposes in plasma and peripheral tissues to yield acrolein and an alkylating metabolite (e.g., phosphoramide mustard). The P450 system also metabolizes metabolites to inactive compounds. Active and inactive metabolites are excreted in urine.

    3. Toxicity

      a. Dose-limiting

        (1) Myelosuppression. Leukopenia develops 8 to 14 days after administration. Thrombocytopenia occurs but is rarely significant.

        (2) Effects on urinary bladder. Degradative products are responsible for hemorrhagic cystitis, which can be prevented by maintaining a high urine output. Hemorrhagic cystitis is more common and can be severe when massive doses are used (e.g., for bone marrow transplantation); under these circumstances, the use of mesna can be preventative. Urinary bladder fibrosis with telangiectasis of the mucosa can occur (usually after long-term oral therapy) without episodes of cystitis. Bladder carcinoma has occurred.

      b. Side effects

        (1) Common. Alopecia, stomatitis, aspermia, amenorrhea; headache (fast onset, short duration). Nausea and vomiting are common after doses of 700 mg/m^2 or more.

        (2) Occasional. Skin or fingernail hyperpigmentation; metallic taste during injection; sneezing or a cold sensation in the nose after injection; abnormal LFTs, dizziness; allergy, fever

        (3) Rare. Transient syndrome of inappropriate secretion of antidiuretic hormone (SIADH, especially if given with a large volume of fluid), hypothyroidism, cataracts, jaundice, pulmonary fibrosis; cardiac necrosis and acute myopericarditis (with high doses); secondary neoplasms (acute leukemia, bladder carcinoma)

    4. Administration. The drug should be administered with a large volume of fluid in the morning or early afternoon to avoid cystitis.

      a. Supplied as 25- or 50-mg tablets; vials contain 100 to 1,000 mg

      b. Dose modification. Hematologic; may be required for hepatic or renal functional impairment

      c. Dose. Cyclophosphamide is frequently employed as part of combination chemotherapy regimens. Some common doses are 0.5 to 1.5 g/m^2 IV every 3 weeks or 50 to 200 mg/m^2 PO for 14 days every 28 days.

      d. Drug interactions. Phenobarbital, phenytoin, and other drugs that stimulate the liver's P450 system may lead to increased production of toxic metabolites.

        (1) Digoxin levels decreased with cyclophosphamide

        (2) Interacts with **warfarin** to prolong the prothrombin time further

        (3) Interacts with **succinyl choline** to increase neuromuscular blockade

E. Dacarbazine [dimethyltriazenoimidazolecarboxamide (DTIC), imidazole carboxamide]

  1. Indications. Hodgkin lymphoma, malignant melanoma, sarcomas, neuroblastoma

  2. Pharmacology

   a. Mechanisms. Inhibits purine, RNA, and protein synthesis. Has some alkylating activity. Causes DNA methylation and direct DNA damage. Cell cycle–nonspecific.

   b. Metabolism. Native drug inactive; requires activation by oxidative N-methylation by the hepatic P450 microsomal system. Excreted in urine predominantly (50% of the drug is unchanged); minor hepatobiliary and pulmonary excretion.

  3. Toxicity

   a. Dose-limiting. Myelosuppression; nadir blood counts occur 2 to 4 weeks after treatment

   b. Common. Nausea and vomiting (often severe), anorexia; pain along the injection site

   c. Occasional. Alopecia, facial flushing, photosensitivity, abnormal LFTs. Flu-like syndrome (malaise, myalgia, chills, and fever) developing 1 week after treatment and lasting several days

   d. Rare. Diarrhea, stomatitis; cerebral dysfunction; hepatic vein thrombosis, hepatic necrosis; azotemia; anaphylaxis

  4. Administration. Dacarbazine is often used in combination chemotherapy regimens. Withdrawing blood into the drug-filled syringe before injecting the mixture reduces the pain of injection. The drug is a vesicant if injected subcutaneously.

   a. Supplied as 100- and 200-mg vials

   b. Dose modification. Necessary for patients with impaired bone marrow, hepatic, or renal dysfunction

   c. Dose

    (1) 375 mg/m^2 every 15 days in ABVD regimen for Hodgkin lymphoma, or

    (2) 220 mg/m^2 IV daily for 3 days every 21 to 28 days

   d. Drug interactions. Phenobarbital, phenytoin, and other drugs that stimulate the liver's P450 system may lead to decreased efficacy of DTIC.

F. Ifosfamide (isophosphamide, Ifex)

  1. Indications. Lymphomas, sarcomas, relapsed testicular tumors, and various carcinomas

  2. Pharmacology

   a. Mechanisms. An alkylating agent (see section I.A); DNA cross-linking and chain breakage. Metabolites are alkylating agents that are similar to cyclophosphamide but are not cross-resistant.

   b. Metabolism. Extensively metabolized by the hepatic P450 microsomal system. Activated at a fourfold slower rate than cyclophosphamide because of a lower affinity for the P450 system. Inactive until activated by hepatic microsomal enzymes. Like cyclophosphamide, the drug undergoes hepatic activation to an aldehyde form that decomposes in plasma and peripheral tissues to yield acrolein and its alkylating metabolite. Acrolein is highly toxic to urothelial mucosa. The chloroacetaldehyde metabolite may be responsible for much of the neurotoxic effects, particularly in patients with renal dysfunction. Drug and metabolites are excreted in urine.

  3. Toxicity

   a. Dose-limiting. Myelosuppression, hemorrhagic cystitis

   b. Common. Alopecia, anorexia, nausea, and vomiting; amenorrhea, oligospermia, and infertility.

   c. Neurotoxicity (especially when given in 1 day rather than for 5 days and when renal dysfunction is present or when sedatives are given); lethargy, dizziness, cranial nerve dysfunction, confusion, ataxia, and, rarely, coma

    d. Occasional. Salivation, stomatitis, diarrhea, constipation; urticaria, hyperpigmentation, nail ridging; abnormal LFTs, phlebitis, fever; hypotension, hypertension, hypokalemia; renal tubular acidosis (at high doses); SIADH

4. Administration. Aggressive concomitant hydration (2 to 4 L/day) and mesna are given to reduce the incidence of hemorrhagic cystitis. Monitor urine for hematuria before each dose. Use antiemetics prophylactically.

    a. Supplied as 1- and 3-g prepackaged vials with mesna

    b. Dose modification. Hematologic and renal dysfunction

    c. Dose. 1,000 to 1,200 mg/m^2 IV over 30 minutes for 3 to 5 days every 3 to 4 weeks

    d. Mesna (sodium 2-mercaptoethanesulfonate, Mesnex) is a uroprotective agent when administering ifosfamide or cyclophosphamide. Alternative dose schedules for mesna, which is given in the same mg dose as the alkylating agent, are:

        (1) Equal doses of ifosfamide and mesna in the same bag when given as a continuous infusion

        (2) Twenty percent of the mesna dose given IV bolus at the time of administration of ifosfamide, then 40% PO at 2 hours and 40% at 6 hours after each dose of ifosfamide/cyclophosphamide

        (3) When given by IV bolus, the total dose of mesna is 60% of the ifosfamide dose. One-third of the mesna dose (20% of the ifosfamide dose) is given 15 minutes before, 4 hours after, and 8 hours after ifosfamide.

    e. Drug interactions. Phenobarbital, phenytoin, and other drugs that stimulate the liver's P450 system may lead to increased production of toxic metabolites.

        (1) Digoxin levels are decreased with cyclophosphamide

        (2) Interacts with **warfarin** to prolong the prothrombin time further

        (3) Interacts with **succinyl choline** to increase neuromuscular blockade

        (4) Cimetidine and **allopurinol** increase ifosfamide toxicity

G. Melphalan (Alkeran, phenylalanine mustard, L-PAM)

  1. Indications. Multiple myeloma. The injection form is used in bone marrow transplantation. Previously used in ovarian and breast carcinomas and polycythemia vera.

  2. Pharmacology

    a. Mechanism. Alkylation (see section I.A)

    b. Metabolism. Acts directly. Ninety percent of the drug is bound to plasma proteins and undergoes rapid hydrolysis in the bloodstream to inert products. Melphalan is excreted in the urine (about 30%) as unchanged drug and metabolites, and the remainder is cleared in feces.

  3. Toxicity

    a. Dose-limiting. Myelosuppression may be cumulative and recovery may be prolonged.

    b. Occasional. Anorexia, nausea, vomiting, mucositis, sterility

    c. Rare. Alopecia, pruritus, rash, hypersensitivity; secondary malignancies (acute leukemia); pulmonary fibrosis, vasculitis, cataracts

  4. Administration

    a. Supplied as 2-mg tablets

    b. Dose modification. Hematologic; administer cautiously in patients with azotemia

    c. Dose. If no myelosuppression is observed after oral dosing, poor oral absorption should be suspected. For continuous therapy: 0.10 to 0.15 mg/kg PO daily for 2 to 3 weeks, no therapy for 2 to 4 weeks, then 2 to 4 mg PO daily. For pulse therapy: 0.2 mg/kg (10 mg/m^2) PO daily for 4 days every 4 to 6 weeks

    d. Drug interactions

        (1) Cimetidine may result in reduced serum melphalan levels.

        (2) Cyclosporine enhances the risk of renal toxicity from melphalan.

H. Nitrogen mustard (mechlorethamine, Mustargen)
1. **Indication.** Hodgkin lymphoma; topical use for T-cell lymphoma
2. **Pharmacology**
   a. **Mechanism.** Rapid alkylation of DNA, RNA, and protein (see section I.A). Cell cycle–nonspecific with activity in all phases of the cell cycle.
   b. **Metabolism.** Native drug is highly active and is rapidly deactivated within the blood by rapid hydrolysis; the elimination half-life is 15 minutes. Metabolites are mostly excreted in urine.
3. **Toxicity**
   a. **Dose-limiting.** Myelosuppression
   b. **Common.** Severe nausea and vomiting beginning 1 hour after administration; skin necrosis if extravasated (sodium thiosulfate may be tried); burning at IV injection site and facial flushing; metallic taste; discoloration of the infused vein; abnormal LFTs within 1 week of therapy (up to 90% of patients)
   c. **Occasional.** Alopecia, sterility, diarrhea, thrombophlebitis, gynecomastia
   d. **Rare.** Neurotoxicity (including hearing loss), angioedema, secondary neoplasms
4. **Administration.** Patients should always be premedicated with antiemetics. The drug should be administered through the tubing of a running intravenous line using extravasation precautions.
   a. **Supplied** as 10-mg vials
   b. **Dose modification.** Hematologic; none required for hepatic or renal impairment
   c. **Dose.** 10 mg/m^2 as a single or divided dose monthly or 6 mg/m^2 on Day 1 and Day 8 of the MOPP regimen (see Appendix D-1).
   d. **Drug interactions.** Sodium thiosulfate inactivates mechlorethamine.

I. Nitrosoureas. Carmustine [BCNU, bischlorethyl nitrosourea (BiCNU)]; lomustine [CCNU, cyclohexyl chlorethyl nitrosourea (CeeNU)]; streptozocin, which is a nitrosourea with a different mechanism of action (see section I.K)
1. **Indications.** Brain cancer, myeloma, melanoma, and some carcinomas
2. **Pharmacology**
   a. **Mechanism.** Alkylation of DNA and RNA (see section I.A); DNA cross-linking; inhibition of DNA polymerase, DNA repair, and RNA synthesis. Cell cycle–nonspecific.
   b. **Metabolism.** Highly lipid-soluble drugs that enter the brain. Rapid spontaneous decomposition to active and inert products; the drugs also are metabolized. Most of the intact drug and metabolic products are excreted in urine; some products have an enterohepatic cycle.
3. **Toxicity**
   a. **Dose-limiting.** Myelosuppression is prolonged, cumulative, and substantially aggravated by concurrent radiation therapy.
   b. **Common.** Nausea and vomiting may last 8 to 24 hours. BCNU causes local pain during injection or hypotension during a too rapid or concentrated injection.
   c. **Occasional.** Stomatitis, esophagitis, diarrhea, LFT abnormalities; alopecia, facial flushing, brown discoloration of skin; interstitial lung disease with pulmonary fibrosis (with prolonged therapy and higher doses, especially with cumulative doses >1,400 mg/m^2); dizziness, optic neuritis, ataxia, organic brain syndrome; renal insufficiency
   d. **Rare.** Secondary malignancies
4. **Administration.** Avoid alcohol at least 1 hour before and after CCNU.
   a. **Supplied** as 100-mg vials of BCNU; 10-, 40-, and 100-mg capsules of CCNU in a dose pack of 300 mg
   b. **Dose modification.** Hematologic and renal
   c. **Dose**
      (1) **BCNU:** 150 to 200 mg/m^2 IV (as a single dose or divided over 2 days) every 6 to 8 weeks. Do not infuse over longer than 2 hours because of incompatibility of the drug with intravenous tubing. If blood and BCNU

are mixed in the syringe before administration, the painfulness of injection may be decreased.

    (2) CCNU: 100 to 130 mg/m^2 PO every 6 to 8 weeks

d. Drug interactions

    (1) With **cimetidine** to decrease nitrosourea metabolism, resulting in increased hematosuppression

    (2) BCNU may lower levels of **digoxin** and **phenytoin**

    (3) Amphotericin B enhances cellular uptake of BCNU, resulting in increased host toxicity

J. Procarbazine (N-methylhydrazine, Matulane)

1. Indications. Hodgkin and non-Hodgkin lymphomas, cutaneous T-cell lymphoma, brain cancer

2. Pharmacology

  a. Mechanism. DNA alkylation and depolymerization. Methylation of nucleic acids. Inhibition of DNA, RNA, and protein synthesis.

  b. Metabolism. Rapidly and extensively metabolized by the hepatic P450 microsomal system. Metabolic activation of the drug is required. Readily enters the cerebrospinal fluid. Degraded in the liver to inactive compounds, which are excreted in urine (70%). Less than 10% of the drug is excreted in unchanged form.

3. Toxicity

  a. Dose-limiting. Myelosuppression, which is most pronounced 4 weeks after starting treatment

  b. Common. Nausea and vomiting, which decrease with continued use; flu-like syndrome (usually with initial therapy); sensitizes tissues to radiation; amenorrhea and azoospermia, sterility

  c. Occasional. Dermatitis, hyperpigmentation, photosensitivity; stomatitis, dysphagia, diarrhea; hypotension, tachycardia; urinary frequency, hematuria; gynecomastia

  d. Neurologic. Procarbazine results in disorders of consciousness or mild peripheral neuropathies in about 10% of cases. These abnormalities are reversible and rarely serious enough to alter drug dosage. Manifestations of toxicity include sedation, depression, agitation, psychosis, decreased deep-tendon reflexes, paresthesias, myalgias, and ataxia.

  e. Rare. Xerostomia, retinal hemorrhage, photophobia, papilledema; hypersensitivity pneumonitis, secondary malignancy

4. Administration. Avoid alcohol, tyramine-containing foods, tricyclic antidepressants, antihistamines, dark beer, wine, cheeses, bananas, yogurt, and pickled or smoked foods.

  a. Supplied as 50-mg capsules

  b. Dose modification. Reduce dose in patients with hepatic, renal, or bone marrow dysfunction.

  c. Dose. 60 to 100 mg/m^2 PO daily for 10 to 14 days in combination regimens

  d. Drug interactions. Procarbazine is a monoamine oxidase inhibitor and thus interacts with numerous prescribed and nonprescribed agents. For the most part, these interacting agents should be avoided for about 2 weeks after stopping procarbazine. Potential reactions from procarbazine interactions with other drugs include the following:

    (1) Disulfiram (Antabuse)-like reactions: Alcohol

    (2) Severe hypertension

      (a) Sympathomimetic amines, levodopa, methyldopa; cocaine, narcotics; buspirone, methylphenidate (Ritalin); dextromethorphan (with hyperpyrexia); caffeine

      (b) Foods and beverages containing amines [e.g., aged cheese, beer, and wine (with or without alcohol); smoked or pickled meats, poultry or fish; fermented sausage; any overripe fruit]

    (3) Hypotension: Hypotension-producing medications, spinal anesthetics

    (4) CNS depression and anticholinergic effects: Antihistamines, phenothiazines, barbiturates, and other CNS depressants

(5) Hyperpyrexia, convulsions, and death: Tricyclic antidepressants, monamine oxidase inhibitors, fluoxetine; sympathomimetic amines; meperidine and other narcotics (also possibly hypotension, respiratory depression, and coma)

(6) Hypoglycemia with insulin or sulfonylureas

(7) Increased anticoagulant effect with coumarin derivatives

(8) Shaking, hyperventilation, confusion, and so forth, with tryptophan

K. Streptozocin (streptozotocin, Zanosar)

1. Indications. Islet cell cancer of the pancreas (in combination with fluorouracil), carcinoid tumors

2. Pharmacology

a. Mechanism. Alkylating agent (see section I.A). A cell cycle–nonspecific nitrosourea analog. Inhibits DNA synthesis and the DNA repair enzyme, guanine-O^6-methyl transferase; affects pyrimidine nucleotide metabolism and inhibits enzymes involved in gluconeogenesis. Selectively targets pancreatic β cells, presumably due to the glucose moiety on the molecule.

b. Metabolism. Drug is a type of nitrosourea that is extensively metabolized by the liver to active metabolites and has a short plasma half-life (<1 hour). Crosses the blood–brain barrier. Excreted in urine as metabolites and unchanged drug.

3. Toxicity

a. Dose-limiting. Nephrotoxicity initially appears as proteinuria and progresses to glycosuria, aminoaciduria, proximal renal tubular acidosis, nephrogenic diabetes insipidus, and renal failure if the drug is continued.

b. Common. Nausea and vomiting (often severe), myelosuppression (mild, but may be cumulative), hypoglycemia after infusion, vein irritation during infusion, altered glucose metabolism with either hypoglycemia or hyperglycemia

c. Occasional. Diarrhea, abdominal cramps, LFT abnormalities

d. Rare. Central nervous system (CNS) toxicity, fever, secondary malignancies

4. Administration. Urinalysis and serum creatinine levels are monitored before each dose. Patients are routinely premedicated with antiemetics. The dose is administered over 30 to 60 minutes to prevent local pain.

a. Supplied as 1-g vials

b. Dose modification. Proteinuria or elevated serum creatinine levels contraindicate use of the drug until the abnormalities resolve.

c. Dose. 1.0 g/m² IV weekly for 6 weeks, then off treatment for 4 weeks, or 0.5 g/m² IV daily for 5 days every 6 weeks

L. Temozolomide (Temodar)

1. Indications. Brain tumors; metastatic melanoma

2. Pharmacology. Structurally and functionally similar to dacarbazine

a. Mechanisms. Structurally and functionally similar to dacarbazine. Metabolic activation to the reactive compound (MTIC) is required for antitumor activity. The drug methylates guanine residues in DNA and inhibits DNA, RNA, and protein synthesis, but does not cross-link DNA strands. Nonclassic alkylating agent, cell cycle–nonspecific.

b. Metabolism. Excreted predominantly by the renal tubules. Because the drug is lipophilic, it crosses the blood–brain barrier.

3. Toxicity

a. Dose-limiting. Myelosuppression

b. Common. Mild to moderately severe nausea and vomiting lasting up to 12 hours, headache, fatigue, mild transaminase elevation

c. Occasional. Photosensitivity

4. Administration. Patients should avoid sun exposure during and for several days after treatment.

a. Supplied as 5-, 20-, 100-, and 250-mg capsules

b. Dose modification. Consider dosage reduction for moderately severe hepatic or renal dysfunction and for elderly patients.

c. Dose. 75 mg/m² PO daily during radiation therapy; 150 mg/m² PO for 5 days each month as maintenance therapy.

M. Thiotepa (triethylenethiophosphoramide, Thioplex)

1. **Indications.** Intracavitary for malignant effusions, intravesicular for urinary bladder, severe thrombocytosis. Also can be used in lymphoma, breast cancer, and ovarian cancer.

2. **Pharmacology.** Ethylenimine analog, chemically related to nitrogen mustard

    a. **Mechanism.** Alkylation (see section I.A). Alkylates the N-7 position of guanine. Cell cycle–nonspecific.

    b. **Metabolism.** Rapidly decomposed in plasma and excreted in urine. Extensively metabolized by the hepatic P450 microsomal system to active and inactive metabolites.

3. **Toxicity**

    a. **Dose-limiting.** Myelosuppression, which may be cumulative

    b. **Common** (for intravesicular administration). Chemical cystitis, abdominal pain, hematuria, dysuria, frequency, urgency, ureteral obstruction; nausea and vomiting 6 hours after treatment

    c. **Occasional.** GI upset, abnormal LFTs, rash, hives; hypersensitivity

    d. **Rare.** Alopecia, fever, angioedema, secondary malignancies

4. **Administration.** Thiotepa has been administered intravenously, intramuscularly, intravesicularly, intrathecally, intra-arterially, intrapleurally, intrapericardially, intraperitoneally, intratumorally, and as an ophthalmic instillation.

    a. **Supplied** as 15-mg vials

    b. **Dose modification.** Necessary for patients with cytopenias

    c. **Dose.** 10 to 20 mg/m^2 IV every 3 to 4 weeks; 30 to 60 mg intravesicularly every week for 4 weeks

    d. **Drug interactions.** Increases neuromuscular blockade with succinyl choline

N. Cisplatin [*cis*-diamminedichloroplatinum (CDDP), Platinol]

1. **Indications.** A wide variety of malignancies

2. **Pharmacology**

    a. **Mechanism.** A heavy metal alkylator of DNA. Covalently bonds to proteins, RNA, and especially DNA, forming DNA cross-linking and intrastrand N-7 adducts. The trans isomer has virtually no antitumor activity. Acquired resistance to cisplatin involves alterations in transmembrane transport of drugs, intracellular levels of glutathione (GSH) or sulfhydryl-containing proteins, and the capacity to repair cisplatin DNA lesions.

    b. **Metabolism.** Widely distributed in the body, except for the CNS. Long half-life in plasma (up to 3 days); may remain bound in tissues for months. Biliary excretion accounts for <10% of the total drug excretion. Approximately 15% of drug is excreted in the urine unchanged, and 10% to 40% of the remainder is excreted in the urine within 24 hours.

3. **Toxicity**

    a. **Dose-limiting**

        (1) **Cumulative renal insufficiency.** The incidence of renal insufficiency is about 5% with adequate hydration measures and 25% to 45% without hydration measures.

        (2) **Peripheral sensory neuropathy** develops after the administration of 200 mg/m^2 and can become dose-limiting when the cumulative cisplatin dose exceeds 400 mg/m^2. Symptoms may progress after treatment is discontinued and include loss of proprioception and vibratory senses, hyporeflexia, and the Lhermitte sign. Symptoms may resolve slowly after many months.

        (3) **Ototoxicity** with tinnitus and high-frequency hearing loss occurs in 5% of patients. Ototoxicity occurs more commonly in patients receiving doses of >100 mg/m^2 by rapid infusion or high cumulative doses.

    b. **Common.** Severe nausea and vomiting (both acute and delayed) occur in all treated patients; preventative antiemetic regimens are required. Hypokalemia, hypomagnesemia (occasionally difficult to correct), and mild myelosuppression occur very frequently; anorexia and metallic taste of foods; alopecia; azoospermia, sterility, impotence.

    c. Occasional. Alopecia, loss of taste, vein irritation, transiently abnormal LFTs, SIADH, hypophosphatemia, myalgia, fever; optic neuritis

    d. Rare. Altered color perception and reversible focal encephalopathy that often causes cortical blindness. Raynaud phenomenon, bradycardia, bundle-branch block, congestive heart failure; anaphylaxis, tetany.

4. Administration

    a. Supplied as 10- and 50-mg vials

    b. Dose modification. Renal function must return to normal before cisplatin can be given. Many physicians avoid using cisplatin when the creatinine clearance is <40 mL/minute. Use with caution in patients with documented hearing impairment.

    c. Dose depends on the chemotherapy regimen, of which there are many. Examples are:

        (1) 40 to 120 mg/m^2 or more IV every 3 to 4 weeks, or

        (2) 20 to 40 mg/m^2 IV daily for 3 to 5 days every 3 to 4 weeks

    d. Method. The principles of cisplatin administration are as follows:

        (1) Monitoring. Serum creatinine, electrolytes, magnesium, and calcium levels should be measured daily during therapy. Audiometry is usually not necessary.

        (2) Antiemetics. Patients should be given prophylactic antiemetics, such as ondansetron and dexamethasone.

        (3) Hydration and diuresis are required when 40 mg/m^2 or more of cisplatin is given to maintain a urine output of 100 to 150 mL/hour before administration of the drug. Furosemide is given to prevent fluid overload. Intravenous fluids are supplemented with KCl and MgSO$_4$.

        (4) Amifostine cytoprotection (see section X.A). Amifostine and mesna may inactivate the nephrotoxic effect of cisplatin.

    e. Drug interactions

        (1) Cisplatin inhibits renal elimination of **bleomycin, etoposide, methotrexate, and ifosfamide**.

        (2) Taxanes should be given before cisplatin when used in combination

        (3) Concomitant use of other **nephrotoxic agents**, such as aminoglycosides, increase the risk of nephrotoxicity

        (4) Phenytoin effect is decreased when given with cisplatin

O. Carboplatin (Paraplatin)

  1. Indications. A wide variety of malignancies

  2. Pharmacology

    a. Mechanisms. Heavy metal alkylating-like agent with mechanisms very similar to cisplatin, but with different toxicity profile. Like cisplatin, it produces predominantly interstrand DNA cross-links rather than DNA–protein cross-links; this effect is apparently cell cycle–nonspecific. Cisplatin and carboplatin exhibit substantial clinical cross-resistance.

    b. Metabolism. Plasma half-life of only 2 to 3 hours. Excreted in urine as unchanged drug (70%) and metabolites.

  3. Toxicity

    a. Dose-limiting. Myelosuppression is significant and cumulative, especially thrombocytopenia. Median nadir hematosuppression at 21 days; increased myelosuppression in patients who have reduced creatinine clearance levels or who have received prior chemotherapy.

    b. Common. Nausea, vomiting, and nephrotoxicity (but less severe less common than with cisplatin), pain at injection site. Cation electrolyte imbalance.

    c. Occasional. Reversible abnormal LFTs, azotemia; peripheral neuropathy (10%); hypersensitivity reactions; amenorrhea, azoospermia, impotence, and sterility

    d. Rare. Alopecia, rash, flulike syndrome, hematuria, hyperamylasemia; hearing loss, optic neuritis; alopecia

  4. Administration

    a. Supplied as 50-, 150-, 450-mg vials

    b. Dose modification. Reduce dosage for creatinine clearance of ≤ 60 mL/minute. Caution is advised when concomitantly administering other myelo-suppressive or nephrotoxic drugs.

    c. Dose by creatinine clearance (Clearance$_{Cr}$), as follows:

Clearance$_{Cr}$ ≥ 60 mL/minute; dose = 360 mg/m^2
Clearance$_{Cr}$ ≥ 41 to 59 mL/minute; dose = 250 mg/m^2
Clearance$_{Cr}$ ≥ 16 to 40 mL/minute; dose = 200 mg/m^2

    d. Dose by Calvert's formula (AUC, area under the curve; GFR, glomerular filtration rate)

Total dose [mg (not per m^2)] = (target AUC) $\times$ (GFR + 25)
Target AUC = 4 to 6 for previously treated patients
Target AUC = 5 to 7 for previously untreated patients

    e. Drug interactions. Taxanes should be administered before carboplatin when given concomitantly.

P. Oxaliplatin (diaminocyclohexane platinum, Eloxatin)

  1. Indications. Stage II, III, and IV colorectal cancer, pancreatic and gastric cancers

  2. Pharmacology

    a. Mechanisms. Binds covalently to DNA with preferential binding to the N-7 position of guanine and adenine; intrastrand and interstrand cross-links.

    b. Metabolism. Undergoes extensive nonenzymatic conversion to its active cytotoxic species; >50% of the drug is cleared through the kidneys. Only 2% of the drug is excreted in feces.

  3. Toxicity

    a. Dose-limiting

      (1) Acute dysesthesias in the hands, feet, perioral area, or throat develop within hours or up to 2 days after dosing, may be precipitated or exacerbated by exposure to cold (cold air or beverages); usually resolves within 2 weeks; frequently recurs with further dosing and may be ameliorated by prolonging the infusion to 6 hours. Dysphagia, dyspnea without stridor or wheezing, jaw spasms, dysarthria, voice changes, or chest pressure may occur. In contrast to cisplatin, ototoxicity occurs rarely.

      (2) Persistent peripheral sensory neuropathy usually characterized by paresthesias, dysesthesias, and hypoesthesias, including deficits in proprioception, which is usually reversible within 4 months of discontinuing oxaliplatin.

    b. Common. Nausea and vomiting, diarrhea; mild myelosuppression

    c. Occasional. Allergic reactions, mild nephrotoxicity

  4. Administration. The drug cannot be mixed with alkaline medications or media [such as basic solutions of fluorouracil (5-FU)]. The patient should avoid exposure to cold.

    a. Supplied as 50- and 100-mg vials

    b. Dose modification. Reduce dose for renal dysfunction

    c. Dose (FOLFOX-4 regimen): 85 mg/m^2 with leucovorin, 200 mg/m^2, both given over 2 hours at the same time through Y-tubing on Day 1. Then, 5-FU is given first as a bolus at a dose of 400 mg/m^2 and then as an infusion of 600 mg/m^2 over 22 hours. On Day 2, leucovorin, 5-FU bolus and 5-FU infusion over 22 hours are repeated. The cycle is repeated every 2 weeks. Several variations of this regimen are available.

II. ANTIMETABOLITES

A. General pharmacology of antimetabolites

  1. Some antimetabolites are structural analogs of normal molecules that are essential for cell growth and replication. Other antimetabolites inhibit enzymes that are necessary for the synthesis of essential compounds. Their major effect is interfering with the building blocks of DNA synthesis (Fig. 4.1). Their activity, therefore, is greatest in the S phase of the cell cycle. In general, these agents have been most effective when cell proliferation is rapid.

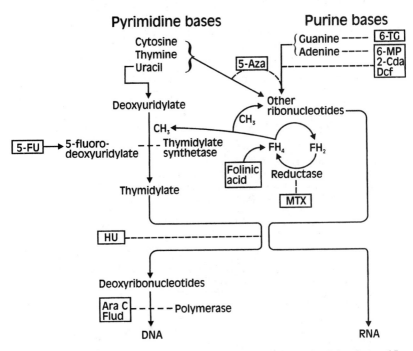

Figure 4.1. Sites of action of antimetabolites. 2-Cda, 2-chlorodeoxyadenosine; 5-Aza, 5-azacytidine; 5-FU, 5-fluorouracil; 6-MP, 6-mercaptopurine; 6-TG, 6-thioguanine; Ara C, cytosine arabinoside; Dcf, deoxycoformycin; Flud, fludarabine; HU, hydroxy-urea; MTX, methotrexate; reductase, dihydrofolate reductase.

2. The pharmacokinetics of these drugs are characterized by nonlinear dose–response curves; after a certain dose, no more are killed with increasing doses (fluorouracil is an exception). Because of the entry of new cells into the cycle, the length of time that the cells are exposed to the drug is directly proportional to the killing potential.

B. Azacitidine (5-azacitidine, Vidaza)
   1. Indication. Acute myelogenous leukemia (experimental); severe myelodysplastic syndromes (MDS) with an anticipated response in 16% of patients.
   2. Pharmacology
      a. Mechanism. Antimetabolite (cytidine analog). Rapidly phosphorylated and incorporated into DNA and RNA, thereby inhibiting protein synthesis; also inhibits pyrimidine synthesis and DNA methylation.
      b. Metabolism. Activated by phosphorylation and deactivated by deamination; similar to cytarabine. Excreted in urine (20% as unchanged drug).
   3. Toxicity
      a. Dose-limiting. Myelosuppression; nausea and vomiting.
      b. Common. Hepatic dysfunction, fatigue, headache, diarrhea, alopecia, fever, injection site erythema
      c. Occasional. Neurotoxicity (dizziness, restlessness, confusion), azotemia (transient), arthralgias, hypophosphatemia with myalgia, stomatitis, phlebitis, rash
      d. Rare. Progressive lethargy and coma, renal tubular acidosis, rhabdomyolysis, hypotension
   4. Administration
      a. Supplied as 100-mg vials

     b. Dose modification. Necessary for patients with impaired liver function. Also reduce dose for patients with renal dysfunction and for serum bicarbonate concentration of <20 mEq/L.

     c. Dose. 75 to 100 mg/m^2 per day SQ for 7 days every 4 weeks for MDS (several cycles may be required for effectiveness)

C. Cladribine [2-chlordeoxyadenosine (2-CdA), Leustatin]

  1. Indications. Hairy cell leukemia, indolent lymphomas, chronic lymphocytic leukemia, Waldenström macroglobulinemia

  2. Pharmacology. An analog of the purine deoxyadenosine

     a. Mechanism. Antimetabolite. The analog accumulates in cells (particularly lymphocytes), blocks adenosine deaminase, and inhibits RNA and DNA synthesis. Inhibits ribonucleotide reductase. Depletes ATP. Induces apoptosis. Active against both dividing and resting cells.

     b. Metabolism. Rapidly metabolized and eliminated through the kidneys.

  3. Toxicity. Patients are at increased risk for opportunistic infections.

     a. Dose-limiting. Myelosuppression

     b. Common. Immunosuppression with decreases in CD4+ and CD8+ cells; nausea, skin reactions at injection site; fever in 50% (most likely due to tumor's releasing pyrogens and cytokines), chills, flulike syndrome.

     c. Occasional. Neurotoxicity (headache, dizziness), hypersensitivity reactions, fatigue

     d. Rare. Neurotoxicity, pancreatitis

  4. Administration

     a. Supplied as 10-mg vials

     b. Dose modification. Hematologic; use with caution with renal dysfunction.

     c. Dose. Either 0.10 mg/kg/day (4 mg/m^2/day) by continuous IV infusion for 7 days, or 0.14 mg/kg daily IV over 2 hours for 5 days

D. Cytarabine (cytosine arabinoside, Cytosar, ara-C)

  1. Indications. Acute leukemia, chronic myelogenous leukemia, lymphoma, meningeal involvement with tumor

  2. Pharmacology. An analog of deoxycytidine

     a. Mechanism. Antimetabolite. Requires intracellular activation to its phosphorylated derivative (ara-CTP), which inhibits DNA polymerases that are involved in the conversion of cytidine to deoxycytidine; some is incorporated into DNA. Ara-CTP inhibits ribonucleotide reductase, which results in decreased levels of deoxyribonucleotides for DNA synthesis and function. Blocks DNA synthesis and repair and terminates DNA chain elongation. Cell cycle–specific (S phase).

     b. Metabolism. Requires activation to ara-CTP by kinase; deactivated by deaminase; ara-C is rapidly and completely deaminated in liver, plasma, and peripheral tissues; ara-C antitumor activity depends on relative amounts of kinase and deaminase in cells. In patients with renal insufficiency, one metabolite (uracil arabinoside) has the ability to produce high concentrations of ara-CTP, which may result in CNS toxicity. Excreted in urine as inactive metabolites.

  3. Toxicity

     a. Dose-limiting. Myelosuppression

     b. Common. Nausea, vomiting, mucositis, diarrhea (potentiated by the addition of an anthracycline); conjunctivitis (usually within the first 3 days of high-dose regimens, but reduced with prophylactic glucocorticoid eyedrops); hydradenitis, arachnoiditis with intrathecal administration.

     c. Neurotoxicity (cerebellar ataxia, lethargy, confusion) begins on the fourth or fifth day of infusion and usually resolves within 7 days. The incidence and severity of toxicity are related to the dose given (especially with total dose of >48 g/m^2), the rate of infusion (least incidence for continuous infusions), age (particularly older than 60 years), sex (especially male), and the degree of hepatic or renal dysfunction (particularly with creatinine clearance of <60 mL/minute). In some cases, it is irreversible or fatal.

   d. Occasional. Alopecia, stomatitis, metallic taste, esophagitis, hepatic dysfunction (mild and reversible), pancreatitis, severe GI ulceration; thrombophlebitis; headache; rash, transient skin erythema without exfoliation. ***Ara-C syndrome,*** described in pediatric patients, is an allergic reaction manifested by fever, flulike syndrome, myalgias, bone pain, maculopapular rash, conjunctivitis, and occasional chest pain (corticosteroids are effective).
   e. Rare. Sudden respiratory distress rapidly progressing to noncardiogenic pulmonary edema; pericarditis, cardiomegaly, tamponade; urinary retention.
 4. Administration. Use prophylactic glucocorticoid eyedrops for patients receiving high-dose regimens.
   a. Supplied as 100-, 500-, 1,000-, and 2,000-mg vials
   b. Dose modification. Use cautiously in patients with liver or renal disease or with risk factors for neurotoxicity.
   c. Dose
     (1) See Chapter 21 for use in patients with lymphoma and Chapter 25 for use in patients with acute leukemia.
     (2) For intrathecal administration: 50 to 100 mg in 10 mL saline for 1 to 3 days weekly
     (3) Low-dose regimen: 10 mg/m^2 SC every 12 to 24 hours for 15 to 21 days
     (4) High-dose therapy should be given over 1 to 2 hours
   d. Drug interactions
     (1) Ara-C antagonizes the efficacy of **gentamycin** and **digoxin**
     (2) Ara-C enhances the cytotoxicity of cisplatin, various alkylating agents, and ionizing radiation
     (3) Fludarabine, hydroxyurea, and **methotrexate** enhance the cytotoxicity of ara-C
     (4) Increased risk of pancreatitis in patients also treated with **L-asparaginase**
E. Decitabine (Dacogen)
 1. Indications. Myelodysplastic syndromes, chronic myelomonocytic leukemia
 2. Pharmacology. Decitabine is an analogue of the natural nucleoside 2'-decoxycytidine.
   a. Mechanisms. Decitabine is believed to exert its antineoplastic effects by inhibition of DNA methyltransferase, causing hypomethylation of DNA and cellular differentiation or apoptosis.
   b. Metabolism. The metabolic fate and route of elimination are not known.
 3. Toxicity
   a. Dose-limiting. Hematosuppression
   b. Common. Hematosuppression, febrile neutropenia, fatigue, pyrexia; nausea, constipation, diarrhea; cough; hypoglycemia.
 4. Administration. Premedicate with antinausea drugs.
   a. Supplied as 50-mg vials as a lyophilized powder
   b. Dose modification: Reduce dose to 11 mg/m^2 if hematologic recovery requires more than 6 weeks. Decitabine should be discontinued if the serum creatinine is ≥2 mg/dL or SGPT or bilirubin is ≥ twice the upper limit of normal. The dose should also be reduced for grade 3 or 4 nonmyelosuppressive toxicities.
   c. Dose. 20 mg/m^2 IV over 1 hour for 5 days. Cycles are repeated every 4 weeks. Responses may require three cycles of treatment.
F. Fludarabine (2-fluoroadenine arabinoside-5-phosphate, Fludara)
 1. Indications. Chronic lymphocytic leukemia, low-grade lymphomas, and cutaneous T-cell lymphomas
 2. Pharmacology. The 5'-monophosphate analog of ara-A (arabinofuranosyladenosine). The 2-fluoro group on the adenosine ring renders this drug resistant to breakdown by adenosine deaminase (compare with cytarabine).
   a. Mechanism. Antimetabolite with high specificity for lymphoid cells. Its active metabolite, 2-fluoro-ara-A, appears to act by inhibiting DNA chain

extension, DNA polymerase-α, and ribonucleotide reductase. It has activity against both dividing and resting cells and induces apoptosis.

    b. Metabolism. Metabolites and unchanged drug (25%) are excreted primarily in urine.

3. Toxicity

    a. Dose-limiting. Myelosuppression, which may be cumulative

    b. Common. Immunosuppression with decreases in CD4+ and CD8+ T cells in most patients and associated with increased risk for opportunistic infections (recovery may take more than a year); mild nausea and vomiting; fever with associated flulike syndrome (25%).

    c. Occasional. Alopecia (mild), abnormal LFTs, tumor lysis syndrome

    d. Rare. Stomatitis, diarrhea; dermatitis; neurotoxicity (usually high doses: somnolence, transient paresthesias, demyelination); chest pain, hypotension, pulmonary infiltrates.

4. Administration

    a. Supplied as 50-mg vials

    b. Dose modification. Decrease dosage by 30% for patients with creatinine clearance of <70 mL/minute.

    c. Dose. 25 mg/m^2 IV over 30 minutes daily for 5 consecutive days every 4 weeks

    d. Drug interactions. Fludarabine may enhance cytotoxicity of cyclophosphamide, cisplatin, and mitoxantrone by inhibiting nucleotide repair mechanisms and of cytarabine by inducing expression of deoxycytidine kinase.

G. 5-Fluorouracil (5-FU, Adrucil)

  1. Indications. Gastrointestinal, breast, pancreatic, and head and neck carcinomas

  2. Pharmacology. A fluoropyrimidine analog

    a. Mechanism. Antimetabolite. Requires activation to cytotoxic metabolite forms. Interferes with DNA synthesis by blocking thymidylate synthetase, an enzyme involved in the conversion of deoxyuridylic acid to thymidylic acid. Metabolites (e.g., FUTP) are incorporated into several RNA species, which thereby interfere with RNA function and protein synthesis. Incorporation of another metabolite (FdUTP) into DNA results in inhibition of DNA synthesis and function. It is cell-cycle S-phase–specific but acts in other cell cycle phases as well and is unique in having a log linear cell-killing action.

    b. Metabolism. 5-FU rapidly enters all tissues, including spinal fluid and malignant effusions. The drug undergoes extensive intracellular activation by a series of phosphorylating enzymes and phosphoribosyl transferase, particularly dihydropyrimidine dehydrogenase. Most of the drug degradation occurs in the liver. Responsive tumors appear to lack degradation enzymes. Metabolism eliminates 90% of 5-FU. Inactive metabolites are excreted in urine, bile, and breath (as carbon dioxide). The elimination half-life is short, ranging from 10 to 20 minutes.

  3. Toxicity is more common and more severe in patients with dihydropyrimidine dehydrogenase deficiency.

    a. Dose-limiting. Myelosuppression (less common with continuous infusion); mucositis (more common with 5-day infusion); diarrhea.

    b. Common. Nasal discharge; eye irritation and excessive lacrimation due to dacryocystitis and lacrimal duct stenosis; dry skin, photosensitivity, and pigmentation of the infused vein.

    c. Neurologic. Reversible cerebellar dysfunction, somnolence, confusion or seizures occurs in about 1% of patients. Symptoms usually disappear 1 to 6 weeks after the drug is discontinued, but they abate after the dose is reduced or even if the same dose is maintained.

    d. Occasional. Esophagitis; hand–foot syndrome with protracted infusion (paresthesia, erythema, and swelling of the palms and soles); myocardial ischemia (particularly in patients with a prior history of myocardial ischemia); thrombophlebitis; nausea, vomiting.

     e. Rare. Alopecia, dermatitis, loss of nails, dark bands on nails; blurred vision, "black hairy tongue" (hypertrophy of filiform papillae), anaphylaxis, fever.

  4. Administration. 5-FU is given by IV bolus, IV infusion over 15 minutes, continuous IV infusion, arterial infusion, intracavitarily, topically, or orally. The use of ice chips in the mouth 15 minutes before and 15 minutes after IV bolus injections of 5-FU may reduce the incidence and severity of mucositis.

     a. Supplied as 500-mg vials

     b. Dose modification. Fluorouracil is withheld if the patient has stomatitis, diarrhea, evidence of infection, leukopenia, or thrombocytopenia; drug is resumed (perhaps at reduced dosage) when these problems have resolved.

       (1) May be contraindicated in patients with active ischemic heart disease or a history of myocardial infarction within the previous 6 months

       (2) Patients who experience unexpected grade 3 or 4 myelosuppression, gastrointestinal and/or neurologic toxicities with initiation of therapy may have an underlying deficiency in dihydropyrimidine dehydrogenase. Further testing to identify this pharmacogenetic syndrome should be considered under these circumstances. If enzyme deficiency is present, therapy with 5-FU must be discontinued immediately.

     c. Dose. Fluorouracil is erratically absorbed orally. Several regimens have been used, including the following:

       (1) 500 to 600 mg/m^2 IV weekly for 6 weeks of every 8 weeks

       (2) 425 to 450 mg/m^2 IV daily for 5 days every 28 days

       (3) 800 to 1,000 mg/m^2/day by continuous infusion for 4 to 5 days every 28 days

       (4) 200 to 400 mg/m^2/day by continuous infusion indefinitely

     d. Drug interactions

       (1) Toxicity is enhanced by leucovorin (along with antitumor activity), methotrexate, trimetrexate, and phosphonacetyl-L-aspartic acid (PALA).

       (2) Allopurinol inhibits activation of 5-FU and may result in decreased effectiveness.

       (3) Thymidine and **uridine** decrease the host toxic effects of 5-FU.

H. Leucovorin (folinic acid, citrovorum factor, 5-formyl tetrahydrofolate)

  1. Indications. Combined with 5-FU in treatment of colorectal and other adenocarcinomas; the rescue agent for antifol toxicity (e.g., methotrexate)

  2. Pharmacology

     a. Mechanism. Leucovorin is a tetrahydrofolic acid derivative that acts as a cofactor for carbon transfer reactions in the synthesis of purines and pyrimidines. It inhibits the effects of methotrexate and other dihydrofolate reductase antagonists. Leucovorin potentiates the cytotoxic effects of fluorinated pyrimidines (i.e., 5-FU and floxuridine) by increasing the binding of folate cofactor and activated 5-FU to thymidylate synthetase (TS) within the cells.

     b. Metabolism. Metabolized intracellularly to the reduced folate, 5, 10-methylenetetrahydrofolate, which forms a ternary complex with the 5-FU metabolite FdUMP and TS. Excreted in urine as metabolites.

  3. Toxicity. Potentiates the toxic effects of fluoropyrimidine therapy

  4. Administration

     a. Supplied as 50-, 100-, and 350-mg vials for IV or IM use and as 5- and 15-mg tablets for oral use

     b. Dose. Depends on combination regimen

       (1) When used as a rescue agent in combination with high-dose methotrexate, leucovorin should be administered 24 hours after methotrexate every 6 hours for up to 12 doses, depending on the serum methotrexate level; continue leucovorin until the methotrexate level falls below 5×10^{-8} M.

       (2) When given in combination with 5-FU, leucovorin should be administered at least 30 to 60 minutes before 5-FU to allow sufficient time for intracellular metabolism to take place.

      c. Drug interactions. Phenobarbital and **phenytoin** may decrease in their efficacy and increase the risk of seizures. Precipitates when mixed in the same solution as 5-FU.

I. Capecitabine (Xeloda)

  1. Indications. Carcinomas of the breast or colon

  2. Pharmacology. Capecitabine is a fluoropyrimidine carbamate that is a systemic prodrug of 5′-deoxy-5-fluorouridine (5′-DFUR), which is converted *in vivo* to 5-FU.

    a. Mechanism. See *fluorouracil*

    b. Metabolism. Hepatic. Catabolism predominantly via dihydropyrimidine dehydrogenase, which is present in liver, leukocytes, kidney, and other extra-hepatic tissues. More than 90% is cleared in the urine (see *5-fluorouracil*).

  3. Toxicity. Similar to 5-FU

    a. Dose-limiting. Diarrhea (50%)

    b. Common. Hand–foot syndrome (palmar–plantar erythrodysesthesia or chemotherapy-induced acral erythema) occurs in 15% to 20% of patients; nausea, vomiting, hematosuppression.

    c. Occasional. Abnormal LFTs, neurotoxicity; cardiac ischemia in patients with a prior history of coronary artery disease; tear duct stenosis, conjunctivitis, blepharitis; confusion, cerebellar ataxia.

    d. Chest pain, EKG changes

  4. Administration. Pyridoxine, 50 mg PO b.i.d. may be used to reduce the incidence and severity of the hand–foot syndrome. Celecoxib (Celebrex), 200-mg b.i.d., or a low-dose nicotine patch may also be effective.

    a. Supplied as 150- and 500-mg tablets

    b. Dose modification. Use with caution with liver dysfunction and in patients taking coumarin derivatives. Reduce dosage in patients with moderate renal dysfunction. Contraindicated in patients with dihydropyrimidine dehydrogenase deficiency or with severe renal impairment.

    c. Dose. 650 to 1,250 mg/m^2 PO b.i.d. (approximately every 12 hours) with a glass of water and within 30 minutes of a meal for 14 days every 3 weeks

    d. Drug interactions

      (1) Warfarin. Patients using warfarin should have dosage monitored closely, even after capecitabine is discontinued.

      (2) Phenytoin toxicity can develop; dosage adjustment may be necessary.

      (3) Liquid antacids may increase the bioavailability of capecitabine.

      (4) Leucovorin enhances the antitumor effect and toxicity of capecitabine.

    e. Treatment of hand–foot syndrome. Hand moisturizers; soak hands and feet in cool to tepid water for 10 minutes, then apply petrolatum jelly onto the wet skin. Bag balm or lanolin-containing salves may help.

J. Gemcitabine (Gemzar)

  1. Indications. Carcinoma of pancreas, bladder, lung, ovary; soft-tissue sarcomas.

  2. Pharmacology. A fluorine-substituted deoxycytidine analog

    a. Mechanisms. Cell-phase specific, primarily killing cells in S phase and also blocking the progression of cells through the G$_1$ phase to S-phase boundary. Metabolized intracellularly to the active diphosphate and triphosphate. Inhibits ribonucleotide reductase; competes with deoxycytidine triphosphate (dCTP) for incorporation into DNA.

    b. Metabolism. Undergoes extensive metabolism by deamination in the liver, plasma, and peripheral tissues. Nearly entirely excreted in urine as active drug and metabolites.

  3. Toxicity

    a. Dose-limiting. Myelosuppression

    b. Common. Nausea, vomiting, diarrhea, stomatitis; fever with flulike symptoms (40%); macular or maculopapular rash; transient LFT elevations; mild proteinuria and hematuria.

    c. Occasional. Hair loss, rash, edema.

    d. Rare. Hemolytic-uremic syndrome; pulmonary drug toxicity; hypersensitivity reactions; alopecia.

  4. Administration. Gemcitabine is a potent radiosensitizer and should be avoided in patients while undergoing radiotherapy.

    a. Supplied as vials of 200 and 1,000 mg

    b. Dose modification. Use with caution in patients with hepatic or renal insufficiency.

    c. Dose. 1,000 mg/m^2 over 30 minutes weekly for 7 weeks or until toxicity, followed by 1 week rest; then for 3 of every 4 weeks.

K. Hydroxyurea (Hydrea)

  1. Indications. Chronic myelogenous leukemia, myeloproliferative disorders, refractory ovarian cancer

  2. Pharmacology. An analog of urea

    a. Mechanism. Antimetabolite. Inhibits DNA synthesis by inhibiting nucleotide reductase, the enzyme that converts ribonucleosides to deoxyribonucleosides. Inhibits DNA repair and thymidine incorporation into DNA. Cell-cycle S-phase–specific, but acts in other phases as well.

    b. Metabolism. Crosses the blood–brain barrier. Half of the drug is rapidly degraded into inactive compounds by the liver. Inactive products and unchanged drug (50%) are excreted in urine.

  3. Toxicity

    a. Dose-limiting. Myelosuppression, which recovers rapidly when treatment is stopped (prominent megaloblastosis)

    b. Occasional. Nausea, vomiting, diarrhea; skin rash, facial erythema, hyperpigmentation; azotemia, proteinuria; transient LFT abnormalities; radiation recall phenomenon.

    c. Rare. Alopecia, mucositis, diarrhea, constipation; neurological events; pulmonary edema; flulike syndrome; painful perimalleolar ulcers; possible acute leukemia in myeloproliferative disorders.

  4. Administration

    a. Supplied as 500-mg capsules

    b. Dose modification. The drug should be given cautiously in the presence of liver dysfunction or when combined with other antimetabolites. Dosages should be reduced for creatinine clearance levels of <50 mL/minute and when given with concomitant radiotherapy.

    c. Dose. 10 to 30 mg/kg PO daily

L. 6-Mercaptopurine (6-MP, Purinethol)

  1. Indication. Acute lymphoblastic leukemia (maintenance therapy)

  2. Pharmacology

    a. Mechanism. Purine analog with activity in the S phase of the cell cycle. Inhibits *de novo* purine synthesis by inhibiting 5-phosphoribosyl-1-pyrophosphate. The parent drug is inactive. Requires intracellular phosphorylation by hypoxanthine-guanine phosphoribosyltransferase (HGPRT) to the monophosphate form, which is eventually metabolized to the triphosphate metabolite. Competes with ribotides for enzymes responsible for conversion of inosinic acid to adenine and xanthine ribotides. Its incorporation into DNA or RNA is of uncertain significance.

    b. Metabolism. Mercaptopurine is slowly degraded in the liver, largely by xanthine oxidase. Allopurinol, a xanthine oxidase inhibitor, causes marked increase in its toxicity. Clearance is primarily hepatic with conventional doses.

  3. Toxicity

    a. Dose-limiting. Myelosuppression

    b. Common. Mild nausea, vomiting, anorexia (25%); usually reversible cholestasis (30%); dry skin, photosensitivity; immunosuppression.

    c. Rare. Stomatitis, diarrhea, dermatitis, fever, hematuria, Budd-Chiari–like syndrome, hepatic necrosis

  4. Administration

    a. Supplied as 50-mg tablets

   b. Dose modification. Dose is reduced by 50% to 75% for patients with hepatic dysfunction.

   c. Dose. 70 to 100 mg/m^2 PO daily until patient responds or toxic effects are seen; then adjust for maintenance therapy.

   d. Drug interactions. If given allopurinol, the 6-MP dose must be reduced by 75%. Dosage may also need to be modified if other hepatotoxic drugs are given. **Warfarin** dosages may be affected by 6-MP. **Bactrim-DS** may enhance myelosuppressive effect of 6-MP.

M. Methotrexate (amethopterin, MTX)

1. Indications. A wide variety of conditions

2. Pharmacology

   a. Mechanism. Cell cycle–specific antifolate analog active in the S phase of the cell cycle. MTX blocks the enzyme dihydrofolate reductase, preventing formation of reduced (tetrahydro-) folic acid; tetrahydrofolic acid is crucial to the transfer of carbon units in a variety of biochemical reactions (Fig. 4.1). MTX thus blocks formation of thymidylate from deoxyuridylate and prevents synthesis of DNA. The drug also inhibits RNA and protein synthesis and prevents cells from entering the S phase of the cell cycle.

   b. Metabolism. MTX is minimally metabolized by the human species. It is converted in the liver and other cells to higher polyglutamate forms. The drug is distributed to body water; patients with significant effusions eliminate the drug much more slowly. Because 50% to 70% of the drug is bound to plasma proteins, displacement by other drugs (e.g., aspirin, sulfonamides) may result in an increase in toxic effects. About 20% of the drug is eliminated in the bile. It is excreted in urine as unchanged drug (80% to 90% within 24 hours). Renal dysfunction results in dangerous blood levels of MTX and possible further renal damage. The half-life of the drug is 8 to 10 hours.

3. Toxicity. Leucovorin can reverse the immediate cytotoxic effects of MTX; generally, 1 mg of leucovorin is given for each 1 mg of MTX.

   a. Dose-limiting. Myelosuppression, stomatitis, renal dysfunction

   b. High-dose regimens. Nausea, vomiting, renal tubular necrosis, cortical blindness

   c. Previously irradiated areas. Skin erythema, pulmonary fibrosis, transverse myelitis, cerebritis

   d. Chronic therapy. Liver cirrhosis (reversible hepatic dysfunction occurs with short-term intermittent therapy); osteoporosis (in children)

   e. Neurotoxicity. MTX neurotoxicity depends on dose and route of administration. Within a few hours after intrathecal administration, MTX can produce an acute aseptic meningitis that is usually self-limited. A subacute encephalopathy and myelopathy can also occur after intrathecal administration.

   High-dose systemic administration can cause a reversible encephalopathy of rapid onset and resolution that lasts from minutes to hours (strokelike episodes). Chronic intrathecal combined with high-dose systemic administration can produce a more serious and irreversible leukoencephalopathy that develops months after treatment, is more likely to occur after brain irradiation, and causes dementia, seizures, spasticity, and ataxia.

   f. Occasional. Nausea, vomiting, diarrhea (GI ulceration, hemorrhage, and perforation can occur if therapy is continued after the onset of diarrhea); dermatitis, photosensitivity, altered pigmentation, furunculosis; conjunctivitis, photophobia, excessive lacrimation, cataracts; fever, reversible oligospermia, flank pain (with rapid intravenous infusion).

   g. Rare. Alopecia, MTX pneumonitis (see Chapter 29, section IV.A)

4. Administration

   a. Supplied as 2.5-mg tablets and 20- to 1,000-mg vials

   b. Dose modification. The drug must not be administered to any patient with a creatinine clearance level of <60 mL/minute (serum creatinine >1.5 mg/dL).

    c. Dose. Varies according to regimen

      (1) High-dose regimens use supralethal doses of MTX followed by adminis-tration of the antidote leucovorin. This treatment is complex and requires experience for the clinician and use of special monitoring techniques.

      (2) Intrathecal administration: 5 to 10 mg/m^2 (maximum, 15 mg) in 7 to 15 mL of preservative-free saline (3 mL if given using an Ommaya reservoir) every 3 to 7 days

    d. Drug interactions

      (1) **Leucovorin** rescues normal tissues from MTX toxicity and may impair its antitumor activity. Folic acid supplements should be discontinued while on therapy.

      (2) **L-Asparaginase and thymidine** also block MTX toxicity and antitumor action.

      (3) **Aspirin, other nonsteroidal anti-inflammatory agents, penicillins, cephalosporins, phenytoin, and probenecid** decrease renal clearance of MTX and increase its toxicity.

      (4) **Sulfonamides and phenytoin** displace MTX from protein-binding sites and may enhance its toxicity.

      (5) **Trimethoprim** is also an inhibitor of dihydrofolate reductase and can enhance MTX toxicity.

      (6) Parenteral **acyclovir** and concomitant intrathecal MTX may result in neurological abnormalities.

      (7) MTX may increase serum levels of **warfarin,** which is displaced from plasma proteins.

      (8) **Omeprazole** (Prilosec) increases serum MTX levels.

N. Mitoguazone [methyl-GAG, methylglyoxal-bis(guanylhydrazone)]

  1. Indications. Investigational agent for lymphomas

  2. Pharmacology

    a. Mechanism. An antimetabolite that inhibits 5′-adenosylmethionine decar-boxylase, which is important in the production of spermidine, which inhibits DNA and RNA synthesis

    b. Metabolism. Triphasic elimination pattern

  3. Toxicity

    a. Dose-limiting. Mucositis (severe); diarrhea (sometimes severe or bloody), nausea and vomiting (rarely severe).

    b. Common. Flushing during infusion, myelosuppression

    c. Other. Polyneuropathy and myopathy; vasculitis, hypoglycemia

  4. Administration

    a. Supplied as 1-g vials

    b. Dose. 500 mg/m^2/week by IV infusion over at least 45 minutes

O. Pemetrexed (Alimta)

  1. Indications. Mesothelioma (with cisplatin) and non–small cell lung cancer (sec-ond line)

  2. Pharmacology

    a. Mechanisms. Pyrrolpyrimidine antifolate analog with activity in the S phase of the cell cycle. Inhibition of the folate-dependent enzyme thymidylate syn-thetase (TS) is the main site of action. It also inhibits dihydrofolate reductase and two formyltransferases.

    b. Metabolism. Metabolized intracellularly to polyglutamates, which are much more potent than the parent monoglutamate. Principally cleared by the kidneys. About 90% of the drug is excreted unchanged in the urine within 24 hours.

  3. Toxicity. Patients with insufficient folate intake may be at increased risk for host toxicity. A baseline homocysteine level >10 predicts for the development of grade 3–4 toxicity.

    a. Dose-limiting. Myelosuppression

    b. Common. Skin rash (usually as the hand–foot syndrome), mucositis, nausea, vomiting, diarrhea; fatigue; transient elevation of LFTs.

4. **Administration.** All patients are given 350 mcg/day PO of folic acid and 1,000 mcg of vitamin B_{12} SC every 3 weeks to reduce drug toxicity. Dexamethasone, 4 mg PO b.i.d. for 3 days before the beginning of treatment, may ameliorate or eliminate the skin rash.
   a. **Supplied** as 100-mg vials
   b. **Dose modification.** Reduce dosage in patients with abnormal renal function
   c. **Dose.** 600 mg/m^2 IV every 3 weeks as monotherapy; 500 mg/m^2 IV every 3 weeks when used with cisplatin.
   d. **Drug interactions.** Nonsteroidal anti-inflammatory drugs may inhibit the renal excretion of pemetrexed, resulting in increased drug toxicity. Thymidine rescues against the host toxic effects, and leucovorin decreases the antitumor effect of pemetrexed.

P. **Pentostatin** [2'-deoxycoformycin (dCF), Nipent]
   1. **Indications.** Chronic lymphocytic leukemia, hairy cell leukemia, and cutaneous T-cell lymphoma
   2. **Pharmacology.** A fermentation product of *Streptomyces antibioticus*
      a. **Mechanism.** Antimetabolite. Both cell cycle–specific and cell cycle–nonspecific. Inhibitor of adenine deaminase, an enzyme that is important for the metabolism of purine nucleosides. Also inhibits ribonucleotide reductase (resulting in inhibition of DNA synthesis and function) and S-adenosyl-L-homocysteine hydrolase (resulting in inhibition of one-carbon dependent methylation reactions).
      b. **Metabolism.** Most dCF is excreted unchanged in urine.
   3. **Toxicity**
      a. **Dose-limiting.** Myelosuppression
      b. **Common.** Immunosuppression; mild nausea and vomiting, diarrhea, altered taste; fatigue, fever.
      c. **Occasional.** Chills, myalgia, arthralgia; abnormal LFTs; keratoconjunctivitis, photophobia; renal failure.
      d. **Rare.** Hepatitis; pulmonary infiltrates and insufficiency.
   4. **Administration.** Hydration with at least 2 L of D5NSS is required to assure a urine output of 2 L on the day of drug administration.
      a. **Supplied** as 10-mg vials
      b. **Dose modification.** Reduce doses for renal impairment.
      c. **Dose.** 4 mg/m^2 IV infusion over 20 minutes every 2 weeks
      d. **Drug interactions.** Pentostatin enhances the toxicity of vidarabine. CNS toxicity may be enhanced with the concomitant use of sedative and hypnotic drugs.

Q. **Raltitrexed** (Tomudex)
   1. **Indications.** Investigational in the United States, but used widely elsewhere for advanced colon cancer, breast cancer, and non–small cell lung cancer.
   2. **Pharmacology**
      a. **Mechanisms.** Quinazoline antifolate analog with activity in the S phase of the cell cycle; metabolized intracellularly to higher polyglutamate forms that are 100-fold more potent than the parent compound and are retained within the cell; inhibits the folate-dependent enzyme thymidylate synthetase.
      b. **Metabolism.** Cleared principally by the kidney as unchanged drug.
   3. **Toxicity**
      a. **Dose-limiting.** Disabling fatigue and malaise (about 50% of patients)
      b. **Common.** Diarrhea and/or mucositis (usually during the second cycle of treatment), myelosuppression, transient elevations of serum transaminases and bilirubin; mild nausea and vomiting.
   4. **Administration.** Advise patients to avoid strenuous physical activity and activities that require mental alertness. Supplement dietary folate.
      a. **Supplied** as 10-mL vials containing 1 mg/mL
      b. **Dose modification.** Use with caution with abnormal renal function.
      c. **Dose.** 3 mg/m^2 IV every 3 weeks

R. **6-Thioguanine** (6-TG, 6-thioguanine, aminopurine-6-thiol-hemihydrate)
   1. **Indication.** Acute myelogenous leukemia

2. **Pharmacology**
    a. **Mechanism.** Purine analog with cell cycle–specific activity in the S phase. The drug requires intracellular phosphorylation by HGPRT to the cytotoxic monophosphate form, which is eventually metabolized to the triphosphate metabolite (see *mercaptopurine*). The drug is incorporated extensively into DNA, resulting in miscoding of transcription and DNA replication, and into RNA.
    b. **Metabolism.** Thioguanine is not degraded by xanthine oxidase and, unlike mercaptopurine, can be given in full doses with allopurinol. Clearance of the drug is primarily hepatic, but also renal.
3. **Toxicity**
    a. **Dose-limiting.** Myelosuppression
    b. **Common.** Stomatitis, diarrhea
    c. **Occasional.** Nausea and vomiting, hepatic dysfunction, hepatic veno-occlusive disease; decreased vibratory sensation, unsteady gait.
4. **Administration**
    a. **Supplied** as 40-mg tablets
    b. **Dose modification.** Dose is reduced with impaired liver function.
    c. **Dose** depends on regimen.
S. **Trimetrexate** (Neutrexin, TMTX)
1. **Indications.** Approved for treatment of *Pneumocystis carinii* pneumonia and toxoplasmosis, but investigational in the United States as an anticancer agent; used widely elsewhere for colon cancer, head and neck cancer, and non–small cell lung cancer.
2. **Pharmacology**
    a. **Mechanisms.** Lipid-soluble, quinazoline antifolate analog with activity in the S phase of the cell cycle; does not undergo polyglutamation (in contrast to MTX); inhibits dihydrofolate reductase, *de novo* thymidylate synthesis, and *de novo* purine synthesis.
    b. **Metabolism.** Undergoes extensive metabolism in the liver by the P450 system to inactive forms.
3. **Toxicity**
    a. **Dose-limiting.** Myelosuppression, mucositis
    b. **Common.** Total alopecia (40%), mild nausea and vomiting, headache; maculopapular rash with pruritus and hyperpigmentation that begins at the neck and upper chest, progresses to the trunk and extremities, develops 5 days after treatment and resolves 7 to 10 days after onset.
4. **Administration**
    a. **Supplied** as 5- and 30-mL multidose vials; incompatible with chloride-containing solutions.
    b. **Dose modification.** Use with caution with abnormal renal or liver function or with hypoalbuminemia.
    c. **Dose.** 8 to 12 mg/m^2 IV for 5 consecutive days every 3 to 4 weeks
    d. **Drug interactions** are possible with other drugs metabolized by the liver **P450** system; leucovorin and thymidine rescue the host toxic effects; trimetrexate enhances antitumor activity of 5-FU.
T. **Uracil/Tegafur (UFT).** Uracil and tegafur are combined in a 4:1 molar ratio and provide an oral prodrug form of 5-FU.
1. **Indications.** Same as 5-FU
2. **Pharmacology.** Tegafur is converted to 5-FU by two metabolic pathways, including one that is mediated by liver microsomal P450 enzymes. Uracil reduces the breakdown of 5-FU by serving as a competitive substrate for the catabolic enzyme dihydropyrimidine dehydrogenase. The antitumor activity is mediated by 5-FU (see section II.F). The drug is well absorbed by the GI tract with nearly 100% bioavailability.
3. **Toxicity**
    a. **Dose-limiting.** Diarrhea (similar to that observed with continuous IV infusion of 5-FU)
    b. **Common.** Similar to that of 5-FU, including hand–foot syndrome

4. Administration
   a. **Supplied** as 100-mg capsules
   b. **Dose.** 100 mg/m^2 every 8 hours PO with a large glass of water, within 1 hour of meals for 28 days, then 1 week of rest
   c. **Drug interactions: Warfarin** and **phenytoin** dosing should be carefully monitored when given with UFT; **sorivudine** never should be given with UFT because a metabolite inhibits 5-FU metabolism.

III. ANTITUMOR ANTIBIOTICS
A. General pharmacology of antitumor antibiotics
   1. Antitumor antibiotics generally are drugs derived from microorganisms. They usually are cell cycle–nonspecific agents that are especially useful in slow-growing tumors with low growth fractions.
   2. They act by a variety of mechanisms. Several of these drugs interfere with DNA through intercalation, a reaction whereby the drug inserts itself between DNA base pairs. Intercalation with DNA prevents DNA replication and messenger RNA production, or both. Other drugs have other actions.
B. Actinomycin D (dactinomycin, Cosmegen)
   1. **Indications.** Trophoblastic neoplasms, sarcomas, testicular carcinoma, Wilms' tumor
   2. **Pharmacology**
      a. **Mechanism.** Intercalates between DNA base pairs and prevents synthesis of messenger RNA; inhibits topoisomerase II.
      b. **Metabolism.** Unknown; extensively bound to tissues, resulting in long half-life in plasma and tissue. Excreted in bile and urine as unchanged drug.
   3. **Toxicity**
      a. **Dose-limiting.** Myelosuppression
      b. **Common.** Nausea and vomiting (often worsening after successive daily doses and lasting several hours); alopecia, acne, erythema, desquamation, hyper-pigmentation; radiation-recall reaction. Drug is a vesicant that can cause necrosis if extravasated.
      c. **Occasional.** Stomatitis, cheilitis, glossitis, proctitis, diarrhea; vitamin K antagonism, elevation of LFTs.
      d. **Rare.** Hepatitis, anaphylaxis, hypocalcemia, lethargy
   4. **Administration.** Premedicate patients with antiemetics. Administer through a running intravenous infusion with extravasation precautions.
      a. **Supplied** as 0.5-mg vials
      b. **Dose modification.** Reduce by 50% in the presence of renal or hepatic functional impairment.
      c. **Dose.** 0.25 to 0.45 mg/m^2 IV daily for 5 days every 3 to 4 weeks
C. Bleomycin (Blenoxane)
   1. **Indications.** Lymphomas, squamous cell carcinomas, testicular carcinoma, malignant effusions
   2. **Pharmacology**
      a. **Mechanism.** Binds to DNA, thereby inhibiting synthesis of DNA and, to a lesser extent, RNA and proteins. Causes DNA strand cleavage by free radicals and inhibits DNA repair by a marked inhibition of DNA ligase. Cell cycle G_2-phase specific; also active in late G_1, S, and M phases.
      b. **Metabolism.** Activated by microsomal reduction; bound to tissues but not to plasma protein; extensive degradation by hydrolysis in nearly all tissues. Both free drug and metabolic products are excreted into the urine.
   3. **Toxicity**
      a. **Dose-limiting.** Bleomycin pneumonitis with dyspnea, dry cough, fine moist rales, interstitial radiographic changes, reduced diffusing capacity, hypoxia, and hypocapnia may be lethal. Pulmonary fibrosis and insufficiency occur in 1% of patients receiving cumulative doses of <200 U/m^2 and in 10% of patients receiving larger doses (see Chapter 29, section IV.A, for further details). Advanced age, underlying pulmonary disease, prior or concomitant

radiotherapy to the chest, and prior exposure to bleomycin predispose patients to pulmonary toxicity.

b. Common

(1) Hypersensitivity reactions with mild to severe shaking chills and febrile reactions are common (25% of patients), frequently occurring within 4 to 10 hours of injection. However, they decrease in incidence and severity with subsequent administrations.

(2) Sensitizes tumor and normal tissues to radiation

(3) Dermatologic (50% of patients): hyperpigmentation of skin stretch areas (e.g., knuckles, elbows), hyperpigmented striae; hardening, tenderness, or loss of fingernails; hyperkeratosis of palms and fingers, scleroderma-like changes; skin tenderness, pruritus, urticaria, erythroderma, desquamation, alopecia.

(4) Anorexia, mucositis; a rancid smell ("like old gym socks") beginning about 10 seconds after injection.

c. Occasional. Nausea, vomiting, unusual tastes; mild reversible myelosuppression, Raynaud phenomenon, phlebitis, pain at injection site.

d. Rare

(1) Hepatotoxicity, pleuropericarditis, arteritis

(2) Anaphylaxis-like reaction develops in 1% to 7% of patients who have lymphoma, usually after the first or second dose and particularly if the dose is 25 U/m^2 or more. This idiosyncratic reaction manifests confusion, faintness, fever, chills, and wheezing that can progress to hypotension, renal failure, and cardiovascular collapse.

4. Administration. A 2-U test dose is given before the first treatment, followed by a 1- to 2-hour observation period to reduce the potential for cardiovascular collapse.

a. Supplied as 15-unit (mg) vials

b. Dose modification. The drug should not be given to patients with symptomatic chronic obstructive lung disease. It must be discontinued in patients who have erythroderma (continued treatment may lead to fatal exfoliative dermatitis). The drug must also be discontinued if there are symptoms or signs of interstitial lung disease. Routine pulmonary function tests are generally not helpful; some authorities recommend monitoring carbon monoxide–diffusing capacity. Dosage should be reduced in patients with renal insufficiency.

c. Dose. Avoid cumulative dosage of > 400 U; some physicians limit the total dose to 300 U.

(1) 10 to 20 U/m^2 IM, IV, or SC once or twice weekly (twice-weekly doses > 20 U each are likely to cause serious toxic reactions of the skin), or

(2) 15 to 20 U/m^2 daily for 3 to 7 days by continuous infusion, or

(3) 60 U/m^2 dissolved in 100 mL of normal saline for intracavitary therapy

d. Drug interactions

(1) Phenothiazines enhance the activity of bleomycin by competing with hepatic P450 enzymes.

(2) Radiation therapy and **high oxygen concentrations** enhance pulmonary toxicity.

D. Daunorubicin (daunomycin, rubidomycin, Cerubidine)

1. Indication. Acute leukemias

2. Pharmacology. Anthracycline antitumor antibiotic. Essentially the same as doxorubicin. Active metabolite, which is formed in the liver, is daunomycinol. Cell cycle–nonspecific. Excreted through the hepatobiliary system, with renal clearance accounting for <20% of drug elimination.

3. Toxicity. Same as doxorubicin. Daunorubicin may also cause precipitous fatal cardiomyopathy months after therapy has stopped; incidence becomes unacceptable after a total dose of 500 to 600 mg/m^2 has been given.

4. Administration. Same as doxorubicin. Use extravasation precautions.

a. Supplied as 20-mg vials

b. Dose modification. Same as doxorubicin

  c. Dose. 45 to 60 mg/m^2 IV daily for 3 days

  d. Drug interactions. Cardiotoxic effects are inhibited by dexrazoxane (Zinecard).

E. Doxorubicin (Adriamycin, hydroxydaunorubicin)

 1. Indications. Effective in a large variety of tumors

 2. Pharmacology

  a. Mechanism. Anthracycline antitumor antibiotic. Intercalates between DNA base pairs, forms free radicals, alters cell membranes, induces topoisomerase II–dependent DNA damage, inhibits preribosomal DNA and RNA. Cell cycle–phase nonspecific.

  b. Metabolism. About 70% of the drug is bound to plasma proteins. Rapidly metabolized by the liver to other compounds, some of which are cytotoxic (including the active metabolite doxorubicinol). The release rate from tissue binding sites is slow compared with the capacity of the liver for metabolism; this results in relatively prolonged plasma levels of drug and metabolites.

  c. Excretion. Metabolites and free drug are extensively excreted in the bile; however, known elimination accounts for only half of the drug. The rate of drug elimination and its toxicity thus is rarely limited by liver function. Some chromogens are excreted through the kidney, occasionally imparting a red tinge to the urine.

 3. Toxicity

  a. Dose-limiting

   (1) Myelosuppression, particularly leukopenia

   (2) Cardiomyopathy with congestive heart failure, which may become refractory (see Chapter 29, section VI.D, for further details). Monitor the left ventricular ejection fraction with radionuclide angiography before initiation of treatment, particularly when the cumulative dose exceeds 300 mg/m^2, and periodically thereafter. Risks and benefits should be considered at total cumulative doses of 550 mg/m^2 (400 mg/m^2 with a history of mediastinal irradiation) or for electrocardiographic changes (voltage reduction, significant arrhythmias, ST-T wave changes). Dexrazoxane (see section X.B), a cardioprotectant, can be considered when the cumulative dose exceeds 300 mg/m^2.

  b. Common

   (1) Alopecia (nearly 100% of patients when administered as a bolus every 3 to 4 weeks, but minimal when the dose is divided and given weekly); nausea and vomiting (mild to severe); stomatitis.

   (2) Doxorubicin is a vesicant; extravasation of the drug results in severe ulceration and necrosis.

   (3) Previously irradiated skin sites may become erythematous and desquamate when the drug is started; this *radiation-recall reaction* can occur years after radiation was given.

  c. Occasional. Diarrhea; hyperpigmentation of nail beds and dermal creases, facial flush, flush along injected vein, skin rash; conjunctivitis, lacrimation; red-colored urine.

  d. Rare. Activation of fibrinolysis, muscle weakness, fever, chills, anaphylaxis

 4. Administration. The drug must be slowly pushed through a running intravenous line using extravasation precautions or continuously infused through a central venous line.

  a. Supplied as 10-, 20-, 50-, 100-, and 150-mg vials

  b. Dose modification. Doxorubicin should not be given to patients with congestive heart failure from any cause. The package insert recommends reduction of dose by 50% for serum bilirubin of 1.2 to 3.0 mg/dL and by 75% for bilirubin of 3 to 5 mg/dL (but see section III.E.2.c).

  c. Dose. 50 to 75 mg/m^2 IV bolus every 3 to 4 weeks or 10 to 20 mg/m^2 IV weekly

  d. Drug interactions

   (1) Dexrazoxane (Zinecard) inhibits doxorubicin's cardiotoxic effects.

   (2) Herceptin and **mitomycin C** increase cardiotoxicity.

(3) Phenobarbital and **phenytoin** increase the plasma clearance of doxorubicin.

(4) 6-MP increases the risk of hepatotoxicity.

F. Doxorubicin, liposomal (Doxil)

1. **Indications.** Kaposi's sarcoma with acquired immunodeficiency syndrome (AIDS), ovarian carcinoma, myeloma

2. **Pharmacology.** Doxorubicin is encapsulated in long-circulating liposomes (microscopic vesicles composed of a phospholipid bilayer). For mechanisms and metabolism, see *doxorubicin*. The plasma clearance is slower than standard doxorubicin.

3. **Toxicity**
   a. **Dose-limiting.** Hematosuppression
   b. **Common.** Fatigue; mucositis, diarrhea, nausea, vomiting; alopecia; infusion reactions (chills, facial swelling, headache, hypotension, shortness of breath), which resolve on interruption of infusion and which do not preclude continued treatment.
   c. **Occasional.** Cardiomyopathy, pain at injection site, radiation-recall reaction; palmar–plantar erythrodysesthesia (ulceration, erythema, and desquamation on the hands and feet with pain and inflammation); red-orange discoloration of urine.
   d. **Rare.** Allergic reaction, hyperglycemia, jaundice, optic neuropathy

4. **Administration**
   a. **Supplied** as 20-mg vials
   b. **Dose modification.** Same as for doxorubicin
   c. **Dose**
      (1) Kaposi's sarcoma in AIDS: 20 mg/m^2 IV over 30 minutes every 2 or 3 weeks
      (2) Ovarian carcinoma: 40 to 50 mg/m^2 IV over 1 to 2 hours every 4 weeks

G. Epirubicin (Ellence) is the 4′-epimer of doxorubicin and is a semisynthetic derivative of daunorubicin. An *epimer* is one of a pair of isomers that differ only in the position of the H- and OH- attached to one asymmetric carbon atom.

1. **Indication.** Breast and gastric cancers

2. **Pharmacology.** Anthracycline antitumor antibiotic. For mechanisms and metabolism, see *doxorubicin*.

3. **Toxicity.** Same as doxorubicin, but with more nausea and vomiting. The risk of developing cardiomyopathy increases substantially after a total dose of 900 mg/m^2.

4. **Administration.** Intravenously over 5 minutes using extravasation precautions
   a. **Supplied as** 50- and 200-mg vials
   b. **Dose modification.** Same as for doxorubicin
   c. **Dose.** 100 to 120 mg/m^2 IV every 3 weeks in combination chemotherapy regimens
   d. **Drug interactions. Cimetidine** increases plasma levels of epirubicin and should be discontinued upon starting epirubicin.

H. Idarubicin (4-demethoxydaunorubicin, Idamycin)

1. **Indication.** Acute leukemia

2. **Pharmacology.** Anthracycline antitumor antibiotic; an analog of daunorubicin. More lipophilic and better cell uptake than other anthracycline antibiotics; otherwise similar to doxorubicin. The active metabolite is 13-epirubicinol.

3. **Toxicity.** Similar to doxorubicin. Myelosuppression is expected. Although idarubicin is less cardiotoxic than doxorubicin and daunorubicin, the same monitoring criteria apply.

4. **Administration.** Intravenously over 15 minutes using extravasation precautions.
   a. **Supplied** as 5- and 10-mg vials
   b. **Dose modification.** Same as doxorubicin
   c. **Dose.** 12 mg/m^2 IV daily for 3 days with induction therapy

I. Mithramycin (plicamycin, Mithracin)
  1. Indication. Refractory hypercalcemia
  2. Pharmacology
    a. Mechanism. Osteoclast inhibitor, antitumor antibiotic. Cytotoxicity probably related to DNA intercalation and adlineation; inhibits DNA-dependent RNA synthesis without affecting DNA synthesis.
    b. Metabolism. Unknown, eliminated in urine (40%)
  3. Toxicity. Renal and hepatic damage are rare with dosage schedules used for hypercalcemia.
    a. Dose-limiting. Thrombocytopenia; coagulation defects may occur in the absence of thrombocytopenia and result in a severe hemorrhagic diathesis (usually with frequent doses).
    b. Common. Nausea, vomiting; hypocalcemia, hypophosphatemia, hypokalemia, hypomagnesemia, rebound hypercalcemia; abnormal LFTs (including prothrombin time); azotemia; skin and soft-tissue necrosis if extravasated.
    c. Occasional. Leukopenia, anemia; stomatitis, diarrhea; hyperpigmentation, acneiform rash; headache, dizziness, drowsiness, nervousness.
    d. Rare. Toxic epidermal necrolysis, fever, lethargy, periorbital pallor
  4. Administration. A running intravenous line using extravasation precautions
    a. Supplied as 2.5-mg vials
    b. Dose modification. Mithramycin must be given cautiously to patients with hepatic or kidney dysfunction.
    c. Dose for hypercalcemia. 15 to 25 mcg (0.025 mg)/kg IV every 3 to 7 days
J. Mitomycin (mitomycin C, Mutamycin)
  1. Indications. A variety of carcinomas
  2. Pharmacology
    a. Mechanism. Antitumor antibiotic. After intracellular activation, functions as an alkylating agent; DNA cross-linking, DNA depolymerization, and free-radical formation.
    b. Metabolism. Metabolized predominantly in the liver by the P450 system and DT-diaphorase. Excreted mainly through the hepatobiliary system.
  3. Toxicity
    a. Dose-limiting. Cumulative myelosuppression, which may be severe and prolonged (particularly thrombocytopenia)
    b. Common. Mild nausea and vomiting, anorexia; a vesicant drug that can cause necrosis if injected subcutaneously (skin erythema and ulceration can occur weeks to months after administration and may appear at a site distant from the site of injection).
    c. Occasional. Alopecia, stomatitis, skin rashes, photosensitivity, pain at site of injection, phlebitis; hemolytic-uremic–like syndrome.
    d. Rare. Hepatic and renal (cumulative) dysfunction, paresthesias, blurred vision, fever; acute interstitial pneumonitis (especially when given with vinblastine or vindesine).
  4. Administration. Administer through a running intravenous infusion using extravasation precautions
    a. Supplied as 5-, 20-, and 40-mg vials
    b. Dose modification. Reduce dose by 50% to 75% for patients who were previously treated with extensive irradiation or who developed a white blood cell count of <2,000/mcL with prior doses of mitomycin. Also reduce dose for liver dysfunction.
    c. Dose
      (1) Single agent: 10 to 20 mg/m^2 IV every 6 to 8 weeks, or
      (2) In combination: 5 to 10 mg/m^2 IV every 5 weeks
K. Mitoxantrone (Novantrone, dihydroxyanthracenedione)
  1. Indications. Breast and prostate cancer, lymphoma, acute leukemia
  2. Pharmacology. Mitoxantrone is in the anthracenedione class of compounds, which are analogs to the anthracyclines. Its mechanism of action and routes of metabolism are similar but not identical to doxorubicin.

a. **Mechanism.** DNA intercalation, single- and double-strand DNA breakage, inhibition of topoisomerase II

b. **Metabolism.** Metabolized by the liver's P450 system; <1% of the drug is excreted in the urine.

3. **Toxicity.** Compared with the anthracyclines, mitoxantrone is associated with less cardiotoxicity, less nausea and vomiting, and decreased potential for extravasation injury.

a. **Dose-limiting.** Myelosuppression

b. **Common.** Mild nausea and vomiting, mucositis; alopecia (usually mild); blue discoloration of urine, sclerae, fingernails, and over venous site of injection that may last 48 hours.

c. **Occasional.** Cardiomyopathy (most well defined for patients who have previously received doxorubicin); appears to be less cardiotoxic than doxorubicin. Pruritus, LFT abnormalities, allergic reactions.

d. **Rare.** Jaundice, seizures, pulmonary toxicity

4. **Administration** as a 30-minute infusion; rarely causes extravasation injury if infiltrated.

a. **Supplied** as 20-, 25-, and 30-mg vials

b. **Dose modification.** Hematologic

c. **Dose.** 10 to 12 mg/m^2 IV given every 3 weeks for solid tumors

IV. MITOTIC SPINDLE AGENTS

A. **General pharmacology of mitotic spindle agents.** Mitotic spindle inhibitors are classically represented by vincristine and vinblastine. These drugs bind to microtubular proteins, thus inhibiting microtubule assembly (M phase of the cell cycle) and resulting in dissolution of the mitotic spindle structure. Taxanes (paclitaxel and docetaxel) not only bind to microtubules but also promote microtubule assembly and resistance to depolymerization, resulting in the production of nonfunctional microtubules.

B. **Paclitaxel** (Taxol)

1. **Indications.** Carcinomas of the breast, ovary, lung, esophagus, and other sites; AIDS-associated Kaposi's sarcoma.

2. **Pharmacology.** Isolated from the bark of the Pacific yew tree, *Taxus brevifolia*

a. **Mechanism.** Plant alkaloid (antimicrotubule agent); see section IV.A.

b. **Metabolism.** Extensively metabolized by the hepatic P450 microsomal system. More than 75% of the drug is excreted in the feces.

3. **Toxicity**

a. **Dose-limiting**

(1) **Neutropenia,** particularly in patients who were previously heavily treated or who receive cisplatin just before paclitaxel

(2) **Hypersensitivity** (3%) is manifested by cutaneous flushing, hypotension, bronchospasm, urticaria, diaphoresis, pain, or angioedema. Reactions usually develop within 20 minutes of starting the treatment; 90% of hypersensitivity reactions develop after the first or second dose.

(3) **Peripheral neuropathy,** particularly in the higher dosage schedules and in patients with concomitant etiologies for peripheral neuropathy. Neurotoxicity occurs less frequently when infused over 24 hours (5%) than when infused over 3 hours (25%). The distribution typically is "stocking-glove" and consists of dysesthesias, paresthesias, and loss of proprioception.

b. **Common.** Alopecia (usually total and sudden, within 3 weeks of treatment); thrombocytopenia (usually not severe); transient arthralgias and myalgias within 3 days of treatment (ameliorated by nonsteroidal anti-inflammatory agents and prednisone), transient bradycardia (usually asymptomatic).

c. **Occasional.** Nausea, vomiting, taste changes, mucositis (cumulative), diarrhea; atrioventricular conduction defects, ventricular tachycardia, cardiac angina; necrosis when extravasated; intoxication when infused over 1 hour (because of high alcohol content in the preparation); onycholysis.

   d. Rare. Paralytic ileus, generalized weakness, seizures; myocardial infarction.

4. **Administration.** Paclitaxel should be given before cisplatin in combination regimens in which both are administered. Cardiac monitoring is recommended for patients with a history of cardiac disease. Use with caution in patients who have a history of myocardial infarction within the previous 6 months or who are on medications known to alter cardiac conduction. Administer with extravasation precautions.

   a. Supplied as 30- and 100-mg vials formulated in polyoxyethylated castor oil (Cremophor EL) and alcohol

   b. Dose modification. Hematologic. Use with caution with abnormal liver function, diabetes mellitus, or prior therapy with neurotoxic drugs, such as cisplatin

   c. Dose

   (1) **Premedications**: Dexamethasone, 20 mg PO or IV is given 12, 6, and 0.5 hours before paclitaxel; diphenhydramine, 50 mg IV, and ranitidine, 50 mg IV, given 30 minutes before administering paclitaxel.

   (2) **Every 3 to 4 weeks:** 135 to 175 mg/m^2 infused over 3 to 24 hours

   (3) **Weekly:** 80 to 100 mg/m^2 for 3 weeks with 1 week rest

   d. Drug interactions

   (1) **Phenobarbital, phenytoin,** and other drugs that the liver's cytochrome P450 CYP3A4 enzyme may affect paclitaxel metabolism (see section VI.A).

   (2) **Radiation therapy.** Paclitaxel is a radiosensitizing agent.

   (3) **Carboplatin, cisplatin, and cyclophosphamide.** Myelosuppression is greater when these compounds are administered before paclitaxel.

C. **Paclitaxel, protein-bound** (Abraxane)

1. **Indications.** Metastatic breast cancer

2. **Pharmacology.** This injectable suspension contains paclitaxel protein-bound particles.

   a. Mechanisms. See *paclitaxel*

   b. Metabolism. See *paclitaxel*

3. **Toxicity**

   a. Dose-limiting. Neutropenia

   b. Common. Hematosuppression, sensory neuropathy, arthralgias/myalgia (usually transient), gastrointestinal disturbances, alopecia, fatigue

   c. Occasional. Abnormal liver function tests, fluid retention

4. **Administration.** Premedication with corticosteroids to prevent hypersensitivity reactions is not required for Abraxane.

   a. Supplied as vials containing 100-mg of paclitaxel and 900 mg of albumin

   b. Dose modification. For neutropenia and sensory neuropathy

   c. Dose. 260 mg/m^2 IV over 30 minutes every 3 weeks

D. **Docetaxel** (Taxotere)

1. **Indications.** Breast cancer after ineffectiveness of anthracycline-based treatment

2. **Pharmacology.** The drug is prepared by semisynthesis beginning with a precursor extracted from the needles of the European yew tree.

   a. Mechanisms. Inhibitor of microtubular depolymerization (see section IV.A). The binding of docetaxel to microtubules does not alter the number of protofilaments in the bound microtubules, which differs from most spindle poisons currently in clinical use.

   b. Metabolism. Extensively metabolized by the hepatic P450 microsomal system. More than 75% is excreted in feces and a small percentage in urine.

3. **Toxicity**

   a. Dose-limiting. Myelosuppression; severe fluid retention.

   b. Common. Alopecia (80% except with the weekly schedule), maculopapular rash and dry itchy skin, discoloration of finger nails; mucositis, diarrhea; fatigue, fever.

  c. Occasional
   (1) Severe hypersensitivity reactions (<5%) despite premedications.
   (2) Fluid retention that is cumulative in incidence and severity (especially after a cumulative dose of 705 mg/m^2) is reversible (usually within 8 months); the fluid retention usually affects the lower extremities but can also result in ascites or pleural or pericardial effusions.
   (3) GI upset, severe nail reactions; hypotension; transiently elevated liver function tests.
   (4) Peripheral neuropathy, which is less common than with paclitaxel, is mainly sensory, but motor or autonomic neuropathy and CNS effects are also seen.
  d. Rare. Cardiac events
 4. Administration
  a. Supplied as 20- and 80-mg vials in polysorbate 80, which is less allergenic than Cremophor EL, which is used for paclitaxel
  b. Dose modification. Patients with elevated serum bilirubin or significantly elevated liver enzymes should generally not receive docetaxel.
  c. Dose
   (1) 60 to 100 mg/m^2 IV over 1 hour every 3 weeks; give dexamethasone, 4 mg PO b.i.d. on the day before, the day of, and the day after docetaxel administration to reduce the incidence and severity of fluid retention and hypersensitivity reactions.
   (2) 35 mg/m^2 weekly for 3 weeks of a 4-week cycle (the weekly schedule is associated with less hematologic toxicity and no hair loss; it requires a maximum of 4 mg dexamethasone on the morning and evening of dosing)
  d. Drug interactions
   (1) Phenobarbital, phenytoin, and other drugs that the liver's cytochrome P450 CYP3A4 enzyme may affect docetaxel metabolism (see section VI.A).
   (2) Radiation therapy. Docetaxel is a radiosensitizing agent.
E. Estramustine (Emcyt, Estracyte)
 1. Indication. Progressive prostate cancer
 2. Pharmacology. Structurally, estramustine is a combination of estradiol phosphate and nornitrogen mustard.
  a. Mechanism. Cell cycle–specific agent with activity in the mitosis (M) phase by binding to microtubule-associated proteins. Although initially designed as an alkylating agent, it has no alkylating activity.
  b. Metabolism. Rapidly dephosphorylated in GI tract and metabolized primarily in the liver. About 20% of the drug is excreted in the urine.
 3. Toxicity. Similar to estrogens
  a. Dose limiting. Thromboembolism
  b. Common. Diarrhea; nausea and vomiting (usually mild); skin rash. Gynecomastia in up to 50% of patients (can be prevented by prophylactic irradiation).
  c. Rare. Myelosuppression, cardiovascular complications
 4. Administration. Contraindicated in patients with active thrombophlebitis or thromboembolic disorders
  a. Supplied as 140-mg capsules
  b. Dose. 600 mg/m^2/day in three divided doses; taken with water 1 hour before meals or 2 hours after meals. Calcium-rich foods may impair drug absorption.
F. Ixabepilone (Ixempra)
 1. Indications. Metastatic breast cancer that is refractory to anthracyclines, taxanes, and capecitabine
 2. Pharmacology. The drug is an epothilone B analog.
  a. Mechanisms. Binds to the β-tubulin subunit of the microtubule, thus arresting the cell cycle at the G$_2$/M phase and inducing apoptosis.
  b. Metabolism. Extensive hepatic metabolism via CYP3A4 into inactive metabolites. Excreted the feces and urine, <10% as unchanged drug.

3. **Toxicity.** Cognitive impairment (due to ethanol content of diluent) or hypersensitivity reactions (related to the Cremophor in the diluent) may occur.
    a. **Dose-limiting.** Myelosuppression (particularly neutropenia) and peripheral neuropathy
    b. **Common.** Alopecia, headache, neutropenia, fatigue, GI disturbance, myalgia/arthralgia
    c. **Occasional.** Edema, fever, dizziness, palmar–plantar dysesthesia (hand–foot syndrome), nail disorders, hyperpigmentation, motor neuropathy, anemia, increased lacrimation, dyspnea
4. **Administration.** Premedicate with an H_1-antagonist drug (e.g., diphenhydramine, 50 mg) and an oral H_2-antagonist (e.g., ranitidine, 150–300 mg). Premedicate with corticosteroids for those with hypersensitivity reactions.
    a. **Supplied** as 15 mg and 45 mg as a powder (diluent contains ethanol and purified polyoxyethylated castor oil [Cremophor® EL])
    b. **Dose modification.** With hepatic dysfunction, reduce dosage when given as monotherapy and *do not use* in combination with capecitabine. Reduce dose for neuropathy or for severe or prolonged neutropenia or thrombocytopenia.
    c. **Dose.** 40 mg/m^2 IV over 3 hours every 3 weeks (maximum 88 mg)
    d. **Drug interactions.** CYP3A4 inducers and inhibitors may decrease or increase the levels or effects of ixabepilone, respectively (see VI.A). If concurrent use of a strong CYP3A4 inhibitor cannot be avoided, reduce dosage to 20 mg/m^2; if the inhibitor is discontinued, allow about 1 week before the ixabepilone dose is increased. Avoid St. John's wort and grape juice.

G. **Vinblastine** (Velban)
1. **Indications.** Lymphomas, testicular carcinoma
2. **Pharmacology**
    a. **Mechanism.** Periwinkle plant alkaloid; see section IV.A. Binds to microtubular proteins. Inhibits RNA synthesis by affecting DNA-dependent RNA polymerases. Cell cycle–phase specific; it arrests cells at the G_2-phase and M-phase interface.
    b. **Metabolism.** Highly bound to plasma proteins and to formed blood elements, especially platelets. Metabolized by the hepatic P450 microsomal system to active and inactive metabolites. Predominantly excreted in bile. Minimal free drug is recovered in urine.
3. **Toxicity**
    a. **Dose-limiting.** Neutropenia
    b. **Common.** Cramps or severe pain in jaw, pharynx, back, or limbs after injection; local vesicant if extravasated.
    c. **Occasional.** Thrombocytopenia, anemia
    d. **Rare.** Nausea, vomiting, diarrhea, mucositis, abdominal cramps, GI hemorrhage; acute interstitial pneumonitis (especially when administered with mitomycin C); ischemic cardiotoxicity.
4. **Administration.** Administered by rapid infusion through the tubing of a running intravenous line with extravasation precautions
    a. **Supplied** as 10-mg vials
    b. **Dose modification.** Decrease dose by 50% for patients with serum bilirubin >3.0 mg/dL.
    c. **Dose.** 5 mg/m^2 IV every 1 or 2 weeks
    d. **Drug interactions**
        (1) Phenobarbital, calcium channel blockers, cimetidine, metoclopramide, and other drugs that inhibit the liver's P450 system (see Section VI.A) may lead to increased production of metabolites. Vinblastine should be used cautiously in patients receiving these medications.
        (2) **Phenytoin** levels are decreased with vinblastine treatment.

H. **Vincristine** (Oncovin, Vcr)
1. **Indications.** A wide variety of malignancies
2. **Pharmacology**
    a. **Mechanism.** Same as vinblastine
    b. **Metabolism.** Same as vinblastine

3. **Toxicity**
   a. **A dose-dependent peripheral neuropathy** universally develops. Cranial nerves and the autonomic system may also be involved. The neuropathies usually reverse within several months. Jaw, throat, or anterior thigh pain occurring within hours of injection disappears within days and usually does not recur.
      (1) **Dose-limiting.** Severe paresthesias, ataxia, foot-drop (slapping gait), muscle-wasting cranial nerve palsies, paralytic ileus, obstipation, abdominal pain, optic atrophy, cortical blindness, seizures
      (2) **Not dose-limiting.** Mild hypoesthesia, mild paresthesias, transient jaw pain (and similar syndromes), loss of deep tendon reflexes
   b. **Common.** Tissue necrosis if extravasated, alopecia (20% to 40%)
   c. **Occasional.** Mild leukopenia (does not have significant effect on erythrocytes or platelets); rash, SIADH
   d. **Rare.** Nausea, vomiting, pancreatitis; fever.
4. **Administration.** Patients receiving Vcr should be given bulk laxatives routinely. Administered by rapid infusion using extravasation precautions.
   a. **Supplied** as 1-, 2-, and 5- mg vials
   b. **Dose modification.** Hepatic dysfunction; same as for vinblastine.
   c. **Dose.** 1.0 to 1.4 mg/m^2 IV every 1 to 4 weeks (often limited to 2 mg per dose in adults); continuous infusion regimens involve 0.4 to 0.5 mg/day for 4 days.
   d. **Drug interactions**
      (1) Phenobarbital, calcium channel blockers, cimetidine, metoclopramide, and other drugs that inhibit the liver's P450 system (see Section VI.A) may lead to increased production of metabolites. Vcr should be used cautiously in patients receiving these medications.
      (2) **Phenytoin** and **digoxin** blood levels are decreased with Vcr treatment.
      (3) **Filgastrim** (Neupogen), when used concurrently with Vcr, may result in severe atypical neuropathy.
      (4) Vcr should be given 12 to 24 hours before **L-asparaginase** because that drug inhibits Vcr clearance.

I. **Vindesine** (Eldisine, desacetylvinblastine amide sulfate)
   1. **Indications.** Experimental for lung cancer, leukemias, and others
   2. **Pharmacology.** Same as vinblastine
   3. **Toxicity.** Same as vinblastine, but alopecia is more common with vindesine. Neurotoxicity is same as for vincristine but is generally less severe.
   4. **Administration.** Same as vinblastine
      a. **Supplied** as 10-mg vials
      b. **Dose modification.** Necessary for patients with hepatic dysfunction; same as for vinblastine.
      c. **Dose.** 3 to 4 mg/m^2 IV every 7 to 14 days

J. **Vinorelbine** (Navelbine)
   1. **Indications.** Non–small cell lung cancer, ovarian cancer, and breast cancer
   2. **Pharmacology.** A semisynthetic alkaloid derived from vinblastine
      a. **Mechanisms.** Inhibits tubular polymerization, disrupting formation of tubules during mitosis (see section IV.A)
      b. **Metabolism.** The majority of the drug is metabolized in the liver by the cytochrome P450 microsomal system. Drug and metabolites are excreted in bile.
   3. **Toxicity**
      a. **Dose-limiting.** Myelosuppression, especially neutropenia
      b. **Common.** Fatigue; nausea, vomiting, constipation, diarrhea.
      c. **Occasional.** Stomatitis; allergic-type pulmonary reactions; peripheral neuropathy; transient abnormalities in LFTs.
      d. **Rare.** Thrombocytopenia; hemorrhagic cystitis.
   4. **Administration.** Same as vinblastine
      a. **Supplied** as 10- and 50-mg vials
      b. **Dose modification.** Reduce dose for hyperbilirubinemia or neutropenia

    c. Dose. 15 to 30 mg/m^2 IV weekly

    d. Drug interactions

      (1) Phenobarbital, calcium channel blockers, cimetidine, metoclopramide, and other drugs that inhibit the liver's P450 system (see Section VI.A) may lead to increased production of metabolites. Vinorelbine should be used cautiously in patients receiving these medications.

      (2) Phenytoin blood levels are decreased with Vcr treatment.

      (3) Acute pulmonary reactions have been reported when given with **mitomycin**.

V. TOPOISOMERASE INHIBITORS

A. General pharmacology of topoisomerase inhibitors. DNA is attached at regular intervals to the nuclear matrix at sites called *domains,* which are wound together with their paired DNA molecules. DNA topoisomerases are enzymes that alter DNA topology by causing and resealing DNA strand breaks. Topoisomerases bind to DNA domains, forming a "cleavable complex," which allows DNA to unwind in preparation for cell division. Topoisomerase I relaxes supercoiled DNA for a variety of crucial cellular processes. Topoisomerase II catalyzes the double-stranded breaking and resealing of DNA, thereby allowing the passage of one double helical segment of DNA through another. They relax superhelical turns, interconvert knotted rings, and intertwist complementary viral sequences into DNA. Topoisomerases are essential for such events as transcription, replication, and mitosis.

    Of all the topoisomerases, groups I and II are the targets of cytotoxic agents. Camptothecin derivatives (irinotecan, topotecan) exert their cytotoxic effect by inhibiting topoisomerase I. Epipodophyllotoxin derivatives (etoposide, teniposide) inhibit topoisomerase II. Drugs from other classes (e.g., amsacrine and the anthracyclines) also inhibit topoisomerases as part of their mechanism of action. Inhibition of topoisomerase interferes with transcription and replication by causing DNA damage, inhibition of DNA replication, failure to repair strand breaks, and, then, cell death.

B. Etoposide (VP-16, VePesid; oral form is etoposide phosphate [Etopophos])

    1. Indications. Testicular carcinoma, lung cancer, lymphoma, and other malignancies

    2. Pharmacology. An epipodophyllotoxin extracted from the *Podophyllum peltatum* mandrake plant

      a. Mechanisms. A topoisomerase II inhibitor (see section V.A); cell cycle–phase specific at G$_2$, late S, and M phases.

      b. Metabolism. Highly bound to plasma proteins (mainly albumin); decreased albumin levels result in potentially greater host toxicity. Metabolized by the liver via glucuronidation to less active metabolites. Excreted in urine (40%) as intact and degraded drug; excretion of the remaining 60% is uncertain.

    3. Toxicity

      a. Dose-limiting. Myelosuppression

      b. Common. Nausea and vomiting (with oral dosing, but uncommon with intravenous dosing); alopecia (usually mild); hypotension if rapidly infused; metallic taste during drug infusion.

      c. Occasional. Anemia, thrombocytopenia, pain at injection site, phlebitis, abnormal LFTs

      d. Rare. Stomatitis, dysphagia, diarrhea, constipation, parotitis, rash, radiation-recall reaction, hyperpigmentation; anaphylaxis, transient hypertension, arrhythmias; somnolence, vertigo, transient cortical blindness; peripheral neuropathy.

    4. Administration. Administer slowly over at least 30 minutes when given intravenously to avoid hypotension.

      a. Supplied as 50-mg capsules and 100-mg vials

      b. Dose modification. Administer with caution in the presence of renal dysfunction; reduce doses by 25% or 50% for creatinine clearance levels of <50 mL/minute and <10 mL/minute, respectively. Dose reduction is also recommended for patients with abnormal liver function.

    c. Dose
- **(1)** 50 mg/m^2 PO daily for 21 days, or
- **(2)** 100 mg/m^2 IV daily for 3 to 5 days, depending on the regimen

    d. Drug interactions
- **(1) Calcium-channel antagonists,** such as verapamil, or methotrexate may increase cytotoxicity of etoposide.
- **(2)** The prothrombin time may be prolonged by etoposide in patients taking **warfarin**.

C. Irinotecan (Camptosar, CPT-11)
  1. Indications. Colorectal cancer, lung cancer
  2. Pharmacology. A water-soluble analog of camptothecin that is a relatively inactive prodrug, which is converted to the active agent
    a. Mechanisms. Inhibits topoisomerase I; see section V.A; cell cycle–phase specific.
    b. Metabolism. Conversion to the active metabolite, SN-38, occurs mainly in the liver, but also in the plasma and intestinal mucosa. The major route of elimination is the bile and feces, with renal clearance playing only a minor role.

      The active form of the drug is metabolized by the polymorphic enzyme UGT1A1. Approximately 10% of the North American population is homozygous for the UGT1A1*28 allele and have reduced UGT1A1 activity and are at increased risk of experiencing grade 4 neutropenia.

  3. Toxicity
    a. Dose-limiting. Profuse diarrhea (especially in patients 65 years of age and older) and myelosuppression
    b. Common. Neutropenia; mild nausea, vomiting, abdominal cramps; flushing during administration; mild alopecia.
    c. Occasional. LFT abnormalities, headache, fever, dyspnea

  4. Administration. Administer as a 90-minute infusion once weekly for 4 weeks in 6-week cycles. If diarrhea, abdominal cramps, or diaphoresis (mostly cholinergic in nature) develops during the infusion of the drug, administer atropine, 0.25 to 1.0 mg IV. For the first poorly formed stool preceding delayed diarrhea, administer loperamide (Imodium), 4 mg PO, then 2 mg every 2 hours (4 mg PO every 4 hours at night) until the patient is free of diarrhea for 12 hours.
    a. Supplied as 100-mg vials
    b. Dose modification. Use with caution for hepatic insufficiency. A diagnostic test is available to detect UGT1A1*1 (normal) and the UGT1A1*28 (variant) alleles in peripheral blood; a lower starting dose is recommended for patients with the variant allele.
    c. Dose. Start at 125 mg/m^2 IV weekly for 4 weeks followed by a 2-week rest.

D. Teniposide (VM-26, Vumon)
  1. Indication. Acute lymphoblastic leukemia
  2. Pharmacology
    a. Mechanism. Plant alkaloid; topoisomerase II inhibitor (see section V.A).
    b. Metabolism. Virtually all of the drug is bound to protein. Systemic metabolism is significant, but metabolites have not been identified. Renal excretion is only a small fraction of its clearance.

  3. Toxicity
    a. Dose-limiting. Neutropenia
    b. Common. Thrombocytopenia, hypotension with too rapid an infusion
    c. Occasional. Nausea and vomiting, alopecia, abnormal LFTs, phlebitis
    d. Rare. Diarrhea, stomatitis; rash, anaphylaxis; azotemia; fever; paresthesias, seizures.

  4. Administration. The drug is administered by slow intravenous infusion over at least 30 minutes.
    a. Supplied as 50-mg vials
    b. Dose. 150 to 250 mg/m^2 once or twice weekly
    c. Drug interactions. Anticonvulsants increase clearance of teniposide.

E. Topotecan (Hycamtin)
  1. **Indications.** Ovarian cancer after failure to respond to previous (cisplatin-based) therapies; cervical cancer in combination with cisplatin; relapsed small cell lung cancer.
  2. **Pharmacology**
     a. **Mechanisms.** A derivative of camptothecin, it inhibits topoisomerase I activity; see section V.A; cell cycle–phase specific. It exerts its cytotoxic effect by blocking DNA repair.
     b. **Metabolism.** Rapid conversion in plasma to the active lactone form. About 60% of the drug is excreted in urine. Metabolism in the liver appears to be minimal and is mediated by the microsomal P450 system.
  3. **Toxicity**
     a. **Dose-limiting.** Myelosuppression
     b. **Common.** Nausea and vomiting; diarrhea, constipation, abdominal pain; alopecia; headache, fatigue, fever; arthralgias and myalgias.
     c. **Occasional.** Transient elevation of LFTs; paresthesia; rash; microscopic hematuria (30%).
  4. **Administration.** The drug is a mild vesicant, and a free-flowing IV site is necessary.
     a. **Supplied** as 4-mg vials and 0.25- and 1-mg capsules
     b. **Dose modification.** None for impaired hepatic function. Reduce dosage by 50% for creatinine clearance levels of 20 to 40 mL/minute.
     c. **Dose.** Usual dose is 1.25 to 1.50 mg/m^2 IV over 30 minutes for 5 consecutive days every 3 weeks; 2.3 mg/m^2 PO for 5 days of 21-day cycle for small cell lung cancer.

VI. TYROSINE KINASES (TK) INHIBITORS
A. CYP3A4 inhibitors and inducers
  1. **Cytochrome P450 (CYP)** families of more than 100 enzymes are located on the endoplasmic reticulum. Although present in all tissues, the highest concentrations are found in the liver and small intestine. These enzymes detoxify ingested substances, such as drugs. The four major enzyme families involved in the metabolism of drugs are CYP1, CYP2, CYP3, and CYP4.
  2. **CYP3A** is a subfamily of the CYP3 enzymes; they are the most abundant cytochrome enzymes in humans, accounting for 30% of the cytochrome enzymes in the liver and 70% of those in the gut. CYP3A3 and CYP3A4 are nearly identical. The relative contribution to drug metabolism in decreasing order of magnitude is CYP3A4 (50%), CYP2D6 (25%), and CYP2C8/9 (15%).

  Many chemotherapeutic agents are metabolized by CYP3A4, particularly among the tyrosine kinase inhibitors. Other related hepatic enzymes also may be operative. Concomitantly prescribed drugs, particularly antimicrobial agents and antiseizure medications, can inhibit or induce CYP3A4 and related enzymes in the liver. Drugs that inhibit CYP3A4 can result in higher levels of the chemotherapeutic agent in the plasma; conversely, drugs that induce CYP3A4 can result in lower levels of the drug in the plasma and indicate higher prescribed dosages of the anticancer drug.
  3. **Inhibitors of CYP3A4** (resulting in higher-than-expected plasma levels of the chemotherapeutic agent and possibly indicating a decrease in dosage):
     a. **Antifungal agents:** Ketoconazole (Nizoral), clotrimazole (Mycelex), fluconazole (Diflucan), itraconazole (Sporanox), voriconazole (Vfend)
     b. **Antibiotics:** Clarithromycin (Biaxin), erythromycin, metronidazole (Flagyl), norfloxacin (Noroxin), telithromycin (Ketek)
     c. **Protease inhibitors:** Atazanavir (Reyataz), delavirdine (Rescriptor), indinavir (Crixivan), nefazodone (Serzone), nelfinavir (Viracept), ritonavir (Norvir), saquinavir (Fortovase)
     d. **Gastrointestinal agents:** Cimetidine (Tagamet), omeprazole (Prilosec)
     e. **Cardiovascular agents:** Diltiazem (Cardizem), nifedipine (Procardia), verapamil (Calan)

f. Psychotropic agents: fluoxetine (Prozac), paroxetine (Paxil), sertraline (Zoloft)

g. Miscellaneous: Grapefruit juice, propoxyphene (Darvon), zafirlukast (Accolate)

4. **Inducers of CYP3A4** (resulting in lower-than-expected plasma levels of the chemotherapeutic agent and possibly indicating an increase in dosage):

   a. Corticosteroids: Dexamethasone (Decadron), prednisone

   b. Antiseizure drugs: Phenytoin (Dilantin), carbamazepine (Tegretol), phenobarbital

   c. Antibiotics: Rifampin (Rifadin), rifabutin (Mycobutin), isoniazid

   d. Nonclassified agents: St. John's wort

B. **Imatinib** (Gleevec)

1. **Indications.** Chronic myelogenous leukemia (CML); gastrointestinal stromal tumors (GIST) expressing *c-kit* TK; consider use in other conditions expressing *c-kit* or platelet-derived growth factor receptor- β (PDGFR-β) activation. Imatinib is also approved by treatment of dermatofibrosarcoma protuberans (DFSP), myelodysplastic/myeloproliferative diseases (MDS/MPD), aggressive systemic mastocytosis (ASM), hypereosinophilic syndrome/chronic eosinophilic leukemia (HES/CEL), and relapsed/refractory Philadelphia chromosome positive acute lymphoblastic leukemias (Ph$^+$ALL).

2. **Pharmacology**

   a. Mechanisms. BCR-ABL encodes a protein, P_{210}BCR-ABL. Imatinib occupies the ATP binding site of the BCR-ABL protein and other related TKs and thus results in subsequent inhibition of substrate phosphorylation. Imatinib is a potent selective inhibitor of the P_{210}BCR-ABL TK, resulting in inhibition of clonogenicity and tumorigenicity and induction of apoptosis of BCR-ABL and Ph+ cells. It also inhibits other activated ABL TKs (including P_{185}BCR-ABL) and other receptor TKs for PDGFR, stem cell factor (SCF), and *c-kit*.

   b. Metabolism. Eliminated mainly in feces. The half-life of the parent drug is 18 hours and of the main metabolites is 40 hours.

3. **Toxicity**

   a. Dose-limiting. Myelosuppression

   b. Common. Transient ankle and periorbital edema that is usually mild to moderate; nausea, vomiting (especially when not taken with food), diarrhea.

   c. Occasional. Fluid retention with pleural effusion, pulmonary edema, ascites (especially in older patients)

4. **Administration.** Drug should be taken with food and a large glass of water.

   a. Supplied as 100-mg capsules

   b. Dose modification. Reduce dose for liver dysfunction.

   c. Dose

      (1) For CML, 400 mg/day in the chronic phase and 600 mg/day for the accelerated phase

      (2) For GIST, 600 mg/day

      (3) For HES/CEL, 400 mg/day; for HES/CEL with demonstrated FIPLI-PDGFR alpha fusion kinase, starting dose 100 mg/day.

      (4) For Ph$^+$ALL, 600 mg/day

      (5) For unresectable, recurrent, or metastatic DFSP, 800 mg/day

      (6) For MDS/MPD associated with PDGFR gene rearrangements, 400 mg/day

      (7) For ASM associated with eosinophilia, starting dose 100 mg/day; for ASM without the D816V *c-kit* mutation or with unknown *c-kit* mutational status, 400 mg/day.

   d. Drug interactions

      (1) Drugs that stimulate or inhibit liver microsomal CYP3A4 affect plasma levels of the drug (see VI.A).

      (2) **Warfarin** dosing must be monitored carefully; imatinib inhibits the metabolism of warfarin.

C. Dasatinib (Sprycel)

1. **Indications.** Chronic, accelerated or blast phase of CML with resistance or intolerance to prior therapy

2. **Pharmacology**

    a. **Mechanisms.** An inhibitor of multiple TK, including BCR-ABL

    b. **Metabolism.** Metabolized in the liver and excreted in the feces

3. **Toxicity**

    a. **Dose-limiting.** Hematosuppression; bleeding events related to thrombocytopenia but also possibly to drug-induced platelet dysfunction.

    b. **Common.** Fluid retention (which can be severe), gastrointestinal disturbances, various dermatoses

    c. **Occasional.** Neurological and muscular disorders, prolongation of QT-interval

4. **Administration.** Avoid the use of antacids, H_2 blockers, and proton pump inhibitors because the drug has pH dependent solubility.

    a. **Supplied** as 20-, 50-, and 70-mg tablets

    b. **Dose modification.** Increase or decrease dose in 20-mg increments per dose based on individual tolerability and blood cell counts.

    c. **Dose.** 100 mg once daily

    d. **Drug interactions.** Inducers or inhibitors of CYP3A4 may respectively decrease or increase plasma concentrations of dasatinib (see VI.A).

D. Erlotinib (Tarceva)

1. **Indications.** Non–small cell lung cancer and pancreatic cancer in combination with gemcitabine

2. **Pharmacology**

    a. **Mechanisms.** A selective small molecule inhibitor of the epidermal growth factor receptor (EGFR) TK that results in inhibition of proliferation, growth metastasis, and angiogenesis

    b. **Metabolism.** Metabolized in the liver primarily by the CYP3A4 microsomal enzyme and, to a lesser extent, by CYP_1A_2. More than 90% of the drugs metabolites are excreted in the bile.

3. **Toxicity**

    a. **Dose-limiting.** Diarrhea

    b. **Common.** Pustular, acneiform rash (oral or gel forms of clindamycin, 2% erythromycin topical gel b.i.d., or minocycline, 100 mg b.i.d. for 5 days, may help)

    c. **Occasional.** Interstitial lung disease (<1% of patients), keratoconjunctivitis

4. **Administration**

    a. **Supplied** as 25-, 100-, and 150-mg tablets

    b. **Dose modification** see package insert for management of skin reactions

    c. **Dose.** 150 mg/day taken 1 hour before or 2 hours after food

    d. **Drug interactions** include those agents that affect the CYP3A4 enzyme (see VI.A) and **warfarin**, which would require careful monitoring.

E. Gefitinib (Iressa)

1. **Indications.** Advanced non–small cell lung cancer after failure of both platinum- and taxane-based chemotherapies

2. **Pharmacology**

    a. **Mechanisms.** Inhibits the TK associated with transmembrane cell surface receptors, including the EGFR TK

    b. **Metabolism.** Extensive binding to plasma proteins, including albumin. The drug undergoes extensive hepatic metabolism by the CYP3A4 microsomal enzyme and is excreted predominantly in feces.

3. **Toxicity**

    a. **Dose-limiting.** Interstitial lung disease (<1%)

    b. **Common.** Diarrhea (50%), nausea, vomiting; mild rash and other skin reactions (60%); mild abnormalities of LFTs

    c. **Occasional.** Anorexia, asthenia; peripheral edema, corneal irritation due to aberrant eyelash overgrowth.

4. Administration
  a. **Supplied** as 250-mg tablets
  b. **Dose modification.** Use with caution with liver dysfunction.
  c. **Dose.** 250 mg PO daily
  d. **Drug interactions.** Inhibitors and inducers of CYP3A4 (see VI.A) and **histamine H$_2$-receptor antagonists** (e.g., ranitidine) alter plasma concentrations of gefitinib.

F. Lapatinib (Tykerb)
  1. **Indications.** In combination with capecitabine for the treatment of patients with advanced or metastatic breast cancers that overexpress human epidermal receptor type 2 (HER2) and who have received prior therapy, including an anthracycline, a taxane, and trastuzumab

  2. **Pharmacology**
  a. **Mechanisms.** Lapatinib is a 4-anilinoquinazoline kinase inhibitor of the intracellular TK domains of both EGFR (ErbB1) and of HER2 (ErbB2). In vitro studies showed an additive effect with 5-FU, the active metabolite of capecitabine.
  b. **Metabolism.** Lapatinib undergoes extensive metabolism, primarily by CYP3A4 and CYP3A5. There is negligible real excretion.

  3. **Toxicity** of lapatinib plus capecitabine
  a. **Dose-limiting.** Diarrhea
  b. **Common.** Diarrhea, nausea, vomiting; palmar–plantar erythrodysesthesia (50%), rash; hematosuppression.
  c. **Occasional**

  4. **Administration.** Capecitabine, 1,000 mg/m^2 PO b.i.d. on days 1 to 14 of each 21-day cycle, is taken with food.
  a. **Supplied** as 250 mg tablets
  b. **Dose modification.** Use with caution in patients with severe liver disease.
  c. **Dose.** 1,250 mg taken once daily PO at least 1 hour before or 1 hour after a meal
  d. **Drug interactions**
  (1) Drugs that induce or inhibit CYP3A4 can result in decreased or increased plasma levels of lapatinib, respectively (see VI.A).
  (2) Drugs that inhibit P-glycoprotein may increase plasma concentrations of lapatinib.

G. Nilotinib (Tasigna)
  1. **Indications.** Chronic, accelerated or blast phase of CML with resistance or intolerance to prior therapy that included imatinib

  2. **Pharmacology**
  a. **Mechanisms.** An inhibitor of multiple TK, including BCR-ABL
  b. **Metabolism.** Metabolized in the liver and excreted in the feces

  3. **Toxicity.** Electrocardiograms should be obtained to monitor the QTc at baseline, 7 days after initiation of therapy, and periodically thereafter, as well as following any dose adjustment. Electrolytes, divalent cations, and other chemistries as suggested below should be followed periodically.
  a. **Dose-limiting.** Myelosuppression. Prolongation of the QT interval, which can result in a type of ventricular tachycardia called *Torsade de pointes*, which may result in syncope, seizure, or sudden death.
  b. **Common.** Prolongation of QT-interval; rash, pruritus; fatigue, headache; musculoskeletal pain; nausea, vomiting, constipation, diarrhea; insomnia, dizziness; hypomagnesemia, hyperkalemia, hyperglycemia; abnormal LFTs; elevated serum lipase/amylase.
  c. **Occasional.** Hypophosphatemia, hypokalemia, hyponatremia, hypocalcemia; hyperthyroidism; interstitial lung disease; pancreatitis; urinary urgency; gynecomastia.

  4. **Administration.** Food increases blood levels of nilotinib; no food should be consumed for at least 2 hours before and 1 hour after the dose is taken.

       a. Contraindications. Patients with long QT syndrome or with hypokalemia or hypomagnesemia (which should be corrected before starting the drug and monitored thereafter)

       b. Supplied as 200-mg capsules

       c. Dose modification. Use with caution in patients with hepatic impairment or with a history of pancreatitis. Avoid drugs known to prolong the QT interval. Consider dose reduction in patients receiving a strong CYP3A4 inhibitor concurrently.

       d. Dose. 400 mg every 12 hours

       e. Drug interactions. Inducers or inhibitors of CYP3A4 may respectively decrease or increase plasma concentrations of dasatinib (see VI.A).

H. Sorafenib (Nexavar)

   1. Indications. Metastatic renal cell carcinoma; unresectable hepatocellular carcinoma.

   2. Pharmacology

       a. Mechanisms. A multiple kinase inhibitor

       b. Metabolism. Metabolized in the liver. Approximately 80% of the drug and its metabolites are excreted in the feces and 20% in the urine.

   3. Toxicity

       a. Dose-limiting. Skin reactions or unacceptable toxicities

       b. Common. Rash/desquamation, hand–foot skin reaction; hypertension; diarrhea, alopecia, hematosuppression.

       c. Occasional. Bleeding, vomiting, myocardial ischemia, increased serum lipase or amylase

   4. Administration

       a. Supplied as 200-mg tablets

       b. Dose. 400 mg b.i.d. taken at least 1 hour before or 2 hours after eating

I. Sunitinib malate (Sutent)

   1. Indications. Metastatic renal cell carcinoma; GIST after progression while on imatinib

   2. Pharmacology

       a. Mechanisms. Inhibition of multiple receptor TKs, which are implicated in tumor growth, pathologic angiogenesis, and metastasis

       b. Metabolism. The drug and its active metabolite are metabolized primarily by the p450 enzyme CYP3A4. More than 80% of the drug is eliminated via feces.

   3. Toxicity

       a. Dose-limiting. Hematosuppression, bleeding

       b. Common. Bleeding events (epistaxis and elsewhere); hypertension; diarrhea, mucositis, nausea/vomiting; fatigue; altered taste; yellow skin discoloration (one-third of patients), rash.

       c. Occasional. Peripheral neuropathy, anorexia, periorbital edema, lacrimation; prolonged QT interval on electrocardiogram; hypothyroidism, adrenal insufficiency, hypophosphatemia, elevated serum lipase or amylase levels.

   4. Administration

       a. Supplied as 12.5, 25-, and 50-mg capsules

       b. Dose modification. Dose changes should be done in 12.5-mg increments.

       c. Dose. 50-mg once daily for 4 weeks on treatment and 2 weeks off treatment, a 6-week schedule. The drug may be taken with or without food.

       d. Drug interactions. Drugs that induce or inhibit CYP3A4 can result in decreased or increased plasma levels of sunitinib, respectively (see VI.A). Dosage modification upward or downward may be warranted under these conditions.

VII. MONOCLONAL ANTIBODIES

A. Monoclonal antibodies have the advantage of relative selectivity for tumor tissue and relative lack of toxicity. Both technical problems and the development of human antimouse antibodies are major problems in using monoclonal antibodies for therapy.

1. **Biological effects.** Monoclonal antibodies can attack certain cells directly (e.g., malignant lymphocytes exposed to a selective monoclonal antibody are lysed in the presence of complement). Various radioactive and chemotherapeutic agents can be conjugated to monoclones, which deliver these agents specifically to cancer cells. Plant toxins (e.g., ricin, abrin), bacterial toxins (*Pseudomonas* endotoxin A, diphtheria toxin), or ribosome-inactivating protein can also be conjugated to monoclonal antibodies as *immunotoxins*. Growth factors (e.g., interleukins, epidermal growth factor, tumor growth factor) can sometimes be used as carriers for toxins; these constructs are called *oncotoxins*.

2. **Clinical uses**
   a. Imaging of tumors using radioisotope-labeled monoclones
   b. Selectively purging bone marrow of cancer cells
   c. Treatment of specific tumors

3. **An *infusion-related cytokine release syndrome*** (IRCRS) develops frequently during infusion of monoclonal antibodies, particularly during the first infusion. Manifestations can include fever or chills, hypotension, bronchospasm with dyspnea, and angioedema. Nausea, vomiting, fatigue, headache, rhinitis, pruritus, urticaria, and flushing also can occur. These symptoms generally develop 30 minutes to 2 hours after beginning the infusion. Symptoms generally respond to slowing the infusion rate or stopping the infusion, which can be resumed at a slower rate after symptoms resolve. Slowing the infusion rate, diphenhydramine and acetaminophen, bronchodilators, or saline infusion may be useful for treating the IRCRS, which must be distinguished clinically from true hypersensitivity and which becomes progressively less of a problem with subsequent infusions.

B. **Alemtuzumab** (Campath-1H)
   1. **Indications.** T-cell prolymphocytic leukemia; relapsed or refractory B-cell chronic lymphocytic leukemia
   2. **Pharmacology**
      a. **Mechanisms.** This recombinant humanized monoclonal antibody is directed against the cell-surface glycoprotein CD52 that is expressed on most normal and malignant B and T lymphocytes, NK cells, monocytes, and macrophages.
      b. **Metabolism.** The half-life is about 12 days with minimal clearance by the liver and kidneys. Steady-state levels are reached by the sixth week. CD4+ and CD8+ counts may take more than 1 year to return to normal.
   3. **Toxicity**
      a. **Dose-limiting.** Significant immunosuppression with increased incidence of opportunistic infections; neutropenia.
      b. **Common.** IRCRS (see VII.A.3) usually occurs within the first week of therapy.
      c. **Occasional.** Pancytopenia
   4. **Administration.** Premedicate with acetaminophen and diphenhydramine.
      a. **Supplied** as 30-mg vials
      b. **Dose modification.** Contraindicated in patients with active systemic infections or underlying immunodeficiency
      c. **Dose.** Initiate therapy with 3 mg over 2 hours and then increase the dose to 10 mg if the 3-mg dose is tolerated. The maintenance dose is 30 mg/day IV three times weekly for a maximum of 12 weeks.
      d. **Prophylactic antibiotics** should include Bactrim DS, one tablet b.i.d. three times per week, and famciclovir, 250 mg PO b.i.d. (or equivalent). Fluconazole can also be given to reduce the occurrence of fungal infections.

C. **Bevacizumab** (Avastin)
   1. **Indications.** Advanced colorectal cancer, breast cancer, nonsquamous non–small cell lung cancer
   2. **Pharmacology.** Bevacizumab is a humanized monoclonal antibody from genetically engineered cells designed to block the action of vascular endothelial growth factor (VEGF). VEGF is a protein that is secreted from malignant and nonmalignant hypoxic cells and stimulates new blood vessel formation by

binding to specific receptors. Metabolism of bevacizumab has not been characterized.

3. Toxicity

    a. Dose-limiting. Thromboembolism, gastrointestinal perforation, wound dehiscence

    b. Common. Hypertension, bleeding (especially epistaxis), IRCRS (see VII.A.3), nephritic syndrome, wound-healing complications

    c. Rare. Bowel perforation, reversible posterior leukoencephalopathy syndrome (RPLS), arterial thrombosis, hypertensive crisis

4. Administration. Bevacizumab should be given at least 28 days after any surgical and/or invasive procedure.

    a. Supplied as 100- and 400-mg vials

    b. Dose. 3 to 15 mg/kg IV every 2 or 3 weeks in combination with other chemotherapeutic drugs

D. Cetuximab (Erbitux)

1. Indications. EGFR-expressing metastatic colon cancer after failure of both irinotecan- and oxaliplatin-based regimens; squamous cell carcinoma of the head and neck.

2. Pharmacology

    a. Mechanisms. Monoclonal antibody that binds to the EGFR (HER1, ErbB-1), which is a transmembrane glycoprotein of the TK growth factor receptor family, and thus inhibits ligand-induced TK autophosphorylation, which affects multiple mechanisms of action (cell growth, apoptosis, production of vascular endothelial growth factor, production of matrix metalloproteinase). There is no evidence to indicate that the level of EGFR expression can predict for the drug's clinical activity.

    b. Metabolism. Metabolism of cetuximab has not been characterized. In steady state, the mean half-life of cetuximab in the serum is approximately 5 days.

3. Toxicity

    a. Dose-limiting. Severe IRCRS (see VII.A.3) characterized by rapid onset of airway obstruction, hypotension, and/or cardiac arrest (particularly during the first infusion); mild or moderate reactions are managed by slowing the infusion rate in subsequent doses. Severe reactions require the immediate and permanent discontinuation of cetuximab therapy. An acneform rash develops in 90% of patients, usually within 2 weeks of starting therapy.

    b. Common. Asthenia/malaise; skin drying and fissuring; abdominal pain, diarrhea, nausea, vomiting; hypomagnesemia (with accompanying hypokalemia and hypocalcemia) during or following infusions.

    c. Rare. Interstitial lung disease

4. Administration. Premedicate with antihistamines (e.g., diphenhydramine, 50 mg IV). Monitor for hypomagnesemia, including for several weeks after treatment is completed.

    a. Supplied as 100-mg vials

    b. Dose modification. For mild or moderate infusion-related reactions, reduce the infusion rate by 50%. Severe acneform rash may require dosage delay or reduction.

    c. Dose. 400 mg/m^2 IV over 2 hours initially and then 250 mg/m^2 IV over 1 hour weekly

E. Gemtuzumab ozogamicin (Mylotarg)

1. Indications. Relapsed CD33-positive acute myelogenous leukemia (AML), especially patients in first relapse who are 60 years of age or older and who are not considered candidates for cytotoxic chemotherapy

2. Pharmacology. The drug is composed of a semisynthetic derivative of calicheamicin covalently linked to a recombinant humanized monoclonal antibody directed against the 67 kDa cell-surface glycoprotein CD33. Calicheamicin is a cytotoxic antibiotic that binds to DNA, resulting in double-strand breaks and inhibition of DNA synthesis. CD33 antigen is expressed on normal myeloid cells, on more than 90% of the leukemia cells in AML, but not on stem cells or nonmyeloid tissues. The metabolism of this drug has not been well characterized, but it appears to undergo hepatobiliary elimination.

3. Toxicity

a. Dose-limiting. Myelosuppression

b. Common. Monitor closely for IRCRS events (see VII.A.3) for at least 6 hours. Abnormal LFTs in 20%; gastrointestinal toxicity.

c. Occasional. Veno-occlusive disease, which can be fatal (especially in patients previously treated with stem cell transplantation)

4. Administration. Premedicate patients with acetaminophen and diphenhydramine 30 minutes before drug infusion. Reduce the WBC to below 30,000/μL with hydroxyurea or leukapheresis to reduce the risk of tumor lysis syndrome and acute respiratory distress syndrome before giving the monoclonal antibody.

a. Supplied as 5-mg vials

b. Dose. 9 mg/m^2 IV over 2 hours; the dose is repeated 14 days later.

F. Panitumumab (Vectibix)

1. Indications. Metastatic colorectal cancer that expresses EGFR and that has progressed with 5-FU-, oxaliplatin-, and irinotecan-containing regimens.

2. Pharmacology. Panitumumab is a recombinant human monoclonal antibody that is produced in genetically engineered mammalian cells.

a. Mechanisms. Panitumumab binds specifically to EGFR on normal and tumor cells and competitively inhibits the binding of ligands for EGFR. The interaction of EGFR with its ligands activates a series of intracellular TKs.

b. Metabolism. Panitumumab concentrations reach a steady state by the third infusion. Its half-life is about 1 week.

3. Toxicity

a. Dose-limiting. IRCRS (see VII.A.3), severe dermatologic toxicity (potentially complicated by infection and septic death)

b. Common. Skin rash (90% of patients), paronychia, fatigue, abdominal pain; nausea, diarrhea, constipation; hypomagnesemia/hypocalcemia; ocular toxicity (conjunctivitis, irritation); mucosal inflammation.

4. Administration. Patients should limit sun exposure while receiving panitumumab as skin reactions could be exacerbated by sunlight.

a. Supplied as 100-, 200-, and 400-mg single-dose vials

b. Dose modification. Discontinue the drug for severe IRCRS, pulmonary infiltration, and severe dermatologic reactions. See manufacturer's recommendations on dosage adjustment for skin reactions.

c. Dose. 6 mg/kg given as a 1-hour intravenous infusion every 2 weeks

G. Rituximab (Rituxan, MabThera)

1. Indications. Relapsed or refractory CD20-positive, B-cell non-Hodgkin lymphoma

2. Pharmacology

a. Mechanisms. The rituximab antibody is a genetically engineered chimeric murine/human monoclonal antibody directed against the CD20 antigen found on the surface of normal and malignant B lymphocytes. CD20 is expressed on more than 90% of all B-cell non-Hodgkin lymphomas. CD20 is not expressed on early pre-B cells, plasma cells, normal bone marrow stem cells, or antigen-presenting dendritic reticulum cells.

In vitro, the Fab domain of rituximab binds to the CD20 antigen on B lymphocytes, and the Fc domain recruits immune effector functions to mediate complement- and antibody-dependent B-cell lysis.

b. Metabolism. Rituximab has been detectable in the serum 3 to 6 months after completion of treatment. Administration results in a rapid and sustained depletion of circulating and tissue-based B cells. B-cell levels return to normal by 12 months after completion of treatment.

3. Toxicity

a. Dose-limiting. Hypersensitivity reactions, serious cardiac arrhythmias

b. Common. IRCRS (see VII.A.3) occurs in 50%.

c. **Occasional.** Severe granulocytopenia or thrombocytopenia; arthralgia, malaise; diarrhea, dyspepsia, taste perversion; hypertension, postural hypotension, tachycardia, bradycardia; lacrimation, paresthesia, hypesthesia, agitation, insomnia; hyperglycemia, hypocalcemia; pain in chest, back, or tumor site.

4. **Administration.** During the first infusion, the initial rate should be 50 mg/hour or less; if hypersensitivity or infusion-related events do not occur, increase the infusion rate in 50-mg/hour increments up to a maximum of 400 mg/hour. Subsequent infusions can be started at 100 mg/hour and escalated by 100 mg/hour at 30-minute intervals. Corticosteroids, epinephrine, and antihistamines should be available for immediate use in the event of a severe hypersensitivity reaction during administration. Watch for tumor lysis syndrome in patients with a high tumor burden.

a. **Supplied** as 10 mg/mL in 10- and 50-mL vials

b. **Dose modification.** Infusion-related reactions respond to stopping the infusion and then resuming at a slower rate. Use with caution in patients with pre-existing heart disease.

c. **Dose.** 375 mg/m^2 IV weekly for 4 weeks

H. **Trastuzumab** (Herceptin, anti-HER-2 antibody)

1. **Indications.** Metastatic breast cancer that overexpresses the HER2 protein

2. **Pharmacology.** The *HER2/neu* (or *c-erb-B2*) protooncogene encodes a transmembrane receptor protein that is structurally related to EGFR. Trastuzumab is a recombinant DNA-derived humanized monoclonal antibody that selectively binds to the extracellular domain of *HER2*. The humanized Ig-Gκ antibody against *HER2* is produced by a mammalian cell (Chinese hamster ovary) suspension culture. It inhibits the proliferation of tumor cells that overexpress *HER2*. The metabolism of trastuzumab is not well characterized.

3. **Toxicity**

a. **Dose-limiting.** Cardiomyopathy

b. **Common.** IRCRS (see VII.A.3) occurs in 40% during the first infusion.

c. **Occasional.** Hematosuppression

4. **Administration.** Monitor electrocardiogram or ejection fraction in these patients during ongoing therapy.

a. **Supplied** as 440-mg vial

b. **Dose modification.** Use with extreme caution in patients with pre-existing cardiac dysfunction or prior cardiotoxic therapy.

c. **Dose.** Initial dose 4 mg/kg over 90 minutes; maintenance dose 2 mg/kg/week or 6 mg/kg every 3 weeks, given over 30 minutes.

d. **Drug interactions.** Increased risk of cardiotoxicity when used in combination with anthracyclines and/or taxanes

VIII. MISCELLANEOUS AGENTS

A. **Anagrelide** (Agrylin)

1. **Indications.** Thrombocytosis in myeloproliferative disorders

2. **Pharmacology**

a. **Mechanisms.** Anagrelide reduces the platelet count by uncertain mechanisms. It does not affect the leukocyte count and does not affect DNA synthesis.

b. **Metabolism.** The drug is extensively metabolized, and <1% is excreted in the urine as unaltered drug.

3. **Toxicity.** Adverse effects are treated symptomatically and usually abate on continuation of therapy. Cardiovascular complications that occur are usually related to underlying diseases.

a. **Dose-limiting.** Thrombocytopenia

b. **Common.** Headache (45%), palpitations, tachycardia, fluid retention, diarrhea, bloating, abdominal pain, asthenia, dizziness

c. **Occasional.** Nausea, vomiting, other GI disturbances; dyspnea, paresthesia, rash, pruritus, fever.

4. **Administration.** Platelet counts should be monitored every 2 to 7 days until maintenance dosage is attained. Propranolol can be helpful for induced arrhythmias.
   a. **Supplied** as 0.5- and 1-mg capsules
   b. **Dose modification.** None for renal dysfunction. Avoid the drug in patients with severe hepatic impairment; reduce dose for patients with moderate hepatic impairment.
   c. **Dose.** Start at 0.5 mg q.i.d. or 1 mg b.i.d. PO; increase dosage weekly by 0.5 mg/day until the desired platelet count is achieved. Maximum recommended dosages are 10 mg/day or 2.5 mg/dose.

B. **Asparaginase** (L-asparaginase, Elspar)
   1. **Indication.** Acute lymphoblastic leukemia
   2. **Pharmacology.** The drug is purified from *Escherichia coli* and/or *Erwinia chrysanthemi*
      a. **Mechanism.** This enzyme hydrolyzes asparagine into aspartic acid and, to a lesser extent, glutamine into glutamic acid. Leads to inhibition of protein synthesis. Kills cells that cannot synthesize asparagine by destroying extracellular asparagine stores. Cell cycle–specific for postmitotic G_1 phase.
      b. **Metabolism.** Plasma half-life (8 to 30 hours) is independent of dose. Metabolism is independent of hepatic and renal function. Only trace amounts are recovered in urine.
   3. **Toxicity**
      a. **Dose-limiting.** Allergic reactions (including chills, urticaria, skin rashes, fever, laryngeal constriction, asthma, and anaphylactic shock) are the most frequent. Allergic reactions develop within 1 hour of dosing and are most likely to occur after several doses are given, particularly if the last dose was given more than 1 month previously and if the drug is administered intravenously rather than intramuscularly. Patients who respond to *Escherichia coli* asparaginase but develop allergic reactions may be treated relatively safely with another source of the enzyme.
      b. **Common**
         (1) **Encephalopathy** in 25% to 50% of patients. Lethargy, somnolence, and confusion tend to occur within the first few days of therapy, reverse after completion of therapy, and are rarely a cause for discontinuing treatment. Hemorrhagic and thrombotic CNS events occur later and are associated with induced imbalances in the coagulation and fibrinolytic systems.
         (2) **GI:** Nausea, anorexia, vomiting (60%)
         (3) **Hepatitis** (abnormal LFTs in more than 50% of treated patients, but rarely severe); pancreatitis (10%).
         (4) **Coagulation defects** associated with decreased synthesis of clotting factors, especially fibrinogen and antithrombin III (usually subclinical but may result in thrombosis or pulmonary embolism)
         (5) **Prerenal azotemia** (65%); a rise in blood urea nitrogen and blood ammonia levels not evidence of toxicity.
         (6) **Hyperglycemia**
         (7) Interferes with **thyroid function tests** for up to 1 month, probably due to marked reduction of thyroxine-binding globulin
      c. **Rare.** Myelosuppression, diarrhea, severe renal failure, hyperthermia
   4. **Administration.** Administer a small (2-U) intradermal test dose to check for hypersensitivity, particularly when the dose is being repeated more than 1 week from the immediately previous dose. Epinephrine (1 mg, 1:1,000), hydrocortisone (100 mg), and diphenhydramine (50 mg) should be readily available to treat anaphylaxis each time the drug is given.
      a. **Supplied** as 10,000-IU vials
      b. **Dose modification.** None for renal dysfunction. Use with caution for hepatic dysfunction. Contraindicated in the presence of pancreatitis.
      c. **Dose.** Usually administered in combination with vincristine and prednisone at a dose of 6,000 IU/m^2 IM every 3 days for nine doses.

    d. Drug interactions

        (1) Asparaginase blocks the action of **methotrexate** and thus rescues the patient from methotrexate toxicity.

        (2) **Vincristine** should be administered 12 to 24 hours before asparaginase, which inhibits the clearance of that drug.

C. Bortezomib (Velcade)

  1. Indication. Multiple myeloma (in patients who have received at least one prior therapy), mantle cell lymphoma

  2. Pharmacology. Bortezomib is a modified dipeptidyl boronic acid.

    a. Mechanisms. Reversible inhibitor of the chymotrypsin-like activity of the 26S proteasome, which is a large protein complex that degrades ubiquitinated proteins, which are involved in regulating the intracellular concentration of specific proteins. Disruption of this pathway affects multiple signaling pathways within the cell, leading to cell death. Down-regulates the NK-κB pathway, leading to inhibition of cell growth.

    b. Metabolism. Metabolized via hepatic P450 enzymes. Elimination is not well characterized.

  3. Toxicity

    a. Dose-limiting. Peripheral neuropathy (predominantly sensory), hematosuppression (especially thrombocytopenia)

    b. Common. Fatigue, fever (up to 40%); gastrointestinal (anorexia, nausea, vomiting, diarrhea, constipation).

    c. Occasional. Orthostatic hypotension (10%); motor neuropathy; congestive heart failure; toxic epidermal necrolysis.

    d. Rare. Interstitial pneumonia and acute respiratory distress syndrome

  4. Administration

    a. Supplied as 3.5-mg vials

    b. Dose modification. Use with caution with hepatic dysfunction.

    c. Dose. 1.3 mg/m^2 IV bolus on days 1, 4, 8, and 11 of each 21-day cycle

    d. Drug interactions

        (1) Patients receiving **oral hypoglycemics** require close monitoring of blood glucose levels.

        (2) Patients who are concomitantly receiving inhibitors of **cytochrome P450** should be closely monitored for toxicities or reduced efficacy.

D. Denileukin diftitox (Ontak, DAB$_{389}$IL-2) is a recombinant fusion protein composed of amino acid sequences of human interleukin-2 (IL-2) and the enzymatic and translocation domains of diphtheria toxin. This protein binds specifically to the CD25 component of the IL-2 receptor and is then internalized via endocytosis. Cellular protein synthesis is inhibited, and apoptosis occurs on release of diphtheria toxin into the cytosol.

  1. Indications. Persistent or recurrent cutaneous T-cell lymphomas whose malignant cells express the CD25 component of the IL-2 receptor (must be confirmed on tumor biopsy)

  2. Toxicity

    a. Hypersensitivity reactions are observed in nearly 70% of patients within the first 24 hours of infusion.

    b. Common. A **vascular leak syndrome** characterized by edema, hypotension, and/or hypoalbuminemia is usually a self-limited process; mild, transient flu-like symptoms; diarrhea, rash.

    c. Occasional. Hyperthyroidism; loss of visual acuity, usually with loss of color vision, has been reported and may be persistent.

  3. Administration. Premedicate with nonsteroidal anti-inflammatory agents and antihistamines. Patients should be monitored closely throughout the entire treatment. Resuscitative medications (epinephrine, corticosteroids) and equipment should be available at bedside before treatment.

    a. Supplied as 150-mcg/mL vials

    b. Dose. 9 or 18 mcg/kg/day IV on days 1 to 5 every 21 days

E. Hexamethylmelamine (altretamine, Hexalen)
   1. Indication. Recurrent ovarian carcinoma
   2. Pharmacology
      a. Mechanism is unknown. It structurally resembles an alkylating agent but does not have alkylating agent activity.
      b. Metabolism. Rapidly demethylated and hydroxylated in the liver by the microsomal P450 system. Excreted in urine and hepatobiliary tract as metabolites.
   3. Toxicity
      a. Dose-limiting. Nausea and vomiting, which may worsen with continued therapy
      b. Common. Myelosuppression (mild) with nadir blood cell counts occurring 3 to 4 weeks after starting treatment
      c. Occasional. Neurotoxicity (25%), including paresthesias, hypoesthesia, hyperreflexia, motor weakness, agitation, confusion, hallucinations, lethargy, depression, coma; abnormal LFTs, flu-like syndrome; abdominal cramps, diarrhea.
      d. Rare. Alopecia, skin rashes, cystitis
   4. Administration
      a. Supplied as 50-mg capsules
      b. Dose modification. Give cautiously to patients with hepatic dysfunction.
      c. Dose. 200 to 260 mg/m^2 PO daily in divided doses for 14 to 21 days of a 28-day schedule when recovery permits
      d. Drug interactions. Cimetidine may inhibit metabolism. Barbiturates may enhance metabolism. Monamine oxidase inhibitors may result in severe orthostatic hypotension.

F. Interferon-α (IFN-α)
   1. Sources. Lymphocytes, macrophages, and other cells
   2. Properties of IFN-α
      a. Antitumor activity
      b. Antiproliferative activity
      c. Inhibition of angiogenesis
      d. Regulation of differentiation
      e. Interaction with growth factors, oncogenes, other cytokines
      f. Enhancement of tumor-associated antigens
      g. Natural killer (NK) cell activation, cytotoxic T-lymphocyte (CTL) activation, induction of major histocompatibility complex (MHC) class I
      h. Antiviral activity
   3. Clinical uses
      a. Response rates reported to be 75% to 90% in previously untreated patients: chronic myelogenous leukemia (chronic phase), hairy cell leukemia, myeloproliferative disorders, cutaneous T-cell lymphomas
      b. Response rates reported to be 40% to 50% in low-grade lymphomas, multiple myeloma
      c. Condylomata acuminata, chronic granulomatous disease, hepatitis C, adjuvant therapy for melanoma
   4. Dose. A wide range of doses and schedules have been used, depending on the condition (from 2- to 10- to 36-million U/m^2 are given SC for 3 to 7 days weekly).
   5. Toxicities (depend on dose and schedule). Flulike symptoms (75% to 100%) may be dose-limiting, develop in 1 to 2 hours, and peak 4 to 8 hours after injection. Malaise, headache, rashes (40% to 50%), GI symptoms (20% to 40%), elevated LFTs (30%); mild leukopenia or thrombocytopenia; neurological symptoms, depression, chronic fatigue (can be dose-limiting).
   6. Supplied as recombinant forms
      a. IFN-α2a (Roferon-A): 3-, 6-, 18-, and 36-million U/mL vials
      b. IFN-α2b (Intron-A): 3-, 5-, 18-, and 50-million U/mL vials

G. Interleukins. IL-2 plays a major role in immune regulation. The primary action of IL-2 is to stimulate growth of activated T cells that bear IL-2 receptors. The binding of antigen in conjunction with IL-1 stimulates T cells to release IL-2, which signals further lymphocyte mitogenesis.

1. **Clinical uses.** Approved by the Food and Drug Administration for the treatment of metastatic renal cell carcinoma and melanoma

2. **Dose.** Up to 75% of patients develop anti-IL-2 antibodies

   a. High-dose regimens administer 600,000 to 720,000 IU/kg every 8 hours for 5 consecutive days for two cycles separated by 7 to 10 days. The course of treatment is repeated for patients who respond.

   b. Low-dose regimens are being investigated. An example for renal cell carcinoma is 6 million U/m^2 by continuous IV infusion (via 48-hour cassettes) for 4 days weekly for 4 weeks in conjunction with IFN-α, 6 million U/m^2 given SC twice weekly.

3. **Toxicity.** High-dose therapy with IL-2 is highly toxic; it induces vascular permeability and promotes secretion of other lymphokines (such as IFN-γ) with their own sets of toxicities. These developments result in fluid retention and interstitial edema in several organ systems that appear to be reversible after administration of IL-2 ceases.

4. **Supplied** as recombinant IL-2 (aldesleukin, Proleukin) in 22-million IU vials

5. **Drug interactions**

   a. **Corticosteroids** decrease the antitumor activity of IL-2.

   b. **Nonsteroidal anti-inflammatory drugs** may enhance the capillary leak syndrome observed with IL-2.

   c. **Antihypertensives** should be stopped at least 24 hours before IL-2 treatment because of IL-2 potentiating the antihypertensive effect.

H. Lenalidomide (Revlimid)

1. **Indications.** Myeloma; myelodysplastic syndrome (MDS) with deletion 5q abnormality

2. **Pharmacology**

   a. **Mechanisms.** Lenalidomide is a thalidomide analogue with immunomodulatory, antiangiogenic, and antineoplastic properties.

   b. **Metabolism.** The majority of the drug is excreted unchanged in the urine.

3. **Toxicity.** Lenalidomide is an analogue of thalidomide, which is a known human teratogen that causes life-threatening human birth defects.

   a. **Dose-limiting.** Neutropenia and thrombocytopenia

   b. **Common.** Diarrhea, other gastrointestinal disturbances, rash, pruritus, fatigue

   c. **Occasional.** Deep vein thrombosis and pulmonary embolism, fever, myalgia/arthralgias, dizziness, headache. Be observant for episodes of thromboembolism based on the experience with thalidomide.

4. **Administration.** The capsules are taken with water and should not be opened, broken, or chewed.

   a. **Supplied** as 5-mg, 10-mg, 15-mg, and 25-mg capsules

   b. **Dose modification.** Use with extreme caution or avoid the drug in patients with impaired renal function.

   c. **Dose.** For MDS, the starting dose is 10 mg daily. For myeloma, the starting dose is 25 mg daily for 21 days of each 28-day cycle.

I. Retinoic acid receptor (RAR) inhibitors

1. **Bexarotene** (Targretin)

   a. **Indication.** Cutaneous T-cell lymphoma (CTCL) that is refractory to at least one prior systemic therapy

   b. **Pharmacology**

      (1) **Mechanisms.** Selectively binds and activates retinoic X receptors (RXRs), which form heterodimers with various other receptors, including RARs, vitamin D receptors, and thyroid receptors. The activated receptors function as transcription factors, which then regulate the expression

of various genes involved in controlling cell differentiation, growth, and proliferation.

(2) Metabolism. Extensively metabolized by the hepatic P450 microsomal system to both active and inactive metabolites. Primarily eliminated through the hepatobiliary system and in feces.

c. Toxicity

(1) Photosensitivity, rash, dry skin

(2) Hypothyroidism (50% of patients), hypoglycemia, hypertriglyceridemia, hypercholesterolemia

(3) Ocular problems: retinal complications, cataracts, xerophthalmia, conjunctivitis, blepharitis

(4) Headache, asthenia

d. Administration. Patients should avoid exposure to sunlight and should be advised to limit vitamin A supplementation to <1,500 IU/day to avoid potential additive toxic effects.

(1) Supplied as 75-mg capsules

(2) Dose modification. Use with caution in patients with liver dysfunction, diabetes (particularly those on hypoglycemic agents), or lipid disorders.

(3) Dose. 300 mg/m^2 PO daily with food as a single dose

(4) Drug interactions. Use with caution in patients who are also taking drugs that inhibit or induce the cytochrome P450 system, such as phenytoin, phenobarbital, and rifampin (see Section VI.A). Avoid concurrent administration of gemfibrozil (Lopid), which inhibits metabolism of bexarotene.

2. Tretinoin (All-Trans-Retinoic Acid, ATRA, Vesanoid)

a. Indication. Acute promyelocytic leukemia

b. Pharmacology

(1) Mechanisms. On entry into cells, tretinoin binds to cellular retinoic acid binding protein, and this complex is transported to the nucleus, where it binds to RARs and/or RXRs. This process induces differentiation of acute promyelocytic cells to normal myelocytes and induces apoptosis by mechanisms that have not been fully elucidated.

(2) Metabolism. Extensively metabolized by the hepatic P450 microsomal system. Excreted both in urine and in feces.

c. Toxicity

(1) Vitamin A toxicity (nearly all patients): headache (which improves after the first week), fever, dryness of skin and mucous membranes, skin rash, mucositis, conjunctivitis, and peripheral edema

(2) Retinoic acid syndrome (25% of patients): Fever, leukocytosis, dyspnea, weight gain, diffuse pulmonary infiltrates, and pleural and/or pericardial effusions. The syndrome usually occurs during the first month of therapy and can be dose-limiting. Development of manifestations of the syndrome mandates discontinuance of the drug and treatment with dexamethasone (10 mg IV q12h for 3 days or until the syndrome has completely resolved). Therapy can be resumed in most cases once the syndrome has completely resolved.

(3) Other common events. Hypercholesterolemia (60%), gastrointestinal symptoms, elevations of serum transaminase and alkaline phosphatase levels (50%), ear discomfort (25%)

(4) Uncommon events. Cardiac ischemia, stroke, myocarditis, pericarditis, pulmonary hypertension; central nervous system toxicity in various forms; renal dysfunction.

d. Administration. Monitor patients closely for retinoic acid syndrome during the first month of therapy.

(1) Supplied as 10-mg capsules

(2) Dose modification. Use with caution in patients who have pre-existing hypertriglyceridemia, diabetes mellitus, obesity, or alcoholism.

(3) Dose. 45 mg/m^2 PO divided in two daily doses for 45 to 90 days

(4) Drug interaction. Use with caution in patients who are also taking drugs that inhibit or induce the cytochrome P450 system.

J. Suramin

1. **Indication.** Investigational agent for prostate cancer
2. **Pharmacology**
   a. **Mechanism.** Suramin is a glycosaminoglycan, an antitrypanosomal agent. Antitumor activity may be related to binding to growth factors and to other mechanisms.
   b. **Metabolism.** Totally bound to plasma proteins; nearly all is excreted in the urine, with an elimination half-life of 40 to 50 days.
3. **Toxicity.** Life-threatening toxicities can usually be avoided by keeping the plasma concentrations <300 mcg/mL.
   a. **Dose-limiting.** Thrombocytopenia
   b. **Neurotoxicity.** Paresthesias, polyradiculoneuropathy (muscle weakness progressing to generalized flaccid paralysis)
   c. **Other.** Leukopenia (mild), elevated clotting times, bleeding; adrenocortical insufficiency, hypocalcemia; nausea, vomiting, abnormal LFTs, metallic taste; nephrotoxicity; keratopathy, photophobia, blurred vision; fever, transient erythematous rash, pruritus.
4. **Administration**
   a. **Supplied** as 1-g vials
   b. **Dose.** 350 mg/m^2/day as a continuous IV infusion until plasma level reaches 250 to 300 mcg/mL, then variable dosing schedules are used

K. Temsirolimus (Torisel)

1. **Indications.** Advanced renal cell carcinoma
2. **Pharmacology**
   a. **Mechanisms.** Inhibitor of mTOR (mammalian target of rapamycin) that controls cell division, resulting in growth arrest in the G_1 phase of the cell cycle and reduced levels of hypoxia-inducible factors (HIF-1 and HIF-2) and of VEGF.
   b. **Metabolism.** Extensively metabolized via the cytochrome P450 3A4 hepatic microsomal pathway into metabolites, including sirolimus (the principle active metabolite). Elimination is primarily through the feces.
3. **Toxicity**
   a. **Dose-limiting.** Hypersensitivity reactions or end-organ damage (see below).
   b. **Common.** Rash, asthenia, mucositis, edema, anorexia; delayed wound healing; anemia, thrombocytopenia; hyperglycemia, hyperlipidemia, hypophosphatemia, elevated serum alkaline phosphatase and/or AST.
   c. **Occasional.** Interstitial lung disease, bowel perforation, renal failure, chest pain, intracerebral hemorrhage (with brain metastasis or anticoagulant therapy)
4. **Administration.** Premedicate with 35 to 50 mg diphenhydramine IV.
   a. **Supplied** as 25 mg/mL vial plus diluent
   b. **Dose modification.** Consider dose modification with concomitant use of other drugs affecting CYP3A4.
   c. **Dose.** 25 mg IV over 30 to 60 minutes weekly
   d. **Drug interactions.** Consider dose modification with concomitant use of other drugs affecting CYP3A4 (see VI.A).

L. Thalidomide (Thalomid)

1. **Indications.** Myeloma; myelodysplastic syndromes; being investigated in a wide variety of malignancies and hematologic disorders.
2. **Pharmacology**
   a. **Mechanisms.** Incompletely understood; inhibits TNF-α, down-modulates certain surface adhesion molecules, may exert an antiangiogenic effect.
   b. **Metabolism.** Not well defined
3. **Toxicity.** Thalidomide's teratogenic effect is its most serious toxicity. All women of childbearing age should have a baseline β-human chorionic gonadotrophin before starting therapy with thalidomide. Women should practice two forms

of birth control throughout treatment: one highly effective form (intrauterine device, hormonal contraception, partner's vasectomy) and one additional barrier method. Men taking the drug must use latex condoms for every sexual encounter with a woman of childbearing potential because the drug may be in the semen.

    a. Dose-limiting. Neurological side effects, including fatigue, sedation, orthostatic hypotension, dizziness, peripheral neuropathy, thrombophlebitis

    b. Common. Constipation, skin rash (maculopapular or urticarial)

    c. Occasional. Stevens-Johnson syndrome has been reported.

  4. Administration

    a. Supplied as 50-, 100-, and 200-mg capsules

    b. Dose modification. Therapy should be discontinued if a rash develops and can be restarted with caution if the rash was not suggestive of a serious skin condition.

    c. Dose. 100 to 400 mg PO at bedtime for myeloma (up to 1,200 mg have been used)

IX. HORMONAL AGENTS

A. Adrenocorticosteroids

  1. Indications. Broad variety of oncological problems that include the following:

    a. Component of combination chemotherapy regimens

    b. Symptomatic lymphangitic lung carcinomatosis; bronchial obstruction by tumor.

    c. Symptomatic brain metastases with or without cerebral edema; spinal cord compression.

    d. Painful liver metastases

    e. Immune-mediated cytopenias

    f. Prevention of chemotherapy-induced vomiting

    g. Appetite stimulant and mood elevator in patients with far-advanced cancer

  2. Toxicity and side effects (usually associated with long-term therapy)

    a. Peptic ulcer disease

    b. Sodium retention (edema, heart failure, hypertension)

    c. Potassium wasting (hypokalemia, alkalosis, muscle weakness)

    d. Glucose intolerance, accumulation of fat on trunk and face, weight gain

    e. Proximal myopathy

    f. Personality changes, including euphoria and psychosis

    g. Osteoporosis, aseptic hip necrosis

    h. Thinning and fragility of the skin

    i. Suppression of the pituitary–adrenal axis

    j. Susceptibility to infection

  3. Administration. Patients receiving high doses of corticosteroids are given prophylactic oral antacid therapy. Methylprednisolone is preferred for patients with severe hepatic dysfunction. Dexamethasone is preferred for peritumoral edema. These drugs are supplied in a wide variety of dosages, as follows:

    a. Prednisone: 1.0-, 2.5-, 5.0-, 10-, 20-, 25-, and 50-mg tablets and 1- and 5-mg/mL oral solutions

    b. Methylprednisolone: 2-, 4-, 8-, 16-, 24-, and 32-mg tablets

    c. Dexamethasone: 0.25-, 0.5-, 0.75-, 1.0-, 1.5-, 2.0-, 4.0-, and 6.0-mg tablets and 0.5 to 1.0 mg/mL elixir

B. Adrenal inhibitors: Mitotane (o,p'-DDD, Lysodren)

  1. Indications. Adrenal carcinoma, ectopic Cushing syndrome

  2. Pharmacology

    a. Mechanism. Causes adrenal cortical atrophy; the exact mechanism is unknown. Blocks adrenocorticosteroid synthesis in normal and malignant cells. Aldosterone synthesis is not affected.

    b. Metabolism. Degraded slowly in the liver and extensively distributed in fatty tissues. Its action is antagonized by spironolactone; the two drugs should not be administered together. Metabolites are excreted in the bile and urine.

    3. Toxicity

      a. Dose-limiting. Nausea and vomiting; adrenocortical insufficiency.

      b. Common. Diarrhea, depression, lethargy, maculopapular rash

      c. Occasional. Orthostatic hypotension; abnormal LFTs; irritability, confusion, tremors; diplopia, retinopathy, lens opacity; myalgia; hemorrhagic cystitis, fever.

    4. Administration. Plasma cortisol levels should be monitored periodically to assess the effectiveness of treatment and the possible development of adrenal insufficiency. Glucocorticoid and mineralocorticoid replacement therapy may be necessary.

      a. Supplied as 500-mg tablets

      b. Dose modification. Reduce dose for patients with hepatic impairment.

      c. Dose. 2 to 10 g PO daily in three or four divided doses

      d. Drug interactions

        (1) Warfarin doses usually have to be increased when mitotane is given.

        (2) Mitotane alters the liver's P450 system and thus may affect the levels of other drugs that are metabolized by this system.

C. Androgens

    1. Indications. Breast carcinoma, short-range anabolic effect, stimulation of erythropoiesis

    2. Toxicity and side effects vary among preparations. Virilization, fluid retention, and hepatotoxicity, which is characterized by abnormal LFTs or cholestasis and is usually reversible, are frequent with certain preparations. May cause hypercalcemia in immobilized patients.

    3. Administration. Use with caution in patients with cardiac, hepatic, or renal disease.

      a. Fluoxymesterone (Halotestin and others): 10 to 40 mg/day in two to four divided doses (supplied as 2-, 5-, and 10-mg tablets)

      b. Methyltestosterone (Android and others): 50 to 200 mg/day in two or three divided doses (supplied as 10- and 25-mg tablets)

D. Antiandrogens (bicalutamide, flutamide, nilutamide)

    1. Indications. Prostate cancer in combination with medical therapy or orchiectomy that reduces testicular but not adrenal androgen production

    2. Pharmacology. Nonsteroidal antiandrogens bind to cytosol androgen receptors and competitively inhibit the uptake or binding of androgens in target tissues. The drugs are almost totally metabolized.

    3. Toxicity (may be contributed to by the combined therapeutic component)

      a. Common. Impotence, gynecomastia, and other manifestations of hypogonadism; diarrhea.

      b. Occasional. Nausea and vomiting, myalgia, depression; mild hypertension or pulmonary disorder (bicalutamide, nilutamide).

      c. Rare. Hepatitis, including cholestatic jaundice (all three), hemolytic anemia or methemoglobinemia (flutamide), iron-deficiency anemia (bicalutamide), interstitial pneumonitis, or visual disturbances (nilutamide)

    4. Administration. Usually given in combination with luteinizing hormone-releasing hormone (LHRH) agonist analogs. Use with caution in patients with hepatic dysfunction.

      a. Bicalutamide (Casodex): 50 mg PO once daily (supplied as 50-mg tablets)

      b. Flutamide (Eulexin): 250 mg t.i.d. PO (supplied as 125-mg capsules)

      c. Nilutamide (Nilandron): 300 mg once daily PO for 30 days, then 150 mg daily (supplied as 50-mg tablets)

E. Estrogens [diethylstilbestrol (DES)]

    1. Indication. Breast carcinoma

    2. Toxicity. Nausea, uterine bleeding; hypercalcemic "flare"; thromboembolic disorders; abnormal LFTs, cholestatic jaundice (rare); chloasma, optic neuritis, retinal thrombosis; rash, pruritus; fluid retention, hypertension, headache, dizziness, hypertriglyceridemia.

3. Administration
    a. Supplied as 0.25-, 0.5-, 1.0-, and 5.0-mg tablets
    b. Dose. 1 to 15 mg PO daily in divided doses

F. Antiestrogens (tamoxifen, toremifene, fulvestrant)
  1. Indication. Breast carcinoma
  2. Pharmacology. Tamoxifen and toremifene are nonsteroidal agents that bind to estrogen receptors and may exert antiestrogenic, estrogenic, or both activities. Fulvestrant is an estrogen receptor antagonist without known agonist effects.
  3. Toxicity (derived from tamoxifen, which is associated with the largest experience)
    a. Common. Hot flashes, menstrual changes, vaginal discharge, uterine bleeding; lowered serum cholesterol (especially low-density cholesterol); thrombocytopenia (mild and transient).
    b. Occasional. Retinopathy or keratopathy (reversible), cataracts; leukopenia, anemia; nausea, vomiting; hair loss (mild), rash; "flare" in first month of therapy of patients with bone metastases; thrombophlebitis or thromboembolism, particularly in patients with cofactors for thrombosis (e.g., inheritance of factor V Leiden).
    c. Rare. Abnormal LFTs; altered mental state; slightly increased occurrence of endometrial adenocarcinoma on prolonged use.
    d. Toxicity of fulvestrant includes transient pain at injection site, gastrointestinal symptoms, headache, back pain, and vasodilatation.
  4. Administration
    a. Tamoxifen (Nolvadex): 20 mg PO once daily (supplied as 10- and 20-mg tablets)
    b. Toremifene (Fareston): 60 mg PO once daily (supplied as 60-mg tablets)
    c. Fulvestrant (Faslodex): 250 mg IM as a 5-mL solution monthly

G. Aromatase inhibitors (anastrozole, letrozole, exemestane, aminoglutethimide)
  1. Indication. Breast cancer in postmenopausal women
  2. Pharmacology. These nonsteroidal inhibitors interfere with aromatase, the enzyme that converts androgens from the adrenals and peripheral tissues to estrogens. Anastrozole and letrozole are competitive inhibitors, whereas exemestane permanently binds to and irreversibly inactivates aromatase. None of these agents inhibit adrenal corticosteroid or aldosterone biosynthesis. All are significantly more potent inhibitors of aromatase than aminoglutethimide (Cytadren), which also inhibits corticosteroid or aldosterone biosynthesis, requires q.i.d. dosing with hydrocortisone, is more toxic than the newer alternatives, and is no longer recommended.
  3. Toxicity. Antiestrogen effects, peripheral edema, thromboembolism, osteopenia, vaginal bleeding
  4. Dose
    a. Anastrozole (Arimidex): 1 mg PO daily (supplied as 1-mg tablets)
    b. Letrozole (Femara): 2.5 mg PO daily (supplied as 2.5-mg tablets)
    c. Exemestane (Aromasin): 25 mg PO daily (supplied as 25-mg tablets)

H. Luteinizing hormone-releasing hormone (LHRH) agonists
  1. Indications. Prostate and breast cancer
  2. Pharmacology. LHRH agonist analogs decrease serum levels of luteinizing hormone and follicle-stimulating hormone and result in castration levels of testosterone in men and of estradiol in women within 2 weeks of treatment.
  3. Toxicity and side effects
    a. Common. Hot flashes, decreased libido; impotence and gynecomastia in men; amenorrhea and uterine bleeding in women.
    b. Occasional. Hypercholesterolemia, local discomfort at site of injection
    c. Rare. GI upset, rash, hypertension, azotemia, headache, depression
  4. Administration
    a. Leuprolide (Lupron)
      (1) Supplied as 7.5-, 22.5-, and 30-mg vials
      (2) Dose. 7.5-, 22.5-, or 30-mg IM every 1, 3, or 4 months, respectively

    b. Goserelin (Zoladex)
      (1) Supplied as 3.6- and 10.8-mg pellets in prefilled syringe
      (2) Dose. 3.6 mg SC monthly or 10.8 mg every 3 months

I. Progestins
  1. Indications. Endometrial and breast carcinomas; or as an appetite stimulant in malignant cachexia; or for hot flashes in patients with breast carcinoma.
  2. Toxicity and side effects
    a. Menstrual changes, uterine bleeding, hot flashes, gynecomastia, galactorrhea
    b. Fluid retention, thrombophlebitis, thromboembolism
    c. Nervousness, somnolence, depression, headache
  3. Administration
    a. Medroxyprogesterone acetate injectable (Depo-Provera)
      (1) Supplied as vials containing 150 or 400 mg/mL
      (2) Dose for hot flashes, 150 mg IM every 3 months
      (3) Dose for endometrial carcinoma. 1 g IM every for six doses, then monthly
    b. Megestrol (Megace)
      (1) Supplied as 20- and 40-mg tablets and 40 mg/mL suspension
      (2) Dose for breast cancer. 40 mg PO q.i.d.
      (3) Dose for endometrial cancer. 20 to 80 mg q.i.d.
      (4) Dose for appetite stimulation. 400 to 800 mg PO daily as a single dose

X. CYTOPROTECTIVE AGENTS
  A. Amifostine (Ethyol)
    1. Indications. Protection against cumulative nephrotoxicity from cisplatin-based therapies. Reduction of xerostomia in patients undergoing postoperative radiation therapy for head and neck cancer.
    2. Pharmacology
      a. Mechanisms. It is a prodrug that is dephosphorylated in tissues to an active free thiol metabolite that acts as a potent scavenger of oxygen free radicals and superoxide anions to inactivate the reactive species of cisplatin and radiation.
      b. Metabolism. Rapidly metabolized to an active free thiol metabolite, which is further converted to a less active disulfide metabolite. The estimated plasma half-life is 8 minutes.
    3. Toxicity
      a. Dose-limiting. Hypotension ($>60\%$ of patients) is treated with fluid infusion and changes in posture.
      b. Common. Hypotension, nausea, and vomiting
      c. Occasional. Hypocalcemia, hiccups; infusion-related reaction with flushing, chills, dizziness, somnolence, and sneezing.
      d. Rare. Transient loss of consciousness, allergic reaction
    4. Administration. Patients should be well hydrated before amifostine is administered. Antiemetics, including dexamethasone and a serotonin receptor antagonist, should be administered before amifostine.
      a. Supplied as 500-mg vials
      b. Dose modification. The infusion should be interrupted if systolic blood pressure decreases significantly.
      c. Dose.
        (1) 910 mg/m^2 over 15 minutes, starting 30 minutes before chemotherapy (740 mg/m^2 if hypotension does not correct itself 5 minutes after interrupting the infusion)
        (2) 200 mg/m^2 once daily 15 to 30 minutes before radiation therapy
      d. Drug interactions. Drugs that could potentiate hypotension should not be administered in conjunction with amifostine.
  B. Dexrazoxane (Zinecard, Totect)
    1. Indications. Zinecard is approved to reduce the incidence and severity of anthracycline cardiotoxicity. Totect is approved as an orphan drug to treat anthracycline extravasation.

2. **Pharmacology.** The drug is converted to a chelating agent that interferes with iron-mediated free-radical generation that is thought to be responsible, in part, for anthracycline-induced cardiomyopathy.

3. **Toxicity.** Added myelosuppression that is usually mild and reversible; pain at injection site.

4. **Administration**

   a. **Cardioprotectant dose.** The Zinecard dose is 10 times the doxorubicin dose, which is given within 30 minutes of starting dexrazoxane. This drug can be begun when the patient has received 300 mg/m^2 of doxorubicin and is expected to be continued on that therapy.

   b. **Extravasation dose.** Totect should be given within 6 hours of extravasation at a dose of 1,000 mg/m^2 every 24 hours twice, then 500 mg/m^2 24 hours later once (maximum body surface area is 2 m^2).

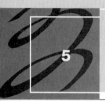

SUPPORTIVE CARE
Eric E. Prommer and Dennis A. Casciato

5

I. PAIN

A. Barriers to optimal pain control. Pain is one of the most common and dreaded symptoms associated with cancer. Its prevalence ranges from 30% to 40% in those getting active therapy to nearly 90% of those with advanced cancer. Uncontrolled pain precludes a satisfactory quality of life. However, advances in pain management techniques have made it possible to control pain in most cancer patients. Barriers that exist to the achievement of optimal analgesia can be divided into patient, physician, and institutional components.

1. Patient-related barriers include

    a. Reluctance to report pain (because of concerns about distracting physicians from treatment of the cancer and fears that pain means that the disease is worse)

    b. Reluctance to follow recommendations (because of concerns about developing tolerance to analgesics)

    c. Fear of addiction (or being thought of as an addict)

    d. Worries about side effects (and the ability to manage them)

    e. Fear of disease progression, injections, and a belief that pain must be accepted

2. Physician barriers include

    a. Failure to appreciate the severity of pain

    b. Knowledge deficit regarding specific treatment for pain (physicians largely underdose patients because of excessive concern about the dose and side effects of narcotics and fear of patient addiction)

3. Institutional barriers for optimal pain management include

    a. Lack of commitment to make pain treatment a priority

    b. Lack of resources

    c. Lack of use of instruments for pain assessment

B. Assessment of pain in cancer patients. Pain is a nonspecific symptom that can result from unrelated benign diseases, effects of treatment, paraneoplastic syndromes, or the direct mechanical effects of the cancer. Pain determined to result from direct mechanical effects of a cancer must be assessed in terms of whether the underlying disease can be treated to relieve the pain. To provide effective pain treatment, an appropriate differential diagnosis must be determined.

1. The following steps should be done in the assessment of cancer pain:

    a. Believe the patient's complaint

    b. Take a history of the pain, which should include the site, quality, onset, exacerbating and relieving features, associated symptoms, impact on quality of life and psychological state, and response to previous and current therapies

    c. Assess the pain as acute, chronic, intermittent, incident, or breakthrough

    d. Prioritize each complaint

    e. Assess for previous history of alcohol or drug dependence

    f. Perform medical and neurologic examinations

    g. Consider diagnostic procedures

    h. Treat and assess response to therapy

    i. Individualize therapy

    j. Communicate with the patient via pain intensity scales

2. **Patient self-assessment** is the most reliable guide to both the cause of the pain and the effectiveness of pain treatment. A log should be kept to track the times that the pain is worst, the intensity of the pain, the times and doses of pain medications or other analgesic measures, and the response to these measures.

   Numeric rating scales are probably the easiest for patients to use. An example is a pain scale of 0 to 10 (0 is for the absence of pain and 10 is for the most severe pain imaginable to the patient). The physician uses the information to adjust dosage and timing of analgesic medications or to change therapy.

3. **Evaluation for depression** is an essential part of pain management. Chronic pain leads to depression, which progressively lowers the pain threshold and creates a positive-feedback cycle of pain and depression. Solicit symptoms of depression, including loss of energy, abnormal sleep patterns, loss of appetite, loss of interest, and decreased ability for cognitive distraction. Some of these symptoms are mistaken for signs of progressive cancer.

C. **Principles of pain management in cancer patients** when the underlying cause cannot be treated effectively

1. **Ideally, the goal of cancer pain management is complete relief of pain.** Even when this is not possible, maximizing pain control improves overall functioning and quality of life.

2. **Pharmacologic step management of cancer pain.** The World Health Organization (WHO) has designed a three-step approach to the systemic management of pain.

   Step 1: Patients with **mild** cancer-related pain can be treated with nonopioid analgesics. These can be combined with other adjuvant analgesics if necessary.

   Step 2: Patients with **moderate** pain, or those who do not get analgesia with the step 1 agent, can be treated with opioids such as hydrocodone or oxycodone conjugated to acetaminophen. Tramadol, a weak opioid with effects on serotonin and norepinephrine uptake, is also a step 2 agent.

   Step 3: Patients with **severe** pain and those who do not get relief with agents appropriate to step 2 should get an opioid designed for moderate to severe pain. This group includes morphine, hydromorphone, methadone, fentanyl, and oxycodone. Newer opioids, such as oxymorphone and its long-acting form (Opana), increase the available step 3 options. These can be combined with a nonopioid analgesic or an adjuvant agent. Sometimes it is necessary to go directly to a step 3 agent.

3. **Intrathecal analgesics** are often used when patients develop intolerable adverse effects to oral opioids or experience inadequate pain relief.

4. **Blocks and neurosurgical procedures** (see section I.I.3)

5. **Localized pharmacologic analgesics and nonpharmacologic interventions for pain,** although not commonly required, are an important part of the armamentarium for pain control. These range from injections of glucocorticoid-lidocaine into isolated painful soft tissue areas to nerve blocks involving ganglia, such as the celiac or hypogastric plexus.

6. **Placebos are never indicated for the treatment of cancer pain** unless the patient is enrolled in a clinical trial in pain management.

7. **Physical dependence and tolerance** are common side effects of prolonged use of opiate analgesics in cancer patients. Terminology is as follows:

   a. **Tolerance** is the need to increase the dose to maintain the same effect. Pharmacologically this is a rightward shift in the dose response curve.

   b. **Physical dependence** is the state where continued administration is necessary to prevent the onset of withdrawal symptoms.

   c. **Psychological dependence** describes compulsive drug-seeking behavior and overwhelming involvement with drug procurement and use.

   d. **Pseudoaddiction** is when the patient with unrelieved pain develops what appears to be drug-seeking behavior to relieve that pain.

8. **Ineffective analgesia** is administered because of the barriers to optimal pain control (section I.A), or persistent pain may mean that the underlying cancer is progressing.

9. **Certain analgesics should be avoided.** Analgesics with mixed agonist and antagonist properties, such as pentazocine (Talwin), should not be used. Likewise, meperidine (Demerol) should not be used because it is not potent, and a risk exists of metabolite accumulation in the setting of renal insufficiency.

D. **Nonnarcotic analgesics,** particularly nonsteroidal anti-inflammatory drugs (NSAID)

1. **Acetaminophen** (AMP, paracetamol, Tylenol and others). As with aspirin, AMP is an antipyretic. Unlike aspirin, AMP has no anti-inflammatory or antiplatelet actions. The starting dose is 650 mg PO q.i.d. and the maximum is 4,000 mg/day.

2. **Salicylates**

   a. **Aspirin** (ASA, acetylsalicylic acid) is the standard against which other NSAIDs are compared. This analgesic is significantly more effective than placebo in patients with pain from cancer. Aspirin should not be used in patients with a history of the syndrome of nasal polyps and asthma, gastritis, peptic ulcer disease, or bleeding diathesis (including severe thrombocytopenia or concomitant use of anticoagulants). Aspirin can inhibit platelet aggregation for 1 week or more.

   b. **Choline magnesium trisalicylate** (Trilisate) is believed to have less gastrointestinal (GI) toxicity than other NSAIDs and no antiplatelet effect, but does have anti-inflammatory properties. The starting dose is 1,500 mg PO once, then 1,000 mg b.i.d. This drug is useful in patients with thrombocytopenia.

3. **Cyclo-oxygenase (COX) inhibitors** can be useful in the treatment of bony metastasis, paraneoplastic fever, and paraneoplastic periosteitis. They are divided into nonselective COX-1 and selective COX-2 inhibitors. COX-1 is present in most tissues, helps maintain gastric mucosa, and influences kidney and platelet function. COX-2 is induced in response to injury and is involved in the inflammatory cascade.

   The nonselective inhibitors can cause gastric ulcers and GI bleeding as well as reversibly affect platelet function. The selective COX-2 inhibitors have relatively reduced the risk of GI toxicity and reduced antiplatelet effect associated with their use. NSAID-induced ulcer disease may be reduced by the coadministration of H_2 blockers or proton pump inhibitors such as omeprazole (Prilosec, 20 mg PO daily). Misoprostol (Cytotec), 100 mcg PO q.i.d. can also ameliorate the GI side effects.

   a. **Nonselective NSAID** that are useful orally include
      (1) **Ibuprofen**, 200 to 800 mg q.i.d. PO
      (2) **Naproxen (Naprosyn)**, 250 to 750 mg b.i.d. PO
      (3) **Ketoprofen (Orudis)**, 50 mg q.i.d. PO
      (4) **Oxaprozin (Daypro)**, 600 to 1,200 mg daily PO
      (5) **Indomethacin (Indocin)**, 25 to 75 mg t.i.d. PO
      (6) **Sulindac (Clinoril)**, 150 to 200 mg b.i.d. PO
      (7) **Diclofenac (Voltaren)**, 50 to 75 mg b.i.d. to t.i.d. PO
      (8) **Piroxicam (Feldene)**, 10 to 20 mg daily PO
      (9) **Nabumetone (Relafen)**, 500 to 1,000 mg b.i.d. PO
      (10) **Etodolac (Lodine)**, 400 to 600 mg b.i.d. PO

   b. **Selective COX-2 inhibitors** include
      (1) **Celecoxib** (Celebrex), 100 to 200 mg once or twice daily PO
      (2) **Rofecoxib** (Vioxx), 50 mg daily PO
      (3) **Meloxicam** (Mobic), 7.5 mg once or twice daily PO

   c. **Ketorolac** (Toradol) is an NSAID available in IM and IV forms. The dose is 30 mg IM or IV once, then 15 mg q6h (not to exceed 5 days).

E. **Adjuvant drugs for cancer pain management**

1. **Corticosteroids** are indicated in refractory neuropathic pain, bone pain, pain associated with capsular distension (painful hepatomegaly), duct obstruction,

headache associated with central nervous system (CNS) metastasis, bowel obstruction, and ascites. The dose in these conditions is largely empiric.

2. **Bisphosphonate infusion** every 4 weeks is the treatment of choice for bone pain and fracture prevention from osteolytic lesions of multiple myeloma. It may also be helpful in controlling bone pain in up to 25% of patients with breast cancer or prostate cancer. Either pamidronate (Aredia, 90 mg IV over 3 hours) or zoledronate (Zometa, 4 mg IV over 15 minutes) can be used.

3. **Anxiolytic agents**

   a. **Benzodiazepines.** Anxious or agitated patients often perceive anxiety as a painful sensation. Diazepam (Valium), alprazolam (Xanax), or lorazepam (Ativan) may be used if narcotic analgesics alone are not effective. These drugs should be avoided in patients with dementia and may produce paradoxical agitated, confusional states in some patients. They may interact with opioids to produce increased somnolence and thus they are looked for first when patients on opioids already develop "opioid" adverse effects, such as increased sedation.

   b. **Antihistamines,** such as hydroxyzine (Atarax, Marax), 25 to 100 mg PO q.i.d., may be useful in the anxious patient as a mild anxiolytic agent with sedating, analgesic, antipruritic, and antiemetic properties.

   c. **Pain can be associated with increased delirium.** Patients with dementia can become agitated and confused when they develop pain. These patients often benefit from a regimen of haloperidol (Haldol), 1 to 3 mg/day, with analgesics. This drug can cause extrapyramidal symptoms, such as Parkinson-like syndromes, torticollis, and swallowing problems. Diphenhydramine (Benadryl) and benztropine mesylate (Cogentin) rapidly reverse extrapyramidal symptoms. Another option in the demented patient who has delirium is to use the newer atypical antipsychotics, such a quetiapine (Seroquel), which have a more favorable side effect profile, at least when it comes to extrapyramidal symptoms.

F. **Neuropathic pain syndromes,** particularly if the pain is lancinating or burning, can often be treated with anticonvulsant drugs alone or in combination with tricyclic antidepressants. These drug combinations are often effective in treatment of peripheral neuralgias, postherpetic neuralgia, and tic douloureux. Gabapentin is considered to be the first-line agent in the treatment of neuropathic pain. Typical doses are as follows:

1. **Antiseizure drugs** used for neuropathic pain

   a. **Gabapentin** (Neurontin), starting dose is 300 mg PO at bedtime (h.s.). The maximal dose is 6,000 mg/day with q.i.d. dosing.

   b. **Phenytoin** (Dilantin), starting dose is 100 mg b.i.d.; titrate upward by 100-mg increments every 3 to 7 days and monitor for side effects.

   c. **Carbamazepine** (Tegretol), starting dose is 100 mg b.i.d.; titrate to toxic level by 100-mg increments every 3 to 7 days.

   d. **Lamotrigine** (Lamictal), 25 mg PO h.s.; increase dose q3d

   e. **Topiramate** (Topamax), 25 mg PO h.s.; increase dose q3d

   f. **Valproic Acid** (Depakote), 200 to 400 mg PO b.i.d. or t.i.d.

   g. **Antidepressant drugs** (see section I.F.2)

2. **Antidepressants** are useful adjuvant analgesics that provide relief at doses below that needed to treat depression. Trials suggesting efficacy have been done in patients with postherpetic neuralgia or diabetic neuropathy. There are few clear studies indicating efficacy in the cancer patient population.

   a. **Tricyclic antidepressants**, which may have lost favor to gabapentin as first-line agents, include amitriptyline (Elavil), desipramine (Norpramin), nortriptyline (Pamelor), doxepin (Sinequan), and imipramine (Tofranil). These are started at 10 to 25 mg h.s. and titrated upward at 10- to 25-mg increments every 5 to 7 days.

   b. **Selective serotonin reuptake inhibitors (SSRIs)** include fluoxetine (Prozac), paroxetine (Paxil), sertraline (Zoloft), citalopram (Celexa), and fluvoxamine (Luvox). These drugs have performed inconsistently in neuropathic pain trials.

    c. **Other antidepressants** include venlafaxine (Effexor), bupropion (Wellbutrin), trazodone (Desyrel), nefazodone (Serzone), and mirtazapine (Remeron). Clinical experience suggests that these agents can be useful, but no controlled clinical trials have established their utility in the treatment of neuropathic pain.

   3. **α-Adrenergic agonists,** such as tizanidine (Zanaflex, 2 mg PO h.s.), may be useful in refractory neuropathic pain but this is based on clinical experience not controlled trials. These agents are most commonly used intrathecally, along with opioids and local anesthetics.

   4. **Systemic local anesthetics**
    a. **IV lidocaine.** Controlled trials suggest that lidocaine is effective in neuropathy associated with diabetes. Response occurs at sub–anti-arrhythmic doses but lasts only a few hours. Response to IV lidocaine may be predictive of a subsequent response to mexiletine.
    b. **Mexiletine** (Mexitil) has been found effective in patients with diabetic neuropathy on the basis of controlled clinical trials. The starting dose is 50 mg t.i.d. PO (taken with meals) with titration upward every 5 to 7 days.

   5. **Topical agents**
    a. **Lidocaine patch, 5%** (Lidoderm). Controlled clinical trials showed efficacy in postherpetic neuralgia. Its use in other conditions is based on anecdotal data. The dose is up to three patches topically (12 hours on and 12 hours off). There are no clinically relevant serum levels.
    b. **Topical capsaicin** (Zostrix) depletes substance P and may act as a counterirritant. Results in trials are mixed for peripheral neuropathy and pain may actually worsen. It is not recommended.
    c. **Topical opioids** are often used for painful ulcerations. Methadone and morphine can be compounded into topical preparations.

G. Opioids alter the unpleasant emotional experience associated with pain and provide pain relief through the interaction with specific opioid receptors. The only significant differences among the various opioids are duration of action and the dose needed to produce the same analgesic effect.

    The best agents are the pure agonists. Agonists or antagonists, such as pentazocine (Talwin), are not effective and should not be used. Meperidine likewise should not be used because it is not potent and its metabolites accumulate in the setting of renal insufficiency. Methadone is being used more often because research has suggested that it works on other receptors involved in pain perception.

    No "ceiling" to opioid doses exists. Doses can be escalated to provide analgesia as long as there are no unacceptable toxicities. Ineffectiveness observed while using opioids usually indicates underdosing; the analgesic effect and the duration of that effect increase as the dose is increased. Ineffectiveness may also reflect progression of the underlying disease.

   1. **Opioids for mild to moderate pain: short-acting opioids** (WHO step 2; there are no step 1 opioids)
    a. **Codeine phosphate:** 60 mg q3–4h PO. Also available as Tylenol #2 (15 mg codeine with AMP), Tylenol #3 (30 mg codeine with AMP), and Tylenol #4 (60 mg codeine with AMP). Do not exceed 4 g/day of AMP. Codeine is rarely used for analgesia as it is especially susceptible to producing constipation. Codeine is one-eighth as potent as morphine.
    b. **Hydrocodone bitartrate** (with ASA or AMP; Lorcet, Lortab, Vicodin): 10 mg q3–4h PO
    c. **Oxycodone hydrochloride** (Roxicodone as single agent or in combination with AMP or ASA as Percocet, Percodan, Tylox): 5 to 10 mg q3–4h PO
    d. **Tramadol (Ultram or Ultracet [with AMP]).** Maximum dose for cancer pain is 300 mg/day. The immediate release form is dosed q6h; the extended release form is dosed q12h.

   2. **Opioids for moderate to severe pain. Short-acting opioids** (WHO steps 2 and 3). Oral immediate release opioids generally have an onset of action of approximately 1 hour and their duration of effect is approximately 4 hours.

a. **Morphine sulfate (MS), immediate release,** is the standard against which all other analgesics are measured. The starting dose of MS in the opioid-naive patient is 4 to 10 mg q3–4h IV and 15 to 30 mg q3–4h PO. MS is available as
  (1) **Tablets and capsules** (MSIR, immediate release MS): 15 and 30 mg
  (2) **Elixirs** (Roxanol): 10 mg/5 mL and 20 mg/mL
  (3) **Rectal suppositories** (RMS): 1, 5, 20, and 30 mg
  (4) **Injectable:** 0.5, 1, 10, and 25 mg/mL concentrations
b. **Hydromorphone** (Dilaudid). Duration of action is 1 to 2 hours, so dosing interval should be q1–3h. Available as
  (1) **Tablets:** 1, 2, 3, 4, and 8 mg
  (2) **Elixir:** 5 mg/5 mL
  (3) **Rectal suppository:** 3 mg
  (4) **Injectables:** 1-, 2-, 3-, 4-, and 10-mg/mL concentrations
c. **Oxycodone hydrochloride:** Considered to be both a step 2 and a step 3 agent. Not available in IV form. Available as:
  (1) **OxyIR, Roxicodone:** 5-mg tablets and capsules
  (2) **Oxyfast:** 20-mg/mL elixir
3. **Long-acting opioids** are usually started after dose titration (achievement of pain relief with short-acting opioids). Analgesic onset is in 3 to 4 hours and lasts for 12 hours. No advantage to q8h dosing, but it is often done. To derive the long-acting opioid dose, divide the total 24-hour immediate-release dose by two. Kadian is the only long-acting opioid that can be crushed, sprinkled, and put in a feeding tube.
  a. **Sustained release morphine:** Available as
    (1) **MS Contin:** 15-, 30-, 60-, 100-, and 200-mg tablets
    (2) **Oramorph SR:** 30-, 60-, and 100-mg tablets
    (3) **Kadian:** 20-, 50-, and 100-mg capsules
  b. **Sustained release oxycodone** is available as **OxyContin** in 10-, 20-, 40-, and 80-mg tablets
  c. **Fentanyl (Duragesic) transdermal patches** : available at delivery rates of 25, 50, 75 and 100 mcg/hour. Therapeutic levels are not reached for 13 to 24 hours. Patches are changed q72h; some patients need the patch changed q48h. The recommended upward dose titration interval is q72h. A 100-mcg patch is equivalent to morphine given IV at 4 mg/hour. Another way to convert fentanyl to morphine and vice-versa is to convert 2 mg of oral morphine for every 1 mcg of fentanyl. Oral transmucosal fentanyl citrate (OTFC) is available in the form of **fentanyl lollipops**. They have a rapid onset of action (minutes) and have been shown to be superior to morphine for "incidental pain." (See below.)
  d. **Methadone** is useful for neuropathic or severe pain. It is also useful when opioids are required in the setting of renal failure. The N-methyl-D-aspartate (NMDA) blocking ability of the drug reverses opioid tolerance. Prospective studies have shown that currently available equianalgesic dosing tables are not accurate when switching from morphine to methadone. The dosing interval should not be less than q8h. The dose may be as little as 5% to 10% of the MS dose, especially in patients on chronic MS therapy.
  e. **Oxymorphone.** Originally used as rectal form (Numorphan suppository), this drug is now available in oral form. The immediate release form is unique in that it has a half-life of approximately 6 hours. A long-acting form is available (Opana). The drug is slightly more potent than morphine (1.2 times),
4. **Side effects of opioids**
  a. **GI effects** include constipation, nausea, and vomiting. Define a prophylactic regimen for constipation and for nausea when the first opioid prescription is written.
    (1) **Constipation** is the most common adverse effect of opioids. It is caused by the opioid effect on motility, as well as decreased pancreatic, biliary,

gastric, and intestinal secretions. Tolerance to this side effect usually does not occur (see section IV.A.5).

(2) Nausea and vomiting caused by opioids is owing to stimulation of the chemoreceptor trigger zone. Thus, antiemetics with antidopaminergic properties are indicated. Agents such as prochlorperazine (Compazine), metoclopramide (Reglan), and haloperidol (Haldol) are good choices.

b. CNS side effects. Morphine-3-glucuronide is the morphine metabolite implicated in the development of CNS toxicity. Other manifestations of CNS toxicity include sedation, hallucinations, delirium, and myoclonus.

(1) Sedation is more common in the opioid naive patient. It rarely lasts more than 48 to 72 hours. If persistent, methylphenidate, 5 mg at 8 AM and at noon, or modafinil 200 mg/day may be useful.

(2) Myoclonus (spontaneous jerking movements) can occur in up to 45% of patients. This is an adverse effect seen with chronic opioid use. Treatment options include opioid dose reduction if pain is well controlled, opioid rotation if pain is poorly controlled, or adding clonazepam (Klonopin, 0.5 to 1 mg) or diazepam (Valium, 2 mg) PO q12h.

c. Respiratory depression is unusual and usually only occurs in patients who are either having rapid dose escalation or are in renal failure (due to accumulation of morphine-6-glucuronide). Respiratory depression is not common because morphine does not have good bioavailability and pain is an antidote to respiratory depression. Respiratory depression can occur when pain is rapidly reduced, such as after a nerve block, or after the addition of adjuvant analgesics. It can also occur when MS is given with other CNS depressants. Treatment is by dose reduction, such as stopping the infusion for 2 hours and then restarting at half the dose, or holding one or two doses of opioids and then restarting at a lower dose if possible.

d. Other side effects of opioids include

(1) Noncardiogenic pulmonary edema occurs with rapid dose escalation and may be related to capillary permeability changes secondary to opioid release of histamine.

(2) Xerostomia is common with concomitant use of antidepressants and anticholinergic agents. Treatment includes sodium bicarbonate rinses or pilocarpine.

(3) Urinary retention is caused by the anticholinergic effects of opioids.

(4) SIADH (syndrome of inappropriate antidiuretic hormone) can be caused by opioids.

(5) Endocrine: hypothyroidism and hypercalcemia potentiate the CNS effects of opioids.

(6) Dermatologic: pruritis is more commonly seen with intrathecal opioids

5. Drug interactions with opioids

a. Potentiators of MS effect generally work by interfering with morphine metabolism. These agents include H_2 blockers, antidepressants, phenothiazines, and antianxiety agents.

b. Agents that decrease MS effect generally induce the metabolism of morphine. These agents include phenytoin, barbiturates, and rifampin.

c. MS effect on other agents. Morphine can increase gabapentin levels and reduce ciprofloxacin levels.

6. Management of narcotic withdrawal. The intensity of withdrawal symptoms is usually proportional to the duration of physical dependence. Symptoms develop within 2 to 48 hours after the last dose and usually peak at 72 hours. Opioid withdrawal is less life-threatening and dangerous than withdrawal from other classes of controlled drugs. Reassurance, education, and perhaps mild sedatives may be all that is required for patients who develop physical dependence during hospitalization and who are not going to continue on the drugs. Small doses of clonidine, 0.05 to 0.1 mg PO t.i.d. (or weekly skin patches), may reduce symptoms of withdrawal, especially tremors, hypertension, anxiety, and fevers.

H. Administration of analgesics

1. **Opioid dosage.** There is no maximum dose or ceiling to MS or other opioids. As the dose is increased, analgesic effects increase. Increments in dosing are always balanced by monitoring for side effects. Once stable drug levels are achieved with immediate-release dosing, the patient can be switched to a long-acting agent. Rescue doses for breakthrough pain with immediate-release agents are made available as needed (p.r.n.). With elderly patients, "go low and go slow" taking into account age-related sensitivity to opioids as well as age-related reductions in renal function.

   a. **Dose-finding for oral opioids.** The oral route is preferred because oral opioids can control pain in patients with advanced cancer 80% to 90% of the time. Doses are given regularly ("around the clock" [ATC]) and supplemental medications are provided p.r.n.

   In the opioid naive patient, the initial dose of MS can be from 5 to 30 mg depending on the severity of pain. This dose is started at q4h. The p.r.n. dose is approximately 50% of the q4h dose and is provided once during the 4-hour dosing interval. The optimal dose is one that relieves the patient's pain (to <4 on a 10-point scale) without causing side effects. In the elderly patient, it is always best to "go low" and "go slow." This means lower starting doses and increased dosing intervals.

   Once the optimal dose is found, the total opioid amount is calculated and then divided by two to yield the q12h, long-acting dose. The q2–4h p.r.n. dose is approximately 10% to 20% of the total 24-hour dose.

   b. **Dose finding for parenteral agents.** In the opioid naive patient with severe pain, initial MS doses of 2 to 4 mg IV or SQ can be given every 15 minutes as necessary to control pain. When pain is controlled, the dose given over a 2- to 4-hour interval becomes the q4h dose and the p.r.n. dose (50% of the ATC dose) is given q1–2h.

   c. **Need for frequent p.r.n. doses.** Patients needing more than four p.r.n. opioid doses per day most likely need an increase in the ATC dose. The ATC dose can be increased by 25% to 50% and adjustments of the p.r.n. dose can be made.

   d. **Incident pain.** Pain with turning, bathing, and transporting can be managed with p.r.n. doses or more generous p.r.n. doses at the time the patient is likely to experience the incident pain.

   e. **Equianalgesic tables** represent rough guidelines that are based on single-dose studies in otherwise healthy patients. The potency ratio of oral MS to oral hydromorphone is 5:1 (5 mg of MS is equivalent to 1 mg of hydromorphone orally). The potency ratio for IV or SQ MS to hydromorphone is 7:1 (7 mg of MS is equivalent to 1 mg of hydromorphone IV or SQ). Oxycodone potency ranges from 1:1 to 1.5:1 compared with MS. Equianalgesic tables are not useful when converting from other step 3 opioids to methadone.

2. **Subcutaneous opioids** are reserved for those who cannot use the oral route for pain administration or who need rapid onset of analgesia. SQ dosing is identical to IV dosing. The limiting feature of this route is the infusion rate; in general, the SQ route can absorb up to 3 mg/hour; with larger volumes, hyaluronidase (Wydase) can be given. The shoulder, abdomen, and thigh are ideal sites for infusion.

3. **Pumps** for patient-controlled analgesia (PCA) are occasionally useful for cancer patients. Begin with a 2- to 5-mg dose of MS with a delay interval of 10 minutes ("lockout"); the patient can thus receive this dose up to six times an hour. The amount given over 4 hours is determined and converted to an hourly dose. The new, every 10 minute *demand dose* becomes 50% of the hourly dose. For patients already on MS, the same method is used except that the 24-hour dose is converted to an hourly dose and then a new demand dose can be formulated.

4. **Intravenous opioids** are reserved for patients who cannot be given opioids by the oral route. It is also ideal for rapid titration of doses. Dosing is based on current analgesic requirements. The usual conversion from oral MS to SQ or

IV MS is to divide the total oral requirement by three with this representing the total IV dose. This amount can be divided by 24 to give hourly rates.

5. Epidural and intrathecal anesthesia are considered when oral and parenteral routes have proven ineffective and/or there is excessive toxicity associated with opioid use.

  a. Epidural analgesia. A catheter is placed close to the involved dermatome. The type of delivery system depends on prognosis of the patient. Tumor invasion of the spine is not a contraindication, because most tumors involve the body of the vertebra and not the spinous process. To calculate the epidural dose from an oral dose, divide the total 24-hour oral dose by 10. To calculate the epidural dose from an SQ dose, divide the total 24 hour SQ dose by 5. Analgesia can be improved when combined with bupivacaine (Marcaine) or clonidine. The addition of these agents is indicated for neuropathic pain, dysesthetic pain, midline pain below the umbilicus, or pain involving the sacral plexus.

  b. Intrathecal analgesia has more effective pain control, uses less opioid, and has less incidence of catheter occlusion than the epidural route. Doses for intrathecal administration are 10% of the epidural doses.

6. Other routes for opioids

  a. Rectal administration can also be used if the oral route is not available. The oral–rectal potency ratio is 1:1.

  b. Sublingual and buccal administration can be used if the oral route is not available. Ideal agents for this route are the more lipophilic opioids such as fentanyl (Actiq) lollipops and methadone. These agents have a greater Buccal or sublingual bioavailability than MS. The buccal–oral potency ratio is 1:1.

  c. Topical opioids have been used for painful ulcerative lesions, cutaneous pain from tumor infiltration, and oral mucositis. It is available in a 1 mg/mL gel vehicle.

I. Other methods of pain management

1. Psychological methods of pain control. Behavioral modification, although not generally effective for moderate to severe chronic cancer pain, may be helpful for mild pain. Operant conditioning, hypnosis, guided imagery, and biofeedback are techniques that can be helpful for chronic mild pain, such as postoperative chest wall pain. *Cognitive distraction* is a useful adjunct for mild pain. These techniques can help patients restore self-control and act in a way that participates in their own care.

2. Physical methods of pain control, such as hot or cold packs for muscle and joint pain, various types of massage therapy, and exercise programs, may be helpful additions to drug therapy in patients with mild to moderate chronic pain syndromes, but are generally ineffective in treatment of severe cancer pain.

  Transcutaneous electrical nerve stimulation (TENS) has demonstrated efficacy in the treatment of malignant disease, but the problems encountered were waning effect and sudden termination of effect. The results of clinical trials on acupuncture have been conflicting; retrospective data suggest that any efficacy of acupuncture for cancer pain is short lived.

3. Neuroablative procedures are considered when standard pain management methods and intraspinal analgesia have failed. These procedures are not for patients who have a short life expectancy or are in poor physical condition.

  a. Unilateral chordotomy is the most effective neuroablative procedure and is particularly useful for patients with unilateral cancer pain below the shoulder. Radiofrequency lesions to spinothalamic tracts of the spinal cord are generally placed at the C-1 to C-2 level.

  Contralateral loss of superficial, deep, and visceral pain is produced in >75% of patients treated with percutaneous chordotomy. The duration of analgesia is limited to only a few months; incapacitating dysesthesia may develop after several months. In experienced hands, unilateral chordotomy is associated with low morbidity and mortality and minimal incidence of motor weakness or loss of bladder function. Sleep apnea, fecal and urinary incontinence, loss of orgasm, and muscle weakness, on the other hand, frequently complicate bilateral chordotomy.

b. Nerve blocks may be useful in patients with pain restricted to a single somatic nerve or adjacent nerves (e.g., postthoracotomy pain may be relieved by subcostal blocks). Short-acting local anesthetics are initially used to determine the location for a permanent procedure.

c. Celiac plexus nerve block is effective in up to 85% of patients for treating upper abdominal visceral pain, particularly from cancers of the pancreas or stomach. The procedure is often accomplished with needle placement under CT or fluoroscopic guidance. It can also be performed endoscopically or at the time of laparotomy. Pretreatment hydration and postoperative observation for 4 to 6 hours (with fluid replacement as necessary) can prevent transient hypotension from this procedure.

d. Lumbar sympathetic blockade can be attempted for pelvic visceral pain. This procedure affects sphincter tone or lower extremity strength uncommonly.

e. Dorsal root entry zone lesions involve the destruction of dorsal horn neurons. It has been used to treat nonmalignant conditions such as brachial plexus avulsions, postparaplegic and postquadraplegic pain, and postamputation pain. Postherpetic neuralgia also responds to this procedure. Its usefulness in cancer pain needs to be studied further.

It is performed under general anesthesia. Proper placement of the lesion (in the cord) is important and can be difficult. Poor performance status, bleeding diathesis, infection, and poor cardiopulmonary reserve are contraindications to the procedure.

f. Intracranial procedures, such as medullary or pontine tractotomy, thalamotomy, cingulotomy, and hypophysectomy, are rarely performed.

II. ORAL SYMPTOMS

A. Stomatitis from chemotherapy can develop 2 to 10 days after treatment with many cytotoxic agents and during RT to the head or neck. Resolution of symptoms usually occurs 2 to 3 weeks after completion of therapy but may persist longer. Sucking on ice chips or popsicles during the short infusion of certain cytotoxic agents (e.g., methotrexate, 5-fluorouracil) or taking oral glutamine preparations may prevent the development of stomatitis.

1. Aggravating factors include poor oral hygiene (gingivitis, poorly maintained dentures), xerostomia, age- or RT-related mucous membrane atrophy, and aerobic or anaerobic bacterial infections. Infection with *Candida* sp. or herpesvirus can complicate or be confused with chemotherapeutic stomatitis; the index of suspicion for the infections is increased in patients with acquired immunodeficiency syndrome (AIDS) and in those taking high-dose or long-term glucocorticoids.

2. Symptoms and signs. Stomatitis is usually first noted by the patient as sensitivity to citrus juice, hot food, or spicy food. Erythema and then aphthous ulcers develop. In severe cases, lesions progress to extensive ulceration and sloughing of the oral mucosa. *Candida albicans* or herpesvirus infection can have a similar appearance and must be considered if the mouth lesions are longer lasting or recognized by their characteristic appearance.

3. Management of stomatitis. The following measures may relieve symptoms:

a. Avoid foods that trigger the pain

b. Abstain from alcohol

c. Suck on popsicles and cold beverages

d. Frequently rinse the mouth with solutions of saline or baking soda

e. Swish and expectorate certain commercial suspensions

    (1) Ulcerease: glycerin, sodium bicarbonate, and sodium borate

    (2) BAX: lidocaine, diphenhydramine, sorbitol, and Mylanta

    (3) Stomafate: sucralfate, Benylin syrup, and Maalox

    (4) Gelclair: contains none of the above ingredients; use undiluted

    f. Formulations: rinse with 15 mL four to six times per day

      (1) Mix 30 mL each of diphenhydramine hydrochloride (Benadryl, 12.5 mg/ 5 mL), viscous xylocaine (2%), and Maalox

      (2) Mix 30 mL of Benadryl (12.5 mg/5 mL), 60 mL of tetracycline or penicillin (125 mg/5 mL), 45 mL of nystatin oral suspension (100,000 U/mL), 30 mL of 2% viscous lidocaine, 30 mL of hydrocortisone suspension (10 mg/5 mL), and 45 mL sterile water for irrigation

  g. Medications

    (1) Viscous 2% lidocaine (Xylocaine), 10 to 15 mL for 30 seconds before meals and q2h p.r.n.

    (2) Sucralfate (Carafate), 1 g q.i.d.

    (3) Opioids, especially parenteral opioids or Fentanyl lollipops (Actiq), may be useful. Elixirs may not be helpful because they contain alcohol, which can exacerbate mucositis.

    (4) Appropriate antimicrobial treatment for bacterial, monilial, or herpesvirus infections

B. Xerostomia

  1. Causes. Xerostomia is a complication of RT to the head and neck area but also may be caused by commonly used medications (e.g., antihistamines and opioids) and by mouth breathing. The severity depends on the volume of exposed salivary glands, dosage, and location. Radiation decreases the amount of saliva produced, and alters the enzymatic content, pH, and viscosity of saliva. This can lead to the development of caries. Therapy consists of the following options:

  2. Management of xerostomia

    a. Maintain good oral hygiene and hydration

    b. Amifostine ethyol, 200 mg/m^2 IV over 15 to 30 minutes before radiation dose. Saliva production at 1 year was greater in those getting the treatment. Adverse effects include nausea and vomiting, but it is not certain whether the cancer may be protected by this drug as well.

    c. Saliva substitutes (e.g., Xerolube, Salivart, synthetic saliva spray) and Biotene chewing gum

    d. Pilocarpine, 5 to 10 mg PO t.i.d. given before radiation starts. Pilocarpine is contraindicated in patients with glaucoma or asthma.

    e. Others: hard candies (e.g., Life Savers, cinnamon, lemon drops), sugarless chewing gum, ice cubes

C. Taste alterations can occur as a reduction in taste sensitivity (hypogeusia), a distortion of taste (dysgeusia), or the absence of taste (ageusia). Patients with advanced cancer frequently lose taste for red meat, even without anticancer therapies.

  1. Causes of taste alterations include carcinomatous involvement of the mouth, head and neck surgery, and CNS lesions. Dental pathology, poor oral hygiene, endocrine factors (hypothyroidism, hypophysectomy, adrenalectomy), stomatitis, xerostomia, malnutrition, drugs, and metabolic disturbances are other causes.

    a. Chemotherapy can cause alterations in taste. Agents reported to cause taste alterations include bleomycin, cisplatinum, gemcitibine, interferon gamma, leuprolide, tamoxifen, docetaxel, and etoposide.

    b. RT can alter taste by reducing and altering salivary gland output. Taste sensitivity to sweets is the least affected; sensitivity to bitter and salty is most affected. At 2,000 cGy and upward, taste loss increases rapidly. Taste acuity can partially return after 20 to 60 days. Taste can be fully restored 2 to 4 months following RT. Zinc, 25 mg PO q.i.d. before RT was reported to lessen hypogeusia, but controlled trials subsequently did not support this finding.

  2. Management of taste dysfunction includes

    a. Maintain good oral hygiene

    b. Search for medications that can alter taste such as amphotericin, allopurinol, β-lactam antibiotics, chlorhexidene mouthwash, and pentamidine

    c. Reduce the urea content (bitterness) of the diet by eating white meats, eggs, and dairy products

d. Mask the bitter taste of urea-containing foods by marinating meats, using more and stronger seasonings, eating food at cold or room temperatures, and drinking more liquids

e. Help overcome general poor taste by eating foods that are tart (lemonade frozen in ice trays, pickles, vinegar) or that leave their own taste (fruit, lemon drops, hard candy)

D. Halitosis occurs when exhaled air is combined with foul-smelling substances from the respiratory or GI tract. The exact incidence is unknown.

  1. Causes of halitosis include diseases of the oral cavity, infections of the respiratory tract, diseases of the digestive tract, metabolic failure (diabetic ketoacidosis, uremia, and hepatic insufficiency), drugs (anything that can cause xerostomia, chemotherapy and RT, opioids), and foods (garlic, onions, meat, and fish).

  2. Management of halitosis includes

  a. Optimal dental hygiene and hydration

  b. Gentle brushing of tongue with a soft toothbrush (the back of the tongue in particular collects malodorous bacteria)

  c. Mouthwash, breath-freshening tablets

  d. Treat infections appropriately

  e. Prokinetic drugs for gastric stasis if indicated

E. Dysphagia is difficulty in transferring solids and liquids from the mouth to the stomach.

  1. Causes of dysphagia include cancer infiltration or fibrosis of the esophagus, external compression, motor neuron damage, cranial nerve involvement by tumor, cerebellar damage, or neuromuscular dysfunction. Treatment (RT, chemotherapy), drugs (neuroleptics, anticholinergic agents), surgery, concurrent disease, and symptoms associated with advanced cancer (dry mouth, candida infections) are other causes of dysphagia. Treatment options depend on the patient's prognosis. In patients with advanced cancer and a very short prognosis it may not be appropriate to subject a patient to IV hydration or feeding tubes. In the patient who has a new diagnosis or who is having a slow decline, the following options are available:

  2. Management of dysphagia. After there is agreement about treatment and feeding goals, treatment possibilities include the following:

  a. Evaluate aspiration for any reason with a videofluoroscopic barium swallow study and fibroendoscopy. Speech therapists could then work with dietitians to design foods with the proper consistency for safe swallowing and sufficient caloric intake.

  b. Palliating an obstructed esophagus from esophageal cancer (See Chapter 9, section VI.B)

  c. If an esophageal stent becomes blocked, the patient should sip small amounts of water and, every 30 minutes, dilute hydrogen peroxide. Alternatively, the tube can be flushed with cola.

  d. Strictures from RT require gradual dilation by experienced gastroenterologists. Antireflux regimens or reduction of stomach acid with famotidine (Pepcid), 10 mg b.i.d., or intermittent 4-week courses of omeprazole (Prilosec), 20 to 40 mg each morning, may be helpful.

  e. Excessive saliva production when total esophageal obstruction produces sialorrhea and drooling can be treated with anticholinergics, alum mouthwashes, or irradiation of the salivary glands (400 to 1,000 cGy).

  f. Nutritional support for chemotherapy or RT can be optimized for the short term with the use of feeding tubes. Patients of advanced age, with CNS disease, and low serum albumin are at high risk for early mortality and a feeding tube may not be appropriate.

III. NAUSEA AND VOMITING
  A. Causes
  1. Differential diagnosis. Nausea and vomiting in cancer patients occur most often as a result of cytotoxic chemotherapy. Other causes of nausea and vomiting

include elevated intracranial pressure, anxiety, bowel obstruction, constipation, opioids, RT, benign gastric disease, metabolic abnormalities (hypercalcemia, renal or hepatic failure), autonomic dysfunction, and other drugs (e.g., NSAIDs and digoxin).

2. Cytotoxic drugs that are highly emetic include cisplatin, dactinomycin, anthracyclines; dacarbazine, nitrosoureas, nitrogen mustard, and high-dose cyclophosphamide (see Appendix B-1). The mechanisms for nausea and vomiting from chemotherapy are poorly defined but appear usually to be mediated by the CNS; some drugs may have peripheral activity. Acute chemotherapy-induced vomiting typically occurs 1 to 2 hours after treatment and usually resolves in 24 hours. Subacute vomiting occurs 9 to 18 hours after giving chemotherapy. Delayed vomiting occurs 48 to 72 hours after giving cisplatin (especially with doses of 100 mg/m^2 or more) and diminishes in 1 to 3 days. Cyclophosphamide can also cause delayed nausea and vomiting; the peak occurs approximately 24 hours after administration.

3. Psychological and behavioral factors may induce or modify vomiting. Patients may vomit even before receiving chemotherapy (anticipatory vomiting) when the IV line is started, the syringe is seen, or even before leaving home on the day chemotherapy is scheduled. Emesis is more easily controlled, on the other hand, in patients with a history of chronic heavy alcohol use.

B. Management of nausea and vomiting

1. Prevention of vomiting. It is best to prevent nausea and vomiting with adequate doses of antiemetics, particularly when chemotherapy drugs known to induce vomiting are used.

  a. Serotonin receptor (5-HT3) antagonists bind to type 3 receptors of serotonin (5-hydroxytryptamine [5-HT]) and are the drugs of choice to prevent emesis generated by highly emetic regimens. 5-HT3 blockers alone achieve complete abrogation of emesis in about 60% of patients and achieve major control of emesis in 75% of patients.

    (1) Dosage. The following agents have about the same effectiveness and improved efficacy with the addition of a corticosteroid, and they are given 30 to 60 minutes before chemotherapy:

      (a) Ondansetron (Zofran), 8 or 32 mg IV (0.125 mg/kg)

      (b) Granisetron (Kytril), 0.01 mg (10 mcg)/kg IV or 1 mg PO

      (c) Dolasetron (Anzemet), 100 mg IV or PO

      (d) Palonosetron (Aloxi), 0.25 mg IV over 30 seconds, for acute *and* delayed nausea and vomiting

    (2) Side effects are mild headache, constipation, and transient transaminase elevations. Extrapyramidal side effects do not occur.

  b. Metoclopramide (Reglan), a procainamide derivative, acts both centrally (at the chemoreceptor trigger zone as a dopamine antagonist) and peripherally (by stimulating gastric and small bowel motility, thereby preventing gastric stasis and dilation). At high doses, metoclopramide also blocks 5-HT receptors.

    (1) Dose: 1 to 3 mg/kg IV q2h for two to six doses

    (2) Side effects include mild sedation, dystonic reactions (especially in young patients), akathisia (restlessness), and diarrhea. The drug is given with lorazepam, diphenhydramine, and corticosteroids to prevent these complications.

  c. Corticosteroids are effective for treating chemotherapy-induced vomiting by themselves or with 5-HT3 blockers. Recommended dosages are as follows:

    (1) Dexamethasone, 10 to 20 mg IV for one or two doses

    (2) Methylprednisolone, 125 mg IV for one or two doses

  d. Lorazepam (Ativan), 1 or 2 mg IV or sublingually q3–6h, is very useful in patients who are treated with emetogenic chemotherapy or who have refractory or anticipatory vomiting. The drug's amnesic effect is also helpful.

2. Agents used for nausea
   a. Cannabinoids. Δ-9-tetrahydrocannabinol (THC) is the main active ingredient in marijuana and can relieve nausea and vomiting in some patients who do not respond to other antiemetic drugs. The drug should be prescribed cautiously for elderly patients and not at all for patients with cardiovascular or psychiatric illness. Cannabinoids are not as effective as serotonin inhibitors and they have frequent side effects.
   (1) Dose
      (a) THC, 2.5 to 10 mg PO q3–4h, is available as Marinol in 2.5-, 5.0-, and 10-mg capsules.
      (b) Nabilone (Cesamet) is a cannabinoid that is now approved by the FDA for patients with nausea and vomiting who have not responded to conventional antiemetics. The dose is 1 mg PO b.i.d. to 2 mg t.i.d., beginning 1 to 3 hours before starting chemotherapy.
   (2) Side effects include orthostatic hypotension, sedation, dry mouth, ataxia, dizziness, euphoria, and dysphoria. Maintaining a "high" is correlated with the antiemetic effect in younger patients.
   b. Scopolamine (Transderm Scop). Patches are changed q3d.
   c. Phenothiazines
      (1) Prochlorperazine (Compazine), 5 to 20 mg PO q4–6h
      (2) Thiethylperazine (Torecan), 10 mg PO t.i.d.
   d. Haloperidol (Haldol), 0.5 to 1.0 mg PO q4–12h
   e. Metoclopramide (Reglan), 10 to 20 mg PO q6–8h (if gastric stasis is suspected)
3. Delayed vomiting, occurring 1 to 2 days after treatment, is most often seen after high doses of cisplatin and is difficult to treat. The following may be tried:
   a. Dexamethasone alone: 8 mg b.i.d. PO for 2 days, then 4 mg b.i.d. for 2 days
   b. Metoclopramide: 0.5 mg/kg q.i.d. PO for 2 days with dexamethasone
   c. Ondansetron: 4 or 8 mg b.i.d. to t.i.d. for 3 days with or without dexamethasone
   d. Aprepitant (Emend) is a NK-1 receptor antagonist that blocks substance P and has been shown to decrease delayed nausea and vomiting by 20%. It is given for 3 days with a 5-HT3 inhibitor and dexamethasone. Give 125 mg PO 1 hour before chemotherapy on day 1, and then give 80 mg PO on the mornings of the second and third days of the chemotherapy cycle.
   e. Palonosetron (Aloxi) (see above for dosing)
4. Anticipatory vomiting is exceedingly difficult to palliate. Prevention of emesis when chemotherapy is first given is the best way to prevent anticipatory vomiting. Antiemetics should be prescribed generously, and chemotherapy should be given as late in the day as possible. Symptoms may improve with the following:
   a. Sedatives, including antihistamines or benzodiazepines
   b. Hypnosis by an experienced psychologist
   c. Progressive muscle relaxation, which involves learning to relax by actively tensing and then relaxing specific muscle groups
   d. Cognitive distraction
   e. Relaxation techniques with guided imagery
   f. Operant conditioning (e.g., patients may be treated in an area and on a day different from their usual place and time)

IV. COLORECTAL SYMPTOMS
A. Constipation is extremely common in patients with advanced cancer. Straining, hard stools, infrequent stools, and abdominal discomfort associated with attempts at having a bowel movement are some of the ways it is described.
   1. Causes of constipation include
      a. Causes directly related to cancer such as bowel obstruction, spinal cord compression, and hypercalcemia

    b. Causes owing to the secondary effects of cancer such as weakness, inactivity, confusion, depression, dehydration, and lack of privacy

    c. Drugs, such as opioids, anticholinergics (antidepressants), antacids, anticonvulsants (Tegretol), antiemetics (5-HT3 inhibitors), chemotherapeutic agents (e.g., vincristine and thalidomide), abused laxatives, and barium from oral contrast radiographic studies

    d. Concurrent disease, such as diabetes, hypothyroidism, anal canal disorders, and diverticulitis

2. Evaluation of the constipated cancer patient requires performing a rectal examination. If hard stools are present, institute stool softeners; manual disimpaction may be needed. If soft stool is present, a stimulatory drug may be needed. If there is no stool, a stimulatory drug may be beneficial. Evidence is that a combination of a softener and a stimulatory drug may be the best approach. Abdominal radiographs may be needed to exclude bowel obstruction.

3. Prophylactic measures include maintaining activity, hydration, fiber in the diet (within reason), and privacy for the patient. Review the patient's medication list for potentially offending agents.

4. Preparations available include the following:

    a. Bulk producers (e.g., Metamucil, Konsyl) are normalizers rather than true laxatives. They must be taken with adequate water; if not, a viscous mass may form leading to obstruction. Their taste is unacceptable. Their effectiveness in severe constipation has not been demonstrated. (We do not use these agents.)

    b. Stool softeners, which are useful in the presence of hard stool, include

        (1) Docusate sodium (Colace): 50- and 100-mg capsules

        (2) Docusate calcium (Surfak): 50- and 240-mg capsules

    c. Bowel stimulants, which are useful if there is soft stool, include

        (1) Senna, sennosides (Senokot): 8.6-mg tablet (or syrup); starting dose is 15 mg h.s.

        (2) Bisacodyl (Dulcolax): 5-mg tablet, 10-mg suppository; starting dose is 10 mg PO h.s.

    d. Commercial combinations include sennosides and docusate sodium (Senokot-S), casanthranol and docusate sodium (Peri-Colace), danthron and docusate sodium (Doxidan), and many others

    e. Lubricant laxatives have little role in chronic constipation and are mainly useful for acute impaction:

        (1) Mineral oil, which is given as enema

        (2) Liquid paraffin, 10 mL PO daily

    f. Osmotic laxatives draw fluid into the bowel:

        (1) Lactulose (Cephulac), starting dose is 15 to 20 mL b.i.d.

        (2) Saline laxatives exert an osmotic effect drawing fluid into the lumen, which can lead to sodium overload, and should not be used in patients with renal failure. Examples are magnesium hydroxide (Milk of Magnesia), magnesium citrate, and sodium phosphates (Fleet Phospho Soda).

    g. Rectal laxatives are undignified for the patient, but often give good results. Their mechanisms of action parallel the oral agents. They consist of

        (1) Lubricant rectal laxatives, such as oil retention enemas, are good for fecal impaction.

        (2) Osmotic laxatives, such as glycerin suppositories

        (3) Saline laxatives, such as Fleet Phospho Soda enema

5. Prevention and management of narcotic-induced constipation. Patients who are receiving regular dosages of narcotics (or neuropathic chemotherapy agents such as vincristine) should be carefully questioned about bowel movements. They should be encouraged to drink liquids (e.g., water, prune juice, coffee) and to eat bran cereal daily.

    These measures plus stool softeners are usually insufficient, however, and bulk producers are poorly tolerated. The combination of a stool softener and a bowel stimulant in parallel increasing doses is recommended to prevent opioid-induced constipation. Brand name preparations (e.g., Senokot-S, Peri-Colace) can cost 10 times more than generic preparations of these agents.

    a. All patients starting on opioids should have senna or Dulcolax available to take h.s. Start all patients on two tablets of senna h.s.

    b. If no response occurs, increase the dosage to two, three, or four tablets b.i.d. or t.i.d. as needed, or switch to Dulcolax, two tablets PO h.s. (or to t.i.d. if needed). Add sorbitol, 15 to 30 mL b.i.d., if needed. Reevaluate patients for other causes of constipation.

    c. If these measures fail, consider a saline laxative.

    d. The management of opioid-induced constipation that is refractory to laxatives has been treated with oral naloxone, methylnaltrexone, and prokinetic agents, such as subcutaneous metoclopramide. Oral naloxone can reverse opioid-induced constipation without precipitating withdrawal because of its extensive hepatic first-pass metabolism, which leads to low plasma levels. Suggested starting doses are

        (1) Oral naloxone, 0.8 mg PO b.i.d. with titration upward every 2 to 3 days, monitoring for laxative effect and withdrawal

        (2) Methylnaltrexone and **alvimopan** (Entrareg) are being evaluated for opioid-induced bowel syndrome

        (3) Metoclopramide, 10 mg SQ q6h

B. Rectal discharge can be caused by hemorrhoids, fecal impaction, tumor, radiation proctitis, and various rectal fistulas. After addressing the primary cause, inflammation may be reduced with corticosteroid suppositories or enemas. The skin of the perineum and genitalia must be protected and kept clean (without soap) and dry.

C. Enterocutaneous fistulas can be managed in the same manner as for surgical stomas with colostomy or ileostomy bags. The direction and advice of a stomal therapist are often warranted.

    1. The skin surrounding the fistulae rapidly breaks down and limits bag attachment. Débrided skin should be kept clean using water with or without a mild soap; detergents and disinfectants aggravate the skin condition. Glucocorticoid creams (not ointments) can be used for local inflammation, and triple-antibiotic cream can be used for infected areas. Several sealants are available to protect the skin from fistula discharge, including newer plastic coverings that permit air but not liquids to reach the skin and sprays, such as Opsite.

    2. Unless the volume of fecal material is large, it is sometimes possible to place a urinary catheter into the stoma, after assessing the anatomy by retrograde barium studies. The catheter can be used as a temporizing measure until abraded skin is sufficiently healed to provide secure attachment for a colostomy appliance.

D. Distal colon and rectal cancerous fistulas involving the bladder or vagina are best managed by a more proximal colostomy. This stops all drainage and allows long-term healing of inflamed tissues.

E. Chemotherapy-induced diarrhea (CID) can be debilitating and potentially life-threatening. The risk for CID is significantly greater with regimens that contain fluoropyrimidines or irinotecan. The cause of diarrhea is most likely a multifactorial process that results in an imbalance between absorption and secretion in the small bowel. Irinotecan causes both an acute and a delayed type of diarrhea. The acute onset type is cholinergic in nature, occurs in the first 24 hours, and responds to atropine (0.25 to 1.0 mg IV). The late onset diarrhea occurs 3 to 11 days after treatment.

    The opioids loperamide (Imodium) and diphenoxylate (Lomotil) are most commonly used for CID. These agents reduce diarrhea by decreasing peristalsis in the small and large intestines. NSAIDs, clonidine, and cyproheptadine control the diarrhea associated with bowel inflammation, bronchogenic carcinoma, and carcinoid syndrome, respectively. Octreotide is effective in controlling the diarrhea associated with islet cell carcinomas, acquired immunodeficiency syndrome (AIDS), and other secretory diarrheal syndromes. Octreotide also controls severe CID, but the optimal dose quantity and duration is unsettled, and the drug is expensive. The basis for treatment of CID is mostly anecdotal. Recommendations are as follows:

    1. Avoid certain food products: milk and dairy products, spicy foods, alcohol, caffeine, prune and orange juices, high-fiber foods, and high-fat foods.

2. **Avoid certain medications:** laxatives, stool softeners, and promotility agents (metoclopramide, cisapride).
3. **Evaluate stool** for the presence of fecal leukocytes and pathogenic microbes in patients with persistent or severe diarrhea; treat accordingly.
4. **Low-grade diarrhea** [National Cancer Institute (NCI) grades 1 and 2; see Appendix B-2].
   a. Observe for and correct any fluid and electrolyte imbalances
   b. Loperamide given as an initial 4-mg dose followed by 2 mg q4h. If diarrhea persists, increase the dose to 2 mg q2h
   c. Octreotide, 100 to 150 mcg SQ t.i.d., is given for patients who are refractory to high-dose loperamide therapy; treatment is continued until diarrhea resolves.
5. **Severe diarrhea** (NCI grades 3 and 4; see Appendix B-2).
   a. Hospitalize patients who have significant dehydration, blood in the stool, or abdominal pain, and treat accordingly
   b. Octreotide, 100 to 150 mcg SQ t.i.d., is given until diarrhea resolves. It is reasonable to increase the dose by 50-mcg increments until diarrhea is controlled. Doses up to 2,000 mcg SQ t.i.d. for 5 days have been used safely in CID.

V. URINARY SYMPTOMS
A. Dysuria
1. **Causes.** Inflammation of the urinary bladder or outlet
2. **Management of dysuria** includes treatment of infection if present and the following:
   a. Phenazopyridine (Pyridium), 100 to 200 mg PO t.i.d.
   b. Amitriptyline, 25 to 50 mg PO h.s. (especially for interstitial cystitis)
B. Bladder spasm
1. **Causes.** Vesicular irritation by cancer, postradiation fibrosis, indwelling catheter, cystitis, or anxiety
2. **Management of bladder spasm.** Cystitis is treated with antibiotics, catheter change, and bladder irrigation if a urethral catheter is present. Drugs of choice are as follows:
   a. Flavoxate (Urispas), 200 to 400 mg PO q.i.d.
   b. Oxybutynin chloride (Ditropan), 5-mg PO t.i.d. or q.i.d.
   c. NSAIDs are reportedly helpful
   d. Hyoscyamine sulfate
      (1) 0.125-mg tablets (Levsin), 1 or 2 tablets PO or SL q4h
      (2) 0.15-mg tablets (Cystospaz), 1 or 2 tablets PO q.i.d.
      (3) 0.375-mg sustained release capsules (Levsinex, Cystospaz-M), 1 capsule q12h
   e. Belladonna-opium suppositories (B & O Supprettes), one q4h
   f. Propantheline bromide (Pro-Banthine), 15 mg PO h.s. or b.i.d.
   g. Blocks of the lumbar sympathetic plexus may be effective for the management of intractable bladder pain.
C. Urinary hesitancy
1. **Causes.** Malignant or benign prostate enlargement, infiltration of the bladder neck, presacral plexopathy, drugs, intrathecal block, bladder denervation by surgery, loaded rectum, inability to stand to void, and asthenia
2. **Management of hesitancy.** Address the specific causes; a urethral catheter may be necessary. Drugs that may be useful include the following:
   a. Terazosin hydrochloride (Hytrin), 1 to 10 mg PO h.s.
   b. Bethanechol (Urecholine), 10 to 30 mg PO b.i.d. to q.i.d.
D. Urinary obstruction by tumor
1. **Causes**
   a. **Upper tract obstruction** can be caused by tumor, stricture, calculi, clots, and retroperitoneal fibrosis.
   b. **Lower tract obstruction** is caused by tumor, benign prostatic enlargement,

clots, calculi, infection, stricture, fecal impaction, detrusor failure from anti-cholinergic side effects of drugs, and neurogenic disease.

2. Management of urinary obstruction

  a. Lower tract obstruction management includes catheter placement in the urethra or suprapubically. Tumor-related obstruction can be treated by surgery, RT, or endoscopic resection depending on the disease stage.

  b. Upper tract obstruction can be treated by nephrostomy tubes, cystoscopically placed stents, or stenting via nephrostomy tube.

  c. Often patients are too debilitated for invasive procedures and supportive care measures become the priority.

E. Discolored urine can be caused by food or drugs and is of no concern, except for the anxiety provoked in the patient.

  1. Pink or red urine: beets, blackberries, rhubarb; doxorubicin (Adriamycin); phenolphthalein (Ex-Lax), senna, cascara, danthron (e.g., in Doxidan); deferoxamine (Desferal); chlorzoxazone (Paraflex); phenothiazines; phenazopyridine (Pyridium)

  2. Brown or black urine: phenacetin, salicylate; metronidazole (Flagyl); nitrofurantoin, chloroquine, quinine quinacrine, sulfonamides (yellow-brown); L-dopa, methyldopa (Aldomet); iron dextran (Imferon)

  3. Blue or green urine: methylene blue, food coloring and other dyes; riboflavin; indomethacin, amitriptyline, danthron, mitoxantrone

  4. Yellow: Suntinib malate (Sutent)

VI. RESPIRATORY SYMPTOMS

A. Cough

  1. Causes

   a. Irritation of airway from dry air, tumor in airway, extrinsic compression, aspiration from vocal cord paralysis, reduced gag reflex, fistula, and gastroesophageal reflux. Infection, medications (e.g., angiotension-converting enzyme [ACE] inhibitors), and excessive sputum must also be considered.

   b. Lung pathology, such as infection, lymphangitic carcinomatosis, radiation pneumonitis, COPD, pulmonary edema, and pleural or pericardial effusion

   c. Irritation of diaphragm, pleura or pericardium

  2. Management of cough is according to the cause

   a. General measures include positioning the patient, and humidifying the air

   b. Antibiotics to treat infection

   c. Bronchodilators for bronchospasm

   d. Drainage is facilitated by physiotherapy and postural drainage.

   e. Mucolytics via steam or nebulized saline, or drugs such as acetylcysteine (Mucomyst)

   f. Antitussives include

    (1) Opioids, such as codeine, hydrocodone, MS, and dihydromorphone, are all options that have equivalent efficacy.

    (2) Benzonatate (Tessalon Perles), 100 mg q4h

    (3) Local anesthetics, such as inhaled lidocaine. The dose is empiric. The starting dose is 5 mL of 2% lidocaine q4h via handheld nebulizer.

    (4) Dextromethorphan (Robitussin DM)

    (5) Inhaled β2 agonists or **anticholinergics** such as ipratropium (Atrovent) for patients with bronchitic component

    (6) Sedation in refractory cases (Valium)

B. Hiccups

  1. Causes

   a. Diaphragmatic irritation from tumor infiltration, subphrenic abscess or empyema, hepatomegaly, and ascites

   b. Phrenic nerve irritation from mediastinal cancers

   c. Gastric distention of any cause

   d. Uremia, esophagitis, or brain tumors

   e. Drugs, such as dexamethasone and barbiturates

2. Management of hiccups
  a. Home remedies are numerous and usually involve pharyngeal stimulation. Methods used have included 2 teaspoons of granulated sugar, two glasses of liquor, a cold key down the back of a hyperextended neck, a nasopharyngeal tube, and drinking a glass of cool water through a straw while plugging both the patient's ears with his or her fingers.
  b. Reduction of gastric distention: nasogastric intubation, peppermint water (relaxes the esophageal sphincter), or antiflatulents (simethicone)
  c. Induction of hypercarbia by breath-holding or using a paper bag
  d. Potentially helpful pharmacologic measures
    (1) Baclofen (Lioresal), 5 to 20 mg PO q6–12h (the only drug tested in a randomized, placebo-controlled manner)
    (2) Chlorpromazine (Thorazine), 25 to 50 mg PO or IV q6h
    (3) Metoclopramide (Reglan), 10 to 20 mg PO q4–6h
    (4) Nifedipine, 10 to 20 mg PO q8–12h
    (5) Benzonatate (Tessalon Perles), 100 mg q.i.d.
    (6) Ondansetron, 8 mg PO t.i.d. or IV bolus
    (7) Anticonvulsants: phenytoin, carbamazepine, valproic acid
    (8) Stimulants: amphetamines, methylphenidate

C. Dyspnea
  1. Causes
    a. Tumor obstruction of trachea or bronchus
    b. Infection of lung tissue or bronchus
    c. Decreased functional lung tissue, such as following resection, tumor involvement, effusion, embolism
    d. Decreased ventilatory movement due to debility, chest wall weakness, elevated diaphragm, ascites, hepatomegaly
    e. Cardiovascular causes, such as congestive heart failure, cardiomyopathy, pericardial effusion
    f. Other: Anemia, anxiety
  2. Management of dyspnea
    a. Oxygen is of benefit in hypoxemic patients
    b. Opioids have shown positive effects in patients with COPD or advanced cancer
    c. Nebulized opioids are controversial
    d. Benzodiazepines when an anxiety component exists
    e. Corticosteroids used in lymphangitic carcinomatosis
    f. Bronchodilators, as indicated
    g. Position the patient comfortably; open windows and use fans
  3. Management of respiratory panic involves the use of anxiolytics together with opioids. Oxygen may be beneficial for the hypoxemic patient.
  4. Management of "death rattle," which results from the weakened patient being too ill to expectorate, includes
    a. Positioning on the left side
    b. Hyoscine (Scopolamine) patch, 1.5 mg q72h
    c. Hyoscine hydrobromide, 0.2 to 0.4 mg SQ q2–4h
    d. Hyoscine butylbromide, 20 mg SQ q2–4h (not available in the United States)
    e. Atropine, 0.4 to 0.8 mg SQ q2–4h
    f. Suctioning is uncomfortable for the patient and should be minimized

VII. SKIN PROBLEMS
  A. Pruritus
    1. Causes. Generalized pruritus can develop as a result of the following:
      a. Scabies, dry flaky skin, or other primary skin conditions
      b. Biliary tract obstruction
      c. Paraneoplastic syndrome, lymphomas, cutaneous metastases
      d. Renal failure

    e. Drugs, such as opioids, amphetamines, intraspinal morphine

    f. Hypersensitivity to drugs

    g. Autoimmune disorders (systemic lupus erythematosus, Sjogren's syndrome)

    h. Iron deficiency, polycythemia vera, systemic mast cell disease

    i. Thyroid disease, hyperparathyroidism

    j. Psychiatric causes

  2. Management of pruritus. Control of the underlying cancer may relieve itching. Drugs suspected of causing hypersensitivity reactions should be stopped. Factors that increase the perception of pruritus include dehydration, heat, anxiety, and boredom.

    a. Instructions to patients. Patients should be told to avoid traumatizing the skin by alcohol rubs, woolen clothing, or frequent bathing. Excessive bathing, especially with detergents and hot water, results in dry skin, which causes itching in itself. The use of baby oil, olive oil, lanolin, bland creams, emollient creams, or petroleum jelly should be encouraged. The skin should be "oiled" after each bath or shower, blotting in the agent while toweling dry. The use of soap should be stopped and situations that result in increased sweating avoided.

    b. Topical therapy. Emollients with camphor and menthol (Sarna lotion), phenol, or pramoxine (PrameGel, Pramosone, or Aveeno anti–itch) can be effective. Cool compresses and oatmeal baths (Aveeno) can be helpful. Topical steroids, such as hydrocortisone 1% or 2.5%, and triamcinolone 0.1%, can be useful provided that they are prescribed in amounts necessary to cover affected skin.

    c. Oral medications include antihistamines, anxiolytics, corticosteroids, and antidepressants

    d. Specific treatments for specific disorders

      (1) Naloxone for intraspinal morphine associated pruritis

      (2) Cholestyramine (4 g PO q6h) for cholestatic pruritis

      (3) Methyltestosterone (25 mg PO q8h) for cholestatic pruritis

      (4) Stenting and anticancer therapy for tumor-related cholestasis

      (5) Topical and systemic steroids for inflammatory skin diseases

      (6) Pruritus associated with polycythemia vera responds to disease therapy, and H_2 blockers

      (7) Pruritus associated with lymphoma can respond to corticosteroids and therapy of the disease

      (8) Urticaria responds to antihistamines and corticosteroids

B. Preventive skin care in dying patients is extremely important to their comfort. The following are recommendations extracted from Twycross RG and Lack SA. *Therapeutics in Terminal Cancer.* London: Pitman, 1984.

  1. Prevent decubiti by redistributing pressure

    a. At home, obtain a camping mattress and fill it with water instead of air to create a waterbed.

    b. For wheelchairs, use an inflatable cushion or egg-crate foam.

    c. Elbow and heel pads, sheepskin mats, self-adhering urethane foam, pillows, and bed cradles may be helpful.

    d. Turn or reposition patients frequently.

    e. Decubitus ulcers are sometimes impossible to prevent or treat in terminal patients, regardless of frequent and meticulous care. Cachexia, skin atrophy, incontinence, and pain on movement are some of the contributing factors. Caring and conscientious nurses may need physician reassurance that decubiti in this setting are impossible to prevent or treat.

  2. Provide optimal hydration and hygiene

    a. Avoid soap on dry, fragile skin; creams and ointments in intertriginous areas; and trauma (from restraints, tape, and so forth).

    b. On normal skin, use mild soaps, pat dry, use gentle massage with bland cream, and use petroleum jelly on elbows and heels.

    c. On dry skin, use fine talc.

   d. On chafed areas, use silicone spray or Opsite.

   e. Change bed linen often.

C. Hair loss

   1. Causes. Irradiation to the scalp and administration of certain cytotoxic drugs result in marked alopecia. Hair loss begins 2 to 3 weeks after these therapies are started. Hair usually regrows after therapy is discontinued. The relative risks of hair loss caused by chemotherapeutic agents are shown in Appendix B-1.

   2. Management

   a. Emotional support. Patients need to be forewarned. Hair loss should be discussed openly and sympathetically and its importance compared with the potential benefits of therapy. Inform patients about the relative risks of the specific regimen for alopecia. Explain that hair loss is preceded by scalp itching or pain and that hair is often curly when it regrows.

   b. Wigs should be obtained as soon as hair loss becomes evident (or before). Complimenting patients' appearance in a wig (if sincere) aids in adjustment. Prescribe a scalp prosthesis for insurance carriers.

   c. Other measures. Suggest the use of hats and colorful scarves, soft-bristle brushes, mild shampoos, and satin pillowcases. Discourage the use of blow-dryers, hot rollers, and exposure of the scalp to the sun.

VIII. NECROTIC, MALODOROUS TUMOR MASSES

   A. Pathogenesis. Progressively growing tumor masses may erode through the overlying skin and ulcerate. The center of the mass becomes necrotic with the formation and release of malodorous polyamines, such as putrescine and cadaverine. These polyamines are reactive and adhere to almost anything with which they come in contact, including skin, clothing, and hospital equipment, leaving a residual nauseating odor in the room. The smell worsens if the mass becomes infected with anaerobic organisms. The stench makes it difficult for others to enter the room. When visitors leave, the smell stays on their clothing and skin; as a result, patients become isolated from contact with others. Patients themselves often do not notice the odor.

   B. Management

   1. RT. Large masses that may invade the overlying skin should be irradiated to prevent skin breakdown.

   2. Amputation may be necessary for tumors that do not respond to RT or chemotherapy (e.g., an extremity that is ravaged with sarcoma).

   3. Skin metastases confined to one small area of the body may be amenable to local resection. However, recurrences are likely.

   4. Chemotherapy or endocrine therapy should be used appropriately for the primary tumor.

   5. Local care

   a. Frequent dressing changes with highly absorbent, nonadhesive material. Alginates can absorb exudates.

   b. Tumor bleeding may be ameliorated with a hemostatic dressing, such as Mepitel, or by applying 1:1,000 epinephrine solutions to the tumor surface before applying the new dressing.

   c. Flushing. Necrotic tumor masses and fistulas should be generously irrigated at least t.i.d. with large volumes of 3% hydrogen peroxide.

   d. Silver nitrate, 1% solution soaked in large gauze pads, may be applied to necrotic areas by a gloved operator every day or two to help reduce oozing and odor. Absorbed silver may cause renal damage.

   e. Maggots actually débride necrotic tissue; however, the sight of maggots in wounds is usually more than nursing staff, physicians, and visitors can tolerate, although patients often do not appear to notice them. Diethyl ether in generous amounts is applied to the tumor surface with 4 × 4 inch gauze; the gauze is wrung out onto the lesion so that it reaches the deeper ulcerated areas. Maggots rapidly recur if treatment with ether is stopped.

6. Measures to control odor

a. Isolate patients with malodorous tumors in private rooms. An outward facing fan is placed to blow air out of the window. Normal areas of skin should be kept clean, and malodorous masses should be kept covered.

b. Room deodorizers should be used. The deodorant aromas should be changed every few days to avoid conditioning of the staff, which soon identify the smell of the product with the rather thinly disguised stench of necrotic cancer.

c. Metronidazole (Flagyl), 250 to 500 mg q.i.d., may be helpful, particularly if anaerobic bacterial infection is present. Crushed metronidazole tablets on soaked gauzes can be applied topically.

d. Chloresium, a 22% chlorophyll–copper complex in isotonic saline, is a true deodorizing agent and can be poured directly onto the necrotic tissues.

e. Disposable protective gowns and gloves should be worn by caregivers.

IX. FEVER

A. Causes. The diagnosis of tumor-induced fever is one of exclusion. It can develop in the course of nearly any malignancy but is especially common in the following conditions:

1. Lymphomas and myeloproliferative disorders
2. Retroperitoneal cancer
3. Metastatic cancer to the liver
4. Hepatocellular and renal cell carcinoma
5. Gastric and pancreatic cancers
6. Osteosarcomas

B. Management

1. Controlling the underlying tumor, when possible, is the most effective means of controlling fever from tumors.
2. Aspirin and acetaminophen may be alternated q2h p.r.n.
3. Indomethacin, 25 to 50 mg PO t.i.d., is often helpful.
4. Corticosteroids may be helpful but are generally not necessary.

X. LYMPHEDEMA is defined as lymphatic production exceeding transport capacity. Most often this is caused by obstruction of lymphatic drainage but also has a component of vascular damage.

A. Patients at risk

1. Breast cancer patients who have had nodal dissection, as well as RT
2. Melanoma patients who have had nodal dissection
3. Prostate cancer patients who have had surgery or whole pelvic radiation

B. Types

1. **Acute, transient, and mild,** occurring a few days after surgery
2. **Acute and painful,** occurring 4 to 6 weeks after surgery as a result of acute lymphangitis or phlebitis
3. **Erysipeloid form,** which occurs after minor trauma and is superimposed on chronic edema
4. **Insidious and painless** is the most common form. There is no erythema and it occurs years after primary treatment.

C. Assessment

1. Attempt to classify the type of edema
2. How does the edema affect the patient in terms of function? Assess for depression.
3. Examine pulses, sensory and motor functions, and document the size of extremities

D. Management of lymphedema

1. Education involves reporting any areas of breakdown, weeping, or erythema to the doctor. The patient should avoid heavy lifting with the affected limb, avoid hot tubs and saunas, and cuts and burns to the extremity, wear gloves while doing gardening, avoid venipuncture and blood pressure checks in the extremity, and

wear a compression sleeve while exercising or traveling. Self-massage should be taught to the patient.

2. **Manual lymphatic drainage** involves lightly massaging the affected limb to move edema fluid through lymphatic anastomoses to functional lymph nodes. Elastic stockings can be applied after the massage.

3. **Extremity pumps** can be helpful.

4. **Exercise and elevation** are never harmful.

5. **Antibiotics** for evidence of infection.

6. **Diuretics** may be helpful if a significant vascular component is thought to be present.

7. **Corticosteroids** are helpful if enlarged nodes are the cause of the edema.

XI. VENOUS ACCESS PROBLEMS

A. Administering chemotherapy to patients with poor venous access

1. **Switching to oral agents.** Many of the available chemotherapeutic agents are absorbed, although incompletely, when given orally.

2. **Difficulty finding veins** may be alleviated by several techniques:

   a. Hang the arms (wrapped in hot, moist towels, with tourniquets lightly applied) for 10 minutes below the level of the heart.

   b. Use a blood pressure cuff expanded halfway between systolic and diastolic pressures. Tight tourniquets are never helpful.

   c. Search other places to find veins, such as the upper arm or legs.

   d. Advise patients to drink plenty of liquids on the day before treatment and to wear a sweater on the day of treatment to keep the arm warm.

   e. Place hot packs over the site before venipuncture.

3. **Vein training.** Patients with inaccessible veins are instructed to sit in a chair with the arms held below heart level and to squeeze tennis balls, Nerf balls, or household sponges t.i.d. for 10 minutes or until fatigued. The arms may be wrapped periodically with warm towels.

4. **Other methods** for securing venous access include arteriovenous fistula (see section XI.C) and right atrial Silastic catheters (see section XI.E).

B. Heparin lock.
A plugged, short catheter may be used in patients requiring intermittent IV infusions. The catheter is flushed regularly with heparin.

C. An arteriovenous fistula
can be established in patients who have inaccessible veins and a reasonably long expected survival. Administration of viscous solutions through the shunt promotes thrombosis.

D. Hypodermoclysis.
Dehydration in patients with difficult venous access can be treated with parenteral fluids administered by clysis. A 21-gauge needle is inserted at a slight angle to the skin of the lateral thigh and then further inserted 1 to 2 inches into the subcutaneous tissue. One vial (150 U) of hyaluronidase (Wydase) is administered through the needle; the enzyme should not be infused into inflamed or cancerous areas. Ringer's lactate solution and mineral additives can then be given at a rate of 100 to 150 mL.

E. Prolonged central venous catheterization.
Polymerized silicone rubber (Silastic) catheters inserted into the right atrium through the cephalic vein can provide prolonged venous access for administering IV fluids, blood products, and drugs, and for sampling blood. Both external and subcutaneously implanted types are available.

1. **A nonfunctioning catheter** is usually the result of obstruction of the catheter tip by either the right atrial wall or a clot. Repositioning the patient usually dislodges the catheter from the atrial wall. A chest radiograph should be taken to evaluate the position of the catheter tip, if it is questionable.

   a. Heparin, 3 mL of 1:1,000 solution, should be injected into the line with a tuberculin syringe to provide extra pressure; leave it in place for 15 to 60 minutes before flushing. Repeat the procedure four more times or until successful.

   b. Urokinase, 5,000 IU (Abbokinase "Open Cath") may also be tried if a clot is suspected.

   c. An infusion of urokinase directly into the dysfunctional catheter may also successfully dissolve clots. The dose is 40,000 U/hour for 1 to 12 hours. Patients should be observed for bleeding for 48 hours.

   d. Alternatively, Alteplase, a tissue plasminogen activator for local fibrinolysis that is manufactured by recombinant DNA technology, can be used. When instilled into a catheter at a dose of 0.5 to 1.0 mg/hour, circulating levels would be expected to return to endogenous circulating levels within 30 minutes of stopping the infusion.

2. Complications. Catheter-related deaths are rare. The most frequent problems are severing the catheter (if external), infections, and clotting. Differences in the incidence of documented infections between external catheters and subcutaneous ports are arguable; if infections do occur, they may be treated successfully with antibiotics without removing the catheter in the appropriate circumstances (see Chapter 35, section III.G). No differences exist in the incidence of clotting between external and subcutaneous catheter devices.

3. Indications for removing venous catheters include persistent fever, unexplained hypotension, entrance-site infection, air leak, axillary; jugular, or superior vena cava thrombosis; or pleural effusion (due to misplacement of the catheter into the pleural space).

XII. NUTRITIONAL SUPPORT

A. Mechanisms of malignant cachexia are poorly understood. The characteristics of cancer cachexia that differ from starvation cachexia include equal mobilization of fat and skeletal muscle (rather than preferential mobilization of fat), normal or increased basal metabolic rate (rather than decreased), increased liver metabolic activity, normal or increased glucose turnover (rather than decreased), and increased protein breakdown (rather than decreased). Related factors include but are not limited to the following:

1. Metabolic abnormalities in cachexia of malignancy

   a. Carbohydrate metabolism: decreased blood glucose levels, glycogen stores, and sensitivity to insulin; increased gluconeogenesis, Cori's cycle activity, glucose turnover, and serum lactate

   b. Fat metabolism: decreased lipoprotein lipase activity, lipid stores; increased lipolysis, serum triglyceride levels, and glycerol turnover

   c. Protein metabolism: decreased skeletal muscle synthesis; increased skeletal muscle catabolism and protein turnover; negative nitrogen balance

   d. Cytokine abnormalities involve tumor necrosis factor, IL-1, IL-6, interferon gamma, leukemia inhibitory factor, and others

2. Decreased intake

   a. Anorexia. Many tumors are associated with anorexia, typically manifested by an aversion to meat. Poorly controlled pain, stomatitis, chemotherapy, RT, and altered sense of taste and smell contribute to the loss of appetite. GI causes of malnutrition or anorexia include decreased gastric reservoir from tumor or extrinsic compression (hepatomegaly), dysphagia from tumor or treatment, and fistula formation. Depression and organ failure are other causes.

   b. Mechanical obstruction of any portion of the intestinal tract makes oral intake impossible. In advanced stages, tumors of the head and neck or ovary frequently make eating impossible.

   c. Nausea and vomiting. See section III.

   d. Diagnostic studies often require fasting; if such studies are not conducted efficiently, patients can become nutritionally further compromised.

3. Increased losses

   a. Biochemical abnormalities. See section XII.A.1.

   b. Diarrhea. Severe diarrhea or malabsorption syndromes are associated with carcinoid syndrome, gastrinoma, medullary thyroid carcinoma, pancreatic carcinoma, small bowel lymphatic obstruction, excessive bowel resection, certain cytotoxic agents, and radiation enteritis.

    c. Lactase deficiency is common in protein starvation and after some chemotherapies, making milk products unsuitable.

  4. Natural history. Increasing loss of body protein leads to progressively worsening anemia, hypoalbuminemia, hypotransferrinemia, loss of cell-mediated immunity, decreased work tolerance, decreased deep-breathing ability, increased risk for pneumonia, inability to ambulate, and then inability to sit up. Other signs include hair loss, scaling skin, brittle nails, and decubitus ulcer. Death occurs when 30% to 50% of body protein stores are lost.

B. Assessment of nutritional status. Serial measurements of the following parameters provide prognostic information about the risk for sepsis and death:

  1. Weight and serum albumin concentration. Substantial protein-calorie malnutrition is characterized by a recent loss of >10% of the stable preillness weight and by significant hypoalbuminemia (<3.0 g/dL). Albumin has a serum half-life of about 3 weeks, and albumin levels change in direct proportion to improvement or deterioration of nutritional status.

  2. Transferrin has a half-life of about 1 week and changes more rapidly than albumin with changes in nutritional state. Serum transferrin is also less affected than albumin by factors unrelated to nutritional state, such as hydration and infection.

  3. Skin tests. Poor nutrition with weight loss of >10% of usual body weight results in anergy and depression of immune competence. Nutritional status and immunocompetence are adequate if two or more of the following skin test antigens produce a positive intradermal reaction: tuberculin, mumps, *Candida* sp., and streptokinase-streptodornase.

  4. Nutritional requirements. The healthy person requires 2,000 to 2,700 (25 cal/kg) calories per day distributed as follows: 15% protein (1 g/kg body weight), 50% carbohydrate (3 g/kg), and 35% fat (1 g/kg). To achieve a positive nitrogen balance and sustain weight, cachectic patients would require hyperalimentation with 2,700 to 4,000 calories and twice the recommended daily allowance of amino acids and essential nutrients. These calculations are for patients with cancer who warrant hyperalimentation (see below).

C. Treatment of anorexia and cachexia

  1. Palliative care of the anorectic or cachectic patient. Progressive weight loss is part of the biology of progressive cancer. Nutritional therapy does not prolong survival if the tumor cannot be controlled. Most patients and families, however, believe that nutritional status is essential, regardless of the underlying disease.

    a. Physician interest in dietary support often provides psychological palliation, especially when active cancer treatment is not helpful. Useful techniques include referral to dietitians, and "folksy" dietary advice, such as the use of caloric supplements and the measures described in section XII.C.2, below, which give patients and families the feeling that they are doing something positive. The physician must recommend against unhealthful diets and potentially toxic doses of "health food" preparations.

    b. It is important that the physician support the wishes of the dying patient who is becoming exhausted by well-meaning family members and friends trying to force food intake. Advise family that, although the intentions are appreciated, pushing a patient to eat is exhausting and adds to that person's misery. The physician should reiterate the futility and harmful psychological effects of forcing food. The refusal to eat is the patient's biology and decision.

  2. Some measures that may be helpful in patients who refuse food include the following:

    a. Provide small, frequent feedings, up to six times a day, as tolerated.

    b. Take a dietary history. Are there times of the day when the patient has an appetite? If so, the major caloric intake should occur at these times.

    c. A small helping looks better on a small plate; do not use large dinner plates.

    d. Have food available whenever the patient is hungry.

    e. Have the patient dress for meals and sit at the table, if possible.

    f. Attend to stomatitis, dry mouth, and foul taste.

    g. Vitamins may be used if not excessive. Vitamin C is ineffective therapy against tumors, but is usually harmless unless substituted for proven therapy or if the doses ingested produce dysuria, diarrhea, or satiety.

    h. Do not routinely weigh the patient.

3. Appetite stimulants that may be helpful include the following:

    a. Megestrol acetate, 400 to 800 mg/day (10 to 20 mL/day of Megace Oral Suspension, which contains 40 mg/mL in 240-mL bottles). Side effects include high cost, venous thrombosis, edema, hypertension, and hyperglycemia.

    b. Dexamethasone, 4 mg in the morning after food. This dose is empirically derived. Side effects include proximal myopathy, fluid retention, mental status changes, and immunosuppression.

    c. Metoclopramide (Reglan), 10 mg PO before meals and bedtime, may be indicated in patients who are experiencing anorexia, nausea, early satiety, and manifestations of dysmotility. Side effects include dystonic reactions and restlessness.

    d. THC, 2.5 to 7.5 mg after breakfast and lunch, starting with the lower dose, which is then escalated. Side effects include dizziness, fluid retention, somnolence, and dissociation, particularly in the elderly. A recent placebo-controlled trial suggests no benefit for cannabinoids in the anorexia-cachexia syndrome.

    e. Antidepressants may be useful with anorexia caused by depression.

    f. Hydrazine sulfate, cyproheptadine, anabolic steroids, dronabinol, and pentoxifylline have been shown to be ineffective for cancer patients in controlled trials.

    g. Psychostimulants, such as methylphenidate (Ritalin), may actually improve appetite when used in the setting of depression.

4. Other measures

    a. Dental relining improves chewing abilities and facial appearance.

    b. An old photograph helps the new caregivers recognize the essential humanness of the emaciated patient.

    c. New photographs of the patient with family, friends, and caregivers help legitimize the value of this "new" person.

    d. The patient should have at least one new set of well-fitting clothes, if affordable.

D. Hyperalimentation in cancer patients. Nutritional deficiency leads to decreased immunocompetence, poor wound healing, and decreased tolerance to antitumor therapy. For cancer patients whose prognosis warrants nutritional support, enteral feeding (EF) or parenteral hyperalimentation (PH) may be given.

    1. Indications for EF. "If the gut works, use it." Patients who have a functional GI tract but are unable to ingest adequate nutrients orally are candidates for EF. EF is far less expensive, more physiologic, and associated with fewer complications than PH.

    2. Indications for PH

        a. The patient has a curable neoplasm, but recovery likely will be protracted from treatment (e.g., extensive bowel resection).

        b. The patient is cured of tumor but is awaiting surgical intervention and has residual nutritional problems (e.g., enterocutaneous fistulas).

        c. The patient requires prolonged postoperative nasogastric suction (>4 to 7 days) for conditions that necessitate avoidance of oral intake.

        d. Patients with severe malabsorption, vomiting, esophageal obstruction from benign causes, or severe dysphagia not amenable to dietary manipulation

        e. Patients with chemotherapy-associated severe diarrhea or prolonged stomatitis leading to weight loss

    3. Contraindications to hyperalimentation

        a. Contraindications to EF are intractable vomiting, upper GI bleeding, or intestinal obstruction.

b. **Hyperalimentation is not useful for** patients with any of the following conditions:

   (1) Minimal nutritional deficits

   (2) Weight loss caused by progressive cancer that is unlikely to respond to therapy

   (3) Aggressive tumors that respond dramatically to therapy (e.g., lymphoma and small cell lung cancer)

c. **PH is strongly discouraged** in most patients receiving chemotherapy because the 12% complication rate is unacceptable. Complications include pneumothorax, thrombosis, and catheter-related septicemia.

E. **Enteral feeding** provides liquid formula diets into the GI tract orally or by means of feeding tubes. Gastrotomy tubes and other tube enterostomies are used when a nasogastric feeding tube cannot be placed or is not tolerated by the patient. Percutaneous endoscopic placement has the advantages of speed and minimal surgical incision.

1. **Preparations.** Many enteral products are available, but a standard formula is usually sufficient for patients with an intact digestive system. Isotonic solutions that contain high nitrogen and a medium caloric density (1 to 2 kcal/mL) are satisfactory in 90% of patients. Preparations that contain a high concentration of amino acids are often unacceptable for patients with cancer-related meat aversion.

   High-calorie preparations are offered as caloric supplements, but they often cause diarrhea and are so rich that many patients refuse them. Asking patients for flavor preference, diluting each can with an equal amount of water, and serving no more than half this amount *on ice* can make these preparations more acceptable to patients. This cooled dilution can provide up to an additional 1,000 cal/day when given *after* patients have eaten what they can of a meal, between meals, and h.s. as tolerated.

2. **Administration.** Start tube feedings with a full-strength solution at about 30 mL. Increase the infusion rate to tolerance by increments of 10 to 25 mL over 12 to 24 hours for 2 to 3 days.

3. **Complications of EF**

   a. **Frequent complications and corrections**

      (1) Vomiting and bloating: reduce the flow rate.

      (2) Diarrhea and cramping: reduce the flow rate; dilute the solution; treat with an antidiarrheal drug; consider a different type of solution. Diarrhea is especially likely in patients who have been given broad-spectrum antibiotics.

      (3) Hyperglycemia: reduce the flow rate; give insulin.

      (4) Edema: usually requires no treatment; diuretics may be used.

      (5) Offensive smell or taste: add flavorings.

      (6) Nasopharyngeal discomfort: encourage the use of sugarless gum, gargling with warm water and mouthwash, topical anesthetics.

      (7) Abnormalities of serum levels of sodium, potassium, calcium, magnesium, or phosphorus: adjust the formula's ingredients.

   b. **Infrequent complications and corrections**

      (1) Congestive heart failure: administer fluids more slowly and treat cardiac decompensation.

      (2) Fat malabsorption: use low-fat formulas; add pancreatic enzymes.

      (3) Elevated serum transaminase: decrease carbohydrate content of formula.

      (4) Acute otitis media: administer antibiotics; change nasogastric tube to other nostril.

      (5) Clogged tube lumen: flush with water or replace tube.

   c. **Rare complications that necessitate discontinuing therapy**

      (1) Aspiration pneumonia (unlikely to occur if the head of the bed is elevated to 45 degrees, volume overload is avoided, and the cough reflex is intact)

      (2) Esophageal erosion from nasogastric tube

(3) Acute purulent sinusitis

(4) Hyperosmolar coma

XIII. CANCER-RELATED FATIGUE

A. Definition. A history of fatigue, diminished energy, increased need to rest disproportionate to any recent change in activity level occurring every day during the same 2-week period in the last month plus five of the following:

1. Weakness

2. Diminished concentration or attention

3. Insomnia or hypersomnia

4. Unrefreshing sleep

5. Need to struggle to overcome inactivity

6. Difficulty completing daily tasks

7. Problems with short-term memory

8. Postexertional malaise lasting several hours

9. Symptoms cause difficulty in everyday functioning

10. Symptoms are a consequence of cancer or cancer-related therapy

11. Symptoms are not a consequence of depression, somatization disorder, or delirium

B. Causes

1. Cancer, cancer therapies, biological response modifiers

2. Systemic disorders, such as anemia, infection, pulmonary infections, liver and renal failure; malnutrition, dehydration, electrolyte disorders, endocrine dysfunction

3. Sleep disorders

4. Immobility and lack of exercise

5. Chronic pain

6. Centrally acting drugs, such as opioids

7. Psychosocial problems

C. Evaluation. Take a history focusing on severity, provocative palliative factors, and impact on quality of life. Look for causes and manifestations of fatigue.

D. Management of cancer-related fatigue

1. Establish reasonable expectations

2. Correct potential causes, such as depression, anemia, fluid and electrolyte disorders, endocrine deficiencies, and hypoxia

3. Treat deconditioning; consider referral to a rehabilitation specialist

4. Pharmacologic interventions

a. Methylphenidate (Ritalin), 2.5 or 5.0 mg PO at 8:00 AM and noon (has been proven not to be helpful)

b. Dextroamphetamine, 2.5 or 5.0 mg PO once or twice daily.

c. Modafinil (Provigil), 100 to 200 mg PO each morning

d. Corticosteroids, such as dexamethasone (1 to 2 mg b.i.d.) or prednisone (5 to 10 mg PO b.i.d.)

5. Nonpharmacologic approaches

a. Educating the patient

b. Individualizing exercise programs if possible

c. Maintaining a diary

d. Educating about sleep, hygiene, stress management, proper nutrition, and hydration may help

Suggested Reading

Bruera E, Kim HN. Cancer pain. *JAMA* 2003;290:2476.

Bruera E, Sweeney C. Methadone use in cancer patients with pain: a review. *J Palliat Med* 2002;5:127.

Bruera E, Valero V, Driver L, et al. Patient-controlled methylphenidate for cancer fatigue: a double-blind, randomized, placebo-controlled trial. *J Clin Oncol* 2006;24:2073.

Caraceni A, Cherny N, Fainsinger R, et al. Pain Measurement Tools and Methods in Clinical Research in Palliative Care: Recommendations of an Expert Working Group of the European Association of Palliative Care. *J P Symptom Manage* 2002;23:239.

Cherny N, Ripamonti C, Pereira J, et al. Strategies to manage the adverse effects of oral morphine: an evidence-based report. *J Clin Oncol* 2001;19:2542.

Davis MP. The opioid bowel syndrome: a review of pathophysiology and treatment. *J Opioid Manag* 2005;1:153.

Estfan B, LeGrand S. Management of cough in advanced cancer. *J Support Oncol* 2004;2: 523.

Foldi E. The treatment of lymphedema. *Cancer* 1998;83(12 Suppl American):2833.

Grocott P. The palliative management of fungating malignant wounds. *J Wound Care* 2000;9(1):4.

Hanks GW, Conno F, Cherny N, et al. Morphine and alternative opioids in cancer pain: the EAPC recommendations. *Br J Cancer* 2001;84(5):587.

Mitchell SA, Berger AM. Cancer-related fatigue: the evidence base for assessment and management. *Cancer J* 2006;12:374.

Navari RM. Prevention of emesis from multiple-day and high-dose chemotherapy regimens. *J Natl Compr Canc Netw* 2007;5:51.

Ngeow WC, Chai WL, Rahman RA, et al. Managing complications of radiation therapy in head and neck cancer patients: Part I. Management of xerostomia. *Singapore Dent J* 2006;28:1.

Stearns L, Boortz-Marx R, Du PS, et al. Intrathecal drug delivery for the management of cancer pain: a multidisciplinary consensus of best clinical practices. *J Support Oncol* 2005;3:399.

Sykes NP. The pathogenesis of constipation. *J Support Oncol* 2006;4:213.

Twycross R, Greaves MW, Handwerker H, et al. Itch: scratching more than the surface. *QJM* 2003;96:7.

Williams CM. Dyspnea. *Cancer J* 2006;12:365.

Yan BM, Myers RP. Neurolytic celiac plexus block for pain control in unresectable pancreatic cancer. *Am J Gastroenterol* 2007;102:430.

Zell JA, Chang JC. Neoplastic fever: a neglected paraneoplastic syndrome. *Support Care Cancer* 2005;13:870.

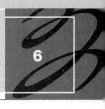

TALKING WITH CANCER PATIENTS AND THEIR FAMILIES

Eric E. Prommer

6

I think the best physician is the one who has the providence to tell to the patients according to his knowledge the present situation, what has happened before, and what is going to happen in the future.

—Hippocrates

I. **INTRODUCTION.** Communication between physicians and patients is a fundamental aspect of cancer care, yet most physicians have had little training in communication. The aspects of communication most valued by patients are those that help patients and their families feel guided, build trust, and support hope. There are a set of concrete skills that can be used to effectively lead to these outcomes. A wide variety of empirical studies document that physician–patient communication is suboptimal. Physicians and nurses typically miss the full range of concerns held by people with cancer. These deficiencies in communication increase the psychological and existential suffering of patients and their loved ones. Compounding these problems is the finding that oncologists lack accuracy in detecting patient distress. Finally, poor communication also hampers a physician's ability to provide pain and symptom management.

The National Cancer Institute named cancer communication as an "extraordinary opportunity" in 1999; the American Society of Clinical Oncology named communication as a key clinician skill. New educational models exist that have been documented to result in physician communication skill improvement. These models are being used in settings ranging from practicing physicians to oncology fellows in training. Communication skills training is associated with less burnout and work-related stress. This chapter highlights some of the techniques useful to improving communication with patients and families.

II. **FUNDAMENTAL COMMUNICATION SKILLS**

A. **Behaviors to avoid**

1. **Blocking** occurs when a patient raises a concern but the physician either fails to respond or redirects the conversation. For example, a woman with metastatic colon cancer might ask, "How long do you think I have?" and the doctor responds, "Don't worry about that," or "How is your breathing?" Blocking is important because physicians typically fail to elicit the range of patient concerns and consequently are unable to address the most important concerns.

2. **Lecturing** occurs when a physician delivers a large chunk of information without giving the patient a chance to respond or ask questions.

3. **Collusion** occurs when patients hesitate to bring up difficult topics and their physicians do not ask them specifically—a "don't ask, don't tell" situation.

4. **Premature reassurance** occurs when a physician responds to a patient concern with reassurance before exploring and understanding the concern.

B. **Behaviors to cultivate**

1. **Ask-Tell-Ask**. Always **ask** about the patient's understanding of the issue. "What have your other doctors been telling you about your illness since the last time we spoke?" "How do you see your health?" **Tell** the patient in straightforward language what you need to communicate—the bad news, treatment options, or other information. Stop short of giving a long lecture or huge amounts of

detail. Information should be provided in short, digestible chunks. A useful rule of thumb is not to give more than three pieces of information at a time. Do not use medical jargon. **Ask** the patient if he or she understood what was said. Consider asking the patient to restate what was said in his or her own words.

2. **Tell me more.** Ask patients if they need more information or if all their questions are being answered. Ask about how they feel about what has transpired and its meaning.

3. **Respond to emotions.** An important mnemonic to help cover emotional responses is **NURSE.** This involves **n**aming, **u**nderstanding, **r**especting, **s**upporting, and **e**xploring the emotional response.

III. BREAKING BAD NEWS. This is perhaps the communication task that has been studied the most extensively. Bad news can be defined as any information that adversely alters one's expectations for the future. Its basic format is the basis for subsequent discussions at various points during the patient's disease trajectory.

Oncologists give bad news thousands of times during the course of a career and it can be highly stressful. In a large survey of oncologists, 20% reported anxiety and strong emotions when they had to tell a patient that their condition would lead to death. In a more detailed study of 73 physicians, 42% indicated that although the stress often peaks during the encounter, the stress from a bad news encounter can last for hours—even up to 3 or more days afterward.

Giving bad news is more difficult when the clinician has a long-standing relationship with the patient, or when the patient is young, or when strong optimism had been expressed for a successful outcome. On the other hand, when bad news is communicated in an empathic manner, it can have an important impact on outcomes such as patient satisfaction and decreased patient anxiety and depression. The physician's caring attitude can be more important than the information or reassurance given. As with any medical procedure, giving bad news requires a coherent strategy. In this case the strategy encompasses a series of six distinct communication steps that can be summarized using the mnemonic **SPIKES.** This protocol includes recommendations endorsed by practitioners and patients.

A. **Setup.** Prepare yourself with the necessary medical facts, take a moment to have a plan in your mind, and find a quiet place if possible. Turn off TVs and pagers. Enlist support for the patient, which means have family there, or if no family is available, find a nurse or social worker or a friend of the patient. Sit down, make eye contact, and sit no closer than 2 feet away from the patient. Have tissues available.

B. **Perception.** Find out if the patient understands the medical situation. What has he or she been told about the disease? What does he or she know about the purpose of the unfavorable test results you are about to discuss? If this is a first contact, what has the patient been told about why he or she should see you in referral? Correct any misconceptions or misunderstandings the patient may have. Try not to talk for at least 1 minute (which is difficult); let the patient tell his or her story.

C. **Invitation.** Find out how much information the patient wants to know. These days most patients want a lot of information but this is not universally true, especially as the disease progresses and patients may want to focus on "What do we do next?" Are you a details person or do you want the general picture?

D. **Knowledge.** Use language that matches the patient's level of education. Be direct. Avoid using jargon as it will confuse the patient. Give a warning that bad news is coming: "I have some serious news to tell you." This will allow the patient to prepare psychologically. If the patient's perception (step 2) was inaccurate, review pertinent information: "After giving this news, stay quiet for at least 10 to 15 seconds—resist the urge to tell the patient how to feel. Give the patient time to absorb the information and respond.

E. **Empathize.** *NURSE!* (see section II.B.3.)

F. **Strategize and plan.** Summarize the clinical information and make a plan for the next step, which may be further testing or discussion of treatment options.

IV. DISCUSSING DIAGNOSIS, TREATMENT, AND PROGNOSIS

A. Decision making.
A number of empirical studies demonstrate that patients are interested in having some role in decision making; the question is, what kind of role does the patient wish to have? Most patients desire some decision-making role for both patient and physician, and a majority prefer shared decision making. One of the reasons for patient interest in the Internet for medical information is to enable them to verify treatment options they are offered and to check about options that were not offered. Shared decision making does not have to take more time and is associated with greater patient satisfaction. Steps to enhance shared decision making include:

1. **Elicit the preferences of the patient for information and decision making.** People vary in how they want to make medical decisions. Inquire about what the patient wants in terms of involvement and decision making. You are inviting the patient to tell you how involved he or she wants to be.

2. **Identify the choices to be made.** Providing the patient with a roadmap of the conversation in a sentence or two can give a sense of what lies ahead. An example would be chemotherapy for lung cancer. First-line therapies differ little in terms of response rates, but toxicities and schedules do differ and may be important to the patient.

3. **Describe treatment options and understanding of them.** Describe the adverse effects, how people handle the therapy. Talk about response rates. Don't use jargon.

4. **Discuss how patient values and concerns relate to treatment options.**

5. **Negotiate a time frame for the decision.**

B. Discussing prognosis

Realism, optimism, and avoidance are the most common strategies physicians use in discussing prognosis. Although these strategies are well intended and commonly used, they also create unintended consequences. None of these strategies is completely satisfactory, but each has useful features.

The useful feature of **realism** is that prognostic information helps patients and physicians to make sound medical decisions. Patients also report that realistic prognostic discussions can be blunt and sometimes brutal. A physician who presents prognosis realistically but without structuring the conversation before the information or responding empathetically afterward can be perceived as uncaring. Moreover, empirical data suggest that roughly 20% of patients, particularly those with advanced, metastatic disease, do not want complete information about their prognosis. Giving these patients realistic information may cause psychological harm, although there are not empirical studies that address this question.

Optimism can play a useful role in supporting a patient's hopes, and many patients report that they want a doctor who is hopeful. In discussions about prognosis, however, physicians who deliberately exaggerate or overemphasize optimistic information may risk losing the trust of patients who later discover that the information they received was not entirely true.

A third strategy is to **avoid prognostication** altogether, often by emphasizing individual differences, unpredictability of disease course, or exceptional outliers. **Collusion** is a variation of this strategy in which physicians avoid providing realistic information by creating a tacit understanding that neither patient nor physician will bring up the topic.

Avoidance is based on reasonable concerns. First, physicians realize that they are often inaccurate when predicting survival for an individual. Second, physicians worry that discussing survival communicates a subtle psychological message that a patient will die at a given time. Third, physicians find that some patients do not want prognostic information. Finally, physicians find that bad news often causes patient distress. Yet physicians who avoid prognostication may seem evasive, and consequently untrustworthy, especially when studies indicate that many patients want to talk about life expectancy.

Strategies to provide a middle-of-the road approach are few, but theoretical proposals include:

1. **Ask explicitly how the patient wants to talk about prognosis.** Because many patients may not understand the term *prognosis*, an alternative is to ask, "How much do you want to know about the likely course of this illness?" This question invites a response that goes beyond "yes" or "no." A physician could even normalize a range of patient interest: "Some people want lots of details, some want the big picture, and others prefer that I talk to their family. What would be best for you?" There will be three kinds of patients:
   a. The patient wants information;
   b. The patient does not want information;
   c. The patient is ambivalent.
2. **Patients who want to know the prognostic information.** Start by negotiating the content of the discussion. Physicians can negotiate information giving by establishing a patient's information needs and proposing ways to meet those needs. Thus, the physician should provide information according to the needs of the patient. Some patients want statistical information; some want the worst-case or best-case scenarios. Again, it is important to acknowledge the emotional responses of patient and family. Check for understanding and have the patient and family write down questions they may have forgotten to ask. This can be covered on subsequent visits. Remember that this is not a one-time conversation.
3. **Patients who do not want information.** Try to elicit an understanding about why the patient does not want to know the information. Include possible emotional level of the patient's' decision by stating, "I know this can be difficult to talk about." This segue might enable the patient to reveal underlying emotional concerns or other practical concerns that he or she may have, such as being fearful, or that the information may affect his or her spouse, or that the patient is sad and worried that the discussion will deepen that sadness. *In the patient who does not want information, it is also important to assess whether the information regarding prognosis is absolutely necessary at that moment.* Inquire about whether the patient would want other people to receive the information or would accept a very limited disclosure.
4. **Patients who are ambivalent.** These patients both want to know and do not want to know. These ambivalent patients can frustrate physicians because the patient may go back and forth in one visit, wanting the opposite of whatever the physician proposes. Ambivalence may also be subtle: patients might say that they wants to talk about prognosis, but simultaneously give other signals— they change the topic or look away. The first step is to acknowledge that the patient has good reasons for wanting to talk and for not wanting to have the information. Ask patients to explain both sides of their dilemma. Let patients know that whatever they want to do, you will be there for them. Sometimes the process involves waiting for the patient to initiate the next step in determining how much information he or she needs.

V. DEALING WITH CANCER TREATMENT
   A. **Preparing the patient for treatment.** Patients who are offered choices in their treatment show better psychologic adjustment, and those who feel they have little control over their disease and treatment have a poorer psychosocial outcome. Studies suggest that patients who believed they were more responsible for treatment decisions and perceived that they had more choice in treatment selection went on to have better health-related quality of life. There is also some evidence to suggest that patients who perceive that their physicians are making an effort to facilitate their involvement in decision making tend to be more involved in that process. Patients who had a physician that employed a participatory decision-making style, including inviting patient assistance in making treatment decisions and giving patients control over their treatment, had higher patient satisfaction and physician loyalty.

   There is a continuum of decision making with informed decision making at one end and the physician making all the decisions for the patient at the other ("You're the doctor!"). In the informed decision-making model, patients make treatment decisions after the physician transfers his or her knowledge of the options, treatment efficacy, and risks to the patient. As the patient's agent, the physician is able to elicit the patient's values and then selects the best treatment for the patient based on the patient's value system. Most clinical decisions appear to be made with the patient and physician meeting somewhere in between these two ends of the decision-making spectrum. Always ask about treatment expectations and the patient's goals.

B. Discussing clinical trials. Research suggests that there is a wide variation in the manner in which physicians talk to patients about clinical trials. No research has established a method that will increase the likelihood of a patient choosing to enter a clinical trial. The possibility of clinical trial participation usually occurs when physicians and patients are discussing treatment options. Recommendations for discussing clinical trials build upon previous discussions regarding treatment options.

1. **Describe a clinical trial as a treatment option.** Describe it as an alternative to the "best standard" therapy.
2. **Always ask the patient his or her understanding of what a clinical trial means.**
3. **Delineate the differences.** Make it clear that the process of a clinical trial is more involved than getting treatment out of the trial. It involves detailed consent forms and special procedures if toxicities develop, and it means that often the doctor or patient do not get to choose therapy.
4. **Right to withdraw.** Emphasize to the patient that he or she may withdraw from the trial at any time.
5. **What happens if a patient withdraws?** The physician should discuss how medical care will be transferred back to the patient's primary oncologist or physician after the participation in the clinical trial has ended or if the patient withdraws.

C. Completing curative therapy. The end of a planned course of anticancer therapy is a source of ambivalent feelings for many patients. Although it is a relief to be finished with anticancer therapy and its side effects, many patients also worry about not being watched as carefully, losing the support of their medical providers, and cancer regrowth if chemotherapy is no longer ongoing. Patients are often unsure about resuming old activities they enjoyed before the cancer diagnosis. Important points to cover at this point are:

1. Support the patient on a job well done.
2. Invite questions about any concerns.
3. Emphasize the follow-up plan.
4. Provide resources. Survivor support groups include the National Coalition for Cancer Survivorship (www.canceradvocacy.org).

D. Discontinuing palliative chemotherapy. One of the most challenging tasks faced by oncologists is talking to a patient with a life-threatening cancer about discontinuing palliative chemotherapy that has proven to be ineffective. Although this is well known to oncologists as a challenge, there has been little empirical study of this task, perhaps because of the difficulty of capturing these conversations. One of the most important things to do when *beginning* palliative chemotherapy is to specifically delineate why it's being given, how a response will be measured, and finally what the indicators for stopping the therapy are. Other important strategies for when palliative chemotherapy is being discontinued include:

1. Structure the discussion like the "bad news" conversation.
2. Assess patient's values and goals at this point as therapy is no longer going to be given.
3. Reframe goals to one of continued support and focus on symptom control.
4. Respond to emotion.
5. Propose a new care plan. This may include discussing treatment limitations and hospice.
6. Follow-up. Use follow-up to address symptoms or items discussed in step 5.

VI. TRANSITIONING TO HOSPICE

A. Introduction. Hospice programs offer unique benefits for patients who are near the end of life and their families. Growing evidence indicates that hospice can provide high-quality care. Despite these benefits, many patients do not enroll in hospice, and those who enroll generally do so very late in the course of their illness.

Some barriers to hospice referral arise from the requirements of hospice eligibility, which will be difficult to eliminate without major changes to hospice organization and financing. However, the challenges of discussing hospice create other barriers that are more easily remedied. The biggest communication barrier is that physicians are often unsure of how to talk with patients clearly and directly about their poor prognosis and limited treatment options (both requirements of hospice referral) without depriving them of hope.

Hospice programs provide a unique set of benefits for dying patients and their families. For instance, hospice patients receive medications related to their hospice diagnosis, durable medical equipment, home health aide services, and care from an interdisciplinary team. Families also receive emotional and spiritual support and bereavement counseling for at least a year after the patient's death. The median length of stay in hospice is approximately 3 weeks, and *10% of patients enroll in their last 24 hours of life.*

It is not known what proportion of patients should enroll in hospice or what the optimal length of stay is. Nevertheless, there is widespread agreement among experts in the field and physicians that more patients could enroll in hospice and many of those who enroll should do so sooner. From the oncologic point of view, the factors that should trigger the consideration of hospice for cancer patients are:

1. Poor performance status
2. Leptomeningeal carcinomatosis
3. Malignant bowel obstruction
4. Malignant pericardial effusion
5. Spinal cord compression
6. Brain metastasis (multiple)
7. Widespread metastatic disease

B. Having the discussion. When patients have a poor prognosis and treatment options are limited, physicians should discuss hospice more directly and recommend it when appropriate. Physicians often find these hospice discussions difficult and uncomfortable because patients are being asked to "give up" on disease-directed treatment. However, just as they can with other "bad news" discussions, physicians can make hospice discussions more compassionate, and more effective, by following a structured approach similar to that first described by Buckman for breaking bad news. The overall aim of a hospice discussion that follows this approach is to define a patient's treatment goals and needs for care and then to present hospice as a way to achieve those goals and meet those needs. Steps in the conversation include:

1. Establish the medical facts. Set the stage. Identify a time and place for an uninterrupted conversation. Because hospice decisions are often shared with family members, they should be present.
2. Assess the patient's understanding of his or her health.
3. Define goals of care. Inquire about patients' hopes and fears, which offer insights into their goals.
4. Identify needs for care. Identify problems that respond particularly well to the multidimensional treatment that hospice can provide, such as dyspnea, depression, anxiety, and existential distress. Important items to examine are availability of caregivers, location of residence, and safety of residence.
5. Introduce hospice as a way to meet the patients' needs but don't forget other programs. Home hospice is poorly equipped to meet the needs of debilitated patients without informal caregivers who want to remain at home, unless they can pay for help. Similarly, frail older adults who require extensive supervision may receive more home care services from a Program of All-inclusive Care for the Elderly (PACE)

     6. Respond to emotion and provide closure.

     7. Make the appropriate referral.

VII. SOCIAL DYNAMICS AFFECTING CANCER TREATMENT

  A. Families. It is no surprise that the family is an important source of support. The type of family support is important. Family members who do not reside with participants and pop in and out of their lives without making particular impacts upon the process of enduring chemotherapy are felt to be more of distraction than a help.

  B. Partners and spouses. Partners or spouses are a source of support, encouragement, and great strength. Living with someone undergoing chemotherapy treatment can cause distress, due to intensity of emotion, anxiety, and the possibility of an unpredictable illness trajectory. The patient and his or her spouse often develop a different set of problems resulting from the chemotherapy situation. Behaviors can change, and spouses can be conscious of their reaction to the disease and treatment in relation to the other.

  C. Children. Research on adolescents identifies that their lives are complicated by the parent's illness, and that some of these complications arise from poor assessment of their information needs. Children of all ages do not like the parent to talk about the futility of the disease and the possible failure of chemotherapy to cure the cancer. They had difficulty coping with parents who had little hope or who had a negative outlook. Children may purposely adopt a position of noninvolvement to protect themselves from the possibility of losing a parent, and sometimes they demonstrate intolerance to ill health. Children wrestle with the possibility of separation during a parent's illness and apparently the feeling of imminent death of a parent is emphasized during chemotherapy.

  D. Friends. Research suggests that support from friends is highly valued. It was regarded almost as important as support from family, and friends were perceived to be significantly more important than care professionals in supporting people with cancer. Unlike family and spouses/partners, friends of our participants appear to be confidantes and motivate patients to socialize.

VIII. DISAGREEMENTS ABOUT THERAPY

  A. Types of conflicts. Physicians often assume that conflict is undesirable and destructive, yet conflict handled well can be productive, and the clarity that results can lead to clearer decision making and greater family, patient, and clinician satisfaction. *Conflict* in medical settings has been defined as "a dispute, disagreement, or difference of opinion related to the management of a patient involving more than one individual and requiring some decision or action." Common sources of conflict include family versus physician, physician versus physician, and family versus family. Brief examples are:

    1. Family versus physician. The son of a patient wants life-preserving therapy yet the medical professionals think that it is futile.

    2. Physician versus physician. Specialist wants to continue with therapy; palliative care physician thinks it's futile.

    3. Family versus family. Daughter wants everything done; son wants patient put in a hospice.

  B. Tools to negotiate conflict

    1. Active listening. "What I hear you say is. . . ." "It sounds like you feel that not all treatment has been offered."

    2. Self-disclosure. "I'm worried that the treatments being discussed are not going to prolong life."

    3. Explaining. "There is a 30% chance that the chemotherapy will cause a response."

    4. Empathizing. "I think anyone in your situation would be frustrated."

    5. Reframing. "Let's take a look at hyperalimentation as part of the bigger picture."

    6. Brainstorming. "Let's come up with some ideas how we can improve her symptoms."

IX. ALTERNATIVE AND COMPLEMENTARY THERAPY

A. Overview. It has been estimated that 83 million Americans used alternative therapies for malignant and nonmalignant disorders. Estimates suggest that from 70% to 90% of patients will not mention alternative therapy visits to their physicians. The reasons why people seek alternative therapies for cancer are broad. Many seek out alternative therapy when options for conventional therapy have been exhausted. There is also the recognition that, for some tumor systems, conventional therapy is of limited effectiveness and that the side effects of chemotherapy, surgery, and radiation are feared. For some tumor systems, no conventional therapy exists and the standard therapy is participation in phase I or phase II trials. Many patients perceive that the conventional approach is emotionally or spiritually empty and provides neither comfort nor solace.

1. **Why do patients seek out alternative therapies?** A large lay literature on alternative therapies suggests that sufficient will and determination can overcome cancer. Many alternative therapies invent a simple etiology explaining all cancers are due to a common etiology, such as a toxin. The use of alternative therapy allows patients to exert autonomy and gives them a sense of participation in their care.

2. **Regulatory status.** Vitamins and herbs are considered to be nutritional supplements and are not regulated by the U.S. Food and Drug Administration (FDA).

3. **How do patients learn about alternative therapies?** A quarter of patients learn about alternative therapies via the lay media, including newspapers, television, magazines, and the hundreds of Web sites that sell bogus cures for cancer. Approximately one-sixth of patients learn about alternative therapy from well-meaning friends and family. One-third learn about alternative therapy from their physician!

4. **What therapies are chosen?** It has been estimated that fewer than half of patients with cancer receive only conventional therapy; approximately 44% use conventional and alternative therapies. Ten percent of patients with cancer use unorthodox therapy only and forgo any form of conventional anticancer treatment.

5. **Is this all harmful?** Usually there is no harm. There are low-risk therapies, such as massage, spiritual healing, therapeutic touch, hypnosis, and relaxation, which do not interfere with conventional therapy. Clearly, any therapy is potentially dangerous if it delays effective or curative conventional therapy. Lack of toxicity does not always mean safety.

B. Role of the oncologist. Many patients who pursue alternative therapy do so because they feel that their alternative practitioner listens to them. Physicians need to recognize that patients have the right to forgo conventional therapy. Common law recognizes the patient's autonomy in making treatment decisions, and this must be respected by the physician.

In most instances, the patient wants the physician's opinion regarding the therapy, but a judgmental or dismissive attitude often drives the patient away. It becomes important to specifically ask during the course of therapy: "Are you considering or are you currently using therapies that are usually considered unconventional or alternative?"

Good communication skills between physician and patient remain the best strategy to combat inappropriate use of alternative medicine. Reassuring patients of continued support no matter what therapy they select remains a key. It is worth remembering that most patients do not have the scientific background to distinguish therapies that have been shown to be effective from completely fraudulent therapies.

A nonjudgmental attitude is important. A particularly useful Web site to which patients can be referred, so that they may get additional information about an alternative therapy, is http://www.quackwatch.com.

X. MANAGING THE DIFFICULT PATIENT

A. Introduction. Most practices include difficult patients; the prevalence is estimated to be 15% of patients. Many physicians enter medicine with the goals of solving medical problems and curing disease. They do not expect to encounter patients who make repeated visits without apparent medical benefit, patients who do not seem to want to get well, patients who engage in power struggles, and patients who focus on issues seemingly unrelated to medical care. The result is often distraction from effective care, waste of physician energy, complaints from patients and staff, and continued health problems for the patient.

A variety of tactics and strategies that reduce common physician–patient communication problems can be applied to difficult encounters. Improving physician communication can lead to increased patient satisfaction, increased health care professional satisfaction, and improved patient health outcomes and a decrease in complaints and lawsuits. Ensuring that patients understand that the physician comprehends their situation and cares about their health is related to better outcomes.

Several factors exist that lead to the generation of the "difficult patient."
1. **Patient factors.** The difficult or frustrating patient, often a "distressed high utilizer of medical services," has unrecognized psychiatric problems. Patients with mood disorders may present with physical symptoms and persistently search for a medical explanation for distress. Patients with alcoholism and borderline personality disorder may present with somatic complaints. Even if the physician recognizes the psychopathology, the patient may reject the diagnosis. Such patients' insistence that the physician pursue somatic symptoms until a medical diagnosis is obtained can be significantly frustrating.
2. **Physician factors.** Physician overwork may be related to greater numbers of patients being considered difficult. Less-experienced physicians more often report encountering more difficult patients. Physicians who have greater need for diagnostic certainty are more likely to consider patients difficult if they present with multiple or vague diagnoses, repeatedly return with poor response to treatment, persistently present with vague physical complaints, or fail to follow through with treatment plans or self-management.

Difficult patients are more likely to identify unmet requests after primary care visits. Patients who feel rushed or ignored may repeat themselves and prolong their visits. These problems may be markers for negative physician attitudes concerning the psychosocial needs of their patients.
3. **System factors.** Managed care has led to increased mistrust between patients and physicians. Attempts to "see more faster" have led to less time with patients. Together, these changes magnify the potential for conflicting expectations between patients and physicians. If expectations are unmet, patients are more likely to be dissatisfied with their visits. Dissatisfied patients may become more demanding, and physicians may feel less able to respond to patient needs, thus transforming the problems of the health care system into interpersonal frustration.
B. **Steps to help manage the difficult patient**
   1. **Psychiatric involvement.** The prevalence of undiagnosed and untreated psychopathology in difficult patients suggests that effective management of such patients routinely should begin with a tactful assessment of the patient's distress. For example, the physician could observe, "You seem quite upset. Could you help me understand what you are going through?" Screen for substance abuse. Targeted psychopharmacology, particularly with selective serotonin reuptake inhibitor (SSRI) therapy, may be considered for patients with symptoms of dysphoria, anxiety, and aggression. Framing medication recommendations in terms of the stress produced by mysterious or intractable medical conditions may facilitate a patient's acceptance of such a prescription. Incorporating a mental health consultant also is helpful.
   2. **Physician responsibility.** Physicians should practice effective self-management. This includes acknowledging and accepting their own emotional responses to patients, as well as seeking help if necessary, be it via colleagues or formal therapy. It may be quite helpful for physicians to elicit feedback on their communication skills. Possible sources include staff, trusted patients, or a review of audiotapes

or videotapes of patient visits. Using the tools described in this chapter such as active listening, empathizing, and reframing can help improve communication.

3. **Counterproductive strategies.** Ignoring the problem or exporting it to another physician does not make the difficulty disappear. Accusing the patient of being problematic may provoke patient anger and counter-blaming. Telling the patient that there is nothing wrong or that there is nothing you can do for him or her may trigger persistent attempts to prove that a problem exists.

Suggested Reading

Back AL, Arnold RM, et al. Approaching difficult communication tasks in oncology. *CA Cancer J Clin* 2005;55:164–177.

Back AL, Arnold RM. Discussing prognosis: "how much do you want to know?" talking to patients who are prepared for explicit information. *J Clin Oncol* 2006;24:4209–4213.

Back AL, Arnold RM. Discussing prognosis: "how much do you want to know?" talking to patients who do not want information or who are ambivalent. *J Clin Oncol* 2006;24:4214–4217.

Back AL, Arnold RM. Dealing with conflict in caring for the seriously ill: "It was just out of the question." *JAMA* 2005;293:1374–1381.

Baile WF, Buckman R, et al. SPIKES—A six-step protocol for delivering bad news: application to the patient with cancer. *Oncologist* 2000;5:302–311.

Buckman R. *How to Break Bad News.* Baltimore: Johns Hopkins University Press; 1992.

Ford S, Fallowfield L, et al. Can oncologists detect distress in their out-patients and how satisfied are they with their performance during bad news consultations? *Br J Cancer* 1994;70:767–770.

Gertz MA, Bauer BA. Caring (really) for patients who use alternative therapies for cancer. *J Clin Oncol* 2003;21(9 Suppl):125–128.

Haas LJ, Leiser JP, et al. Management of the difficult patient. *Am Fam Physician* 2005; 72:2063–2068.

Leighl N, Gattellari M, et al. Discussing adjuvant cancer therapy. *J Clin Oncol* 2001;19: 1768–1778.

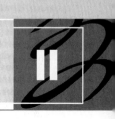

Solid Tumors

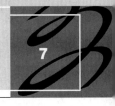

HEAD AND NECK CANCERS

Robert G. Parker, Eric J. Sherman, Steve P. Lee,
Dale H. Rice, and Dennis A. Casciato

7

I. GENERAL ASPECTS OF HEAD AND NECK CANCERS

Head and neck cancers include a heterogeneous group of malignant tumors arising in all structures cephalad to the clavicles, except for the brain, spinal cord, base of the skull, and usually the skin. A meaningful understanding of these malignant tumors requires anatomic separation into those cancers arising in the oral cavity, oropharynx, hypopharynx, nasopharynx, larynx, nasal fossa, paranasal sinuses, thyroid and salivary glands, and vermilion surfaces.

A. Epidemiology and etiology

1. **Incidence.** Cancers arising in the head and neck constitute about 3% of all newly diagnosed cancers in humans. In 2007, an estimated 45,500 newly diagnosed cancers of the oral cavity, pharynx, and larynx resulted in 11,200 related deaths.

2. **Etiology.** Cigarette smoking and substantial alcohol intake are the major risk factors. *Field cancerization* is a concept based on the prolonged exposure of the oral and pharyngeal mucosa to carcinogens. Of the survivors of one cancer of the head and neck, 20% develop another primary head and neck cancer.

B. Pathology

1. **Histology.** Nearly all cancers of the oral cavity and pharynx are squamous cell carcinomas of varying differentiation. Adenoid cystic and mucoepidermoid cancers arise from salivary glands. A range of histologically different cancers, such as papillary, follicular giant cell, Hürthle cell carcinomas, and lymphomas, arise in the thyroid gland.

2. **Metastases.** Most primary cancers of the head and neck spread by invasion of adjacent tissues and metastases to regional lymph nodes. Metastases to distant sites are infrequent.

C. Diagnosis

1. **Common symptoms and signs**
   a. Painless mass
   b. Local ulceration with or without pain
   c. Referred pain to teeth or ear
   d. Dysphagia, mechanical or painful
   e. Alteration of speech, such as difficulty pronouncing words (tongue) or change in character (larynx, nasopharynx)
   f. Persistent hoarseness (larynx)
   g. Unilateral tonsillar enlargement in an adult
   h. Persistent unilateral "sinusitis"
   i. Persistent unilateral nosebleed or obstruction
   j. Unilateral hearing loss often with serous otitis
   k. Cranial nerve palsies

2. **Biopsy and imaging.** Primary cancers of the head and neck must be documented by biopsy. In some circumstances, when epidermoid carcinoma has been identified in a cervical lymph node and no obvious primary tumor found on physical or imaging examinations, "blind" biopsies of Waldeyer's ring are appropriate. Magnetic resonance imaging (MRI) and computed tomography (CT) from the base of the skull to the thoracic inlet are essential in establishing the local or

regional extent of the tumor. Chest x-rays remain part of the evaluation, although intrathoracic metastases are infrequent.

3. **Endoscopy.** Visualization of the oral cavity, nasal cavity, nasopharynx, oropharynx, hypopharynx, larynx, cervical esophagus, and proximal trachea is essential in establishing the presence and extent of tumor. These examinations have been facilitated by development of flexible, small caliber, bright-light endoscopes. Biopsies can be done at the time of endoscopy. It is useful for all oncologists likely to be involved in the management of a specific patient to be present at the endoscopy.

4. **Evaluation of masses in the neck.** A new, firm, usually nontender mass or masses, in the neck, either unilateral or bilateral, especially in adults should be considered metastatic (or primary in the thyroid) cancer until proved otherwise. Before direct biopsy, search for a primary cancer is important. This search may include "blind" biopsies of Waldeyer's ring and should include MRI and CT examinations. Initial direct biopsy of a suspicious, enlarged cervical lymph can be done by fine-needle aspiration. Open biopsy should be done as a last resort.

D. **Staging.** Staging can be based on clinical information or information found at surgery. Clinical staging is important because many patients are treated by radiation therapy (RT). Clinical staging is based on physical examination and information from MRI, CT, or both examinations. All primary cancers must be documented histologically.

The TNM system proposed by the American Joint Committee on Cancer (AJCC) is the most frequently used system in the United States (Table 7.1). T reflects primary tumor size and extension; N is based on the size, number, and location of cervical lymph node metastases; and M represents more distant metastases. The T staging classification varies slightly with the specific anatomic site and will be discussed with each cancer. The N and M classifications and stage groupings are the same for all head and neck cancers except nasopharyngeal carcinoma.

Stage IV is divided into three groups representing locally advanced but still resectable disease (IVA), unresectable locally advanced disease (IVB), and distant metastases (IVC).

E. **Prognostic factors.** The most important prognostic factors for patients with primary cancers of the head and neck are primary tumor site, size and extent, and regional or distant metastases. Histologic differentiation of epidermoid carcinomas is less important. A major risk factor is a previous head and neck cancer. Continued cigarette smoking and consumption of alcoholic beverages expose the mucosa to known carcinogens.

F. **Prevention.** The main preventatives for cancer of the head and neck are abstinence from the use of alcoholic beverages and tobacco. Also avoidance or elimination of chronic irritants, such as an irregular sharp tooth or ill-fitting denture, is desirable. Isoretinoin (13-*cis*-retinoic acid) can reverse severe leukoplakia and possibly reduce the development of squamous cell carcinomas in the oral cavity, but it has no influence on the recurrence of previously treated cancers.

G. **Management principles of head and neck cancers.** Before commitment to a therapy program for a specific patient, there should be input from all members of the multidisciplinary oncology group who will be involved. Included are surgeons, radiation oncologists, medical oncologists, dentists, nurses, social workers, and rehabilitation personnel. Proper management includes frequent, periodic examinations after treatment. Persistent or "recurrent" cancers usually can be recognized within 2 years of the completion of treatment.

1. **Surgery** has long been a mainstay of the treatment of patients with cancers of the head and neck. Treatment of the primary tumor requires removal of the tumor and its local and regional extensions. Sometimes anatomic barriers, such as the base of the skull, make such complete removal unlikely. In such situations, adjuvant RT, chemotherapy, or both may facilitate or even negate the need for radical surgery. Recent advances have promoted adequate resection of some tumors involving the base of the skull.

TABLE 7.1	TNM Staging for Head and Neck Cancers[a,b]

Primary tumor (T)[c,d]

TX	Primary tumor cannot be assessed
T0	No evidence of primary tumor
Tis	Carcinoma *in situ*
T1	Tumor $\leq$2 cm in greatest dimension
T2	Tumor >2 cm but $\leq$4 cm
T3	Tumor >4 cm
T4	Tumor invades adjacent structures (defined under specific site)
T4a	Tumor invades adjacent structures, but is potentially resectable
T4b	Tumor invades adjacent structures, but is unresectable

Regional lymph nodes (N)

NX	Regional lymph nodes cannot be assessed
N0	No regional node metastasis
N1	Metastasis in a single ipsilateral lymph node, $\leq$3 cm
N2a	Metastasis in a single ipsilateral lymph node, >3 cm but $\leq$6 cm
N2b	Metastasis in multiple ipsilateral lymph nodes, none >6 cm
N2c	Metastasis in bilateral or contralateral lymph nodes, none >6 cm
N3	Metastasis in a lymph node >6 cm in greatest dimension

Distant metastases (M)

MX	Distant metastasis cannot be assessed
M0	No distant metastasis
M1	Distant metastasis

Stage groupings

0	Tis	N0	M0		
I	T1	N0	M0		
II	T2	N0	M0		
III	T1–3	N1	M0,	T3 N0	M0
IVA	T4a	N0–2	M0,	T1–3 N2	M0 (advanced, resectable disease)
IVB	Any T	N3	M0,	T4b any N	M0 (advanced, unresectable disease)
IVC	Any T	any N	M1 (advanced, distant metastatic disease)		

[a]Excludes nasopharynx cancers.
[b]N staging, M staging, and stage groupings are identical for the other carcinomas of the head and neck (lip, oral cavity, oropharynx, hypopharynx, larynx, nasal cavity, paranasal sinuses, and major salivary glands).
[c]T staging for carcinomas of the hypopharynx and major salivary glands has the same definitions for tumor size but also depends on local tumor extension.
[d]Carcinomas of the larynx and paranasal sinuses have specific definitions for all T stages that depend on tumor location rather than on tumor size.
Adapted from the *AJCC Cancer Staging Manual.* 6th ed. New York: Springer-Verlag, 2002.

a. **Preservation of functions,** such as swallowing, voice or vision, and cosmesis, must be considered in any management plan. Tumor extension into bone, such as the mandible or maxilla, usually requires resection. Often reconstruction can minimize the long-term morbidity.

b. **Metastases to cervical lymph nodes,** particularly from the oral cavity, paranasal sinuses, hypopharynx, and thyroid, are best treated surgically, although postoperative irradiation frequently is indicated. Removal of cervical nodes containing metastatic cancer can be accomplished by *en bloc* resection (radical neck dissection) or a limited procedure, such as suprahyoid dissection.

2. **RT** can control many cancers of the head and neck, usually with better consequent function and cosmesis than following radical resection. No anatomic barriers to RT exist, although specific tissue tolerance limitations do. Basic radiobiological principles must be observed in devising specific treatment approach (see Chapter 3).

   a. **Primary treatment.** RT is used as the initial and possibly only therapy. This is done mainly to either preserve organs and functions or substitute for surgery for unresectable tumors.

   b. **Adjuvant treatment.** RT is planned for use before or after surgery. The irradiated volume can be the preoperative or the postoperative tissue volume at risk, or it can be separate from the operative site, such as the treatment of cervical nodes after surgical removal of the primary tumor.

   c. **Volume treated.** RT should include all known tumor-bearing anatomic sites plus any sites of suspected tumor spread, such as the neck in a patient with aggressive oral tongue or pharyngeal cancers.

   d. **RT doses.** Included are incremental doses (usually in daily *fractions*) and total doses. Both relate to the probabilities of tumor control and treatment-related sequelae. In general, daily doses should be 180 to 200 cGy/fraction. For epidermoid carcinomas of the head and neck without surgery, the total doses are usually 6,500 to 7,500 cGy. When used as a postoperative adjuvant, the total doses can be lower (5,500 to 6,000 cGy), and when used preoperatively even lower doses (4,500 to 5,000 cGy) are appropriate.

   e. **Altered fractionation schemes.** Special fractionation regimens have been created to exploit certain radiobiological advantages for the treatment of head and neck cancers. (See Chapter 3, section III.E.) They have been tested in numerous international phase-III multicenter randomized trials, and the results have in general been favorable as compared with conventional fractionation practice, especially for locoregionally advanced disease.

   f. **Hyperfractionation** delivers more fractions with smaller dose per fraction to a higher total dose than conventional fractionation, over the same length of overall treatment time. It aims to enhance tumor cell killing while maintaining the same level of late normal tissue damage.

   g. **Accelerated fractionation** aims to overcome the therapy-induced *accelerated repopulation* of cancer cells, and delivers a conventional amount of total dose while shortening the overall treatment time with more intensely fractionated patterns.

   h. **Combined chemoradiotherapy.** In recent years, cytotoxic chemotherapy as well as biologic response modifiers have been shown to augment the therapeutic effect of RT. Most randomized trials have shown the benefit of concurrent chemo-RT (CCRT; see section I.J.3), while induction or neoadjuvant chemotherapy before definitive RT continues to be tested.

   i. **Precision-oriented RT.** Recent advances in computer technology have enabled the development of ultraprecision treatment techniques, such as *stereotactic irradiation* and *intensity modulated RT (IMRT)*. *Particle therapy* with protons and heavy ions are also available in a few centers worldwide (see Chapter 3, sections IV.C, D).

H. Management of the primary cancer

1. **Most T1 and T2 primary cancers** can be controlled equally well by surgery or RT. Therefore, the choice of treatment may be influenced by tumor site, accessibility, histologic grade, the patient's health status, vocation, or preference. Organ or functional preservation may be provided by RT for cancers of the oral and pharyngeal tongue, floor of the mouth, larynx, orbit, or tonsil. Surgery is preferable when tumor involves bone.

2. **Most T3 and T4 primary cancers** often require combinations of surgery and RT. If resection is not possible, high-dose RT may still be effective and adjuvant chemotherapy may be useful. Although preoperative irradiation may reduce the tumor size and theoretically facilitate the surgery, postoperative irradiation is nearly always preferable because the extent of tumor can be better determined and tissue healing is less impaired. The total radiation doses after complete

resection of the primary and regional tumors may be reduced to 5,500 to 6,000 cGy. Indications for postoperative RT include

    a. Close or inadequate resection margins

    b. Poorly differentiated cancers

    c. Involvement of lymphatics, including cervical nodes

    d. Perineural invasion

  3. When cancer reappears clinically at the initial site following a complete response to the primary treatment, this is considered local recurrence of cancer. If a tumor arises at a different site, especially if the histology is different, it is considered a new cancer. The retreatment of cancers can be difficult, with reduced effectiveness and increased morbidity, although surgery may "rescue" failures of RT, and irradiation may control surgical failures.

    a. Recurrence of a tumor usually indicates a biologically aggressive cancer and the prognosis is worse than before the initial treatment.

    b. If the local failure is at the margin of the treatment site, it may be a direct result of "geographical miss," and additional focal salvage treatment may still provide effective cure.

I. Treatment of metastases to cervical lymph nodes is related to extent of the metastases (massive, fixed, or bilateral), the location of the metastases, the histology, and the primary tumor site. The most frequent treatment is surgery either at the time of resection of the primary cancer or later.

  1. The types of neck dissection (ND) are

    a. Classic radical ND. Removes *en bloc* all tissues from the clavicle to the mandible and from the anterior margin of the trapezius muscle to the midline strap muscles between the superficial layer of the deep cervical fascia (platysma) and the deep layer of the deep cervical fascia. Included are the sternocleidomastoid muscle, internal jugular vein, and accessory (11th) cranial nerve.

    b. A **modified radical ND** usually spares the accessory (11th) nerve, the sternocleidomastoid muscle, or both. This operation is usually used when the neck is "clinically negative," but at high risk for metastases or when the metastases to cervical nodes are minimal and when RT is to be used. A variant is the **supraomohyoid dissection** that removes nodes only from the upper neck.

    c. When a **partial neck dissection** is done, only a limited number of lymph nodes are removed. This might be a single, suspicious node.

  2. The risk of clinically undetected metastases varies with primary tumor site and size and the histology. For example, approximately 40% of patients with squamous cell carcinomas of the oral tongue will eventually develop cervical adenopathy. This risk is higher, and often bilateral, for patients with carcinomas of the pharyngeal tongue. In contrast, cervical metastases do not develop in patients with cancers limited to the true vocal cords because there are no lymphatics.

  3. Selection of treatment. When metastases to cervical lymph nodes are present at the time of diagnosis, treatment of the neck is usually dictated by the treatment modality selected for the primary tumor. For squamous cell carcinomas, primary in the oral cavity and paranasal sinuses, surgery may be preferable. When the cancers arise in the nasopharynx, RT is the choice because these tumors are radioresponsive; they often are bilateral and may not be resectable because of anatomic barriers. Other pharyngeal and laryngeal primary tumors would require both surgery and RT, but with cervical nodal metastases primary, RT with or without chemotherapy is preferable, often followed by planned neck dissection.

J. Role of chemotherapy in squamous cell carcinomas of the head and neck (SCCHN). Chemotherapy does not have a role in most early stage (I and II) SCCHN. The greatest benefit derived from chemotherapy is in patients with locally advanced disease when chemotherapy is used either sequentially with RT or concurrently with RT (CCRT), with or without surgery. It has been shown in this setting to increase the possibility of larynx preservation and improve survival. In the metastatic setting, it may be used as a palliative measure and has also been shown to improve overall survival.

1. **Effective agents.** Many drugs have shown activity as single agents in the metastatic setting with potentially high response rates (RR) in phase II studies. Examples include methotrexate (RR 10% to 45%), cisplatin (RR 15% to 40%), bleomycin (RR 5% to 45%), 5-fluorouracil (5-FU; RR 0% to 33%), paclitaxel (RR 30%–40%), docetaxel (RR 30% to 40%), carboplatin (RR 10% to 30%), ifosfamide (RR 25%), cetuximab (RR 16%), and erlotinib (RR 4%). These response rates often decrease significantly in phase III studies.

2. **Induction chemotherapy** (before surgery or RT) has been evaluated extensively. Despite very high RR, early studies did not show survival benefit with this approach. A meta-analysis has shown, however, a small but significant survival benefit when cisplatin and 5-FU are used in combination.

   Several randomized studies in the United States and Europe have also shown a benefit when a taxane (usually docetaxel) is added to cisplatin/5-FU, given either before RT or CCRT. The Dana Farber group (TAX 324) showed a significant improvement in 3-year overall survival from 48% to 62% when docetaxel was added to cisplatin/5-FU, then followed by carboplatin given concurrently with RT. What is not known is whether the addition of any induction chemotherapy will improve survival compared with the optimal CCRT.

3. **Induction chemotherapy regimens for SCCHN** include:
   a. Given in 21-day cycles
      Docetaxel, 75 mg/m^2, IV on day 1
      Cisplatin, 75 mg/m^2, IV on day 1
      5-FU, 750 mg/m^2/day by continuous IV infusion over 24 hours on days 1 through 5
   b. Given in 21-day cycles
      Docetaxel, 75 mg/m^2, IV on day 1
      Cisplatin, 100 mg/m^2, IV on day 1
      5-FU, 1,000 mg/m^2/day by continuous IV infusion over 24 hours on days 1 through 4

4. **Concurrent chemoradiotherapy** has been shown to improve larynx preservation rates in intermediate, locally advanced laryngeal cancer by the Radiation Therapy Oncology Group (RTOG 91-11). A meta-analysis of CCRT used in patients with locally advanced SCCHN has shown a statistically significant improvement in overall survival (absolute improvement 8%). Survival benefits have been seen in randomized studies using various chemotherapy regimens, such as cisplatin alone, cisplatin with 5-FU, and carboplatin with 5-FU.

   A study with cetuximab, a monoclonal antibody to the epidermal growth factor receptor, in combination with RT, has shown a significant survival benefit compared with RT alone (55% vs. 45% 3-year overall survival). Although CCRT using conventional cytotoxic agents will increase mucosal toxicity compared with RT alone, this increase in toxicity was not seen with cetuximab. A small (21 patients) single institution phase II study done at Memorial Sloan-Kettering Cancer Center evaluated the combination of cisplatin, cetuximab, and RT and showed an impressive 3-year overall survival rate of 76% in a group of patients with very advanced disease; however, five significant adverse events, including two deaths, occurred. This regimen is being tested in a phase III cooperative group study (RTOG 05-22), but because of the potential toxicity, is not recommended outside of a clinical trial.

5. **CCRT regimens for SCCHN** include
   a. Given in 21-day cycles for three cycles with RT
      Cisplatin, 100 mg/m^2, IV on day 1
   b. Given in 21-day cycles for 3 cycles with RT
      Carboplatin, 70 mg/m^2, IV on days 1 through 4
      5-FU, 600 mg/m^2/day by continuous IV infusion over 24 hours on days 1 through 4
   c. Cetuximab, 400 mg/m^2 IV loading dose given on the week before RT starts, then 250 mg/m^2 IV weekly for 7 weeks

6. **Adjuvant chemotherapy** is not recommended as standard of care after RT, with the single exception of nasopharyngeal carcinoma. In the Intergroup Study 0099, patients with stage III/IV nasopharyngeal carcinoma were randomized to RT alone or concurrent cisplatin and RT followed by three cycles of adjuvant cisplatin and 5-FU. The 3-year overall survival was 47% and 78%, respectively ($P = 0.005$), establishing this regimen with CCRT followed by adjuvant chemotherapy as the standard of care.

   Although no benefit was seen with the use of RT alone (e.g., Intergroup 00-34) in the postoperative setting, several studies have evaluated CCRT in "high risk" patients. The two largest phase III randomized studies that have been completed were done by the European Organization for Research of Cancer (EORTC 22931) and the RTOG (RTOG 95-01). Both studies randomized patients to either high dose cisplatin as CCRT or RT alone and showed significant improvement in disease-free survival with cisplatin added. However, only EORTC 22931 showed a significant improvement in overall survival (absolute 13% survival benefit at 5 years). Subset analyses of both studies have shown that *significant improvement in survival is seen only for patients with either extracapsular lymph node extension or positive surgical margins.*

   a. **CCRT plus adjuvant regimen for nasopharyngeal carcinoma:**

   Cisplatin, 100 mg/m^2, IV on day 1 of 21-day cycles for three cycles concurrently with RT

   Followed by three 28-day cycles (after RT is completed) of Cisplatin, 80 mg/m^2 IV on day 1, and

   5-FU, 1,000 mg/m^2/day by continuous IV infusion over 24 hours on days 1 through 4

   b. **Postoperative CCRT regimen:**

   Cisplatin, 100 mg/m^2, IV on day 1 of 21-day cycles for three cycles concurrently with RT

7. **Reirradiation.** The standard of care for patients with recurrent unresectable disease in a previously irradiated field is palliative chemotherapy. Several investigators, however, have evaluated the use of reirradiation concurrently with chemotherapy with overall 2- to 5-year survival rates ranging from 15% to 25%.

   RTOG 99-11 evaluated hyperfractionated RT with cisplatin (15 mg/m^2) and paclitaxel (20 mg/m^2), both given daily for 5 days every 14 days for four cycles; treatment resulted in a 27% 2-year overall survival. The use of granulocyte colony-stimulating factor is routinely required between cycles.

   An early phase II study (RTOG 96-10) evaluated reirradiation using hyperfractionated RT with concurrent hydroxyurea (1.5 g) and 5-FU (300 mg/m^2), both given daily for 5 days every 14 days for four cycles; treatment resulted in a 16% 2-year overall survival.

   A phase III study to determine if this approach is superior to standard chemotherapy had to close early because of poor accrual. At this time, this highly toxic approach should be considered investigational and should not be done outside of a clinical trial or a center with extensive experience with this treatment.

8. **Metastatic SCCHN** is treated with chemotherapy alone and is not curable. Multiple chemotherapy agents have shown activity in this setting.

   a. Although combination regimens have shown superior improvement in responses compared with single agents, no randomized study has ever demonstrated an improvement in overall survival. During this time, single agent methotrexate (40 to 60 mg/m^2 IV weekly) should have been considered standard of care because no other regimen had been shown to be superior.

   b. **Cetuximab** is a promising agent for the treatment of SCCHN.

   (1) The EXTREME trial was presented in June of 2007, which compared cisplatin (100 mg/m^2 on day 1) or carboplatin (AUC 5 on day 1) plus 5-FU (1,000 mg/m^2/day by continuous infusion on days 1 through 4), both

with and without cetuximab (400 mg/m^2 loading dose followed by 250 mg/m^2 weekly). This study showed a significant improvement in median survival with the addition of cetuximab from 7 months to 10 months. No crossover to cetuximab was allowed in the study.

(2) A randomized phase III trial by the Eastern Cooperative Oncology Group compared cisplatin and placebo with cisplatin and cetuximab in 117 eligible patients. The median and progression-free survivals were 8 months and 3 months in the control group versus 9 months ($P = 0.21$) and 4 months ($P = 0.07$) in the experimental arm. Crossover was allowed in this study.

(3) Many investigators have interpreted the results of these important studies to mean that cetuximab should be used in the treatment of metastatic SCCHN. This is not necessarily so as the first-line regimen. It is always appropriate, when available, to treat on a clinical trial, even if this means cetuximab is held until for second- or third-line treatment.

K. Adverse effects of treatment. All treatments of cancer, even when properly administered by current standards, may have unintended adverse consequences.

1. Radical surgery
   a. Interference with swallowing
   b. Loss or change in quality and forcefulness of voice
   c. Aspiration
   d. Shoulder or upper limb weakness
   e. Localized cutaneous sensory change or loss
   f. Need for thyroid replacement
   g. Diplopia, visual loss
   h. Cosmetic changes

2. Radiation therapy
   a. Acute, self-limiting effects
      (1) Erythema of skin
      (2) Conjunctivitis
      (3) Mucositis in oral cavity, oropharynx, hypopharynx, nasopharynx, larynx, nasal fossa
      (4) Epilation, dose related, involving scalp, facial hair, eyelashes, eyebrows. Returning hair may be more sparse and even of a different color and texture.
      (5) Edema. Laryngeal is the most serious
      (6) Lhermitte syndrome is an infrequent problem manifested as an "electric shocklike" sensation, usually in the upper limbs precipitated by flexion of the neck. This syndrome is secondary to radiation-induced change, probably temporary demyelination. It is not a precursor of permanent myelopathy.
      (7) Alteration of taste
      (8) Xerostomia, which may be minimized by total radiation dose reduction through use of techniques such as intensity modulated radiation therapy (IMRT). Medications, such as pilocarpine (Salagen), have been tried without scientifically documented success.
      (9) Infection, the most frequent of which is candidiasis controllable by fluconazole.
   b. Long-term or permanent
      (1) Xerostomia. Recovery from acute change may be minimal with long-term adverse consequences, including tooth decay, oral infections, and problems swallowing and associated weight loss. Xerostomia also may be associated with autoimmune disorders (Sjögren's syndrome), diabetes, scleroderma, and many medications, including antidepressants, antihypertensives, and medication for allergies.
      (2) Altered taste: usually for salt or sweet
      (3) Cataract: develops slowly (more frequent in diabetics)

(4) Osteoradionecrosis, usually of the mandible (worse with poor oral hygiene)

(5) Cervical myelopathy appears over several months and is permanent

(6) Soft tissue change: atrophy, telangiectasia, rarely ulceration

(7) Skin cancer: described in literature but is very rare

(8) Epilation

3. **Chemotherapy** as an adjunct can increase acute side effects of RT.

4. **Toxicity of CCRT.** The addition of chemotherapy to RT increases toxicity of treatment, particularly mucositis. RTOG 91-11 compared CCRT with induction chemotherapy followed by RT and with RT alone. The incidence of grade 3 to 4 stomatitis was 73% in the CCRT arm and about 40% in the other two arms. At 1 year after treatment, the proportions of patients who could swallow only soft foods or liquids and who could not swallow at all were 23% and 3%, respectively, for CCRT; 15% and 3%, respectively, for RT alone; and 9% and 0%, respectively, for induction chemotherapy. No difference was noted in the three arms with regards to speech. Late grade 3 to 4 toxic effects were also reported to be 30% in the CCRT group compared with 36% in the RT only group. Treatment-related deaths were 5% in the CCRT compared with 3% in the induction chemotherapy and RT only arms.

L. Supportive care

1. **Acute mucositis.** Discomfort can be decreased by use of bland foods at room temperature, ice chips, topical analgesics or anesthetics, preparations (e.g., Ulcerease or Gelclair), and pain medications.

2. **Opportunistic infections,** most frequently candidiasis, can be controlled by specific medications.

3. **Adequate nutrition** is very important. Frequent meals, diet supplements, and high-calorie intake usually are adequate. Hyperalimentation is rarely used.

4. **Dental care**

   a. All patients who plan to receive high-dose RT to the head and neck region, especially if major salivary glands are in the irradiated fields, should have dental consultation before the start of treatment.

   b. Fluoride gel treatment should be used before, during, and after RT. Continuation of treatment should be based on consultation with the involved dentist.

   c. Dentures should not be worn during treatment or until healing of the oral mucosa is complete (several months). Special dentures may be advisable.

   d. Prophylactic tooth extraction may need to be performed before RT, and 1 to 2 weeks of recovery time may be necessary before any irradiation begins.

   e. Special devices, such as intraoral shielding or bite opener, may need to be constructed by a specialty dentist before the RT planning session.

   f. Chemotherapy can exacerbate significantly the dental sequelae of RT.

M. Special clinical problems

1. **Local or regional regrowth** of the previously treated cancer needs to be distinguished from the side effects of treatment. Cancer usually increases in mass and firmness and the overlying skin may become brawny, purple in color, and fixed to adjacent tissue. There may be associated ulceration. Although radiation side effects may persist or temporarily increase, usually there is tissue decrease with fibrosis and atrophy. Secondary radiation changes will be limited to the irradiated volume, whereas the regrowing cancer may extend outside the treatment volume. Biopsies of radiation-induced changes may be hazardous with the development of poorly or nonhealing ulceration and infection. Therefore, treatment, if potentially useful, usually can be instituted based on clinical appearance.

2. **Cosmetic defects** may be devastating to the patient. These usually are distortions such as secondary to seventh nerve palsy, reduction in size of the oral cavity, loss of portions of the nose or ear, loss or alteration of orbital contents, permanent absence of dentures, and unsightly grafts. Often reconstructive surgery is indicated. Psychological support is imperative. Interactions with support groups with similar problems may be useful.

3. **Massive facial edema** is an infrequent problem. The underlying cause is extensive venous or lymphatic obstruction secondary to uncontrolled cancer. Management is symptomatic and usually unsatisfactory. This usually is an end-stage problem with death secondary to cerebral edema, hemorrhage, or inanition.

4. **Arterial rupture with rapid exsanguination** owing to disruption of the carotid artery secondary to cancer or necrosis is a rare problem. Prevention is based on local tumor control, avoidance of progressive infection with necrosis, and proper technique of neck dissections.

5. **Upper airway obstruction** may be secondary to progressive cancer, edema, or a combination. The edema can be treated with high doses of prednisone (40 to 60 mg/day orally). Tracheostomy may bypass the obstruction and produce temporary relief. Associated infection should be vigorously treated. For patients who have tumor regrowth after irradiation, chemotherapy may provide tumor reduction.

6. **Obstructive dysphagia.** If this is secondary to progressive, previously treated cancer, there probably are accompanying adverse findings, such as airway obstruction and pain. Management usually accomplishes very little.

7. **Infection** associated with progressive, necrotic cancer can be treated with broadspectrum antibiotics, although the effect usually is minimal and temporary.

N. Specific head and neck cancer sites. The relative occurrence, sex predominance, most common site, and histology of the constituents of head and neck cancers are compared in Table 7.2.

II. LIP

A. Definition. Cancers of the lip arise on the vermilion surfaces and mucosa. Cancers arising on the skin of the lower lip are considered separately as primary skin cancers.

B. Pathology. Nearly all lip cancers are squamous cell carcinomas, usually well differentiated.

C. Natural history

1. **Presentation.** Of primary lip cancers, 95% arise on the lower vermilion surface. The gross appearances range from minimal erythematous change, through dryscaling to ulcerated masses, occasionally with destruction of underlying muscle and bone. The prognosis may be worse with a need for more aggressive treatment when the lateral commissure is involved by tumor.

2. **Risk factors.** Long-time exposure to sun or wind; chronic irritation.

TABLE 7.2 Features of Head and Neck Cancers by Site of Origin

Primary tumor	Most common site	Relative occurrence (%)	Cervical lymph node metastases at time of presentation (%)
Lip[a]	Lower lip (90%)	15	5
Oral cavity[a]	Tongue (lateral border)	20	40
Oropharynx[a]	Tonsillar region	10	80 for tonsillar fossa and base of tongue 40 for other sites
Hypopharynx[a]	Pyriform sinus	5	80
Larynx[a]	True vocal cord	25	<5 for early glottic, 35 for other sites
Nasopharynx[a]	Roof	3	80
Nasal cavity and sinuses	Maxillary antrum	4	15
Salivary glands	Parotid (80%)	15	25

[a]At least 97% are squamous cell carcinomas.

3. **Lymphatic drainage.** From the upper lip primarily to the submandibular lymph nodes; from the lower lip to the submental, submandibular, and subdigastric nodes. The risk of metastases to regional lymph nodes increases with less differentiated tumors, large size, and extension of tumor to the lateral commissures. Of patients, 5% to 10% are likely to have spread to regional lymph nodes at the time of diagnosis and another 5% to 10% will develop adenopathy later.

D. **Differential diagnosis**
   1. Keratoacanthoma is an exophytic lesion that arises rapidly and usually resolves spontaneously within a few months. Small doses of RT accelerate this resolution, but usually are not advisable.
   2. Hyperkeratosis, often with irritation, infection, or both
   3. Leukoplakia
   4. Chancre when syphilis was more frequent

E. **TNM staging.** See Table 7.1 for regional lymph node (N) and metastasis (M) classifications and for stage groupings. Primary tumor (T) classification for lip cancers is as follows:

T_{is} Carcinoma *in situ*
T_1 Tumor ≤ 2 cm in largest dimension
T_2 Tumor >2 cm, but not >4 cm in greatest dimension
T_3 Tumor >4 cm in greatest dimension
T_4 Tumor invades through cortical bone, alveolar nerve, floor of mouth, or skin of chin or nose

F. **Management of the primary cancer.** Lip cancer, when detected early, can be cured equally well by limited surgery, RT, or chemosurgery (Moh's method)
   1. **Vermilionectomy** (lip shave) can be used to treat leukoplakia, severe dysplasia, and limited carcinoma *in situ*.
   2. **T_{is} and T_1 carcinomas** (≤ 1.0 cm). RT (external beam, isotope surface application or implantation) or surgery (minimal resection with primary closure without reduction of oral stoma) are highly effective with good resulting cosmesis.
   3. **T_{1-4} carcinomas** (>1.0 cm). RT has some cosmetic and functional advantages over surgery if no destruction of underlying normal tissues. If bone is involved or there is substantial loss of normal tissue, surgery with reconstruction is preferable.
   4. **Commissure involvement.** RT has advantage over surgery.
   5. **Local tumor control rate.** Failure rates are related to tumor size and extent. For the primary cancer, the failure rate is $<10\%$ for T_1 lesions. Failure rate in the neck is $<10\%$ when the neck initially is N_0, but may increase to 45% when there is gross metastatic adenopathy.

G. **Treatment of regional lymph nodes**
   1. **Clinically negative neck.** Observation is preferable. RT can be used for primary cancers that are large or histologically poorly differentiated.
   2. **Clinically involved nodes.** Surgery is preferable. When the primary cancer crosses the midline, both sides of the neck are at risk. The major adenopathy is best treated surgically. Subclinical tumor on the other side of the neck can be irradiated or treated with a limited neck dissection.
   3. **Delayed neck dissections** can effectively treat metastatic adenopathy that appears clinically after previous treatment of the primary cancer.

H. **Treatment of locally "reappearing" cancer** can be effective. Surgery is preferable for the treatment of RT failures and additional resections can be used for surgical failures.

III. ORAL CAVITY

A. **Definition.** Includes primary cancers of the oral tongue, floor of the mouth, buccal mucosa (including the retromolar tigone), gingiva, alveolar ridge, hard palate, and anterior tonsillar pillar.

B. **Pathology.** Nearly all primary cancers are squamous cell carcinomas. Less than 5% are adenocarcinomas (adenoid cystic, mucoepidermoid carcinomas arising from minor salivary glands).

C. Natural history

1. **Risk factors** include use of tobacco products, long-time ingestion of alcoholic beverages, poor oral hygiene, and prolonged focal irritation from teeth or dentures.

2. **Presentation**

   a. Patients with **oral tongue cancers** may notice a local mucosal irritation or a mass that may become ulcerated, infected, and painful. A foul odor or taste may be associated with infection. Pain may be local or referred to the ear. Infiltration of muscle can give rise to problems transporting boluses or speaking.

   b. Early **buccal mucosa cancers** may be asymptomatic or felt by the tongue. Ulceration can result in local pain. Obstruction of Stensen's duct may be the basis of tender enlargement of the parotid gland. Pain referred to the ear follows tumor involvement of the lingual or dental nerves. Local tumor extension can cause trismus.

   c. **Gingival cancers** may be noted as local mucosal changes, often with accompanying leukoplakia. More extensive cancers cause loosening of teeth, interference with denture use, bleeding, or pain. Underlying bone may be invaded. Tumor may extend to involve adjacent anatomic structures, such as floor of mouth, buccal mucosa, hard and soft palate, or maxillary sinus.

   d. Cancers of the **retromolar trigone** can cause trismus by involving the pterygomandibular space, pterygoid, and buccinator muscles.

   e. Cancers arising on the **hard palate** are likely to invade bone.

   f. Cancers arising from the mucosa of the **floor of the mouth** may be seen as a localized mucosal change, often with leukoplakia, or felt as a mass by the patient. When localized with ulceration and tenderness, these lesions initially may be misdiagnosed as canker sores. With local extension, there may be a submandibular mass, obstruction of the submaxillary ducts with gland enlargement, and invasion of the oral tongue or mandible.

3. **Lymphatic metastases** most often involve subdigastric, upper jugular, and submandibular nodes. The frequency varies with site, extent, and differentiation of the primary cancer, but may range up to 30% to 35% at the time of diagnosis with a later increase in untreated necks secondary to the growth of initial subclinical metastases. The risk of bilateral metastases increases as the primary tumor approaches or involves the anatomic midline.

4. **Metastases** below (caudad) the clavicles or above (cephalad) the base of the skull are infrequent, whether lymphatic or hematogenous.

D. Diagnosis.
Establishment of a diagnosis of cancer arising in the oral cavity should be relatively straightforward because patients usually have distinctive symptoms and signs and the tumors can easily be visualized and palpated. A diagnosis must be established by biopsy. Imaging examinations (CT, MRI) have become a major part of the appraisal of tumor extent, bone involvement, and lymph node metastases.

E. TNM staging.
See Table 7.1 for primary tumor (T), regional lymph node (N), and metastasis (M) classifications.

F. Management of the primary tumor

1. **Oral tongue and floor of mouth carcinomas**

   a. **Small tumors (<1.0 cm).** Resection with primary closure; interstitial RT; or external beam RT using oral cone (rarely used)

   b. **T_1 or T_2 tumors.** Resection if minimal deformity or combination of external beam RT and interstitial RT. The choice can vary with patient preference, health status, and occupational, social or psychological factors.

   c. **Extensive tumors.** Resection followed by external beam RT. Surgery is preferable when the mandible is invaded by tumor, and for verrucous carcinomas and unreliable patients.

   d. **Local tumor control rate with RT** (approximate)

   T_1 tumors, 80%
   T_2 tumors, 65% to 70%
   T_3 tumors, 25%

2. **Gingival and hard palate carcinomas**
   a. **Small tumors.** Resection
   b. **Extensive tumors.** Resection and postoperative RT
   c. **Local control rate of T$_1$ tumors.** 60%
3. **Buccal mucosal carcinomas**
   a. **Small tumors (<1.0 cm).** Resection and primary closure
   b. **T$_{1-3}$.** RT or resection, probably with a graft
   c. **Larger superficial cancers (T$_{1-2}$).** RT effective
   d. **Extensive tumors (T$_{3-4}$) with invasion of muscle.** Resection and postoperative RT
   e. **Tumor extension to commissure.** RT should be considered
   f. **Local tumor control rate** with RT (approximate)

   T$_1$ tumors, >95%
   T$_2$ tumors, 70%
   T$_3$ tumors, 70%
   T$_4$ tumors, 50%

4. **Retromolar trigone.** (faucial pillar carcinomas)
   a. **T1 to T2 tumors.** RT or resection with or without RT
   b. **T3 superficial tumors.** RT
   c. **Large tumors, deep infiltration.** Resection and postoperative RT (special problems exist with extension of tumor into the pharyngeal tongue or bone)
   d. **Local tumor control rate**

   T1 tumors, 75%
   T2 tumors, 70% to 75%
   T3 tumors, 70% to 75%

5. **Management of the neck.** When the primary cancer is controlled, death caused by uncontrolled metastatic cancer in the neck should be uncommon. The risk of subclinical involvement of neck nodes is related to the T stage and histologic differentiation. Although adenopathy usually can be treated successfully after observation of an N$_0$ neck, elective treatment may lessen the risk of uncontrolled tumor in the neck and development of distant metastases. *Some general guidelines are as follows:*
   a. **Clinically "negative" neck**
      (1) T$_1$, low-grade primary cancers. Observation if the patient is reliable
      (2) T$_2$ to T$_4$ or poorly differentiated primary cancers
         (a) If the primary tumor is treated surgically, perform elective neck dissection
         (b) If the primary cancer is irradiated, the neck should be concurrently irradiated
         (c) If the primary cancer is managed by combined treatment methods, either treatment method may be used
   b. **Clinical lymphadenopathy**
      (1) If the primary tumor is treated surgically, add ND
      (2) If the primary tumor is treated with RT, irradiate the neck and follow with ND for residual adenopathy after adequate observation or if an initially enlarged node was large (i.e., >3.0 cm)
      (3) When the tumor-involved nodes are "fixed," start with RT. If the adenopathy becomes resectable, perform ND after about 5,000 cGy. If not, give RT to full total dose.

IV. OROPHARYNX
   A. **Definition.** Includes pharyngeal ("base of") tongue, tonsillar region (fossa and pillars although anterior pillar often included in oral cavity), soft palate, and pharyngeal walls between the pharyngoepiglottic fold and the nasopharynx.
   B. **Pathology.** Ninety-five percent are squamous cell carcinomas, usually less histologically differentiated than those of the oral cavity. A few tumors may be adenocarcinomas arising in the minor salivary glands or primary lymphomas.

C. Natural history

1. **Risk factors** include prolonged intake of alcoholic beverages, especially for primary carcinomas of the anterior tonsillar pillar and posterior pharyngeal wall.

2. **Clinical presentation**

   a. May be clinically "silent," especially those cancers arising in the pharyngeal tongue where the tumor may be submucosal, but indurated.

   b. Pharyngeal tongue and tonsillar carcinomas may appear clinically as cervical adenopathy.

   c. Symptoms include localized pain aggravated by swallowing, ipsilateral otalgia, difficulty swallowing secondary to pain, or decreased mobility of the tongue. The patient may feel a mass at the primary site or in the neck.

3. **Lymphatic drainage.** The lymphatics of the pharyngeal tongue, tonsil, and pharyngeal wall are abundant. The lymphatics of the pharyngeal tongue drain into the deep cervical nodes and involvement often is bilateral. The lymphatics of the tonsillar region and faucial arch drain into the subdigastric, upper and middle cervical, and parapharyngeal nodes. Metastases usually are ipsilateral unless the primary tumor approaches the midline. Lymphatic drainage from the pharyngeal wall is to the retropharyngeal and level II–III cervical nodes.

D. Diagnosis. Cancers arising in the oropharynx can be visualized and palpated. The diagnosis must be documented by biopsy. Differential diagnoses on physical examination include tonsillar abscess, benign lymphoid hyperplasia, and benign ulceration with induration.

E. TNM staging. See Table 7.1 for primary tumor (T), regional lymph node (N), and metastasis (M) classifications and for stage groupings.

Staging includes epithelial malignant tumors arising in the sites defined above. Nonepithelial tumors arising in lymphoid tissue, soft tissue, bone, and cartilage are not included. Clinical staging often is used because many of these cancers are treated by primary RT. Assessment for clinical staging is based on inspection, palpation, CT, and MRI examination. Pathologic staging adds information found at surgery.

F. Management of the primary tumor

1. **Pharyngeal tongue**

   a. **Small tumors.** Surgery if lateralized or RT

   b. **Larger tumors.** Especially if approaching midline, RT

   c. **Local tumor control**

   T_1 tumors, 85% to 90%
   T_2 tumors, 75%
   T_3 tumors, 65%

2. **Tonisllar region**

   a. **Small tumors.** Surgery or RT

   b. **Extensive primary tumors.** Surgery plus postoperative RT

   c. **Local tumor control**

   T_1 tumors, 95%
   T_2 tumors, 85%
   T_3 tumors, 50%
   T_4 tumors, 20%

3. **Soft palate**

   a. **Small tumors.** Usually RT or surgery if minimal resulting dysfunction

   b. **Large tumors.** RT

   c. **Local tumor control**

   T_1 tumors, 95%
   T_2 tumors, 65% to 90%
   T_3 tumors, 50% to 75%
   T_4 tumors, 20%

4. **Pharyngeal wall**
    a. **Small tumors.** RT can be effective with minimal morbidity
    b. **Extensive tumors.** RT and surgery if applicable
    c. **Local tumor control rate for T_{2-3} tumors.** 35% to 50%
G. **Management of the neck.** Primary carcinomas arising in the pharyngeal tongue, soft palate, and pharyngeal wall are likely to metastasize to nodes in both sides of the neck. Limited primary cancers of the tonsillar region may metastasize only to ipsilateral nodes.

   For primary carcinomas managed by RT, the neck should be part of the initial treatment plan. As the cervical adenopathy becomes larger or more nodes are involved, ND becomes part of the management. If the initial treatment of the primary site and the neck is surgery, postoperative RT is advisable when the primary tumor is extensive, the histology is poorly differentiated, the adenopathy is large (i.e., >3.0 cm), multiple nodes are involved, or when tumor extends through the capsule of the node. CCRT may also be considered under these circumstances.
H. **Treatment of "recurrence."** Repeated thorough examinations at intervals of a few months are an important part of patient management. Most persistence or regrowth of tumor can be recognized within 2 years of treatment of the initial cancer. Salvage treatment by either surgery or RT or both may be successful. These patients are also at high risk to develop other cancers.

V. NASOPHARYNX

A. **Definition.** Carcinomas of the nasopharynx arise in a small anatomic site bordered by the nasal fossae, the posterior wall continuous with the posterior wall of the oropharynx (first and second cervical vertebrae), the body of the sphenoid and basilar part of the occipital bones, and the soft palate.
B. **Pathology.** About 90% of malignant tumors are squamous cell carcinoma, whereas 5% are lymphomas and 5% are of other various subtypes. The squamous cell carcinomas are 20% well-differentiated, 40% to 50% moderately differentiated, and 40% to 50% undifferentiated (lymphoepitheliomas).
C. **Natural history**
    1. **Risk factors**
        a. Incidence higher in Asians, particularly those from southern China, Eskimos, and Icelanders. This risk prevails in first generation immigrants to other parts of the world.
        b. Nonkeratinizing nasopharyngeal carcinomas are uniformly associated with Epstein-Barr virus (EBV); patients usually have increased levels of immunoglobulin A antibody to the viral capsid antigen and early antigen. Monitoring EBV DNA in the serum of affected patients using real-time polymerase chain reaction technology appears to be useful tool for gauging responses to therapy.
        c. Can occur in the pediatric age group.
    2. **Presentation**
        a. Often initially noted as high posterior cervical adenopathy, which may be bilateral
        b. Epistaxis, nasal obstruction
        c. Change in voice
        d. Unilateral hearing loss or "fullness" in one ear, serous otitis
        e. Trismus
        f. Headache
        g. Proptosis
        h. Cranial nerve syndromes secondary to tumor invasion of base of skull
            (1) **Retrosphenoidal syndrome** from involvement of cranial nerves II through VI manifests as unilateral ophthalmoplegia, ptosis, pain, trigeminal neuralgia, and unilateral weakness of muscles of mastication.
            (2) **Retroparotid syndrome** from compression of cranial nerves IX through XII and sympathetic nerves manifests as mechanical dysphagia, problems with taste, salivation, or respiration, weakness of the trapezius, sternocleidomastoid muscles, or tongue muscles, and Horner's syndrome.

  i. Distant metastases more frequent with nasopharyngeal carcinoma than with any other head and neck cancer

 3. Lymphatic drainage. The abundant lymphatics drain to the retropharyngeal and deep cervical lymph nodes (internal jugular and spinal accessory nerve chains). Drainage is bilateral. Lymphadenopathy is present in 80% of patients at presentation with 50% being bilateral.

 4. Prognostic factors
  a. Tumor extent, particularly invasion of the base of the skull
  b. Size and level of cervical node metastases
  c. Age (prognosis is better with age <40 to 50 years)
  d. Tumor type

D. Diagnosis
 1. Endoscopy to identify the primary cancer, which may be a minimal mucosal alteration or mass
 2. Palpation of the neck for adenopathy, which usually is high posterior cervical and often is bilateral
 3. CT or MRI to identify the extent of primary tumor and adenopathy and involvement of the base of the skull
 4. Cranial nerve examination
 5. Differential diagnoses include benign adenopathy of Waldeyer's ring, nasopharyngitis, and cervical adenopathy of other etiology.

E. TNM staging for nasopharyngeal carcinoma differs from that of other head and neck cancers and definitions are as follows:

Primary tumor (T)

T_1	Tumor confined to nasopharynx
T_2	Tumor extends to tissues of oropharynx or nasal fossa
T_{2a}	without parapharyngeal extension
T_{2b}	with parapharyngeal extension
T_3	Tumor invades bony structure or paranasal sinuses
T_4	Tumor with intracranial extension or involvement of cranial nerves, infratemporal fossa, hypopharynx, masticator space or orbit

Regional lymph nodes (N)

N_x	Cannot be assessed
N_0	No regional metastases to nodes
N_1	Unilateral metastases in lymph node or nodes, ≤ 6 cm in greatest dimension, above the supraclavicular fossa
N_2	Bilateral metastases in lymph nodes ≤ 6 cm in greatest dimension above the supraclavicular fossa
N_{3a}	Metastasis >6 cm in greatest dimension
N_{3b}	Extension to supraclavicular fossa

Distant metastasis (M)

M_x	Cannot be assessed
M_0	No distant metastases
M_1	Distant metastases

Stage groupings

I	T1	N0	M0	
II	T1,2	N1	M0	
III	T1-3 N2 M0; T3		N0,1	M0
IV	Any T4 or any N3 or M1			

F. Management of the primary tumor. Surgery usually is not applicable because tumor-free margins cannot be obtained at the base of the skull. RT with high-energy x-rays, often combined with chemotherapy, is the treatment of choice.

1. **Local tumor control rate** at 5 years after initial treatment can be related to T stage

   T_1 90%
   T_2 80%
   T_3 70%
   T_4 50%

2. **Treatment sequelae** may be severe after RT with the necessary high total doses. These include local ulceration, occasionally with necrosis, retinopathy, fibrosis of soft tissues in the neck, and middle ear changes. These sequelae can be reduced with modern treatment planning.

G. Management of regional lymph nodes. External beam RT is the choice because the adenopathy frequently is bilateral in the neck and often involves the retropharyngeal lymph nodes. Control of regional adenopathy also is related to N stage but has not been well documented. Neck dissection may be useful for tumor that persists or regrows after primary irradiation.

H. Chemotherapy for nasopharyngeal carcinoma. About 60% of patients have stage III or IV disease and often develop distant metastases. Induction chemotherapy has resulted in high response rates, but no change in overall survival and is not recommended. CCRT involving cisplatin with or without 5-FU (see section I.J.3) for three cycles is considered standard therapy in the Western world. CCRT appears to double the 5-year survival rate to 67%, but about half of the patients cannot complete planned therapy because of toxicity.

I. Treatment of local recurrence. Retreatment is more often successful for nasopharyngeal carcinoma than after failure of treatment of other head and neck cancers. Reirradiation of the primary tumor site still requires a high total dose, and may be done with precision-oriented external beam treatment, such as intensity modulated RT (IMRT) or brachytherapy. Limited post-RT failures in the neck may be controlled by surgery.

VI. HYPOPHARYNX

A. Definition. The "low pharynx" is between the level of the hyoid bone and the entry to the esophagus at the level of the lower border of the cricoid cartilage. It contains the piriform sinuses, aryepiglottic folds, postcricoid region, and lateral pharyngeal walls.

B. Pathology. Of malignant tumors, >95% are squamous cell carcinomas. Histologic differentiation varies with the anatomic site. For example, squamous cell carcinomas of the aryepiglottic fold are twice as likely to be well differentiated than are tumors arising in the piriform sinus.

C. Natural history
   1. **Risk factors**
      a. Use of tobacco and alcoholic beverages
      b. Having had other cancers in the aerodigestive tract
      c. Women more likely to develop postcricoid carcinomas than are men
   2. **Clinical presentation**
      a. May be asymptomatic and notice mass in the neck
      b. Pain aggravated by swallowing
      c. Blood-streaked saliva
      d. Mechanical dysphagia
      e. Ear pain
      f. Voice change
      g. Aspiration with pneumonia
      h. Cervical adenopathy in >50% (in 25%, a mass in the neck will be the initial finding)
   3. **Lymphatic drainage**
      a. Extensive lymphatics with frequent metastases to midcervical chain (jugulodigastric nodes may be first affected), posterior cervical triangle and paratracheal lymph nodes.

   b. Frequency of metastases to cervical nodes related to primary tumor site and extent
      (1) Piriform sinus. 60%
      (2) Aryepiglottic fold. 55%
      (3) Pharyngeal wall. 75%
4. Prognostic factors
   a. Anatomic site and extent of primary tumor
   b. Cervical node metastases
   c. Distant metastases (20% at diagnosis)
D. Diagnosis. These cancers usually are locally advanced at diagnosis.
   1. History and physical examination to include palpation and direct and indirect laryngoscopy
   2. CT and MRI are essential to determine extent of primary tumor and cervical node metastases
E. TNM staging. See Table 7.1 for regional lymph node (N) and metastasis (M) classifications and for stage groupings. Definition of the primary tumor (T) classification is similar to the other head and neck cancers but differs by the inclusion of local tumor extension as follows:

T_1 Tumor limited to one subsite and measuring <2.0 cm in greatest dimension

T_2 Tumor involves more than one subsite of hypopharynx or an adjacent site, does not fix the hemilarynx and measures >2.0 cm but not >4.0 cm in greatest dimension

T_3 Tumor measures >4.0 cm in largest dimension or fixes the hemilarynx

T_4 Tumor invades adjacent structures

F. Management of the primary tumor
   1. Piriform sinus
      a. T_1 and some T_2 tumors. RT might be preferable. Partial laryngopharyngectomy with neck dissection is effective but with greater morbidity.
      b. Advanced carcinoma extending into apex or outside piriform sinus often with invasion of larynx, thyroid cartilage, soft tissues of neck. Total laryngopharyngectomy, radical ND, and postoperative RT. If resection not possible, RT for palliation.
      c. Local tumor control rate

      T_{1-2} 65% to 80%
      T_{3-4} 50%

   2. Aryepiglottis
      a. T_{1-2} tumors. RT or supraglottic resection
      b. T_{3-4} tumors. Surgery with laryngeal conservation if possible, followed by RT
      c. Local tumor control rate for T_{1-2} tumors. 90%.
   3. Hypopharyngeal walls
      a. RT or resection with unilateral neck dissection plus postoperative RT
      b. Local tumor control rate

      T_1 90%
      T_2 70%
      T_3 60%
      T_4 35%

   4. Management of local recurrence at the primary site. RT if patient only had surgery; further RT is not effective in previously irradiated patients.
G. Management of the neck
   1. No clinical adenopathy. RT to primary site and neck, with or without planned ND
   2. Clinical cervical node metastases. RT plus planned ND

3. Management of recurrence in the neck. ND if failure of RT, or RT if failure of ND. The patient, however, often has already had both ND and RT.

VII. LARYNX

A. Definition. Laryngeal cancer involves three anatomic sites
   1. Glottis—paired true vocal cords
   2. Supraglottis—epiglottis, false vocal cords, ventricles, aryepiglottic folds (laryngeal surface), arytenoids
   3. Subglottis—arbitrarily begins 5.0 mm below free margin of true vocal cord and extends to inferior border of cricoid cartilage

B. Pathology. Of malignant tumors arising from the epithelium, >95% are squamous cell carcinomas. The remainder are sarcomas, adenocarcinomas, and neuroendocrine tumors.

C. Natural history
   1. Risk factors
      a. Use of tobacco
      b. Prior occurrence of other carcinomas of aerodigestive tract
   2. Presentation
      a. Vocal cord. Persistent hoarseness
      b. Supraglottis. Often no symptoms; sore throat; intolerance to hot or cold food; ear pain
      c. Subglottis. Usually no symptoms until locally extensive
   3. Lymphatic drainage
      a. True vocal cords. None (the true vocal cords are devoid of lymphatics)
      b. Supraglottis. Rich network draining to subdigastric and midinternal jugular nodes
      c. Subglottis. Sparse network draining to inferior jugular nodes

D. Diagnosis
   1. Palpation of neck for cervical adenopathy and laryngeal crepitus
   2. Endoscopy
   3. CT and MRI to assess site and extent of primary tumor and cervical adenopathy

E. TNM staging. See Table 7.1 for definitions of regional lymph node (N) and metastasis (M) classifications and for stage groupings, which are the same as for other head and neck cancers. Classification of the primary tumor (T) is as follows:

   1. Supraglottis

T_1	Tumor limited to one anatomic subsite; normal vocal cord mobility
T_2	Tumor invades mucosa of more than one adjacent subsite of supraglottis or glottis or region outside the supraglottis; normal vocal cord mobility
T_3	Tumor limited to larynx with vocal cord fixation or invasion of postcricoid or pre-epiglottic tissues
T_{4a}	Tumor invades through thyroid cartilage or invades tissues beyond the larynx (e.g., trachea, soft tissues of neck, including deep extrinsic muscles of the tongue, strap muscles, thyroid, or esophagus)
T_{4b}	Tumor invades prevertebral space or mediastinal structures, or encases carotid artery

   2. Glottis

T_1	Tumor limited to vocal cord(s) with normal mobility—may involve anterior or posterior commissure
T_{1a}	Tumor limited to one vocal cord
T_{1b}	Tumor involves both vocal cords
T_2	Tumor extends to supraglottis and/or subglottis and/or with impaired vocal cord mobility
T_3	Tumor limited to larynx with vocal cord fixation and/or invasion of the paraglottic space, and/or minor thyroid cartilage erosion
$T_{4a,4b}$	Same as supraglottis

3. Subglottis

T_1 Tumor limited to subglottis

T_2 Tumor extends to vocal cord(s) with normal or impaired mobility

T_3 Tumor limited to larynx with vocal cord fixation

T_{4a} Tumor invades through cricoid or thyroid cartilage and/or invades tissues beyond the larynx (e.g., trachea, soft tissues of neck, including deep extrinsic muscles of the tongue, strap muscles, thyroid, or esophagus)

T_{4b} Same as supraglottis

F. Management of the primary tumor

1. **Principles.** After the initial objective of tumor control with preservation of the patient's life, preservation of voice and the swallowing reflex become of major importance. RT alone or limited surgery can accomplish these objective in many laryngeal cancers.

   a. **Partial laryngectomy** for selected situations may result in tumor control and preservation of a useful voice.

   b. **Salvage (total) laryngectomy** may be successful after failure of conservative treatment.

   c. **Locally extensive cancers,** especially with edema, usually require total laryngectomy often followed by RT.

   d. **Chemotherapy.** Induction chemotherapy followed by definitive RT achieves laryngeal preservation in a high percentage of patients with advanced cancer, but does not improve overall survival. CCRT (section I.J.3) has been more successful for both laryngeal preservation and survival than induction chemotherapy, however, and is recommended as the treatment of choice for locally extensive cancers. High total radiation doses with modern techniques, such as IMRT, conformal planning, accelerated fractionation, and hyperfractionation, may be comparably successful.

   e. **Sequelae of treatment**

      (1) **RT.** Edema, usually temporary, and chondritis, which is rare; infrequent persistent minimal voice change

      (2) **Partial laryngectomy.** Some voice deterioration, interference with swallowing reflex

      (3) **Total laryngectomy.** Loss of voice; >50% of patients can develop effective speech with a prosthesis (speaking fistula)

2. **True vocal cords** including anterior or posterior commissures

   a. **T_{is}.** RT or "cord stripping"

   b. **T_{1-2}.** RT preferable; cordectomy and vertical hemilaryngectomy have more sequelae

   c. **T_3, limited tumors.** May respond to RT, surgical salvage can follow

   d. **T_3, extensive tumors.** Surgery, usually followed by RT; or CCRT

   e. **T_4.** Total laryngectomy and postoperative RT; or CCRT for larynx preservation

   f. **Persistent or recurrent cancer**

      (1) Surgery for RT failure

      (2) RT or more extensive surgery or both for failure of limited surgery

      (3) RT for failure after total laryngectomy

   g. **Local tumor control rates**

      (1) **T_1.** 90% to 95% with RT and most failures can be salvaged surgically; voice preservation in 95%

      (2) **T_2.** 75% to 80% with RT and most failures can be salvaged by surgery; voice preservation in 80% to 85%

      (3) **T_3. favorable tumors** with minimal fixation of vocal cords. 60% by RT increased to 85% by salvage surgery

      (4) **T_3 more extensive tumors.** 40% with RT, increased to 60% by salvage surgery; total laryngectomy—55% to 70%

   (5) T$_{4a}$ favorable with early invasion of thyroid cartilage. 65% with RT; extensive with involvement of piriform sinus 20% with RT; laryngectomy, 40% to 50%

3. Supraglottic carcinoma
   a. T$_{1-2}$. RT or supraglottic laryngectomy
   b. T$_3$. RT often controls exophytic tumors; surgery can be reserved for salvage; for infiltrating tumors, surgery is preferable often with postoperative RT
   c. T$_4$. Surgery followed by postoperative RT. In a group of medically inoperable patients, RT resulted in a 35% local tumor control.
   d. Local tumor control rate

T$_1$	95% to 100%
T$_2$	80% to 85%
T$_3$	65% to 75%
T$_4$	<50%

   e. Treatment of recurrent cancer
      (1) Surgery for RT failures
      (2) RT for surgery failures
      (3) Chemotherapy
4. Subglottic carcinoma
   a. Usually extensive when discovered; treat with surgery + RT
   b. Local tumor control <25%
G. Management of the neck
   1. Glottic carcinomas. When tumor limited to true vocal cords, there are no metastases to be treated.
   2. Extensive glottic tumors and supraglottic carcinomas. The neck can initially be managed by the method used for treatment of the primary tumor. Persistent adenopathy after primary RT should be treated surgically. Surgical failures can be irradiated.

VIII. NASAL CAVITIES AND PARANASAL SINUSES
   A. Definition. Knowledge of the complex anatomy is basic to understanding these tumors. The *nasal vestibule* is the entrance to the *nasal fossa*. It is bounded by the columella, nasal ala, and floor of the nasal cavity. The nasal fossa extends from the vestibule (limen nasi) to the choana posteriorly, communicating with the nasopharynx, paranasal sinuses, lacrinal sac, and conjunctiva. The boundaries of the *maxillary sinus* are the orbit, lateral wall of the nasal fossa, hard palate (the roots of the first two molar teeth may project into the floor), infratemporal fossa, and pterygoplatine fossa. The multiple *ethmoidal sinuses* are in the ethmoid bone between the nasal cavity and orbit. The left and right *frontal sinuses* in the frontal bone are separated by a septum. The dual *sphenoid sinuses* are surrounded by the pituitary fossa, cavernous sinuses, ethmoidal sinuses, nasopharynx, and nasal cavities.
   B. Pathology
      1. Nasal vestibule. Nearly all are squamous cell carcinomas; a few are basal cell or adnexal carcinomas; <1% are melanomas.
      2. Nasal cavity and paranasal sinuses. Most are squamous cell carcinomas; 10% to 15% arise in minor salivary glands; 5% are lymphomas. Other tumors include chondrosarcoma, osteosarcoma, Ewing's tumor, giant cell tumor of the bone.
      3. Esthesioneuroblastomas arise from neuroepithelium. (See Chapter 19, section VII.)
      4. Inverting papilloma
      5. Midline lethal granuloma (extranodal NK/T-cell lymphoma, nasal type)
   C. Natural history
      1. Risk factors. Causes are unknown, but carcinoma is more frequent in workers exposed to nickel or wood dust and, historically, in patients exposed to radioactive thorium as an x-ray contrast agent.
      2. Presentation
         a. Nasal vestibule. Small, crusted plaques, ulceration, bleeding
         b. Nasal fossa. Unilateral discharge, bleeding, obstruction

   c. Maxillary sinus. Findings may mimic inflammation, pain, upper dental problems, proptosis

   d. Ethmoid sinuses. Anatomic distortion, pain, local extension

   e. Sphenoid sinus. Ill-defined headache, neuropathy of cranial nerves III, IV, V, and VI

3. Lymphatic drainage

   a. Nasal fossa, ethmoidal and frontal sinuses—to submaxillary nodes; to nodes at base of skull when olfactory region involved

   b. Maxillary sinus—to ipsilateral subdigastric and submandibular nodes

   c. Sphenoid sinus—to jugulodigastric nodes

4. Prognostic factors

   a. Anatomic site (i.e., cancers of nasal fossa nearly always are cured, whereas cancers of the sphenoid sinus are rarely controlled)

   b. Tumor extent

   c. Patient's general health (treatment usually is demanding)

D. Diagnosis

   1. Clinical symptoms and signs

   2. Direct visualization of nasal vestibule and fossa, palate, alveolar ridge, external orbit (proptosis)

   3. Endoscopy of nasopharynx for tumor extension

   4. Cranial nerve evaluation

   5. MRI and CT examinations of primary site and neck

   6. Differential diagnoses

   a. Nasal polyps (inverting papillomas)

   b. Inflammatory disease

   c. Upper dental problems

   d. Destructive mucoceles

E. TNM staging. The AJCC staging system is limited to the maxillary and ethmoidal sinuses and excludes nonepithelial tumors. Clinical staging includes inspection, palpation; examination of orbits, nasal and oral cavities, nasopharynx, and of cranial nerves; MRI and CT. Pathologic staging includes clinical data plus information from the surgical specimen and the surgeon's observations.

   See Table 7.1 for regional lymph node (N) and metastasis (M) classifications and for stage groupings. Primary tumor (T) classification is as follows:

1. Maxillary sinus

T_1	Tumor limited to antrum without erosion or destruction of bone
T_2	Tumor causing bone erosion or destruction (except for posterior wall of maxillary sinus and pterygoid plates), including extension into hard palate or middle nasal meatus
T_3	Tumor invading any of the following: bone of the posterior wall of the maxillary sinus, subcutaneous tissues, floor or medial wall of orbit, infratemporal fossa, pterygoid plates, or ethmoid sinuses
T_{4a}	Tumor invades anterior orbital contents, skin of cheek, pterygoid plates, infratemporal fossa, cribriform plates, sphenoid sinus, or frontal sinuses
T_{4b}	Tumor invades any of the following: orbital apex, dura, brain, middle cranial fossa, cranial nerves other than V_2, nasopharynx, or clivus

2. Ethmoid sinus and nasal cavity

T_1	Tumor confined to any one subsite, with or without bony invasion
T_2	Tumor invades two subsites in a single region or extends to involve an adjacent region within the nasoethmoidal complex, with or without bony invasion
T_3	Tumor invades the medial wall or floor of the orbit, maxillary sinus, palate, or cribriform plate
T_{4a}	Tumor invades any of the following: anterior orbital contents, skin of nose or cheek, minimal extension to anterior cranial fossa, pterygoid plates, sphenoid, or frontal sinuses
T_{4b}	Same as maxillary sinus

3. **Nasal vestibule.** Same as for skin of face
F. **Management of primary tumors**
   1. **Nasal vestibule**
      a. **Small tumors.** RT if surgery will produce deformity; chemosurgery or laser surgery
      b. **Large tumors.** RT or surgery + RT (plastic surgery repair if possible)
      c. **Persistence of tumor.** Surgery for RT failures; more extensive surgery or RT for surgery failures; chemosurgery, laser surgery
   2. **Nasal fossa**
      a. **Small tumors.** RT if surgery will produce deformity; surgery with or without RT if bone involved
      b. **Large tumors.** Combined surgery and RT; RT for lymphomas and melanomas
      c. **Esthesioneuroblastomas.** Probably combined surgery and RT; chemotherapy (i.e., cisplatin + etoposide) may be helpful
   3. **Maxillary sinus.** Fenestration of the palate allows direct inspection and access for biopsy and drainage
      a. **Small tumors.** Surgery alone except for infrequent highly radiation responsive tumors such as lymphomas
      b. **Advanced tumors.** Surgery and postoperative RT; chemotherapy and radiotherapy may be used preoperatively in an attempt to make resection possible
      c. **Unresectable tumors.** RT and chemotherapy
      d. **Local treatment failure.** Usually all modalities have been used; trial of chemotherapy, cautery, or cryosurgery
   4. **Ethmoid sinus**
      a. **Limited lesions.** Surgery
      b. **Most tumors.** Surgery and postoperative RT
   5. **Sphenoid sinus.** RT, possibly with chemotherapy (nearly always extensive when recognized)
   6. **Local tumor control rates**
      a. **Nasal vestibule.** Most tumors are small and nearly 100% controlled
      b. **Nasal fossa.** Stage I, nearly 100%; control decreases with increasing extent
      c. **Esthesioneuroblastoma.** 90% for Kadish stage A tumors
      d. **Ethmoid sinuses.** ~60%
      e. **Maxillary sinus.** 75% to 80%
      f. **Sphenoid sinuses.** Usually extensive when discovered with very infrequent local tumor control
G. **Management of the neck**
   1. **Nasal vestibule.** Small tumors; observation with ND if adenopathy develops
   2. **Nasal fossa.** Observation and ND if adenopathy develops (for tumors <5 cm, <10% ever develop adenopathy)
   3. **Esthesioneuroblastoma.** ND, usually as part of primary surgery
   4. **Maxillary sinus.** ND, usually as part of primary surgery
H. **Treatment of local recurrence**
   1. **Small tumors** may be salvaged by surgery after RT failures or additional surgery after failure of initial surgery
   2. **Extensive tumors** usually have received both surgery and RT and re-treatment usually not feasible; palliative chemotherapy

IX. SALIVARY GLANDS
A. **Definition**
   1. **Major salivary glands.** Parotid, submandibular, sublingual
   2. **Minor salivary glands.** Widespread in mucosa of upper aerodigestive tract
B. **Pathology.** A range of histological tumor types arise from ductal and acinar cells of the epithelium. The most frequently involved site is the parotid gland with tumors being 10-fold more frequent than in the submaxillary or minor salivary glands. The histologic subtypes and approximate frequencies are:

Mucoepidermoid, 35%
Adenocarcinoma, 25%
Adenoidcystic, 25%
Acinic cell, 10%
Epidermoid, 5% to 10%
Other, 1% to 5%

C. Natural history
   1. Risk factors
      a. Previous exposure to ionizing radiations
      b. Skin cancer of face
   2. Clinical presentations
      a. Mass, often painless, in salivary gland
      b. Neurologic changes with involvement of facial nerve
      c. Younger women, older men
   3. Lymphatic drainage
      a. Parotid gland to preauricular, jugulodigastric, intraglandular nodes
      b. Submaxillary gland to submental, jugulodigastric, intraglandular nodes
   4. Prognostic factors
      a. Tumor type and grade
      b. Tumor site and extent
      c. Tumor involvement of surgical margins; attempts to spare facial nerve resulting in inadequate resection
      d. Regional node metastases
D. Diagnosis. Differentiate from inflammatory changes with tenderness of mass and warmth of overlying skin plus hematologic changes.
   1. Mass in salivary gland, usually painless, often fixed
   2. Paresis and/or numbness related to involvement of facial nerve
   3. Biopsy
   4. CT or MRI of primary site and neck
E. TNM staging. The AJCC staging system includes malignant tumors of the parotid, submandibular, and sublingual glands. Clinical staging includes inspection, palpation, neurologic evaluation of cranial nerves, MRI, and CT. Pathologic staging includes clinical staging data, plus findings in the resected tissue and the surgeon's observations.
   See Table 7.1 for regional lymph node (N) and metastasis (M) classifications and for stage groupings. Primary tumor (T) classification is as follows:

T_X Primary tumor cannot be assessed
T_0 No evidence of tumor
T_1 Tumor ≤ 2.0 cm without extraparenchymal extension
T_2 Tumor >2.0 but not >4.0 cm in greatest dimension without extraparenchymal extension
T_3 Tumor >4.0 cm or with extraparenchymal extension
T_{4a} Tumor may invade skin, mandible, ear canal, and facial nerve
T_{4b} Tumor may invade base of skull and pterygoid plates, and encases carotid artery

F. Management of primary tumor
   1. Surgery is the treatment of choice, if the tumor is resectable. Minimal surgery for parotid tumors is superficial parotidectomy with preservation of the facial nerve. Unwelcome sequelae, if extensive surgery is performed, include facial nerve palsy and auriculotemporal syndrome with gustatory sweating.
   2. RT has a secondary role as postoperative adjuvant therapy when the histology is poorly differentiated, when significant perineural invasion is seen, or the surgical margins are not tumor-free. RT is also used when the tumor has recurred. Primary irradiation for medically inoperable patients has had some success. Salivary gland tumors seem responsive to fast neutron teletherapy.

3. Local tumor control rates
a. Surgery alone
Stages I–II: 95% to 100%
Stages III–IV: 40% to 50%
Low grade: 90%
High grade: 40%

b. Surgery plus RT
Stages I–II: 95% to 100%
Stages III–IV: 75%
Low grade: 90%
High grade: 80%

c. RT for nonresectable disease
Using photons 25%
Using fast neutrons 65%

G. Management of the neck
1. Small, low-grade tumors. Surgery when adenopathy is present
2. Extensive, poorly differentiated tumors. Surgery plus postoperative RT

X. METASTASES OF UNKNOWN ORIGIN (MUO) TO NECK LYMPH NODES

A. Definition. MUO are metastatic solid tumors (hematopoietic malignancies and lymphomas are excluded) for which the site of origin is not identified despite a thorough history, physical examination, chest radiograph, routine blood and urine studies, and a thorough histologic evaluation.

B. Pathology. Metastases are located in the upper jugular chain in most patients. The histologic type of metastasis to neck nodes varies in incidence according to anatomic location (Table 7.3); the probability for squamous carcinoma rises the higher the node is on the chain. Involved nodes are single in 75% of patients, multiple but ipsilateral in 15%, and bilateral in 10%. Multiplicity is often associated with adenocarcinoma or metastases from the nasopharynx or infraclavicular sites.

C. Natural history. MUO account for 3% to 9% of head and neck cancers. The occurrence of MUO to cervical lymph nodes is six times higher in men than in women. Patients are usually heavy smokers and heavy drinkers who have noted the mass for several months. Despite the absence of a detected primary site, both long-term survival and cures are observed in a significant percentage of patients.

1. Upper cervical nodes. The primary site is the upper respiratory passages for most squamous tumors that present as MUO in the upper half of the neck. About 35% of these patients can potentially be cured. With CT or MRI scanning and skillful endoscopic evaluation, a primary site can be determined in at least 30% of cases.

Carcinomas of the nasopharynx, hypopharynx, base of the tongue, and tonsil present with cervical node metastasis as the first manifestation of disease

TABLE 7.3 **Histology of Neck Node Metastases from Unknown Primary Site**

Lymph nodes	Histopathology: relative fequencies (%)			
	Squamous cell carcinoma	Undifferentiated carcinoma	Adenocarcinoma	Other[a]
Upper to middle cervical	60	25	10	5
Lower cervical	45	40	5	10
Supraclavicular	20	45	35	

[a]Malignant melanoma accounts for most cases with other histologies.

in 30% to 50% of cases. These sites or the larynx harbor the primary tumor 95% of the time when the primary site is ultimately found after initially manifesting as MUO to cervical nodes.

2. **Lower cervical nodes.** About 65% of metastases to the low cervical nodes originate in sites below the clavicle, most commonly in the lung. Thus, this presentation is usually associated with a poor prognosis.

3. **Supraclavicular nodes.** Involvement of this group of lymph nodes with malignancy nearly always indicates disease that is far advanced. The primary site is usually the lung, breast, or gastrointestinal tract. The expected survival time is <6 months.

4. **Prognostic factors.** Prognosis is predominantly affected by the N stage of neck disease, by the location in the neck (see above), by the histopathology, and by whether the primary site is ever found (the prognosis is much better if the primary tumor never becomes manifest).

D. Diagnosis. Excisional biopsy of cervical nodes should not be performed because it distorts surgical planes and may result in poor outcomes if it proved to be a squamous cell carcinoma originating in an occult site in the head and neck. Supraclavicular lymphadenopathy, on the other hand, rarely represents curable disease; these nodes may be excised directly for histologic examination. **The recommended sequence of evaluation of cases of potentially cancerous cervical nodes** is as follows:

1. **Initial evaluation.** Carefully inspect and palpate all accessible areas of the mouth and nose. Then evaluate the upper airways, especially the nasopharynx, with mirrors or Hopkin's laryngoscope.

2. **Imaging.** Obtain a CT or MRI scan of the neck and paranasal sinuses to search for a primary tumor. Positron emission tomography with CT (PET/CT) before obtaining biopsies is often useful if the CT or MRI fails to identify the primary site.

3. **Fine-needle aspiration** (FNA) is performed if these efforts fail to demonstrate any hint of a primary cancer. The results of cytologic evaluation direct further evaluation, as follows:

    a. **Squamous cell or undifferentiated carcinoma.** Perform panendoscopy and manage the patient for a primary head and neck cancer.

    b. **Indeterminate or equivocal histology.** Excise the node, and perform immunoperoxidase stains and other special studies on the tissue as necessary.

    c. **Adenocarcinoma.** Manage as for MUO to viscera (see Chapter 20). The outlook is nearly hopeless unless originating in a major salivary gland (which is rare).

    d. **Melanoma.** Manage as discussed in section V.A of Chapter 20.

    e. **Lymphoma.** Manage accordingly (see Chapter 21).

4. **Panendoscopy** (nasopharyngoscopy, laryngoscopy with tracheoscopy, bronchoscopy, and esophagoscopy) is performed under general anesthesia. All suspected lesions and random areas of apparently normal tissue at the base of tongue, pyriform sinus, and nasopharynx are subjected to biopsy in search of a primary source. Ipsilateral tonsillectomy has a better yield than tonsillar fossa biopsy and is often performed as well. If a primary tumor is found, treatment is planned with consideration of the primary site and neck metastasis.

5. **Biopsy of the suspect node should be done only when**

    a. Thorough physical examination fails to reveal a primary tumor

    b. CT or MRI examination does not disclose a primary tumor

    c. FNA cytology fails to reveal the diagnosis

    d. Panendoscopy fails to reveal a primary site

    e. Lymphoma is suspected (excluded in the definition of MUO)

E. Treatment alternatives. Treatment should follow the guidelines for locally advanced SCCHN. Treatment must be comprehensive at the outset because salvage therapy has a low yield.

1. **Comprehensive RT** (encompassing the nasopharynx, oropharynx, hypopharynx, and both sides of the neck) achieves a high rate of local control in the neck.

In theory, RT fields should encompass the undiscovered primary tumor. Less extensive RT, however, has been shown to be associated with the same good results and less morbidity.

2. Surgery. The use of surgical treatment alone should be discouraged in these patients because primary sites in the head and neck become manifest in approximately 40% of patients treated with ND alone. Furthermore, 20% to 50% of patients treated with surgery alone develop contralateral neck disease or subsequently manifest a primary tumor site. The incidences of subsequent manifestation of a primary site or development of contralateral neck disease are both much less after RT than after ND.

3. Chemotherapy. Randomized trials have demonstrated the superiority of cisplatin-based CCRT in patients with known primary site SCCHN at high risk for local recurrence. The application of CCRT to MUO involving cervical lymph nodes in appropriately selected patients appears to be a logical extension of those findings. In general, subjects with SCCHN MUO in the neck do better when the primary site is not found. It is generally agreed that N1 tumors should be treated without chemotherapy. Several single institutional studies have shown impressive survival rates with CCRT for N2-N3 disease. Most randomized studies do not include MUO, however.

F. Recommended treatment. Many centers use RT for all cases and CCRT for patients at particularly high risk for local recurrence.

1. Stage N1 involving upper or middle neck node. Treat patients with RT alone. Alternatively, perform ND (particularly if the metastasis is <3 cm in diameter); if the specimen reveals other involved nodes (stage N2b) or extracapsular invasion, administer postoperative RT or CCRT.

2. Stage N2 involving upper or middle neck nodes. Use RT or CCRT followed by ND or after ND.

3. Stage N3 (massive nodes). Use RT alone or CCRT in medically suitable patients. ND should be performed either before or after RT or CCRT.

4. Squamous cell carcinoma of lower cervical or supraclavicular nodes or adenocarcinomas. Administer RT alone (survival rates are poor no matter what is done; the goal of treatment is control of local disease).

G. Results of treatment

1. Patients with upper cervical lymph node metastasis. The 5-year survival rate for all patients is 30% if the primary tumor is eventually found and 60% if it is never found.

a. Stage N1 or N2a. The 5- and 10-year survival rates are both 70% to 80%. At 10 years after treatment, the risk of finding a primary site is about 30%, which is the same as the odds of developing a second cancer after successful treatment.

b. Stage N2b. The reported survival rates are variable.

c. Stage N3. The 5-year survival is about 20%.

2. Patients with low cervical or supraclavicular lymph node metastasis. The 5-year survival rate is 5% (median survival time is 7 months).

Suggested Reading

Adelstein DJ, et al. An intergroup phase III comparison of standard radiation therapy and two schedules of concurrent chemoradiotherapy in patients with unresectable squamous cell head and neck cancer. *J Clin Oncol* 2003;21:92.

Al-Sarraf M, et al. Post-operative radiotherapy with concurrent cisplatin appears to improve locoregional control of advanced, resectable head and neck cancers: RTOG 88–24. *Int J Radiat Oncol Biol Phys* 1997;37:777.

Al-Sarraf M, et al. Chemoradiotherapy versus radiotherapy in patients with advanced nasopharyngeal cancer: phase III randomized intergroup study 0099. *J Clin Oncol* 1998;16:1310.

American Joint Committee on Cancer. *AJCC Cancer Staging Manual.* 6th ed. New York: Springer-Verlag; 2002.

Balz V, et al. Is the p53 inactivation frequency in squamous cell carcinomas of the head and neck underestimated? Analysis of p53 exons 2–11 and human papillomavirus 16/18 E6 transcripts in 123 unselected tumor specimens. *Cancer Res* 2003;63:1188.

Bernier J, Bentzen SM. Altered fractionation and combined radio-chemotherapy approaches: pioneering new opportunities in head and neck oncology. *Eur J Cancer* 2003;39:560.

Bonner JA, et al. Radiotherapy plus cetuximab for squamous-cell carcinoma of the head and neck. *N Engl J Med* 2006;354:567.

Browman GP, et al. Choosing a concomitant chemotherapy and radiotherapy regimen for squamous cell head and neck cancer: a systematic review of the published literature with subgroup analysis. *Head Neck* 2001;23:579.

Chan AT, et al. Concurrent chemotherapy-radiotherapy compared with radiotherapy alone in locoregionally advanced nasopharyngeal carcinoma: progression-free survival analysis of a phase III randomized trial. *J Clin Oncol* 2002;20:1968.

Clark JR, et al. Induction chemotherapy with cisplatin, fluorouracil, and high-dose leucovorin for squamous cell carcinoma of the head and neck: long term results. *J Clin Oncol* 1997;15:3100.

Cohen EE, Lingen MW, Vokes EE. The expanding role of systemic therapy in head and neck cancer. *J Clin Oncol* 2004;22:1743.

Forastiere AA, et al. Concurrent chemotherapy and radiotherapy for organ preservation in advanced laryngeal cancer. *N Engl J Med* 2003;349:2091.

Fu KK, et al. A Radiation Therapy Oncology Group (RTOG) phase III randomized study to compare hyperfractionation and two variants of accelerated fractionation to standard fractionation radiotherapy for head and neck squamous cell carcinomas: first report of RTOG 9003. *Int J Radiat Oncol Biol Phys* 2000;48:7.

Haas I, et al. Diagnostic strategies in cervical carcinoma of an unknown primary (CUP). *Eur Arch Otorhinolaryngol* 2002;259:325.

Horiot JC, et al. Accelerated fractionation (AF) compared to conventional fractionation (CF) improves loco-regional control in the radiotherapy of advanced head and neck cancers: results of the EORTC 22851 randomized trial. *Radiother Oncol* 1997;44:111.

Kramer NM, et al. Toxicity and outcome analysis of patients with recurrent head and neck cancer treated with hyperfractionated split-course reirradiation and concurrent cisplatin and paclitaxel chemotherapy from two prospective phase I and II studies. *Head Neck* 2005;27:406.

Lo YMD, et al. Molecular prognostication of nasopharyngeal carcinoma by quantitative analysis of circulating Epstein-Barr virus DNA. *Cancer Res* 2000;60:6878.

Parker RG, Janjan NA, Selch MT. Cancers of the head and neck. In: *Radiation Oncology for Cure and Palliation.* New York: Springer-Verlag; 2003:187.

Pignon JP, et al. Chemotherapy added to locoregional treatment for head and neck squamous-cell carcinoma: three meta-analyses of updated individual data. MACH-NC Collaborative Group Meta-Analysis of Chemotherapy on Head and Neck Cancer. *Lancet* 2000;355:949.

Staar S, et al. Intensified hyperfractionated accelerated radiotherapy limits the additional benefit of simultaneous chemotherapy: results of a multicentric randomized German trial in advanced head-and-neck cancer. *Int J Radiat Oncol Biol Phys* 2001;50:1161.

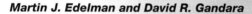
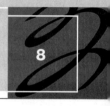

LUNG CANCER

8

Martin J. Edelman and David R. Gandara

I. EPIDEMIOLOGY AND ETIOLOGY

A. Incidence. Lung cancer is the most common visceral malignancy, accounting for roughly one-third of all cancer deaths, and it is the most common cause of cancer-related death in both men and women. Annually there are 200,000 new cases in the United States. This appears to be an increase, but a revised methodology has been utilized. Although rates for men are decreasing, there is a continued increase for women. Even more disturbing is a possibly increased incidence of non–small cell lung cancer (NSCLC) in relatively young nonsmoking women.

B. Etiology

1. **Smoking.** Cigarette smoking is the cause of 85% to 90% of lung cancer cases; the risk for lung cancer in smokers is 30 times greater than in nonsmokers. Smoking cigars or pipes doubles the risk for lung cancer compared with the risk in nonsmokers. Passive smoking probably increases the risk of lung cancer about twofold, but because a proportion of the risk associated with active inhalation is about 20-fold, the actual risk is small.

   a. The risk for lung cancer is related to cumulative dose, which for cigarettes is quantified in "pack-years." One in seven people who smoke more than two packs per day die from lung cancer. The incidence of death from lung cancer begins to diverge from the nonsmoking population at 10 pack-years.

   b. After cessation of smoking, the risk steadily declines, approaching, but not quite reaching, that of nonsmokers after 15 years of abstinence for patients who smoked for <20 years. With the decline in smoking in the United States, a large percentage of new diagnoses of lung cancer occur in former smokers.

   c. The risk of the major cell types of lung cancer is increased in smokers. Some adenocarcinomas, especially in women, are unrelated to smoking (see I.B.7 below).

   d. Small cell lung cancer (SCLC) is almost always associated with smoking. The diagnosis should be questioned in patients who deny a smoking history.

2. **Asbestos** is causally linked to malignant mesothelioma. Asbestos exposure also increases the risk for lung cancer, especially in smokers (three times greater risk than smoking alone).

3. **Radiation exposure** may increase the risk for SCLC in both smokers and non-smokers. Radon has been associated with up to 6% of lung cancer cases.

4. **Other substances** associated with lung cancer include arsenic, nickel, chromium compounds, chloromethyl ether, and air pollutants.

5. **Lung cancer** is itself associated with an increased risk for a second lung cancer occurring both synchronously and metachronously. Other cancers of the upper aerodigestive tract (head and neck, esophagus) are associated with an increased risk for lung cancer because of the "field cancerization" effect of cigarette smoking.

6. **Other lung diseases.** Lung scars and chronic obstructive pulmonary disease are associated with an increased risk for lung cancer.

7. **Never and minimal smokers and lung cancer.** A substantial portion of the lung cancer population has no obvious toxic exposure. It is estimated that approximately 10% of patients with NSCLC are never-smokers. This number

appears to be rising. Many of these cases are associated with abnormalities of the epidermal growth factor receptor (EGFR). Mutations of the EGFR have been described as have increases in gene copy number (as measured by fluorescence in situ hybridization, FISH) or protein expression (as measured by immunohistochemistry). The etiology of these abnormalities is unknown.

II. PATHOLOGY AND NATURAL HISTORY

Fine-needle aspiration (FNA), through bronchoscopy or transthoracic CT guided biopsy, makes specific histological classification of lung cancer difficult. Although FNA can usually distinguish between SCLC and NSCLC, it is difficult to distinguish between the histologic subtypes of NSCLC, and this can occasionally result in misdiagnosis of carcinoid as SCLC. A needle core biopsy or paraffin fixation of FNA material is preferable as these allow for better histologic analysis as well as immunohistochemistry or other special diagnostic techniques. These are of increasing importance as targeted therapies for specific subsets of patients are validated.

A. Small cell lung cancer (SCLC; 15% of all lung cancers). SCLC comprises several histologic subtypes: oat cell, polygonal cell, lymphocytic, and spindle cell carcinoma. The natural histories of these subtypes are virtually identical.

    1. Location. More often central or hilar (95%) than peripheral (5%)

    2. Clinical course. Patients with SCLC often have widespread disease at the time of diagnosis. Rapid clinical deterioration in patients with chest masses often indicates SCLC.

        a. Hematogenous metastases commonly involve the brain, bone marrow, or liver. Pleural effusions are common.

        b. Relapse after radiation therapy (RT) or chemotherapy occurs in the sites initially affected as well as in previously uninvolved sites.

    3. Associated paraneoplastic syndromes include the syndrome of inappropriate antidiuretic hormone (SIADH; most common), hypercoagulable state (common), ectopic adrenocorticotropic hormone (ACTH) syndrome (uncommon), and Eaton-Lambert (myasthenic) syndrome (rarely seen with any other tumor). Hypercalcemia occurs rarely in SCLC, even in the presence of extensive bony metastases.

B. Non–small cell lung cancer (NSCLC; 85% of all lung cancers). The other histological variants (squamous, adenocarcinoma, large cell) of lung cancer are grouped together as NSCLC because of similarities in presentation, treatment, and natural history.

    1. Squamous cell carcinoma (20% to 25% of NSCLC)

        a. Location. Previously, adenocarcinomas were thought to occur in a predominantly peripheral location, whereas squamous cell cancers occurred centrally. Studies indicate a changing radiographic presentation, with the two cell types now having similar patterns of location.

        b. Clinical course. Compared with other kinds of lung cancers, squamous cell lung cancers are most likely to remain localized early in the disease and to recur locally after either surgery or RT.

        c. Associated paraneoplastic syndromes. Hypercalcemia resulting from ectopic production of parathyroid hormone–related peptide (PTH-RP) is the more frequent syndrome. Hypertrophic osteoarthropathy (occasional), paraneoplastic neutrophilia (sometimes associated with hypercalcemia), prominent joint symptoms (occasional), or hypercoagulability is also seen.

    2. Adenocarcinoma (50% to 60% of NSCLC). Adenocarcinoma is the most common cell type occurring in nonsmokers, especially young women. Most cases, however, are smoking associated. The incidence of this histology has increased in recent years.

        a. Location. These tumors present as peripheral nodules more commonly than squamous cell carcinoma.

        b. Clinical course. More than half of patients with adenocarcinoma, apparently localized as a peripheral nodule, have regional nodal metastases. Adenocarcinomas and large cell carcinomas have similar natural histories and spread widely outside the thorax by hematogenous dissemination, commonly involving the bones, liver, and brain.

  c. **Associated paraneoplastic syndromes** include hypertrophic osteoarthropathy, hypercoagulable state, hypercalcemia due to PTH-RP or cytokines, and gynecomastia (large cell).

  d. **Bronchioloalveolar carcinoma** (BAC) is a subtype of adenocarcinoma with distinct histological, biological, epidemiological, clinical, and therapeutic characteristics. Pure bronchioloalveolar carcinoma is characterized by a spreading ("lepidic") pattern within the bronchioles without evidence of invasion. The disease is characterized radiographically by an infiltrative pattern and is frequently multicentric. It is frequently misdiagnosed as pneumonia on initial presentation. The most common type of BAC is adenocarcinoma with a BAC component. This implies invasiveness through the basement membrane. Epidemiologically, it seems to occur more frequently in young, female nonsmokers and reportedly is more responsive than other lung cancer types to the tyrosine kinase inhibitor erlotinib.

  3. **Large cell and "not otherwise specified" lung cancer.** The remainder of NSCLC consists of large cell and other histologies. Large cell NSCLC with neuroendocrine features is increasingly diagnosed on the basis of immunohistochemical features of neuroendocrine differentiation (e.g. chromogrannin, neuron specific enolase).

C. **Uncommon tumors of the lung**

  1. **Bronchial carcinoids** may present with local symptoms from airway obstruction, ectopic ACTH production, or carcinoid syndrome (see Chapter 15, section II). These tumors demonstrate neuroendocrine differentiation and are occasionally confused with SCLC.

  2. **Cystic adenoid carcinomas** ("cylindromas") are locally invasive cancers. Locoregional recurrence is most common, but they may also metastasize to other areas of the lung and to distant sites (see Chapter 19, section V).

  3. **Carcinosarcomas** are large lesions that have a tendency to remain localized and are more often resectable than other lung malignancies.

  4. **Mesotheliomas** are caused by exposure to asbestos and occur in the lung, pleura, peritoneum, or tunica vaginalis or albuginea of the testis. A history of asbestos exposure of any duration at any time is *prima facie* evidence that it caused the mesothelioma.

    a. **Histopathology.** Mesotheliomas consist of several histological variants: sarcomatous, epithelioid, and others that have the histological appearance of adenocarcinoma. The latter type can be distinguished from other adenocarcinomas by the absence of mucin staining and the loss of hyaluronic acid staining after digestion by hyaluronidase.

    b. **Clinical course.** The diffuse (usual) form of mesothelioma spreads rapidly over the pleura and encases the lung. It may develop multifocally and invade the lung parenchyma. Distant metastases are not common and usually occur late in the course. If there is a sarcomatous pattern, liver, brain, and bone may be involved.

III. **DIAGNOSIS AND FURTHER EVALUATION.** The diagnostic evaluation should proceed in an orderly manner to establish an accurate diagnosis and stage of disease. If lung cancer is suspected on the basis of the signs and symptoms described in the following subsections, an initial limited laboratory and radiological evaluation is indicated. The primary effort should be directed at establishing a histological diagnosis because this will determine the need for, and type of, additional tests as well as therapeutic options.

   If NSCLC is diagnosed, the subsequent staging evaluation is directed to determine which modalities of therapy (surgery, radiotherapy, or chemotherapy) should be employed. In the past, surgery has been the mainstay of therapy for NSCLC and remains the primary mode in early stage (I and II) disease. Therefore, the initial evaluation determines whether the tumor is potentially **resectable** (the tumor can be surgically removed with clear margins) and **operable** (the patient is physiologically capable of withstanding such a procedure).

The fundamental question must also be asked: What are the long-term results for surgical resection of any given stage of NSCLC? If surgery is not warranted, then the next question is whether the patient is a potential candidate for nonsurgical management with curative intent (i.e., chemoradiotherapy).

If SCLC is diagnosed, the evaluation is directed at determining whether the patient has limited- or extensive-stage disease because stage dictates prognosis and the appropriate therapeutic approach. Generally, the therapeutic approach to SCLC involves chemotherapy with or without radiotherapy. Only occasionally does surgery play a role in this disease.

A. Symptoms and signs

1. **Symptoms.** The majority of patients present with symptomatic disease. Symptoms may be referable to the primary disease in the chest (new or changing cough, hoarseness, hemoptysis, chest pain, dyspnea, pneumonia), metastatic disease (new nodal masses, bone pain, pathologic fracture, headache, seizure), or paraneoplastic manifestations (anorexia, weight loss, nausea due to hypercalcemia, etc.). These symptoms frequently inspire a smoker to quit just before the diagnosis of lung cancer. Patients may also be completely asymptomatic and present as a consequence of an incidental finding on a radiographic study obtained for another reason. Even asymptomatic patients may have advanced disease.

   a. Patients with cancers located in the lung apices or superior sulcus (Pancoast tumor) may have paresthesias and weakness of the arm and hand as well as Horner syndrome (ptosis, miosis, and anhidrosis) caused by involvement of the cervical sympathetic nerves.

   b. Evidence of metastatic disease includes bone pain; neurological changes; jaundice, bowel, and abdominal symptoms with a rapidly enlarging liver; subcutaneous masses; and regional lymphadenopathy.

2. **Physical findings.** In addition to local findings in the chest and lungs, physical examination should be directed at determining whether there is metastatic disease, which would both provide staging information and, in the case of superficial cutaneous or lymph node involvement, allow for easier biopsy. Particular attention should be paid to the head and neck for concomitant cancers; to lymph node areas in the supraclavicular fossa, neck, and axilla for metastases; and to the abdomen for hepatomegaly.

B. Laboratory studies

1. **Radiographs**

   a. **Chest radiograph.** If a mass is present, old x-ray films should be obtained for comparison. Persistent infiltrates, particularly in the anterior segments of the upper lobes, are suggestive of cancer.

   b. **Computed tomography (CT) scan of the chest and abdomen** through the level of the adrenal glands. CT of the chest for the staging of lung cancer is clearly superior to chest radiographs and has been reported to have an overall accuracy of 70%. Mediastinal lymph nodes are generally considered abnormal when larger than 1.5 cm in diameter and normal when smaller than 1.0 cm; nodes between these two limits are indeterminate. If 1.5 cm is used to categorize mediastinal lymphadenopathy as abnormal, sensitivity of CT is relatively poor, but specificity is excellent. CT scanning provides information about the extent of invasion of the primary tumor, the presence of pleural effusion, and lymph node status. Magnetic resonance imaging (MRI) rarely adds additional information.

      (1) **Adrenal masses.** Unsuspected adrenal metastases are common in NSCLC and alter management if the patient otherwise appears to have early stage disease. Nonmalignant adrenal masses are also common (adrenal adenomas), however, and care must be taken not to deprive a patient of an otherwise curative procedure based on an isolated adrenal mass. It is sometimes possible to distinguish between metastatic disease

and adenomas based on the density characteristics on CT or MRI. If the diagnosis is unclear and the adrenal is the only site of suspected metastases, biopsy is indicated.

    (2) Other single areas that are suspect for, but not diagnostic of, malignancy (i.e., liver, brain) warrant a similar approach. See also section VII.B.

C. Obtaining pathological proof of lung cancer. Before embarking on other studies, a diagnosis of lung cancer must be proved histologically. Pursuit of the diagnosis should start with the least invasive procedure that gives histological proof of malignancy.

    1. Sputum cytology, which was once routine practice, has been largely replaced by the flexible fiberoptic bronchoscope. Even in the best series, repeated sputum cytology is positive in only 60% to 80% of centrally located NSCLC and 15% to 20% of peripheral NSCLC.

    2. Flexible fiberoptic bronchoscopy if symptomatic or radiologic evidence indicates a central and accessible cancer or nodal disease. Most cancers can be directly visualized. Additional tumors are evident only as extrinsic bronchial narrowing, which may be diagnosed through the bronchoscope by transbronchial biopsy in some cases. Inspection of the airways by bronchoscopy also rules out endobronchial lesions from a second bronchogenic carcinoma. Bronchoscopy is unnecessary if histologic or cytologic diagnosis of metastatic lung cancer has already been made.

    3. Suspicious cutaneous nodules may undergo biopsy to establish a histological diagnosis and for staging.

    4. Lymph nodes. Enlarged, hard, peripheral lymph nodes represent another potential site for biopsy. Blind biopsy of nonpalpable supraclavicular nodes is positive for cancer in less than 5% of cases. The finding of granuloma in lymph nodes can be misleading; some patients have cancer concomitant with sarcoidosis or granulomatous infections.

D. Subsequent evaluation. After the histological diagnosis of lung cancer, the evaluation should focus on determining whether disease is confined to the chest and may therefore be treated with curative intent (limited-stage SCLC and stages I to III NSCLC) or whether the patient has distant disease. In appropriately selected patients, the following diagnostic studies may assist in making this determination. *In the absence of abnormalities evident from history, physical examination, and routine blood studies, these studies are likely to be normal.*

    1. Positron emission tomography (PET). PET scanning is an established technology based on the differential uptake of radiolabeled glucose [fluorodeoxyglucose (FDG)] by neoplastic tissues compared with normal tissue. Although PET scanning has demonstrated superiority to CT scanning and is complementary to mediastinoscopy in the evaluation of mediastinal nodes, it is most useful in excluding distant occult metastases. PET may also be useful in restaging after a preoperative therapy (i.e., chemotherapy or chemoradiotherapy) or in follow-up. The precise criteria for what constitutes a "response" by PET scan are in evolution. PET-CT scanners are now becoming available and may further improve the ability to accurately stage patients. False-positive PET scans may occur in the setting of infection, inflammation, or after chemoradiotherapy. False-negative scans are frequently seen in well-differentiated adenocarcinoma with BAC features.

    2. Spinal MRI for patients who have suspected epidural metastases in the spinal canal or suspected lung cancer with back pain or brachial plexopathy. In patients with back pain and suspected lung (or any other) cancer, the workup should be performed on an urgent or emergent basis to allow for rapid therapeutic intervention with steroids, RT, or surgery.

    3. Brain CT or MRI should be obtained as part of routine staging for patients with SCLC, which is associated with a 10% incidence of neurologically asymptomatic brain metastases. These studies are not recommended for staging most patients with stage I or II NSCLC in the absence of clinical signs. For patients with histologies characterized by frequent spread to the central nervous system (CNS; e.g., large cell with neuroendocrine differentiation or adenocarcinoma), CNS imaging for localized disease should be considered. Patients with stage III and IV NSCLC who are under consideration for aggressive multimodality therapy or chemotherapy should undergo CNS scanning.

4. **Mediastinoscopy** is useful in the following circumstances:

   a. For *routine* preoperative staging of NSCLC (radiological assessment alone of the mediastinum is inadequate)

   b. In patients with mediastinal masses, negative sputum cytology, and negative bronchoscopy

   c. To evaluate mediastinal lymphadenopathy. Hyperplastic nodes related to postobstructive infection are common. Mediastinoscopy may permit the patient to be considered for curative resection if enlarged nodes on CT scan are demonstrated to be pathologically negative.

5. **Percutaneous and transbronchial needle biopsy** are frequently used to diagnose lung cancer. Some argue that if NSCLC is found by these techniques and medical resectability is assumed, mediastinoscopy or thoracotomy inevitably follows in the absence of evidence of metastatic disease, and therefore the procedure is unnecessary. Furthermore, if cancer is suspected and the needle biopsy reveals a granuloma, the cancer may have been missed. If the diagnosis is SCLC, however, thoracotomy may be avoided. Additionally, medically inoperable patients with negative bronchoscopy still require a tissue diagnosis.

6. **Bone scans** have largely been supplanted by PET. However, the bone scan offers complementary information regarding bone disease to PET and is substantially less expensive. There may be value for obtaining a bone scan in a patient with known metastatic disease in whom new bone involvement is suspected.

7. **Bone radiographs** (plain films) of painful areas

8. **Bone marrow aspiration and biopsy.** Bone marrow examination remains a standard part of the evaluation for patients with apparently limited-stage SCLC because of the relatively high incidence of subclinical involvement. Some believe that it is unnecessary if the patient has a normal lactate dehydrogenase level. It is rarely indicated in NSCLC.

E. Evaluation of the solitary pulmonary nodule requires a diagnostic strategy that maximizes the chance of detecting cancer and minimizes the chance of performing a needless thoracotomy if the nodule is benign. *The diagnostic approach must be individualized.* Facts that should be considered include:

1. **Characteristics that define a solitary pulmonary nodule** are as follows:

   a. *A peripheral lung mass* measuring <6 cm in diameter

   b. The nodule is asymptomatic.

   c. Physical examination is normal.

   d. CBC and LFTs are normal.

2. **Calcification** of the nodules has little bearing on the diagnostic approach. Calcified nodules are more likely to be malignant unless the pattern is circular, crescentic, or completely and densely calcified.

3. **Risk that a solitary pulmonary nodule is malignant**

   a. According to age

   (1) Younger than 35 years of age: <2%

   (2) 35 to 45 years of age: 15%

   (3) Older than 45 years of age: 30% to 50%

   b. According to tumor volume doubling time (DT)

   (1) DT of 30 days or less: <1%

   (2) DT of 30 to 400 days: 30% to 50%

   (3) DT of >400 days: <1%

   c. According to smoking history. The risk of a solitary nodule being cancerous in a smoker compared with a nonsmoker is not known. The incidence is generally higher for smokers in the older age group.

4. **Needle biopsies** of solitary nodules are falsely negative in 15% of cases. In a patient with a high likelihood of cancer (e.g., a smoker who is older than 40 years of age), who is also a good surgical candidate, proceeding directly to thoracotomy without a tissue diagnosis is reasonable.

5. **PET scanning** has recently demonstrated considerable value in the diagnostic evaluation of the solitary pulmonary nodules, with sensitivity and specificity exceeding all other diagnostic modalities short of thoracotomy.

IV. STAGING SYSTEM AND PROGNOSTIC FACTORS

A. **Staging system.** The "TNM" system is applied primarily to NSCLC. Table 8.1.A presents the proposed staging system for the 7th edition of *AJCC Cancer Staging Manual,* based on the recommendations of an expert panel and review of >67,000 lung cancer cases. This system provides for additional cutoffs for tumor size, reassigns the category for pulmonary nodules in some locations, and reclassifies effusions as substage M. This table also shows the current stage groupings (from the 6th edition, 2002).

Table 8.1.B shows the proposed new stage groupings; bolded stages indicate changes from the last edition. In the proposed system, stages IA to IIIA represent disease for which a surgical approach (in physiologically appropriate patients) should be considered in the management plan.

B. **Performance status** (PS) has direct bearing on patient survival and should be accounted for in studies evaluating treatment modalities for lung cancer. Criteria for assessment of functional PS are described on the inside of the back cover. Patients who feel well and have few symptoms of disease (PS of 0 to 1) survive longer than ill patients (PS of 2 or more) and are more likely to tolerate chemotherapy, independent of other prognostic factors.

C. **Weight loss.** Involuntary weight loss of 5% or more is an independent and negative prognostic factor.

D. **Tumor histology.** Survival is not greatly influenced by cell type if PS and extent of disease are taken into account. In NSCLC, specific histology appears to be of importance in the selection of specific chemotherapy regimens on the basis of both patterns of toxicity and efficacy. Patients with SCLC, however, have debility and extensive disease more often than those with the other cell types. A few patients with indolent but unresectable squamous lung cancer may live for several years.

E. **Molecular prognostic factors.** Suppressor oncogene alterations are common in NSCLC and are associated with a poor prognosis; mutated *p53* (17p) oncogene occurs in half of patients with NSCLC and in almost all with SCLC. Dominant oncogene overexpression (*c-myc, K-ras, erb-B2*) is associated with a poor prognosis.

1. **EGFR mutation** and other abnormalities are increasingly recognized as important features of lung cancer. EGFR abnormalities appear to be associated with a better overall prognosis as well as to predict for benefit from anti-EGFR therapies.

2. **ERCC1,** a component of the nucleotide excision and repair system, may be of use in selecting patients who can benefit from platinum agents. Overexpression of ERCC1 as determined by immunohistochemistry is associated with lack of benefit from platinum agents. At this time, this has not yet been established in clinical practice.

V. PREVENTION AND EARLY DETECTION

A. **Prevention** is the best way to reduce the death rate from lung cancer. More than 90% of patients with lung cancer would not have developed the disease if they had not smoked. Every smoking patient should be advised of the enormous risks. Several ongoing studies are evaluating the role of retinoids and other compounds in preventing secondary tumors. Trials of vitamin A analog supplementation and beta-carotene have failed to demonstrate benefit. Epidemiologically, aspirin use in individuals who have quit smoking has been associated with reduced risk of developing lung cancer.

TABLE 8.1A   Proposed Staging System for Lung Cancer[a]

Primary tumor (T)	Regional lymph nodes (N)
TX Primary tumor cannot be assessed, or tumor proved by the presence of malignant cells in sputum or bronchial washings but not visualized radiographically or bronchoscopically	**NX** Regional lymph nodes cannot be assessed.
T0 No evidence of primary tumor	**N0** No regional lymph node metastasis
Tis Carcinoma *in situ*	**N1** Metastasis in ipsilateral peribronchial, ipsilateral hilar, and/or intrapulmonary nodes, including involvement by direct extension
T1 A tumor that is ≤3 cm in greatest dimension, and is ■ surrounded by lung or visceral pleura, and ■ without evidence of invasion proximal to a lobar bronchus at bronchoscopy (i.e., not in the main bronchus) *T1a Tumor ≤2 cm in greatest dimension* *T1b Tumor >2 cm but ≤3 cm in greatest dimension*	**N2** Metastasis in ipsilateral mediastinal and/or subcarinal lymph nodes **N3** Metastasis to contralateral mediastinal lymph nodes, contralateral hilar lymph nodes, ipsilateral or contralateral scalene or supraclavicular lymph nodes
T2 A tumor >3 cm *but ≤7 cm* with any of the following features: ■ involves main bronchus ≥2 cm distal to the carina, or ■ invades into visceral pleura, or ■ is associated with atelectasis or obstructive pneumonitis that extends to the hilar region but does not involve the entire lung *T2a Tumor >3 cm but ≤5 cm in greatest dimension* *T2b Tumor >5 cm but ≤7 cm in greatest dimension*	**Distant metastases (M)** **MX** Distant metastasis cannot be assessed **M0** No (known) distant metastasis **M1** Distant metastasis present **M1a** ■ *Separate tumor nodule(s) in a contralateral lobe; or* ■ *Tumor with pleural nodules or malignant pleural (or pericardial) effusion* **M1b** *Distant metastases*
T3 A tumor *> 7 cm or* one that directly invades chest wall (including superior sulcus tumors), diaphragm, *phrenic nerve,* mediastinal pleura, parietal pericardium; or ■ involves the main bronchus <2 cm distal to the carina but not the carina; or ■ has associated atelectasis or obstructive pneumonitis of the entire lung; or ■ has separate tumor nodule(s) within the same lobe	
T4 A tumor of any size with: ■ invasion of the mediastinum, heart, great vessels, trachea, carina, recurrent laryngeal nerve, esophagus, or vertebral body; or ■ separate tumor nodule(s) in a different ipsilateral lobe	

Changes of descriptors from the 6th edition of the *AJCC Cancer Staging Manual* (2002) are shown in italics.
[a]Adapted from Goldstraw P, Crowley J, Chansky K, et al. The IASLC Lung Cancer Staging Project: Proposals for the revision of the TNM Stage Groupings in the forthcoming (seventh) edition of the TNM classification for malignant tumors. *J Thor Oncol* 2007;2:706–714. Note that the seventh edition is due to be published in 2009.

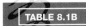

| TABLE 8.1B | Proposed Stage Groupings for Lung Cancer[a] | | | | |

T/M Descriptor in 6th Edition	Proposed T/M	N0	N1	N2	N3
T1 (≤2 cm)	T1a	IA	IIA	IIIA	IIIB
T1 (>2–3 cm)	T1b	IA	IIA	IIIA	IIIB
T2 (≤5 cm)	T2a	IB	**IIA**	IIIA	IIIB
T2 (>5–7 cm)	T2b	**IIA**	IIB	IIIA	IIIB
T2 (>7 cm)	T3	**IIB**	**IIIA**	IIIA	IIIB
T3 (invasion)	T3	IIB	IIIA	IIIA	IIIB
T4 (same lobe nodules)	T3	**IIB**	**IIIA**	**IIIA**	IIIB
T4 (extension)	T4	**IIIA**	**IIIA**	IIIB	IIIB
M1 (ipsilateral lung)	T4	**IIIA**	**IIIA**	**IIIB**	**IIIB**
T4 (pleural effusion)	M1a	**IV**	**IV**	**IV**	**IV**
M1 (contralateral lung)	M1a	IV	IV	IV	IV
M1 (distant)	M1b	IV	IV	IV	IV

Bold print indicates a change from the 6th edition for a particular TNM category.
[a]Reprinted with permission from Goldstraw P, Crowley J, Chansky K, et al. The IASLC Lung Cancer Staging Project: Proposals for the revision of the TNM Stage Groupings in the forthcoming (seventh) edition of the TNM classification for malignant tumours. *J Thor Oncol* 2007;2:706–714. Note that the seventh edition is due to be published in 2009.

B. Early detection of lung cancer by screening high-risk populations with chest radiographs and sputum cytology has not been clearly demonstrated to improve survival rates. The role of chest radiography is being re-evaluated. New antibody tests and fluorescent bronchoscopy are also under study.

Spiral CT scan can increase the number of cancers detected. However, this increased rate of detection has not yet been demonstrated to reduce the overall or lung cancer–specific death rate. It is therefore not established as an effective screening tool. The National Lung Screening Trial (NLST) has completed accrual of 50,000 subjects considered to be at high risk of lung cancer. This study compares CT with CXR. The preliminary results of this study may become available in late 2009. Because the value of a screening test is dependent on the prevalence of a disease in a population, the determination that smokers with minimal degrees of obstructive disease are at substantially higher risk for lung cancer may improve the sensitivity and specificity of screening tests.

VI. MANAGEMENT

A. NSCLC. Surgery, the previous mainstay of management, is still the primary mode of therapy in stage I and II disease. Stage III disease (characterized by mediastinal nodal disease or involvement of major structures) is frequently resectable but almost invariably relapses, resulting in the patient's death within 5 years (90% to 95%) when managed by surgery alone. Therefore, multimodality therapy is increasingly employed in this large subset (about 40,000 patients per year). Patients with only a single mediastinal nodal "station" positive for disease or with incidentally discovered stage III disease (i.e., patients who undergo surgery for stage I or II disease and who are found to have microscopic mediastinal nodal disease) fare substantially better than other stage III patients.

After histological proof of NSCLC is obtained, resectability is determined by the extent of the tumor and operability according to the overall medical condition of the patient. About half of patients with NSCLC are potentially operable. About half of tumors in operable patients are resectable (25% of all patients), and about half of patients with resectable tumors survive 5 years (12% of all patients or 25% of operable patients).

The following recommendations are consistent with those of the American Thoracic Society and the European Respiratory Society.

1. **Determinants of resectability. Signs of unresectable NSCLC** are as follows:
   a. Distant metastases, including metastases to the opposite lung. If solitary adrenal, hepatic, or other masses are detected by scans, these areas should be evaluated by biopsy because there is a significant incidence of benign masses that masquerade as tumor. See also section VII.B.
   b. Persistent pleural effusion with malignant cells. Cytological examination of 50 to 100 mL of fluid is positive for malignant cells in about 65% of patients. Repeat thoracentesis may provide the diagnosis in most of the remaining patients. In the event of negative cytology and in the absence of other contraindications to surgery, thoracoscopy should be undertaken at the time of surgery. Pleural involvement with malignant cells would preclude surgery. Transudative and parapneumonic effusions that clear do not contraindicate surgery. Most exudative effusions in the absence of pneumonia are malignant, regardless of cytological findings.
   c. Superior vena cava obstruction
   d. Involvement of the following structures:
      (1) Supraclavicular or neck lymph nodes (proved histologically)
      (2) Contralateral mediastinal lymph nodes (proved histologically)
      (3) Recurrent laryngeal nerve
      (4) Tracheal wall
      (5) Main-stem bronchus <2 cm from the carina (resectable by sleeve resection technique)

2. **Determinants of operability**
   a. **Age and mental illness** per se are not factors in deciding operability. Elderly patients, arbitrarily defined as individuals >70 years of age, experience the same degree of benefit from therapy as younger patients provided that they have adequate nutritional and performance status. Clear distinction should be made between the "fit" elderly and those who have multiple comorbidities. The appropriate treatment of the "frail elderly" is unclear.
   b. **Cardiac status.** The presence of uncontrolled cardiac failure, uncontrolled arrhythmia, or a recent myocardial infarction (within 6 months) makes the patient inoperable.
   c. **Pulmonary status.** The patient's ability to tolerate resection of part or all of a lung must be determined. The presence of pulmonary hypertension or inadequate pulmonary reserve makes the patient inoperable. *It is critical that any patient for whom surgery is contemplated stop smoking for at least several weeks before the operation.*
      (1) **Routine pulmonary function tests** (PFT). Arterial blood gases and spirometry should be obtained in all patients before surgery. PFTs must be interpreted in the light of optimal medical management of pulmonary disease and patient cooperation. The patient with PFT abnormalities should receive a trial of bronchodilators, antibiotics, chest percussion, and postural drainage before inoperability is concluded. The following results suggest inoperability:
         (a) A $PaCO_2$ that is >45 mm Hg (that cannot be corrected) or a PaO_2 that is <60 mm Hg, or
         (b) Forced vital capacity (FVC) <40% of predicted value, or
         (c) Forced expired volume at 1 second (FEV_1) ≤ 1 L. Patients with an FEV_1 of >2 L or >60% of predicted value can tolerate pneumonectomy.
      (2) **Special PFTs**
         (a) **The quantitative perfusion lung scan** is done when patients with impaired pulmonary function are suspected of not being able to tolerate excision of lung tissue. The FEV_1 is measured before the scan. The percentage of blood flow to each lung is calculated from the

results of the scan. The percentage of flow in the noncancerous lung is multiplied by the FEV_1, giving a measure of the anticipated postoperative FEV_1. Pneumonectomy is contraindicated if the calculated postoperative FEV_1 is <700 mL because the patient is likely to develop refractory cor pulmonale and respiratory insufficiency.

   (b) Exercise testing. If maximal oxygen consumption is >20 mL/kg, perioperative morbidity is low; if it is <10 mL/kg, morbidity and mortality are high.

B. NSCLC: Management of stage I and II disease

1. **Surgery.** Surgical resection of the primary tumor is the treatment of choice for patients who can tolerate surgery and who have stage I or II NSCLC. The selection of the operative procedure varies with the surgeon's criteria for patient selection, the extent of disease, and the patient's ventilatory function.

   Definition of nodal involvement during surgical resection is mandatory to determine prognosis and to evaluate the results of treatment; the anatomic boundaries of 13 nodal stations have been described. Although considered technically resectable, most patients with stage IIIa disease (predominantly N2 disease) do poorly (see section VI.C). An exception is the patient with malignant involvement of a single mediastinal nodal station.

   a. **Incomplete resections** are rarely, if ever, indicated.

   b. **Lobectomy** is the procedure of choice in patients whose lung function permits it. Conservative resection (segmentectomy) has been associated with a significantly worse disease-free survival and an increased local recurrence rate.

   c. **Bilobectomy, sleeve lobectomy, or pneumonectomy** with or without lymph node dissection are used in other clinical presentations.

   d. **Video-assisted thoracoscopic surgery** (VATS) is increasingly employed in thoracic surgery. Its utilization for resection of lung cancer is associated with results comparable to open procedures.

   e. **Surgical mortality.** A multicenter study of contemporary operative mortality due to lung surgery documented the following death rates within 30 days of operation: pneumonectomy, 7.7%; lobectomy, 3.3%; and segmentectomy or wedge resection, 1.4%. Advanced age, weight loss, coexisting disease, reduced FEV_1, and more extensive resection are significant risk factors.

2. **Pancoast tumor.** Historically, RT has been employed as the preliminary treatment for Pancoast tumors (T3 N0 M0, stage IIb) before surgical resection of the primary tumor and involved chest wall. Mature results from a national intergroup trial using preoperative chemotherapy and RT (chemoradiotherapy) in the treatment of this disease entity, however, demonstrated a median survival of 37 months and 5-year survival of 42%, far exceeding the historical approach of radiation followed by surgery. Given the relative rarity of this entity, the use of preoperative chemoradiotherapy can now be considered the standard of care.

3. **Adjuvant chemotherapy.** The majority of patients undergoing complete resections for NSCLC relapse and die within 3 years of resection. Adjuvant therapy failed to improve outcome in early studies, but they were flawed by the use of ineffective chemotherapy or poor trial design.

   Platinum-based adjuvant chemotherapy has now been unequivocally established on the basis of large randomized trials in Europe and North America. Patients were randomized to adjuvant chemotherapy or observation. The International Adjuvant Lung Trial (IALT) detected a 4% to 5% absolute benefit in long-term survival for patients treated with adjuvant platinum-based chemotherapy. Although this trial was characterized by heterogeneous chemotherapy regimens and premature closure, it was the largest trial ever performed studying this question. The results of this trial have now been confirmed by the North American Intergroup trial (JBR-10) and another European trial (ANITA). The latter two studies employed cisplatin/vinorelbine as the adjuvant regimen and demonstrated an approximately 10% absolute reduction in mortality. This level of benefit is comparable to the degree of benefit seen in breast and colon adjuvant studies. Routine use of adjuvant therapy with a cisplatin-based, two-drug regimen is now recommended for patients with resected stage IIa, IIb, and IIIa disease.

The role of adjuvant chemotherapy in patients with resected stage Ib is controversial. Only one trial has specifically addressed this issue, and although it demonstrated improved disease-free survival, overall survival was not significantly improved. Retrospective analysis indicates that patients with tumors >4 cm may enjoy a benefit comparable to that of stage II and III patients, but this is not established. Adjuvant therapy should be discussed on an individual basis with patients with stage Ib disease. Preoperative chemotherapy in localized NSCLC is an alternative approach.

4. **Adjuvant RT** has also been frequently employed in the treatment of resected stage I, II, and III disease. Its use clearly results in improved local control. As documented in a recent meta-analysis, however, improved local control may come at the expense of diminished survival. Hence, the routine use of adjuvant RT in completely resected NSCLC cannot be recommended.

5. **Resectable but inoperable.** Definitive RT should be the primary treatment for medically inoperable but resectable patients. The overall survival rate at 5 years is about 20%, depending on the size of the primary tumor and associated comorbidities. The sterilization rate for small tumors ranges from 25% to 50%. Chemoradiotherapy may also be considered for these patients, particularly those with N1 disease, for whom the outcome is very poor with RT alone.

C. **NSCLC: Management of stages IIIa and IIIb**

1. **Combined-modality therapy.** In the past, the standard treatment for most of these patients was RT or surgery alone, with modest evidence of survival benefit over supportive care alone. Historical data suggest that RT results in a median survival of 9 months, a 2-year survival rate of 10% to 15%, and a 5-year survival rate of 5% (worse for stage IIIb). Clinical trials indicate a survival advantage at 1, 2, and 3 years with the use of chemoradiotherapy in this setting (with or without surgery); the 2-year survival rate has been reported to be 25% to 40%. Several randomized trials have demonstrated that the use of concurrent chemoradiotherapy is superior to sequential therapy.

    a. A number of different drug combinations and approaches have been evaluated. Conceptually, there are two major approaches: "systemic full dose chemotherapy" with concurrent radiotherapy and "radiosensitizing" chemotherapy concurrent with radiation and followed by consolidative chemotherapy. For the former approach, the most mature data utilize cisplatin/etoposide and concurrent radiation to 61 Gy. For the latter, the most commonly utilized approach combines weekly low doses of carboplatin (AUC 2 mg/mL x min) and paclitaxel (45 to 50 mg/m^2) concurrent with 61 Gy followed by full doses of carboplatin/paclitaxel. These regimens are detailed in Table 8.2.

    b. Most chemoradiotherapy trials entered patients with good PS, minimal weight loss, and little comorbid illness. The use of chemoradiotherapy is also appropriate, however, in many poor-risk patients, defined by weight loss and other medical problems. A multicenter study demonstrated a median survival of 13 months in these patients, comparable to that of more favorable patients. These sicker patients, not surprisingly, do not experience the same long-term survival.

    c. An emerging problem in stage III–disease patients treated with combined modality therapy is the occurrence of CNS metastases, which may be the sole site of relapse in 10% to 20% of patients. The role of prophylactic cranial irradiation for patients with stage III disease treated with chemoradiotherapy has been addressed in a multicenter trial. Though the study failed to reach its anticipated accrual, >300 patients were enrolled. The results are not yet available. See section VII.B.

2. **Preoperative "neoadjuvant" chemotherapy** (with or without RT) for patients with locally advanced disease may down-stage the malignancy and make it resectable. Adjuvant surgical resection after chemoradiotherapy was compared

TABLE 8.2 First-Line Chemotherapy Regimens for Advanced Non–Small Cell Lung Cancer

Regimen	Dose (mg/m²)[a]	Days given	Cycle length (days)
Cisplatin	100	1	28
Vinorelbine	25	1, 8, 15	
Carboplatin	AUC = 6	1	21
Paclitaxel	225 (over 3 h)	1	
Carboplatin	AUC = 5.5	1	21
Gemcitabine	1,000	1, 8	
Cisplatin	75	1	21
Docetaxel	75	1	
Carboplatin	AUC = 6	1	21
Paclitaxel	200	1	
Bevacizumab	15 mg/kg	1	
Cisplatin	75	1	21
Pemetrexed	500	1	

[a]AUC, area under the curve.

with chemoradiotherapy alone in stage IIIa (N2), which was addressed in a North American Intergroup trial. Preliminary results indicate that an increase in early mortality in the surgical group, primarily in patients undergoing pneumonectomy, offsets a possible long-term advantage from surgery. At this time, the role of surgical resection after chemoradiotherapy remains to be established and should not be done outside of centers with substantial expertise in this approach.

3. **Technical aspects of RT** are important, both as a single modality and in combination with chemotherapy. Issues of dose, schedule, and fields are crucial. Evidence indicates that hyperfractionated accelerated RT (two or three times a day) may be superior to conventional, daily fractionation when used alone. A randomized trial failed to demonstrate an advantage for twice-a-day fractions when combined with chemotherapy over standard chemoradiotherapy. Additionally, the use of three-dimensional conformal techniques may reduce or prevent toxicity to normal lung within the radiation field and allow dose escalation.

4. **Concurrent versus sequential treatment.** Several randomized controlled trials in the United States, Europe, and Japan have demonstrated the superiority of concurrent chemoradiotherapy over sequential therapy. A Japanese study utilized mitomycin, vindesine, and cisplatin concurrent with RT. A trial by the Radiation Therapy Oncology Group used cisplatin and vinblastine concurrent with 6,100 cGy of RT administered over 6 weeks. Significant differences in median survival times (17 vs. 14 months) and in survival at 2 and 3 years strongly favored concurrent treatment.

5. **Specific management recommendations** should be individualized. In the absence of a clinical trial, patients with documented N2 or N3 disease should receive concurrent chemoradiotherapy. Patients with T4 N0 disease may be considered for induction chemotherapy with or without RT followed by surgery.

6. **Radiographic responses.** In all cases, patients treated with multimodality therapy may have variable radiographic responses. Except for those who demonstrate progressive disease (and consequently have a dire prognosis), there is no

correlation between degree of radiographic response (complete response, partial response, or stable disease) and outcome. It is unclear that PET scanning improves the ability to assess these patients noninvasively.

D. NSCLC: Management of stage IV disease

1. **Fully ambulatory patients** have increased survival, and symptoms are often palliated by the use of platinum-containing (cisplatin or carboplatin) chemotherapy. A clear advantage for the use of chemotherapy has now been conclusively demonstrated in patients with stage IV disease and PS of 0 to 1. The median survival of such patients is 4 months, and the 1-year survival rate is 10% with *best supportive care*. With platinum-based chemotherapy (either as single agents or combined with etoposide, vinblastine, vindesine, or mitomycin), these survivals are improved to about 6 to 8 months and 20% to 25%, respectively.

   Newer regimens (carboplatin plus paclitaxel, cisplatin plus vinorelbine, cisplatin plus gemcitabine, cisplatin plus pemetrexed) have resulted in median survivals of 9 to 10 months and 1-year survival rates of 30% to 40% in large multicenter randomized trials. Bevacizumab, an antibody to the vascular endothelial growth factor (VEGF), has been demonstrated to result in superior survival in selected patients with advanced NSCLC. Studies with bevacizumab have excluded patients with squamous carcinoma, bleeding disorders, significant cardiovascular or thrombotic disease, CNS metastases, or cavitary lesions. The approved dose is 15 mg/kg q 21 days. A recent report from Europe indicates the 75 mg/kg q 21 days may be equally efficacious and less toxic. However, this was based on progression-free as opposed to overall survival, and the data are not yet fully mature. The role of newer inhibitors of the VEGF receptor tyrosine kinase domain (including agents approved for other indications, such as sorafenib and sunitinib) are under active investigation.

   Several studies and meta-analyses have demonstrated improved quality of life for patients treated with chemotherapy as opposed to best supportive care. Economic analysis has demonstrated that it is more cost-effective to treat patients with chemotherapy because of the reduced need for hospitalization, RT, and other interventions.

2. **Patients who are less than fully ambulatory** (PS of ≥ 2) have poor outcomes. Emerging evidence indicates that such patients do benefit from therapy. The best current evidence indicates that carboplatin-based two-drug therapy is superior to single-agent treatment and to best supportive care. However, management must be individualized, and options are ultimately dependent on the presence of comorbid disease and the patient's wishes.

3. **Patients who have progressed after initial chemotherapy** and who have good PS (0 to 1) may respond to second-line therapy with docetaxel (75 mg/m^2 IV over 1 hour q 21 days). Two multicenter randomized trials have demonstrated an advantage for docetaxel in this setting (compared with best supportive care in one study and with either ifosfamide or vinorelbine in the other). Pemetrexed (500 mg/m^2 q 21 days) (multitargeted antifolate, Alimta) was compared with docetaxel in a randomized phase III trial and was demonstrated to have similar efficacy with a favorable toxicity profile.

4. **Erlotinib** (Tarceva), 150 mg PO daily, has been approved for second- and third-line therapy of NSCLC. This agent appears to benefit a small fraction of patients (radiographic response rate of 5% to 10%), but this benefit has been reported to be dramatic when it occurs. Retrospective analyses indicate that female patients with adenocarcinoma (particularly those with bronchioloalveolar features), young age, and minimal smoking history are most likely to benefit.

   The value of potential predictive markers such as EGFR mutational analysis, EGFR gene copy number by FISH, or EGFR expression by immunohistochemistry are under investigation. None of these markers can be recommended for routine clinical use at this time.

   a. **The major toxicities** of this therapy are skin rash, diarrhea, and, rarely, interstitial pneumonitis. Interstitial pneumonitis is predominantly seen in Asians and may be fatal; the incidence in <1%. Cessation of drug, steroid therapy, and hospitalization (as appropriate) should be undertaken in the patient with worsening dyspnea and radiographic changes consistent with interstitial pneumonitis. It is frequently difficult to distinguish pneumonitis from disease progression.

b. **Skin rash** is a very common toxicity, and its occurrence may correlate with tumor response. At present, there are no established guidelines in either the dermatologic or ophthalmologic literature for treatment of rash-related side effect from the EGFR inhibitors. The following is an algorithm that was adopted from data on file at Genentech, Inc. *Prescriptions for topical 1% or 2.5% hydrocortisone cream and 1% clindamycin gel should be provided at the time of the initial erlotinib prescription so that they may be used at the first sign of rash*, which may be before the 2-week follow-up visit.

(1) **For mild rash** (grade 1), use topical hydrocortisone 1% or 2.5% cream and/or clindamycin 1% gel b.i.d. to affected areas. Make sure to apply the topicals at least 1 hour apart. Continue the EGFR inhibitor at current dose, and monitor for change in severity. If after 2 weeks the reactions do not improve, then proceed to treatment for moderate rash.

(2) **For moderate rash** (grades 2 or 3), use either hydrocortisone 2.5% cream and/or clindamycin 1% gel or pimecrolimus 1% cream *plus* doxy-cycline 100 mg PO b.i.d. or minocycline 100 mg b.i.d. Continue the EGFR inhibitor at the current dose, and monitor for change in severity. If there is no improvement in 2 weeks and symptoms worsen, then treat as above with the addition of a methylprednisolone dose pack. If reaction continues to worsen, then dose interruption or discontinuation may be necessary.

(3) For the patients who report pruritic, dry, erythematous eyes when the onset could be attributed to treatment with EGFR inhibitors, use prednisolone sodium phosphate ophthalmic (0.125%), 1 to 2 drops to the affected eyes b.i.d.–q.i.d. If condition increases in severity, it is recommended that the patient follow up with an ophthalmologist.

(4) Topical preparations of mTOR (e.g., sirolimus) may be of use, if available.

c. **Diarrhea** should be managed with Imodium or Lomotil. If toxicities persist despite adequate management (i.e., > grade I), dose interruption followed by reductions of erlotinib are indicated.

5. **Duration of therapy.** The maximum benefit from any specific chemotherapy regimen is achieved in six cycles. Fewer cycles may be adequate. Two studies have demonstrated equivalent response and survival when three or four cycles of a platinum-based regimen were compared with more cycles of the same regimen.

6. **The choice of which platinum-based chemotherapy** regimen to use as first-line therapy can be based on several considerations. The considerations include convenience of administration, cost, and toxicity profiles. Cisplatin-based regimens are less expensive and in one recent randomized trial demonstrated a survival advantage compared with a carboplatin-based treatment. However, these cisplatin regimens are less convenient and cause more nausea, vomiting, renal toxicity, and ototoxicity. Taxane-based regimens universally result in alopecia and have significant cumulative neurotoxicity. Gemcitabine-platinum regimens are more myelotoxic, but usually do not cause alopecia. Bevacizumab has been safely combined with carboplatin/paclitaxel and cisplatin/gemcitabine in large phase III studies. Data regarding the ability to combine bevacizumab with other commonly utilized regimens (e.g., carboplatin/gemcitabine, carboplatin/docetaxel) should be available shortly. There is a choice of regimens, but no regimen of choice. Table 8.2 provides the details of a few of the most commonly utilized regimens for advanced NSCLC.

7. **Problems with phase II trials** . New chemotherapy agents and combinations are undergoing evaluation. Performance status, age, sex, degree of weight loss, and staging of the patients govern the response to and toxicity of these regimens. Some phase II trials include patients with stage IIIb (without pleural effusion) disease. Additionally, small numbers (25 to 50) of patients are accrued to such trials, as opposed to the hundreds of patients accrued to phase III trials. As

TABLE 8.3	Regimens for Small Cell Lung Cancer		
Regimen	**Dose (mg/m²)**	**Days given**	**Cycle length (days)**
Cisplatin	60	1	21
Etoposide	120	1, 2, 3	
Chest RT	1.5 Gy (45 Gy total)	Twice daily	For 5 weeks
PCI	2.5 Gy (25 Gy total)	Daily	For 3 weeks (after completion of other therapy)[a]
Cisplatin	100	1	21
Etoposide	100	1, 2, 3	
Cisplatin	60	1	28
Irinotecan	60	1, 8, 15	
Topotecan	1.5	1, 2, 3, 4, 5	21

[a]PCI (prophylactic cranial irradiation) is indicated in patients with limited disease who have obtained a good partial response or a complete response after the completion of other therapy. Chest RT and PCI are administered Monday to Friday.

a result, early reports of phase II data frequently overstate the activity and underestimate the toxicity of new regimens.

E. Small cell lung carcinoma: Management

1. **Limited stage (I, II, III)** is confined to one hemithorax, including contralateral supraclavicular adenopathy. Less than 5% of patients with SCLC have stage I or II disease. About one-third, however, have disease that is clinically confined to the hemithorax and draining regional nodes at presentation (stages IIIa and IIIb).

    a. **Combined-modality therapy.** The available data indicate that these patients should receive concurrent chemotherapy and thoracic RT. Sequential chemotherapy followed by RT results in inferior long-term survival and should be discouraged. At this time, the most accepted chemotherapy regimen is cisplatin and etoposide (Table 8.3). RT given twice daily (hyperfractionated) has been demonstrated to be superior to once-daily therapy (4,500 cGy). It is unclear whether conventionally fractionated RT to a higher dose would be equal or superior to hyperfractionated 4,500 cGy treatment. If given concurrently as induction, combined-modality therapy yields a median survival of 23 months and a 5-year survival rate of 25%.

    b. **Prophylactic cranial irradiation** (PCI) decreases the rate of brain metastases. The use of PCI is controversial because the occurrence of synchronous metastases has made it difficult to demonstrate a survival advantage. The best evidence is that the use of PCI results in about a 5% improvement in survival. When PCI is administered in low-dose fractions (≤200 cGy/day, to a dose of 3,000 cGy), the incidence of neurocognitive dysfunction is not increased.

2. **Extensive stage (ESLC).** Fully ambulatory patients with extensive disease have a good response to PE or cyclophosphamide, doxorubicin (Adriamycin), and vincristine (CAV regimen), or alternation of PE and CAV regimens (Table 8.3). Only 15% to 20% of such patients achieve complete response. The median survival of fully ambulatory patients is about 1 year, and the 2-year survival rate is 20%. Survival for 5 years, however, is unusual.

    a. randomized trial from Japan comparing cisplatin/irinotecan with PE demonstrated superior survival for cisplatin/irinotecan. A U.S. trial comparing platinum/etoposide with platinum/irinotecan failed to demonstrate an advantage for the latter regimen. Either PE or cisplatin/irinotecan can be considered an acceptable regimen for the treatment of ESCLC. In elderly or compromised patients, carboplatin is frequently substituted for cisplatin.

b. Topotecan has demonstrated activity as second-line therapy for SCLC. Other agents (paclitaxel, gemcitabine, vinorelbine, and docetaxel) also have activity in extensive-stage disease.

c. Patients with SCLC who are less than fully ambulatory may still be appropriate candidates for chemotherapy. Patients who respond may have significant improvement in performance status.

d. PCI has recently been demonstrated to reduce the risk of CNS metastases and improve event-free and overall survival in patients with ESCLC who have had any degree of response (including stable disease) to initial chemotherapy.

VII. SPECIAL CLINICAL PROBLEMS

A. Positive sputum cytology with a negative chest radiograph (TX N0 M0) and no other evidence of disease is an occasional problem, usually occurring in screening programs. Patients should be examined by CT scan of the chest and fiberoptic bronchoscopy with selective washings. Bronchial washings may not be helpful in localizing the malignancy because multiple sites may have tumors or suspected dysplastic change.

1. When these measures fail to identify a lesion, patients must be informed that the likelihood that they have a cancer too small to be detected is significant. Such patients should be followed with monthly chest radiographs and should be strongly advised to stop smoking. Repeated sputum cytology is not helpful if the original cytology findings were diagnostic of malignancy and laboratory errors were not suspected.

2. The cytological discovery of an unequivocal small cell cancer in the absence of other findings should be confirmed by repeat sampling and solicitation of a second pathologist's opinion at another institution. After the diagnosis is confirmed, patients should be treated as described previously.

B. Solitary brain metastasis. Patients with NSCLC who present with a single site of metastatic disease, most commonly in the brain, can be treated with curative intent. There are two situations in which this occurs: patients who have received definitive therapy and relapse with a single CNS metastasis (and no other disease), and those who at initial presentation have chest disease and the CNS as the sole site of metastasis.

For the relapsed patients, resection of the CNS metastasis may lead to long-term survival. For patients with synchronous disease, resection of the primary chest tumor and resection or the use of radiosurgery for the CNS disease is appropriate. If the patient has locally advanced disease (stage IIIa or IIIb), one could consider resection of the CNS disease followed by chemoradiotherapy with or without surgery for the chest disease in selected patients.

1. The use of postoperative whole-brain RT (WBRT) after surgical resection of a solitary metastasis is recommended because of the frequency of occult micrometastases. Although the use of WBRT in patients who have been treated either with surgery or with radiosurgery has failed to demonstrate a survival advantage, the neurological event-free survival is clearly superior with WBRT. Most patients who do not initially receive WBRT after treatment of a solitary lesion will receive therapy at the time of relapse.

2. If brain metastasis is anatomically unresectable, stereotactic radiosurgery is superior to whole-brain RT alone.

VIII. FOLLOW-UP

A. After primary therapy. Although most cases of SCLC and NSCLC recur, there is little evidence that frequent laboratory or radiological studies detect disease before the development of symptoms or that early detection improves outcome. In the nonprotocol setting, we recommend history and physical examination every 2 to 3 months and chest radiograph twice yearly for the first few years after resection. The follow-up visit is an excellent opportunity to reinforce the importance of smoking cessation in individuals who continue to abuse tobacco.

B. Radiological abnormalities. Patients who undergo chemoradiotherapy frequently demonstrate scarring and infiltrates on radiological studies, which may evolve with time. These abnormalities are frequently misinterpreted as progressive disease. Proper interpretation of these studies requires determination of RT ports and comparison of initial and follow-up studies.

C. Patients undergoing therapy for metastatic disease should have periodic reassessments of the known sites of disease. Progression of disease (>20% increase in the sum of unidimensional measurements of indicator lesions or the appearance of new disease) or deteriorating performance status is a reason to stop therapy. The appearance of new lesions, even if other disease is smaller or has resolved, constitutes progression.

Suggested Reading

Albain KS, Crowley JJ, LeBlanc M, et al. Determinants of improved outcome in small-cell lung cancer: an analysis of the 2,580-patient Southwest Oncology Group Data Base. *J Clin Oncol* 1990;8:1563.

Albain KS, Rusch VW, Crowley JJ, et al. Concurrent cisplatin/etoposide plus chest radiotherapy followed by surgery for stages IIIA (N2) and IIIB non–small cell lung cancer: mature results of Southwest Oncology Group Phase II Study 8805. *J Clin Oncol* 1995;13:1880.

Al-Sugair A, Coleman RE. Applications of PET in lung cancer. *Semin Nucl Med* 1998;28:303.

American Society of Clinical Oncology. Clinical practice guidelines for the treatment of unresectable non-small-cell lung cancer. ASCO Special Article. *J Clin Oncol* 1997;15:2996.

American Thoracic Society/European Respiratory Society. Pretreatment evaluation of non-small-cell lung cancer. *Am J Respir Crit Care Med* 1997;156:320.

Auperin A, Arriagada R, Pignon JP, et al. Prophylactic cranial irradiation for patients with small cell lung cancer in complete remission. *N Engl J Med* 1999;341:476.

Dillman RO, Herndon J, Seagren SL, et al. Improved survival in stage III non-small-cell lung cancer: seven year follow-up of Cancer and Leukemia Group B (CALGB) 8433 trial. *J Natl Cancer Inst* 1996;88:1210.

Edelman MJ, Gandara DR, Roach M, et al. Multimodality therapy in stage III non-small cell lung cancer. *Ann Thorac Surg* 1996;61:1564.

Fossella FV, DeVore R, Kerr RN, et al. Randomized phase III trial of docetaxel versus vinorelbine or ifosfamide in patients with advanced non-small cell lung cancer previously treated with platinum containing regimens. *J Clin Oncol* 2000;18:2354.

Furuse K, Fukuoka M, Kawahara M. Phase III study of concurrent versus sequential thoracic radiotherapy in combination with mitomycin, vindesine, and cisplatin in unresectable stage III non-small cell lung cancer. *J Clin Oncol* 1999;17:2692.

Hanna N, Shepherd FA, Fossella FV, et al. Randomized phase III trial of pemetrexed versus docetaxel in patients with non-small cell lung cancer previously treated with chemotherapy. *J Clin Oncol* 2004;22(9):1589.

Johnson DH, Einhorn LH, Bartolucci A, et al. Thoracic radiotherapy does not prolong survival in patients with locally advanced, unresectable non-small cell lung cancer. *Ann Intern Med* 1990;113:33.

Kaneko M, Eguchi K, Ohmatsu H, et al. Peripheral lung cancer: screening and detection with low-dose spinal CT versus radiography. *Radiology* 1996;201:798.

Kelly K, Bunn PA Jr. Is it time to reevaluate our approach to the treatment of brain metastases in patients with non–small cell lung cancer? *Lung Cancer* 1998;20:85.

Kelly K, Crowley J, Bunn PA Jr. Randomized phase III trial of paclitaxel plus carboplatin versus vinorelbine plus cisplatin in the treatment of patients with advanced non–small-cell lung cancer: a Southwest Oncology Group trial. *J Clin Oncol* 2001;19:3210.

Mountain CF. Revisions in the International System for Staging Lung Cancer. *Chest* 1997;111:1710.

Noda K, Nishiwaki Y, Kawahara M, et al. Irinotecan plus cisplatin compared with etoposide plus cisplatin for extensive small cell lung cancer *N Engl J Med* 2002;346:85.

Non-small Cell Lung Cancer Collaborative Group. Chemotherapy in non–small cell lung cancer: a meta-analysis using updated data on individual patients from 52 randomized clinical trials. *BMJ* 1995;311:899.

Ost D, Fein AM, Feinsilver SH. The solitary pulmonary nodule. *N Engl J Med* 2003;348: 2535.

Paez JG, Janne PA, Lee JC, et al. EGFR mutations in lung cancer: correlation with clinical response to gefitinib therapy. *Science* 2004;304:1497.

Pieterman RM, van Putten JWG, Meuzelaar JJ, et al. Preoperative staging of non–small cell lung cancer with positron emission tomography. *N Engl J Med* 2000;343:254.

Quinn D, Gianlupi A, Broste S. The changing radiographic presentation of bronchogenic carcinoma with reference to cell types. *Chest* 1996;110:1474.

Rosell R, Gomez-Codina J, Camps C, et al. A randomized trial comparing preoperative chemotherapy plus surgery with surgery alone in patients with non–small cell lung cancer. *N Engl J Med* 1994;330:153.

Sandler A, Gray R, Perry MC, et al. Paclitaxel-carboplatin alone or with bevacizumab for non–small-cell lung cancer. *N Engl J Med* 2006;355:2542.

Schiller JH, Harrington D, Belani CP, et al. Comparison of four chemotherapy regimens for advanced non–small cell lung cancer. *N Engl J Med* 2002;346:92.

Shepherd FA, Pereira JR, Ciuleanu T, et al. Erlotinib in previously treated non–small-cell lung cancer. *N Engl J Med* 2005;353:123.

Turrisi AT, Turisi AT III, Kim K, et al. Twice-daily compared with once-daily thoracic radiotherapy in limited small-cell lung cancer treated concurrently with cisplatin and etoposide. *N Engl J Med* 1999;340:265.

Von Pawel J, Schiller JH, Shepherd FA, et al. Topotecan versus cyclophosphamide, doxorubicin, and vincristine for the treatment of recurrent small-cell lung cancer. *J Clin Oncol* 1999;17:658.

Walsh GL, O'Connor M, Willis KM, et al. Is follow-up of lung cancer patients after resection medically indicated and cost-effective? *Ann Thorac Surg* 1995;60:1563.

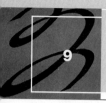

GASTROINTESTINAL TRACT CANCERS
Steven R. Alberts and Richard M. Goldberg

Cancers of the gastrointestinal (GI) tract account for 19% of all new visceral cancers and 24% of cancer deaths in the United States. The frequency and mortality of cancers of the various GI organs are shown in Table 9.1.

 ESOPHAGEAL CANCER

I. EPIDEMIOLOGY AND ETIOLOGY
A. Epidemiology. The incidence of esophageal cancer is noted in Table 9.1.
1. Squamous cell esophageal cancer is the foremost malignancy in the Bantu of Africa. South Africa, Japan, China, Russia, Scotland, and the Caspian region of Iran also have relatively high incidence rates.
2. Incidence rates of squamous cell esophageal cancer can vary 100- to 200-fold among different populations living in geographic adjacency.
3. In many Western countries and in some portions of Asia the incidence of adenocarcinoma of the esophagus (distal esophagus and gastroesophageal junction) is rapidly rising and the incidence of squamous cell cancers is declining.

B. Etiology
1. **Carcinogens**
   a. Long-term use of tobacco and alcohol increases the incidence of both squamous cell carcinoma and adenocarcinoma of the esophagus.
   b. Human papillomavirus (HPV) infection is associated with squamous cell carcinoma of the esophagus.
   c. Dietary carcinogens relevant to the development of squamous cell esophageal cancers include the following:
      (1) Plants growing in soil deficient in molybdenum have reduced vitamin C content and cause hyperplasia of esophageal mucosa, a precursor of cancer.
      (2) Elevated nitrates in the drinking water and soup kettles that concentrate the nitrate
      (3) Food containing fungi: *Geotrichum candidum* (pickles, air-dried corn), *Fusarium* sp., and *Aspergillus* sp. (corn)
      (4) Bread that is baked once a week and eaten when moldy (*G. candidum*)
      (5) Dried persimmons, a rough food that injures the esophageal mucosa when eaten (China)

2. **Predisposing factors for squamous cell esophageal cancer**
   a. Howel-Evans syndrome or tylosis (hyperkeratosis of the palms and soles) is a rare genetic disease that is transmitted as a mendelian-dominant trait (nearly 40% develop esophageal cancer).
   b. Lye stricture (up to 30%)
   c. Esophageal achalasia (30%)
   d. Esophageal web (20%)
   e. Plummer-Vinson syndrome (iron-deficiency anemia, dysphagia from an esophageal web, and glossitis, 10%)
   f. Short esophagus (5%)
   g. Peptic esophagitis (1%)

TABLE 9.1 Occurrence of Digestive Tract Cancers in the United States (2007)[a,b]

	Proportion of digestive tract cancers		
Primary site	Frequency of new cases (%)	Frequency of cancer deaths (%)	Male/female ratio
Esophagus	5.7	10.4	3.5
Stomach	7.8	8.3	1.6
Small bowel	2.1	0.8	1.0
Colon	41.4	38.7[c]	1.0
Rectum	15.3		1.4
Anus and anorectum	1.7	0.5	0.7
Liver and intrahepatic bile ducts	7.1	12.5	2.5
Gallbladder, bile ducts	3.4	2.4	0.9
Pancreas	13.7	24.8	1.0
Other digestive organs	1.8	1.6	0.4
TOTAL	100	100	

[a]Extracted from Jamal A. Cancer statistics 2007. *Cancer J Clin* 2007;57:45.
[b]Gastrointestinal tract malignancies account for about 271,250 new cancers and 134,710 cancer deaths annually.
[c]Death rates from colon cancer and rectal cancer are combined.

  h. Other conditions associated with squamous cell esophageal cancer
    (1) Patients with head and neck cancer (Field's cancerization theory)
    (2) Patients with celiac disease
    (3) Chronic esophagitis without Barrett esophagus (see section II.A)
    (4) Thermal injury to the esophagus because of drinking boiling hot tea or coffee (Russia, China, and Middle East)
  3. Predisposing factors for adenocarcinoma of the esophagus
    a. Barrett esophagus is metaplastic replacement of squamous with intestinalized columnar epithelium.
      (1) Adenocarcinomas associated with Barrett esophagus constitute the cancer whose incidence is most rapidly increasing worldwide, but particularly in white men.
      (2) In the United States, the incidence of adenocarcinoma of the esophagus has increased six- to sevenfold since 1970. Patients with Barrett esophagus have a 30- to 125-fold increased risk for esophageal adenocarcinoma compared with the average U.S. population.
    b. Obesity
    c. Reflux esophagitis

II. PATHOLOGY AND NATURAL HISTORY
  A. Histology. While squamous cell tumors once constituted the majority of esophageal cancers, particularly in the upper and middle esophagus, adenocarcinomas are now the predominant form of esophageal cancer. A small portion of esophageal cancers will be sarcomas, small cell carcinomas, or lymphomas. Adenocarcinoma may arise from esophageal continuation of the gastric mucosa (Barrett esophagus) or may represent extension of a gastric adenocarcinoma.
  B. Location of cancer in the esophagus
    1. Cervical: 10%
    2. Upper thoracic: 40%
    3. Lower thoracic: 50%
  C. Clinical course. Esophageal cancer is highly lethal; >80% of affected patients die from the disease. About 75% present initially with mediastinal nodal involvement

or distant metastasis. Death is usually caused by local disease that results in malnutrition or aspiration pneumonia.

III. DIAGNOSIS

A. Symptoms and signs. Dysphagia is the most common complaint. Patients become unable to swallow solid foods and eventually liquids. Symptoms rarely develop until the esophageal lumen is greatly narrowed and metastasis has occurred. Pain may or may not be present. Physical findings other than cachexia, palpable supraclavicular lymph nodes, or hepatomegaly are rare.

B. Diagnostic studies

1. **Preliminary studies** include physical examination, CBC, LFT, chest radiograph, esophagoscopy, and barium esophagogram. Brushings can be obtained and lesions can undergo biopsy using endoscopy.

2. **CT** scan staging predicts invasion or metastases with an accuracy rate of >90% for the aorta, tracheobronchial tree, pericardium, liver, and adrenal glands; 85% for abdominal nodes; and 50% for paraesophageal nodes.

3. **Endoscopic ultrasound** (EUS) is more accurate than CT in assessing tumor depth and paraesophageal nodes. Transesophageal biopsy to sample enlarged lymph nodes is possible under EUS guidance.

4. **Positron emission tomography** (PET) is a potentially useful diagnostic tool for the preoperative assessment of patients with esophageal cancer. It has a greater sensitivity for the detection of nodal metastases when compared with CT.

5. **Laparoscopy** allows assessment of subdiaphragmatic, peritoneal, liver, and lymph node metastases. In patients who are getting chemotherapy and radiation, either preoperatively or in lieu of surgery, placement of a jejunostomy tube for enteral alimentation during laparoscopy is clinically useful. Thoracoscopy can allow patients who are noted to have intrathoracic dissemination to be spared radical resections.

6. **Bronchoscopy** for tumors of the upper or middle esophagus can diagnose direct tumor extension into the tracheobronchial tree and synchronous primary sites.

IV. STAGING SYSTEM AND PROGNOSTIC FACTORS

A tumor-lymph node-metastasis (TNM) staging classification is available. Patients with earlier disease stage, particularly N0 and M0, have a better prognosis. Readers should consult an up-to-date staging manual because of the frequent revisions of staging systems. Most patients die from their disease within 10 months of diagnosis. The 5-year survival rate is <10% despite all efforts at treatment.

V. SCREENING AND EARLY DETECTION

In high-risk populations, such as in portions of Asia, mass screening using balloon-assisted brushings or endoscopy has been used. Early detection by these methods is of uncertain benefit. In the United States, screening for esophageal cancer is not effective in the general population, but patients such as those with lye-induced strictures or Barrett esophagus, who are at higher risk, should undergo periodic screening via upper endoscopy.

VI. MANAGEMENT

A variety of options exist for the treatment of esophageal cancer depending on its stage.

A. Resection of primary tumor. Results of surgical resection in cancer of the esophagus are poor. The operative mortality rate is about 5% to 10%. In the United States, the 5-year survival rate in patients undergoing R0 (complete) tumor resection is <20%. Aggressive surgery, however, may be justified, particularly for some patients with lesions in the lower half of the esophagus.

B. Palliating an obstructed esophagus can be accomplished by several procedures and permits enteral nutrition.

1. **Laser therapy** may relieve obstruction and bleeding. Endoscopic laser therapy has a <1% mortality rate but may require prior mechanical dilation. Although

successful, laser therapy may require multiple endoscopic sessions, it can be done on an outpatient basis, and its overall cost is still much lower than the cost of palliative surgery. Photosensitization of esophageal tumors using an injectable porphyrin derivative can beneficially increase the laser energy absorbed by the tumor but is associated with generalized dermal photosensitivity to sunlight lasting 4 to 6 weeks.

2. **Esophageal stenting.** At least 17 devices are available for esophageal intubation. About 15% of patients with malignant esophageal obstruction are candidates for tube placement. The tube may be introduced with a pusher tube, which is loaded either onto a bougie or over an endoscope and expands after placement. The latter method permits visualization of the obstructed lumen. The success rate is 90% to 97%.

   a. **Advantages** of tube placement are improved ability to swallow saliva, pleasure of oral alimentation, relief from pulmonary aspiration related to esophagopulmonary fistula, independence from physician or hospital for constant care, and ability to spend time with family and friends in relative comfort.

   b. **Contraindications** to placement of endoprosthesis are carcinoma <2 cm below the upper sphincter, limited life expectancy (<6 weeks), and uncooperativeness.

   c. **Complications** include perforation, dislocation, tumor overgrowth, reflux symptoms with stricturing, pressure necrosis, foreign body impaction with obstruction, bleeding, and failure of intubation. The complication rate (early and late) is 10% to 25%.

3. **Feeding gastrostomy** is not advisable because it does not palliate dysphagia, which forces patients with complete or nearly complete esophageal obstruction to expectorate saliva and secretions, does not increase life expectancy, and has its own morbidity and mortality.

4. **Colonic interposition** to bypass the obstructed segment is recommended only for surgical candidates in whom a suitable gastric remnant cannot be fashioned because of prior gastric resection, extent of disease, or underlying esophageal disease.

5. **External-beam irradiation** or endoluminal brachytherapy can result in tumor regression with palliation in some cases. Up to 70% to 80% of patients with dysphagia may note improved swallowing after external-beam irradiation. Endoluminal brachytherapy can be useful in previously irradiated patients with local tumor regrowth causing dysphagia.

C. **Single-modality treatment**

1. **Radiotherapy (RT) alone** to a dose of 6,000 cGy resulted in 1-, 2-, 3- and 5-year survival rates of 33%, 12%, 8%, and 7%, respectively, of patients treated on the radiation arm of a randomized trial in which responding patients were permitted to proceed to resection at physician discretion.

2. **Surgery alone.** The surgical procedures employed in esophagectomy depend on the location and preference of the surgeon and include principally transhiatal esophagectomy or the Ivor-Lewis procedure, which requires both thoracotomy and laparotomy. In the 25% to 30% of patients in whom complete resection is possible, 5-year survival rates are 15% to 20%.

3. **Chemotherapy alone** is seldom an effective palliative modality of the primary tumor in patients with esophageal cancer. When chemotherapy is employed, it should be coupled with mechanical or radiotherapeutic approaches for palliation of dysphagia. As in gastric cancer, discussed later, multiagent chemotherapy-induced responses tend to be short-lived.

D. **Combined-modality therapy**

1. **Primary combined therapy without surgery.** In patients not planning to undergo esophageal surgery because of comorbid disease or patient or physician choice, combined chemotherapy and RT can lead to long-term survival in some, as compared with surgery alone.

   a. Currently, the following regimen is most commonly used and is given during the first and fourth weeks of RT:

Cisplatin, 75 mg/m² IV on day 1 of the cycle, and 5-fluorouracil (5-FU), 1,000 mg/m²/day by continuous IV infusion for 4 days. Several other multiagent regimens have resulted in higher response rates, but have increased toxicity without a clear overall survival benefit.

b. In a prospective randomized trial of patients with squamous cell or adenocarcinoma of the thoracic esophagus, combined-modality treatment (5-FU plus cisplatin plus 5,000 cGy) resulted in improved median survival (9 months vs. 12.5 months) when compared with RT alone (6,400 cGy). The 2-year survival rate for patients randomized to combined chemotherapy and radiation was 38%, compared with 10% for those randomized to radiation alone. The patients receiving the combined-modality treatment experienced decreased local and distant recurrences but significantly more toxicity, much of which was serious or life-threatening. Only half of these patients received all of the planned cycles of chemotherapy.

2. Preoperative or postoperative RT alone may reduce the local recurrence rate but has no apparent affect on median survival.

3. Perioperative chemotherapy alone. Similarly, neither preoperative (as reported in six randomized trials) nor postoperative chemotherapy alone has improved outcomes in patients with esophageal cancer. Response rate to multiagent neoadjuvant chemotherapy can be as high as 40% to 50%, and up to 25% of treated patients may have apparent pathologic complete remissions. Preoperative chemotherapy using cisplatin and 5-FU, however, did not improve overall survival when compared with surgery alone in a randomized trial of 440 patients with squamous esophageal cancer.

4. Triple-modality therapy. The combination of preoperative chemotherapy and RT has led to an increase in the 3-year survival rates and prolonged median disease-free survival in several randomized studies compared with surgery alone. In one trial of stage I and II squamous cell cancers, the overall survival was not improved by triple-modality therapy. In a separate trial in which both squamous and adenocarcinoma patients were entered, there was a statistically significant survival benefit for triple-modality treatment. A variety of trials are now exploring new chemotherapy regimens, in combination with RT, to enhance the response rate. Patients with complete pathologic response at surgery have about a 50% likelihood of long-term survival.

E. Advanced disease. The responses using single chemotherapeutic agents (15% to 20%) are usually partial and of brief duration (2 to 5 months). Combination chemotherapy, usually including cisplatin with 5-FU, a taxane, or both, is associated with reported response rates ranging from 15% to 80%, a median duration of response of 7 to 10 months, and many times with substantial toxicity. Higher response rates, however, do not necessarily translate into significant benefit for these patients, and the outcome remains poor.

 GASTRIC CANCER

I. EPIDEMIOLOGY AND ETIOLOGY

A. Incidence. The prevalence and death rates of gastric carcinoma (particularly distal cancers) have been markedly and significantly decreasing in all regions of the world and in all age groups by about 2% to 7% per year. Deaths due to gastric cancer have decreased to 20% of that seen in the 1930s in the United States, although it remains the second leading cause of cancer death worldwide. However, an increase in cardia and gastroesophageal tumors has been observed in the United States.

Dietary factors and improvement in food storage are believed to be the major factors causing this decline. Improvements include reduction in toxic methods of food preservation (such as smoking and pickling), a decline in salt consumption, greater use of refrigeration, and increased consumption of fruits and vegetables.

Mortality from gastric cancer is highest in Costa Rica (61 deaths per 100,000 population) and East Asia (Hong Kong, Japan, and Singapore) and lowest in the United States (5 deaths per 100,000). Of interest, the Nordic and Western European countries have incidence rates 2 to 3 times higher than the United States. The incidence remains high in Japan and is intermediate in Japanese immigrants to the United States; first-generation Japanese Americans have an incidence comparable with other Americans. The average age of onset is 55 years.

B. Etiology. Two gastric cancer entities can be distinguished by their risk factors and histology. *Diffuse gastric cancer* is associated with hereditary factors and a proximal location and does not appear to occur in the setting of intestinal metaplasia or dysplasia. *Intestinal-type gastric cancer* is more distal, occurs in younger patients, is more frequently endemic, and is associated with inflammatory changes and with *Helicobacter pylori* infection.

1. **Diet.** Gastric cancer has been linked to the ingestion of red meats, cabbage, spices, fish, salt-preserved or smoked foods, a high-carbohydrate diet, and low consumption of fat, protein, and vitamins A, C, and E. Selenium dietary intake may be inversely proportional to the risk of gastric cancer but not to that of colorectal cancer.

2. ***Helicobacter pylori* infection** is associated with an increased risk for gastric adenocarcinoma and may be a cofactor in the pathogenesis of noncardiac gastric cancer. The *H. pylori* organism was identified in the malignant and nearby inflammatory tissue of 89% of patients with intestinal-type cancer, whereas it was present in 32% of tissues taken from patients with diffuse-type cancers. This raises the possibility now under investigation in prospective randomized trials that eradicating *H. pylori* through antibiotic treatment and bismuth administration may be preventive of both atrophic gastritis and intestinal-type gastric cancer.

3. **Heredity and race.** African, Asian, and Hispanic Americans have a higher risk for gastric cancer than whites. The diffuse histologic pattern is the predominant pathologic type seen in families with multiple affected members.

4. **Pernicious anemia, achlorhydria, and atrophic gastritis.** Pernicious anemia carries an increased relative risk for gastric cancer that is said to be 3 to 18 times that of the general population, based on retrospective studies. Although some controversy surrounds this finding, follow-up endoscopy is generally suggested for patients known to have pernicious anemia.

5. **Previous gastric resection.** Gastric stump adenocarcinomas, which occur with a latency period of 15 to 20 years, are more common in patients after surgical treatment for benign peptic ulcer disease, particularly in those who have hypochlorhydria and reflux of alkaline bile. These cancers are associated with dysplasia of gastric mucosa, elevated gastrin levels, and a poor prognosis. Two meta-analyses have supported this increased risk. Some population-based studies do not support this finding.

6. **Mucosal dysplasia** is graded from I to III, with grade III showing marked loss in cell differentiation and increased mitosis. The finding of high-grade dysplasia by experienced pathologists in two separate sets of endoscopic biopsies is considered to be a marker for future gastric cancer. Intestinal metaplasia, replacement of gastric glandular epithelium with intestinal mucosa, is associated with intestinal-type gastric cancer. The risk for cancer appears to be proportional to the extent of metaplastic mucosa.

7. **Gastric polyps.** As many as half of adenomatous polyps show carcinomatous changes in some series. Hyperplastic polyps (>75% of all gastric polyps) do not appear to have malignant potential. Patients with familial adenomatous polyposis (FAP) have a higher incidence of gastric cancer. Patients with adenomatous polyps or FAP should have endoscopic surveillance.

8. **Chronic gastritis.** In chronic atrophic gastritis of the corpus or antrum, *H. pylori* infection and environmental and autoimmune (as in pernicious anemia) causes are thought to be associated with an increased risk for gastric cancer.

In Ménétrier disease (hypertrophic gastritis), an increase in the incidence of gastric cancer is also observed.

9. **Other risk factors.** Gastric cancer is more common in men older than 50 years of age and in people with blood group A. Gastric cancer is consistently seen more commonly among those of lower socioeconomic class across the world.

II. PATHOLOGY AND NATURAL HISTORY

A. **Histology and classification.** About 95% of gastric cancers are adenocarcinomas; 5% are leiomyosarcomas, lymphomas, carcinoids, squamous cancers, or other rare types.

1. **Useful characteristics of gastric cancer**

   a. **Histologic classification (Lauren):** Diffuse (scattered solitary or small clusters of small cells in the submucosa), intestinal (polarized columnar large cells with inflammatory infiltrates localized in areas of atrophic gastritis or intestinal metaplasia), and mixed types. This classification has proved to be the most useful for adenocarcinomas because the two major types (diffuse and intestinal) represent groups of patients with differing ages, sex ratios, survival rates, epidemiology, and apparent origin. Studies have shown that diffuse histology affects younger patients, with slight predominance among women. Diffuse histology occurred in 50% of all cases and in 55% of unresectable cases. Intestinal type predominates in high-risk regions of the world and among older people, and affects more men than women.

   b. **Clinical classification (gross anatomy):** Superficial (superficial spreading), focal (polypoid, fungate, or ulcerative), and infiltrative (linitis plastica) types.

   c. **Japanese Endoscopic Society (JES) classification:** Type I (polypoid or masslike), type II (flat, minimally elevated, or depressed), and type III (cancer associated with true ulcer)

2. **Location of cancers**

   a. Distal location: 40%

   b. Proximal: 35%

   c. Body: 25%

B. **Clinical course.** About 20% of gastric cancer patients are long-term survivors in the United States. Gastric carcinoma spreads by the lymphatic system and blood vessels, by direct extension, and by seeding of peritoneal surfaces. The ulcerative and polypoid types spread through the gastric wall and involve the serosa and draining lymph nodes. The scirrhous type spreads through the submucosa and muscularis, encasing the stomach, and in some instances spreads to the entire bowel. The physical examination is often normal.

Widespread metastatic disease may affect any organ, especially the liver (40%), lung (may be lymphangitic, 40%), peritoneum (10%), supraclavicular lymph nodes (Virchow node), left axillary lymph nodes (Irish node), and umbilicus (Sister Mary Joseph nodule). Sclerotic bone metastases, carcinomatous meningitis, and metastasis to the ovary in women (Krukenberg tumor) or rectal shelf in men (Blumer shelf) may also occur.

C. **Associated paraneoplastic syndromes**

1. Acanthosis nigricans (55% of cases that occur in malignancy are associated with gastric carcinoma)

2. Polymyositis, dermatomyositis

3. Circinate erythemas, pemphigoid

4. Dementia, cerebellar ataxia

5. Idiopathic venous thrombosis

6. Ectopic Cushing syndrome or carcinoid syndrome (rare)

7. Leser-Trélat sign

III. DIAGNOSIS

A. **Symptoms and signs.** Gastric cancer often progresses to an advanced stage before symptoms and signs develop. Symptoms of advanced disease include anorexia, early satiety, distaste for meat, weakness, and dysphagia. Abdominal pain is present in about 60% of patients, weight loss in 50%, nausea and vomiting in 40%, anemia in 40%, and a palpable abdominal mass in 30%. The abdominal pain is similar to ulcer pain, is gnawing in nature, and may respond initially to antacid treatment but remains unremitting. Hematemesis or melena occurs in 25% and, when present, is seen more often with gastric sarcomas.

B. Diagnostic studies

1. **Preliminary studies** include CBC, LFT, esophagogastroduodenoscopy (EGD) or upper GI barium studies, and chest radiographs.

2. **CT of the abdomen** is useful for assessing the extent of disease. At laparotomy, however, half of patients are found to have more extensive disease than predicted by CT. Laparoscopy can identify patients with regionally advanced or disseminated disease who are not candidates for immediate potentially curative surgical intervention.

3. **EUS** is up to 6 times more accurate in staging the primary gastric tumors than CT, but differentiation between benign and malignant changes in the wall is often difficult. EUS is useful in imaging the cardia, which may be difficult to evaluate by CT. Lymph node biopsy can also be obtained by EUS guidance.

4. **Endoscopy.** The combination of flexible upper GI endoscopy with biopsy of visible lesions, exfoliative cytology, and brush biopsy is able to detect >95% of gastric cancers. Biopsy of a stomach lesion alone is accurate in only 80% of cases. Positive gastric cytology with no endoscopic or radiographic abnormalities indicates superficial spreading gastric cancer.

C. Differential diagnosis and gastric polyps. The differential diagnosis of gastric cancer includes peptic gastric polyps, ulcer, leiomyoma, leiomyoblastoma, glomus tumor, malignant lymphoma (and pseudolymphoma), granulocytic sarcoma, carcinoid tumors, lipoma, fibrous histiocytoma, and metastatic carcinoma. Gastric polyps rarely undergo malignant transformation (3% after 7 years), but many contain independent carcinoma.

1. **Inflammatory gastric polyps** are not true neoplasms. They are usually located in the pyloroantrum and are associated with hypochlorhydria but not with carcinoma.

2. **Hyperplastic gastric polyps** (Ménétrier's polyadenome polypeux) are the most common polyps (75%). Randomly distributed throughout the stomach, these polyps are usually small and multiple. Coexisting carcinoma is present in 8% of cases.

3. **Adenomatous polyps** are usually located in the antrum of the stomach and are frequently single and large. Coexisting carcinoma is present in 40% to 60% of patients.

4. **Villous adenomas** rarely occur in the stomach but are more often malignant.

5. **Polyposis syndromes**

   a. **Familial gastric polyposis** presents with multiple gastric polyps but no skin or bone tumors. The gastric wall is usually invaded with atypical carcinoma.

   b. **FAP** is associated with gastric involvement in more than half of patients. The gastric polyps are adenomatous, hyperplastic, or of the fundic gland hyperplasia type. Gastric carcinoma and carcinoid tumor may occur.

IV. STAGING AND PROGNOSTIC FACTORS

A. Staging system. The TNM staging system developed for gastric cancer is shown in Table 9.2. The current TNM system does not take into account the location of the tumor within the stomach, the histologic type (Lauren classification), the pattern of growth (linitis plastica), or whether all disease could be resected (and if so, the type of resection).

B. Prognostic factors. Previously, data using three grave prognostic signs (serosal involvement, nodal involvement, and tumor at the line of resection) have shown that if none of these signs is present, the 5-year survival rate is 60%, and if all are present, the 5-year survival rate is <5%.

1. **Stage.** Multivariate analysis indicates that stage, invasion, and lymph node involvement are the most significant prognostic factors. The most important

TABLE 9.2 TNM Staging System for Cancers of the Stomach[a]

Primary tumor (T)		Regional lymph nodes (N)	
TX	Primary tumor cannot be assessed	NX	Regional lymph nodes cannot be assessed
T0	No evidence of primary tumor		
Tis	Carcinoma *in situ* (intraepithelial tumor without invasion of lamina propria)	N0	No regional lymph node metastasis
		N1	Metastases in 1–6 regional lymph nodes
T1	Tumor invades lamina propria or submucosa	N2	Metastases in 7–15 regional lymph nodes
T2a	Tumor invades muscularis propria	N3	Metastases in >15 regional lymph nodes
T2b	Tumor invades subserosa		
T3	Tumor penetrates serosa (visceral peritoneum) without invasion of adjacent structures[b]	**Distant metastases (M)**	
		MX	Distant metastasis cannot be assessed
T4	Tumor invades adjacent structures[b]	M0	No distant metastasis
		M1	Distant metastasis is present

Stage groupings

Stage	TNM classification							
0	Tis	N0	M0					
IA	T1	N0	M0					
IB	T1	N1	M0,	T2a/b	N0	M0		
II	T1	N2	M0,	T2a/b	N1	M0,	T3	N0	M0
IIIA	T2a/b	N2	M0,	T3	N1	M0,	T4	N0	M0
IIIB	T3	N2	M0					
IV	T4	N1–3	M0;	T1–3	N3	M0;	any T	any N	M1

[a]Adapted from the *AJCC Cancer Staging Manual.* 6th ed. New York: Springer-Verlag; 2002.
[b]Intramural extension to the duodenum or esophagus is classified by the depth of the greatest invasion in any of these sites, including the stomach.

prognostic determinant appears to be the number of positive lymph nodes. Interestingly, patients with one to three lymph nodes involved with metastasis have as good a prognosis as those without nodal involvement.

2. **Clinical classification.** Survival is better with superficial than with focal cancer and worst with infiltrative types of cancer.

3. **JES classification.** Survival is better with type II (flat) than with type III (associated with ulcer) tumors and worst with type I (polypoid) tumors.

4. **Grade.** Tumors with high histologic grade have a poor prognosis.

5. **Flow cytometry.** The median disease-free survival is 18 months for patients with diploid tumors and 5 months for those with aneuploid tumors. Aneuploid tumors constitute 96% of gastroesophageal junction–cardia carcinomas and only 48% of body–antrum tumors. Women are more likely to have diploid tumors.

6. **Nature and extent of resection.** Survival is better with curative resection (a resection with uninvolved margins, or R0 resection) versus palliative resection, distal gastrectomy versus proximal gastrectomy, and subtotal gastrectomy versus total gastrectomy.

V. SCREENING AND EARLY DETECTION. Early detection of gastric cancers is clearly improved with relentless investigation of persistent upper GI symptoms. In Japan, mobile screening stations equipped with video gastrocameras have resulted in early detection of gastric cancer. Gastric cancer, which was detected in 0.3% of those screened, was associated with a 95% 5-year survival rate (50% of the patients had involvement of mucosa and submucosa only). Despite such screening programs, gastric cancer remains the most common cause of cancer death in Japan. Screening of populations with routine risk factors for gastric cancer is not recommended, however, in the United States.

VI. MANAGEMENT

A. Surgery

1. **Curative resection.** Subtotal gastrectomy with adequate margins of grossly uninvolved stomach (3 to 4 cm) and regional lymph node dissection is the treatment of choice, and is generally considered the only potentially curative approach for patients with gastric cancer. Total gastrectomy is not superior to subtotal gastrectomy for achieving cures and should be used only when indicated by the local extent of the disease. More extensive lymphatic dissection, known as D-2 resections (e.g., of the celiac lymph nodes), omentectomy, and splenectomy are of uncertain benefit, but do not appear to be advisable outside its use in Japan.

2. **Palliative resections** are performed to rid patients of infected, bleeding, obstructed, necrotic, or ulcerated polypoid gastric lesions. For these purposes, a limited gastric resection may suffice. Palliative resections succeed in ameliorating symptoms about half the time.

3. **Vitamin B_{12} deficiency** develops in all patients who undergo total gastrectomy within 6 years and in 20% of patients who undergo subtotal gastrectomy within 10 years unless parenteral B_{12} injections are administered.

B. Chemotherapy

1. **Neoadjuvant, adjuvant, or perioperative chemotherapy**

   a. **Neoadjuvant chemotherapy.** Patients with potentially resectable disease treated in phase II studies with preoperative chemotherapy RT, or both have shown a high response rate, and some have had pathologically negative resection specimens. There have not been any randomized trials published to help discern whether response translates into resectability, time to progression, or survival advantage over no neoadjuvant therapy.

   b. **Adjuvant chemotherapy.** Nearly all trials involving 5-FU in combination with other agents (doxorubicin, epirubicin, mitomycin, or cytarabine) as adjuvant therapy have failed to show any benefit. A meta-analysis of data from 14 trials published since 1980 on adjuvant chemotherapy after resection of gastric cancer versus surgery alone concluded that postoperative chemotherapy cannot be considered standard treatment.

   c. **Perioperative chemotherapy.** In a randomized phase III trial of perioperative ECF chemotherapy (epirubicin, cisplatin, and infusional 5-FU), with three cycles of preoperative and three cycles of postoperative therapy, a significant improvement was seen in overall survival compared with surgery alone. While this trial enrolled primarily patients with stomach cancer, similar benefit appeared to extend to those with adenocarcinoma of the gastroesophageal junction or lower esophagus. Cycles are given every 3 weeks as follows:

      Epirubicin, 50 mg/m^2 IV on day 1
      Cisplatin, 60 mg/m^2 IV on day 1
      5-FU, 225 mg/m^2/day by continuous IV infusion on days 1 to 21

2. **Combined-modality therapy**

   Several clinical trials for potentially resectable gastric cancer have assessed sequential chemotherapy and radiation. A previously completed Intergroup trial (Intergroup 0116) involving nearly 600 patients undergoing potentially curative resection randomized patients to either observation alone or to combined-modality therapy. Patients randomized to adjuvant therapy received one cycle of 5-FU and leucovorin followed by a combination of bolus 5-FU and RT. After the RT was completed, two additional cycles of 5-FU and leucovorin were given. Significant 3-year relapse-free and overall survival were seen in the patients randomized to adjuvant therapy. The benefit of this approach appeared to be in a reduction of locoregional failures. Less benefit was seen with treatment in reducing distant failures.

3. **Chemotherapy for advanced disease.** Single agents produce low response rates. Combination regimens produce higher response rates but are more toxic and more costly. Cisplatin has been increasingly used in new combinations that also yield higher response rates, but the incidence of important toxic events exceeds 10%. The reported response rates are about 20% for 5-FU alone and 10% to 50% for combination chemotherapy; the median survival times range from 5 to 11 months.

After nearly two decades of using combination chemotherapy, including mitomycin, doxorubicin, epirubicin, etoposide, methotrexate, nitrosoureas, irinotecan, taxanes, or cisplatin, there is no regimen considered standard in the setting of advanced disease.

a. **ECF.** The chemotherapy regimen of epirubicin, cisplatin, and continuous infusion 5-FU (ECF) was shown to have superior activity over 5-FU, doxorubicin, and methotrexate (FAMtx) in a phase III trial. Dosages for ECF are shown in section VI.B.1.c.

b. **EOX.** A newer version of ECF, EOX (epirubicin, oxaliplatin, and capecitabine) showed an improvement in overall survival and less toxicity compared with ECF. The dosage schedule for EOX is as follows; cycles are repeated every 3 weeks:

Epirubicin, 50 mg/m^2 IV on day 1
Oxaliplatin, 130 mg/m^2 IV on day 1
Capecitabine, 625 mg/m^2/dose twice daily days 1 to 21

c. **DCF.** The use of docetaxel (Taxotere) has also been of benefit. As assessed in a trial comparing docetaxel, cisplatin (DCF), and 5-FU versus cisplatin and 5-FU (CF), the combination of DCF provided improved overall survival. However, this combination also produced moderately significant toxicity. DCF is given in 3-week cycles as follows:

Docetaxel, 75mg/m^2 IV on day 1
Cisplatin 75 mg/m^2 IV on day 1
5-FU, 750 mg/m^2/day by continuous IV infusion on days 1 to 5

C. **RT**

1. **Localized disease.** RT alone has not proved useful for treating gastric cancer. RT (4,000 cGy in 4 weeks) in combination with 5-FU (15 mg/kg IV on the first 3 days of RT), however, appears to improve survival over RT alone in patients with localized but unresectable cancers. Intraoperative radiation therapy (IORT) allows high doses of radiation to the tumor bed or residual disease while permitting the exclusion of mobile radiosensitive normal tissues from the area irradiated. Trials are limited to single institutional experiences; therefore, generalizing from such trials is difficult. Selected patients may benefit from IORT, particularly when combined with supplemental external-beam radiation and chemotherapy. Long-term survival has been reported in some patients treated in this fashion for residual disease after surgery.

2. **Advanced disease.** Gastric adenocarcinoma is relatively radioresistant and requires high doses of radiation with attendant toxic effects to surrounding organs. RT may be useful for palliating pain, vomiting due to obstruction, gastric hemorrhage, and metastases to bone and brain.

COLORECTAL CANCER

I. EPIDEMIOLOGY AND ETIOLOGY

A. **Incidence.** Colorectal cancer is the second most common cause of cancer mortality after lung cancer in the United States and ranks third in frequency among primary sites of cancer in both men and women. Nearly one million cases are diagnosed annually worldwide, accounting for 9% to 10% of human cancers. Peak incidence rates are observed in Europe, the United States, Australia, and New Zealand. The lowest incidence rates are noted in India and South America and among Arab Israelis. A 10-fold variability is noted from highest to lowest regional incidence rates. Both the incidence and the mortality rates have declined since they peaked in 1985, a phenomenon thought to be a consequence of increased screening for and removal of premalignant polyps. Studies of migrant populations have discerned that the incidence of colorectal cancer reflects country of residence and not the country of origin. This suggests that overall environmental influences outweigh genetic trends for populations in which the experiences of those people with inherited special risk are pooled with those of lesser risk. Rural dwellers have a lower incidence of colorectal cancer than do urbanites. In the United States, cancer of the colon/rectum is more common in the East and the North than in the West and the South.

The risk for colorectal cancer increases with age, but 3% of colorectal cancers occur in patients younger than 40 years of age. The incidence is 19 per 100,000 population for those younger than 65 years of age and 337 per 100,000 among those older than 65 years of age. It was estimated that, in the United States in 2007, 147,500 new cases of colorectal cancer would develop and an estimated 57,000 persons would die from the disease. In the United States, a person of average risk has a 5% lifetime risk for developing colorectal cancer.

B. Etiology. Multiple forces drive the transformation of healthy colorectal mucosa to cancer. Inheritance and environmental factors, such as maintaining a low body mass index and exercising regularly, correlate with lower incidence rates, but the extent of the interdependence of these two factors as causative variables remains unknown.

1. Polyps. The main importance of polyps is the well-recognized potential of a subset to evolve into colorectal cancer. The evolution to cancer is a multistage process that proceeds through mucosal cell hyperplasia, adenoma formation, and growth and dysplasia, to malignant transformation and invasive cancer. Environmental carcinogens may result in the development of cancer regardless of a patient's genetic background, but patients with genetically susceptible mucosa inherit a predisposition to abnormal cellular proliferation. Oncogene activation, tumor suppressor gene inactivation, deficient DNA mismatch repair processes, and chromosomal deletion may lead to adenoma formation, growth with increasing dysplasia, and invasive carcinoma.

a. Types of polyps. Histologically, polyps are classified as neoplastic or nonneoplastic. Nonneoplastic polyps have no malignant potential and include hyperplastic polyps, mucous retention polyps, hamartomas (juvenile polyps), lymphoid aggregates, and inflammatory polyps. Neoplastic polyps (or adenomatous polyps) have malignant potential and are classified according to the World Health Organization system as tubular (microscopically characterized by networks of complex branching glands), tubulovillous (mixed histology), or villous (microscopically characterized by relatively short, straight glandular structures) adenomas, depending on the presence and volume of villous tissue. Polyps larger than 1 cm in diameter, those with high-grade dysplasia, and those with predominantly villous histology are associated with higher risk for colorectal cancer and are termed *screen-relevant neoplasias.* Colonoscopic polypectomy and subsequent surveillance can reduce the incidence of colon cancer by 90%, compared with that observed in unscreened controls.

b. Frequency of polyp types. About 70% of polyps removed at colonoscopy are adenomatous, 75% to 85% of which are tubular (no or minimal villous tissue), 10% to 25% are tubulovillous (<75% villous tissue), and fewer than 5% are villous (>75% villous tissue). The incidence of synchronous adenomas in patients with one known adenoma is 40% to 50%.

c. Dysplasia may be classified as low and high grade. About 6% of adenomatous polyps exhibit high-grade dysplasia and 5% contain invasive carcinoma at the time of diagnosis.

d. The malignant potential of adenomas correlates with increasing size, the presence and the degree of dysplasia in a villous component, and the patient's age. Small colorectal polyps (smaller than 1 cm) are not associated with increased occurrence of colorectal cancer; the incidence of cancer, however, is increased 2.5- to fourfold if the polyp is large (larger than 1 cm) and five- to sevenfold in patients who initially have multiple polyps. The study of the natural history of untreated polyps larger than 1 cm showed that the risk for progression to cancer is 2.5% at 5 years, 8% at 10 years, and 24% at 20 years. The time to malignant progression depends on the severity of dysplasia, averaging 3.5 years for severe dysplasia and 11.5 years for mild atypia.

e. Management of polyps. Because of the adenoma–cancer relationship and the evidence that resecting adenomas prevents cancer, newly detected polyps should be excised and additional polyps should be sought through colonoscopy. There are data to show that the miss rate for polyps that are potentially detectable during colonoscopy is lower when the operator exceeds a withdrawal time of 6 minutes. A minority of polyps are flat and lack an easily detectable profile in the absence of special techniques, such as instillation of dye, to accentuate mucosal irregularities during screening.

The accuracy of colonoscopic examinations (94%) exceeds that of barium enema (67%), which is seldom used as a screening tool currently. Additionally, with colonoscopy, therapeutic polypectomy can be accomplished during the diagnostic examination. CT colonography (virtual colonoscopy) is increasingly sensitive and specific, with refinements in software and radiologist expertise leading to sufficient improvements in the technique such that many centers offer this as a screening option. Fecal DNA assays that target genetic abnormalities specific to the malignant transformation of mucosal cells are now commercially available and continuously being refined to improve their performance. The year 2000 recommendations of the American College of Gastroenterology for the management of colorectal polyps are discussed by Bond and colleagues (see Suggested Reading).

f. Intestinal polyposis syndromes. Table 9.3 summarizes familial polyposis syndromes and their histology distribution, malignant potential, and management (see section V.B.3 for discussion of the potential benefit of anti-inflammatory drugs).

2. Diet. Populations with high intake of fat, higher caloric intakes, and low intake of fiber (fruits, vegetables, and grains) characterized as a westernized diet tend to have increased risk for colorectal cancer in most but not all studies. Higher calcium intake, calcium supplementation, vitamin D supplementation, and regular aspirin use are associated with a lower risk for colorectal polyps and cancer in some studies. Fewer tumors that overexpress Cox-2 occur in individuals who regularly use aspirin, which is known to be reduce the incidence of both polyps and cancers. Increased intake of vitamins A, C, and E and beta-carotene do not appear to decrease the risk for polyp formation. The higher incidence of rectal and sigmoid cancer in men may be related to their greater consumption of alcohol. Women who have taken postmenopausal estrogen replacement therapy appear to have a lower risk for colorectal cancer than those who have not.

3. Inflammatory bowel disease

a. Ulcerative colitis is a clear risk factor for colon cancer. About 1% of colorectal cancer patients have a history of chronic ulcerative colitis. The risk for the development of cancer in these patients varies inversely with the age of onset of the colitis and directly with the extent of colonic involvement and duration of active disease. The cumulative risk is 2% at 10 years, 8% at 20 years, and 18% at 30 years. Individuals with colon cancers associated with ulcerative colitis have a similar prognosis to sporadic cases.

The recommended approach to the increased risk for colorectal cancer in ulcerative colitis has been annual or semiannual colonoscopy to determine the need for total proctocolectomy in patients with extensive colitis of >8 years' duration. This strategy is based on the assumption that dysplastic lesions can be detected before invasive cancer has developed. An analysis of prospective studies concluded that immediate colectomy is essential for all patients diagnosed with a dysplasia-associated mass or lesion. Most important, the analysis

TABLE 9.3 Polyp Syndromes and Colorectal Cancer

Disease	Histology	Distribution of polyps	Malignant potential	Associated manifestations	Age for first FOB test (years)	Age for first colonoscopy (years)	Surgery
Discrete polyps and CC	Few AP	Colon	High	None	≥45	≥45	Same as for general population
Hereditary discrete common polyps and CC	AP	Proximal colon	High	Lynch I[a]	30–35	35	Same as for general population
HNPCC	AP → Ac	Proximal colon	High	Lynch II[a]	None (ES)	20	Subtotal colectomy[d]
Familial CC	AP	Proximal colon; may be distal	High	None	30–35	35	Same as for general population
FAP and Turcot syndrome	Scattered AP → Ac	Colon	High	Central nervous system tumors	None (ES)	Teens	Prophylactic subtotal colectomy[d]
FAP and Oldfield syndrome	Scattered AP → Ac	Colon	High	Skin tumors	None (ES)	Teens	Prophylactic subtotal colectomy[d]
FAP and Gardner syndrome	Scattered AP → Ac	Usually colon; also stomach and SB	High	See footnote[b]	None (ES)	Teens	Prophylactic subtotal colectomy[d,e]
Peutz-Jeghers syndrome	Hamartomas	Stomach, SB, colon, ovary	Low	Buccal and cutaneous pigmentation	≥45	≥45	None
Generalized GI juvenile polyposis	JP	Stomach, SB, colon	Low	None	None	≥45	None
Juvenile polyposis coli of infancy	JP	Stomach, SB, colon	None	Protein-losing enteropathy	None	No special indications	None
Cronkhite-Canada syndrome	JP	Stomach, SB, colon	None	Protein-losing enteropathy[c]	None	No special indications	None

FOB, fecal occult blood; CC, colorectal cancer; AP, adenomatous polyps; HNPCC, hereditary nonpolyposis colorectal cancer ("cancer family syndrome"); Ac, adenocarcinoma; ES, endoscopic surveillance; FAP, familial adenomatous polyposis; SB, small bowel; JP, juvenile (retention) polyps.

[a] **Lynch syndrome I:** autosomal-dominant inheritance with susceptibility to early onset of colorectal cancer proximal to the splenic flexure in the absence of diffuse polyps; **Lynch syndrome II:** contains most of the features of Lynch I with excess incidence of carcinomas of the endometrium, ovary, kidney, ureter, bladder, bile duct, and small bowel and of lymphoma. (Lynch HT. The surgeon and colorectal cancer genetics. *Arch Surg* 1990;125:699.)

[b] Epidermoid cysts, fibromas, desmoids, dental and osseous abnormalities, intraperitoneal and retroperitoneal fibrosis, ampullary carcinoma, and tumors in other glandular structures. Follow with ophthalmoscopy for associated congenital hypertrophy of the retinal pigment epithelium.

[c] And hyperpigmentation, alopecia, and nail dystrophy.

[d] Prophylactic colectomy should be considered if 5 to 10 adenomatous polyps are present or if polyps recur.

[e] Or, total colectomy with pouch reconstruction. Nonsteroidal anti-inflammatory drugs decrease the number and size of polyps (see "Colorectal Cancer" section V.B.3).

demonstrated that the diagnosis of dysplasia does not preclude the presence of invasive cancer. The diagnosis of dysplasia has inherent problems with sampling of specimens and with variation in agreement among observers (as low as 60%, even with experts in the field).

b. Crohn's disease. Patients with colorectal Crohn's disease are at increased risk for colorectal cancer, but the risk is less than that of those with ulcerative colitis. The risk is increased about 1.5 to 2 times.

4. Genetic factors

a. Family history may signify either a genetic abnormality or shared environmental factors or a combination of these factors. About 15% of all colorectal cancers occur in patients with a history of colorectal cancer in first-degree relatives. Individuals with a first-degree relative who has had colorectal cancer are more than twice as likely to develop colon cancer than those individuals with no family history.

b. Gene changes. Specific inherited (adenomatous polyposis coli [*APC*] gene) and acquired genetic abnormalities (*ras* gene point mutation; *c-myc* gene amplification; allele deletion at specific sites of chromosomes 5, 8, 17, and 18) appear to be capable of mediating steps in the progression from normal to malignant colonic mucosa. About half of all carcinomas and large adenomas have associated point mutations, most often in the *K-ras* gene. Such mutations are rarely present in adenomas smaller than 1 cm. Allelic deletions of 17p– are demonstrated in three-fourths of all colorectal carcinomas, and deletions of 5q– are demonstrated in more than one-third of colonic carcinoma and large adenomas.

Two major syndromes and several variants of these syndromes of inherited predisposition to colorectal cancer have been characterized. The two syndromes, which predispose to colorectal cancer by different mechanisms, are FAP and hereditary nonpolyposis colorectal cancer (Lynch syndrome or HNPCC).

(1) FAP. The genes responsible for FAP, *APC* genes, are located in the 5q21 chromosome region. Inheritance of defective *APC* tumor-suppressor gene leads to a virtually 100% likelihood of developing colon cancer by 55 years of age, leading to the recommendation of a total proctocolectomy for affected individuals during their 20s or 30s. Screening for polyps should begin during early teenage years. The FAP syndrome is associated with the development of gastric and ampullary polyps, desmoid tumors, osteomas, abnormal dentition, and abnormal retinal pigmentation. Variants of FAP include Gardner and Turcot syndromes.

(2) HNPCC. The autosomal-dominant pattern of HNPCC includes Lynch syndromes I and II, both of which are associated with an increased incidence of predominantly right-sided colon cancer. This genetic abnormality in the mismatch repair mechanism leads to defective excision of abnormal repeating sequences of DNA known as *microsatellites* (microsatellite instability). Retention of these sequences leads to expression of a mutator phenotype characterized by frequent DNA replication errors (also called the *RER+* phenotype), which predispose affected people to a multitude of primary malignancies, including cancers of the endometrium, ovary, bladder, ureter, stomach, and biliary tract.

(a) Specific mutated genes on chromosomes 2 and 3, known as *hMSH2, hMLH1, hPMS1,* and *hPMS2,* have been linked to HNPCC. Patients with the RER+ phenotype may not have a germ line abnormality and may instead have acquired abnormal methylation of DNA as the source of the absence of expression of the genes previously noted. Abnormal methylation, which silences the promoter region of mismatch repair genes preventing protein synthesis, is more common in older patients and women. Germ line testing to determine if the RER+ phenotype is inherited or acquired is necessary as a part of genetic counseling when an individual is found to have a mismatch repair defect.

Immunohistochemical stains can be used to determine if a tumor manifests microsatellite instability, and then patients with absent gene expression should undergo germ line testing to enable appropriate counseling of family members.

(b) Patients with HNPCC have a tendency to develop colon cancer at an early age, and screening should begin by 20 years of age or 5 years earlier than the age at diagnosis of the earliest affected family member for relatives of HNPCC patients. The median age of HNPCC patients with colon cancer at diagnosis was 44 years, versus 68 years for control patients in one study.

(c) The prognosis for HNPCC patients appears to be better than for those patients with sporadic colon cancer; the death rate from colon cancer for HNPCC patients is two-thirds that for sporadic cases over 10 years. One study suggests that patients with HNPCC may derive less benefit from adjuvant chemotherapy based on fluorouracil combinations than patients without this abnormality. Correlation with additional data from patients treated in the adjuvant setting and from patients with advanced disease is needed.

  c. Tumor location. Proximal tumors appear to represent a more genetically stable form of the disease and may arise through the same mechanisms that underlie inherited nonpolyposis colon cancer. Distal tumors show evidence of greater genetic instability and may develop through the same mechanisms that underlie polyposis-associated colorectal cancer.

5. Smoking. Men and women smoking during the previous 20 years have 3 times the relative risk for small adenomas (<1 cm) but not for larger ones. Smoking for >20 years was associated with 2.5 times the relative risk for larger adenomas. It has been estimated that 5,000 to 7,000 colorectal cancer deaths in the United States can be attributed to cigarette use.

6. Other factors. Personal or family history of cancer in other anatomic sites (such as breast, endometrium, and ovary) is associated with increased risk for colorectal cancer. Exposure to asbestos (e.g., in brake mechanics) increases the incidence of colorectal cancer to 1.5 to 2 times that of the average population. Other than this association, there appears to be little relationship between occupational exposures and the incidence of colon cancer. Data indicate that HPV infection of the columnar mucosa of the colon may cause benign and malignant neoplasia.

II. PATHOLOGY AND NATURAL HISTORY

  A. Histology. Ninety-eight percent of colorectal cancers above the anal verge are adenocarcinomas. Cancers of the anal verge are most often squamous cell or basaloid carcinomas. Carcinoid tumors cluster around the rectum and cecum and spare the rest of the colon, and are distinguished from small cell tumors of the colon by their tendency to be both well differentiated and indolent in their behavior.

  B. Location. Two-thirds of colorectal cancers occur in the left colon and one-third in the right colon, although women more often develop right-sided tumors. About 20% of colorectal cancers develop in the rectum. Rectal tumors are detected by digital rectal examination in 75% of cases. Nearly 3% of colorectal adenocarcinomas are multicentric, and the risk for developing a second primary tumor in the colon is estimated to be approximately 1% per year.

  C. Clinical presentation. The common clinical complaints of patients with colorectal cancer relate to the size and location of the tumor. Right-sided colonic lesions are often asymptomatic but when symptoms are manifested, these tumors most often result in dull and ill-defined abdominal pain, bleeding, and symptomatic anemia (causing weakness, fatigue, and weight loss), rather than in colonic obstruction. Left-sided lesions lead commonly to changes in bowel habits, bleeding, gas pain, decrease in stool caliber, constipation, increased use of laxatives, and colonic obstruction.

  D. Clinical course. Metastases to the regional lymph nodes are found in 40% to 70% of cases at the time of resection. Venous or lymphatic invasion is found in up to

60% of cases. Metastases occur most frequently in the liver, peritoneal cavity, and lung, followed by the adrenals, ovaries, and bone. Metastases to the brain, while rare, are noted more commonly as survival with distant disease is extended by better treatments. Rectal cancers are 3 times more likely to recur locally than are proximal colonic tumors, in part because the anatomic confines of the rectum preclude wide resection margins and in part because the rectum lacks an outer serosal layer through most of its course. Because of the venous and lymphatic drainage of the rectum into the inferior vena cava (as opposed to the venous drainage of the colon into the portal vein and variable lymphatic drainage), rectal cancer often recurs first in the lungs. Colon cancer more frequently recurs first in the liver.

III. DIAGNOSIS
A. Diagnostic studies.
After the clinical diagnosis of colorectal cancer is made, several diagnostic and evaluative steps should be taken.
1. **Biopsy confirmation** of malignancy via colonoscopy or via CT-guided fine-needle aspiration is important. If an obstructing lesion cannot undergo biopsy, brush cytology may be feasible.
2. **General evaluation** includes a complete physical examination with digital rectal examination, CBC, LFT, and chest imaging.
3. **Carcinoembryonic antigen (CEA) screening** is recommended by the American Society of Clinical Oncology (ASCO) as a means of identifying early recurrence despite the lack of elevation in 40% of individuals with metastatic disease. A preoperative CEA can be useful as a prognostic factor and in determining if the primary tumor is associated with CEA elevation. Preoperative CEA elevation implies that CEA may aid in early identification of metastases because metastatic tumor cells are more likely to result in CEA elevation in this circumstance.
4. **CT or MRI** with contrast of the chest, abdomen, and pelvis may identify small lung, liver, or intraperitoneal metastases.
5. **Endoscopy or CT colonography** is indicated to assess the entire colonic mucosa because about 3% of patients have synchronous colorectal cancers and a larger percentage have additional premalignant polyps.
6. **EUS** significantly improves the preoperative assessment of the depth of invasion of large bowel tumors, especially rectal tumors. The accuracy rate is 95% for EUS, 70% for CT, and 60% for digital rectal examination. In rectal cancer, the combination of EUS to assess tumor extent and digital rectal examination to determine mobility should enable precise planning of surgical treatment and definition of those patients who may benefit from preoperative chemoradiation (T3,4 and N+). Transrectal biopsy of perirectal lymph nodes can often be accomplished under EUS direction.
7. **PET scanning** is of increasing utility to help distinguish if anatomic lesions of unclear origin are malignant or benign. Such scans are also useful to determine if localized metastatic disease is potentially respectable.
B. Biological markers
1. **CEA** is a cell-surface glycoprotein that is shed into the blood and is the best-known serologic marker for monitoring colorectal cancer disease status and for detecting early recurrence and liver metastases. CEA is too insensitive and nonspecific to be useful for screening of colorectal cancer. Elevation of serum CEA levels, however, does correlate with a number of parameters. Higher CEA levels are associated with histologic grade 1 or 2 tumors, more advanced stages of the disease, and the presence of visceral metastases. Although serum CEA concentration is an independent prognostic factor, its putative value lies in serial monitoring after surgical resection.
2. **Other markers,** such as CA 19-9, may be of value in monitoring recurrences and complement CEA. Monoclonal antibodies (anti-CEA, anti–TAG-72) may also be useful in immunohistologic chemical staining of tissues. The presence of an abnormal number of chromosomes in the tumor cells (aneuploidy) confers a worse prognosis than is observed in patients with diploid tumors. Light microscopic features and stage, however, remain the most reliable prognostic measures. Early

TABLE 9.4	TNM Staging System for Cancers of the Colon And Rectum

Primary tumor (T)		Regional lymph nodes (N)	
TX	Primary tumor cannot be assessed	NX	Regional lymph nodes cannot be assessed
T0	No evidence of primary tumor		
Tis	Carcinoma *in situ:* intraepithelial or invasion of the lamina propria	N0	No regional lymph node metastasis
T1	Invasion of the submucosa	N1	Metastases in 1–3 regional lymph nodes
T2	Invasion of the muscularis propria	N2	Metastases in 4 or more regional lymph nodes
T3	Invasion through the muscularis propria into subserosa or into nonperitonealized pericolic or perirectal tissues	**Distant metastases (M)**	
		MX	Distant metastasis cannot be assessed
T4	Perforation of visceral peritoneum or direct invasion into adjacent organs or tissues	M0	No distant metastasis
		M1	Distant metastatic disease

Stage groupings

Stage	TNM classification			Duke's system	MAC system	5-year survival rate (%)
0	Tis	N0	M0	—	—	100
I	T1	N0	M0	A	A	95
	T2	N0	M0	A	B1	90
IIA	T3	N0	M0	B	B2	80
IIB	T4	N0	M0	B	B3	75
IIIA	T1–2	N1	M0	C	C1	79
IIIB	T3–4	N1	M0	C	C2/C3	56
IIIC	any T	N2	M0	C	C1/C2/C3	50
IV	any T	any N	M1	—	D	5

MAC, Modified Astler-Coller classification.

reports suggest that tumor DNA and circulating tumor cells may also have utility both as initial diagnostic tools and for early diagnosis of recurrent disease.

IV. STAGING AND PROGNOSTIC FACTORS

- **A. Staging system.** Staging using the TNM system has been recommended over the Astler-Coller modification of the Dukes system. Readers should consult an up-to-date staging manual because of frequent revisions of staging systems. The current staging system is delineated in Table 9.4.
- **B. Prognostic factors**
  - **1. Stage** is the most important prognostic factor (see section IV.A)
  - **2. Histologic grade** significantly influences survival regardless of stage. Patients with well-differentiated carcinomas (grades 1 and 2) have a better 5-year survival than those with poorly differentiated carcinomas (grades 3 and 4).
  - **3. The anatomic location of the tumor** appears to be an independent prognostic factor. For equal stages, patients with rectal lesions have a worse prognosis than those with colon lesions, and transverse and descending colon lesions result in poorer outcomes than ascending or rectosigmoid lesions.
  - **4. Clinical presentation.** Patients who present with bowel obstruction or perforation have a worse prognosis than patients who present with neither of these problems.

5. **Chromosome 18.** The prognosis of patients with an allelic loss of chromosome 18q is significantly worse than that of patients with no allelic loss. The survival of patients with stage II (B) disease is the same as that for stage I (A) when there is no allelic loss and the same as for stage III (C) when there is allelic loss. Other abnormalities that have been identified and that are of potential value for determining prognosis are located on chromosomes 1, 5, 8, 17, and 22. Identification of these genes or their products is possible using gel electrophoresis or immunohistochemical probes. These observations may ultimately prove to be helpful in selecting patients with stage II (B) disease for adjuvant therapy or stage III (C) patients with better-than-average prognoses who can avoid the potential toxicity and expense of adjuvant therapy.

6. **Other tumor characteristics.** Investigators have examined a number of tumor characteristics as judged by immunohistochemical or polymerase chain reaction-based assays for use either as factors for predicting prognosis or as characteristics that could potentially predict the likelihood of an individual patient's response to a specific regimen. These evaluations include levels in the tumor of thymidylate synthetase, dihydropyrimidine dehydrogenase (DPD), proliferation markers (Ki-67 or MIB-1), and tumor-suppressor deletions (such as 18q deletions), among others. None have yet been determined to be standard parameters that should be ordered outside the context of a research study.

V. SCREENING AND PREVENTION

A. **Screening.** The National Cancer Institute (NCI), the American College of Surgeons, the American College of Physicians, and the American Cancer Society (ACS) recommend a number of potential screening tests as alternatives for asymptomatic patients who are 50 years of age and older. One option is to have a sigmoidoscopic examination every 3 to 5 years. An annual digital rectal and three-sample fecal occult blood (FOB) test examination are recommended by the ACS, American College of Gastroenterology, and NCI for people 50 years of age and older. Screening colonoscopy has also been recommended for average-risk individuals every 10 years. Screening colonoscopy for high-risk patients with a family history of colorectal cancer in first-degree relatives but no clear evidence of FAP or HNPCC should begin at 40 years of age.

1. Three large randomized trials in which >250,000 patients were tested for FOB or followed according to the usual patterns of care have been reported. In the largest trial and the only one conducted in the United States, annual testing of a rehydrated fecal smear was associated with a 33.4% decrease in risk for death from colorectal cancer in 46,551 adults older than 50 years of age. Better markers for colorectal cancer are being sought because of the high false-positive and false-negative rates associated with FOB.

2. There has been burgeoning interest in the isolation of specific DNA sequences such as those in the *APC* or *p53* genes and long segments of DNA that can be obtained from colonocytes shed into the stool and assayed using techniques for amplifying the amount of DNA present. These markers appear to be sensitive and specific for screening for malignancy in the aerodigestive tract. These technologies continue to undergo refinement and large-scale randomized trials of FOB versus these DNA-based assays are under way.

B. **Prevention.** The management of patients with ulcerative colitis is discussed in section I.B.3.a.

1. **Periodic sigmoidoscopy or colonoscopy** identifies and removes precancerous lesions (polyps) and reduces the incidence of colorectal cancer in patients who undergo colonoscopic polypectomy. However, no prospective randomized clinical trials have yet demonstrated that sigmoidoscopy is effective in the prevention of colorectal cancer death, although trials to test this strategy are in progress. The presence of even small rectosigmoid polyps is associated with polyps beyond the reach of the sigmoidoscope, and their presence should lead to full colonoscopy.

2. **Diets** that are high in fiber and low in fat or that contain calcium supplements, or both, may deter polyp progression to cancer.

3. **Nonsteroidal anti-inflammatory drugs (NSAIDs).** In a randomized, double-blind, placebo-controlled study of patients with familial polyposis, the NSAID sulindac at a dose of 150 mg b.i.d. significantly decreased the mean number and mean diameter of polyps as compared with those in patients given placebo. The size and number of the polyps, however, increased 3 months after the treatment was stopped but remained significantly lower than at baseline. Data further suggest that aspirin reduces the formation, number, and size of colorectal polyps and reduces the incidence of colorectal cancer, whether familial or nonfamilial. These protective effects appear to require continuous exposure to at least 325 mg of aspirin per day for years. Selective Cox-2 inhibitors have also been shown to be preventive for colon cancer but have been associated with an increased risk of cardiac events such that these are not routinely recommended.

VI. MANAGEMENT

A. **Surgery** is the only universally accepted potentially curative treatment for colorectal cancer. Curative surgery should excise the tumor with wide margins and maximize regional lymphadenectomy such that at least 12 lymph nodes are available for pathologic evaluation. For lesions above the rectum, resection of the tumor with a minimum 5-cm margin of grossly negative colon is considered adequate, although the ligation of vascular trunks required to perform an adequate lymphadenectomy may necessitate larger bowel resections. Laparoscopic colectomy approaches have been developed and appear to be equally effective staging and therapeutic approaches to open colectomy, with modest decreases in hospital stay and pain medication use and improved cosmetic results. Subtotal colectomy and ileoproctostomy may be advisable for patients with potentially curable colon cancer and with adenomas scattered in the colon or for patients with a personal history of prior colorectal cancer or a family history of colorectal cancer in first-degree relatives.

1. **Arterial supply.** Excision of a tumor in the right colon should include the right branch of the middle colic artery as well as the entire ileocolic and right colic artery. Excision of a tumor at the hepatic or splenic flexure should include the entire distribution of the middle colic artery.

2. **Avoidance of permanent colostomy** in middle and low rectal cancers has been encouraged by the emergence of new surgical stapling techniques as well as the use of preoperative chemotherapy and radiation to shrink tumors prior to resection.

3. **Rectal tumors** may be treatable by primary resection and more distal anastomosis, usually without even a temporary (anastomosis-protective) colostomy, if the lower edge is above 5 cm from the anal verge. Treatment options for rectal tumors include the following:

   a. **Middle and upper rectum** (6 to 15 cm): anterior resection of rectum

   b. **Lower rectum** (0 to 5 cm): coloanal anastomosis, with or without a pouch, transanal excision, transsphincteric and parasacral approaches, diathermy, primary radiation therapy, or abdominoperineal resection (APR)

   c. **Total mesorectal excision (TME).** The mesorectum is defined as the lymphatic, vascular, fatty, and neural tissues that are circumferentially adherent to the rectum from the level of the sacral promontory to the levator ani muscles. Data from Europe suggest that local recurrence rates may be decreased with *en bloc* sharp dissection of the entire mesorectum at the time of tumor extirpation, and this procedure has now become standard.

4. **Obstructing tumors** in the right colon are usually managed by primary resection and primary anastomosis. Obstructing tumors in the left colon may be managed with initial decompression (proximal colostomy) or stent insertion followed by resection of the tumor and deferred closure of the colostomy. Recent trends, however, favor extending resection and primary anastomosis to include obstructing tumors in the transverse, descending, and even sigmoid colon.

5. **Perforated colon cancer** requires initial excision of the primary tumor and a proximal colostomy, followed later by reanastomosis and closure of the colostomy.

B. **Adjuvant chemotherapy for stage III colon cancer** (lymph node involvement) with 5-FU plus levamisole (mainly of historical interest) or 5-FU plus leucovorin (FU/L) has reduced the incidence of recurrence by 41% (p <0.001) in a number of large prospective randomized trials. The MOSAIC study in Europe randomized 2,200 patients (40% stage II, 60% stage III) to receive 5-FU infusion and leucovorin without or with oxaliplatin (FOLFOX). The primary end point of this trial is 3-year overall disease-free survival (DFS) rather than the more conventional end point of 5-year overall survival. There was a 73% 3-year DFS for the standard 5-FU/leucovorin arm and a 78% 3-year DFS for the FOLFOX regimen, with a 7.5% statistically significant advantage for stage III disease. Recently presented data have shown a 2.6% benefit in 6-year overall survival for FOLFOX over the two-drug regimen and the difference was 4.4% for stage III disease. The National Surgical Adjuvant Breast Project (NSABP) C-07 study showed a similar outcome for DFS but mature overall survival data have not yet been reported. In that trial, a bolus-based 5-FU plus oxaliplatin regimen called *FLOX* was employed.

Three randomized trials have failed to show an advantage to irinotecan-containing regimens in the adjuvant setting. The use of irinotecan alone or in combinations is not recommended in the adjuvant setting.

As a consequence, the standard treatment for stage III colon cancer is now an oxaliplatin-containing regimen, most commonly FOLFOX, unless there are contraindications to its use, such as pre-existing sensory neuropathy. In that case FU/L is recommended. In a large study known as the EXACT trial, capecitabine, an oral 5-FU prodrug, was compared with FU/L and outcomes were essentially equivalent. Adjuvant chemotherapy is begun 3 to 5 weeks after surgery.

1. **FU/L regimens** Two bolus 5-FU regimens commonly employed in the United States are as follows:

   a. **Dosage, Mayo Clinic regimen:** leucovorin, 20 mg/m^2 by 30-minute IV infusion, followed by 5-FU, 425 mg/m^2 by rapid IV injection, daily for 5 consecutive days for two 4-week cycles and then every 5 weeks thereafter

   b. **Dosage, Roswell Park Memorial Institute (RPMI) regimen:** leucovorin, 500 mg/m^2 by 30-minute IV infusion, followed by 5-FU, 500 mg/m^2 by rapid IV injection, weekly for 6 of every 8 weeks

   c. **The side effects of the Mayo and RPMI regimens and capecitabine** are similar. Toxicity of grade III or more is based on the NCI common toxicity criteria (see Appendix B-2). The principal difference in toxicity between the two regimens relates to rates of severe stomatitis and diarrhea. The Mayo regimen is associated with more grade III stomatitis and the RPMI regimen with a higher rate of grade III diarrhea. Hematologic toxicity seen with both regimens is mainly neutropenia. Grade III or greater neutropenia afflicts about one-third of patients at some time during the course of therapy. Nausea and vomiting are generally not severe. Dermatologic side effects are generally limited to erythema and desquamation of sun-damaged skin.

   Capecitabine is able to be administered orally and is associated with less GI toxicity and neutropenia than bolus FU regimens. However, it does cause hand-foot syndrome in which the skin of the palms and soles can become tender, erythematous, and if the drug is continued, exfoliation of the overlying skin may follow.

   d. **Dihydropyrimidine (DPD)** is the rate-limiting enzyme in the breakdown of 5-FU. Less than 1% of the U.S. population has a deficiency of DPD. Such patients have severe toxicity and often die after exposure to standard doses because of profound and prolonged neutropenia and mucositis. Cerebellar toxicity occurs relatively commonly in DPD-deficient patients. An assay for DPD levels is commercially available and can be selectively ordered if DPD deficiency is suspected based on history or clinical parameters.

2. **FOLFOX and FLOX** are the preferred regimens

   a. **Dosage, FOLFOX4.** Leucovorin, 200 mg/m^2, is given preceding a bolus of 5-FU of 400 mg/m^2. A 22-hour infusion of 600 mg/m^2 is then administered via infusion pump. The FU/L infusion is given on 2 consecutive days. Oxaliplatin is given at a dose of 85 mg/ m^2 on day 1. The cycle is repeated every 2 weeks. Other FOLFOX regimens including FOLFOX 6, modified FOLFOX 6, and FOLFOX 7 explore variations on the oxaliplatin dose and have eliminated the 5-FU bolus.

   b. **Dosage, FLOX.** Leucovorin 500 mg/m^2 is given preceding a bolus of 5-FU of 500 mg/m^2 weekly for 6 weeks in three 8-week cycles. Oxaliplatin, 85 mg/m^2, is given on weeks 1, 3, and 5 of each 8-week cycle. No pumps or prolonged infusions are used.

   c. **The side effects of FOLFOX4.** This regimen is commonly associated with grade 3-4 neutropenia (41% in the MOSAIC trial) but seldom causes neutropenic fever (1.8%). GI tract toxicity is less problematic than in the bolus-based 5-FU regimens, with 2.7% having stomatitis, 5.9% vomiting, and 10.8% diarrhea. Alopecia is relatively rare at 5%. Chronic sensory neuropathy, which is often aggravated by cold exposure and can limit the amount of oxaliplatin that can be administered over time, afflicted 12.3% of patients, but most patients with grade 3 neuropathy had recovered 1 year after the agent was stopped.

   d. **The side effects of FLOX.** The bolus 5-FU in the FLOX regimen is associated with a 38% rate of grade 3-4 diarrhea but is seldom associated with significant neutropenia (4%).

C. Adjuvant chemotherapy for stage II colon cancer (no lymph node involvement) is controversial. Investigators from the NSABP advocate for adjuvant therapy in this setting because it has produced a small but consistent benefit in patients with stage II disease in serial NSABP trials. Conversely, a meta-analysis of five trials involving about 1,000 patients showed a statistically insignificant difference in 5-year survival rates of 82% versus 80%, treated versus untreated, respectively, for patients with stage II disease. The QUASAR group did show a 3% survival advantage at 5 years for FU/L over observation in a trial that enrolled >3,200 patients. There was no survival advantage for the 40% of stage II patients enrolled in the MOSAIC trial. The ASCO recommends against the routine use of chemotherapy in stage II colon cancer.

   Intense efforts have focused on differentiating stage II patients with higher risk for recurrence from those with lower risk through examination of molecular markers such as tumor ploidy (number of chromosomes), p53 status, levels of thymidylate synthesis, presence or absence of individual chromosomal mutations, and other parameters. Although none of these is accepted as a standard prognostic determinant, in one trial, patients with aneuploid tumors had a 5-year survival rate of 54%, compared with patients with diploid tumors who had a 74% 5-year survival rate. Although some preliminary data suggest that high-risk stage II patients with obstruction or perforation may have benefited from FU/L more than the overall populations, these data have not yet been published.

D. Neoadjuvant therapy for rectal cancer. Because of the anatomic confines of the pelvic bones and sacrum, surgeons often cannot achieve wide, tumor-free margins during the resection of rectal cancer. Almost half of recurrences in rectal cancer are in the pelvis. This observation led a German group to compare preoperative chemotherapy with 5-FU and radiation to postoperative therapy in order to determine if the preoperative strategy could improve outcomes and reduce the number of APRs that result in a permanent colostomy. The trial randomized >800 patients and the outcomes favored preoperative therapy, which showed a lower local recurrence rate, less anastomotic stenosis, and fewer APRs. Patients who have a complete pathologic response to preoperative therapy have a favorable long-term prognosis. In general, postoperative adjuvant therapy with FOLFOX or FU/L based on preoperative staging is indicated for patients with known or suspected positive nodes. This trial has led to a widespread shift in practice to embrace preoperative chemotherapy plus RT.

   1. **Variations** in the use of RT alone or combined with chemotherapy and in surgical technique have been investigated in attempts to improve local control rates. Numerous randomized controlled studies of both preoperative and postoperative

RT alone have demonstrated no improvement in survival; at best, there has been a small decrease in the rate of local recurrence. In the United States, radiation is generally given over 6 weeks to a dose approaching 5,000 cGy and surgery is performed 4 to 6 weeks later. In Europe, it is common to give 2,500 cGy in five fractions without chemotherapy and proceed promptly to surgery. These approaches have not been compared in a randomized trial.

A number of European surgeons have advocated TME and it has now become the standard of care. A Dutch trial showed that TME is associated with a lower local recurrence rate than conventional rectal resection but have also noted that rectal stump devascularization results in a higher rate of postoperative anastomotic site leakage. RT after TME reduces the rate of local recurrence at 2 years from the time of surgery, suggesting that RT is still a valuable tool in reducing local recurrence even after the more extensive *en bloc* resection done with TME.

2. **The current standard therapy** for stage III rectal cancer, and sometimes for stage II disease, is preoperative chemotherapy using 5-FU and RT, followed by surgery, and then followed by adjuvant chemotherapy.

E. **Postoperative follow-up.** About 85% of all recurrences that are destined to occur in colorectal cancer are evident within 3 years after surgical resection, and nearly all recurrences are noted within 5 years. High preoperative CEA levels usually revert to normal within 6 weeks after complete resection.

1. **Clinical evaluation.** After curative surgical resection, patients with stage II and III colon or rectal cancer are commonly seen more frequently during the first 2 postoperative years and less frequently thereafter. After 5 years, follow-up is mainly targeted at detection of new primary tumors. The primary goal of follow-up is to detect metastatic disease early. Some patients with colorectal cancer develop a single or a few metastatic sites (known as *oligometastases*) in the liver, in the lungs, or at the anastomotic site from which the primary bowel cancer was removed that can be resected with curative intent (see section VI.F).

2. **Chest CT scanning has largely replaced chest radiographs** for detecting recurrence. They are advocated annually or semiannually.

3. **Colonoscopy.** Patients who presented with obstructing colon lesions that preclude preoperative imaging of the colon should have colonoscopy 3 to 6 months after surgery to ensure the absence of a concurrent neoplastic lesion in the remaining colon. The purpose of endoscopy done thereafter is to detect a metachronous tumor, suture line recurrence, or colorectal adenoma. In the absence of obstruction, colonoscopy is performed annually for 1 to 3 years after surgery and, if negative, at 5-year intervals thereafter.

4. **Rising CEA levels** call for further studies to identify the site of recurrence and are most often helpful in identifying hepatic recurrences. An elevated CEA calls for further testing using CT of the abdomen, pelvis, and chest as well as other studies as dictated by symptoms. If pelvic recurrence of a rectal cancer is suspected, MRI may be more helpful than CT. The use of hepatic imaging by CT, ultrasound, or MRI at regular intervals is now advocated by ASCO. PET scans may also be of value in identifying early signs of recurrent disease and for quantifying the number if metastatic deposits of disease visible at the time of recurrence.

F. **Management of isolated recurrence.** Early detection and surgical resection of isolated intrahepatic or pulmonary recurrence may be curative or result in improved survival. Those patients most likely to do well have a single lesion in a single site and a disease-free interval of 3 or more years between the primary diagnosis and evidence of metastatic disease. Resection of an isolated hepatic metastasis that involves one lobe of the liver may result in a 60% 5-year survival rate. Resection of an isolated pulmonary metastasis may result in 5- and 10-year survival rates of 40% and 20%, respectively. Even patients with multiple lesions can be resected and cured, although cure rates decrease with more widespread, albeit resectable, disease. In selected patients, multiple resections may be performed even for disease in lung and liver with favorable outcomes. As more effective chemotherapy and biologic therapy is developed, the possibility of converting patients who were initially unresectable into resection candidates is more and more common. Restaging with an eye toward resection when possible should be done on a frequent basis in patients who may be resection candidates.

G. Management of advanced colorectal cancer: local measures

1. **Surgery.** About 85% of patients diagnosed with colorectal cancer can undergo surgical resection. Patients with incurable cancer may benefit from palliative resection to prevent obstruction, perforation, bleeding, and invasion of adjacent structures. However, in the absence of symptoms, surgery can often be avoided when metastatic disease is present. It is common with newer CT scans to note the primary tumor on the scan and to observe shrinkage with chemotherapy treatment. The use of colonic stents and laser ablation of intraluminal tumors can often obviate the need for surgery even in symptomatic cases.

2. **RT** may be used as the primary and only treatment modality for small, mobile rectal tumors or in combination with chemotherapy after resection of rectal tumors (see earlier discussion). RT in palliative doses relieves pain, obstruction, bleeding, and tenesmus in about 80% of cases. In selected cases with locally advanced disease, the use of IORT may provide an advantage. However, no randomized trials of external-beam versus IORT or IORT plus external-beam therapy have been reported.

3. **Hepatic arterial infusion** takes advantage of the dual nature of hepatic blood supply. Metastases in the liver derive their blood supply predominantly from the hepatic artery, whereas hepatocytes derive blood principally from the hepatic vein. The installation of floxuridine (FUDR) into the hepatic artery has been advocated and appears to improve the response rate over 5-FU administered systemically. Problems with this approach include variable anatomy, which makes placement of a single catheter impossible; catheter migration; biliary sclerosis; and gastric ulceration. Progression of extrahepatic disease is a common pattern of failure with this modality. Randomized trials of systemic versus intrahepatic therapy have shown modest advantages to this approach but the practical difficulties of managing these lines and ever-improving systemic therapies have kept this approach from widespread usage.

H. Management of advanced colorectal cancer: chemotherapy. The most commonly used chemotherapeutic agents are 5-FU (alone or in combination with leucovorin, FU/L), capecitabine (the oral 5-FU prodrug), irinotecan, and oxaliplatin.

1. **Biochemical modulation of 5-FU with leucovorin.** The combination of 5-FU and leucovorin increases the activity as well as the toxicity of 5-FU, results in significant improvement in regression rate, and according to some studies, culminates in improved survival. The partial response rate is about 25%. The dose-limiting toxicities are diarrhea, mucositis, and hematosuppression. Regimens being used with essentially the same response rate involve:
   a. 5-FU plus low-dose or high-dose leucovorin given weekly, or
   b. 5-FU plus low-dose or high-dose leucovorin given for 5 days every 4 to 5 weeks, or
   c. 5-FU plus leucovorin by infusion over 24 to 48 hours or for longer intervals.

2. **Continuous IV infusion of 5-FU** changes the toxicity profile from hematologic to predominantly mucositis and dermatologic (hand-foot syndrome) when compared with bolus administration. Multiple randomized trials, however, have shown that continuous infusion of 5-FU using an ambulatory infusion pump, as compared with rapid injection, results in marginally improved survival, prolonging life on average for <1 month. Because of its favorable toxicity profile, the use of short-term infusion as the backbone of the FOLFOX and FOLFIRI regimens, and improvements in infusion pumps, has become common practice to treat advanced colorectal cancer.

3. **Therapy with irinotecan** has been shown to improve survival and quality of life in patients with advanced colorectal cancer. In patients with recurrent disease refractory to at least one 5-FU regimen, the survival at 1 year of patients treated with supportive care alone or with 5-FU was about 15%, compared with 36% when patients were treated with irinotecan. In the United States, a commonly used regimen for irinotecan is 125 mg/m^2 weekly for 4 of every 6 weeks or

2 of every 3 weeks. Irinotecan can also be administered as 350 mg/m^2 every 3 weeks.

About 10% of the population in the United States has an inherited polymorphism of the *UGT1A1* gene that results in diminished activity of the enzyme that detoxifies irinotecan. Such patients have a higher risk of neutropenia, especially with the every-3-week higher dose regimen. A test for this abnormality is now commercially available, and testing is recommended in the package insert. In second-line therapy, there are no clear data supporting better outcomes from combinations of irinotecan with FU/L over single-agent irinotecan if a patient has had prior 5-FU exposure.

4. **Oxaliplatin** is a diaminocyclohexane-containing platinum agent with broad activity in cisplatin-resistant human tumor xenografts. It has been used in Europe for a decade and has been approved in the United States in combination with 5-FU and leucovorin for patients with metastatic colorectal cancer in the first- and second-line settings, as well as the adjuvant setting. It is generally administered in combination with 5-FU and leucovorin using one of a number of regimens called *FOLFOX 1 to FOLFOX 7* as data suggest greater efficacy in combination.

5. **First-line chemotherapy.** A number of randomized studies have compared three-drug regimens to FU/L as first-line therapy.

   a. **Combination regimens being compared** include:
      (1) **IFL:** irinotecan, 125 mg/m^2, with 5-FU, 500 mg/m^2, and leucovorin, 20 mg/m^2
      (2) **FOLFIRI:** irinotecan, 180 mg/m^2, followed by folinic acid (leucovorin), 200 mg/m^2, and then 5-FU, 2.4 g/m^2 infused over 24 hours. Recent data have shown that the FOLFIRI regimen has advantages in both activity and toxicity over bolus 5-FU or capecitabine-based combinations.
      (3) **FOLFOX4:** folinic acid (leucovorin), 5-FU (given with a loading dose and 22-hour infusion repeated on consecutive days), and oxaliplatin (dosing schedule is defined in section VI.B.2)
      (4) **FOLFOX6:** folinic acid (leucovorin), 5-FU (given with a loading dose and 46-hour infusion), and oxaliplatin
      (5) **FUFOX:** 5-FU given in high dose as a 24-hour infusion, folinic acid (leucovorin), and oxaliplatin
      (6) **IROX:** irinotecan plus oxaliplatin

   b. **Results of randomized studies** are shown in Table 9.5.
      (1) Both the IFL and FOLFIRI regimens have been shown in randomized trials to offer an advantage to patients in median survival (MS), median time to progression (MTP), and response rate (RR) over FU/L regimens.
      (2) Several studies have compared oxaliplatin plus FU/L to FU/L alone. Both the FOLFOX and FUFOX regimens have been shown in randomized trials to offer a statistically significant advantage to patients with respect to MTP and RR but showed no statistically significant difference in MS over FU/L regimens.
      (3) Studies have compared regimens in which FU/L is coupled to either irinotecan or oxaliplatin. In one large trial, 795 patients were randomly assigned to IFL versus FOLFOX versus IROX. The FOLFOX regimen was superior to both IFL and IROX with respect to overall MS, MTP, and RR. Toxicity also favored the FOLFOX regimen as patients had fewer episodes of severe diarrhea, febrile neutropenia, vomiting, and dehydration.
      (4) A comparison of FOLFOX followed by FOLFIRI versus the reverse sequence has shown no significant differences in outcomes with respect to MS (21 months), RR in first-line therapy (55%), or MTP (8 months for first-line and 3 to 4 months for second-line therapy) based on the two sequences. Toxicity patterns were similar between the two regimens.

6. **Monoclonal antibodies**
   a. **Bevacizumab (Avastin)** is a monoclonal antibody that targets the vascular endothelial growth factor receptor. Bevacizumab plus IFL was compared with IFL alone in a randomized trial involving 815 patients (Table 9.5). The results for IFL alone were very similar to those reported in other phase III studies.

| TABLE 9.5 | Randomized Trials of Combination Chemotherapy Regimens In Advanced Colorectal Cancer |

Compared regimens[a]	Median survival (months)	Median time to progression (months)	Response rate (%)
Randomized trials vs. FU/L			
IFL vs. FU/L	14 vs. 13	7 vs. 4	39 vs. 21
FOLFIRI vs. FU/L	17 vs. 14	7 vs. 4	41 vs. 23
FOLFOX vs. FU/L	16 vs. 15	9 vs. 6	49 vs. 22
FUFOX vs. FU/L	21 vs. 16	8 vs. 5	49 vs. 23
Randomized trial of 795 patients[b]			
IROX[b]	17	7	35
IFL[b]	15	7	31
FOLFOX[b]	20	9	45
Randomized trial of 815 patients[c]			
IFL vs. IFL + Bev[c]	16 vs. 20	6 vs. 11	35 vs. 45

[a]Regimens are defined in "Colorectal Cancer" section VI.H.5. FU/L (5-fluorouracil/leucovorin) regimen is defined in "Colorectal Cancer" section VI.B.1.a.
[b]Study compared IROX vs. IFL vs. FOLFOX for 795 patients.
[c]Bev, bevacizumab (Avastin); study involved 815 patients.

The patients receiving IFL plus bevacizumab in this study achieved a better RR and MS compared with those receiving IFL alone. Toxicity was increased only modestly by the addition of bevacizumab, which led to hypertension and rare episodes of bowel perforation. Additional trials of bevacizumab with FOLFIRI and FOLFOX, and capecitabine chemotherapy combinations have shown improvements in activity of lesser magnitude than that observed in IFL and bevacizumab study with similar toxicity profiles to the base regimens.

b. Cetuximab (Erbitux) and panitumumab (Vectibix) are two other monoclonal antibodies that target the epidermal growth factor and have been approved for use in refractory colorectal cancer. They are being tested in lower stages of disease, including the adjuvant setting. Both have single-agent activity resulting in response rates of <10% in third-line therapy. In second-line treatment, the combination of either antibody with irinotecan is more active than irinotecan alone. Combinations of both agents with FOLFOX and FOLFIRI in phase II trials look promising, and phase III trials are underway.

Cetuximab has been combined with bevacizumab and shown activity in heavily pretreated patients. Cetuximab is a mouse monoclonal antibody and panitumumab is fully humanized. Both commonly cause an acnelike skin rash and paronychia in some patients, and development of this rash seems to correlate with benefit from the agents. Anaphylactic reactions are more common with cetuximab than with panitumumab.

7. FOLFOXIRI. A study comparing a 5-FU plus irinotecan regimen to all three chemotherapy agents given together has shown an advantage for the FOLFOXIRI regimen, including a median survival for patients enrolled in the multidrug arm of 23 months and a high rate of liver resections among patients initially judged to be unresectable.

8. Serial sequential single agents versus combined chemotherapy. Two trials done in Europe, the FOCUS study and the CAIRO study, have compared serial single agents with combinations. While trends favored combination therapies, neither study showed a significant advantage for combinations over serial single agents. However, median survivals were 15 to 17 months in all arms of both studies, which does not compare to the nearly 2-year median survivals seen with combinations. In addition, exposure to all three chemotherapy agents over the entire course of treatment for advanced disease is associated with better outcomes than less intensive therapy.

9. **Summary of chemotherapy recommendations for patients with advanced disease.** It appears that combination therapy with either irinotecan or oxaliplatin coupled to FU/L is better than serial single-agent treatment with respect to overall survival. There are no clear data to favor FOLFOX, FOLFIRI, FOLFOXIRI, or FLOX as the best first-line therapy. However, the infusion of 5-FU seems to be better tolerated than does bolus 5-FU, and use of the IFL regimen is not generally recommended. The toxicity profiles of the two regimens do differ, with FOLFOX causing more neutropenia and neuropathy and FOLFIRI more GI toxicity and alopecia; the side effect profiles should be considered when choosing therapy on a patient-by-patient basis. Capecitabine can be substituted for 5-FU infusion with similar outcomes.

Most oncologists tend to begin patients on FOLFOX or FOLFIRI plus bevacizumab as first-line therapy in the United States. Recent pooled analyses have suggested that patients older than 70 years and those with a performance status of 2 can tolerate and benefit from combination therapy similar to younger and asymptomatic patients.

 ANAL CANCER

I. EPIDEMIOLOGY AND ETIOLOGY

A. Incidence. Anal cancers constitute 1% to 2% of large bowel cancers, and 4,000 new cases are diagnosed annually in the United States. Anal canal cancer most commonly develops in patients 50 to 60 years of age and is more frequent in women than in men (female-to-male ratio, 2:1). Cancer of the anal margin is more frequent in men. During the 1990s, however, the incidence of anal canal cancer in men younger than 35 years of age increased, and the gender ratio is reversed in this age group. Anal cancer more frequently afflicts urban than rural populations.

B. Etiology. In most patients with carcinoma of the anus, HPV appears to play a causal role.

1. **Infectious agents.** HPV, particularly types 16 and 18, is a prime suspect as a causative agent for anal cancer (see Chapter 36, section V and VI). >70% of tumor tissues show HPV DNA by polymerase chain reaction techniques. An HPV-produced protein, E6, inactivates the tumor-suppressor gene *p53*. The presence of genital warts increases the relative risk by a factor of 30.

Although human immunodeficiency virus (HIV) has been suggested as a causative agent, anal tumors are extremely rare in IV drug abusers. The relative risk for homosexuals with acquired immunodeficiency syndrome (AIDS) is 84 and for heterosexuals with AIDS is 38. Other associated infections include herpes simplex virus type 2, *Chlamydia trachomatis* infection in women, and gonorrhea in men.

2. **Diseases associated with anal cancer** include AIDS, prior irradiation, anal fistulas, fissures, chronic local inflammation, hemorrhoids, Crohn disease, lymphogranuloma venereum, condylomata acuminata, carcinoma of cervix, and carcinoma of the vulva. The relative risk for anal cancer development after a diagnosis of AIDS is 63. Sexual activity, particularly with multiple partners, is associated with an increased risk for anal canal cancer.

3. **Immune suppression.** Kidney transplant recipients have a 100-fold increase in anogenital tumors.

4. **Cigarette smoking** is associated with an eightfold increase in the risk for anal cancer.

5. **Anal-receptive intercourse in men** but not in women is strongly associated with anal cancer at a risk ratio of 33. Studies have shown that the incidence of anal cancer (squamous and transitional cell carcinomas) is 6 times greater in single men than in married men. Single women are not at an increased risk.

II. PATHOLOGY AND NATURAL HISTORY

A. Anatomy. The anal canal is a tubular structure 3 to 4 cm in length. The junction between the anal canal and perineal skin is known as the anal verge (Hilton's line). The pectinate (or dentate) line is located at the center of the anal canal.

The lining of the anal canal is composed of columnar epithelium in its upper portion and keratinized and nonkeratinized squamous epithelium in its lower portion. Intermediate epithelium (also known as *transitional* or *cloacogenic* epithelium, which resembles bladder epithelium) lines a middle zone (0.5 to 1 cm in length) that corresponds to the pectinate line. Anal tumors appear to originate near the mucocutaneous junction and grow either upward into the rectum and surrounding tissue or downward into the perineal tissue.

B. Lymphatics. Some of the upper lymphatics of the anus communicate with those of the rectal ampulla that lead to the sacral, upper mesocolic, and para-aortic lymph nodes. The lower lymphatics communicate with those of the perineum that lead to the superficial inguinal lymph nodes. Of patients undergoing abdominal perineal (AP) resection, 25% to 35% manifest pelvic lymph node metastases.

C. Histology. Squamous cell carcinoma accounts for 63% of cases; transitional cell (cloacogenic) carcinoma, 23%; and mucinous adenocarcinoma, 7% (often with multiple fistulous tracts). Basal cell carcinoma (2%) is curable either by local excision or by irradiation. Paget disease (2%) is a malignant neoplasm of the intraepidermal portion of the apocrine glands. Malignant melanoma (2%) usually begins at the pectinate line and progresses as single or multiple polypoid masses; the prognosis is poor and depends on tumor size and depth of invasion. Other forms include small cell carcinoma (rare but extremely aggressive), verrucous carcinoma (a polypoid neoplasm closely related to giant condyloma acuminata), Bowen disease, embryonal rhabdomyosarcoma (infants and children), and malignant lymphoma (in patients with AIDS).

III. DIAGNOSIS

A. Symptoms. Bleeding occurs in 50% of patients, pain in 40%, sensation of a mass in 25%, and pruritus in 15%. About 25% of patients do not have symptoms.

B. Physical examination should include digital anorectal examination, anoscopy, proctoscopy, endoscopic ultrasound if available, and palpation of inguinal lymph nodes. Anorectal examination may have to be performed under sedation or general anesthesia in patients with severe pain and anal spasm.

C. Biopsy. An incisional biopsy is necessary and preferable to confirm the diagnosis. Excisional biopsy should be avoided. Suspicious inguinal lymph nodes should undergo biopsy to differentiate inflammatory from metastatic disease. Needle aspiration of these nodes may establish the diagnosis; if aspiration is negative, surgical biopsy should be performed. Sentinel node biopsy is advocated by some surgeons in order to improve staging accuracy.

D. Staging evaluation should include physical examination, chest radiograph, and LFT. Pelvic CT and EUS of the anal canal may be useful. HIV testing is appropriate when warranted by individual patient risk factors.

IV. STAGING AND PROGNOSTIC FACTORS

A. Staging system. The TNM staging system may be used. Readers should consult an up-to-date staging manual because of frequent revisions of staging systems. Anal margin tumors are staged as for skin cancer. The T stage of anal canal tumors is determined by size and by invasion into adjacent organs, as follows:

TX	Primary tumor cannot be assessed
Tis	Anal intraepithelial neoplasm or carcinoma *in situ*
T1	Tumor 2 cm or smaller in greatest dimension
T2	Tumor larger than 2 cm but 5 cm or smaller in greatest dimension
T3	Tumor larger than 5 cm in greatest dimension
T4	Tumor of any size that invades adjacent organ or organs (e.g., vagina, urethra, bladder [involvement of rectal wall, perirectal skin or subcutaneous tissue, or the sphincter muscle alone is not classified as T4])

B. Prognostic factors

1. TNM stage. Patients with Tis have a propensity to progress to higher T stages and to have widespread superficial spread of disease, particularly among those that are HIV-positive. Patients with T1 cancer (lesions smaller than 2 cm in diameter) have a significantly better prognosis than those with larger lesions. Five-year survival rates are >80% for patients with T1 and T2 cancers and <20% for those with T3 and T4 cancers. The survival is poor even with aggressive therapy for lesions larger than 6 to 10 cm in diameter. In a multivariate analysis, T stage was the only significant independent prognostic factor for anal cancers. Metastasis to lymph nodes also results in a poor outcome. Anal canal cancers tend to remain regionally localized, with distant metastases noted in <10% of cases.

2. Other factors

a. Histology. The histologic type (i.e., cloacogenic vs. epidermoid) has not been found to be prognostically relevant. Keratinizing carcinoma is associated with a better outcome than nonkeratinizing cancers. Patients with mucoepidermoid carcinoma and small cell anaplastic carcinoma have a worse prognosis.

b. Symptoms. Patients without symptoms do better than those with symptoms. Symptoms are usually directly related to the size of the tumor.

c. Tumor grade. Patients with low-grade tumors have a better 5-year survival rate than patients with high-grade tumors (75% vs. 25%, respectively). DNA ploidy may or may not have prognostic significance.

V. PREVENTION AND EARLY DETECTION.
Early detection depends on the patient's and physician's awareness of the disease, the presence of risk factors, and the histologic examination of all surgical specimens, even those removed from minor anorectal surgery. Yearly anoscopy may be indicated in high-risk patients. Anal examination should be performed routinely in patients with cervical and vulvar cancer.

VI. MANAGEMENT.
Small tumors of the anal verge or the anal canal (<2 cm) can be cured in 80% of cases by simple excision with 1-cm margins, and cure by repeat local excision may be possible after local recurrence. An approach derived from Mohs surgery in which involved tissue is shaved and examined by a pathologist at the bedside until negative margins have been obtained is commonly done for Tis lesions. Combined chemotherapy and RT are the primary therapeutic modalities for more advanced anal verge or anal canal carcinoma. AP resection is now used as salvage treatment for chemoradiation-resistant disease (i.e., patients who fail to respond or who relapse after a complete response) and for patients who have fecal incontinence at presentation. Considering the rarity of anal canal cancer, randomized trials have led to considerable advances, shifting the standard of therapy from surgery, in which colostomy was routinely necessary as a first approach, to combined-modality chemoradiotherapy, leaving surgery as a last resort.

A. Combined chemoradiation therapy is the primary treatment of choice for anal carcinoma. This combination resulted in higher rates of both local control and survival (82%) and preserved anal function when compared with surgery. The administration of high-dose RT reduced the incidence of persistent carcinoma and eliminated the need for surgical lymphadenectomy. The radiation dose, the number of chemotherapy cycles required to improve the local control rate, and the role (if any) of invasive restaging after completion of therapy remain controversial.

1. Primary therapy. External-beam RT appears to be superior to interstitial implants. RT doses of >5,000 cGy do not appear to be necessary. Using mitomycin C plus 5-FU with RT is superior to using 5-FU alone with RT at 4 years of median follow-up with respect to colostomy-free survival (71% vs. 59%), locoregional control (82% vs. 64%), and DFS (73% vs. 51%). The combination of these two drugs when administered concurrently with RT is superior to RT alone. RT regimens vary among institutions; 5-FU is given by continuous IV infusion in each case. Two useful regimens are as follows:

a. Radiation Therapy Oncology Group (RTOG)

Mitomycin C: 10 mg/m^2 IV bolus (day 2)

5-FU: 1,000 mg/m^2/24 hours by continuous IV infusion (days 2 to 4 and days 28 to 32)

RT: 170 cGy/day between days 1 and 28
Total RT dose: 4,500 to 5,000 cGy

b. National Tumor Institute (Milan)

Mitomycin C: 15 mg/m^2 IV bolus (day 1)
5-FU: 750 mg/m^2/24 hours by continuous IV infusion (days 1 to 5)
RT: 180 cGy/day for 4 weeks with a 2-week rest
Total RT dose: 5,400 cGy (in patients with locally advanced disease, the boost dose is increased but the total dose does not exceed 6,000 cGy)

  2. Follow-up therapy. Additional 6-week cycles of chemotherapy with mitomycin C and 5-FU are given depending on tumor control or treatment toxicity. Full-thickness biopsy at the original tumor site is often performed 6 to 8 weeks after the completion of therapy. Patients are examined via digital examination and anoscopy at 3-month intervals for the first year and at 6-month intervals thereafter. AP resection is performed for biopsy-proven carcinoma during the follow-up period. Second-line chemotherapy with 5-FU plus cisplatin and AP resection are potentially curative salvage approaches after relapse.

B. Surgery alone. Wide, full-thickness excision is sufficient treatment for discrete, superficial, anal margin tumors and results in an 80% 5-year survival rate unless the tumor is large and deep. AP resection of the anorectum as the exclusive treatment for anal canal tumors and large anal margin tumors results in only a 55% 5-year survival rate.

C. Follow-up of patients with anal cancer every 3 months with digital rectal examination, anoscopy or proctoscopy, and biopsy of suspicious lesions is especially important during the first 3 years after initial treatment because salvage therapy may be curative.

PANCREATIC CANCER

I. EPIDEMIOLOGY AND ETIOLOGY

A. Incidence. In the United States, the incidence of pancreatic cancer has remained stable for several decades. There are approximately 31,000 new cases diagnosed annually in the United States and 30,000 deaths from pancreatic cancer, making it the fifth leading cause of U.S. cancer deaths. The disease has a male-to-female ratio of 1:1 and is rare before the age of 45 years; the peak incidence occurs between the ages of 65 and 79 years.

  In India, Kuwait, and Singapore, the rate is <2 per 100,000 population. In Japan, the incidence has risen sharply from 2 to 5 per 100,000 since the early 1980s.

B. Etiology and risk factors. The cause of pancreatic adenocarcinoma remains unknown, but several factors show a modest association with its occurrence.

  1. Cigarette smoking is a consistently noted risk factor for pancreatic cancer, with a relative risk of at least 1.5. The risk increases with increasing duration and amount of cigarette smoking. The excess risk levels off 10 to 15 years after cessation of smoking. The risk is ascribed to tobacco-specific nitrosamines.

  2. Diet. A high intake of fat, meat, or both, is associated with increased risk, whereas the intake of fresh fruits and vegetables appears to have a protective effect.

  3. Partial gastrectomy appears to correlate with a 2 to 5 times higher than expected incidence of pancreatic cancer 15 to 20 years later. The increased formation of N-nitroso compounds by bacteria that produce nitrate reductase and proliferate in the hypoacidic stomach has been proposed to account for the increased occurrence of gastric and pancreatic cancer after partial gastrectomy.

  4. Cholecystokinin is the primary hormone that causes growth of exocrine pancreatic cells; others include epidermal growth factor and insulinlike growth factors. Pancreatic cancer has been induced experimentally by long-term duodenogastric reflux, which is associated with increased cholecystokinin levels. Some clinical evidence suggests that cholecystectomy, which also increases the circulating cholecystokinin, may increase the risk for pancreatic cancer.

5. **Diabetes mellitus** may be an early manifestation of pancreatic cancer or a predisposing factor. It is found in 13% of patients with pancreatic cancer and in only 2% of controls. Diabetes mellitus that occurs in patients with pancreatic cancer may be characterized by marked insulin resistance, which moderates after tumor resection. Islet amyloid polypeptide, a hormonal factor secreted by pancreatic β cells, reduces insulin sensitivity *in vivo* and glycogen synthesis *in vitro* and may be present in elevated concentrations in patients with pancreatic cancer who have diabetes.

6. **Chronic and hereditary pancreatitis** is associated with pancreatic cancer. Chronic pancreatitis is associated with a 15-fold increase in the risk for pancreatic cancer.

7. **Toxic substances.** Occupational exposure to 2-naphthylamine, benzidine, and gasoline derivatives is associated with a fivefold increased risk for pancreatic cancer. Prolonged exposure to DDT and two DDT derivatives (ethylan and DDD) is associated with a fourfold to sevenfold increased risk for pancreatic cancer.

8. **Socioeconomic status.** Pancreatic cancer occurs in a slightly higher frequency in populations of lower socioeconomic status.

9. **Coffee.** Analysis of 30 epidemiologic studies showed that only one case-control study and none of the prospective studies confirmed a statistically significant association between coffee consumption and pancreatic cancer.

10. **Idiopathic deep-vein thrombosis** is statistically correlated with the subsequent development of mucinous carcinomas (including pancreatic cancer), especially among patients in whom venous thrombosis recurs during follow-up.

11. **Dermatomyositis and polymyositis** are paraneoplastic syndromes associated with pancreatic cancer and other cancers.

12. **Tonsillectomy** has been shown to be a protective factor against the development of pancreatic cancer, an observation that has been described for other cancers as well.

13. **Familial pancreatic cancer.** It is estimated that 3% of pancreatic cancers are linked to inherited predisposition to the disease.

II. PATHOLOGY

A. **Primary malignant tumors** of the pancreas involve either the exocrine parenchyma or the endocrine islet cells (the latter are discussed in Chapter 15, section VI). Nonepithelial tumors (sarcomas and lymphomas) are rare. Ductal adenocarcinoma makes up 75% to 90% of malignant pancreatic neoplasms: 57% occur in the head of the pancreas, 9% in the body, 8% in the tail, 6% in overlapping sites, and 20% in unknown anatomic subsites. Uncommon but reasonably distinctive variants of pancreatic cancer include adenosquamous, oncocytic, clear cell, giant cell, signet ring, mucinous, and anaplastic carcinoma. Anaplastic carcinomas often involve the body and tail rather than the head of pancreas. Reported cases of pure epidermoid carcinoma (a variant of adenosquamous carcinoma) probably are associated with hypercalcemia. Cystadenocarcinomas have an indolent course and may remain localized for many years. Ampullary cancer (which carries a significantly better prognosis), duodenal cancer, and distal bile duct cancer may be difficult to distinguish from pancreatic adenocarcinoma.

B. **Metastatic tumors.** Autopsy studies show that for every primary tumor of the pancreas, four metastatic tumors are found. The most common tumors of origin are the breast, lung, cutaneous melanoma, and non-Hodgkin lymphoma.

C. **Genetic abnormalities.** Mutant *c-K-ras* genes have been found in approximately 95% of all specimens of human pancreatic carcinoma and their metastases.

III. DIAGNOSIS

A. **Symptoms.** Most patients with pancreatic cancer have symptoms at the time of diagnosis. Predominant initial symptoms include abdominal pain (80%); anorexia (65%); weight loss (60%); early satiety (60%); xerostomia and sleep problems (55%); jaundice (50%); easy fatigability (45%); weakness, nausea, or constipation (40%); depression (40%); dyspepsia (35%); vomiting (30%); hoarseness (25%);

taste change, bloating, or belching (25%); dyspnea, dizziness, or edema (20%); cough, diarrhea because of fat malabsorption, hiccup, or itching (15%); and dysphagia (5%).

B. Clinical findings. At presentation, patients with pancreatic cancer have cachexia (44%), serum albumin concentration of <3.5 g/dL (35%), palpable abdominal mass (35%), ascites (25%), or supraclavicular lymphadenopathy (5%). Metastases are present in at least one major organ in 65% of patients, to the liver in 45%, to the lungs in 30%, and to the bones in 3%. Carcinomas of the distal pancreas do not produce jaundice until they metastasize and may remain painless until the disease is advanced. Occasionally, acute pancreatitis is the first manifestation of pancreatic cancer.

C. Paraneoplastic syndromes. Panniculitis-arthritis-eosinophilia syndrome that occurs with pancreatic cancer appears to be caused by the release of lipase from the tumor. Dermatomyositis, polymyositis, recurrent Trousseau syndrome or idiopathic deep-vein thrombosis, and Cushing syndrome have been reported to be associated with cancer of the pancreas.

D. Diagnostic studies

   1. Ultrasonography. Abdominal ultrasound is technically adequate in 60% to 90% of patients and is noninvasive, safe, and inexpensive. Ultrasound can detect pancreatic masses as small as 2 cm, dilation of the pancreatic and bile ducts, hepatic metastases, and extrapancreatic spread. Intraoperative ultrasound facilitates surgical biopsy and may detect unsuspected liver metastases in 50% of patients.

   2. CT is less operator-dependent than ultrasound and is not limited by air-containing abdominal organs, as is ultrasound. CT is favored over ultrasound because of its superior ability to demonstrate retroperitoneal invasion and lymphadenopathy. A pancreatic tumor must be at least 2 cm in diameter to become visible. *Dynamic CT* with continuous infusion of IV contrast is the best test for assessing the size of the tumor and its extension. At least 20% of pancreatic tumors believed to be resectable may not be detectable by CT.

   3. MRI has no demonstrated advantage over CT in the diagnosis and staging of pancreatic cancer.

   4. Endoscopic retrograde cholangiopancreaticography (ERCP) is the mainstay in the differential diagnosis of the tumors of the pancreatobiliary junction, 85% of which originate in the pancreas (about 5% each in the distal common bile duct, ampulla, and duodenum). Ampullary and duodenal carcinoma can usually be visualized and biopsy performed with ERCP. The pancreatogram typically shows the pancreatic duct to be encased or obstructed by carcinoma in 97% of cases.

   It may be difficult to distinguish between pancreatic cancer and chronic pancreatitis because both diseases share clinical and radiologic characteristics. Pancreatic duct stricture usually does not exceed 5 mm in chronic pancreatitis; strictures longer than 10 mm (especially if irregular) indicate pancreatic cancer. Cytologic examination of cells in samples of pancreatic juice obtained during ERCP with secretin stimulation has been reported to be highly specific for the diagnosis of carcinoma and 85% sensitive. Brush biopsy of the pancreatic stricture (when possible) increases the diagnostic yield.

   5. EUS. Prospective studies showed that EUS is more accurate than standard ultrasound, CT, and ERCP for diagnosis, staging, and predicting resectability of pancreatic tumors. EUS detected 100% of malignant lesions <3 cm, whereas angiography, CT, and ultrasound were of limited value for these small lesions. EUS can detect tumors smaller than 2 cm; ERCP cannot. The additional information obtained from EUS has been reported to result in a major change in the clinical management in one-third of patients and to aid in the clinical decision in three-fourths of patients.

   The current limitations of EUS include a short optimal focal range of only 4 cm, inability to differentiate focal chronic pancreatitis from carcinoma reliably, and inability to differentiate chronic lymphadenitis from metastatic lymph node involvement. The ability to biopsy lymph nodes using EUS does allow assessment of lymph nodes for malignancy in some cases.

6. **Percutaneous fine-needle aspiration cytology** is safe and reliable, with a reported sensitivity of 55% to 95% and no false-positive results for the diagnosis of pancreatic cancer. This procedure should be performed for histologic confirmation on all patients with unresectable or metastatic disease unless a palliative surgical procedure is planned. Needle aspiration cytology distinguishes adenocarcinoma from islet cell tumors, lymphomas, and cystic neoplasms of the pancreas, permitting therapy to be tailored to the specific diagnosis in each case.

The drawbacks to percutaneous aspiration biopsy include potential tumor seeding along the needle tract, potential to enhance intraperitoneal spread, and negative biopsy results that do not exclude the diagnosis of malignancy. Furthermore, the diagnosis of early and smaller tumors is most likely to be missed by this technique.

7. **Angiography** is excellent for assessing major vascular involvement but is not useful in determining the size and location of tumor (pancreatic cancer is hypovascular). In most cases, spiral CT scanning with proper administration of IV contrast allows resectability to be judged preoperatively.

8. **Laparoscopy** can demonstrate extrapancreatic involvement in 40% of patients without demonstrable lesions on CT.

9. **Tumor markers.** No available serum marker is sufficiently sensitive or specific to be considered reliable for screening of pancreatic cancer.
   a. **CA 19-9** is widely used for the diagnosis and follow-up of patients with pancreatic cancer but is not specific for pancreatic cancer.
   b. **CEA** is of minimal value in pancreatic cancer.

IV. STAGING AND PROGNOSTIC FACTORS

A. **Staging system.** The TNM system is most commonly used. Readers should consult an up-to-date staging manual because of frequent revisions of staging systems. T1 and T2 tumors are potentially resectable tumors. T1 tumors are localized to the pancreas, and T1a tumors are <2 cm in diameter. T2 indicates that there is a limited direct extension into the duodenum, bile duct, or stomach. T3 indicates advanced direct extension that is incompatible with surgical resection.

B. **Preoperative evaluation.** Identifying patients with unresectable pancreatic tumor or with metastasis or vessel involvement would spare many patients a major operation. Operative mortality and morbidity for pancreatic surgery remain high, except in specialized centers. Modern diagnostic methods have reduced unnecessary laparotomies from 30% to 5% and have increased the resectability rate on patients judged to be potentially resectable on the basis of preoperative imaging from 5% to 20%. Accuracy in determining resectability before exploration has become even more important because of the availability of effective decompression of biliary obstruction endoscopically for palliation of obstructive jaundice without the need for laparotomy.

CT, angiography, and laparoscopy assess different aspects of resectability and are complementary. In general, if one of these studies indicates vascular invasion or local or regional spread, the resectability rate is about 5%, whereas if all are negative, the resectability rate is 78%. Gross nodal involvement is usually associated with other signs of unresectability and may be identified by CT or EUS.

C. **Prognostic factors.** Fewer than 20% of patients with adenocarcinoma of the pancreas survive the first year, and only 3% are alive 5 years after the diagnosis.

1. **Resectable disease.** The 5-year survival rate of patients whose tumors were resected is poor; the reported range is 3% to 25%. The 5-year survival is 30% for patients with small tumors (≤2 cm in diameter), 35% for patients with no residual tumor or for patients in whom the tumor did not require dissection from major vessels, and 55% for patients without lymph node metastasis.

2. **Nonresectable or metastatic disease.** The median survival of patients with such disease is 2 to 6 months. Performance status and the presence of four symptoms (dyspnea, anorexia, weight loss, and xerostomia) appear to influence

survival; patients with the higher performance status and the least number of these symptoms lived the longest.

V. MANAGEMENT

A. Surgery. Only 5% to 20% of patients with pancreatic cancer have resectable tumors at the time of presentation.

1. **Surgical procedures**

   a. **Pancreaticoduodenal resection** (Whipple procedure or a modification) is the standard operation. This implies that only cancer involving the head of the pancreas is resectable.

   b. **A pylorus-preserving variation of Whipple procedure** is a commonly used operation in the United States, in part because it has resulted in a significant reduction of postgastrectomy syndrome with no decrease in survival.

   c. **An extended Whipple procedure,** with a more extensive lymph node dissection, is used commonly in Japan but has not been widely accepted in the United States because of higher morbidity and lack of data from randomized trials to suggest that the procedure results in better survival.

   d. **Regional pancreatectomy** confers no survival advantage over conventional Whipple procedure.

   e. **Total pancreatectomy** produces exocrine insufficiency and brittle diabetes mellitus and should be performed only when necessary to achieve clear surgical margins.

2. **Surgical mortality and morbidity.** The perioperative mortality rate from pancreatic resection is <5% when the operation is performed by expert surgeons. Nationally, however, the surgical mortality rate is about 18%. The major complication rate is 20% to 35% and includes sepsis, abscess formation, hemorrhage, and pancreatic and biliary fistulae.

3. **Relief of obstructive jaundice by surgical biliary bypass** (cholecystojejunostomy or choledochojejunostomy) is effective, but the average survival time is 5 months, and the postoperative mortality rate in large collected series is 20%. Jaundice can be relieved endoscopically by the placement of stents with a success rate of up to 85%, a procedure-related mortality rate of 1% to 2%, and significant reduction in the length of hospitalization and recovery compared with palliative surgery. Randomized trials showed no difference in survival between endoscopic stent placement and surgical bypass, but patients treated with stents had more frequent readmissions for stent obstruction, recurrent jaundice, and cholangitis.

B. Adjuvant therapy appears to be a reasonable approach to the patient who has undergone curative resection.

1. **Chemotherapy.** Prior trials assessing the potential benefit of adjuvant chemotherapy have shown mixed results. However, in a phase III trial 368 patients were randomized to either observation alone or six cycles of gemcitabine following gross complete resection. Significant improvement was noted in DFS, but only a trend toward benefit in overall survival.

2. **Combined-modality therapy.** There is one prospective randomized study of 43 patients (completed by the Gastrointestinal Study Group in the 1980s) that showed that adjuvant RT and 5-FU after a curative Whipple procedure improved survival. In that study, the median survival was 20 months for patients treated, and 3 of 21 patients survived 5 years or more. For patients not treated, the median survival was 11 months, and only 1 of 22 patients survived 5 years. The 5-year survival rate was 40% for patients with no lymph node involvement and <5% for patients with lymph node metastasis.

   An RTOG trial randomized patients to either gemcitabine or infusional 5-FU after surgery. Both groups also received radiation. The results of this trial showed improved significant improvement in survival for patients receiving gemcitabine, but only those with cancer arising from the head of the pancreas.

C. Therapy for locally advanced disease

1. **External-beam RT combined with 5-FU** (15 mg/kg IV on the first 3 and last 3 days of RT) significantly improves survival as compared with RT alone

(10 months vs. 5.5 months, respectively). Some favor the use of continuous-infusion 5-FU during irradiation, although there are no randomized trials to suggest incremental benefit to infusion over bolus 5-FU in pancreatic cancer.

2. **Intraoperative electron-beam RT** delivered to a surgically exposed tumor from which radiosensitive bowel has been excluded by insertion of a field-limiting cone increased the median survival compared with historical controls in selected patients to 13 months, with excellent local control (5% of patients have lived 3 to 8 years). Intraoperative RT relieves pain in 50% to 90% of patients.

D. Chemotherapy for metastatic disease. 5-FU has a response rate of 0% to 20% in pancreatic cancer. Weekly gemcitabine at a dose of 1,000 mg/m^2 for 3 of every 4 weeks has been shown to have activity and to provide palliative benefit exceeding that of 5-FU in a randomized trial of 126 patients with advanced disease. The median survival times were 5.6 versus 4.4 months ($p = 0.002$) for gemcitabine versus 5-FU, respectively. A potentially promising alternative schedule for the administration of gemcitabine using fixed-dose rate infusion, compared with the standard 30-minute infusion did not show benefit in a phase III trial. The administration of multiagent chemotherapy has generally not resulted in better outcomes than single-agent therapy. Several phase III trials comparing gemcitabine alone with gemcitabine and either oxaliplatin, bevacizumab, or cetuximab have all failed to show benefit. However, a significant improvement was seen in overall survival (6.2 vs. 5.9 months) when erlotinib was added to gemcitabine. The addition of capecitabine has also improved outcome when added to gemcitabine based on the preliminary presentation of a recently completed phase III trial.

E. Neuroablation for pain control. The relentless, boring, posterior abdominal and back pain caused when the celiac nerve plexus becomes invaded by pancreatic cancer can be extremely distressing and frequently requires the use of large doses of narcotics, particularly sustained-release morphine. Chemical splanchnicectomy (celiac axis nerve block) should be performed at the time of operation in nonresectable cases. Either 6% phenol or 50% alcohol (25 mL is injected on each side of the celiac axis) is used. This procedure results in relief of pancreatic cancer-related pain in >80% of patients. Percutaneous chemical neurolysis of the celiac ganglion, which may be attempted in patients who did not have an intraoperative splanchnicectomy or were not explored, is reported to be equally effective. Transient postural hypotension may occur. Celiac plexus block may be repeated if initially unsuccessful or if pain recurs.

F. Other supportive measures. Appetite suppression, decreased caloric intake, and malabsorption can all lead to cancer cachexia in patients with pancreatic cancer. Megestrol acetate (Megace) suspension in doses up to 800 mg/day can be an effective appetite stimulant for treatment of anorexia. Calorie supplements are also potentially valuable. Fat malabsorption resulting from loss of the exocrine function of the pancreas responds to pancreatic enzyme replacement. Ascites can be managed with diuretics when possible and paracentesis when necessary. Removal of protein-rich ascitic fluid, however, can become an additional contributor to the negative protein balance in these already malnourished patients.

LIVER CANCER

I. EPIDEMIOLOGY AND ETIOLOGY

A. Incidence. Liver cancer is among the most common neoplasms and causes of cancer death in the world, occurring most commonly in Africa and Asia. Up to one million deaths due to hepatocellular carcinoma (HCC) occur each year worldwide. In the United States, 17,000 new cases of cancer of the liver and biliary passages develop annually. Incidence throughout the world varies dramatically, with 115 cases per 100,000 people noted in China and Thailand, compared with 1 to 2 cases per 100,000 in Britain. In countries with high incidence rates, there are often subpopulations also with high incidence rates living nearby lower risk subpopulations. For example, the incidence rates in black South Africans and Alaska Natives far exceeds those of nearby white populations. HCC is 4 to 9 times more common in men than in women.

B. Conditions predisposing to HCC

1. **Hepatitis B virus (HBV).** High titers of hepatitis B surface antigen (HBsAg) and core antibody (HBcAb) are frequently found in patients with HCC. HBsAg was found in the serum of 50% to 60% of patients with HCC and in 5% to 10% of the general population. In the United States, HCC is increased by 140-fold in HBsAg carriers. Anti-HBcAb was found in 90% of black South African and 75% of Japanese patients with HCC, as compared with 35% and 30% of matched controls, respectively. When HCC develops, the patient usually has had chronic HBV infection for three to four decades. The risk factors for the development of HCC in HBsAg carriers are the presence of cirrhosis, family history of HCC, increasing age, male sex, Asian or African race, cofactors (such as alcohol, aflatoxin, and perhaps smoking), and the duration of the carrier state. In Asia, HBV is transmitted vertically from mother to infant in the first few months of life; in Africa, HBV is transmitted horizontally.

2. **Cirrhosis.** HCC often develops in a cirrhotic liver. Autopsy studies showed that 60% to 90% of HBsAg-positive subjects have associated cirrhosis and 20% to 40% of patients with cirrhosis have HCC. Studies show that in Taiwan, the annual estimated incidence of HCC is 0.005% in HBsAg-negative patients, 0.25% in HBsAg-positive patients, and 2.5% in HBsAg-positive patients with liver cirrhosis (500 times higher than in HBsAg-negative patients). In France, the development of HCC in the presence of alcoholic cirrhosis was nearly always associated with HBV infection, and alcoholism was thought to hasten the development of HCC. In Italy, the prevalence of HCC in patients with cirrhosis was nearly 7%, with a yearly crude incidence of 3%; hepatitis C virus (HCV) chronic infection was the cause of cirrhosis in 45% of these patients. A clear association between alcohol-induced cirrhosis and HCC exists; associations between alcohol and HCC in the absence of cirrhosis are less clear.

3. **HCV infection** is a risk factor for the development of HCC. Apparently, HCV induces cirrhosis and to a lesser extent increases the risks for HCC in patients with cirrhosis. HCV infection acts independently of HBV infection, alcohol abuse, age, and gender. The ratios for HCC risk factors in patients with chronic liver disease, adjusted for age, sex, and other factors, are as follows:
   a. Risk ratio six- to sevenfold: age, 60 to 69 years; HBsAg-positive
   b. Risk ratio fourfold: high-titer anti-HBcAb, anti-HCV positivity
   c. Risk ratio twofold: presence of liver cirrhosis, currently smoking

4. **Aflatoxins** are produced by the ubiquitous fungi *Aspergillus flavus* or *Aspergillus parasiticus,* which commonly colonize peanuts, corn, and cassava in all except extremely cold climates. Aflatoxin B1 has been proved to be a potent hepatocarcinogen in experimental animals, and the amount of exposure is correlated with increased HCC risk in humans. For example, the daily intake of aflatoxin in Mozambique is 4 times greater than in Kenya, and the incidence of HCC is 8 times greater.

5. **Mutations of tumor-suppressor gene** *p53* have been reported in half of patients with HCC. These mutations, specifically of 249^{ser} *p53*, are correlated both with geographic areas where the ingestion of aflatoxin is common and with the prevalence of HBV infection.

6. **Sex hormones.** The risk for liver cell adenomas and HCC is increased in women who have used oral contraceptives for 8 or more years. Although liver cell adenomas regress with discontinuation of oral contraceptives in most cases, adenomas must be considered premalignant. Close and prolonged follow-up is necessary for women with adenomas who continue to use oral contraceptives. HCC has also been observed in people with a history of anabolic steroid use.

7. **Cigarette smoking, alcohol intake, diabetes, and insulin intake.** A study performed in Los Angeles showed that in non-Asian populations that have a low risk for HCC, cigarette smoking, heavy alcohol consumption, and diabetes mellitus,

especially with insulin administration, appear to be significant risk factors for HCC.

8. **Other factors.** A relatively small number of HCCs develop in patients with various other diseases. The most common of these are α_1-antitrypsin deficiency, tyrosinemia, and hemochromatosis. Phlebotomy therapy can deplete hepatic iron and induce regression of hepatic fibrosis but does not prevent the development of HCC in hemochromatosis. Clonorchiasis, vinyl chloride exposure, and administration of thorium dioxide (an x-ray contrast agent used between 1930 and 1955) or methotrexate are also associated with the development of HCC.

II. PATHOLOGY AND NATURAL HISTORY
A. Pathology

1. **Liver cell adenoma** has low malignant potential. True adenomas of the liver are rare and occur mostly in women taking oral contraceptives. Most adenomas are solitary; occasionally multiple (10 or more) tumors develop in a condition known as *liver cell adenomatosis*. These tumors are smooth, encapsulated masses and do not contain Kupffer cells. Patients usually have symptoms; hemoperitoneum occurs in 25% of cases.

2. **Focal nodular hyperplasia** (FNH) has no malignant potential. FNH occurs with a female-to-male ratio of 2:1. The relationship of oral contraceptives to FNH is not as clear as for hepatic adenoma; only half of patients with FNH take oral contraceptives. FNH tumors are nodular, are not encapsulated, but do contain Kupffer cells. Patients usually do not have symptoms; hemoperitoneum rarely occurs.

3. **HCC** may present grossly as a single mass, as multiple nodules, or as diffuse liver involvement; these are referred to as *massive, nodular,* and *diffuse* forms. The growth pattern microscopically is trabecular, solid, or tubular, and the stroma, in contrast to bile duct carcinoma, is scanty. A rare sclerosing or fibrosing form has been associated with hypercalcemia. Fibrolamellar carcinoma, another variant, occurs predominantly in young patients without cirrhosis, has a favorable prognosis, and is not associated with elevation of serum α-fetoprotein (FP) levels. In the United States, almost half of HCCs in patients younger than 35 years of age are fibrolamellar, and more than half of them are resectable.

   Table 9.6 depicts the clinical and pathologic differences between HCC, bile duct carcinoma, and metastatic adenocarcinoma. Appendix C-4.IV shows immunohistochemical phenotypes of HCC and bile duct carcinomas as well as other adenocarcinomas.

B. Natural history.
Most patients die from hepatic failure and not from distant metastases. The disease is contained within the liver in only 20% of cases. HCC invades the portal vein in 35% of cases, hepatic vein in 15%, contiguous abdominal organs in 15%, and vena cava and right atrium in 5%. HCC metastasizes to the lung in 35% of cases, abdominal lymph nodes in 20%, thoracic or cervical lymph nodes in 5%, vertebrae in 5%, and kidney or adrenal gland in 5%.

C. Associated paraneoplastic syndromes
include fever, erythrocytosis, hypercholesterolemia, gynecomastia, hypercalcemia, hypoglycemia, and virilization (precocious puberty).

III. DIAGNOSIS

A. Symptoms and signs.
Pain in the right subcostal area or on top of the shoulder from phrenic irritation is common (95%). Severe symptoms of fatigue (31%), anorexia (27%), weight loss (35%), and unexplained fever (30% to 40%) are not uncommon. Many patients have vague abdominal pain, fever, and anorexia for up to 2 years before the diagnosis of carcinoma is made. Hemorrhage into the peritoneal cavity is often seen in patients with HCC and may be fatal. Ascites or the presence of an upper abdominal mass noticeable by the patient is an ominous prognostic sign. Any sudden deterioration in a patient with known liver disease or with positive HbsAg or hepatitis C serology should raise the suspicion of HCC. Physical findings include

| TABLE 9.6 | Differential Diagnosis of Hepatocellular Carcinoma (HCC) Versus Adenocarcinoma | |

Characteristics	HCC	Adenocarcinoma[a]
Clinical features		
Sex predilection	Male	None
Presence of cirrhosis	Common	Exceptional
Preferential spread	Venous	Lymphatics
Pathologic features		
Gross features	Soft and hemorrhagic	Hard and whitish
Main growth pattern	Trabecular	Glandular
Growth at tumor margin	Replacement	Often sinusoidal
Fibrous stroma	Minimal[b]	Often prominent
Microscopic features		
Tumor cell nucleus		
Intranuclear inclusions	Common	Uncommon
Prominent nucleolus	Typical	Often
Tumor cell cytoplasm	Often abundant	Variable
Hyaline globules	Occ present	Rare
Mallory bodies	Occ present	Absent
Bile	Occ present	Absent
Mucin	Absent	Often present
Hepatocyte dysplasia	May be present	Absent
Immunohistochemistry		
α-Fetoprotein	Often present	Occ present (metastases)
β-Antitrypsin	Often present	Absent
Villin	Often present	Absent
Hb$_s$Ag	Often present	Absent
Polyclonal CEA (canalicular)	Often present	Absent
Monoclonal CEA (cytoplasmic)	Rarely present	Often present
Erythropoiesis associated	Often present	Absent

Occ, occasionally; CEA, carcinoembryonic antigen.
[a]Adenocarcinoma, cholangiocarcinoma, and metastatic adenocarcinoma.
[b]The fibrolamellar and sclerosing variants of HCC are exceptions because they contain prominently fibrous stroma.
Adapted from Sternberg SS, eds. *Diagnostic Surgical Pathology.* 2nd ed. New York: Raven Press; 1994:1543, and other sources.

hepatomegaly (90%), splenomegaly (65%), ascites (52%), fever (38%), jaundice (41%), hepatic bruit (28%), and cachexia (15%).

B. Diagnostic studies

  1. LFTs may be normal or elevated and are affected by liver cirrhosis. Elevated serum bilirubin and lactate dehydrogenase values and lowered serum albumin are associated with poor survival. Serum γ-glutamyl transferase (GGT) isoenzyme II (of 11 isoenzymes) was positive in 90% of patients with HCC. GGT-II was negative in most patients with acute and chronic viral hepatitis or extrahepatic tumors, in pregnant women, and in healthy controls. GGT-II was found to be valuable for the detection of small or subclinical HCC.

  2. Biopsy of liver nodules. Some authors believe that percutaneous liver biopsy carries a high risk and has little or no role in the workup of liver tumors, whereas others believe that it can be performed without any significant risk. Nevertheless, liver biopsy is needed to establish the diagnosis and may be obtained either at operation or percutaneously.

3. **Serum tumor markers.** Serum α-FP is often elevated in patients with HCC but can also be elevated in patients with benign chronic liver disease. In patients with liver cirrhosis and no HCC, serum α-FP may be normal or elevated, with values ranging from 30 to 460 ng/mL (median, 30 to 70 ng/mL). In patients with HCC, the serum α-FP concentrations may range from 30 to 7,000 ng/mL (median, 275 ng/mL). Measurement of α-FP fractions L3, P4, and P5 (different sugar-chain structures) may allow the differentiation of HCC from cirrhosis in some cases. It may also be predictive for the development of HCC during follow-up of patients with cirrhosis. Serum ferritin levels are also frequently elevated in patients with HCC.

4. **Radiologic studies**

   a. **Ultrasound.** HCC is usually well circumscribed, hyperechogenic, and associated with diffuse distortion of the normal hepatic parenchyma. Metastatic deposits are usually hyperechogenic but may be hypoechogenic.

   b. **CT.** HCC typically appears as an area of low attenuation on CT. Lesions may occasionally be isodense with normal hepatic parenchyma, however. Metastatic tumors with low attenuation (close to the density of water) include mucin-producing tumors of the ovary, pancreas, colon, and stomach and tumors with necrotic centers, such as sarcomas. Mucin-producing metastases may have nearly normal attenuation values because of diffuse microscopic calcifications within the tumor.

   c. **MRI** has been reported to be superior to CT scanning and ultrasound for the detection of liver tumors.

   d. **Selective hepatic, celiac, and superior mesenteric angiography** can confirm portal vein involvement, define the arterial supply, and identify vascular lesions that are as small as 3 mm in diameter. Intra-arterial epinephrine injection can differentiate normal hepatic arteries from tumor vessels, which do not constrict because of the absence of smooth muscles in their walls.

   e. **Radionuclide scans**

      (1) **Liver–spleen scan.** All primary and metastatic liver tumors, except for FNH and regenerating nodules, are devoid of Kupffer cells and appear as "cold" areas in liver scans. However, the liver-spleen scan has now been replaced by MRI, ultrasound, and CT.

      (2) **Gallium scan** of liver may be able to differentiate primary hepatic tumors from metastatic carcinoma because gallium is taken up by the HCC.

IV. STAGING AND PROGNOSTIC FACTORS

A. **Staging.** The initial step is to establish whether the HCC is resectable. Indications of unresectability may be determined either at exploratory laparotomy, by laparoscopy, or by CT, MRI, or angiography. Unresectable disease includes bilobar or four-segment hepatic parenchymal involvement, portal vein thrombus, and vena caval involvement with tumor or tumor thrombus. Metastatic disease includes involvement of regional lymph nodes, which is proved by biopsy at surgery. Liver failure or portal hypertension alone does not contraindicate surgery. Readers should consult an up-to-date staging manual because of frequent revisions of staging systems.

B. **Prognostic factors.** The number of liver lesions and the presence of vascular involvement are the most significant prognostic determinants in patients with disease limited to the liver. Neither the presence nor the degree of α-FP elevation has any prognostic importance. The prognostic factors that relate to survival in patients with resectable HCC are as follows:

   1. **Number, size, and location of liver lesions.** The 5-year survival rate for patients with a solitary tumor is 45%, and it is 15% to 25% for those with multiple liver lesions. The 5-year survival rate is 40% to 45% for patients with small tumors (2 to 5 cm) and 10% for patients with tumors larger than 5 cm. Patients without cirrhosis with tumors located in the left lobe of the liver or in the right inferior segments (anteriorly or posteriorly) have the best prognosis.

   2. **Vein involvement.** All patients with gross tumor thrombi involving the portal vein or the hepatic vein die within 3 years, whereas the 5-year survival rate for patients with no vascular involvement of any kind is 30%.

3. **Extent and type of resection.** The 5-year survival rate for patients undergoing curative resection is 55%, compared with 5% for those undergoing noncurative resections. The 5-year survival rate is 85% for hepatic lobectomy, 50% for sub-segmentectomy, and 20% for wedge enucleation. In patients with resected HCC, the liver is the site of disease recurrence in 90% of cases.

4. **Hepatic reserve.** Patients who have better hepatic reserve, as determined by retention rate of indocyanine green dye at 15 minutes, have better survival.

V. PREVENTION AND EARLY DETECTION

A. Prevention. Avoidance of the risk factors for HCC is difficult in those parts of the world where socioeconomic conditions are poor and where HBV infection is endemic. The widespread use of HBV vaccine may affect the incidence of HCC, but with a considerable lag time.

1. Almost four billion people (75% of the world population) live in areas of intermediate or higher prevalence of HBV. Infections with HBV and HCV can be treated with interferons, although prevention of initial infection is preferable. Protection against HBV, if attempted, is best done in infancy. In the United States, vaccination with recombinant HBsAg is recommended for health workers in contact with blood, for people residing for >6 months in areas that are highly endemic for HBV, and for all others at risk. Interferon-α treatment of patients with chronic active hepatitis and cirrhosis lowered the rate of progression to hepatocellular carcinoma twofold in one trial.

2. Steps should be taken to reduce the high levels of aflatoxin food contaminations that occur in many areas of Asia and southern Africa, as has been done in the Western world.

B. Early detection. Two recent reports describe attempts for early detection of HCC in patients with liver cirrhosis. A study from Italy shows that patients with persistently elevated serum α-FP have a higher incidence of HCC (3% per year) than those with fluctuating levels. This screening program did not appreciably increase the rate of detection of potentially curable liver tumors, however. In a study from Japan, higher percentages of α-FP L3, P4, and P5 fractions allowed the differentiation of HCC in some cases.

VI. MANAGEMENT

A. Liver anatomy. The liver is anatomically divided into four lobes: a larger right lobe, which is separated from a smaller left lobe by the attachment of the falciform ligament, and two small lobes (the quadrate lobe on the anterior inferior aspect and the caudate lobe). Practical surgical anatomy divides the liver into nearly equal halves, and each half is divided into two segments. The right half is divided into anterior (ventrocranial) and posterior (dorsocaudal) segments. The left half is divided into medial and lateral segments by a visible left sagittal accessory fissure. Each of the four segments is subdivided into superior and inferior subsegments. The French literature labels the eight liver subsegments with Roman numerals.

B. Localized and resectable HCC. Only 10% of HCCs are resectable with solitary or unilobar hepatic lesions at the time of diagnosis. The survival in resectable lesions depends on the prognostic factors discussed in section IV.B. In the United States, the median survival after surgical resection is about 22 months for patients with cirrhotic livers and 32 months for patients with normal livers (range, 2 months to 15 years). The perioperative morbidity is minimal and is slightly higher in the cirrhotic group. Morbidity includes subphrenic abscess, subhepatic abscess, pneumothorax, and wound infection. Total hepatectomy with orthotopic liver transplantation may be of benefit in patients with unresectable nonmetastatic fibrolamellar HCC, intrahepatic bile duct cancers, or hemangiosarcoma and is under investigation as a strategy for patients with poor underlying hepatic function or bilobar disease limited to the liver.

C. Localized and nonresectable disease

1. **Preoperative multimodality treatment followed by surgery.** There are no current preoperative approaches that have been shown to be of benefit.

2. **Transcatheter arterial chemoembolization (TACE)** of unresectable HCC using a mixture of Gelfoam powder, Lipiodol, and contrast media with

chemotherapeutic drugs has been used with some success. TACE may also be used preoperatively to reduce intraoperative bleeding or as a palliative measure in patients with far advanced HCC. Recent trials with TACE suggest that there may be a survival advantage with its use.

3. Transcatheter arterial radioembolization (TARE) is a newer modality that uses tumor ablation by transarterial injection of Y90 radioactive microspheres following the principles of transarterial chemoembolization. TARE has not been as rigorously studied as TACE. Early uncontrolled studies suggest that there is a risk of progressive long-term liver decompensation in patients with more advanced liver disease at the time of treatment initiation.

4. Other treatments. Percutaneous intralesional installation of absolute ethanol under ultrasound guidance has resulted in a reported 5-year survival rate of nearly 80% in highly selected patients, particularly those with small tumors who are not surgical candidates. The use of radiofrequency ablation has become a common alternative to ethanol ablation. Radiofrequency ablation is performed by applying a high-frequency electrical current through a treatment probe that is inserted into the HCC. Cryosurgery has been reported to have similar efficacy in highly selected patients.

D. Nonresectable and metastatic disease

1. Targeted and antiangiogenic therapy has shown early evidence of promise. In a randomized phase III trial comparing sorafenib with best supportive care, a significant increase in overall survival of approximately 2.5 months was seen with the use of sorafenib. A number of trials are underway to better assess this drug and other similar drugs when used alone or in combination with other agents.

2. Hormonal therapy. About 40% of patients with HCC have estrogen receptor protein in the cell cytosol. Large tumors are commonly estrogen receptor-negative. In a prospective, randomized study of tamoxifen (40 mg/day) plus best supportive care versus best supportive care alone, there was no difference in median survival (16 vs. 15 months). Similar negative results have been observed in trials with flutamide, megestrol acetate, and octreotide.

3. Systemic chemotherapy has a response rate of 10% or less and does not affect median survival (3 to 6 months). Doxorubicin as a single agent or in combination with other drugs has been used. Other than in highly selected circumstances, the use of chemotherapy is generally not recommended.

 GALLBLADDER CANCER

I. EPIDEMIOLOGY AND ETIOLOGY

A. Incidence. Primary gallbladder carcinoma (GBC) is the most common malignant tumor of the biliary tract and the fifth most common cancer of the digestive tract. There are 6,000 to 7,000 cases annually in the United States. GBCs were found in 1% to 2% of operations on the biliary tract.

B. Risk factors. The cause of GBC remains unknown. Reported risk factors include the following:

1. Sex. The female-to-male ratio is 3:1 to 4:1. Acalculous carcinoma is also more common in women.

2. Race. The incidence of GBC is doubled in southwestern American Indians, who also have a two- to threefold greater incidence of cholelithiasis. The incidence of GBC is also high in Peru and Ecuador among populations with Native American genealogy.

3. Older age. The mean age for the occurrence of GBC is 65 years; the disease is rare before 40 years of age.

4. Chronic cholecystitis and cholelithiasis are associated with the development of GBC in 50% and 75% of cases, respectively. Latency periods are lengthy; 1% of patients known to have gallstones for >20 years develop GBC. Those with larger stones are more prone to GBC than those with stones smaller than 1 cm. The incidence of GBC is decreasing among populations in the world where cholecystectomy is becoming more common. Calcification of the wall of the gall-bladder (porcelain gallbladder) increases the risk for GBC by 10% to 60%. Chole-cystitis associated with liver flukes and in chronic typhoid carriers is linked to the increased incidence of GBC.

5. **Benign neoplasms.** Both inflammatory and cholesterol polyps are associated with appreciable risk. Papillary and nonpapillary adenomas of the gallbladder may contain carcinoma *in situ.* Malignant transformation is rare, however.

6. **Ulcerative colitis** increases the risk for extrahepatic biliary cancer by a factor of 5 to 10; 15% of these cancers occur in the gallbladder.

7. **Carcinogens.** Rubber industry employees have a higher incidence and earlier onset of GBC.

II. PATHOLOGY AND NATURAL HISTORY

A. **Pathology.** Most GBCs are adenocarcinomas (80%) showing varying degrees of differentiation. The mucus secreted by this cancer is typically of the sialomucin type, in contrast to the sulfomucin type secreted by the normal or inflamed mucus-secreting glands. Other types of GBC include adenoacanthoma, adenosquamous carcinomas, and undifferentiated (anaplastic, pleomorphic, sarcomatoid) carcinomas. Some adenocarcinomas have choriocarcinomalike elements, and others have morphology equivalent to small cell carcinoma.

B. **Natural history.** GBC has a propensity to involve the liver, stomach, and duodenum by direct extension. The common sites of metastasis are the liver (60%), adjacent organs (55%), regional lymph nodes (35%), peritoneum (25%), and distant visceral organs (30%).

C. **Clinical presentation.** GBC may present as one of the following clinical syndromes:

1. **Acute cholecystitis** (15% of patients). These patients appear to have less advanced carcinoma, a higher rate of resectability, and longer survival.

2. **Chronic cholecystitis** (45%)

3. **Symptoms suggestive of malignant disease** (e.g., jaundice, weight loss, generalized weakness, anorexia, or persistent right upper quadrant pain; 35%)

4. **Benign nonbiliary manifestations** (e.g., GI bleeding or obstruction; 5%)

III. DIAGNOSIS

A. **Symptoms.** The lack of specific symptoms prevents detection of GBC at an early stage. Consequently, the diagnosis is usually made unexpectedly at the time of surgery because the clinical signs commonly mimic benign gallbladder disease. Pain is present in 79% of patients; jaundice, anorexia, or nausea and vomiting in 45% to 55%; weight loss or fatigue in 30%; and pruritus or abdominal mass in 15%.

B. **Physical examination.** Certain combinations of symptoms and signs may suggest the diagnosis, such as an elderly woman with a history of chronic biliary symptoms that have changed in frequency or severity. A right upper quadrant mass or hepatomegaly and constitutional symptoms suggest GBC.

C. **Laboratory examination.** Elevated serum alkaline phosphatase is present in 65% of patients, anemia in 55%, elevated bilirubin in 40%, leukocytosis in 40%, and leukemoid reaction in 1% of patients with GBC. The association of elevated alkaline phosphatase without elevated bilirubin is consistent with GBC; about 40% of these patients have resectable lesions.

D. **Radiologic examination**

1. **Abdominal ultrasound** is abnormal in about 98% of patients. Cholelithiasis, thickened gallbladder wall, a mass in the gallbladder, or a combination of these constitutes the most common finding. Ultrasound is diagnostic of GBC in only 20% of cases, however.

2. **CT of the abdomen** may be diagnostic in half of patients.

3. **MRI** can differentiate gallbladder tumors from adjacent liver. Use of magnetic resonance cholangiography can help determine whether biliary tract encasement is present, and vascular enhancement techniques often permit preoperative diagnosis of portal vein involvement.

4. **Percutaneous transhepatic cholangiography (PTHC)** is abnormal in 80% of cases and diagnostic in 40%.
5. **ERCP** is abnormal in about 75% of cases and yields a tissue diagnosis in 25%.
6. **Laparoscopic exploration** may allow assessment of the peritoneal surfaces, liver, and tissues adjacent to the gallbladder to determine potential resectability.

IV. STAGING AND PROGNOSTIC FACTORS

A. Staging. There are two commonly used staging systems: the American Joint Commission on Cancer staging system (stages 0 to IV) and the Nevin system (stages 1 to 5). Readers should consult an up-to-date staging manual because of frequent revisions of staging systems.

Stage I: An intramuscular lesion or muscular invasion unrecognized at operation and later discovered by the pathologist
Stage II: Transmural invasion
Stage III: Lymph node involvement
Stage IV: Involvement of two or more adjacent organs, or >2 cm invasion of liver, or distant metastasis

B. Prognostic factors. The overall median survival of patients with GBC is 6 months. After surgical resection, only 27% are alive at 1 year, 19% at 3 years, and 13% at 5 years. Disease stage is the most significant prognostic factor. The 5-year survival rate after surgical resection is 65% to 100% for stage I, 30% for stage II, 15% for stage III, and 0% for stage IV disease. Poorly differentiated (higher grade) tumors and the presence of jaundice are associated with poorer survival. Ploidy patterns do not correlate with survival.

V. PREVENTION. Cholecystectomy has been recommended to prevent GBC. For every 100 gallbladders removed, there is one patient with GBC. However, the overall mortality rate of cholecystectomy is also about 1% (including patients with diabetes and gangrenous gallbladder as well as patients with cholangitis or gallstone pancreatitis).

VI. MANAGEMENT. Despite the improvement of diagnostic capabilities, better perioperative care, and a more aggressive surgical approach, GBC remains a fatal illness in most patients.

A. Cholecystectomy is the only effective treatment. The best chance for long-term survival is the serendipitous discovery of an early cancer at the time of cholecystectomy. Radical cholecystectomy or resection of adjacent structure has not resulted in better survival.

B. RT appears to have no added benefit in the adjuvant setting, although the only reports of such therapy have been small retrospective series. Intraoperative RT has been reported to be of benefit in several small series of highly selected patients. RT may be useful as a primary treatment (without surgical resection) using either external-beam RT alone or external-beam RT plus ^{192}Ir implants. RT may relieve pain in a small number of patients.

C. Chemotherapy. The data on adjuvant systemic chemotherapy are anecdotal. 5-FU–based combinations are most commonly used, but the response rates are poor. Phase II trials have shown potential benefit to the use of gemcitabine.

⟨⟩ BILIARY TRACT (INTRAHEPATIC AND EXTRAHEPATIC) CANCER

I. EPIDEMIOLOGY AND ETIOLOGY

A. Epidemiology. Biliary tract carcinomas (BTCs, cholangiocarcinomas) are rare and occur with equal frequency in men and women at the average age of 60 years. In American Indians, Israelis, and Japanese, the incidence of BTC is 6 to 7 per 100,000 population, compared with 1 per 100,000 among the U.S. population. However, cancer of the intrahepatic bile ducts appears to be increasing in incidence in both the

United States and elsewhere. In a review of incidence data for intrahepatic cholangiocarcinoma from the Surveillance, Epidemiology, and End Results Program of the NCI, there was a 165% increase in incidence between 1975 and 1999. This increase is likely partly a result of more accurate diagnosis causing a shift from a classification of "unknown primary" to cholangiocarcinoma. Despite this possible shift, there appears to be a meaningful increase in the incidence of cholangiocarcinoma. The reasons for the observed increase have not been identified.

Extrahepatic bile duct cancers accounts for less than one-third of BTCs. When BTC is combined with GBC, GBC accounts for two-thirds of all BTCs. Half of patients with BTC have undergone cholecystectomy for cholelithiasis.

B. Etiology and risk factors. An increased incidence of BTC has been reported in patients with Crohn disease, choledocholithiasis, cystic fibrosis, chronic long-term ulcerative colitis, primary sclerosing cholangitis, and *Clonorchis sinensis* infestation. The incidence is also reportedly increased in patients with congenital anomalies of the intrahepatic and extrahepatic bile ducts (e.g., cysts, congenital dilation of the bile ducts, choledochal cyst, Caroli disease [congenital cystic dilation of multiple sections of the biliary tree], congenital hepatic fibrosis, polycystic disease, abnormal pancreaticocholedochal junction). Conditions that cause chronic bile duct stasis and infection are linked to increased risk for BTC. A history of exposure to the outmoded contrast agent Thorotrast has also been associated with BTC.

II. PATHOLOGY
A. Histology
1. **Malignant tumors** of the bile ducts are adenocarcinoma in 95% of cases. Microscopically, BTCs generally extend to 1 to 4 cm beyond the gross margin of the tumor. Multiple foci of carcinoma *in situ* may be noted. Malignant tumors of intrahepatic bile ducts are less common than HCC and have no relation to cirrhosis. Mixed hepatic tumors with elements of both HCC and cholangiocarcinoma do occur; most of these cases are actually HCC with focal ductal differentiation. Table 9.6 depicts the clinical and pathologic differences between HCC, bile duct carcinoma, and metastatic adenocarcinoma. Appendix C-4.IV shows immunohistochemical phenotypes of HCC and bile duct carcinomas as well as other adenocarcinomas.

   Other malignant tumors that involve the bile ducts include anaplastic and squamous carcinomas, cystadenocarcinomas, primary malignant melanoma, leiomyosarcoma, carcinosarcoma, and metastatic tumors (particularly breast cancer, myelomas, and lymphomas).

2. **Biliary tract adenomas** are solitary in 80% of cases and may grossly resemble metastatic carcinoma. Most are <1 cm in diameter and are located under the capsule.

3. **Biliary tract cystadenoma and cystadenocarcinoma.** Benign and malignant cystic tumors of biliary origin arise in the liver more frequently than in the extrahepatic biliary system.

4. **Biliary tract carcinoma** (cholangiocarcinoma; see Extrahepatic Bile Duct Cancer, later). Malignant tumors of intrahepatic bile ducts are less common than HCC and have no relation to cirrhosis. Mixed hepatic tumors with elements of both HCC and cholangiocarcinoma do occur; most of these cases are actually HCC with focal ductal differentiation. Table 9.6 depicts the clinical and pathologic differences between HCC, bile duct carcinoma, and metastatic adenocarcinoma. Appendix C-4.IV shows immunohistochemical phenotypes of HCC and bile duct carcinomas as well as other adenocarcinomas.

B. Location.
BTCs are divided anatomically into those that arise from the intrahepatic upper third of the biliary tract, including the hilum (50% to 70% of all tumors); the middle third (10% to 25%); the lower third (10% to 20%); and the cystic duct (<1%). Tumors found near the junction of the right and left hepatic duct (Klatskin tumors) are usually small and may be inconspicuous at laparotomy. Adenocarcinomas located in the right and left hepatic ducts or common hepatic duct are frequently scirrhous, constricting, diffusely infiltrating, or nodular and may mimic sclerosing

cholangitis or stricture. Adenocarcinomas of the common bile duct or cystic duct are more often fungating and may have a better prognosis. Carcinoma of the cystic duct is rare, and distention of the gallbladder occurs before jaundice becomes apparent.

III. DIAGNOSIS

A. Symptoms. Jaundice is present in the majority of patients. Abdominal pain, weight loss, fever, malaise, or hepatomegaly occurs in half of cases, but generally in patients with advanced BTC. Patients with proximal tumors in the upper third of the biliary tract usually have symptoms for twice as long as those with tumors in the lower third.

B. Laboratory studies

1. **Serum chemistries.** Serum bilirubin levels greater than 7.5 mg/dL are found in 60% of cases, alkaline phosphatase greater than twice normal in 80%, and increased transaminase level and prothrombin time in 25%.

2. **Tumor marker.** Serum CA 19-9 is elevated in 90% of patients.

3. **Radiologic examination**

   a. **Abdominal ultrasound** shows dilation of the common bile duct or intrahepatic biliary ducts.

   b. **CT or MRI** may reveal a mass and suggest the site or origin of carcinoma.

   c. **PTHC** is the most specific test for proximal bile duct lesions.

   d. **ERCP** is the best diagnostic test for distal bile duct tumors.

   e. **Angiography and portovenography** are useful in determining the extent of the disease for the preoperative evaluation of resectability.

IV. STAGING AND PROGNOSTIC FACTORS

A. Staging. Readers should consult an up-to-date staging manual because of frequent revisions of staging systems. All patients should be initially staged so that those with unresectable tumors are not subjected to needless surgery. If PTHC shows that the tumor extends into the parenchyma of both the right and left lobes of the liver, the tumor is unresectable and no surgery is performed. If angiography shows encasement of the main portal vein or hepatic artery, the tumor is also unresectable. If, however, the tumor extends into only one lobe, or if there is involvement of one branch of the portal vein or hepatic artery, surgical exploration is considered with the possibility of adding hepatic lobectomy to the hepatic duct resection. The criteria (Blumgart) for unresectability are as follows:

1. Bilateral intrahepatic duct involvement
2. Entrapment of the main trunk of the portal vein
3. Bilateral invasion of the branches of the portal vein or hepatic artery
4. Ductal involvement in the contralateral lobe

B. Prognostic factors. The poor prognostic variables with statistical significance are mass lesion, cachexia, poor performance status, serum bilirubin 9 mg/dL or greater, multicentric disease, hilar or proximal sites, high tumor grade, sclerotic histology, liver invasion, lymph node involvement, and advanced stage.

V. MANAGEMENT

A. Surgical resection is the only treatment that may result in long-term survival. In specialized medical centers, about 45% of patients who undergo exploratory surgery also undergo complete resection with no gross tumor left behind, 10% undergo incomplete resection, and 45% have tumors that are not resectable. Tumors in the middle and distal ducts have a higher resectability rate than tumors in the proximal ducts, which have a maximal resectability rate of 20%. The median survival of patients with intrahepatic tumors following resection is 18 to 30 months, while that for patients with extrahepatic tumors is 12 to 24 months. The 5-year survival rate is about 10% to 45%. The 30-day operative mortality rate may be as high as 25%. The high postoperative complication rate includes wound infection, cholangitis, liver abscess, subphrenic abscess, pancreatitis, and biliary fistulas.

B. Adjuvant therapy has been advocated to reduce the high incidence of local recurrence (up to 100%), but it does not appear to improve survival after curative resection. The role of adjuvant RT remains unclear. Cholangiocarcinoma is radiosensitive, but bile duct tolerance to radiation is limited. The complications of RT include biliary and duodenal stenosis. The results of small series of selected patients treated with 5-FU combined with RT have led some authors to advocate this as an adjuvant to surgery or in cases with locally advanced and unresectable disease.

C. Biliary tract bypass

1. **Surgical biliary tract bypass** is carried out predominantly in those patients whose tumors are found to be unresectable at operation. Biliary-enteric anastomosis is usually performed using a Roux-en-Y jejunal loop. The operative mortality rate ranges from 0% to 30%, and the median survival varies from 11 to 16 months. The theoretical advantage of operative drainage is the decreased potential for recurrent cholangitis.

2. **Surgical stenting.** T-tube or U-tube catheters can be passed through the obstruction. A T-tube is hard to replace when it becomes clogged. The advantage of a U-tube is that both of its ends are externalized separately, easing replacement when the tube becomes obstructed. The 30-day mortality rate for operative stenting varies from 10% to 20%.

3. **Endoscopic stenting** has two advantages: a decreased morbidity and no creation of external fistulization. This method is more successful with distal bile duct tumors and is associated with a 30-day mortality rate of 10% to 20%.

4. **Percutaneous stenting** to provide drainage, either as an externalized stent or as an endoprosthesis, is associated with a 30-day mortality rate of 15% to 35%.

D. Other methods of treatment

1. **Liver transplantation** is generally not considered appropriate because of the high incidence of local recurrence. With orthotopic liver transplantation used alone, long-term survival is only 20% of highly selected patients with disease limited to the liver. The use of pretransplant chemotherapy and radiation has increased 5-year survival to 70% to 80%, making transplant a more meaningful option in selected patients.

2. **RT** appears to have some effect on the tumor size and may relieve jaundice in patients without biliary stenting. RT may be used (usually with biliary stenting) either as primary treatment or as adjuvant therapy. Conventional external-beam RT has the advantage of giving a moderately high dose of radiation (5,000 to 6,000 cGy) to a relatively large volume of tissue and is more effective in treating bulky tumor masses. Implantation with ^{192}Ir seeds (effective radius of 1 cm from the seeds) delivers high-dose RT to localized residual disease after surgical resection or may provide palliation to patients with bile ducts obstructed by tumor. The typical dose with ^{192}Ir seeds is 2,000 cGy.

3. **Chemotherapy** is of limited benefit. 5-FU has a response rate of 15%. Gemcitabine has been shown to have meaningful activity with an approximately 20% to 40% response rate and improved overall survival of 8 to 14 months. Combination chemotherapy may provide a higher response rate, but is of unclear long-term benefit.

CANCER OF THE AMPULLA OF VATER

I. PATHOLOGY

Carcinoma of the ampulla of Vater is a papillary neoplasm arising in the last part of the common bile duct where it passes through the duodenum. Distinction between true ampullary tumor and periampullary tumors originating in the duodenal mucosa or pancreatic ducts is important because the periampullary cancers have a poor prognosis compared with ampullary cancers. The differentiation may be made by examination of the mucins they produce. Ampullary cancer produces sialomucins, whereas periampullary cancers produce sulfated mucins.

II. STAGING SYSTEM AND PROGNOSTIC FACTORS

The TNM staging system is used to stage ampullary cancer. The prognosis of patients with ampullary carcinoma is better than that of patients with cancer arising in any other site in the biliary tree. Pancreatic invasion and lymph node metastasis are the two most important prognostic factors. The 5-year survival rate is in excess of 50% when no nodal metastasis and no invasion of the pancreas have occurred. Nodal metastasis occurs much more frequently in patients with tumors larger than 2.5 cm.

III. MANAGEMENT

Surgery is the only curative treatment modality for ampullary carcinoma. Pancreatico-duodenal resection (Whipple procedure or a modification) is the surgical procedure of choice. The 5-year survival rate ranges from 5% to 55% depending on lymph node involvement, invasion of the pancreas, and histologic differentiation. Ampullectomy (local ampullary excision) performed on poor-risk patients with apparently localized disease is associated with a 10% 5-year survival rate.

Suggested Reading

Esophageal and Gastric Cancer

Carneiro F, Chaves P. Pathologic risk factors of adenocarcinoma of the gastric cardia and gastroesophageal junction. *Surg Oncol Clin N Am* 2006;15:697.

Cunningham D, Allum WH, Stenning SP, et al. Perioperative chemotherapy versus surgery alone for resectable gastroesophageal cancer. *N Engl J Med* 2006;355:11.

Das P, Fukami N, Ajani JA. Combined modality therapy of localized gastric and esophageal cancers. *J Natl Canc Netw* 2006;4:375.

Enzinger PC, Mayer RJ. Esophageal cancer. *N Engl J Med* 2003;349:2241.

Herskovic A, Martz K, al-Sarraf M, et al. Combined chemotherapy and radiotherapy compared with radiotherapy alone in patients with cancer of the esophagus. *N Engl J Med* 1992;326:1593.

Macdonald JS, Smalley SR, Benedetti J, et al. Chemoradiotherapy after surgery compared with surgery alone for adenocarcinoma of the stomach or gastroesophageal junction. *N Engl J Med* 2001;345:725.

Van Cutsem E, Moiseyenko VM, Tjulandin S, et al. Phase III study of docetaxel and cisplatin plus fluorouracil compared with cisplatin and fluorouracil as first-line therapy for advanced gastric cancer: a report of the V325 Study Group. *J Clin Oncol* 2006;24:4991.

Wagner AD, Grothe W, Haerting J, et al. Chemotherapy in advanced gastric cancer: a systematic review and meta-analysis based on aggregate data. *J Clin Oncol* 2006;24:2903.

Walsh TN, Noonan N, Hollywood D, et al. A randomized trial of multimodality therapy versus surgery for esophageal adenocarcinoma. *N Engl J Med* 1996;335:462.

Webb A, Cunningham D, Scarffe JH, et al. Randomized trial comparing epirubicin, cisplatin, and fluorouracil versus fluorouracil, doxorubicin, and methotrexate in advanced esophagogastric cancer. *J Clin Oncol* 1997;15:261.

Colorectal Cancer

André T, Boni C, Mounedji-Boudiaf L, et al. Oxaliplatin, fluorouracil, and leucovorin as adjuvant treatment for colon cancer. *N Engl J Med* 2004;350:2343.

Bertagnolli MM, Eagle CJ, Zauber AG, et al. Celecoxib for the prevention of sporadic colorectal adenomas. *N Engl J Med* 2006;355:873.

Bond JH. Polyp guideline: diagnosis, treatment and surveillance for patients with nonfamilial colorectal polyps. *Ann Intern Med* 1993;119:836.

Cunningham D, Humblet Y, Siena S, et al. Cetuximab monotherapy and cetuximab plus irinotecan in irinotecan-refractory metastatic colorectal cancer. *N Engl J Med* 2004;351:337.

de Gramont A, Figer A, Seymour M, et al. Leucovorin and fluorouracil with or without oxaliplatin as first-line treatment in advanced colorectal cancer. *J Clin Oncol* 2000;18:2938.

Falcone A, Ricce S, Brunetti I, et al. Phase III trial of infusional fluorouracil, leucovorin, oxaliplatin, and irinotecan (FOLFOXIRI) compared with infusional fluorouracil, leucovorin, and irinotecan (FOLFIRI) as first-line treatment for metastatic colorectal cancer: the Gruppo Oncologico Nord Ovest. *J Clin Oncol* 2007;25:1670.

Goldberg RM, Fleming TR, Tangen CM, et al. Surgery for recurrent colon cancer: strategies for identifying resectable recurrence and success rates after resection. *Ann Intern Med* 1998;129:27.

Goldberg RM, Sargent DJ, Morton RF, et al. A randomized controlled trial of fluorouracil plus leucovorin, irinotecan and oxaliplatin combinations in patients with previously untreated colorectal cancer. *J Clin Oncol* 2004;22:23.

Kabbinavar F, Hurwitz HI, Fehrenbacher L, et al. Phase II, randomized trial comparing bevacizumab plus fluorouracil (FU)/leucovorin (LV) with FU/LV alone in patients with metastatic colorectal cancer. *J Clin Oncol* 2003;21:60.

Mandel JS, Bond JH, Church TR, et al. Reducing mortality from colorectal cancer by screening for fecal occult blood. Minnesota Colon Cancer Control Study. *N Engl J Med* 1993;328:1365.

Moertel CG. Chemotherapy for colorectal cancer. *N Engl J Med* 1994;330:1136.

O'Connell MJ, Laurie JA, Kahn M, et al. Prospectively randomized trial of postoperative adjuvant chemotherapy in patients with high-risk colon cancer. *J Clin Oncol* 1998;16: 295.

Ratto C, Sofo L, Ippoliti M, et al. Prognostic factors on colorectal cancer: literature review for clinical application. *Dis Colon Rectum* 1998;41:1033.

Rothenberg ML, Oza AM, Bigelow RH, et al. Superiority of oxaliplatin and fluorouracil-leucovorin compared with either therapy alone in patients with progressive colorectal cancer after irinotecan and fluorouracil-leucovorin: interim results of a phase III trial. *J Clin Oncol* 2003;21:2059.

Rougier P, Van Cutsem E, Bajetta E, et al. Randomised trial of irinotecan versus fluorouracil by continuous infusion after fluorouracil failure in patients with metastatic colorectal cancer. *Lancet* 1998;352:1407.

Saltz LB, Cox JV, Blanke C, et al. Irinotecan Study Group. Irinotecan plus fluorouracil and leucovorin for metastatic colorectal cancer. *N Engl J Med* 2000;343:905.

Tournigand C, André T, Achille E, et al. FOLFIRI followed by FOLFOX 6 or the reverse sequence in advanced colorectal cancer: a randomized GERCOR study. *J Clin Oncol* 2004;22:229.

Twelves C, Wong A, Nowacki MP, et al. Capecitabine as adjuvant treatment for stage III colon cancer. *N Engl J Med*. 2005;352:2696.

Van Cutsem E, Peeters M, Siena S, et al. Open-label phase III trial of panitumumab plus best supportive care compared with best supportive care alone in patients with chemotherapy-refractory metastatic colorectal cancer. *J Clin Oncol* 2007;25:1658.

Winawer SJ, Zauber AG, Ho MN, et al. Prevention of colorectal cancer by colonoscopic polypectomy. *N Engl J Med* 1993;329:1977.

Anal Cancer

Flam M, John M, Pajak TF, et al. Role of mitomycin in combination with fluorouracil and radiotherapy, and salvage chemoradiation in the definitive nonsurgical treatment of epidermoid carcinoma of the anal canal: results of a phase III randomized intergroup study. *J Clin Oncol* 1996;14:2527.

Klas JV, Rothenberger DA, Wong WD, et al. Malignant tumors of the anal canal: the spectrum of disease, treatment, and outcomes. *Cancer* 1999;85:1686.

Martenson JA Jr, Gunderson LL. External radiation therapy without chemotherapy in the management of anal cancer. *Cancer* 1993;71:1736.

UKCCR Anal Cancer Trial Working Party. Epidermoid anal cancer: results of the UKCCR randomised trial of radiotherapy alone versus radiotherapy, 5-fluorouracil, and mitomycin. *Lancet* 1996;348:1049.

Pancreatic Cancer

Burris HA 3rd, Moore MJ, Andersen J, et al. Improvements in survival and clinical benefit with gemcitabine as first-line therapy for patients with advanced pancreas cancer: a randomized trial. *J Clin Oncol* 1997;15:2403.

Gastrointestinal Study Group. Further evidence of effective adjuvant combined radiation and chemotherapy following curative resection of pancreatic cancer. *Cancer* 1987;59:2006.

Moore MJ, Goldstein D, Hamm J, et al. Erlotinib plus gemcitabine compared with gemcitabine alone in patients with advanced pancreatic cancer: A phase III trial of the National Cancer Institute of Canada Clinical Trials Group. *J Clin Oncol* 2007;25:1960.

Neoptolemos JP, Stocken DD, Friess H, et al. A randomized trial of chemoradiotherapy and chemotherapy after resection of pancreatic cancer. *N Engl J Med* 2004;350:1200.

Oettle H, Post S, Neuhaus P, et al. Adjuvant chemotherapy with gemcitabine vs observation in patients undergoing curative-intent resection of pancreatic cancer: a randomized controlled trial. *JAMA* 2007;297:267.

Liver Cancer

Farazi PA, DePinho RA. Hepatocellular carcinoma pathogenesis: from genes to environment. *Nature Rev Cancer* 2006;6:674.

Louvet JM, Bruix J. Systematic review of randomized trials for unresectable hepatocellular carcinoma: chemoembolization improves survival. *Hepatology* 2003;37:429.

Marrero JA, Pelletier S. Hepatocellular carcinoma. *Clin Liver Dis* 2006;10:339.

Yeo W, Mok TS, Zee B, et al. A randomized phase III study of doxorubicin versus cisplatin/interferon alpha-2b/doxorubicin/fluorouracil (PIAF) combination chemotherapy for unresectable hepatocellular carcinoma. *J Natl Cancer Inst* 2005;97:1532.

Cholangiocarcinoma and Gallbladder Cancer

Dingle BH, Rumble RB, Brouwers MC, et al. The role of gemcitabine in the treatment of cholangiocarcinoma and gallbladder cancer: a systematic review. *Can J Gastroenterol* 2005;19:711.

Heimbach JK, Gores GJ, Nagomey DM, et al. Liver transplantation for perihilar cholangiocarcinoma after aggressive neoadjuvant therapy: a new paradigm for liver and biliary malignancies? *Surgery* 2006;140:331.

Hejna M, Pruckmayer M, Raderer M. The role of chemotherapy and radiation in the management of biliary cancer: a review of the literature. *Eur J Cancer* 1998;34:977.

Jarnagin WR, Shoup M. Surgical management of cholangiocarcinoma. *Semin Liver Dis* 2004;24:189.

Lillemoe KD. Tumors of the gallbladder, bile ducts, and ampulla. *Semin Gastrointest Dis* 2003;14:208.

Reid KM, Ramos-De la Medina A, Donohue JH. Diagnosis and surgical management of gallbladder cancer: a review. *J Gastrointest Surg* 2007;11:671.

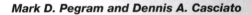

BREAST CANCER

Mark D. Pegram and Dennis A. Casciato

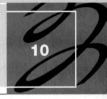

10

I. EPIDEMIOLOGY AND ETIOLOGY

A. Incidence

1. The American Cancer Society (ACS) estimated that breast cancer would be diagnosed in 178,480 women and 2,030 men in the United States during 2007. Another 62,030 women were diagnosed with *in situ* breast carcinoma. Breast cancer was estimated to be the cause of death in 40,640 women and 450 men during that year.

    The death rate from breast cancer in North America has been declining, with a 1.7% annual reduction in mortality since 1992. This decline has occurred despite an increased incidence of the disease over the same time period. Over the last 10 years, mortality caused by breast cancer in the European Union has fallen by 9.8%. These reductions are most likely owing to increased early detection and improved efficacy of adjuvant therapies.

2. Although breast cancer is the most common neoplasm in women, accounting for 26% of all cancers diagnosed annually, it is overall the second leading cause of cancer death (following lung cancer). Breast cancer, however, is the leading cause of cancer death in women aged <65 years.

3. The incidence of breast cancer is highest among women of higher socioeconomic background. Although the incidence of breast cancer is higher in whites, black women are more likely to die from their disease. This disparity may be owing both to delay in diagnosis because of restricted access to health care and to differing biology of the disease (e.g., higher frequency of *HER2*-positive disease or variations in the incidence of estrogen receptor [ER] or progesterone receptor [PR] activity) in these populations.

B. Genetic predisposition.

Most breast cancers diagnosed are sporadic and not associated with any clear familial genetic predisposition. Approximately 10% of breast cancer patients, however, have tumors that can be attributed to inherited germline mutations in genes that control DNA repair, cell growth regulation, or cell cycle control.

1. **Germline genetic defects** associated with an increased risk of breast cancer are as follows:

    a. **BRCA-1.** The *BRCA-1* gene, assigned to chromosome 17q21, was first identified in 1990. The gene product is a 1,863 amino acid nuclear protein with pleotropic activities including sensing or signaling DNA damage, transcriptional regulation, transcription-coupled DNA repair, and ubiquitin ligase activity. Several hundred different mutations have been identified by DNA sequence analysis. Particular *BRCA-1* mutations are prevalent in specific populations (e.g., del 185 mutation among patients of Ashkenazi Jewish ancestry). Mutation of *BRCA-1* accounts for about 20% of all familial breast cancers.

    (1) *BRCA* mutations are inherited in an autosomal-dominant fashion with variable penetrance, and are associated with an increased risk of breast, ovarian, colorectal, and prostate cancers.

    (2) Breast tumors harboring *BRCA-1* mutations frequently lack expression of both ER and PR, and lack amplification of the *HER2* gene. These

237

tumors very frequently also have somatic mutations in the *P53* tumor suppressor gene.

(3) Molecular classification of *BRCA-1* mutant tumors by gene expression profiling frequently demonstrates a "basal" breast cancer phenotype (see section II.B.).

(4) Patients with inherited mutation of *BRCA-1* can expect a lifetime risk of breast cancer in the range of 50% to 85%, and a 15% to 45% risk for ovarian cancer.

b. *BRCA-2*. The *BRCA-2* gene, assigned to chromosome 13q12, was first sequenced in 1995. The gene encodes a 3,418 amino acid protein involved in DNA repair. As with *BRCA-1*, many different mutations have been described in the *BRCA-2* gene in affected individuals.

Germline mutations in *BRCA-2* are associated with an increased risk of a unique spectrum of human neoplasms, including melanoma, breast cancer (in both men and women), ovarian cancer, and pancreatic cancer. Breast cancers associated with *BRCA-2* mutation are frequently ER positive and tend to occur at an older age than with *BRCA-1*.

c. Li-Fraumeni syndrome is caused by germline mutations in the *P53* tumor suppressor gene found on chromosome 17p13. In addition to breast cancer, there is an increased risk of other tumor types (sarcomas, brain tumors, leukemia, and adrenal tumors). The lifetime risk of breast cancer associated with this syndrome is about 50%.

d. The *PTEN* gene is assigned to chromosome 10q22-23 and encodes a tumor suppressor. **Cowden syndrome** is the clinical phenotype resulting from mutations in *PTEN*. The syndrome is a rare autosomal-dominant disorder characterized by multiple benign hamartomas and malignant tumors (breast and thyroid cancers). The syndrome is recognized by the pathognomonic presentation of facial trichilemmomas and fibromas of the oral mucosa that cause cobblestone appearance of the tongue and acral palmoplantar keratoses. The risk of breast cancer is increased by approximately 50% in subjects with mutation of the gene.

e. *CHEK-2*. This cell cycle checkpoint kinase gene is an important component of the cellular DNA repair pathway. Mutation of the gene increases the risk of breast cancer in women by twofold and in men by tenfold.

f. Mutations in other genes have been associated with an increased risk of breast cancer (e.g., ATM and STK11—Puetz-Jeghers syndrome). In approximately half of subjects with an apparent familial association with breast cancer based on analysis of the pedigree, no specific gene mutation can be found.

2. Genetic testing for *BRCA-1* and *BRCA-2* is commercially available, but should ideally be interpreted in consultation with a genetic counselor. Factors that indicate an increased likelihood of having germline *BRCA* mutations include

a. Multiple cases of early onset breast cancer

b. Ovarian cancer with a family history of breast or ovarian cancer

c. Breast and ovarian cancer in the same individual

d. Bilateral breast cancer

e. Male breast cancer

f. Ashkenazi Jewish ancestry

3. American Society of Clinical Oncology (ASCO) guidelines recommend that cancer predisposition genetic testing should be offered when (*a*) there is a personal or family history suggestive of a genetic cancer susceptibility condition, (*b*) the test can be adequately interpreted, and (*c*) the test result will influence medical management. Once a proband has been identified as a carrier for a heritable cancer predisposition condition, it is important that patients and their family members be counseled regarding additional screening and prevention strategies, and be alerted to the risk of other primary neoplasms.

4. Prophylactic surgery. Prophylactic bilateral mastectomy reduces the risk of breast cancer among *BRCA* mutation carriers by more than 90%. Prophylactic bilateral salpingo-oopherectomy reduces the risk of ovarian cancer (although not primary peritoneal carcinoma) by 90% and also reduces the risk of breast cancer by approximately 65% in premenopausal women with *BRCA* abnormalities.

5. **Insurance issues.** The United States Health Insurance Portability and Accountability Act (HIPAA) of 1996 states that genetic information may not be treated as a pre-existing medical condition for the purposes of denying insurance coverage or basing the cost of insurance. In addition to federal policy, many states have additional laws to prevent discrimination owing to genetic information. Consequently, most insurance companies will pay for genetic testing and any subsequent treatment that is indicated.

C. Etiologic factors

1. **Endogenous estrogen exposure.** The following factors affecting endogenous estrogen exposure have been associated with an increased risk of breast cancer in epidemiologic studies.
   a. Nulliparity
   b. Late first full-term pregnancy (women who completed their first full-term pregnancy after age 30 are two to five times more likely to develop breast cancer compared with those who had had term pregnancies <18 years of age).
   c. Early menarche (<12 years)
   d. Late menopause (>55 years)
   e. Lactation may reduce the risk of breast cancer

2. **Exogenous estrogen and progestin use:** Hormone replacement therapy (HRT) following menopause. A preponderance of the evidence from previous historical cohort studies suggested that the risk of breast cancer was increased modestly by long-term estrogen use alone, and that women on estrogen plus progestin were more likely to have tumors with more favorable biological characteristics (hormone receptor positive disease) and lower tumor stage.

   The Women's Health Initiative (WHI) study was begun in 1993 with the following results and effects:
   a. The WHI was a placebo-controlled study that enrolled 10,739 patients with a history of prior hysterectomy and 16,608 patients with an intact uterus. The former were randomized to receive conjugated equine estrogen (CEE, 0.625 mg/day) versus placebo, and the latter to CEE (0.625 mg/day) plus medroxyprogesterone acetate (MPA, 2.5 mg/day) versus placebo. The hypothesis being tested in this trial was that long-term CEE + MPA would have more benefit than risk on chronic diseases, such as coronary heart disease.
   b. Published in 2003, the study demonstrated a 24% increase in the risk of breast cancer among the women with an intact uterus randomized to receive CEE + MPA ($P = 0.003$). Moreover, tumors detected in the CEE + MPA group had a larger mean tumor size (1.7 vs. 1.5 cm, $P = 0.038$) and were more likely to have lymph node metastasis (25.9% vs. 15.8%, $P = 0.033$). In addition, more women in the CEE + MPA group had abnormal mammograms at 1 year (9.4% vs. 5.4%, $P < 0.0001$). The study further demonstrated that the risk both of ER/PR positive as well as ER/PR negative disease was increased similarly, contrary to previous reports from non-placebo-controlled cohort studies. Finally, the use of CEE + MPA was found to decrease the risk of colorectal cancer, although the colorectal cancers that were diagnosed were of more advanced stage.
   c. The WHI study concluded that combined CEE + MPA increases the number of abnormal mammograms and the risk of invasive breast cancer, and that breast cancers are diagnosed at a later stage. This increased risk of invasive breast cancer was not seen in the women with prior hysterectomy who were randomized to receive CEE alone. The use of CEE alone increased the risk of stroke, decreased the risk of hip fracture, and did not affect the risk of coronary heart disease.
   d. It is important to note that patients with prior hysterectomy in this study were more likely to report past or current hormone use, had a higher body mass index, and that 41% had prior bilateral oophorectomy.

e. Together, these data led to a revised view of postmenopausal HRT because use of CEE + MPA potentially leads to delay in diagnosis of two of the three most common cancers in postmenopausal women:

   (1) HRT with CEE + MPA should be used at the lowest possible dose and shortest duration sufficient to control vasomotor or vaginal symptoms

   (2) Women with prior hysterectomy treated with short-term CEE therapy have no significant increase in breast cancer risk, although the risk of stroke was increased

f. Subsequent to publication of findings from the WHI study, there has been a sharp decline in the number of new prescriptions for HRT in the United States from 22.8 million in the first quarter of 2001 to 15.2 in the first quarter of 2003. Coincident with this practice was a sharp (7%) decrease in the breast cancer incidence, especially among older women with HR positive disease, suggesting a possible link between decreased incidence and decreased exogenous estrogen and progestin exposure in the form of HRT.

3. Age. The incidence of breast cancer increases steadily with age. Approximately 75% of all cases are diagnosed in postmenopausal women. The risk of developing breast cancer at age 25 years is 1 of 19,608, whereas the lifetime risk is 1 of 8 for women living into their 80s.

4. Benign breast disease. Most forms of benign breast disease, such as fibrocystic disease, are not associated with increased risk. Hyperplasia with atypia, papillomas, sclerosing adenosis, and lobular carcinoma *in situ* have been reported to be associated with an increased risk. **Hyperplasia with atypia** is felt to be a proliferative disease that is associated with an 8% risk of developing invasive breast cancer in patients with a negative family history and a 20% risk in patients with a positive family history of breast cancer.

5. Physical activity. Most cohort studies suggest an inverse association between physical activity and breast cancer risk, regardless of the age at which the physical activity occurred.

6. Ionizing radiation. Exposure to radiation increases the risk of breast cancer. Medical RT to the chest, for example to a mantle field for Hodgkin lymphoma, can increase subsequent risk of breast cancer. Exposure to fallout from nuclear weapons appears to increase risk. Breast cancers following radiation exposure are typically long latency, often a decade or more following the exposure.

7. Ethanol. Studies have shown a positive linear relationship between incremental alcoholic beverage intake and increasing breast cancer risk.

II. PATHOLOGY, MOLECULAR CLASSIFICATION, AND NATURAL HISTORY. Breast cancer is a highly heterogeneous disease. Classification based on clinical and pathologic features have historically been used to guide in the treatment of patients. Although classic histopathologic classification of breast cancer remains important, molecular characterization of the disease is rapidly emerging as a vital tool for understanding clinical prognosis, as well as predicting response to systemic therapies.

A. Classic histopathologic classification. Based on cellular morphology, breast tumors can be broadly categorized as tumors composed of cells of ductal origin (ductal adenocarcinomas) or of lobular origin (lobular carcinomas). Breast malignancies are further classified into invasive (infiltrating) carcinomas capable of metastasizing, and noninvasive disease that can invade beyond the basement membrane (ductal carcinoma *in situ*, [DCIS], also known as intraductal carcinoma).

   1. Ductal adenocarcinoma (70% to 80%) is the most common histology. The clinical prognosis is highly variable, ranging from indolent to rapidly progressive. Prognosis may be estimated by evaluation of cellular morphologic characteristics and molecular markers, such as expression of ER, PR, Ki67 (a marker of cell proliferation, see section V.B.5), and HER2.

   2. Lobular carcinoma (10% to 15%). Lobular carcinoma *in situ* (LCIS) is associated with an increase risk of developing subsequent invasive disease, either ductal or lobular. LCIS, in and of itself, is of no clinical consequence, however.

Invasive lobular carcinoma is capable of metastasis and has a stage-adjusted prognosis similar to infiltrating ductal carcinoma. Invasive lobular carcinomas may be especially difficult to diagnose because of their unique single cell radial pattern of tissue invasion (so called *Indian-filing* on light microscopy) rendering them frequently nonpalpable or mammographically silent. Invasive lobular carcinomas are somewhat more likely to be bilateral compared with infiltrating ductal carcinomas. Metastases from lobular breast carcinomas have a predilection for pleuropericardial surfaces.

3. **Special subtypes with a favorable prognosis** (<10%) include papillary, tubular, mucinous, and pure medullary carcinomas.

4. **Inflammatory breast cancer** (~1%) is a particularly aggressive subtype that can be recognized microscopically based on presence of dermolymphatic invasion. Clinically, this is often associated with cutaneous erythema of the breast (which can mimic mastitis) and cutaneous edema "peau d'orange."

5. **Paget's disease of the breast**, which is characterized by unilateral eczematous change of the nipple, is frequently seen in association with underlying DCIS.

6. **Cystosarcoma phylloides** is a rare, predominantly benign tumor comprising less than 1% of all breast neoplasms. About 90% of phylloides tumors are benign and about 10% are malignant. Although these tumors rarely metastasize, they can recur locally. Surgical resection with ample margins is necessary to optimize local control.

7. **Rare tumors** include squamous cell carcinoma, lymphoma, and sarcoma.

B. **Molecular classification of breast malignancy.** Molecular classification of breast tumors can be based on single gene assays, such as ER, PR, *HER2* gene copy numbers, proliferation index, and Ki67; or on multigene expression platforms, which can measure dozens to even thousands of gene transcripts simultaneously. Multigene transcript profiles use either real-time quantitative polymerase chain reaction (RT-PCR) or gene chip expression microarray. An example of the former is the Oncotype DX assay (see section VIII.A.2.b), and Mammaprint is an example of the latter (see section VIII.A.2.c).

The classification of breast cancer based on gene expression profiling has not yet been completely reconciled with classic histopathologic classification. Gene expression profiling using DNA microarrays have, however, defined new molecular subtypes of breast cancer associated with the cell-of-origin distinction. Recent reports indicate distinct gene expression profiles for inflammatory breast cancer, lobular breast cancer, *HER2*-positive breast cancer, and *BRCA*-mutant breast cancer. Based on these observations, breast cancer has been divided into five subgroups with distinct biological features and clinical outcomes.

1. **Luminal A.** The luminal tumors express cytokeratins 8 and 18, have the highest levels of ER expression, tend to be low grade, will most likely respond to endocrine therapy, and have a favorable prognosis. They tend to be less responsive to chemotherapy.

2. **Luminal B.** Tumor cells are also of luminal epithelial origin, but with a gene expression pattern distinct from luminal A. Prognosis is somewhat worse than luminal A.

3. **Normal breastlike tumors.** These tumors have a gene expression profile reminiscent of nonmalignant "normal" breast epithelium. Prognosis similar to the luminal B group.

4. **HER2-amplified.** These tumors have amplification of the *HER2* gene on chromosome 17q, and frequently exhibit coamplification and overexpression of other genes adjacent to *HER2*. *HER2*-positive cases have significantly decreased expression of ER and PR and have upregulation of vascular endothelium growth factor (VEGF). Historically, the clinical prognosis of such tumors was poor. With the advent of trastuzumab, however, the clinical outcome for patients with *HER2*-positive tumors is markedly improving.

5. **Basal.** These ER- or PR-negative and *HER2*-negative tumors (so called *triple negative*) are characterized by markers of basal or myoepithelial cells. They tend to be high grade, and express cytokeratins 5/6 and 17 as well as vimentin, p63,

CD10, smooth muscle actin, and epidermal growth factor receptor (EGFR). It is likely that the basal group is still somewhat heterogeneous; for example, patients with *BRCA-1* mutant tumors also fall within this molecular subtype. Overall, basal breast cancers have a poor clinical prognosis, although they likely benefit to some extent from chemotherapy.

C. **Location and mode of spread.** The most common anatomic presentation of breast cancer is in the upper outer quadrant. Breast cancers spread by contiguity, lymphatic channels, and blood-borne metastases. The most common organs involved with symptomatic metastases are regional lymph nodes, skin, bone, liver, lung, and brain. Internal mammary nodes have evidence of tumor in 25% of patients with inner quadrant lesions and 15% with outer quadrant lesions. Internal mammary node metastases rarely occur in the absence of axillary node involvement.

D. **Clinical course.** The clinical course of breast cancer is heterogeneous at best, but, generally, there are trends based on stage. Early breast cancer is curable, but has a 10% to 20% chance of distant metastases occurring even 10 to 20 years after treatment. Locally advanced cancer has an increased risk of latent distant metastasis. In some women, the course is quite rapid, particularly in women with aggressive tumors having indicators of a poor prognosis. Metastatic breast cancer is not curable but typically has a course of stable disease on therapy and then progression in a stepwise fashion.

III. SCREENING AND EARLY DETECTION

A. **Mammography** detects about 85% of breast cancers. A distinction should be made between diagnostic mammography and screening mammography. A screening mammogram is an x-ray study of the breast used to detect breast changes in women who have no signs or symptoms of breast cancer. A diagnostic mammogram is an x-ray study of the breast that is used to check for breast cancer after a lump or other sign or symptom of breast cancer has been found. Although 15% of breast cancers cannot be visualized with mammography, 45% of breast cancers can be seen on mammography before they are palpable. A normal mammographic result must not dissuade the physician from obtaining a biopsy of a suspicious mass.

Digital mammography is gradually replacing film mammography. Digital mammography takes an electronic image of the breast and uses less radiation than film mammography. Digital mammography allows improvement in image storage and transmission because images can be stored and sent electronically. Diagnostic software may also be used to help interpret digital mammograms. Digital systems, however, currently cost approximately one and a half to four times more than film systems.

1. **The American College of Radiology BI-RADS System** for reporting mammographic findings is as follows:

Category 1: Negative
Category 2: Benign finding
Category 3: Probably benign finding. Short interval follow-up is suggested. The findings have a very high probability of being benign, but the radiologist would prefer to establish stability.
Category 4: Suspicious abnormality: biopsy should be considered. These are lesions that do not have characteristic findings of breast cancer, but have a definite probability of being malignant.
Category 5: Highly suggestive of malignancy.

2. **Meta-analysis** of eight randomized mammogram screening trials has shown a 24% reduction in the mortality rate of breast cancer. Mortality reductions have been observed in trials of women aged 40 to 69 years with mammography performed at intervals of 12 and 24 months.

3. **The ACS recommends** an annual mammogram for women at average risk beginning at age 40. Breast cancer mammographic screening should continue annually regardless of age as long as the woman is in reasonably good health,

has a life expectancy of at least 3 to 5 years, and would be willing to undergo therapy. Chronologic age alone should not be used as a reason to discontinue screening mammography.

B. Breast physical examinations. Despite the lack of data showing a reduction in risk of death from breast cancer owing to clinical breast examination (CBE) or breast self-examination (BSE), the ACS has maintained recommendations related to both of these screening modalities.

    1. CBE is recommended for women at average risk of breast cancer beginning in their 20s. CBE should be part of a periodic health examination and should occur at least every 3 years. Women aged 40 years and older should receive CBE, preferably annually, and, ideally, before, or in conjunction with, the annual screening mammogram.

    2. Women should be told about the benefits and limitations of BSE in their 20s. Women who choose to do BSE should receive instruction and have their technique reviewed on the occasion of a periodic health examination.

C. High-risk patients. The ACS reported that women at increased risk for breast cancer might benefit from additional screening strategies beyond those offered to women at average risk. These interventions may include initiation of screening at a younger age, shorter screening intervals, or the addition of other radiologic investigations in addition to mammography, including magnetic resonance imaging (MRI) or ultrasound.

    1. ACS guidelines recommend MRI screening in addition to mammograms for women who have at least one of the following conditions:

        a. A *BRCA1* or *BRCA2* mutation

        b. A first-degree relative (parent, sibling, child) with a *BRCA1* or *BRCA2* mutation, even if they have yet to be tested themselves

        c. A lifetime risk of breast cancer that has been scored at 20% to 25% or greater based on one of several accepted risk assessment tools that evaluate family history and other factors

        d. A history of radiation to the chest between the ages of 10 and 30 years

        e. Germline p53 mutation (Li-Fraumeni syndrome), or hamartoma syndromes associated with *PTEN* mutation (Cowden syndrome or Bannayan-Riley-Ruvalcaba syndrome), or one of these syndromes based on a history in a first-degree relative

    2. The ACS guideline indicates that sufficient evidence still does not exist to recommend for or against MRI screening in women who have

        a. A 15% to 20% lifetime risk of breast cancer, based on one of several accepted risk assessment tools that evaluate family history and other factors

        b. LCIS or atypical lobular hyperplasia (ALH)

        c. Atypical ductal hyperplasia (ADH)

        d. Very dense breasts or unevenly dense breasts (when viewed on a mammogram)

        e. Already had breast cancer, including DCIS

    3. Contralateral breast cancer. A newly published study in the *New England Journal of Medicine* shows that MRI scans can be a useful adjunct for finding contralateral breast tumors in women with newly diagnosed disease. In this report, 969 newly diagnosed breast cancer patients were studied; MRI found 30 early-stage tumors that mammograms and physical examinations could not detect, and missed only 3 tumors (see Lehman, et al. in *Suggested Reading*).

IV. DIAGNOSIS

A. Physical findings and differential diagnosis

    1. Breast lumps are detectable in many patients with breast cancer and constitute the most common sign on history and physical examination. The typical malignant breast mass tends to be solitary, unilateral, solid, hard, irregular, and nontender.

    2. Spontaneous nipple discharge through a mammary duct is the second most common sign of breast cancer. Nipple discharge develops in about 3% of women and 20% of men with breast cancer, but is a manifestation of benign disease in 90% of patients. Discharge in patients >50 years of age is more likely to represent cancer rather than benign conditions. Milky or purulent discharges are associated with a negligible chance of cancer.

   3. Other presenting manifestations include skin changes, axillary lymphadenopathy, or signs of locally advanced or disseminated disease. A painful breast is a common symptom, but it is usually a result of something other than the cancer. Paget's carcinoma appears as unilateral eczema of the nipple. Inflammatory carcinoma appears as skin erythema, edema, and underlying induration in the absence of infection.

B. Evaluation of a breast mass

   1. Breast lump or mass in women < 30 years of age. Ultrasound is the preferred diagnostic modality for young women with a breast mass. If the mass is solid and suspicious, then mammography followed by tissue diagnosis is recommended. If the mass is thought to be benign ultrasonographically, then the option of tissue diagnosis versus observation with frequent physical and ultrasonographic surveillance is appropriate. If the breast mass is cystic on ultrasound and appears to be a simple cyst, no intervention is required. If it appears to be a complex cyst, then aspiration is appropriate. If the mass disappears with aspiration and the aspirate is not bloody, then routine screening can again begin.

   2. Breast lump or mass in women > 30 years of age. Diagnostic mammography should be performed. If the mammographic features are indeterminate, then ultrasonography should be performed. If the mammogram or ultrasound shows a suspicious lesion, tissue sampling is required.

   3. Breast biopsy. When a tissue diagnosis is required, then a choice must be made among the differing techniques.

      a. Fine-needle aspiration (FNA) cytology may be performed if both technical and cytopathologic expertise are available. The method is easy, quick, and safe. *Seeding tumor cells along the needle track* is not a consideration in breast cancer. The sensitivity in diagnosing malignancy has been reported to be 90% to 95%, with 98% specificity. It is, however, impossible to distinguish invasive from *in situ* carcinoma because only cells are obtained; the architecture of the tissue cannot be assessed with FNA.

      b. Ultrasound or stereotactic core biopsy. These techniques are increasingly used as an alternative to excisional biopsy or FNA and are the standard for mammographic changes without accompanying mass; wire- or needle-guided lumpectomies can follow the procedure. In addition, the core biopsy allows sufficient tissue to be removed to appropriately characterize the histology of the specimen. ER, PR, and *HER2* testing may be performed if an invasive malignancy is diagnosed.

      c. Excisional biopsy is the standard technique for diagnosis of a breast mass if stereotactic or ultrasound-guided core biopsy is unavailable. If excisional biopsy is performed, an adequate amount of normal tissue should be removed around the suspicious lesion so that the biopsy serves as a segmental mastectomy in the event that a malignancy is found. This tactic allows for complete excision with clear margins and full histologic evaluation.

C. Pretreatment staging procedures for invasive breast cancer. Should an invasive breast cancer be found on tissue sampling, as recommended above, pretreatment staging may be considered before definitive surgical therapy of the breast and axillary lymph nodes.

   1. Complete blood count, liver function tests

   2. Chest radiograph, diagnostic bilateral mammography

   3. Bone scan and radiologic evaluation of the liver may be considered if the patient is symptomatic or is found to have an elevated alkaline phosphatase.

   4. Bone marrow aspiration if there is unexplained cytopenia or a leukoerythroblastic blood smear

   5. The role of positron emission tomography (PET), with or without computed tomography, in the initial staging of breast cancer is being evaluated. In general,

PET can accurately detect sites of distant disease with a sensitivity of 80% to 97% and specificity of 75% to 94%.

V. STAGING AND PROGNOSIS

A. Staging system. The American Joint Committee on Cancer (AJCC) implemented the current TNM staging system for breast cancer in 2003. The T and M descriptors and stage groupings are shown in Table 10.1. The N substage descriptors are shown in Table 10.2.

TABLE 10.1   **Postoperative-Pathologic TNM Staging System for Breast Cancer**

Primary tumor (T)

TX:	*Primary* tumor cannot be assessed
Tis:	Carcinoma *in situ* (CIS)
Tis (DCIS)	Ductal CIS
Tis (LCIS)	Lobular CIS
Tis (Paget)	Paget's disease of the nipple with no tumor
T0:	No demonstrable tumor in breasts
T1:	Size: ≤2.0 cm in greatest dimension
T1mic:	Microinvasion ≤0.1 cm
T1a:	>0.1 cm and ≤0.5 cm
T1b:	>0.5 cm and ≤1.0 cm
T1c:	>1.0 cm and ≤2.0 cm
T2:	Size: >2 cm and ≤5 cm
T3:	Size: >5 cm
T4:	Any size with direct extension to chest wall or skin, only as described below.
T4a:	Extension to chest wall, not including pectoralis muscle
T4b:	Skin ulceration, edema (including peau d'orange), or satellite nodules confined to the same breast
T4c:	Both T4a and T4b
T4d:	Inflammatory carcinoma

Regional lymph nodes (N) descriptors are defined in Table 10.2

Distant metastases (M)

M0:	Absent
M1:	Present

Stage grouping

Stage	TNM classification		
0	Tis	N0	M0
I	T1	N0	M0
IIA	T0,1	N1	M0
	T2	N0	M0
IIB	T2	N1	M0
	T3	N0	M0
IIIA	T0,1,2	N2	M0
	T3	N1,2	M0
IIIB	T4	Any N	M0
IIIC	Any T	N3	M0
IV	Any T	Any N	M1

Adapted from the *AJCC Cancer Staging Manual.* 6th ed. New York: Springer-Verlag; 2002.

TABLE 10.2 Posteroperative-Pathologic TNM Staging System for Breast Cancer: Regional Lymph Nodes (N)[a]

pNX:	RLN cannot be assessed
pN0:	No RLN metastases histologically; no additional examination for *isolated tumor cells*[b] performed
pN0(i–/+):	Negative/positive IHC with no IHC cluster >0.2 mm
pN0(mol–/+):	Negative/positive molecular findings (e.g., polymerase chain reaction)
pN1:	Metastases in 1–3 ALN and/or IMLN.
pN1mi:	Micrometastases (>0.2 mm, none >2.0 mm) in ALN
pN1a:	Metastases in 1–3 ALN
pN1b:	Metastases in IMLN with microscopic disease detected by SNLD but not "clinically apparent" (by clinical exam or imagery, excluding lymphoscintography).
pN1c:	pN1a + pN1b
pN2:	Metastases in 4–9 ALN, or in clinically apparent IMLN in the absence of ALN metastases.
pN2a:	Metastases in 4–9 ALN (at least one tumor deposit >2.0 mm)
pN2b:	Metastases in clinically apparent IMLN in the absence of ALN metastases.
pN3:	Metastases in ≥10 ALN; or in clinically apparent ipsilateral IMLN in the presence of >1 ALN; or in >3 ALN with clinically negative microscopic metastases in IMLN; or in infraclavicular lymph nodes, or in ipsilateral supraclavicular lymph nodes.
pN3a:	Metastases in ≥10 ALN (at least one tumor deposit >2.0 mm), or metastases to the infraclavicular lymph nodes.
pN3b:	Metastases in clinically apparent ipsilateral IMLN in the presence of ≥1 positive ALN; or in >3 ALN and in IMLN with microscopic disease detected by SNLD but not clinically apparent.
pN3c:	Metastases in ipsilateral supraclavicular lymph nodes.

ALN, axillary lymph nodes; IHC, immunohistochemistry; IMLN, internal mammary lymph nodes (in the intercostal spaces along the edge of the sternum); pN, pathologically evaluated nodes; RLN, regional lymph nodes [axillary, internal mammary, and transpectoral ("Rotter's")]; SLND, sentinel lymph node dissection.
[a]Node classification is based on ALN dissection with or without SLND. Classification based solely on SLND without subsequent ALN dissection is designated (sn) for sentinel node (e.g., pN0[sn]).
[b]Lymph node involvement identified by IHC only is designated by "i" (e.g., pN0[i+][sn]).

B. Prognostic factors

1. **Tumor grade** is an important prognostic variable; the higher the grade, the more guarded the prognosis. The Nottingham combined histologic grade (Elston-Ellis modification of the Bloom-Scarff-Richardson grading system) is recommended by the AJCC staging system. A tumor is graded by assessing three morphologic features (tubule formation, nuclear pleomorphism, and count of mitoses). A value of 1 (favorable) to 3 (unfavorable) is assigned to each feature. A combined score of 3 to 5 points is designated grade 1, 6 to 7 points is grade 2, and 8 to 9 points is grade 3.

2. **Pathologic stage** has a clear impact on expected survival.
   a. **Tumor size.** The risk of recurrence increases linearly with tumor size for patients with fewer than four lymph nodes involved with metastases; thereafter, the prognostic weight of lymph node metastases generally supercedes tumor size. The effect of tumor size on prognosis is reflected by the

following SEER 5-year survival data (adapted from Carter C, et al. in *Suggested Reading*).

Tumor size	5-year survival rate according to the number of axillary lymph nodes with metastases	
	None	**1–3 nodes**
T1a: <0.5 cm	99%	95%
T1b: 0.5–0.9 cm	98%	94%
T1c: 1.0–1.9 cm	96%	87%

The 20-year breast cancer-specific, disease-free survival for node-negative patients treated with mastectomy alone is about 92% for pT1a–b tumors and 75% to 80% for patients for pT1c tumors. Tumor grade affects these probabilities.

- **b. Lymph node involvement** is the greatest prognostic indicator for breast cancer recurrence. Because of the recent change in staging systems for breast cancer, the potential exist for confusion regarding the long-term prognosis for patients by pathologic stage. The 1988 staging system did not differentiate cancer stage by numbers of lymph nodes involved. The 2003 revised TNM staging system shown in Table 10.2 does address this issue.
- **c. Distant metastases.** Many patients with stage IV disease survive 2 to 4 years, depending on sites of metastases, their rate of progression, and response to therapy. Prolonged survival can be achieved, particularly in patients with HR-positive disease with bone-only metastasis.

3. **Hormone receptor status.** Patients with tumors that are negative for both ER and PR have a slightly worse prognosis than those patients who have cancers with either ER or PR being positive. These data, however, are based on the National Surgical Adjuvant Breast Project (NSABP) B-06 trial, where ER and PR were measured by biochemical methods. It is felt that ER and PR as measured by current immunohistochemical (IHC) techniques represent very strong predictive factors for response to hormone therapy rather than being strong prognostic factors for survival.

4. *HER2* **overexpression.** All normal cells, including breast epithelial cells, carry two copies of the human epidermal growth factor receptor-2 gene (*HER2*; also known as the *c-erbB2* gene). In about 20% to 25% of breast cancers, multiple copies of the gene are found owing to gene amplification. *HER2* gene amplification results in increased expression of the gene product, a 185-kDa transmembrane receptor tyrosine kinase. Pathologic overexpression of p185^{HER2} leads to constitutive activation of the *HER2* kinase, resulting in increased proliferation, survival, and metastasis of tumor cells.

- **a. Tumors that overexpress *HER2*** tend to metastasize earlier and to have a worse prognosis. Tumors that exhibit amplification of the *HER2* gene by fluorescent *in situ* hybridization (FISH) are among the most likely to benefit from systemic humanized monoclonal antibody therapy with trastuzumab (Herceptin).
- **b. The methods of identifying *HER2* alteration** are IHC and FISH. To develop guidelines to improve the accuracy of *HER2* testing and its utility as a predictive marker, ASCO and the College of American Pathologists convened an expert panel, which developed recommendations for optimal *HER2* testing performance. The panel recommends that *HER2* status should be determined for all invasive breast cancers. Laboratories performing the test must show 95% concordance with another validated test for positive and negative assay results. The recommended algorithm for defining results for both *HER2* protein expression and gene amplification is as follows:
  - **(1)** A positive *HER2* result is IHC staining of 3+ (uniform, intense membrane staining of >30% of invasive tumor cells), a FISH result of >6 *HER2* gene

copies per nucleus, or a FISH ratio (*HER2* gene signals to chromosome 17 signals) of more than 2.2

(2) A negative result is an IHC staining of 0 or 1+, a FISH result of <4.0 *HER2* gene copies per nucleus, or a FISH ratio of <1.8

(3) Equivocal results require additional action for final determination

5. Other biomarkers

a. Ki-67 protein is a cellular marker for proliferation. It is strictly associated with cell proliferation. Ki-67 protein is present during G1, S, G2, and mitosis phases of the cell cycle, but is absent in resting cells (G0). The fraction of Ki-67-positive tumor cells (the Ki-67 labeling index) has been correlated with the clinical course.

b. DNA flow cytometry can be performed on tumor biopsy material following fluorescent staining with propidum iodide. From this analysis, total DNA content (and thus DNA ploidy) and the percentage of cells undergoing S-phase can be measured.

c. Mutation of the p53 tumor suppressor gene frequently (although not always) leads to aberrant accumulation of dysfunctional p53 protein in the nucleus. Nuclear accumulation of p53 protein can be visualized using IHC staining and has been used as a surrogate marker for p53 gene mutation. Overexpression of normal p53 protein can sometimes be seen in breast cancer cells, even in the absence of p53 gene mutation. Conversely, some tumors harbor p53 mutations that result in protein truncation, which cannot be accurately measured by IHC. Therefore, p53 IHC staining is not an accurate measure of p53 genotype and has limited clinical utility.

VI. MANAGEMENT OF NONINVASIVE BREAST CANCER

A. Ductal carcinomas *in situ*, although noninvasive, is clearly a malignant disease and it recurs in about 35% of cases within 10 to 15 years if treated with excisional biopsy alone. The recurrence, if it occurs, is invasive carcinoma in >25% of cases. When axillary node dissection has been performed, metastases have been found in <3% of DCIS cases. When mastectomy has been performed, the disease is often found to be *multicentric* (additional CIS lesions >2 cm away from the main lesion).

1. Local treatment. Patients often have DCIS found by mammography alone without an accompanying mass. Stereotactic core biopsy is frequently used to make the diagnosis.

a. For women with multicentric DCIS, mastectomy, with or without reconstruction, should be performed. For women with unicentric disease, total mastectomy, without lymph node dissection, or excisional biopsy with adequate negative margins are both acceptable options. Mastectomy cures at least 98% of patients with DCIS.

b. The NSABP B-17 trial randomized 818 women with DCIS treated by lumpectomy to no further therapy or breast RT (see Fisher ER, et al. in *Suggested Reading*). The trial demonstrated a reduction in ipsilateral recurrence (invasive plus noninvasive) from 27% to 12% with the use of RT at 8 years of follow-up. Half of the ipsilateral breast tumor recurrences were invasive for those who did not receive radiation. The incidence of all noninvasive tumors was reduced from 13% to 8% ($P = 0.007$), and all invasive tumors were reduced from 13% to 3%.

c. The European Cooperative Group Study randomized 1,010 women to receive either 5,000 cGy of RT or observation following surgery (see Julien JP, et al. in *Suggested Reading*). The relapse rate was 16% without RT and 9% with RT. A select group of women with DCIS might be considered for excision without radiation. These include women with low-grade DCIS with negative surgical margins by at least 1.0 cm in all directions.

2. Adjuvant systemic therapy for DCIS. Data from the NSABP B-24 trial involved 1,804 women who had lumpectomy and RT and randomized them to receive either tamoxifen (20 mg/day for 5 years) or placebo (see Fisher B, et al. in

Suggested Reading). The cumulative incidence of breast cancer events was 8% and 13%, respectively. These data were elaborated in 2002 as follows:

a. The tumors were tested for ER status in 676 of the 1,804 women. The DCIS tumors were ER positive in 75% of those on the placebo arm (344 women) and in 80% of those on the tamoxifen arm (332 women).

b. For the women with ER-negative DCIS, 18% developed an ipsilateral recurrence regardless of the randomization to tamoxifen or placebo. Also, no difference was noted in the incidence of contralateral breast cancer.

c. For women with ER-positive DCIS, 13% of those on placebo and 7% of those on tamoxifen developed an ipsilateral recurrence, and 8% and 3% developed a contralateral breast cancer, respectively. There was no difference in survival.

d. The data support the use of adjuvant tamoxifen for treatment of ER-positive DCIS. The use of adjuvant tamoxifen for ER-positive DCIS must be carefully weighed against the known toxicities of the drug because there was no survival benefit.

B. Lobular carcinoma *in situ* is also called *lobular neoplasia.* LCIS is considered by many authorities to be a nonmalignant disease. This tumor tends to be multicentric and is commonly bilateral (~30%). The presence of LCIS is a marker for increased risk of subsequent invasive breast cancer. About 20% of patients with lobular CIS develop invasive breast cancer over 15 years.

1. Surgical therapy is not routinely recommended for LCIS. Annual diagnostic mammography is recommended to follow women who do not undergo mastectomy. In very select circumstances, bilateral mastectomy might be considered for risk reduction.

2. Patients should be counseled regarding the potential benefit of tamoxifen for risk reduction in this circumstance. The NSABP P-1 prevention trial demonstrated a 56% reduction in developing invasive breast cancer among women with a history of a prior LCIS after 5 years of tamoxifen.

VII. MANAGEMENT OF EARLY INVASIVE BREAST CANCER: SURGERY AND RT. Removal of the primary tumor does not substantially alter the risk of metastases. Variation in local therapies (radical, modified radical, or simple mastectomies, with or without RT) does not alter survival results.

Regional lymph nodes are harbingers of systemic disease and not barriers to tumor spread. Lymph nodes are removed because of the strong prognostic information gained by learning of their involvement. Removal of axillary nodes at surgery does not affect the frequency of recurrence, the development of distant metastases, or survival rates.

A. Surgical management

1. Breast conservation therapy involves the total gross removal of tumor by limited surgery followed by RT to eradicate any residual tumor left in the remaining breast tissue. An axillary node dissection or *sentinel node* procedure should be done for staging purposes.

Contraindications to lumpectomy involve those that make radiation impossible or preclude a cosmetically acceptable result as follows:

a. Absolute contraindications for breast conservation

(1) Prior radiation to the breast or chest wall resulting in excessive exposure of radiation to the chest wall

(2) Radiation to be delivered during pregnancy

(3) Multicentric breast cancer

(4) Diffuse malignant-appearing microcalcifications on mammography

b. Relative contraindications for breast conservation

(1) Multifocal breast cancer requiring two separate incisions

(2) Active connective tissue disease involving the skin, such as scleroderma or lupus erythematosus

(3) T3 disease, or a sizable tumor in a smaller breast where the subsequent cosmetic outcome is unacceptable

2. **Modified radical mastectomy** is the standard surgical procedure for patients who choose surgery as their only local treatment (e.g., to avoid radiation) or for those patients for whom breast conservation therapy is contraindicated. This procedure includes complete removal of the breast as well as axillary lymph node resection. A number of randomized trials have shown survival equivalence for women undergoing modified radical mastectomy versus breast-conserving surgery. The cosmetic deformity that results can be managed by reconstruction or the use of a prosthesis.

3. **Axillary lymph nodes.** Standard pathologic evaluation of the axillary lymph nodes includes a level I and level II (lower and middle) axillary dissection.
   a. Lymphedema develops in about 5% of patients (see section X.B). Nerve damage may occur, but is rare.
   b. The significance of minimally involved (≤0.2 mm) axillary nodes is unresolved whether further axillary or systemic treatment is indicated. Such findings should not by themselves be used to upstage the patient or to justify giving local, regional, or systemic therapy.

4. **Sentinel lymph nodes (SLN).** Most centers have replaced lymph node dissection with the *SLN technique*, which allows a more limited removal of lymph nodes for staging purposes and results in a lower rate of complications (particularly lymphedema). Women with clinically negative axillae are candidates for SLN technique if a surgeon experienced with the technique is available. Surgeon experience that indicates adequate training and case volume improves the results of SLN biopsy.
   a. **Completion axillary dissection** at present should be offered to most patients with SLN metastases >0.2 mm. Patients who choose to omit completion axillary lymph node dissection following the finding of positive SLN should be informed of the potential increased risk of axillary nodal recurrence and its consequences.
   b. **The routine use of cytokeratin IHC for detection of SLN micrometastases should be discouraged** until the results of prospective trials are available to determine the prognostic significance of IHC-detected nodal micrometastases.

5. **Breast reconstruction**
   a. **Indications for breast reconstruction** include the availability of adequate skin and soft tissue for a reasonable cosmetic result and realistic expectations on the part of the patient.
   b. **Contraindications to breast reconstruction** include inflammatory carcinoma, the presence of extensive radiation damage to the skin from prior treatment, unrealistic expectations on the part of the patient, and the presence of comorbid diseases that render surgery dangerous.

B. **Radiation therapy.** RT is used as an adjunct to breast conservation therapy in early stage disease, for patients with four or more axillary lymph node metastases (including RT to the supraclavicular fossa), for local control of metastatic disease, and for locally advanced disease with positive margins. For women who undergo breast conservation, most of the radiation is given as external-beam megavoltage γ-irradiation to the entire breast (~4,500 to 5,000 cGy), and the remainder is given as a boost to the area of the biopsy (1,000 to 2,000 cGy). Newer products currently in clinical trials involve implanted devices that deliver the radiation in the lumpectomy cavity in a shorter period of time and then are removed *in lieu* of giving whole-breast radiation.

VIII. MANAGEMENT OF EARLY INVASIVE BREAST CANCER: ADJUVANT CHEMOTHERAPY

A. **Principles.** An overview of the randomized trials of adjuvant chemotherapy has been reported by the Early Breast Cancer Trialists' Collaborative Group. Application of about 6 months of polychemotherapy reduces the annual breast cancer death rate by about 38% for women <50 years of age, and by ~20% for those aged 50 to 69. Table 10.3 shows the approximate reductions for mortality rate by

TABLE 10.3 Approximate Reduction of Mortality at 10 Years With Adjuvant Chemotherapy for Breast Cancers That are ER-Negative and PR-Negative Treated With Doxorubicin-Based Regimens

	Reduction in mortality with adjuvant chemotherapy[a]			
	Age 35 years		Age 60 years	
Stage	Grade 1	Grade 2/3	Grade 1	Grade 2/3
I (T1b N0)	1	2	1	2
I (T1c N0)	3	6	2	4
IIA	6	12	4	8
IIB	9	15	6	10
IIIA	14	20	10	13
IIIC	18	21	12	14

[a]"Mortality" is the number of deaths caused by breast cancer among 100 patients; "Reduction" is the fewer number of deaths caused by breast cancer among 100 patients. Data do not account for *HER2* positivity or treatment with trastuzumab.
Adapted From *Adjuvant! Online* and Woodward WA, Strom EA, Tucker SL, et al. Changes in the 2003 American Joint Committee on Cancer Staging for breast cancer dramatically affect stage-specific survival. *J Clin Oncol* 2003; 21:3244.

chemotherapy for patients who are 35 or 60 years of age and whose tumors are negative for hormone receptor activity. Table 10.4 shows the approximate rate reductions in mortality by chemotherapy followed by hormonal therapy for patients who are 35 or 60 years of age and whose tumors are positive for hormone receptor activity.

TABLE 10.4 Approximate Reduction of Mortality at 10 Years With Adjuvant Chemotherapy for Breast Cancers That are ER-Positive or PR-Positive Treated With Doxorubicin-Based Regimens With or Without Hormonal Therapy

	Reduction in mortality with adjuvant chemotherapy[a]							
	Age 35 years				Age 60 years			
	Grade 1		Grade 3		Grade 1		Grade 3	
Stage	H	C-H	H	C-H	H	C-H	H	C-H
I (T1b N0)	<1	<1	2	3	<1	<1	2	2
I (T1c N0)	1	2	4	8	1	1	4	6
IIA	3	5	8	15	3	4	7	11
IIB	6	16	12	25	4	6	10	13
IIIA	9	18	14	30	7	12	13	22
IIIC	12	26	14	35	11	14	13	20

C-H, chemotherapy followed by hormonal therapy for 5 years; H, hormonal therapy alone.
[a]"Mortality" is the number of deaths caused by breast cancer among 100 patients; "Reduction" is the fewer number of deaths caused by breast cancer among 100 patients. Data do not account for *HER2* positivity or treatment with trastuzumab.
Adapted from *Adjuvant! Online* and Woodward WA, Strom EA, Tucker SL, et al. Changes in the 2003 American Joint Committee on Cancer Staging for breast cancer dramatically affect stage-specific survival. *J Clin Oncol* 2003; 21:3244.

1. **Candidates for adjuvant systemic therapy.** Women at sufficiently high risk to warrant adjuvant chemotherapy include nearly all women with positive axillary lymph nodes and many with high-risk, node-negative disease as well. Historically, node-negative patients with sufficiently high risk to be considered as candidates for adjuvant chemotherapy tend to be those with tumors that (a) are hormone receptor negative, high grade, or poorly differentiated; (b) overexpress *HER2*; (c) have markers of increased proliferation (e.g., mitotic index, high Ki67, or elevated S-phase fraction); or (d) have evidence of angio-lymphatic invasion. The relative benefit of chemotherapy depends on the woman's age at diagnosis and her hormone receptor status.

2. **Patient selection for adjuvant chemotherapy.** If a woman's risk of recurrence is 100%, a relative risk reduction of 30% would reduce her risk to 70%; however, if a woman's risk is only 10%, a relative risk reduction of 30% will reduce it to a 7% risk of recurrence. Thus, for early breast cancer but with poor prognostic markers, treatment recommendations must be made with a blend of the science and art of medicine. Moreover, patients with favorable prognostic features may be spared the toxicities of chemotherapy and treated appropriately with adjuvant endocrine therapy alone.

   a. ***Adjuvant! Online.*** Patient selection for appropriate systemic adjuvant therapy has been revolutionized by computerized decision-making tools such as *Adjuvant! Online* (www.adjuvantonline.com). Breast cancer outcome estimates made by *Adjuvant! Online* are for patients who have (a) unilateral, unicentric, invasive adenocarcinoma of the breast, (b) undergone definitive primary breast surgery and axillary node staging, and (c) no evidence of metastatic or known residual disease.

   In this online algorithm, professionals enter age, comorbidities, ER status, tumor grade, tumor size, and the number of positive lymph nodes. Then that person selects for type of adjuvant endocrine therapy (i.e., tamoxifen, aromatase inhibition) and adjuvant chemotherapy regimen (first, second or third generation). A report is then generated estimating 10-year recurrence risk or 10-year mortality (a) with no systemic adjuvant therapy, (b) with adjuvant endocrine therapy alone, (c) with adjuvant chemotherapy alone, or (d) both endocrine and chemotherapy. Graphic printouts of the results are available for counseling patients on both the risks and the benefits of adjuvant chemotherapy.

   Potential shortcomings of *Adjuvant! Online* include the relative lack of clinical data for patients who have very small lymph node-negative tumors or who are elderly, and the absence of important known risk factors such as *HER2* (although a new version will include data on *HER2* and adjuvant trastuzumab). An important update to *Adjuvant! Online* now includes a genomic version that does include Oncotype DX recurrence scores.

   b. **Oncotype DX assay** quantifies the *likelihood* of breast cancer recurrence in women with newly diagnosed, early stage, lymph node-negative, ER-positive breast cancer. The assay is performed using formalin-fixed, paraffin-embedded tumor tissue. This multiplex PCR assay measures messenger RNA (mRNA) transcripts of a panel of 16 breast cancer-associated genes that correlate with distant metastases and 5 control genes. The calculation of the Recurrence Score (RS) then combines the gene expression data into a single result (0 to 100).

      (1) The Oncotype DX gene panel and RS calculation were validated in a large, independent, multicenter clinical trial of adjuvant tamoxifen treatment (NSABP Study B-14). Patients treated adjuvantly with tamoxifen in this trial could be classified according to recurrence scores into high risk (RS $\geq$31), intermediate risk (RS =18 and <31), or low risk (RS <18) based on 10-year distant disease free survival.

      (2) In addition to prognostic information, the Oncotype DX assay may indicate the probability of response to adjuvant therapies. In the B-14 study,

patients with low or intermediate risk had a significant benefit from the use of adjuvant tamoxifen, whereas the high risk group did not. Moreover, retrospective subset analysis of the NSABP B-20 study (a randomized trial of adjuvant chemotherapy with CMF-like regimens), patients in the high risk recurrence score strata significantly benefited from adjuvant chemotherapy, whereas the intermediate and low risk groups did not achieve statistical significance.

(3) An ongoing, randomized clinical trial is prospectively evaluating whether patients with intermediate recurrence scores (defined by RS 11-25) benefit from adjuvant chemotherapy.

c. MammaPrint analyzes a DNA microarray consisting of 70 genes regulating cell cycle, invasion, metastasis, and angiogenesis. This assay requires the use of fresh tumor tissue preserved in a special buffer designed to preserve RNA integrity.

By performing DNA microarray analysis on primary breast tumors of patients, a gene expression signature that was strongly prognostic for development of distant metastasis in lymph node-negative patients was identified. The gene expression profile was validated on a consecutive set of >1,000 patients and has been demonstrated to be superior to commonly used *clinical* parameters in predicting disease outcome. A potential advantage of the MammaPrint assay is its inclusion of both ER-negative and ER-positive early stage patients.

B. Chemotherapy regimens. The National Comprehensive Cancer Network (NCCN) intermittently reviews the available published clinical trial data regarding benefits from adjuvant systemic treatments for breast cancer. In their 2007 Breast Cancer Practice Guidelines, recommendations were made concerning the chemotherapy options to offer women depending on their *HER2* status (see www.nccn.org , Breast cancer, v.2, 2007). These options are shown in Table 10.5. Drug dosing and schedules for these options are shown in Table 10.6.

 TABLE 10.5   **Adjuvant Chemotherapy Options for Breast Cancer**

Nontrastuzumab containing regimens
CMF
FAC or CAF
FEC or CEF
EC
AC with or without sequential D or P
DAC
A or E → CMF
AC × 4 cycles then sequential P × 4 cycles
(regimen every 2 weeks with filgrastim support)
A → P → C (regimen every 2 weeks with filgrastim support)
Trastuzumab-containing regimens
AC → P + concurrent H
AC → D + concurrent H
D + H → FEC
H+ D-Carb
Chemotherapy followed by H sequentially

Key: →, followed by
A, Adriamycin (doxorubicin); C, cyclophosphamide; Carb, carboplatin; D, docetaxel (Taxotere); E, epirubicin; F, 5-fluorouracil; H, Herceptin (trastuzumab); P, paclitaxel (Taxol).

TABLE 10.6   **Combination Chemotherapy Regimens for Breast Cancer[a]**

Regimen (cycle frequency)	Alkylator	5-Fluorouracil	Other
CMF (3 wks)	Cyc 600 (d 1)	600 (d 1)	Mtx 40 (d 1)
Classic CMF (4 wks)	Cyc 100 PO (days 1 to 14)	600 (d 1 & 8)	Mtx 40 (d 1 & 8)
AC (3 wks)	Cyc 600 (d 1)		Adr 60 (d 1)
FAC (4 wks)	Cyc 400–500 (d 1)	400–500 (d 1 & 8)	Adr 40–50 (d 1)
CAF (4 wks)	Cyc 100 PO days (days 1 to 14)	600 (d 1 & 8)	Adr 30 (d 1 & 8)
EC (3 wks)	Cyc 600 (d 1)		Epi 100 (d 1)
CEF120 (4 wks)	Cyc 75 PO (days 1 to 14)	500 (d 1 & 8)	Epi 60 (d 1 & 8), Abx
FEC 100 (3 wks)	Cyc 500 (d 1)	500 (d 1)	Epi 50 (d 1 & 8) or 100 (d 1)
PC (weekly)	Carb AUC 2		Pac 80
DAC (3 wks)	500 (d 1)		Adr 50 (d 1)
			Doc 75 (d 1)
Dose dense			
AC (2 wks × 4)[b]	Cyc 600 (d 1)		Adr 60 (d 1)
Then, (2 wks × 4)[b]			Pac 175 (d 1)
BCIRG-006			
DC/H (3 wks × 6)	Carb AUC 6 (d 1)[c]		Doc 75 (d 1),[c] and Her 4 mg/kg d 1, then 2 mg/kg wkly × 18 wks, then 6 mg/kg every 3 wks for 1 yr from d 1
AC-D/H (AC 3 wks × 4) (Then, D 3 wks × 4)	Cyc 600 (d 1)[c]		Adr 60 (d 1)[c] Doc 100, and Her 4 mg/kg d 1, then 2 mg/kg wkly × 12 wks, then 6 mg/kg every 3 wks for 1 yr from d 1

Abx, prophylactic antibiotics; Adr, Adriamycin (doxorubicin); AUC, Area under the curve by Calvert's formula; Carb, carboplatin; Cyc, cyclophosphamide, Doc, docetaxel (Taxotere); Epi, epirubicin (Ellence); Her, Herceptin (trastuzumab); Mtx, methotrexate; Pac, paclitaxel (Taxol); wks/wkly, weeks/weekly..
[a]Drug doses are in mg/m² body surface area (days on which drugs are given intravenous [IV] in each cycle are in parentheses); all drugs are given IV except PO where indicated.
[b]Granulocyte colony-stimulating factor (filgastrim, 300 or 480 mcg subcutaneous [SQ] on days 2 through 10, or pegfilgastrim, 6 mg SQ on day 2) is given during each 2-week cycle.
[c]Given on day 2 of first cycle

C. Role of taxanes in the adjuvant setting

    1. Three clinical trials, individually and together, strongly suggest an additional benefit to adding a taxane to an anthracycline-based chemotherapy regimen for women with lymph node-positive breast cancer.

        a. Cancer and Acute Leukemia Group B (CALGB 9344) showed a 17% reduction in risk of recurrence and an 18% reduction in risk of death at a median follow-up of 69 months with the addition of paclitaxel given every 3 weeks for four cycles after four cycles of Adriamycin–cyclophosphamide (AC).

        b. NSABP B-28 showed a 17% reduction in risk of recurrence at a median of 65 months by adding paclitaxel sequentially to AC in a manner similar to the CALGB 9344.

    c. Breast Cancer International Research Group (BCIRG 001) showed that do-
cetaxel/AC (DAC) delivered every 3 weeks for six cycles resulted in a 28%
improvement in disease-free survival (DFS) compared with six cycles of CA-
fluorouracil (CAF) with a median follow-up of 55 months. In addition, a
30% improvement in overall survival (OS) was noted during this same time
period.

2. Because all ER-positive breast cancers respond less well to chemotherapy compared with ER-negative tumors, the additional benefit of adding a taxane for
ER-positive patients is not as pronounced compared with ER-negative patients.

3. What these studies do not tell us is which is the best regimen and which taxane or
taxane dosing schedule is superior. In an attempt to address this shortcoming,
the Eastern Cooperative Oncology Group (ECOG) conducted a randomized,
prospective clinical trial (E1199) designed to compare taxanes (docetaxel versus
paclitaxel) and taxane dosing schedules (weekly versus every 3 weeks) head to
head. In this 2 × 2 factorial study design, patients received four cycles of AC
every 3 weeks followed by (a) paclitaxel every 3 weeks for four cycles, (b)
docetaxel every 3 weeks for four cycles, (c) paclitaxel weekly for 12 weeks, or
(d) docetaxel weekly for 12 weeks.

    a. The primary comparisons failed to demonstrate any significant advantage of
one taxane over another, or the weekly schedule over the every-3-week schedule. This finding was potentially confounded because a significant fraction
of patients randomized to the weekly docetaxel regimen could not feasibly
complete all planned cycles because of untoward toxicity.

    b. In planned secondary comparisons, both the weekly paclitaxel arm and the
every-3-week docetaxel arm were significantly superior to the every-3-week
paclitaxel arm. The weekly paclitaxel arm had a significant survival advantage compared with the every-3-week paclitaxel control arm. Moreover, considering toxicities, the weekly paclitaxel arm had a superior therapeutic index, although it was associated with a higher risk of neurotoxicity (peripheral
neuropathy).

D. Adjuvant trastuzumab (Herceptin). Trastuzumab is a humanized, monoclonal antibody with specificity for the extracellular domain of the human *EGFR-2* (*HER2*;
HER2/neu).

    1. Randomized trials. Results from five prospective randomized trials testing ad-
juvant trastuzumab have been reported. Together, the adjuvant trastuzumab
trials are remarkably consistent, with most analyses indeed reporting an overall
survival benefit with trastuzumab treatment.

    a. In NSABP B-31, patients with *HER2*-positive, node-positive breast cancer
were randomly assigned to AC for four cycles every 3 weeks followed by
paclitaxel given every 3 weeks for four cycles or the same regimen with 52
weeks of trastuzumab commencing with the paclitaxel. In the North Central
Cancer Treatment Group (NCCTG) N9831 intergroup trial, patients who
were *HER2*-positive with early stage cancer were similarly randomized except that paclitaxel was given by a low dose weekly schedule for 12 weeks;
a third arm testing sequential chemotherapy followed by trastuzumab was
added.

        Because of their similarities, the B-31 and NCCTG N9831 trials with
3,351 patients together were analyzed jointly. With a median follow-up of
2 years, trastuzumab resulted in a 52% reduction in the risk of recurrence
($P < 0.001$) and a 33% reduction in the risk of death ($P = 0.015$). Similar
beneficial effects on DFS were observed when results of the NSABP B-31 and
NCCTG N9831 trials were analyzed separately.

    b. A third trial (HERA) involving 5,081 patients tested trastuzumab for 1 ver-
sus 2 years (compared with no further treatment) following all local therapy
and a menu of standard chemotherapy regimens. With early follow-up, 1
year of trastuzumab resulted in a 46% reduction in the risk of recurrence
($P < 0.0001$). The data for 2 years of adjuvant trastuzumab are not yet reported.

c. The BCIRG 006 study randomized 3,222 women with *HER2*-amplified, node-positive or high-risk node-negative breast cancer to AC followed by docetaxel, AC followed by docetaxel plus trastuzumab (DH) for 1 year, or carboplatin plus docetaxel plus trastuzumab. At 36 months of follow-up, patients receiving AC followed by docetaxel with trastuzumab had a hazard ratio for disease-free recurrence of 0.61 (*P* <0.0001) when compared with the non-trastuzumab control arm. The hazard ratio for DFS was 0.67 (*P* = 0.0003) for patients in the carboplatin/docetaxel/trastuzumab (CDH) arm. No statistically significant difference in the hazard ratio for DFS was observed between the two trastuzumab-containing arms. A significant survival benefit was observed in both trastuzumab-containing arms. Importantly, the non-anthracycline arm (TCH) had significantly less cardiac toxicity than the AC followed by the TH arm. Dosages and schedules for these regimens are shown in Table 10.6.

d. A fifth trial (FinHer) randomized 1,010 women to either 9 weeks of vinorelbine followed by three cycles of FEC (defined in Table 10.6) versus docetaxel for three cycles followed by three cycles of FEC. Patients (*N* = 232) with *HER2*-positive cancers were further randomized to receive trastuzumab or not for 9 weeks during the vinorelbine or docetaxel treatment. With a median follow-up of 3 years, the addition of trastuzumab was associated with a reduction in risk of recurrence (hazard ratio 0.42; *P* = 0.01).

2. **Cardiac adverse events** from adjuvant trastuzumab. In the adjuvant trastuzumab trials, the rates of grade III/IV congestive heart failure (CHF) or cardiac-related death for patients receiving treatment regimens containing trastuzumab ranged from 0% (FinHer trial) to 4.1% (NSABP B-31 trial). The risk of cardiac dysfunction appears to be related to age, baseline left ventricular ejection fraction (LVEF), prior anthracycline treatment, and use of concomitant antihypertensive medications. It is worth noting that patients in all of these trials had *rigorous monitoring of LVEF every 3 months* while on trastuzumab treatment, and strict guidelines for withholding trastuzumab, even for asymptomatic declines in LVEF, were followed. Moreover, the median age of patients enrolled in all of these trials was about 50 years, and virtually any significant cardiac history was exclusionary.

Candidates for treatment with trastuzumab should undergo thorough baseline cardiac assessment, including history and physical examination and assessment of LVEF by echocardiogram or radionuclide scan. Monitoring may not identify all patients who will develop cardiac dysfunction. Caution should be exercised in treating patients with pre-existing cardiac dysfunction. Discontinuation of trastuzumab treatment should be strongly considered in patients who develop a clinically significant decrease in LVEF.

3. **HER2 status, topoisomerase II, and the role of anthracyclines.** Numerous large retrospective studies have linked *HER2* status with response to anthracyclines. Transfection and overexpression of *HER2* in breast cancer cell lines does not, however, increase sensitivity to doxorubicin *in vitro*. This observation suggests that some factor other than *HER2* confers drug sensitivity to anthracyclines.

The topoisomerase IIα gene is in close physical proximity to the *HER2* gene on the long arm of chromosome 17, and in 35% of patients with *HER2* gene amplification, the topoisomerase II gene is coamplified. The current hypothesis is that amplification of topoisomerase II confers sensitivity to anthracyclines, and not *HER2* gene amplification per se. Of note, topoisomerase II gene amplification is seen rarely (if ever) in the absence of *HER2* gene amplification. Thus, it is arguable whether or not anthracyclines are of any benefit in *HER2*-negative early stage breast cancers.

The US Oncology Network is currently testing docetaxel plus cyclophosphamide for six cycles, versus the DAC regimen for six cycles in *HER2*-negative early stage patients. Moreover, in the BCIRG 006 adjuvant trastuzumab trial, no apparent advantage was seen to an anthracycline-based adjuvant trastuzumab regimen above and beyond a non-anthracycline-based trastuzumab regimen (regardless of topoisomerase II status), suggesting that so long as trastuzumab is used, anthracyclines may be dispensable.

E. Dose-dense therapy. Delivering identical doses of chemotherapy on a more frequent basis is described as *dose-dense* therapy. One large clinical trial (CALBG 9741) showed a 26% improvement in DFS and a 31% improvement in OS for women with lymph node-positive breast cancer receiving chemotherapy on an every-2-week basis with growth factors when compared with the same regimen delivered every 3 weeks without growth factor support. AC (every 2 weeks for four cycles) was followed by paclitaxel (every 2 weeks for four cycles).

Although this trial's data are compelling, they do not differentiate the benefit of dose-dense chemotherapy employing AC versus paclitaxel, either of which could be responsible for the improvement in DFS and OS. One possible explanation is the more frequent dosing of the paclitaxel, which has been shown to be superior to every 3 weeks of paclitaxel in the metastatic setting. The NSABP has recently completed accrual to a large randomized trial (NSABP B-38) comparing two-dose dense adjuvant therapy regimens (one including gemcitabine) versus DAC.

F. Adjuvant chemotherapy is <u>not</u> indicated in the following circumstances:

1. In women with a good prognosis without such treatment, including those with the following conditions:

   a. Noninvasive CIS of any size in women of any age

   b. Very small primary tumors (<0.5 cm; T1a) and negative axillary lymph nodes, irrespective of the status of hormone receptors

   c. Comorbid medical conditions that make survival beyond 5 years unlikely or that make the potential adverse effects of therapy unacceptable

2. Controversy exists regarding the use of adjuvant systemic chemotherapy for women whose tumors are 0.6 to 1.0 cm with negative hormone receptors or with a grade interpreted as moderately or poorly differentiated.

G. Radiation and chemotherapy. For women who are prescribed both chemotherapy and RT, it is recommended that these modalities be used sequentially with chemotherapy delivered first. RT may be used concurrently with CMF chemotherapy, but not with other published regimens.

H. Adjuvant endocrine therapy

1. Selective ER modifiers. Tamoxifen has been considered the standard of care for all women with an invasive breast cancer that expresses either ER or PR. The benefit of tamoxifen is seen regardless of the patient's age, the number of involved lymph nodes, and whether or not chemotherapy is used. Trials have demonstrated that patients did the best when taking 20 mg of tamoxifen daily for 5 years. One large trial in women with ER-positive, lymph node-negative breast cancer comparing 5 versus 10 years of tamoxifen in the adjuvant setting has demonstrated a detrimental effect on DFS for those women taking tamoxifen for 10 years.

2. Aromatase inhibitors block the peripheral conversion of the adrenal androgens (androstenedione and testosterone) into estradiol and estrone in women. Aromatase inhibitors should not be considered in those women who have any ovarian function because blockage of peripheral aromatization will not block the ovarian production of estrogen and progesterone.

   a. The ATAC trial randomized 9,366 postmenopausal women with early invasive breast cancer to one of three arms: anastrozole (Arimidex) 1 mg daily for 5 years, tamoxifen 20 mg daily for 5 years, and the combination of both drugs daily for 5 years (see ATAC Trialists' Group in *Suggested Reading*). The outcome of those women taking the combination of anastrozole and tamoxifen was the same as that of the women taking tamoxifen alone. At a median follow-up of 48 months, however, findings were an 18% improvement in DFS and a 22% improvement in time to recurrence for those patients with ER-positive tumors who were randomized to anastrozole compared with tamoxifen. In addition, an additional 44% reduction was noted in new contralateral breast tumors for women receiving 5 years of anastrozole. Because of this trial, postmenopausal women with hormone receptor-positive invasive breast cancer now have the option of taking either tamoxifen for 5 years or anastrozole for 5 years as their adjuvant hormonal therapy.

b. The MA 17 trial randomized 5,187 postmenopausal women with ER-positive and ER-negative invasive breast cancer who had received from 4.5 to 5.5 years of tamoxifen in the adjuvant setting. These women were randomized to 5 years of further therapy with either placebo or letrozole (Femara). At the first interim analysis at a median follow-up of 2.4 years, it is estimated that the DFS for those randomized to letrozole is 93% compared with 87% for those randomized to placebo. Additionally, letrozole decreased the incidence of contralateral breast cancer by 46%. These benefits were seen for women who were originally lymph node positive or negative. Thus, for postmenopausal women, the addition of letrozole after 5 years of tamoxifen may be considered.

c. Finally, a double-blind, randomized trial to test whether, after 2 to 3 years of tamoxifen therapy, switching to exemestane (Aromasin) was more effective than continuing tamoxifen therapy for the remainder of the 5 years of treatment has been conducted. Exemestane therapy after 2 to 3 years of tamoxifen therapy significantly improved DFS as compared with the standard 5 years of tamoxifen treatment. Contralateral breast cancer occurred in 20 patients in the tamoxifen group and 9 in the exemestane group ($P = 0.04$).

d. In summary, aromatase inhibition is superior to tamoxifen in postmenopausal ER-positive patients whether used first line in place of tamoxifen, following 2 to 3 years of tamoxifen, or following 5 years of tamoxifen. The optimal duration of aromatase inhibitor therapy remains unknown. Ongoing trials will address this issue.

3. Ovarian ablation. Ovarian ablation via surgical oophorectomy, or suppression with agonists of luteinizing hormone-releasing hormone (LHRH) are effective therapy for premenopausal ER-positive early stage breast cancer. Available data suggest similar benefit from surgical ovarian ablation as there is with the use of CMF chemotherapy in such patients. Trials currently underway will address whether ovarian ablation plus an aromatase inhibitor will be superior to adjuvant tamoxifen in premenopausal women who are ER positive.

4. Combination chemohormonal therapy. When chemotherapy and tamoxifen are both used in the adjuvant setting, they should be used sequentially, rather than in combination, because of a detrimental outcome when comparing concurrent versus sequential chemohormonal therapy. Whether this will also hold true for aromatase inhibitors is unknown.

I. Preoperative (neoadjuvant) therapy

1. The use of preoperative cytoreductive chemotherapy for those who desire breast conservation therapy may be considered. No survival advantage exists to the delivery of the chemotherapy preoperatively compared with its postoperative use. No randomized clinical trials have been performed to evaluate the benefit of adjuvant chemotherapy in women who have received both anthracyclines and taxanes in the preoperative setting.

2. For patients with inoperable locally advanced disease at presentation, the initial use of preoperative chemotherapy with an anthracycline and a taxane is standard treatment. Following neoadjuvant therapy measures aimed at local control usually consist of total mastectomy with axillary lymph node dissection, with or without delayed breast reconstruction, or lumpectomy and axillary dissection. Both local treatment groups are considered to have sufficient risk of local recurrence to warrant the use of chest wall (or breast) and supraclavicular node irradiation. Involved internal mammary lymph nodes should also be irradiated. Tamoxifen (or an aromatase inhibitor if postmenopausal) should be added for those with hormone receptor positive tumors.

3. In selected ER-positive patients, neoadjuvant endocrine therapy may be used; for example in elderly or frail patients, or patients with a contraindication to neoadjuvant chemotherapy.

4. For *HER2*-positive patients, neoadjuvant chemotherapy regimens incorporating trastuzumab have been shown to have very impressive pathologic complete response rates. Thus, trastuzumab-based regimens are considered the standard of care for *HER2*-positive locally advanced disease.

IX. MANAGEMENT: DISSEMINATED DISEASE (STAGE IV).

Except in rare cases, stage IV breast cancer is considered incurable. Thus, the focus of treatment for advanced disease should be on palliation of disease-related symptoms.

A. Hormone receptor–positive metastatic breast cancer. For women who have non-life-threatening, ER-positive or PR-positive metastatic breast cancer, single-agent hormone therapy is recommended. Chemotherapy is reserved for hormone-resistant disease, or patients with symptomatic or life-threatening metastases, such as lymphangiitic pulmonary metastases or progressive liver metastases.

1. For postmenopausal women, the following hormones can be used in a sequential manner:

   a. Aromatase inhibitors
   - **(1)** Anastrozole (Arimidex), 1 mg PO daily, or
   - **(2)** Exemestane (Aromasin), 25 mg PO daily, or
   - **(3)** Letrozole (Femara), 2.5 mg PO daily

   b. Tamoxifen (20 mg PO daily) or toremifene (Fareston, 60 mg PO daily)

   c. Fulvestrant (Faslodex), 250 mg IM monthly

   d. Megestrol acetate (Megace), 40 mg PO q.i.d.

   e. Fluoxymesterone (Halotestin), 10 mg PO b.i.d. or t.i.d

   f. Diethylstilbestrol, 5 mg PO t.i.d.

2. For premenopausal women, options include the following:

   a. Tamoxifen

   b. LHRH agonist or surgical or radiotherapeutic oophorectomy

   c. Megestrol acetate

   d. Fluoxymesterone

   e. Diethylstilbesterol

B. Chemotherapy. No gold standard chemotherapy regimen exists for metastatic breast cancer. Chemotherapy combinations are shown in Table 10.6; although somewhat more active than single agents, the combinations are associated with more treatment-related side effects. Consequently, sequential single agent chemotherapy (except in cases where rapid response is required) is most commonly used to manage advanced ER-negative (or hormone-refractory ER-positive) disease.

1. *HER2*-negative, ER-negative metastatic breast cancer

   a. Preferred single agents include the anthracyclines (doxorubin [Adriamycin], epirubicin [Ellence], or liposomal doxorubicin [Doxil]), the taxanes (paclitaxel [Taxol], docetaxel [Taxotere], or albumin-bound paclitaxel [Abraxane]), capecitabine [Xeloda], or vinorelbine (Navelbine). Effective treatment options for patients with metastatic breast cancer resistant to anthracyclines and taxanes are limited.

   b. Other active agents include gemcitabine, platinoids, vinblastine, irinotecan, mitomycin, and ixabepilone. One study showed that ixabepilone plus capecitabine prolonged median progression-free survival (6 *vs.* 4 months), and increased objective response rate (35% *vs.* 14%; $P <0.0001$) compared with capecitabine alone.

   c. Bevacizumab. A randomized trial of weekly paclitaxel with or without bevacizumab (Avastin) as first-line treatment for patients with metastatic breast cancer has been conducted by ECOG (E2100). A significant improvement in progression-free survival was demonstrated, but no significant benefit seen in terms of OS. In another study, patients with metastatic disease previously treated with anthracyclines and taxanes were randomized to capecitabine alone versus capecitabine plus bevacizumab. The response rate was increased with bevacizumab, but no significant difference was found in time-to-progression or OS.

2. *HER2*-positive metastatic breast cancer

a. Trastuzumab. Data support the use of single-agent trastuzumab (Herceptin) or the combination of trastuzumab with chemotherapy drugs. The anthracyclines are to be avoided, however, because of the risk of cardiotoxicity when trastuzumab is combined with these agents. Two randomized trials in women with metastatic breast cancer have shown a survival benefit for women who were placed immediately on trastuzumab therapy with concurrent chemotherapy.

b. Lapatinib is a small molecule, orally bioavailable tyrosine kinase inhibitor of *HER2* and EGFR. It is active (in combination with capecitabine) in women with *HER2*-positive metastatic breast cancer that has progressed after trastuzumab-based therapy.

In a randomized pivotal trial of lapatinib, patients with *HER2*-positive advanced or metastatic breast cancer that had progressed after treatment with regimens that included an anthracycline, a taxane, and trastuzumab were randomly assigned to receive either combination therapy (lapatinib at a dose of 1,250 mg/day continuously plus capecitabine at a dose of 2,000 mg/m^2 on days 1 through 14 of a 21-day cycle) or capecitabine alone. An interim analysis of time to progression met specified criteria for early reporting on the basis of superiority in the combination-therapy arm. The median time to progression of 8 months in the combination-therapy group as compared with 4 months in the capecitabine alone arm. Notable toxicities of lapatinib include rash and diarrhea (similar to other EGFR kinase inhibitors), and only infrequent reports of cardiotoxicity. In combination with capecitabine, an increase in frequency of diarrhea was seen, but other capecitabine-associated toxicities, such as palmar-plantar erythrodysaesthesia, were not significantly increased.

C. Bisphosphonates are recommended for women with breast cancer metastatic to bones. Both pamidronate (Aredia, 90 mg IV monthly) and zoledronate (Zometa, 4 mg IV monthly) are effective in reducing bone pain and pathologic fractures. Zoledronate may be superior to pamidronate for reducing (*a*) bony fracture, (*b*) spinal cord compression, (*c*) hypercalcemia of malignancy, and (*d*) the need for palliative RT in patients with metastatic disease. Cancer patients taking bisphosphonate drugs for the prevention of fractures caused by bone metastases appear more likely to develop osteonecrosis of the jaw than patients who do not take the drugs.

D. Local therapy for metastatic disease. Metastatic disease is generally treated systemically, but some local problems benefit from local RT.

1. Bony metastases can be followed as markers of disease, but if they are painful or show impending signs of fracture, these usually respond to local RT. If in the axial skeleton, RT should include the vertebrae above and below the involved vertebra. In addition, all patients with bony metastases should receive a bisphosphonate (see section IX.C). Patients with spinal cord compression should be considered for early surgical intervention based on data that demonstrated a higher percentage of ambulatory patients, but no change in OS, if surgical decompression was undertaken before RT.

2. All cervical spine and femoral neck lesions, with or without symptoms, should usually be treated with local RT because of the potential for fracture. Femoral neck lesions may also require surgical fixation.

3. Brain and orbital metastases. Patients who present with headache or nausea and vomiting and metastatic disease should alert the clinician to promptly investigate for brain metastases or meningeal carcinomatosis. Brain MRI, with and without gadolinium, is necessary to diagnose metastatic disease. Solitary lesions may be excised surgically or radiated with new modalities, such as cyberknife or gamma knife. Multiple lesions must be given whole-brain radiation.

4. Chest wall recurrence. These patients are generally treated first with systemic therapy. In some cases, RT may be used, especially when the patient is otherwise without evidence of disease.

X. SPECIAL CLINICAL PROBLEMS

A. Postsurgical edema of the arm without pain was regularly associated with the traditional radical mastectomy but also occurs with less extensive surgery. The incidence is increased in patients who receive postoperative RT. The edema usually develops within 6 months after surgery, but may be delayed much longer. Therapy is not always helpful but includes elevation of the arm, arm compression sleeves, compression pump, lymphomassage, and physical therapy. Physical therapists or occupational therapists trained in lymphatic massage often benefit the patient.

B. Edema of the arm with pain or paresthesias occurring >1 month after surgery may reflect recurrent tumor. The cancer is often not clinically discernible because it resides high in the apex of the axilla or lung and involves the brachial plexus. Patients may complain of tingling or pain in the hands and progressive weakness and atrophy of the hand and arm muscles. If sufficient time passes, a tumor mass becomes palpable in the axilla or supraclavicular fossa, but the patient is usually left with a paralyzed hand unresponsive to therapy. These patients may receive RT to the axilla and supraclavicular fossa, if radiation has not previously been delivered to this region. The recurrence to the brachial plexus may not be easily seen on MRI or CT scanning. PET scanning may be useful in this circumstance. Occasionally, the pain of this nerve involvement is so severe that nerve blocks by a pain management specialist are necessary.

C. Breast implants can create a special challenge in both diagnosis and treatment of breast cancer. No relationship exists between breast implants and the development of breast cancer. In fact, women with breast augmentation with breast implants appear to be less likely to develop breast cancer in their lifetime than women who choose to not have implants placed for cosmetic augmentation. Mammography techniques have been developed to assess the breast tissue in women with implants, and they appear to have the same sensitivity for picking up early breast cancers as in women without implants.

1. When an abnormality is seen on a mammogram in a woman with breast implants, special consideration is given to the type of biopsy techniques that must be used. Stereotactic techniques may be avoided to lessen the likelihood of puncturing the implant. Each case is taken on an individual basis depending on the proximity of the abnormality to the implant.

2. When a woman elects to have a mastectomy as part of her local breast cancer management and subsequently requires chest wall RT, placement of breast implants is frequently avoided. A greater risk exists of scar tissue contracting around the implant with radiation, thus significantly reducing an optimal cosmetic benefit of breast reconstruction. If chest wall radiation is to be considered, most plastic surgeons would prefer to bring a flap of tissue from outside the radiation field to accomplish optimal reconstruction and cosmesis.

D. Breast cancer during pregnancy. In a California registry study, there were 1.3 breast cancers diagnosed per 10,000 live births. Breast cancer during pregnancy is most often associated with larger tumor size and with lymph node metastasis. Histologically, these tumors are often poorly differentiated, more frequently ER-negative and PR-negative, and are frequently *HER2*-positive. Delay in diagnosis is typical because tumor masses can be masked by breast engorgement owing to lactation, and inflammatory changes may be mistaken for mastitis.

1. Mammography with shielding can be performed safely, although interpretation can be difficult because of increased breast density. Ultrasonography of the breast and regional lymph nodes is used to assess the extent of disease and also to guide biopsy.

2. Core needle biopsy is preferred for histologic diagnosis and biomarker analysis.

3. Staging assessment of the pregnant patient can be problematic. In addition to complete blood count and serum chemistries, including hepatic function testing, a chest radiograph (with shielding) is feasible. Additionally, in patients who have clinically node-positive or T3 breast lesions, an ultrasound of the liver and directed screening MRI of the thoracic and lumbar spine without contrast can be used. Documentation of metastases may alter the treatment plan and influence the patient's decision regarding maintenance of the pregnancy.

4. Assessment of the pregnancy should include a maternal fetal medicine consultation.

5. Indications for systemic chemotherapy do not differ for the pregnant patient with breast cancer, although chemotherapy is to be avoided during the first trimester of pregnancy because of the risk of fetal malformation. Fetal malformation risks in the second and third trimester fall to approximately 1.3%, no different than that of unexposed fetuses.

   a. The greatest treatment experience in pregnancy has been with anthracycline and alkylating agent chemotherapy. Limited data are found on the use of taxanes during pregnancy.

   b. Chemotherapy during pregnancy should be avoided following week 35 to avoid hematologic complications at the time of delivery. Ondansetron, lorazepam, and dexamethasone may be used for the antiemetic regimen.

   c. There are two case reports of trastuzumab use during pregnancy. Oligohydramnios was reported in both cases. Trastuzumab should be delayed until the postpartum period.

   d. Endocrine therapy and radiation therapy are contraindicated during pregnancy, and should not be initiated until the postpartum period.

Suggested Reading

ATAC Trialists' Group. Anastrozole alone or in combination with tamoxifen versus tamoxifen alone for adjuvant treatment of postmenopausal women with early breast cancer: first results of the ATAC randomised trial. *Lancet* 2002;359:2131.

Bear HD, Anderson S, Smith RE, et al. Sequential preoperative or postoperative docetaxel added to preoperative doxorubicin plus cyclophosphamide for operable breast cancer: National Surgical Adjuvant Breast and Bowel Protocol B-27. *J Clin Oncol* 2006;24: 2019.

Carlson RW, McCormick B. Update: NCCN Breast Cancer Clinical Practice Guidelines. *J Natl Compr Canc Netw* 2005(Suppl);1:S7.

Carter C, Allen C, Henson D. Relation of tumor size, lymph node status, and survival in 24,740 breast cancer cases. *Cancer* 1989;63:181.

Citron ML, Berry DA, Cirrincione C, et al. Randomized trial of dose-dense versus conventionally scheduled and sequential versus concurrent combination chemotherapy as postoperative adjuvant treatment of node-positive primary breast cancer: first report of Intergroup trial C9741/Cancer and Leukemia group B trial 9741. *J Clin Oncol* 2003;21: 1431.

Coombes RC, Hall E, Gibson LJ, et al. A randomized trial of exemestane after two to three years of tamoxifen therapy in postmenopausal women with primary breast cancer. *N Engl J Med* 2004;350:1081.

Early Breast Cancer Trialists' Collaborative Group. Effects of chemotherapy and hormonal therapy for early breast cancer on recurrence and 15-year survival: an overview of the randomised trials. *Lancet* 2005;365:1687.

Fan C, Oh DS, Wessels L, et al. Concordance among gene expression-based predictors for breast cancer. *N Engl J Med* 2006;355:560.

Fisher B, Dignam J, Wolmark N, et al. Tamoxifen in treatment of intraductal breast cancer: National Surgical Adjuvant Breast and Bowel Project B-24 randomised controlled trial. *Lancet* 1999;353:1993.

Fisher ER, Dignam J, Tan-Chiu E, et al. Pathologic findings from the National Surgical Adjuvant Breast Project (NSABP) eight-year update of protocol B-17. Intraductal carcinoma. *Cancer* 1999;86:429.

Geyer CE, Forster J, Lindquist D, et al. Lapatinib plus capecitabine for HER2-positive advanced breast cancer. *N Engl J Med* 2006;355(26):2733.

Goss PE, Ingle JN, Martino S, et al. Randomized trial of letrozole following tamoxifen as extended adjuvant therapy in receptor-positive breast cancer: updated findings from NCIC CTG MA-17. *J Natl Cancer Inst* 2005;97:1262.

Greene FL, Page DL, Fleming ID, et al. *AJCC Cancer Staging Manual.* 6th ed. New York: Springer-Verlag; 2002.

Hillner BE, Ingle JN, Chlebowski RT, et al. American Society of Clinical Oncology 2003 update on the role of bisphosphonates and bone health issues in women with breast cancer. *J Clin Oncol* 2003;21:4042.

Jemel A, Siegel E, Ward T, et al. Cancer statistics, 2007. *CA Cancer J Clin* 2007;57:45.

Julien JP, Bijker N, Fentiman IS, et al. Radiotherapy in breast-conserving treatment for ductal carcinoma in situ: first results of the EORTC randomised phase III trial 10853. EORTC Breast Cancer Cooperative Group and EORTC Radiotherapy Group. *Lancet* 2000;355:528.

Lehman CD, Gatsonis C, Kuhl CK, et al. ACRIN Trial 6667 Investigators Group. MRI evaluation of the contralateral breast in women with recently diagnosed breast cancer. *N Engl J Med* 2007;356(13):1295.

Mansel RE, Fallowfield L, Kissin M, et al. Randomized multicenter trial of sentinel node biopsy versus standard axillary treatment in operable breast cancer: the ALMANAC Trial. *J Natl Cancer Inst* 2006;98:599.

Morrow M, Strom EA, Bassett LW, et al. Standard for the management of ductal carcinoma in situ of the breast (DCIS). *CA Cancer J Clin* 2002;52:256.

Morrow M, Strom EA, Bassett LW, et al. Standard for breast conservation therapy in the management of invasive breast cancer. *CA Cancer J Clin* 2002;52:277.

NCCN Clinical Practice Guidelines in Oncology. *Breast Cancer* V.2.2007. www.nccn.org

Olivotto IA, Bajdik CD, Ravdin PM, et al. Population-based validation of the prognostic model ADJUVANT! for early breast cancer. *J Clin Oncol* 2005;23:2716.

Paik S, Tang G, Shak S, et al. Gene expression and benefit of chemotherapy in women with node-negative, estrogen receptor-positive breast cancer. *J Clin Oncol* 2006;24: 3726.

Piccart-Gebhart MJ, Procter M, Leyland-Jones B, et al. Trastuzumab after adjuvant chemotherapy in HER2-positive breast cancer. *N Engl J Med* 2005;353:1659.

Recht A, Edge SB, Solin LJ, et al. Postmastectomy radiotherapy: clinical practice guidelines of the American Society of Clinical Oncology. *J Clin Oncol* 2001;19:1539.

Romond EH, Perez EA, Bryant J, et al. Trastuzumab plus adjuvant chemotherapy for operable HER2-positive breast cancer. *N Engl J Med* 2005;353:1673.

Slamon D, Eiermann W, Robert NJ, et al. Phase III randomized trial comparing doxorubicin and cyclophosphamide followed by docetaxel (AC → T) with doxorubicin and cyclophosphamide followed by docetaxel and trastuzumab (AC → TH) with docetaxel, carboplatin and trastuzumab (TCH) in HER2 positive early breast cancer patients: BCIRG 006 study [Abstract]. Presented at the San Antonio Breast Cancer Symposium, San Antonio, TX, December 8–11, 2005; Abstract 1.

Slamon DJ, Leyland-Jones B, Shak S, et al. Use of chemotherapy plus a monoclonal antibody against HER2 for metastatic breast cancer that overexpresses HER2. *N Engl J Med* 2001;344:783.

Sorlie T, Perou CM, Tibshirani R et al. Gene expression patterns of breast carcinomas distinguish tumor subclasses with clinical implications. *Proc Natl Acad Sci USA* 2001; 98:10869.

Sparano JA, Wang M, Martino S, et al. Phase III study of doxorubicin-cyclophosphamide followed by paclitaxel or docetaxel given every 3 weeks or weekly in patients with axillary node-positive or high-risk node negative breast cancer [Abstract]. Presented at the San Antonio Breast Cancer Symposium, San Antonio, TX, December 8–11, 2005; Abstract 48.

Tan-Chiu E, Yothers G, Romond E, et al. Assessment of cardiac dysfunction in a randomized trial comparing doxorubicin and cyclophosphamide followed by paclitaxel, with or without trastuzumab as adjuvant therapy in node-positive, human epidermal growth factor receptor 2-overexpressing breast cancer: NSABP B-31. *J Clin Oncol* 2005;23:7811.

van de Vijver MJ, He YD, van't Veer LJ et al. A gene-expression signature as a predictor of survival in breast cancer. *N Engl J Med* 2002;347:1999.

Warner E, Yaffe M, Kimberly S. et al. American Cancer Society Guidelines for Breast Screening with MRI as an Adjunct to Mammography. *CA Cancer J Clin* 2007;57:75.

Weiss RB, et al. Natural history of more than 20 years of node-positive primary breast carcinoma treated with cyclophosphamide, methotrexate, and fluorouracil-based adjuvant chemotherapy: a study by the Cancer and Leukemia Group B. *J Clin Oncol* 2003;21:1825.

Woodward WA, Strom EA, Tucker SL, et al. Changes in the 2003 American Joint Committee on Cancer Staging for breast cancer dramatically affect stage-specific survival. *J Clin Oncol* 2003;21:3244.

Wooster R, Weber BL. Genomic medicine: breast and ovarian cancer. *N Engl J Med* 2003;348:2339.

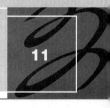

GYNECOLOGIC CANCERS
Sanaz Memarzadeh and Jonathan S. Berek

11

 GENERAL ASPECTS

I. EPIDEMIOLOGY. Malignancies of the genital tract constitute about 20% of visceral cancers in women. The incidence and mortality rates according to primary site are shown in Table 11.1.

II. DIAGNOSTIC STUDIES
   A. Staging evaluation is necessary regardless of the site of the primary lesion after cancer of the female genital tract is proved histologically. Potentially valuable studies include the following:
   1. Pelvic and rectal examinations (to determine whether the adnexa, vagina, or pelvic wall is involved)
   2. CBC, serum electrolytes, creatinine, and LFTs
   3. Chest radiograph: plain chest x-ray or CT as indicated (for pulmonary metastases)
   4. Abdominal-pelvic ultrasonography, CT scans, including evaluation of the ureters, or MRI (to delineate abnormal areas)
   5. Sigmoidoscopy with biopsy of abnormal areas is optional, as indicated (for mucosal involvement or mass lesions)
   6. Cystoscopy with biopsy of abnormal areas for cancers of the vulva, vagina, cervix, or endometrium is optional as indicated (to look for bladder mucosal involvement)
   7. Cytological evaluation of effusions
   8. The use of positron emission tomography (PET) in gynecologic malignancies is being evaluated.
   B. Immunohistochemical tumor markers pertaining to gynecologic cancers are shown in Appendix C.

III. LOCALLY ADVANCED CANCER IN THE PELVIS
   A. Pathogenesis. Massive pelvic metastases commonly develop in the course of gynecologic and urologic cancers, rectal carcinomas, and some sarcomas. Locally advanced cancers in the pelvis produce progressive pelvic and perineal pain, ureteral obstruction with uremia, and lymphatic and venous obstruction with pedal and genital edema. Invasion of the rectum or bladder can lead to erosion with bleeding, sloughing of tumor into the urine or bowel, and bladder or bowel outlet obstruction.
   B. Management
   1. **Drug therapy** is preferred initially in some tumors, depending on the primary site.
   2. **Radiation therapy** (RT) frequently relieves symptoms and is useful when the tumor does not respond to chemotherapy.
   3. **Surgery.** A bowel resection, colostomy, or suprapubic cystostomy may relieve bowel or urethral obstruction. Ureteral bypass can be accomplished by placement of ureteral stent catheters or by nephrostomy.
   4. **No therapy.** Patients with progressive pelvic disease unresponsive to irradiation or chemotherapy usually die from uremia. Uremia is usually the least painful death possible. Urinary stream bypass techniques are not recommended for patients with progressive, unresponsive pelvic pain syndromes or relentlessly eroding tumors.

265

Primary site	New cases	Percentage (%)	Deaths from cancer
TABLE 11.1		Yearly Rates for Cancers of the Female Genital Tract in the United States[a]	
Cervix	11,150	14.2	3,670
Uterine corpus	39,080	50	7,400
Ovary	22,430	28.6	15,280
Vulva	3,490	4.5	880
Vagina	2,140	2.7	790
Total	78,290	100%	28,020

[a]Extracted from Jemal A, et al. Cancer statistics. *CA Cancer J Clin* 2007;57(1):43.

IV. ADVERSE EFFECTS OF RADIATION TO THE PELVIS
A. Radiation cystitis
1. **Acute transient cystitis** may occur during RT to the pelvis. The possibility of urinary tract infection should be investigated. Urinary tract analgesics and antispasmodics may be helpful for pain (see Chapter 5, section V).
2. **Late radiation cystitis** occurs when high-dose curative RT to the urinary bladder has been preceded by extensive fulgurations. The bladder becomes contracted, fibrotic, and subject to mucosal ulcerations and infections. Urinary frequency and episodes of pyelonephritis or cystitis (often hemorrhagic) are the clinical findings. If symptomatic management is not successful, cystectomy may be required.
B. Radiation vulvitis of a moist and desquamative type usually begins at about 2,500 cGy and may require temporary discontinuation of treatment for 1 to 2 weeks in up to half of patients.
C. Radiation proctitis. See Chapter 30, section VI.D.
D. Vaginal stenosis. See "General Aspects," section V.B.1.c.
E. Effects on gonads. See Chapter 26.

V. MANAGING TREATMENT-RELATED SEXUAL DYSFUNCTION. Patients treated for cancers of the female genital tract often have difficulty performing sexual intercourse.
A. Broaching the subject
1. Address changes in sexual function directly, preferably before therapy is undertaken; the patient's sexual partner should also be included.
2. Inquire about current sexual activities and about fears the patient or sexual partner might have about the cancer or therapy. Patients should be specifically reassured that the cancer is not contagious, that a small amount of bleeding after intercourse is not hazardous, and that a reasonably normal sex life is expected and desirable for most patients after therapy. See Chapter 26 for discussion of these issues.
B. Specific sexual problems
1. **After radiation therapy** (RT)
   a. **External-beam RT.** Patients receiving external-beam RT should be advised to continue their normal sexual activity; continued intercourse may help prevent vaginal stenosis. Should vaginal dryness develop, the patient should be advised to use water-soluble lubricants. Estrogen is also useful for treating vaginal dryness in patients with cervical cancer.
   b. **Radiation implants.** Patients with radiation implants should be advised against intercourse until several weeks after treatment. Implants are usually removed before discharge from the hospital. Manual foreplay to the point of orgasm is advised as a temporary substitute for intercourse.
   c. **Vaginal stenosis secondary to RT** may make penile penetration difficult. This complication is often preventable by using dilation and lubrication during

the course of irradiation. Manual foreplay, anogenital sex, and orogenital sex are alternatives. Surgical reconstruction by excision of scar tissue and placement of a split-thickness skin graft may yield good results.

2. **After radical hysterectomy,** the vaginal cuff may be foreshortened, resulting in dyspareunia. Vaginal reconstruction usually has good results. Alternatively, the woman can place her hips on a pillow to provide a better angle for penetration. The man can approach from the rear, which may be more comfortable. If these measures are unsatisfactory, lubricated hands placed at the base of the penis may give the sensation of a longer vagina.

3. **After radical vulvectomy,** vulvar sensation may be diminished. The patient and her partner should be counseled.

4. **After pelvic exenteration,** the physician should emphasize the need to allow adequate time for healing of the wound and adjustment to the ostomies. Thereafter, sexual management is as recommended for the stenotic vagina (see section V.B.1.c). Patients can be advised that vaginal reconstruction can be accomplished during exenteration.

5. **After vaginectomy.** Reconstruction is performed at the time of primary surgery. Both sexual and reproductive function can often be preserved after treatment of vaginal cancer. The gynecologist determines when intercourse can be resumed.

CANCER OF THE UTERINE CERVIX

I. EPIDEMIOLOGY AND ETIOLOGY

A. Incidence (Table 11.1). The mortality rate of cervical cancer has declined by 50% since the 1950s, largely as a result of early detection and treatment.

B. Relationship to sexual history. The common denominator for increased risk for cervical cancer is early age at first sexual intercourse. The incidence is also higher in patients with an early first pregnancy, multiple sexual partners, and venereal disease, especially human papillomavirus (HPV) infection.

C. Relationship to HPV. A large body of evidence supports the relationship among HPV, cervical intraepithelial neoplasia (dysplasia), and invasive carcinoma. DNA transcripts of HPV have been identified by Southern blot analysis in >60% of cervical carcinomas. The viral DNA is typically integrated into the human genome rather than remaining in an intact viral capsid. More than 60 HPV subtypes have been identified. Types 6 and 11 are usually associated with benign condyloma acuminata, whereas types 16, 18, 31, and 33 are more likely to be associated with malignant transformation. Type 18 has been associated with poorly differentiated histology and a higher incidence of lymph node metastases.

D. Relationship to smoking. There is evidence that a personal history of smoking significantly increases the risk for cervical cancer.

II. PATHOLOGY AND NATURAL HISTORY

A. Histology. About 80% of cervical carcinomas are squamous cancers, and 20% are adenocarcinomas. Sarcomas are rare. The disease is believed to start at the squamo-columnar junction. A continuum from cervical intraepithelial neoplasia (CIN) to invasive squamous cell carcinoma is apparent. The average age of women with CIN is 15 years younger than that of women with invasive carcinoma, suggesting a potentially slow progression. The natural history of HPV infection is in part influenced by the host immune system; that all stages of CIN may regress spontaneously, remain unchanged, or progress to invasive carcinoma reflects this fact. A small percentage of lesions appear to bypass this progression and may evolve over a substantially shorter period of time.

B. Metastases. After invasive cancer is established, the tumor spreads primarily by local extension into other pelvic structures and sequentially along lymph node chains. Uncommonly, patients with locally advanced tumors may have evidence of blood-borne metastases, most often to the lung, liver, or bone.

III. PREVENTION AND EARLY DETECTION OF CERVICAL CANCER

A. Vaccination. Bivalent (HPV 16/18) and quadrivalent HPV 6/11/16/18 vaccines have shown efficacy by demonstrating protection against CIN, persistent HPV, and external genital warts in double-blind, randomized, placebo-controlled trials. The vaccines are well tolerated, and the American College of Obstetricians and Gynecologists (ACOG), in conjunction with the Advisory Committee on Immunization Practices (ACIP), recommends administration of approved vaccines from ages 9 to 26. The duration of immunity offered by this vaccine is unknown. The HPV vaccine does not eliminate the need for cervical cytology screening.

B. Screening with Pap testing

Most patients with cervical cancer do not have symptoms, and cases are detected by routine Pap test screening.

1. Frequency. For >50 years, the Papanicolaou, or Pap, test has been used as the main screening tool for cervical diseases. Early detection has greatly reduced the morbidity and mortality of cervical cancer. The conventional Pap smear has been shown to have a sensitivity of approximately 50%. Overall, it is estimated that about two-thirds of the false-negative rates are due to sampling error, and the remaining one-third are due to laboratory detection error. The American Cancer Society's recommendations for Pap testing are as follows:

a. Women should have yearly Pap smears starting at age 21 or after the onset of sexual activity,

b. Women at low risk for cervical cancer and who have never had a significant abnormality may have the test less often, for example, every 2 to 3 years, if she has had three normal tests in a row.

c. Women who have had their uterus removed do not need to have regular Pap tests. In postmenopausal patients who are ≥70 years of age, screening may be stopped in the presence of three consecutively normal and satisfactory Pap smears and in the absence of an abnormal Pap test over the last 10 years.

2. Technique. There are many problems that contribute to the low sensitivity of Pap tests. Some of these include sample adequacy, slide preparation, and slide interpretation. The new technologies are aimed at improving the quality of the samples and reducing the false-negative rate. The squamocolumnar junction, where cervical cancer arises, recedes upward and inward with advancing age. This process decreases the usefulness of scrapings alone to make the diagnosis.

a. Conventional Pap smears. When performing the conventional Pap smear, the cytobrush, used together with an extended tip spatula, is the most effective combination for cell collection. The specimens are smeared on clean glass slides and fixed immediately.

b. Liquid-based Pap smears. This technique involves thin-layer, liquid-based systems. The cervical sample is taken and suspended in an alcohol-based preservative solution. In this liquid, the blood, mucus, and inflammatory cells are filtered out. In the laboratory, a representative sample of cells is then deposited by an automatic device on the slide. The slide is then stained and screened in the usual manner. This specimen can be used for detection of HPV, and "reflex" HPV testing can be performed if cytology reveals evidence of atypical squamous cells of undetermined significance (ASC-US). ThinPrep and SurePath are the two liquid-based cytology systems that are approved by the Federal Drug Administration (FDA).

3. Pap smears are graded using the 2001 Bethesda system as follows:

> **Negative for Intraepithelial Lesion or Malignancy**
> **Epithelial Cell Abnormalities**
> > **Squamous Cell**
> > > Atypical squamous cells (ASC)
> > > Of undetermined significance (ASC-US)
> > > Cannot exclude HSIL (ASC-H)
> > > Low-grade squamous intraepithelial lesion (LSIL)
> > > Encompassing: human papillomavirus (HPV)/mild dysplasia/ cervical intraepithelial neoplasia type 1 (CIN 1)

High-grade squamous intraepithelial lesion (HSIL)
　　Encompassing: moderate and severe dysplasia, carcinoma *in situ* (CIS)/CIN 2 and CIN 3
　　With features suspicious for invasion
Squamous cell carcinoma
Glandular Cell
Atypical
　　Endocervical cells (not otherwise specified, NOS)
　　Endometrial cells (NOS)
　　Glandular cells (NOS)
Atypical
　　Endocervical cells, favor neoplastic
　　Glandular cells, favor neoplastic
Endocervical adenocarcinoma *in situ*
Adenocarcinoma
　　Endocervical
　　Endometrial
　　Extra-uterine
　　Not otherwise specified (NOS)
Other Malignant Neoplasms

IV. DIAGNOSIS
A. Symptoms and signs
1. **Symptoms** of early stage invasive cervical cancer include vaginal discharge, bleeding, and particularly postcoital spotting. More advanced stages often present with a malodorous vaginal discharge, weight loss, or obstructive uropathy.
2. **Signs.** Findings on pelvic examination include the appearance of obvious masses on the cervix; gray, discolored areas; and bleeding or evidence of cervicitis. If a tumor is present, the extent should be noted; involvement of the vagina or parametria is an important prognostic factor.

B. Biopsy.
Biopsy specimens should be taken of all visibly abnormal areas, regardless of the findings on the Pap smear. Diagnostic conization may be required if the biopsy shows microinvasive carcinoma, if endocervical curettage shows high-grade dysplasia, or if adenocarcinoma *in situ* is suspected from cytology.

C. Patients with a positive Pap smear and no visible lesion
generally undergo colposcopy, which can detect 90% of dysplastic lesions. The purpose of colposcopy is the examination of the uterine cervix and lower genital tract epithelium under magnification, identification of potentially dysplastic or cancerous areas, and performance of directed biopsies of abnormal areas to provide a histological diagnosis.

D. Endocervical curettage
(ECC) is required when the Pap smear shows a high-grade lesion but colposcopy does not reveal a lesion, when the entire squamocolumnar junction cannot be visualized, when atypical endocervical cells are present on the Pap smear, or when women previously treated for CIN develop new high-grade findings on cytology. If the ECC reveals a high-grade squamous intraepithelial lesion, patients should undergo cervical conization with a knife or a loop electrosurgical excision procedure (LEEP).

E. Further diagnostic studies
in patients whose biopsy reports show cancer depend on the depth of invasion.
1. For early CIS, other studies are not necessary.
2. If blood or lymphatic vessels are invaded, or if the tumor penetrates >3 mm below the basement membrane, pretherapy staging studies are required (see "General Aspects," section II.A).

V. STAGING SYSTEM AND PROGNOSTIC FACTORS
A. The staging system is clinical as outlined in Table 11.2.
B. Prognostic factors
in each stage include size of primary tumor, presence of lymph node metastasis, tumor grade, and histological cell type.

TABLE 11.2	**Staging System for Cervical Cancer**	

Stage	Extent	5-yr survival rate (%)
0	Carcinoma *in situ* (no stromal invasion)	100
I	Strictly confined to cervix (disregard extension to the corpus)	80
Ia	Preclinical carcinoma (diagnosed only by microscopy)	
Ia1	Lesions with ≤3 mm depth of stromal invasion	
Ia2	Lesions detected microscopically that can be measured (>3–5 mm in depth of invasion from the originating epithelial base *and* ≤7 mm in horizontal spread)	
Ib	Lesions with greater dimensions than Ia2, whether seen clinically or not	
Ib1	Lesion ≤4 cm in greatest dimension	
Ib2	Lesion >4 cm in greatest dimension	
II	Tumor extends beyond the cervix but not onto the pelvic sidewall	60
IIa	Lesion involves the proximal vagina (upper two-thirds)	
IIb	Obvious parametrial involvement	
III	Tumor extends to the pelvic sidewall or to the lower one-third of vagina, or causes hydronephrosis or a nonfunctioning kidney	30
IV	Tumor extends beyond true pelvis, or biopsy-proved involvement of bladder or rectal mucosa	5
IVa	Spread to adjacent organs	
IVb	Distant metastases	

VI. MANAGEMENT

A. Dysplasia/cervical intraepithelial neoplasia (CIN) 1–3. Treatment modalities include superficial ablative therapies, LEEP, cone biopsy, and hysterectomy (Fig. 11.1).

1. CIN 1 lesions may be observed if the patient has good follow-up because of the high rate of spontaneous regression of these lesions, or lesions may be treated with ablative therapy. In young patients, especially adolescents, CIN 2 may be followed expectantly.

2. Patients with high-grade (CIN 2 and 3) squamous lesions are suitable for ablative or resection therapies, provided the entire transformation zone is visible on colposcopy, the histology of the biopsies is consistent with the Pap smear, the ECC is negative, and there is no suspicion of occult invasion.

3. For high-grade lesions, we recommend LEEP, which involves the use of wire loop electrodes with radiofrequency alternating current to excise the transformation zone under local anesthesia. This has become the preferred treatment for high-grade CIN that can be adequately assessed by colposcopy. Ablative techniques include cryosurgery, carbon dioxide laser therapy, and electrocoagulation diathermy, which are now less frequently employed.

4. Cone biopsy with a scalpel is preferred for lesions that cannot be assessed colposcopically or when adenocarcinoma *in situ* is suspected.

5. If the patient has other gynecologic indications for hysterectomy, a vaginal or an extrafascial (type I) abdominal hysterectomy may be performed.

B. Invasive cervical cancer: Stage I disease (Table 11.3). The management of patients with early carcinoma of the cervix is diagrammed in Figure 11.1 and summarized in Table 11.3.

1. **Stage Ia1 disease** with <3-mm invasion may be treated with excisional conization, provided the lesion has a diameter of <7 mm and no lymph or vascular

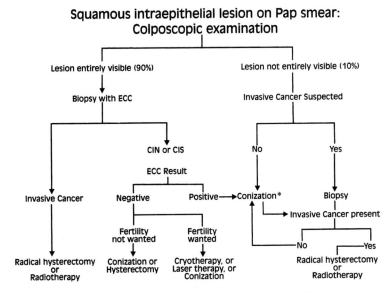

Figure 11.1. Management of patients with positive Pap smear cytology and early carcinoma of the uterine cervix. CIN, cervical intraepithelial neoplasia; CIS, carcinoma *in situ*; ECC, endocervical curettage. *If invasion is not found on conization, patients are followed with Pap smears, biopsies, or repeat conization, depending on the patient and patient's age.

    space invasion. A vaginal or extrafascial hysterectomy is also appropriate if further childbearing is not desired.

2. **Stage Ia2 disease.** For patients with stage Ia2 disease and 3 to 5 mm of stromal invasion, the risk for nodal metastases is 5% to 10%. Bilateral pelvic lymphadenectomy should be performed in conjunction with a modified radical (type II) hysterectomy. If future childbearing is desires, in selected cases with well-differentiated tumors, radical trachelectomy with pelvic lymphadenectomy may be considered.

3. **Stage Ib disease** carries a 15% to 25% risk for positive pelvic lymph nodes and should be treated with a type II or radical (type III) hysterectomy, bilateral pelvic

TABLE 11.3	Treatment of Stage I Cervical Carcinoma
Stage	**Typical treatment options**
Ia1 with ≤3 mm invasion but without lymph–vascular space invasion	Therapeutic cone or type I hysterectomy
Ia1 with 1–3 mm invasion and with lymph–vascular space invasion	Type I or II hysterectomy with pelvic lymph node dissection
Ia2 with >3–5 mm invasion	Type II hysterectomy and bilateral pelvic lymphadenectomy or radiation therapy for inoperable patients
Ib and IIa	Type II or III hysterectomy with bilateral pelvic lymphadenectomy with para-aortic lymph node evaluation or radiation therapy for inoperable patients

lymphadenectomy, and para-aortic lymph node evaluation. In patients who are poor surgical candidates or in whom the tumor is large (generally >4 cm), RT in conjunction with cisplatin chemosensitization is preferred. In patients with high-risk features (e.g., lymph node metastasis), postoperative RT with concurrent chemotherapy (CCT) with cisplatin as a radiation sensitizer should be given. Fertility preservation with a radical trachelectomy and pelvic lymphadenectomy may be considered if tumors are <2 cm and well differentiated with no evidence of lymph-vascular space invasion.

C. **Concurrent chemotherapy (CCT) with RT** reduces recurrence by 30% to 50% and improves 3-year survival rates by 10% to 15% over adjuvant treatment with RT alone.

  1. **CCT is indicated** in the following circumstances:
     a. High-risk stages I to IIa (e.g., with lymph node involvement or positive margins)
     b. Stages IIb, III, and IVa
  2. *Point A* and *point B* are common terms used in the management of cervical cancer. Point A is 2 cm proximal and 2 cm lateral to the cervical os. Point B is 3 cm lateral to point A.
  3. **Regimens.** Several combination chemotherapy regimens involving cisplatin and 5-fluorouracil (5-FU) have been effective. Representative regimens are as follows:
     a. Cisplatin, 40 mg/m^2 weekly for 6 weeks (with or without 5-FU infusions)
     b. Cisplatin, 50 mg/m^2 on Days 1 and 29, and 5-FU, 1,000 mg/m^2 per day by continuous IV infusion for 4 days beginning on Days 1 and 29. Extension of treatment to four courses is being investigated.

D. **Stage II disease.** Stage IIa disease is treated in the same manner as stage Ib disease. When the tumor extends to parametrium (IIb), patients should be treated with RT and CCT involving cisplatin (see section VI.C).

E. **Stage IIb and III disease.** When the parametrium (IIb), the distal vagina (IIIa), or the pelvic sidewall (IIIb) is involved, clear surgical margins are not possible to achieve, and patients should be treated with maximum-dose (8,500 cGy) RT delivered both externally and by brachytherapy. CCT with cisplatin as radiation sensitizers improves survival rates when compared with RT alone (see section VI.C).

F. **Recurrent and stage IV disease.** Advanced cancer in the pelvis is discussed in "General Aspects," section III, and obstructive uropathy is discussed in Chapter 31.

  1. **Lower vaginal recurrence** can occasionally be cured by RT or exenteration.
  2. **Pelvic exenteration.** A pelvic exenteration may also be considered for central pelvic recurrent disease after primary RT when spread is confined to the bladder or rectum. Exenteration carries a higher morbidity rate. Metastatic cancer outside the pelvis and poor medical condition of the patient are contraindications to exenteration. Ureteral obstruction, leg edema, and sciatic pain usually suggest sidewall disease. Surgery should be abandoned if there is more extensive cancer than was clinically suspected.
  3. **RT** alone or with chemotherapeutic sensitizers can occasionally cure stage IVA disease. External-beam RT is combined with intracavitary or interstitial radiation to a total dose of about 8,500 cGy. If disease persists after chemoradiation, pelvic exenteration can be performed.
  4. **Chemotherapy** for metastatic disease is not curative. Distant metastases or incurable local disease should be treated as for any advanced malignancy. A number of chemotherapeutic drugs (e.g., cisplatin, carboplatin, paclitaxel, topotecan) produce short-term responses in 10% to 30% of patients.

G. **Complications of surgery or RT**

  1. **LEEP.** Bleeding occurs in 1% to 8% of cases, cervical stenosis occurs in 1%, and pelvic cellulitis or adnexal abscess occurs rarely.
  2. **Conization.** Hemorrhage, sepsis, infertility, stenosis, and cervical incompetence occur rarely.

3. **Radical hysterectomy.** Acute complications include blood loss (average, 800 mL), urinary tract fistulas (1% to 3%), pulmonary embolus (1% to 2%), small bowel obstruction (1%), and febrile morbidity (25% to 50%). Subacute complications include transient bladder dysfunction (30%) and lymphocyst formation (<5%). Chronic complications include bladder hypotonia or atonia (3%) and, rarely, ureteral strictures.

4. **Pelvic exenteration.** The surgical mortality rate is <1%. The postoperative recuperative period may be as long as 3 months, and the massive fluid shifts and hemodynamic status that sometimes occur may require monitoring. Most postoperative morbidity and mortality result from sepsis, pulmonary embolism, wound dehiscence, and intestinal complications, including small bowel obstruction and fistula formation. A reduction in gastrointestinal complications can be achieved by using unirradiated segments of bowel and closing pelvic floor defects with omentum. The 5-year survival rate for patients undergoing total pelvic exenteration is 30% to 50%.

5. **Pelvic irradiation.** Radiation proctitis and enteritis with intractable diarrhea or obstruction, cystitis, sexual dysfunction because of vaginal stenosis and loss of secretions, loss of ovarian function, fistula formation, and 0.5% mortality either from intractable small bowel injury or from pelvic sepsis (see "General Aspects," section IV).

VII. SPECIAL CLINICAL PROBLEMS

A. **Chance finding of cancer at hysterectomy.** Cancer found in hysterectomy specimens removed for other reasons carries a poor prognosis unless treated with additional surgery or postoperative RT soon after surgery.

B. **Uncertainty of recurrent cancer.** Recurrent cancer is usually manifested by pelvic pain, particularly in the sciatic nerve distribution; vaginal bleeding; malodorous discharge; or leg edema. Recurrence must be demonstrated by biopsy specimen because these symptoms and even physical findings are similar to radiation changes. If no tumor is found using noninvasive measures, a surgeon experienced in pelvic cancer should perform exploratory laparotomy.

C. **Postirradiation dysplasia.** Abnormal Pap smears on follow-up examinations may represent postirradiation dysplastic changes or a new primary cancer. Suspected areas should undergo biopsy. If the biopsy findings show cancer, surgical removal may be necessary.

CANCER OF THE UTERINE BODY

I. EPIDEMIOLOGY AND ETIOLOGY

A. **Incidence** (Table 11.1). Endometrial cancer is the most common malignancy of the female genital tract in the United States. The peak incidence is in the sixth and seventh decades of life; 80% of patients are postmenopausal. Most premenopausal women with endometrial carcinoma have the Stein-Leventhal syndrome. <5% of all cases are diagnosed before the age of 40 years.

B. **Risk factors**

1. **Estrogen exposure** that is unopposed by progesterone increases the risk for endometrial carcinoma by four- to eightfold. Tamoxifen acts as a weak estrogen. Data suggest that the use of tamoxifen is associated with a twofold increased risk for endometrial cancer.

2. **Medical conditions producing increased exposure to unopposed estrogens** and associated with increased risk of endometrial carcinoma are:

   a. Polycystic ovarian disease (anovulatory menstrual cycles with or without hirsutism and other endocrine abnormalities)

   b. Anovulatory menstrual cycles

   c. Obesity

   d. Granulosa cell tumor of the ovary, or any other estrogen-secreting tumor

   e. Advanced liver disease

3. **Other medical conditions** associated with increased risk for endometrial carcinoma
   a. Infertility, nulliparity, irregular menses
   b. Diabetes mellitus
   c. Hypertension
   d. History of multiple cancers in the family
   e. Patient history of breast or rectal cancer
4. **Hereditary factors** resulting from germ line mutations in DNA mismatch repair (MMR) genes. Mutations in MMR genes (MSH2, MLH1, or MSH6) can result in Lynch syndrome II (hereditary nonpolyposis colorectal cancer). By age 70, up to 40% of these individuals maybe diagnosed with endometrial cancer.

II. PATHOLOGY AND NATURAL HISTORY

A. **Histology.** About 95% of uterine cancers arise from the endometrium, and the most common histological subtype is endometrioid adenocarcinoma. Clear cell, papillary serous, and squamous cell carcinoma account for the other 10% of endometrial cancers.

B. **Role of estrogens.** Classically, unopposed estrogens cause a continuum of endometrial changes from mild hyperplasia to invasive carcinoma. Progestin therapy is very effective in reversing endometrial hyperplasia without atypia, but less effective for endometrial hyperplasia with atypia. The most reliable method for reversing hyperplasia is continuous progestin therapy (megesterol acetate).

C. **Mode of spread.** Tumors are confined to the body of the uterus (stage I) in 75% of cases. Endometrial cancer most commonly spreads by direct extension. Deep myometrial invasion and involvement of the uterine cervix are associated with a high risk for pelvic lymph node metastases. It is rare to find positive para-aortic nodes in the absence of positive pelvic nodes. The presence of cells in peritoneal washes suggests retrograde flow of exfoliated cells along the fallopian tubes. Hematogenous spread is an uncommon late finding in adenocarcinoma but occurs early in sarcoma. The lungs are the most frequent site of distant metastatic involvement.

III. DIAGNOSIS

A. **Symptoms and signs**
   1. **Abnormal vaginal bleeding** is the most common symptom (97%).
      a. **Premenopausal women** with prolonged menses, excessive menstrual bleeding, or intermenstrual bleeding must be evaluated for endometrial cancer, particularly if they have a history of irregular menses, diabetes mellitus, hypertension, obesity, or infertility.
      b. **All postmenopausal women with vaginal bleeding** >1 year after the last menstrual period are considered to have endometrial cancer unless proved otherwise. Even women who have been on estrogens to control postmenopausal symptoms must have histological proof that withdrawal bleeding is not the result of an unrelated endometrial cancer.
   2. **Patients without symptoms** and with atypical endometrial cells on Pap smears should undergo endometrial sampling.
   3. **Women with AGC** (atypical glandular cells) on Pap smears who are >35 years, as well as younger women with AGC who have unexplained vaginal bleeding, must undergo an endometrial biopsy in addition to colposcopy.
   4. **Locally extensive tumors** may be palpable on pelvic examination.
   5. **Advanced disease** is the original manifestation of cancer in 5% of cases. Presenting problems include ascites, jaundice, bowel obstruction, or respiratory distress from lung metastases.

B. **Endocervical curettage and office endometrial biopsy** should be performed in all patients suspected of having endometrial carcinoma. The preferred technique is to use a small flexible plastic catheter (e.g., Pipelle). An endometrial biopsy should be made for optimal interpretation. The accuracy of endometrial sampling is 95% to 98%. All patients with symptoms and a negative biopsy must undergo dilation and curettage.

C. Fractional curettage is the diagnostic method of choice for endometrial cancer. The technique involves scraping the endocervical canal and then, in a set sequence, the walls of the uterus. If cancer is found by histological evaluation, the fractional scrapings help to locate the tumor site. The gross appearance of the scrapings often suggests cancerous tissue, which is gray, necrotic, and friable.

D. Pap smears. Conventional Pap smears from endocervical aspiration or brushing have a much lower yield than fractional curettage or jet washout. Pap smears alone should not be used to exclude suspected endometrial cancer. Only half of patients with endometrial cancer have abnormal cells on Pap smear.

E. Transvaginal ultrasound with and without color-flow imaging is under investigation. Early data suggest a strong association between thickness of the endometrial stripe and endometrial disease. Normal endometrium is usually less than 5 mm thick, and false-positive results based on this criterion alone may be excessively high.

F. Staging evaluation. See "General Aspects," section II.A.

IV. STAGING SYSTEM AND PROGNOSTIC FACTORS

A. The staging system is surgical as shown in Table 11.4. Staging for endometrial cancer involves total abdominal hysterectomy, bilateral salpingo-oophorectomy, peritoneal cytology, pelvic and para-aortic lymphadenectomy, and sampling of any suspicious peritoneal implants.

B. Prognostic factors

1. **Histological grade and myometrial invasion.** Increasing tumor grade and myometrial penetration are associated with increasing risk for pelvic and para-aortic lymph node metastases, positive peritoneal cytology, adnexal metastases, local vault recurrence, and hematogenous spread and thus have great prognostic value.

2. **Tumor histology.** Histological types ranked from best to worst prognosis are adenocanthoma, adenocarcinomas, adenosquamous carcinomas, clear cell carcinomas, papillary serous carcinomas, and small cell carcinomas.

 TABLE 11.4 **Surgical Staging System for Cancer of the Uterine Body**

Stage	Extent	5-yr survival rate (%)
I	Cancer confined to the corpus	81–91
Ia	Tumor limited to endometrium	91
Ib	Invasion to less than one half the myometrium	90
Ic	Invasion to more than one half the myometrium	81
II	Cancer involves corpus and cervix but does not extend outside the uterus	71–79
IIa	Endocervical glandular involvement only	79
IIb	Cervical stromal invasion	71
III	Cancer extends outside the uterus but not outside the true pelvis	30–60
IIIa	Tumor invades serosa and/or adnexa or positive peritoneal cytology	60
IIIb	Vaginal metastases	30
IIIc	Positive pelvic and/or para-aortic nodes	52
IV	Cancer extends outside true pelvis or invades bladder or rectal mucosa	10
IVa	Tumor invasion of bladder and/or bowel mucosa	15
IVb	Distant metastases including intra-abdominal and/or inguinal lymph nodes	17

Table adapted from Creaseman WT, et al. Carcinoma of the corpus uteri: FIGO annual report. *Int J Gynaecol Obstet* 2003;83:79.

3. **Vascular space invasion.** Vascular space invasion is an independent prognostic factor for recurrence and death from endometrial carcinoma of all histological types.
4. **Hormone receptor status.** The average estrogen receptor (ER) and progesterone receptor (PgR) levels are, in general, inversely proportional to the histological grade. However, ER and PgR levels have also been shown to be independent prognostic indicators, with higher levels corresponding to longer survival.
5. **Nuclear grade.** Criteria for nuclear atypia vary, and intraobserver and interobserver reproducibility is poor. Despite these difficulties, a number of researchers have shown that nuclear grade is a more accurate prognosticator than histological grade.
6. **Tumor size.** The larger the tumor, the larger the risk for lymph node metastases, and, therefore, the worse the prognosis.
7. **DNA ploidy.** Aneuploid tumors constitute a fairly small percentage (25%) of endometrial carcinomas as compared with ovarian and cervical cancers. Aneuploidy is, however, associated with increased risk for early recurrence and death.

V. PREVENTION AND EARLY DETECTION
A. **Prevention.** Unopposed exogenous estrogen administration should be avoided in postmenopausal women, and women who are anovulatory or who have endometrial hyperplasia should be treated with cyclic progestins.
B. **Early detection.** Patients in whom evaluation for endometrial carcinoma is necessary include postmenopausal women who have abnormal bleeding on exogenous estrogens; obese postmenopausal women, particularly with a strong family history of endometrial, breast, bowel, or ovarian cancer; and premenopausal women with chronic anovulatory cycles (i.e., polycystic ovarian disease). Women in whom endometrial carcinoma must be excluded include all postmenopausal women with significant bleeding or with pyometra; perimenopausal women with severe intermenstrual or increasingly heavy periods; and premenopausal women with unexplained abnormal uterine bleeding, especially if chronically anovulatory.

VI. MANAGEMENT
A. **Early disease**
1. **Surgery.** Total abdominal hysterectomy with bilateral salpingo-oophorectomy (TAH/BSO), pelvic and para-aortic lymphadenectomy is the treatment for patients with early stage endometrial cancer. Patients with an expanded (enlarged) cervix may be treated with a type II (modified radical) hysterectomy; those with microscopic involvement of the cervix may be treated with an extrafascial hysterectomy. Optimal tumor debulking is recommended for patients with metastatic extrauterine disease. Patients with persistent atypical hyperplasia after adequate progestin treatment are adequately treated with TAH/BSO in the absence of endometrial cancer. Notably, 40% of these patients will have coexisting endometrial cancer, and complete surgical staging is essential in this population. Any peritoneal fluid should be sent for cytology; if no fluid is found, a peritoneal wash with 50 mL normal saline should be performed. Any enlarged pelvic or para-aortic lymph nodes are resected.
   a. If the lymph nodes are negative and the patient has stage Ia or Ib disease with grade 1 or 2 histology and the tumor measures <2 cm, no further treatment is necessary.
   b. In young women who have well-differentiated lesions, the use of high-dose progestin hormones can be curative. We recommend medroxyprogesterone (Megace), 80 to 320 mg/day for 3 to 9 months with endometrial sampling every 3 months to assess response. After the disease is gone, the patient must undergo cyclic hormonal therapy to avoid anovulatory hyperplasia. Hysterectomy is recommended in this group of patients after completion of childbearing.

2. RT
   a. RT alone is used only for patients at high risk for surgical mortality because of concomitant medical conditions. The survival rate of patients with stage I or II disease treated with RT alone is significantly inferior to the rates associated with surgery alone or surgery combined with RT.
   b. Postoperative RT. To facilitate accurate risk stratification and selection for RT, surgical staging and the histopathologic finding in the uterine specimen and the status of lymph nodes is essential. Based on the relative risk of recurrent disease, patients are categorized into three groups.
      (1) Low-risk disease is defined as well-differentiated tumors (grade 1 or 2) with minimal or less than one-half myometrial invasion or grade 3 tumors with no myometrial invasion, with negative lymph nodes and absence of lymph vascular space invasion in the primary tumor. These patients do not require any further treatment.
      (2) Intermediate-risk disease includes patients with grade 1 or 2 tumors invading greater than one-half of the myometrium, or patients with grade 1, stage II disease (cervical involvement). This group precludes any disease in the lymph nodes or involvement of the lymph vascular spaces. We recommend adjuvant RT in the form of brachytherapy in this subset of patients. If this group of patients has not undergone a thorough lymphadenectomy, external pelvic irradiation (about 5,000 cGy) should be considered.
      (3) High-risk disease is defined by grade 3 tumor with any evidence of invasion, extrauterine disease, evidence of lymph vascular space invasion in the primary tumor, and grade 2 and beyond stage II disease. These groups of patients are at high risk of recurrence and must receive adjuvant treatment in the form or radiation, chemotherapy, or a combination of these two modalities.
3. Chemotherapy has a role in the management of early endometrial cancers. Randomized studies comparing platinum-based chemotherapy (platinum, taxane, and/or anthracycline) to pelvic radiation in intermediate- and high-risk low-stage endometrial cancer suggest that chemotherapy may be an effective adjuvant in endometrial cancer, and perhaps as effective as radiation. It is unclear whether the sequence of chemotherapy followed by radiation is more effective than chemotherapy alone. In patients with papillary serous or clear cell carcinomas, we prefer the use of carboplatin and paclitaxel (see "Ovarian Cancer," section VI.E.2 for regimen dosages).

B. Advanced disease
1. Stage III or IV disease is treated best with optimal cytoreduction. Surgery should be followed with systemic multiagent chemotherapy. Efficacious regimens in this setting include combination of doxorubicin and cisplatin or carboplatin and paclitaxel.
   a. Removed tumor should be assayed for ER and PgR levels, because hormonal treatments with progestins, tamoxifen, or aromatase inhibitors can also be utilized in an adjuvant setting.
   b. Pelvic exenteration may be considered for the occasional patients with recurrent disease extension limited to the bladder or rectum.
2. Drug therapy. Patients with widespread metastases or with previously irradiated, recurrent local disease are treated with hormones and cytotoxic agents.
   a. Hormonal therapy. Response to progestins occurs in 20% to 40% of patients. The average duration of response is 1 year, and expected survival in responding patients is twice that of nonresponders. A few patients survive in excess of 10 years. Hormone receptor studies are of predictive value. The following drugs are most frequently used:
      (1) Repository form of medroxyprogesterone acetate (Depo-Provera), 1.0 g IM weekly for 6 weeks and monthly thereafter
      (2) Megestrol acetate (Megace), 40 mg PO four times daily
      (3) Tamoxifen, 20 mg PO daily
   b. Chemotherapy. Drug regimens containing platinum and doxorubicin can be effective; response may be produced in up to 40% of patients, which improves

their expected survival by several months. We prefer carboplatin and pacli-taxel, and the patients should be treated as if they have advanced ovarian carcinoma (see "Ovarian Cancer," section VI.E.2 for regimen dosages).

VII. SPECIAL CLINICAL PROBLEMS

Daily estrogen replacement therapy for younger patients with stage I disease is impor-tant to protect against osteoporosis and to improve quality of life. This treatment has not been associated with deleterious effects; however, it should be individualized for each patient considering all their pre-existing medical conditions. Other complications are discussed in "General Aspects."

 VAGINAL CANCER

I. EPIDEMIOLOGY AND ETIOLOGY

A. Incidence. Primary carcinoma of the vagina constitutes 1% to 2% of cancers of the female genital tract. Dysplastic changes of the vaginal mucosa appear to be precursors of VAIN (*vaginal intraepithelial neoplasia*). The likelihood of vaginal carcinoma is increased in women with a history of cervical carcinoma. About 80% to 90% of cases of vaginal cancer are metastatic in origin and are treated according to the primary lesion.

B. HPV. HPV is associated with VAIN. The exact potential of VAIN to progress to frankly invasive carcinoma is unknown but appears to be in the range of 3% to 5% when the dysplasia is treated with various methods.

C. Estrogens

1. The two million daughters of women treated with diethylstilbestrol (DES) dur-ing the first 18 weeks of gestation are at risk for developing vaginal clear cell adenocarcinomas. As of February 1992, 580 cases of clear cell vaginal and cer-vical carcinomas had been reported by the Registry for Research on Hormonal Transplacental Carcinogenesis. DES exposure accounted for two-thirds of the reported cases. The actual risk for clear cell adenocarcinoma in DES-exposed women is estimated to be 1 in 1,000, with the highest risk in women exposed before 12 weeks' gestation.

2. Vaginal adenosis is present in nearly 45% of women exposed to DES, and 25% have structural abnormalities of the uterus, cervix, or vagina. Almost all women with vaginal clear cell carcinoma also have vaginal adenosis.

3. This tumor is decreasing in incidence owing to the discontinuation of DES circa 1970.

II. PATHOLOGY AND NATURAL HISTORY

A. Histology. About 85% of vaginal carcinomas are squamous carcinomas, and the remainder are adenocarcinomas, melanomas, and sarcomas.

B. Location. Primary vaginal cancers most commonly arise on the posterior wall of the upper one-third of the vagina. If the cervix is involved, the disease is defined as cervical rather than vaginal cancer. If the vulva is involved, the disease is defined as vulvar cancer.

C. Mode of spread

1. **Direct extension** to adjacent soft tissues and bony structures, including para-colpos and parametria, bladder, urethra, rectum, and bony pelvis, usually occurs when the tumor is large.

2. **Lymphatic dissemination** occurs to pelvic and then para-aortic nodes from the upper vagina, whereas the posterior wall is drained by inferior gluteal, sacral, and deep pelvic nodes. The anterior wall drains into lymphatics of the lateral pelvic walls, and the distal one-third of the vagina drains into the inguinal and femoral nodes.

3. **Hematogenous spread** occurs late and is most often to lung, liver, bone, and supraclavicular lymph nodes.

III. DIAGNOSIS

A. Symptoms and signs. The most frequent presenting symptoms are vaginal discharge and bleeding. Vaginal adenosis is usually asymptomatic but may produce a chronic watery discharge. Bladder pain and urinary frequency may occur early on. Advanced posterior tumors may cause tenesmus or constipation.

B. Diagnostic studies

1. Diagnosis of vaginal carcinoma is often missed on initial examination, especially when the tumor is located in the distal two-thirds of the vagina, where the blades of the speculum may obscure the lesion. The speculum should always be rotated as it is withdrawn and the vaginal mucosa inspected carefully.

2. Vaginal Pap smears and biopsy of abnormal areas on pelvic examination are the mainstays of diagnosis. If no lesion is detected with an abnormal Pap smear, application of Lugol's iodine and inspection with a colposcope may be helpful in identifying lesions.

3. Staging procedures are discussed in "General Aspects," section II.A.

IV. STAGING SYSTEM AND PROGNOSTIC FACTORS

A. Staging system. Several staging systems are used. Despite their clear influence on prognosis, however, tumor bulk and location of the primary lesion in the vagina are not included. Because expected survival depends on clinical stage, variable survival rates have been reported. A representative staging system and approximate survival rates are shown in Table 11.5.

B. Prognostic factors. Generally, the greater the tumor size, the worse the prognosis. Cancers located in the upper vagina, however, have a better prognosis than those located in the lower vagina (upper posterior tumors can become large before invading the muscularis and changing the stage of disease).

V. PREVENTION AND EARLY DETECTION

A. Cytology and routine examination are the basis of screening the general population. Up to 30% of patients with vaginal cancer have a history of *in situ* or invasive cervical cancer; these patients should be screened with annual Pap smears.

B. Females with a history of *in utero* exposure to DES should have a pelvic examination and Pap smear yearly from the time of menarche. Younger girls who have been exposed to DES should be examined at the first sign of bleeding or discharge because clear cell carcinomas can occur in childhood. All suspected areas should undergo biopsy, and careful palpation of all mucosal surfaces is extremely important.

VI. MANAGEMENT

A. Early disease

1. Surgery. The close proximity of bladder, urethra, and rectum restricts the surgical margins that can be obtained without an exenterative procedure. In addition,

TABLE 11.5 Staging System for Vaginal Cancer

Stage	Extent	5-yr survival rate (%)
0	Carcinoma *in situ*	100
I	Limited to vagina	70
II	Invasion of subvaginal tissues but not extending to pelvic wall	50
III	Extension to pelvic wall	20
IV	Extension beyond true pelvis or biopsy proof of bladder or rectal involvement	<10

attempts to maintain a functional vagina and the associated psychosocial issues play an important role in treatment planning.

a. Vaginal mucosa stripping has been used for CIS.

b. Stage I disease involving the upper posterior vagina may be managed with radical hysterectomy, partial vaginectomy, and bilateral pelvic lymphadenectomy. In a patient with prior hysterectomy, radical upper vaginectomy with bilateral pelvic lymphadenectomies can be used.

c. Pretreatment exploratory laparotomy in patients requiring radiation allows for the following:

(1) More precise determination of disease involvement

(2) Resection of bulky involved lymph nodes

(3) Ovariopexy (ovarian transposition) to minimize the chance of radiation-induced infertility

d. Vaginal reconstruction may be performed using split-thickness skin grafts from the thighs or with myocutaneous flaps, usually with gracilis muscle.

2. RT is an alternative treatment for patients with stage I disease; there are no controlled studies to prove that RT is as effective as surgery. Radiation is the treatment of choice for all higher stages, usually using combined external-beam and intravaginal RT. When the distal vagina is involved, the inguinal nodes are also treated.

3. Chemotherapy. Topical fluorouracil, applied twice daily, has been used for VAIN. Intense vaginal burning results. The long-range benefits of topical fluorouracil are not yet proved; this modality cannot be recommended as standard practice.

4. Laser therapy is useful for stage 0.

B. Advanced disease is managed as for cancer of the cervix (see "Cancer of the Uterine Cervix," section VI). In otherwise healthy patients with stage IV disease or central recurrence after previous RT, an exenterative procedure may be performed.

VII. SPECIAL CLINICAL PROBLEMS

Loss of genitalia and vaginal stenosis are discussed in "General Aspects," section V.

 VULVAR CANCER

I. EPIDEMIOLOGY AND ETIOLOGY

A. Incidence. Carcinomas of the vulva constitute 3% to 4% of malignant lesions of the female genital tract. The disease is most common in women >50 years of age, with a mean age at diagnosis of 65 years.

B. Etiology

1. HPV viruses play a role in the development of vulvar cancer. High risk subtypes of HPV (16, 18, and 31) have been isolated from invasive vulvar cancer.

2. Intraepithelial neoplasia of the vulva (VIN) and CIN increase a woman's risk for carcinoma of the vulva. Vaccination with the quadrivalent HPV virus will provide protection against VIN, commonly a precursor lesion to invasive vulvar cancer.

3. Medical history associated with increased risk of vulvar cancer includes obesity, hypertension, diabetes mellitus, arteriosclerosis, menopause at an early age, and nulliparity.

II. PATHOLOGY AND NATURAL HISTORY

A. Histology. Malignant tumors of the vulva are squamous cell carcinoma in >90% of cases and melanoma in 5% to 10%. Adenocarcinoma, sarcoma, basal cell carcinoma, and other tumors constitute the remainder.

B. Location. The sites of tumor in order of decreasing frequency are labia majora, labia minora, clitoris, and perineum.

C. Natural history

1. **Squamous cell carcinomas** in the vulva have not been shown to develop as a continuum from vulvar intraepithelial neoplasia to CIS to invasive carcinoma. Most studies report that only about 2% to 4% of vulvar intraepithelial neoplasia lesions become invasive cancer. These cancers tend to grow locally, spread to superficial and deep groin lymph nodes, and then spread to pelvic and distant nodes. Hematogenous spread usually occurs after lymph node involvement, and death usually results from cachexia or respiratory failure secondary to pulmonary metastases.

2. **Malignant melanoma** of the vulva accounts for 5% of all melanoma cases, despite the comparatively small surface area involved and the paucity of nevi at this site (see Chapter 16, "Malignant Melanoma"). Therefore, all pigmented vulvar lesions should be removed.

3. **Paget disease of the vulva** is a preinvasive lesion with thickened epithelium infiltrated with mucin-rich Paget cells, which are derived from the stratum germinativum of the epidermis. Approximately 10% to 12% of patients have invasive vulvar Paget disease, and 4% to 8% have an underlying adenocarcinoma. Underlying adenocarcinomas are usually clinically apparent. The natural course of this disease is characterized by local recurrence over many years, and recurrences are almost always *in situ*. These patients are also predisposed to developing extragenital glandular cancers and need careful clinical evaluation and follow-up.

4. **Bartholin gland adenocarcinoma** is extremely rare and is usually seen in older women. Inflammation of this gland is uncommon in women >50 years of age and is virtually nonexistent in postmenopausal women; gland swelling in women in these age groups should arouse suspicion for the presence of cancer.

5. **Basal cell carcinomas and sarcomas** of the vulva have natural histories similar to that of primary tumors located elsewhere.

III. DIAGNOSIS
A. Signs and symptoms
1. Squamous cell carcinomas most often present with a vulvar lump or mass, often with a history of chronic vulvar pruritus. The tumors often ulcerate or become fungating. Bleeding, superinfection, and pain can develop with continued growth.
2. Paget disease has a characteristic lesion that is velvety red, with raised, irregular margins. Lesions are pruritic, with secondary excoriation and bleeding.
3. Basal cell carcinomas and melanomas are discussed in Chapter 16.
4. Lymph node enlargement may be palpable in the inguinal or femoral regions or in the pelvis.

B. Indications for vulvar biopsy
1. Patches of skin that appear red, dark brown, or white
2. Areas that are firm to palpation
3. Pruritic or bleeding lesions
4. Any nevus in the genital region
5. Enlargement or thickening in the region of Bartholin glands, particularly in patients >50 years of age

C. Staging evaluation. See "General Aspects," section II.A.

IV. STAGING SYSTEM AND PROGNOSTIC FACTORS FOR SQUAMOUS CELL CARCINOMA
A. Staging system. FIGO (the International Federation of Gynecology and Obstetrics) has adopted a surgically based TNM (tumor, nodes, metastases) staging system to avoid the problems associated with clinical assessment of lymph nodes (see Table 11.6.).
B. Prognostic factors and survival. Survival is determined by stage, structures invaded, and tumor location.
1. **Lymph node involvement** is exceedingly important. Metastases to pelvic or periaortic nodes are rare in the absence of inguinal or femoral lymph node metastases.

TABLE 11.6	Staging Systems for Vulvar Squamous Cell Carcinoma	
FIGO stage	**TNM stage**	**Clinical/pathological findings**
I	T1 N0 M0	Tumor confined to the vulva or perineum, <2 cm in greatest dimension, lymph nodes negative
II	T2 N0 M0	Tumor confined to the vulva and/or perineum, >2 cm in greatest dimension, lymph nodes negative
III	T3 N0 M0 T1,2,3 N1 M0	Tumor of any size with adjacent spread to lower urethra or anus (T3) or unilateral regional lymph node spread (N1)
IVA	T1,2,3 N2 M0 T4 Any N M0	Tumor invades upper urethra, bladder mucosa, rectal mucosa, or pelvic bone (T4) or bilateral regional lymph node spread (N2)
IVB	Any T Any N M1	Any distant metastasis, including pelvic lymph nodes

FIGO, International Federation of Gynecology and Obstetrics; TNM, tumor, nodes, metastases.

2. **The 5-year survival rate** in patients with negative or one microscopically positive lymph node is 95%. In contrast, the 5-year survival rate for patients with two positive nodes is 80%, and that for patients with three or more positive nodes is 25%. Note that the risk for hematogenous spread with three or more positive nodes is 66%, in contrast to the risk with two or fewer nodes, which is only 4%.

V. PREVENTION AND EARLY DETECTION. The routine history and physical examination of all postmenopausal women should include specific questioning regarding vulvar soreness and pruritus followed by careful inspection and palpation of the vulva and palpation for firm or fixed groin nodes. All suspicious lesions should undergo biopsy.

VI. MANAGEMENT
  A. Surgery is the treatment of choice for early stage lesions.
    1. **Vulvar intraepithelial neoplasia.** Wide local excision for small lesions. Carbon dioxide laser of the warty variety is acceptable. Alternative treatments include topical administration of 5-fluorouracil, resulting in a chemical sloughing of the skin, or imiquimod (Aldara), leading to a local inflammatory reaction. Before the use of either agent, the existence of invasive disease has to be ruled out.
    2. **Paget disease.** As the Paget cells may invade the underlying dermis, this dermal layer should also be removed during surgical excision. Recurrent lesions may be treated with local excision in the absence of adenocarcinoma. If invasive adenocarcinoma is present, it should be treated in the same manner as an invasive squamous cell vulvar cancer.
    3. **Invasive carcinoma with <1 mm invasion.** Radical wide local excision
    4. **Stage I disease with >1 mm invasion.** Radical local excision with ipsilateral groin lymphadenectomy for lateralized lesions and bilateral lymphadenectomy for centralized lesions
    5. **Stage II lesions** may be treated with bilateral groin lymphadenectomy and radical local excision (or modified radical vulvectomy) provided that at least 1 cm of clear margins in all directions can be achieved while preserving critical midline structures.
    6. **Complications of modified radical vulvectomy** include wound breakdown, local infection, sepsis, thromboembolism, and chronic edema of the lower extremities. Using separate incisions for the groin lymphadenectomies reduces the incidence of wound breakdown and leg edema.
    7. **Stage III or IV disease.** These lesions should be treated RT and chemosensitization (with cisplatin or 5-FU). Selected cases can be treated with radical vulvectomy,

Rare cases of persistent or recurrent disease can be salvaged with exenterative surgery.

B. RT
   1. RT may be used to shrink stage III and IV tumors that involve the anus, rectum, rectovaginal septum, or proximal urethra preoperatively to improve resectability.
   2. RT has been shown to improve survival and decrease groin recurrence when there is evidence of ≥3 micrometastases or macrometastasis (≥10 mm) in the groin nodes.
   3. Postoperative RT to the vulva may be used to reduce local recurrence when tumors exceed 4 cm or there are positive surgical margins.
   4. External-beam RT to 5,000 cGy with follow-up biopsy should be considered for small anterior tumors involving the clitoris, especially in young women, to prevent the psychosocial issues involved with surgery.
   5. Patients who have medical conditions precluding surgery may be treated with RT alone.

C. Chemotherapy
   1. 5-FU or cisplatin chemotherapy can be used as a radiation sensitizer.
   2. Systemic treatment with agents active against cervical squamous cell carcinomas, such as cisplatin, carboplatin, paclitaxel, and topotecan, may be used for metastatic disease, but partial response rates are low (10% to 15%) and usually last only a few months.

 OVARIAN CANCER

I. EPIDEMIOLOGY AND ETIOLOGY
   A. Incidence (Table 11.1). About 22,430 American women will be diagnosed with ovarian cancer this year, and 15,280 deaths will be expected due to this disease. It is the leading cause of death among all gynecologic cancers, the fifth most common female cancer in the United States, with a lifetime risk of 1.4% to 1.8%. Despite the advances in surgical and chemotherapeutic management of this disease, the 5-year survival rate for women with stage III/IV epithelial ovarian cancer has remained as low as 12% over the past 30 years.
   B. Predisposing factors are listed below.
       1. **Geographical.** The highest rates of ovarian cancer are recorded in industrialized countries.
       2. **Genetic.** Germ line mutations in DNA repair genes (BRCA1, BRCA2, MLH-1, MSH-2, PMS1, and PMS2) account for 10% to 15% of ovarian cancer cases. Identification of this group of women by genetic testing is essential as prophylactic risk reduction surgery with a bilateral salpingo-oophorectomy can decrease the risk of gynecologic cancers by 96%. Patients with the following family pedigrees and family history should be considered for genetic testing:
           a. Two or more women with ovarian or breast cancer or both, especially if diagnosed premenopausally
           b. Women who have separate diagnoses of breast and ovarian cancer
           c. Women who have had breast cancer in both breasts
           d. Male relatives who have had breast cancer in both breasts
           e. Women of Ashkenazi Jewish ancestry with ovarian cancer at any age
       3. **Personal history of breast or endometrial cancer** results in an increased risk for ovarian cancer.
       4. **Reproductive history** such as nulliparity with "incessant ovulation" is a risk factor. Endometriosis in now found to be an independent risk factor for ovarian cancer. The use of oral contraceptives reduces the risk of ovarian cancer, and postmenopausal estrogens may increase the risk.
       5. **Environmental.** Intraperitoneal exposure to talc has been associated with a slight increase in the risk of ovarian cancer. Cigarette smoking may increase the risk of certain subtypes of ovarian cancer.

TABLE 11.7 Histology of Ovarian Neoplasms

A. Epithelial tumors (approximate frequency)
Serous cystadenocarcinoma (75%–80%)
Mucinous cystadenocarcinoma (10%)
Endometrioid carcinoma (10%)
Clear cell (mesonephroma) (<1%)
Undifferentiated carcinoma (<1%)
Brenner tumor (<1%)
Mixed epithelial tumor
Unclassified

C. Sex cord stromal tumors
Sertoli-Leydig cell tumor
Granulosa–stromal cell tumor
Gynandroblastoma
Androblastoma
Unclassified

B. Germ cell tumors
Dysgerminoma
Endodermal sinus tumor
Embryonal carcinoma
Polyembryoma
Choriocarcinoma
Teratoma
Mixed

D. Other tumors
Lipid cell tumors
Gonadoblastoma
Nonspecific soft-tissue tumors
Unclassified

II. PATHOLOGY AND NATURAL HISTORY

A. Histology. The World Health Organization (WHO) classification of neoplasms of the ovary is shown in Table 11.7.

B. Histological grade. The percentage of undifferentiated cells present in tissue determines the grade of the tumors.

Grade	Percentage of undifferentiated cells
G1	0–25
G2	25–50
G3	>50

C. Biological behavior

1. **Borderline tumors,** also called "tumors of low malignant potential," tend to occur in premenopausal women and remain confined to the ovary for long periods of time. Metastatic implants may occur, and some may be progressive, leading to bowel obstruction and death.

2. **Other histological subtypes** behave similarly when grade and stage are considered. Even in early stages, careful exploration frequently reveals subdiaphragmatic and omental implants. Organ invasion and distant metastases are less likely than is spread over serosal surfaces. The lethal potential of ovarian cancer is most frequently related to encasement of intra-abdominal organs. Death usually results from intestinal obstruction and inanition.

D. Associated paraneoplastic syndromes

1. Neurological syndromes are common. Peripheral neuropathies, organic dementia, amyotrophic lateral sclerosis–like syndrome, and cerebellar ataxia are the most frequent occurrences.

2. Peculiar antibodies that cause difficulties in cross-matching blood can be corrected with prednisone.

3. Cushing syndrome

4. Hypercalcemia

5. Thrombophlebitis

III. DIAGNOSIS

A. Symptoms and signs. Early ovarian carcinoma is typically asymptomatic. The majority of patients with advanced ovarian cancer present with vague symptoms of abdominal discomfort, such as bloating, constipation, gas, irregular menses if premenopausal, urinary frequency, or abnormal vaginal bleeding. Physical findings include ascites and abdominal masses. Any pelvic mass in a woman who is more than 1-year postmenopausal is suspicious for ovarian cancer.

B. Tissue diagnosis. Diagnosis requires biopsy of ovarian or other suspected abdominal masses.

    1. Masses that are smaller than 8 cm in premenopausal women are most commonly benign cysts. Patients should undergo ultrasound to confirm the cystic nature of the mass and receive suppression with oral contraceptives for 2 months. Benign lesions should regress.

    2. Surgical evaluation is necessary for masses with the following characteristics:

        a. Less than 8 cm in diameter and cystic but still present after 2 months of observation in premenopausal women

        b. Smaller than 8 cm in premenopausal women and solid on ultrasound

        c. Larger than 8 cm in premenopausal women

        d. Present in any postmenopausal patient

C. Serum tumor markers. CA-125 is useful to monitor the response to therapy in epithelial ovarian tumors. β-human chorionic gonadotropin (β-hCG), α-fetoprotein (α-FP), and LDH are useful in germ cell malignancies. None of these markers is useful for screening purposes.

D. Staging evaluation (see "General Aspects," section II.A)

IV. STAGING SYSTEM AND PROGNOSTIC FACTORS. Staging for ovarian cancer is surgical.

    A. Staging system and 5-year survival rate for epithelial tumors are shown in Table 11.8.

TABLE 11.8   **Staging System for Ovarian Epithelial Tumors**

Stage	Extent (proportion of cases)	5-yr survival rate (%)
I	Cancer limited to ovaries (15%)	80
Ia	Limited to one ovary, no ascites	
Ib	Both ovaries involved, no ascites	
Ic	Ia or Ib with ascites or positive peritoneal washings	
II	Cancer of one or both ovaries with extension limited to pelvic tissue (15%)	60
IIa	Extension to uterus or tubes	
IIb	Extension to other pelvic tissues	
IIc	IIa or IIb with ascites or positive peritoneal washings	
III	Cancer involving one or both ovaries with peritoneal implants outside the pelvis and/or positive retroperitoneal or inguinal nodes. Tumor is limited to the true pelvis but with histologically proved extension to small bowel or omentum (65%).	30
IIIa	Tumor grossly limited to the true pelvis with negative nodes but with histologically confirmed microscopic seeding of abdominal peritoneal surfaces	40
IIIb	Same as IIIa, but abdominal peritoneal implants do not exceed 2 cm in diameter.	25
IIIc	Abdominal implants >2 cm in diameter and/or positive retroperitoneal or inguinal lymph nodes	23
IV	Distant metastases present [including cytology-positive pleural effusions, metastasis to liver parenchyma or peripheral superficial lymph nodes (5%)].	10

B. Prognostic factors. Extent, stage, and grade of disease are more important than specific histological types. The extent to which the disease can be surgically debulked also affects prognosis.

V. PREVENTION AND EARLY DETECTION

Women with strong family histories of epithelial ovarian cancer are at a twofold increased risk for epithelial ovarian cancer compared with other women, and women with family histories of breast or ovarian cancer or a personal history of breast cancer also are at a twofold increased risk. The risk for developing ovarian cancer by age 70 is 20% to 60% for women with a mutation in *BRCA1* and 10% to 35% for women with *BRCA2* mutations. Mutations in the *MMR* genes responsible for the Lynch Type II syndrome (see Chapter 9, Table 9.3) portend a lifetime risk of 9% to 12% for ovarian cancer.

All of these groups should undergo proper genetic counseling and consider prophylactic oophorectomy when childbearing has been completed. Women should be advised that prophylactic oophorectomy does not offer absolute protection because peritoneal carcinomas occasionally occur after bilateral oophorectomy. The value of CA-125 for screening and transvaginal ultrasound in these women has not been clearly established.

VI. MANAGEMENT OF EPITHELIAL OVARIAN CANCERS (see part A in Table 11.7 for subtypes of epithelial ovarian cancers)

A. Surgical staging evaluation
1. The ovarian tumor should be removed intact, if possible, and sent for frozen section. If the tumor is confined to the pelvis, a thorough surgical evaluation should be carried out.
2. Any free fluid, especially in the pelvic cul-de-sac, should be sent for cytological evaluation. If no free fluid is found, peritoneal washings should be obtained with 50 to 100 mL normal saline from the cul-de-sac, from each paracolic gutter, and from beneath each hemidiaphragm.
3. Systematic exploration of all peritoneal surfaces and viscera is performed. Any suspicious areas or adhesions of peritoneal surfaces should undergo biopsy.
4. The diaphragm should be sampled by biopsy or by scraping and preparation of a cytological smear.
5. The omentum should be resected from the transverse colon (an infracolic omentectomy).
6. The retroperitoneal surfaces are then explored to evaluate the pelvic and para-aortic lymph nodes. Any enlarged lymph nodes are submitted for frozen section. If frozen section is negative, a formal pelvic and para-aortic lymphadenectomy is performed.

B. Borderline tumors. Treatment is surgical resection of the primary tumor. There is no evidence that subsequent chemotherapy or radiation improves survival. Even in most patients who have multifocal disease, adjuvant therapy probably has no role. Chemotherapy can be used for patients with invasive implants.

C. Stage Ia and Ib, grade 1
1. **Premenopausal patients** in this category may, after staging laparotomy is completed, undergo unilateral oophorectomy to preserve fertility. Follow-up should include regular pelvic examinations and determinations of CA-125 levels. Generally, the other ovary and uterus are removed when childbearing is completed.
2. **Postmenopausal patients** and women in whom childbearing is not an issue should undergo TAH/BSO and staging.

D. Stage Ia and Ib (grades 2 and 3) and stage Ic are treated with TAH/BSO and staging followed by chemotherapy. Carboplatin plus paclitaxel for three to six cycles is recommended for most patients (see section VI.E.4 for regimen dosages). It may be preferable to give older patients a course of single-agent chemotherapy with carboplatin for four to six cycles.

E. Stages II, III, and IV

1. **Surgery** with exploration and removal of as much disease as possible should be carried out. Removal of the primary tumor and as much metastatic disease as possible is referred to as *cytoreductive surgery* or *debulking.* "Optimal debulking" is defined as having residual tumor diameters <1 cm in diameter.

2. **Chemotherapy.** Platinum-based combination regimens have been the mainstay of treatment for advanced ovarian cancer. Combination of a platinum agent (carboplatin or cisplatin) with paclitaxel is the standard treatment for epithelial ovarian cancer. This regimen can be administered intravenously or intraperitoneally (in selected patients).

   a. **The intravenous regimen** is given to patients every 3 weeks for six to eight cycles as follows:

   Paclitaxel (Taxol), 135 to 175 mg/m^2 (given before carboplatin or cisplatin)
   Carboplatin, AUC 5 to 6

   b. **The intraperitoneal (IP) regimen** is an option in patients with microscopic residual disease after cytoreductive surgery. In this subset of patients, a significant improvement in progression-free and overall survival was noted compared with intravenous therapy. Due to increased side effects, such as abdominal pain, gastrointestinal discomfort, fatigue, hematologic toxicities, and neuropathy, many patients are not able to tolerate the full six courses of IP therapy. This regimen is administered in six cycles every 21 days as tolerated:

   Day 1 IV Paclitaxel 135 mg/m^2 over 24 hours
   Day 2 IP Cisplatin 100 mg/m^2
   Day 8 IP Paclitaxel 60 mg/m^2

   c. **Relative toxicities.** Carboplatin has fewer gastrointestinal, neurological, and renal side effects than cisplatin but more hematotoxicity. When paclitaxel is infused over 3 hours, it is associated with more neurological toxicity and less hematologic toxicity than when it is infused over 24 hours.

   d. **Maintenance therapy with paclitaxel** every 28 days for a 12-month period may improve progression-free survival, but the overall survival is not affected. Therefore, maintenance chemotherapy in patients with advanced ovarian cancer who have achieved complete remission with standard induction chemotherapy is not the standard of care.

3. **Serial CA-125 determinations** should be followed. Rising CA-125 levels to a level >20 to 35 U/mL are associated with persistent or recurrent disease.

F. Second-line therapy

1. **Cytotoxic drugs.** If disease relapses later than 12 months or more after completion of primary therapy, the original drugs may be retried. If disease progresses on first-line therapy or relapses a short time after completion of primary therapy, other drugs should be used.

   a. Chemotherapeutic agents that may be helpful after failure of first-line therapy include liposomal doxorubicin, topotecan, gemcitabine and carboplatin, oral etoposide (100 mg/day for 14 days of each 21-day cycle), and hexamethylmelamine. In most cases, single-agent therapy appears to be as effective as combinations. Response rates are about 15% to 25%.

   b. Hormonal treatment with tamoxifen has demonstrated 10% to 20% efficacy in this setting.

   c. Recently, bevacizumab (Avastin), a monoclonal antibody against vascular endothelial growth factor, has been used alone or in combination with cytotoxic agents in the treatment of recurrent epithelial ovarian cancer and is being investigated as a primary treatment with carboplatin and paclitaxel.

2. **High-dose chemotherapy** with autologous stem cell support has been disappointing for the treatment of ovarian cancer. More dose-intense approaches have not yielded better results than standard intravenous schedules.

3. **Second-look laparotomy.** A second-look operation is one performed to determine the response to therapy on a patient who has no clinical evidence of

disease after a prescribed course of chemotherapy. Second-look laparotomy has not been shown to influence patient survival, although the information obtained at second look is highly prognostic. The operation should only be performed in a research setting, such as in patients receiving therapy in a setting where second-line therapies are undergoing clinical trial.

4. **Secondary cytoreductive surgery**

   a. May be beneficial for patients who have isolated residual disease at relapse, such as a persistent pelvic mass. This benefit depends on the ability to completely resect the residual disease.

   b. Is not beneficial for patients with disease that is unresponsive to chemotherapy

5. **Palliative surgery** may be considered in patients who develop bowel obstruction and resistance to chemotherapy but have a reasonably good performance status; this is usually a difficult recommendation to make for all concerned. The goal is to allow the patient sufficient oral intake to maintain hydration or some nutrition at home. If successful, the procedure may allow 3 to 6 months of relief. Unfortunately, the complication and mortality rates from surgery are high, and the success rate is low. The patient and her family must clearly understand these limitations when decisions are made.

G. **Patient follow-up** after disease-free second-look operations is clinical because there are no reliable means of surveillance. CA-125 levels should be followed, but CT and ultrasound have proved too insensitive to detect early recurrent disease. CT may be used to follow known masses.

VII. **PERITONEAL TUMORS** of müllerian histology (primary peritoneal cancers)

The histology of peritoneal mesothelium is identical to that of germinal epithelium. The peritoneum may transform into malignant müllerian epithelial patterns that resemble advanced epithelial ovarian carcinoma and present as implants throughout the peritoneal cavity (including ovarian surfaces). Management is the same as for stage III epithelial ovarian carcinoma.

VIII. **GERM CELL TUMORS** (see part B in Table 11.7 for subtypes)

A. **General aspects of germ cell tumors**

   1. **Epidemiology.** Germ cell tumors make up 20% to 25% of all ovarian neoplasms, but only 3% of these tumors are malignant. These malignancies constitute <5% of all ovarian cancers in Western countries and up to 15% in Asian and African populations. Germ cell tumors constitute >70% of ovarian neoplasms in the first two decades of life, and in this age range, one-third are malignant.

   2. **Signs and symptoms.** These tumors grow rapidly and often present with subacute pelvic pain and pressure and menstrual irregularity. Acute symptoms related to torsion or adnexal rupture are often confused with acute appendicitis. Adnexal masses >2 cm in premenarchal girls and in premenopausal women are suspicious; they usually require surgical investigation.

   3. **Diagnosis**

      a. Young patients should be tested for serum LDH, β-hCG, and α-FP titers along with other routine blood work.

      b. A **karyotype** should be obtained because of the propensity of these tumors to arise from dysgenetic gonads.

      c. A **chest radiograph** is essential because germ cell tumors may metastasize to lungs or mediastinum.

B. **Dysgerminoma**

   1. **Natural history.** Dysgerminomas are the most common germ cell malignancy and represent up to 10% of ovarian cancers in patients <20 years of age. Three-fourths of dysgerminomas occur between the ages of 10 and 30 years. About 5% are found in dysgenic gonads. Three-fourths of cases are stage I, and 10% to 15% are bilateral. Unlike other ovarian malignancies, dysgerminomas often spread earlier through the lymphatics than to peritoneal surfaces. These tumors secrete LDH.

2. **Treatment** is primarily surgical; the minimal operation is unilateral oophorectomy with complete surgical staging. The chance of recurrence in the other ovary during the next 2 years is 5% to 10%, but these lesions are sensitive to chemotherapy. When fertility is an issue, the uterus and contralateral ovary should be preserved even in the presence of metastatic disease. If fertility is not an issue, TAH/BSO should be performed. If a Y chromosome is found by karyotyping, both ovaries should be removed, but the uterus may be left in place.

   a. **Chemotherapy** is the adjuvant treatment of choice for metastatic disease. A combination of bleomycin, etoposide, and cisplatin (BEP regimen) is most often used. BEP dosages are as follows:

   Bleomycin, 15 U/m^2 per week for 5 weeks; then on Day 1 of the fourth course
   Etoposide, 100 mg/m^2 per day for 5 days every 3 weeks
   Cisplatin, 20 mg/m^2 per day for 5 days, or 100 mg/m^2 on 1 day, every 3 weeks

   b. **RT.** If fertility is not an issue, metastatic disease may be treated with radiation because these tumors are extremely radiosensitive.

3. **Prognosis.** The 5-year survival rate for patients with stage Ia disease is >95% when the disease is treated with unilateral oophorectomy alone. Recurrence is most likely in patients with lesions larger than 10 to 15 cm in diameter, who are younger than 20 years of age, and who have an anaplastic histology. Patients with advanced disease that is treated with surgery followed by BEP chemotherapy have a 5-year survival rate of 85% to 90%.

C. Immature teratoma

1. **Natural history.** Pure immature teratomas account for less than 1% of all ovarian cancers but are the second most common germ cell malignancy. They constitute 10% to 20% of ovarian malignancies in patients younger than 20 years of age and account for 30% of ovarian cancer deaths in this group. Serum tumor markers (β-hCG, α-FP) are not found unless the tumor is of mixed type. The most common site of spread is the peritoneum; hematogenous spread is uncommon and occurs late.

2. **Treatment.** In premenopausal women in whom the lesion is confined to one ovary, a unilateral oophorectomy with surgical staging is warranted. In postmenopausal women, TAH/BSO is performed.

   a. For patients with stage Ia, grade 1 tumors, no adjuvant therapy is required. For stage Ia, grade 2 or 3, or for higher stages with gross residual disease, adjuvant chemotherapy with BEP should be used. Chemotherapy is also indicated for patients with ascites, regardless of grade.

   b. RT is reserved for patients with localized disease after chemotherapy.

   c. Second-look laparotomy is best reserved for patients at high risk for treatment failure (i.e., patients with macroscopic disease at the start of chemotherapy) because there are no reliable tumor markers for this disease.

3. **Prognosis.** The most important prognostic feature of immature teratomas is their histological grade. The 5-year survival rate is 80% to 100%. Patients whose lesions cannot be completely resected before chemotherapy have a 5-year survival rate of only 50%, as compared with 94% for completely resected disease.

D. Endodermal sinus tumors (yolk sac carcinomas) are rare. The median age at diagnosis is 18 years. Pelvic or abdominal pain is the most common presenting symptom. Most of these lesions secrete α-FP, and serum levels are useful in monitoring response to treatment.

1. **Treatment** consists of surgical staging, unilateral oophorectomy, and frozen section for diagnosis.

2. **All patients** are given adjuvant or therapeutic chemotherapy. BEP appears to be most effective. Other cisplatin-containing regimens include POMB-ACE (cisplatin, vincristine, methotrexate, bleomycin, actinomycin D, cyclophosphamide, etoposide), which may be used for high-risk cases with extensive metastatic disease, such as for those with lung or liver metastasis.

   E. Embryonal carcinoma is an extremely rare tumor that occurs in young women and girls, with a median age of 14 years. These tumors may secrete estrogens, producing symptoms of precocious pseudopuberty or irregular bleeding. Two-thirds are confined to one ovary at presentation, and they frequently secrete α-FP and β-hCG, which are useful to follow response to therapy. Treatment is unilateral or bilateral oophorectomy followed by chemotherapy with BEP.

   F. Choriocarcinoma of the ovary is extremely rare; most patients are younger than 20 years of age. β-hCG is often a useful tumor marker. Half of premenarchal patients present with isosexual precocity. The prognosis is usually poor, but complete responses have been reported with combination methotrexate, actinomycin D, and cyclophosphamide (Cytoxan) (MAC III regimen; see "Gestational Trophoblastic Neoplasia," section VI.B.3.b).

   G. Mixed germ cell tumors most commonly have a dysgerminoma or endodermal sinus component. Secretion of α-FP or β-hCG depends on component parts. Lesions should be managed with unilateral oophorectomy and chemotherapy with BEP. A second-look laparotomy may be indicated when macroscopic disease is present at the start of chemotherapy to determine response to therapy in components that do not produce tumor markers.

IX. SEX CORD STROMAL TUMORS (see part C in Table 11.7 for subtypes) account for 5% to 8% of all ovarian cancers. Most tumors are a combination of cell types derived from the sex cords and ovarian stroma or mesenchyme.

   A. Granulosa–stromal cell tumors include granulosa cell tumors, thecomas, and fibromas. Thecomas and fibromas are rarely malignant and are then called *fibrosarcomas*. Granulosa cell tumors are low-grade, estrogen-secreting malignancies that are seen in women of all ages. Endometrial cancer occurs with granulosa cell tumors in 5% of cases, and 25% to 50% are associated with endometrial hyperplasia. Inhibin, which may be secreted by some granulosa cell tumors, may be a useful tumor marker. Surgery alone is usually sufficient therapy; RT and chemotherapy are reserved for women with recurrent or metastatic disease. Granulosa cell tumors have a 10-year survival rate of about 90%. DNA ploidy correlates with survival.

   B. Sertoli-Leydig tumors have a peak incidence between the third and fourth decades. These rare lesions are usually low-grade malignancies. Most produce androgens, and virilization is seen in 70% to 85% of patients. Usual treatment is unilateral salpingo-oophorectomy with evaluation of the contralateral ovary. TAH/BSO is appropriate for older patients. The utility of radiation or chemotherapy is yet to be proved.

X. OTHER TUMORS (see part D in Table 11.7)

   A. Lipoid cell tumors are extremely rare, with only slightly more than 100 cases reported. They are thought to arise from adrenal cortical rests near the ovary. Most are virilizing and are benign or low-grade malignancies. Treatment is surgical extirpation.

   B. Ovarian sarcomas are also extremely rare, and most occur in postmenopausal women. They are aggressive lesions with no effective treatment. Most patients die within 2 years.

   C. Lymphoma can involve the ovaries, usually bilaterally, especially with Burkitt lymphoma. A hematologist-oncologist should be consulted intraoperatively when lymphoma is found to determine the need for special studies; plans for cytoreductive surgery should be abandoned. Treatment is as for lymphomas elsewhere in the body.

XI. SPECIAL CLINICAL PROBLEMS

   A. Pseudomyxoma peritonei occurs in the setting of mucinous cystadenocarcinoma or "benign" mucinous adenomas. The peritoneum becomes filled with jellylike material that compresses the bowel and produces painful abdominal distention. Chemotherapy may impede cellular production of the mucoid material but usually has little direct effect on the tumor. Periodic surgical debulking may be the only way to provide relief of abdominal symptoms. It is now believed that these lesions are typically associated with mucinous adenocarcinomas of the appendix.

B. Fallopian tube cancers account for 0.3% of all cancers of the female genital tract. They are seen most frequently in the fifth and sixth decades of life. The classic triad of symptoms is a prominent watery vaginal discharge, pelvic pain, and pelvic mass; however, this triad is seen in <15% of patients. The histological features, evaluation, and treatment are similar to those of ovarian cancer.

C. Pregnancy with ovarian cancer (see Chapter 26). Pregnancy is rarely complicated by the development of ovarian cancer. All pregnant patients have luteal cysts, which should be <5 to 6 cm in diameter. Masses that are larger or continue to enlarge over several weeks should be examined by laparoscopy at 16 weeks of gestation. Management of pregnant patients with ovarian cancer is the same as for nonpregnant patients who desire childbearing.

D. Obstructive complications. Intestinal obstruction is discussed in Chapter 30, section II. Rectal or urinary tract obstruction or dyspareunia in patients with advanced pelvic cancers may respond to either systemic chemotherapy or local irradiation (see "General Aspects," section III).

 GESTATIONAL TROPHOBLASTIC NEOPLASIA

I. EPIDEMIOLOGY AND ETIOLOGY. Gestational choriocarcinoma accounts for <1% of malignancies in women. The etiology is unknown, but certain risk factors and the relationship with hydatidiform mole are well recognized.

A. Hydatidiform mole develops in about 1 in 1,500–2,000 pregnancies in North America and Europe. The incidence is 5 to 10 times greater in Asia, Latin America, and other countries.

B. Other factors that are associated with the occurrence of hydatidiform mole include the following:

1. Patients who have had a prior molar pregnancy

2. Extremes of reproductive age

3. Presence of twin pregnancy

II. PATHOLOGY AND NATURAL HISTORY

A. Classification. Molar pregnancies are classified as partial or complete based on morphology, histopathology, and karyotype. *Complete moles* have diploid karyotype, tend to have grapelike structures with diffuse hydropic villi, and can be accompanied with paraneoplastic sequellae. *Partial moles* have triploid karyotype, can resemble hydropic abortion with recognizable fetal tissue, and have focal trophoblastic hyperplasia.

B. Malignant transformation. Persistent gestational trophoblastic disease (GTD) is diagnosed when there is clinical, hormonal, pathological, and/or radiological evidence of gestational trophoblastic tissue. About 20% of patients with complete molar pregnancy will develop persistence; 15% will have localized uterine disease, whereas 4% have evidence of metastatic disease. In contrast, partial moles develop nonmetastatic persistence in 2% to 4% of cases. Choriocarcinoma results from the malignant transformation of the trophoblast and is characterized by the absence of villi. The clinical course determines whether the growth is benign or malignant. Occasionally, malignant growth may not become clinically evident until years after the last gestation.

C. Dissemination. Persistent GTD disseminates locally to the vagina and pelvic organs. Choriocarcinoma disseminates rapidly and widely through the bloodstream. The lungs are the most common site of metastases, followed by the vaginal metastases. Hepatic and cerebral metastases are seen less commonly.

III. DIAGNOSIS

A. Symptoms of molar pregnancy or malignant trophoblastic disease include the following:

1. Vaginal bleeding during pregnancy (nearly all cases of molar pregnancy or malignant trophoblastic disease cause bleeding)

2. Hyperemesis gravidarum
3. Passage of grapelike villi from the uterus
4. Sweating, tachycardia, weight loss, and nervousness resulting from paraneoplastic hyperthyroidism (see section VII.A)
5. Pulmonary symptoms as a consequence of lung metastases
6. Right upper quadrant pain or jaundice as a consequence of liver metastases
7. Any neurological abnormality resulting from brain metastases
8. Abdominal (uterine) pain early in pregnancy

B. Physical findings
1. The uterus is usually, but not always, larger than expected for the duration of pregnancy.
2. Fetal heart tones are absent (the coexistence of a viable fetus and a partial hydatidiform mole is uncommon).
3. The patient develops signs of toxemia of pregnancy (hypertension, retinal sheen, sudden weight gain, proteinuria, or peripheral edema). If signs occur in the first or second trimester, a molar pregnancy is strongly suspected.

C. Preliminary laboratory studies
1. CBC, platelet count, alkaline phosphatase level, LFTs
2. β-hCG production is maximal in early pregnancy and decreases thereafter. Normal hCG values for pregnancy depend on the assay method used by the laboratory. hCG is elevated in all patients with choriocarcinoma; the serum concentration directly reflects the tumor volume. The serum half-life of hCG is 18 to 24 hours.

D. Special diagnostic studies
1. Ultrasonography of the uterus and Doppler examination reveal no evidence of fetal parts or heartbeat in trophoblastic disease. If these examinations show no fetus, plain radiographs of the pelvic organs are obtained for confirmation.
2. A chest radiograph should be obtained in patients with molar pregnancy.
3. Radionuclide and CT scans are used to detect brain, liver, or other abdominal metastases. Scans and films of the abdomen and pelvis must be avoided until the absence of a fetus is proved.
4. Thyroid studies (serum thyroxine concentration and tri-iodothyronine-resin uptake) are obtained in patients with clinical evidence of hyperthyroidism.

IV. STAGING SYSTEMS AND PROGNOSTIC FACTORS
A. The FIGO staging system for GTD is shown in Table 11.9.
B. The World Health Organization (WHO) scoring system for GTD is summarized in Table 11-10. *High-risk* patients are those with a score of ≥7 and *low-risk* patients are those with score of ≤6. In addition, another scoring system can be assigned by determining the risk of resistance to single-agent chemotherapy.

V. PREVENTION AND EARLY DETECTION. Early detection depends on careful attention to the signs and symptoms of trophoblastic disease in pregnant and postpartum patients.

TABLE 11.9   **FIGO Staging System for Gestational Trophoblastic Disease**

Stage	Description
I	Confined to the uterus
II	Extension to adnexa or vagina, confined to the genital structures
III	Lung metastasis
IV	All other sites of metastasis

FIGO, International Federation of Gynecology and Obstetrics.

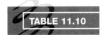

| TABLE 11.10 | WHO Prognostic Scoring System for Gestational Trophoblastic Disease | | | |

	Score			
Parameter	**0**	**1**	**2**	**4**
Age (years)		$\leq$39	>39	
Antecedent pregnancy	Mole	Abortion	Term	
Interval (months)	<4	4–6	7–12	>12
Pretreatment hCG	<10^3	10^3–10^4	>10^4–10^5	>10^5
Largest tumor (cm)		3–4	>5	
Site of metastasis		Spleen, kidney	Gut	Brain, liver
Number of metastases	0	1–4	5–8	>8
Prior chemotherapy drugs failed			1	$\geq$2

WHO, World Health Organization.

VI. MANAGEMENT. All forms of gestational trophoblastic neoplasia, from hydatidiform mole to choriocarcinoma, are almost invariably lethal if not treated.

  A. Early disease signifies a molar pregnancy without evidence of distant metastases by history, physical examination, LFTs, chest radiograph, or scans.

    1. Surgery. Molar tissue is removed by suction curettage while oxytocin is being administered, and then by sharp curettement. Hysterectomy is recommended for women >40 years of age. Disappearance of hCG is achieved within 8 weeks in 80% of patients treated by surgery; virtually all of these patients are cured. The patient is followed with weekly blood assays for hCG.

    2. RT has no role in early disease.

    3. Chemotherapy. After surgical treatment of a molar pregnancy with no suggestion of metastatic disease, weekly serum hCG titers are obtained. Chemotherapy is started for histological diagnosis of choriocarcinoma, rising hCG titer (for 2 weeks), plateau of hCG titer (for 3 weeks), documentation of metastatic disease, or return of titers with no other explanation after achieving a zero titer. So long as titers continue to decrease, treatment is usually not started; in the past, treatment was started after a predetermined number of weeks.

      a. Methotrexate is the drug of choice in early gestational trophoblastic neoplasia. It can be administered in the following three ways:

        (1) Pulse methotrexate, 40 mg/m^2 IM weekly

        (2) 5-day methotrexate, 0.4 mg/m^2 IV or IM daily for 5 days; with response, re-treat at same dose every 2 weeks

        (3) Methotrexate, 100 mg/m^2 IV in 250 mL of normal saline over 30 minutes or 200 mg/m^2 IV in 500 mL normal saline over 12 hours; leucovorin (15 mg PO or IM every 12 hours for 4 doses) is given 24 hours after starting methotrexate.

      b. Actinomycin D is used instead of methotrexate in patients with renal function impairment or when there is resistance to methotrexate. This drug can be administered every 2 weeks either as 12 mcg/kg IV push daily for 5 days or as a pulse of 1.25 mg/m^2 IV.

  B. Advanced disease

    1. Surgery is used to evacuate or excise the uterus for the same indications outlined in early disease (see section VI.A.1).

    2. RT, in combination with chemotherapy, is clearly indicated for the primary management of patients with liver or brain metastases.

    3. Chemotherapy is the mainstay of management for metastatic trophoblastic disease. All patients undergo the restaging evaluation described in section III.

    a. Low-risk patients are treated with methotrexate or actinomycin D, as for early disease patients. Patients not responding to one of these agents are switched to the alternative drug.

    b. High-risk patients are treated with combination chemotherapy regimens, such as EMA-CO or EMA-CE (described subsequently). RT is given if the liver or brain is involved by metastases. Chemotherapy dosage schedules are as follows (cycle intervals should not be extended without good cause):

        (1) EMA-CO is given in 14-day cycles:

        Etoposide, 100 mg/m^2 IV on Days 1 and 2

        Methotrexate, 100 mg/m^2 IV push, followed by 200 mg/m^2 by continuous IV infusion over 12 hours on Day 1; leucovorin, 15 mg PO or IM, every 12 hours for four doses beginning 24 hours after the start of methotrexate

        Actinomycin D, 0.5 mg (*not* per m^2) IV push on Days 1 and 2

        Cyclophosphamide, 600 mg/m^2 IV on Day 8

        Vincristine (Oncovin), 1.0 mg/m^2 IV push on Day 8 (maximum 2 mg)

        (2) EMA-CE is given in 14-day cycles:

        Etoposide, 100 mg/m^2 IV on Days 1 and 2

        Methotrexate, 100 mg/m^2 IV push, followed by 1,000 mg/m^2 by continuous IV infusion over 12 hours on Day 1; leucovorin, 30 mg PO or IM, every 12 hours for six doses beginning 32 hours after starting methotrexate

        Actinomycin D, 0.5 mg (*not* per m^2) IV push on Days 1 and 2

        Cisplatin, 60 mg/m^2 IV on Day 8 with prehydration

        Etoposide, 100 mg/m^2 IV on Day 8

    c. Duration of treatment. Chemotherapy should be continued until no hCG is demonstrable in the serum for 3 consecutive weekly assays. If the hCG titer rises or plateaus between any two measurements, the chemotherapy regimen must be changed.

C. Patient follow-up

    1. The hCG level is the single most important tumor marker in trophoblastic neoplasia. For stage I, II, and III disease weekly hCG levels are recommended until normal for 3 consecutive weeks. Then, monitor hCG levels monthly until they are normal for 12 consecutive months. The duration is increased to 24 months for stage IV disease. Effective contraception during the entire interval of hormonal follow-up is essential.

    2. Other studies that demonstrated disease at the start of therapy should be repeated monthly until complete remission is documented.

VII. SPECIAL CLINICAL PROBLEMS

A. Thyrotoxicosis and even "thyroid storm" may result from the thyroid-stimulating hormone–like effect of high concentrations of hCG. Clinical evidence of hyperthyroidism in choriocarcinoma occurs in the presence of widespread metastases and is associated with a poor prognosis. Laboratory confirmation requires a serum thyroxine concentration and tri-iodothyronine-resin uptake levels compatible with hyperthyroidism. If the symptoms are mild, propylthiouracil or methimazole can be used. In severe cases, patients must be given propranolol and Lugol's solution.

B. Development of choriocarcinoma can occur long after the last pregnancy or even hysterectomy. This development serves to emphasize that histological diagnosis is necessary in metastatic cancer when the primary tumor is not evident. The diagnosis of choriocarcinoma can lead to lifesaving therapy.

C. Subsequent pregnancies. Patients should be reassured that they can anticipate normal subsequent pregnancy outcomes. They are, however, at increased risk for repeat molar pregnancy. This risk is 1% after one molar pregnancy and 20% after two molar pregnancies.

Suggested Reading

Berek JS. *Berek & Novak's Gynecology*. 14th ed. Philadelphia: Lippincott Williams & Wilkins; 2007.

Berek JS, Hacker NF, eds. *Practical Gynecologic Oncology*. 4th ed. Philadelphia: Lippincott Williams & Wilkins; 2005.

Cancer of the Uterine Cervix

Abu-Rustum NR, et al. Fertility-sparing radical abdominal trachelectomy for cervical carcinoma: technique and review of the literature. *Gynecol Oncol* 2006;103(3): 807.

Berek JS. Simplification of the new Bethesda 2001 classification system. *Am J Obstet Gynecol* 2003;188(3 Suppl):S2.

Im SS, Monk BJ. New developments in the treatment of invasive cervical cancer. *Obstet Gynecol Clin North Am* 2002;29:659.

Morris M, et al. Pelvic radiation with concurrent chemotherapy compared with pelvic and paraaortic radiation for high-risk cervical cancer. *N Engl J Med* 1999;340:1137.

Rose PG, et al. Concurrent cisplatin-based radiotherapy and chemotherapy for locally advanced cervical cancer. *N Engl J Med* 1999;340:1144.

Saslow D, et al. 2002 American Cancer Society guideline for the early detection of cervical neoplasia and cancer. *CA Cancer J Clin* 2002;52(6):342. Review.

Sedlis A, et al. A randomized trial of pelvic radiation therapy versus no further therapy in selected patients with stage 1B carcinoma of the cervix after radical hysterectomy and pelvic lymphadenectomy: a Gynecologic Oncology Group Study. *Gynecol Oncol* 1999;73:177.

Thigpen T. The role of chemotherapy in the management of carcinoma of the cervix. *Cancer J* 2003;9(5):425. Review.

Villa LL, et al. 2005 Prophylactic quadrivalent human papillomavirus (types 6, 11, 16, and 18) L1 virus-like particle vaccine in young women: a randomised double-blind placebo-controlled multicentre phase II efficacy trial. *Lancet Oncol* 2005;6(5):271.

Wright TC Jr, et al. 2001 consensus guidelines for the management of women with cervical intraepithelial neoplasia. (American Society for Colposcopy and Cervical Pathology.) *Am J Obstet Gynecol* 2003;189:295.

Cancer of the Uterine Body

Ackerman I, et al. Endometrial carcinoma: relative effectiveness of adjuvant radiation vs therapy reserved for relapse. *Gynecol Oncol* 1996;60:177.

Carey MS, et al. Good outcome associated with a standardized treatment protocol using selective postoperative radiation in patients with clinical stage I adenocarcinoma of the endometrium. *Gynecol Oncol* 1995;57:138.

Chi DS, et al. The role of surgical cytoreduction in stage IV endometrial carcinoma. *Gynecol Oncol* 1997;67(1):56.

Creasman WT, et al. Carcinoma of the corpus uteri. *Int J Gynaecol Obstet* 2003;83(Suppl 1):79.

Hirsch M, Lilford RJ, Jarvis GJ. Adjuvant progestogen therapy for the treatment of endometrial cancer: review and metaanalysis of published, randomized controlled trials. *Eur J Obstet Gynecol Reprod Biol* 1996;65:201.

Levine DA, Hoskins WJ. Update in the management of endometrial cancer. *Cancer J* 2002;8(Suppl 1):S31.

Mohan DS, et al. Long-term outcomes of therapeutic pelvic lymphadenectomy for stage I endometrial carcinoma. *Gynecol Oncol* 1998;70:165.

Morrow CP, et al. Relationship between surgical-pathological risk factors and outcome in clinical stage I and II carcinoma of the endometrium: a Gynecologic Oncology Group study. *Gynecol Oncol* 1991;40(1):55.

Randall TC, Kurman RJ. Progestin treatment of atypical hyperplasia and well-differentiated carcinoma of the endometrium in women under age 40. *Obstet Gynecol* 1997;90: 434.

Schmeler KM, et al. Prophylactic surgery to reduce the risk of gynecologic cancers in the Lynch syndrome. *N Engl J Med* 2006;354(3):261.

Trimble CL, et al. Concurrent endometrial carcinoma in women with a biopsy diagnosis of atypical endometrial hyperplasia: a Gynecologic Oncology Group study. *Cancer* 2006;106(4):812.

Vaginal Cancer

Stock RG, Chen ASJ, Seski J. A 30-year experience in the management of primary carcinoma of the vagina: analysis of prognostic factors and treatment modalities. *Gynecol Oncol* 1995;56:45.

Vulvar Cancer

Berek JS, et al. Concurrent cisplatin and 5-fluorouracil chemotherapy and radiotherapy for advanced stage squamous carcinoma of the vulva. *Gynecol Oncol* 1991;42:197.

Bruchim I, Gottlieb WH, Mahmud S, et al. HPV-related vulvar intraepithelial neoplasia: outcome of different management modalities. *Int J Gynaecol Obstet* 2007;99(1):23.

Farias-Eisner R, et al. Conservative and individualized surgery for early squamous carcinoma of the vulva: the treatment of choice for stages I and II (T1–2;N0–1, M0) disease. *Gynecol Oncol* 1994;53:55.

Jones RW, Rowan DM. Vulvar intraepithelial neoplasia. III. A clinical study of the outcome of 113 cases with relation to the later development of invasive vulvar carcinoma. *Obstet Gynecol* 1994;84:741.

Markowitz LE, Dunne EF, Saraiya M, et al. Quadrivalent human papillomavirus vaccine: recommendations of the Advisory Committee on Immunization Practices (ACIP). *MMWR Recomm Rep* 2007 Mar 23;56(RR-2):1.

Rhodes CA, Cummings C, Shafi MI. The management of squamous cell vulval cancer: a population-based retrospective study of 411 cases. *BJOG* 1998;105:200.

Ovarian Cancer

Armstrong DK, et al. Intraperitoneal cisplatin and paclitaxel in ovarian cancer. *N Engl J Med* 2006;354(1):34.

Berchuck A, et al. Role of BRCA1 mutation screening in the management of familial ovarian cancer. *Am J Obstet Gynecol* 1996;175:738.

Berek JS. Interval debulking of ovarian cancer: an interim measure. *N Engl J Med* 1995;332:675.

Bristow RE, Lagasse LD, Karlan BY. Secondary surgical cytoreduction for advanced epithelial ovarian cancer: patient selection and review of the literature. *Cancer* 1996;78:2049.

Cannistra SA, et al. Progress in the management of gynecologic cancer: consensus summary statement. *J Clin Oncol* 2003;21(10 Suppl):129.

Farias-Eisner R, et al. The influence of tumor grade, distribution and extent of carcinomatosis in minimal residual epithelial ovarian cancer after optimal primary cytoreductive surgery. *Gynecol Oncol* 1994;55:108.

Frank TS, et al. Sequence analysis of BRCA1 and BRCA2: correlation of mutations with family history and ovarian cancer risk. *J Clin Oncol* 1998;16:2417.

Goff BA. Development of an ovarian cancer symptom index: possibilities for earlier detection. *Cancer* 2007;109(2):221.

Hoskins WJ, et al. The influence of cytoreductive surgery on recurrence-free interval and survival in small volume state III epithelial ovarian cancer: a Gynecology Oncology Group Study. *Gynecol Oncol* 1992;47:159.

Kalil NG, McGuire WP. Chemotherapy for advanced epithelial ovarian carcinoma. *Best Pract Res Clin Obstet Gynaecol* 2002;16:553.

Markman M. New, expanded, and modified use of approved antineoplastic agents in ovarian cancer. *Oncologist* 2007;12(2):186.

Markman M, et al. Gynecologic Oncology Group Phase III randomized trial of 12 versus 3 months of maintenance paclitaxel in patients with advanced ovarian cancer after complete response to platinum and paclitaxel-based chemotherapy: a Southwest Oncology Group and Gynecologic Oncology Group trial. *J Clin Oncol* 2003;21:2460.

Memarzadeh S, Berek JS. Advances in the management of epithelial ovarian cancer. *J Reprod Med* 2001;46:621.

NIH Consensus Development Panel on Ovarian Cancer. Ovarian cancer: screening, treatment and follow-up. *JAMA* 1995;273:491.

Struewing JP, et al. The risk of cancer associated with specific mutations of BRCA1 and BRCA2 among Ashkenazi Jews. *N Engl J Med* 1997;336:1401.

Van der Burg MEL, et al. The effect of debulking surgery after induction chemotherapy on the prognosis in advanced epithelial ovarian cancer. *N Engl J Med* 1995;332:629.

Gestational Trophoblastic Disease

Kohorn EI. Negotiating a staging and risk factor scoring system for gestational trophoblastic neoplasia: a progress report. *J Reprod Med* 2002;47:445.

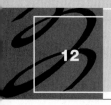

12 TESTICULAR CANCER
Lawrence H. Einhorn

I. EPIDEMIOLOGY AND ETIOLOGY
A. Epidemiology
1. **Incidence.** Testicular cancer constitutes only 1% of all cancers in men but is the most common malignancy that develops in men between the ages of 20 and 40 years. About 8,000 new cases are diagnosed annually in the United States.
2. **Racial predilection.** The incidence of testicular cancer in blacks is one-sixth that in whites. Asians also have a lower incidence than whites.
3. Bilateral cancer of the testis occurs in about 2% of cases.

B. Etiology
1. **Cryptorchidism.** Male patients with cryptorchidism are 10 to 40 times more likely to develop testicular carcinoma than are those with normally descended testes. The risk for developing cancer in a testis is 1 in 80 if retained in the inguinal canal and 1 in 20 if retained in the abdomen. Surgical placement of an undescended testis into the scrotum before 6 years of age reduces the risk for cancer. However, 25% of cancers in patients with cryptorchidism occur in the normal, descended testis.
2. **Testicular feminization syndromes** increase the risk for cancer in the retained gonad by 40-fold. Tumors in these patients are often bilateral.
3. **Other risk factors.** The magnitude of other suggested risk factors, such as a history of orchitis, testicular trauma, or irradiation, is not known.

II. PATHOLOGY AND NATURAL HISTORY
A. Histology. Immunophenotypes of germ cell tumors are shown in Appendix C.3.VI.
1. Nearly all cancers of the testis in members of the younger age groups originate from germ cells (seminoma, embryonal cell, teratoma, and others). Other types, which account for <5% of cases, include rhabdomyosarcoma, lymphoma, and melanoma. Rarely, Sertoli cell tumors, Leydig cell tumors, or other mesodermal tumors develop.
2. In men >60 years of age, 75% of neoplasms are not germinal cancers. Lymphomas are the most common testicular tumors in this age group.
3. Metastatic cancer to the testis is most often associated with prostatic carcinoma, small cell lung cancer, melanoma, or leukemia.

B. Histogenesis. Each type of germinal cancer is thought to be a counterpart of normal embryonic development (Fig. 12.1). Seminoma is the neoplastic counterpart of the spermatocyte. The tissues of the early cleavage stage are the most undifferentiated and pluripotential, and give rise to both the embryo and the placenta; the malignant counterpart is embryonal cell carcinoma. Teratomas are the neoplastic counterparts of the developing embryo. Choriocarcinoma is actually a more highly undifferentiated cancer; its aggressive biological behavior reflects the capacity of its normal counterpart (the placenta) to invade blood vessels. The histologic similarity between germ cell cancer and normal embryology is illustrated by the following observations:
1. Pure choriocarcinomas metastasize only as choriocarcinomas.
2. Seminomas usually metastasize as seminomas; those that do not are believed to represent mixed tumors undetected on the original histologic examination.

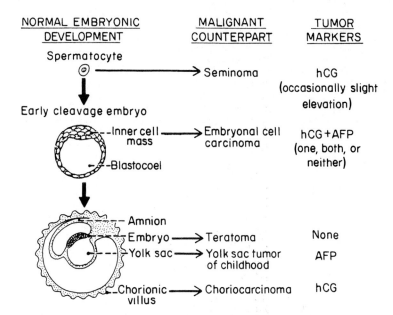

Figure 12.1. Histogenesis of testicular neoplasms. Embryonic *counterparts* and tumor marker production are shown. hCG, human chorionic gonadotropin; AFP, α-fetoprotein.

3. Metastases from embryonal carcinomas may be found to consist of teratoma or choriocarcinoma elements.

4. In metastases from mixed tumors, chemotherapy destroys the rapidly growing, drug-sensitive cell elements. The drug-resistant teratomatous elements persist after chemotherapy and require surgical resection.

C. **Natural history.** The natural history of testis cancer varies with the histologic subtype. Both blood-borne and lymphatic metastases occur. Lymphatic drainage usually occurs in an orderly progression involving ileal and para-aortic lymphatic chains as well as more lateral nodes near the kidneys; inguinal and femoral nodes are normally not affected. Previous surgery, such as scrotal contamination with scrotal orchiectomy, disrupts normal lymphatic drainage patterns.

1. **Seminoma** (40% to 50% of testicular cancers) occurs in an older age group than other germ cell neoplasms, most commonly after the age of 30 years. Sixty percent of patients with cryptorchidism who develop testicular cancer have seminoma. Seminomas tend to be large, show little hemorrhage or necrosis on gross inspection, and metastasize in an orderly, sequential manner along draining lymph node chains. About 25% of patients have lymphatic metastases, and 1% to 5% have visceral metastases at the time of diagnosis. Metastases to parenchymal organs (usually lung or bone) can occur late. Seminoma is the type of testicular cancer most likely to produce osseous metastases.

   a. **Spermatocytic seminoma** (4% of seminomas) occurs mostly after the age of 50 years and is the most common germ cell tumor after the age of 70 years. It is more often bilateral (6% compared with 2%) and appears to have a much lower incidence of both lymphatic and parenchymal metastases (even to draining lymph nodes) when compared with typical seminoma. These patients are usually cured with orchiectomy alone.

2. **Pure choriocarcinoma** (<0.5% of testicular cancers) metastasizes rapidly through the bloodstream to lungs, liver, brain, and other visceral sites. They have very high serum human chorionic gonadotropin (hCG) levels with normal α-fetoprotein (AFP) levels.

3. **Yolk sac tumors** are common cancers in children and have a relatively unaggressive clinical course. Yolk sac elements in testicular cancer found in adult patients, on the other hand, portend a worse prognosis compared with that of children. Pure yolk sac tumors have elevated AFP and normal hCG.

4. **Embryonal cell carcinoma** can be associated with elevated serum hCG, AFP, both, or neither tumor marker. When patients have clinical stage I testicular cancer with predominantly embryonal cell carcinoma, they are more likely to have occult microscopic disease in the retroperitoneum or elsewhere.

5. **Teratoma** appears pathologically inert as it is associated with cartilage, glandular, and glial tissue. Teratoma of and by itself does not have the capacity to metastasize, but it is often associated with embryonal cell carcinoma, choriocarcinoma, yolk sac tumor, and seminoma in the testis and can metastasize as a template. In that situation, chemotherapy will often completely eliminate the nonteratomatous elements, but the teratoma will remain and require surgical resection for cure. When teratoma remains after postchemotherapy, it can and will grow by local extension and can even cause death from teratoma alone. In addition, because teratoma is pluripotential tissue that can differentiate along endodermal, ectodermal, or mesoderm elements, it can undergo malignant transformation. The most common of these is mesodermal differentiation to sarcomatous elements associated with teratoma. Malignant transformation of teratoma does have the potential to metastasize. These elements can sometimes briefly respond to chemotherapy directed at the dominant cell type of malignant transformation.

6. **Rare testicular tumors**
   a. **Sertoli cell and Leydig cell tumors** are not germ cell tumors and are not associated with elevated serum hCG or AFP. They vary in malignant potential, but all can metastasize. Size, necrosis, and mitotic index predict potential for spread and need for retroperitoneal lymph node dissection. Leydig cell tumors rarely respond to chemotherapy. Sertoli cell tumors may benefit from platinum combination chemotherapy.
   b. **Rhabdomyosarcoma** of the testis occurs most often before 20 years of age. Its clinical behavior is similar to that of embryonal carcinoma; metastases to draining lymph nodes and lung are common at the time it first appears. They are usually paratesticular.

III. DIAGNOSIS

A. **Symptoms and signs.** Postorchiectomy, most patients will have an otherwise normal history and physical examination.
   1. **Symptoms**
      a. **Mass and pain.** The most common symptom of testicular cancer is a painless enlargement, usually noticed during bathing or after a minor trauma. Painful enlargement of the testis occurs in 30% to 50% of patients and may be the result of bleeding or infarction in the tumor. Acute pain in a patient with a cryptorchid testis suggests the possibility of torsion of a testicular cancer.
      b. **Acute epididymitis.** Nearly 25% of patients with mixed teratoma and embryonal cell tumor present with findings indistinguishable from acute epididymitis. The testicular swelling from tumor may even decrease somewhat after antimicrobial therapy.
      c. **Gynecomastia** due to high levels of serum hCG is rarely a presenting sign.
      d. **Infertility** is the primary symptom in about 3% of patients.
      e. **Back pain** from retroperitoneal node metastases is a presenting feature in 10% of patients.
      f. **Other presenting symptoms.** Thoracic symptoms are rare even when extensive pulmonary metastases are present. When there is extensive replacement of pulmonary parenchyma, patients may develop hemoptysis, chest pain, or dyspnea.
   2. **Physical findings**
      a. **Scrotum.** A testicular mass is nearly always present. The testis should be palpated using bimanual technique; the finding of irregularity, induration, or

nodularity is indication for further evaluation, including a testicular ultrasound to look for a hypoechogenic mass.

  b. Lymph nodes. Patients must be carefully examined for lymphadenopathy, particularly in the supraclavicular region. Scrotal contamination, such as following testicular biopsy, vasectomy, or herniorrhaphy, alters the normal lymphatic drainage; as a result, ipsilateral inguinal nodes may become involved. Large retroperitoneal masses may be palpable on abdominal examination.

  c. Breasts. Gynecomastia is associated with tumors that secrete high levels of hCG.

B. Differential diagnosis

  1. Hydroceles are usually benign, but about 10% of testicular cancers are associated with coexisting hydroceles. The finding of a hydrocele in a young man should increase suspicion for an associated neoplasm.

  a. Benign hydroceles extend along the spermatic cord, often cause groin swelling, and can give the penis a foreshortened appearance. Hydroceles can be transilluminated.

  b. If the fluid prevents adequate palpation of the testis, a testicular ultrasound should be performed.

  2. Epididymitis produces acute enlargement of the testis with severe pain, fever, dysuria, and pyuria. The same symptoms may be caused by an underlying testicular cancer.

  a. Persistent pain or swelling after treatment may result from a supervening testicular abscess or a coexisting tumor; testicular ultrasound is indicated.

  b. Recurrent epididymitis with a completely normal testis occasionally occurs. Surgical exploration should not be considered if physical examination between episodes is completely normal and there is no evidence of a tumor on testicular ultrasound. Recurrent epididymitis per se does not necessarily indicate cancer.

  3. Varicoceles are swollen veins in the pampiniform plexus of the spermatic cord. The scrotum feels like it contains a "bag of worms." The veins collapse when the patient is in Trendelenburg position.

  4. Spermatoceles are translucent masses that are located posterior and superior to the testis, and feel cystic.

  5. Inguinal hernias generally are not a diagnostic problem.

  6. Other masses include gummatous and tuberculous orchitis, hematoma, and acute swelling from testicular torsion. None of these can be distinguished clinically from cancer, and all require exploratory surgery.

C. Tumor markers are the most crucial and sensitive indicators of testicular cancer (Fig. 12.1). Serum hCG and α-AFP are the quintessential markers in oncology. One or both of these serum markers are present in more than 90% of patients with metastatic nonseminomatous germ cell cancer of the testis. The incidence rates of these markers according to tumor histology are shown in Table 12.1.

  1. hCG is markedly elevated with pure choriocarcinoma and also elevated in embryonal cell carcinoma and may be mildly elevated in patients with pure seminoma. The blood half-life of hCG is 18 to 24 hours.

  a. hCG may also be found in patients with a variety of other tumors, including melanoma, large cell lung cancer, breast, ovary, or pancreatic cancer.

  b. Nonmalignant conditions associated with elevated hCG levels may occur with marijuana use or with testicular dysfunction due to cross-reactivity with luteinizing hormone. This may occasionally occur after chemotherapy. A repeat serum hCG level 2 weeks after the administration of 300 mg of depotestosterone intramuscularly will resolve this dilemma.

  c. In testicular cancer, the presence of hCG after orchiectomy constitutes proof that the patient has residual cancer and requires further treatment. The absence of hCG, however, does not exclude the presence of active cancer, particularly in previously treated patients.

  2. AFP is produced by yolk sac elements and is most commonly associated with embryonal carcinomas and yolk sac tumors. Elevated levels of AFP are never found

TABLE 12.1   Incidence of Tumor Markers in Testicular Cancers

| | Proportion of cases (%) | |
| | hCG | AFP |
Neoplasm	Normal levels: < 3 mIU/mL	< 25 ng/mL
Seminoma	10	0
Embryonal carcinomas with or without teratomas	65	>70
Choriocarcinoma	100	0

hCG, human chorionic gonadotropin; AFP, α-fetoprotein.

in patients with pure seminoma or pure choriocarcinoma. The blood half-life of AFP is 5 days, but may be much longer after successful chemotherapy.

a. Elevated levels may also be explained by hepatocellular carcinoma, other cancers (occasionally), fetal hepatic production in pregnant women, infancy, and nonmalignant liver diseases (e.g., hepatitis, cirrhosis, necrosis).

b. Elevated levels of AFP after surgery or cytotoxic agent therapy for testicular cancer indicate the presence of residual disease and the need for further therapy.

D. Laboratory evaluation

1. Routine preoperative studies

a. Complete blood count, liver function tests (especially lactate dehydrogenase [LDH] and alkaline phosphatase levels), and renal function tests

b. Chest radiograph, including posteroanterior (PA) and lateral projections

c. Blood levels of hCG and AFP

2. Routine postoperative studies are undertaken after the diagnosis of testicular cancer is proved. Studies performed in patients with all cell types include the following:

a. Chest computed tomography (CT) scan can detect occult posterior mediastinal or pulmonary parenchymal metastases. This is not usually a necessary test if the PA and lateral chest x-rays are abnormal.

b. Abdominal and pelvic CT scans assist assessment of retroperitoneal or rarely pelvic adenopathy.

c. Positron emission tomography (PET scan) is never indicated in the initial staging. It can be of assistance in deciding the necessity of postchemotherapy surgery, especially in patients with pure seminoma. A PET scan will not be "positive" when a residual mass is teratoma, and it will not detect microscopic disease.

IV. STAGING SYSTEM AND PROGNOSTIC FACTORS

A. Staging system and survival. The system presented is a pathologic staging system for nonseminomatous tumors, for which lymphadenectomy is a standard practice. The system is also used for clinical staging of seminomas, for which lymph node sampling is not part of management.

The survival statistics for testicular tumors have been drastically altered by modern therapy. The 5-year survival rate in patients with seminoma treated with radiation therapy (RT) alone is 95% to 99% for stage A disease and 80% to 90% for stage B; most patients with stage C disease are cured with chemotherapy. The 5-year survival rate in patients with stage C nonseminomatous tumors is 70% to 80%.

Stage	Extent of disease
A	Disease confined to the testis
B	Metastases to the retroperitoneal lymph nodes
B1	Five or fewer encapsulated lymph nodes positive for tumor
B2	More than five lymph nodes positive for tumor
B3	Massive retroperitoneal lymph node disease
C	Tumor involving supradiaphragmatic nodes, lungs, liver, bone, or brain

B. Prognostic factors
   1. Elevated serum levels of AFP or hCG after orchiectomy is prima facie evidence that the patient has residual cancer.
   2. Serum LDH levels correlate fairly well with tumor burden.
   3. Nonseminomatous tumor patients receiving chemotherapy are categorized as having advanced (poor-risk) disease, with a 50% cure rate in the presence of:
      a. Very high markers (serum hCG >50,000 IU/mL, AFP >10,000 ng/mL) or LDH levels >10 times the upper limits of normal,
      b. Nonpulmonary visceral metastases (such as liver, bone, or CNS), or
      c. Primary mediastinal nonseminomatous germ cell tumors.

V. PREVENTION AND EARLY DETECTION. Cryptorchidism should be surgically corrected before puberty, usually before age 4 years, because the risk for malignancy is substantial. Prophylactic removal of undescended testes should be performed in postpubertal patients; the complication rate is minuscule, the testes are functionless, and prostheses are available to fill the empty scrotum.

The effectiveness of early detection by screening programs has not been tested. Most patients have symptoms or signs of a scrotal mass; few cases are detected by routine history and physical examination.

VI. MANAGEMENT
A. Transinguinal orchiectomy is performed to make the diagnosis for all testicular cancers in all stages and is the treatment for stage A disease. A transinguinal approach is essential; the blood supply of the spermatic cord is immediately controlled. Transscrotal orchiectomy has been proved to result in tumor seeding to the scrotum and inguinal nodes. Likewise, transscrotal needle biopsy of a suspected testicular mass is *absolutely contraindicated*.

The subsequent management of early-stage testicular tumors depends on whether the histopathology shows pure seminoma or nonseminomatous elements.
B. Management of seminomas: stages A and B
   1. **Surgery.** No further surgery is necessary after orchiectomy.
   2. **RT.** Abdominal CT and often chest CT are performed postoperatively in patients with seminoma. Many patients with clinical stage A seminoma are managed with just para-aortic RT rather than the older *hockey stick* field that included pelvic nodes. The ipsilateral retroperitoneal lymph nodes are irradiated for patients with stage B seminoma with lymph nodes that are <3 cm in diameter. Seminomas are exquisitely sensitive to RT. Prophylactic mediastinal irradiation should not be used. Total dosage should be 2,000 to 2,500 cGy. Surveillance or single-agent carboplatin are also options (*vide infra*).
   3. **Chemotherapy** with single-agent carboplatin has been found to be equivalent to RT for clinical stage A seminoma. Patients with bulky stage B (>3 cm disease) or stage C disease are treated the same as those with nonseminomatous germ cell cancer, and the results are similar (see section VI.D). Seminoma confers a favorable prognosis because none of these cases, even those with nonpulmonary visceral disease, is classified as poor-risk disease. Results with salvage chemotherapy are better for seminomatous than nonseminomatous patients.
   4. **Surveillance.** The cure rate with orchiectomy alone for clinical stage A seminoma is 80% to 85%. Therefore, surveillance (*vide infra*) is often a preferred option in compliant patients.

C. Management of nonseminomatous germ cell cancer: stages A and B

  1. Surgery. Retroperitoneal lymphadenectomy has been the standard of practice at most centers in the United States when staging evaluation does not reveal distant metastases, *and when there is no lymph node with a maximal transverse diameter of 3 cm on abdominal CT.* If lymph node metastases are demonstrated at surgery, patients either may be treated with two courses of adjuvant chemotherapy or observed without treatment and achieve the same nearly 100% cure rate. Lymphadenectomy previously interrupted the sympathetic pathways and invariably resulted in sterility from failure of ejaculation, but not impotence. Modern nerve-sparing retroperitoneal lymph node dissections, however, now routinely preserve fertility and allow antegrade ejaculation.

  2. Chemotherapy. The agents used are discussed in section VI.D. Indications for chemotherapy include the following:

  a. Rising serum levels of hCG or AFP after primary treatment or elevated levels of hCG or AFP with normal abdominal CT scan.

  b. The presence of bulky retroperitoneal disease (>3 cm in maximal transverse diameter of a node on abdominal CT) requires chemotherapy. If the abdominal CT scan becomes normal, retroperitoneal lymphadenectomy is not necessary. Otherwise, postchemotherapy retroperitoneal lymph node dissection is usually performed.

  c. A recent phase III study comparing one course of bleomycin and etoposide and cisplatin (BEP; see section VI.D.1) with retroperitoneal lymph node dissection demonstrated superiority for chemotherapy for clinical stage A disease, with a relapse rate of only 1%.

  3. Surveillance is an appropriate strategy for compliant patients with clinical stage A disease (normal markers, physical examination, and radiographic studies after orchiectomy). It is crucial that both the physician and the patient understand the necessity for close observation. Relapses are usually treated with chemotherapy. Surveillance is even appropriate in high-risk clinical stage A disease (embryonal predominant, vascular and/or lymphatic invasion, or absence of yolk sac tumor).

  If surveillance is chosen, history and physical examinations, serum markers, and chest radiographs (PA and lateral views) are obtained every 2 months during the first year. The same studies are obtained every 4 months during the second year, every 6 months during the third, fourth, and fifth years after orchiectomy, and then annually. Abdominal CT is performed every 4 months during the first and second years, and then every 6 months during the third, fourth, and fifth years. If serum markers were significantly elevated before orchiectomy, they should be measured monthly for the first year.

D. Management of disseminated disease: stage C

  1. Combination chemotherapy with etoposide and cisplatin (EP regimen) or with EP plus bleomycin (BEP regimen) produces complete remission in 70% to 80% of patients. Complete remissions are obtained with all cell types and are long lasting. Relapses may occur within 1 year of initiating therapy. Maintenance chemotherapy after achieving a complete remission is not necessary.

  a. Standard chemotherapy for good-risk patients is either BEP for three courses or EP for four courses. Patients with poor-risk (advanced) disease are treated with four courses of BEP.

  b. BEP is administered every 3 weeks for three or four cycles. Dosages are as follows:

  Bleomycin, 30 U IV weekly on days 1, 8, and 15
  Etoposide, 100 mg/m^2 IV daily for 5 days
  Cisplatin, 20 mg/m^2 IV daily for 5 days

  2. Resection of residual disease. After completion of chemotherapy, many patients who do not achieve a complete remission can become candidates for surgical resection of the residual localized disease in the chest or retroperitoneum. Radiologic findings cannot distinguish benign from malignant processes in these patients. PET scans can sometimes be helpful, but should not be used to dissuade the clinician from recommending surgery as normal PET scans are seen in the presence of microscopic cancer or gross teratoma.

  a. The presence of elevated levels of tumor markers always signifies the continued presence of carcinoma and the need for further chemotherapy. The absence of tumor markers signifies that the residual disease in the thorax or retroperitoneum is either a benign process (fibrosis, inflammation), teratoma, or carcinoma.

  b. Surgical resection of residual disease defines the subsequent treatment strategy in all of these patients and is therapeutic in some.

  (1) If surgical resection of residual disease reveals fibrosis or teratoma, no further treatment is required.

  (2) If surgical resection reveals carcinoma, two more cycles of cisplatin and etoposide therapy are given.

  3. Salvage chemotherapy. Patients who do not achieve a complete remission with BEP are still curable with salvage chemotherapy. Options include cisplatin plus ifosfamide plus either vinblastine or paclitaxel followed by tandem peripheral blood stem cell transplant or four courses of a cisplatin–ifosfamide combination triplet regimen. Occasionally patients may be cured with a nonplatinum salvage regimen such as paclitaxel plus gemcitabine, even after progression following high-dose chemotherapy.

VII. SPECIAL CLINICAL PROBLEMS

  A. Gynecomastia and elevated blood hCG levels are occasionally found in patients with clinically normal testes and no other evidence of cancer. A number of other cancers can also produce hCG. Patients should be evaluated with ultrasonography of the testes and CT of the abdomen and chest. Thereafter, it is best to follow such patients clinically until there is demonstrable cancer or rising hCG levels. Blind or random biopsies in this setting are not likely to reveal a diagnosis, can expose patients to unnecessary morbidity, and are contraindicated.

  B. Extragonadal germ cell neoplasms can occur in any anatomic site through which the normal germ cells migrate in the embryo. Such sites include the pineal gland, anterior mediastinum, and middle retroperitoneal areas. Tumor markers (hCG and AFP) should be measured. Chemotherapy with BEP should be used for nonseminomatous germ cell cancers. Results of treatment are less successful than for primary testicular cancer, especially for primary mediastinal nonseminomatous germ cell tumors.

  C. Solitary mediastinal or retroperitoneal masses with undifferentiated histology may represent germ cell cancer. Diagnosis by histopathology may be impossible. If differentiation is impossible and the patient is in the correct age group (15 to 45 years), a reasonable approach would be to treat the patient for disseminated nonseminomatous germ cell cancer. Mediastinal germ cell tumors are discussed in Chapter 19, section I.B.4.

Suggested Reading

Albers P, Siener R, Krege S, et al. One course of adjuvant BEP chemotherapy versus retroperitoneal lymph node dissection in patients with stage I non-seminomatous germ cell tumors; results of the German prospective multicenter trial. *Proc Am Soc Clin Oncol* 2006;15:1377.

Bhatia S, Porcu P, Cornetta, et al. High dose chemotherapy as initial salvage chemotherapy in patients with relapsed testicular cancer. *J Clin Oncol* 2000;18:3346.

Einhorn LH. Curing cancer. Testicular cancer. *Proc Nat Acad Sci U S A* 2002;99:4592.

Einhorn LH, Brames MJ, Juliar B, et al. : Phase II study of paclitaxel plus gemcitabine salvage chemotherapy for germ cell tumors after progression following high dose chemotherapy with tandem transplant. *J Clin Oncol* 2007;25:513.

Feldman DR, Bosl GJ, Sheinfeld J, et al. Medical treatment of advanced testicular cancer. *JAMA* 2008;299:672.

Fossa SD, Horwich A, Russell JM, et al. Optimal planning target volume for stage I testicular seminoma: a Medical Research Council randomized trial. *J Clin Oncol* 1999;16:1146.

International Germ Cell Collaborative Group. International germ cell consensus classification: a prognostic factor-based staging system for metastatic germ cell cancers. *J Clin Oncol* 1997;15:594.

Jones WG, Fossa SD, Mead GM, et al. Randomized trial of 30 versus 20 Gy in the adjuvant treatment of stage I testicular seminoma: a report on the Medical Research Council Trial TE 18, European Organization for the Research and Treatment of Cancer Trial 30942. *J Clin Oncol* 2005;23:1200.

Kondagunta GV, Bacik J, Bajorin D, et al. Etoposide and cisplatin chemotherapy for metastatic good-risk germ cell tumors. *J Clin Oncol* 2005;23:9290.

Kondagunta GV, Bacik J, Donadio A, et al. Combination of paclitaxel, ifosfamide and cisplatin is an effective second-line therapy for patients with relapsed testicular germ cell tumors. *J Clin Oncol* 2005;23:6549.

Loehrer PJ, Gonin R, Nichols CR, et al. Vinblastine plus ifosphamide plus cisplatin as initial salvage therapy in recurrent germ cell tumors. *J Clin Oncol* 1998;16:2500.

Oliver RTD, Mason MD, Mead GM, et al. Radiotherapy versus single-dose carboplatin in adjuvant treatment of stage I seminoma: a randomized trial. *Lancet* 2005;366:293.

Schmoll HJ, Souchon R, Krege S, et al. European consensus on diagnosis and treatment of germ cell cancer: a report of the European germ cell cancer consensus group. *Ann Oncol* 2004;15:1377.

Williams SD, Birch R, Einhorn LH, et al. Treatment of disseminated germ cell tumors with cisplatin, bleomycin, and either vinblastine or etoposide. *N Engl J Med* 1987;316:1435.

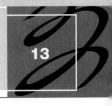

URINARY TRACT CANCERS

Amnon Zisman, Przemyslaw Twardowski, Dan Leibovici, and Robert A. Figlin

13

RENAL CANCER

I. EPIDEMIOLOGY AND ETIOLOGY

A. Incidence (Table 13.1). Renal cell carcinoma (RCC) constitutes 3% of adult malignancies. The worldwide incidence is increasing at an annual rate of about 2%, with 32,000 new cases per year in the United States and 12,000 associated deaths. Men are affected twice as often as women. RCC is a tumor of adults, occurring primarily in those in their fourth and sixth decades. The incidence and mortality rates for blacks appear to be increasing in excess to those for whites in the United States.

B. Etiology. Approximately 70% of sporadic cases of clear cell RCC (the most common histologic variant) are associated with inactivating mutations of both copies of the Von Hippel-Lindau (VHL) tumor suppressor gene. This results in overexpression of hypoxia inducible factor-1 (HIF-1) and vascular endothelial growth factor (VEGF), leading to defective regulation of angiogenesis, which is of major importance in the pathophysiology of RCC.

  1. Factors that increase the risk for RCC include the following:

   a. Smoking (relative risk is 2.3 for heavy smokers)

   b. Urban living

   c. Family history of renal cancer

   d. Thorotrast exposure

   e. Genetic syndromes include:

    (1) Von Hippel-Lindau disease (associated with germline mutations of the *VHL* gene; 35% to 45% of these patients have RCC, mostly multiple and bilateral)

    (2) Hereditary type 2 papillary RCC: associated with mutations in MET proto-oncogene

    (3) Birt-Hogg-Dube (BHD) syndrome

  2. Unproven factors that may increase the risk for RCC include polycystic kidney disease, diabetes mellitus, and chronic dialysis.

II. PATHOLOGY AND NATURAL HISTORY

A. Adenocarcinomas (historically named *hypernephromas* or *Grawitz's tumors*) make up nearly all renal cancers in adults. They are typically round and have a pseudocapsule of condensed parenchyma and connective tissue. Bilateral tumors occur in 2% of sporadic cases, either synchronous or asynchronous.

  1. The most common histologic types include clear cell (60%), papillary (10%), chromophobe (10%), and unclassified RCC. Sarcomatoid tumors can arise from any cell subtype.

  2. These tumors originate from proximal tubular cells, invade local structures, and frequently extend into the renal vein. Metastasis occurs through the lymphatics and bloodstream. The most common sites of distant metastases are the lungs, liver, bones, and brain. Adenocarcinomas may present with metastases to unusual sites, such as the fingertips, eyelids, and nose. A primary renal cancer may be diagnosed based on the characteristic histology of a metastatic deposit.

  3. The natural history of RCC is more unpredictable than that of most solid tumors. The primary tumor has variable growth patterns and may remain localized for

TABLE 13.1 Cancer of the Urinary Tract in the United States for 2007

Primary site		Incidence[a]	Mortality[b]
Kidney and renal pelvis cancer	All	51,190	12,890
	Men	31,590	8,080
	Women	19,600	4,810
Urinary bladder cancer	All	67,160	13,750
	Men	50,040	9,630
	Women	17,120	4,120
Prostate cancer		218,890	27,050

[a]Estimated new cases.
[b]Estimated deaths.
From Jemal A, et al. Cancer statistics: 2007. CA 2007; 57:45, with permission.

many years. Metastatic foci may have long periods of indolent or apparently arrested growth and may be detected many years after removal of the primary tumor.

B. Transitional cell carcinomas are uncommon tumors that arise in the renal pelvis and often affect multiple sites of urothelial mucosa, including the renal pelvis, ureters, and urinary bladder (see "Urinary Bladder Cancer," section II). These tumors usually are low grade, but are being discovered late in the course of the disease. Transitional cell carcinomas occasionally have a peculiar disposition to spread over the posterior retroperitoneum in a sheetlike fashion, encasing vessels and producing urinary tract obstruction. Hematogenous dissemination occurs, particularly to lung and bone.

C. Rare renal tumors

1. **Nephroblastomas** (Wilms' tumors) appear as large, bulky masses in children, but rarely occur in adults (see Chapter 18, "Wilms' Tumor").

2. **Lymphomas and sarcomas** arising in the kidney have clinical courses similar to their counterparts elsewhere in the abdomen.

3. **Juxtaglomerular tumors** (reninomas) are rare causes of hypertension and are usually benign.

4. **Hemangiopericytomas** are renin-secreting tumors associated with severe hypertension and are occasionally malignant (15% of cases).

5. **Oncocytomas** (7%) are benign tumors originating from a subtype of collecting ducts.

6. **Bellini tumors** (collecting duct RCC, <1%) are aggressive cancers originating from collecting ducts.

7. **Medullary cancer** (<1%)

8. **Benign renal adenomas.** The existence of benign renal adenoma is controversial because it is not possible to determine malignant or benign biological behavior only by histology on any lesion <3 cm in diameter.

D. Metastatic tumors. The kidney is a frequent metastatic landing site for many malignancies, mainly cancers of the lung, ovary, colon, and breast.

E. Paraneoplastic syndromes commonly occur with renal adenocarcinomas.

1. **Erythrocytosis.** Renal adenocarcinomas are associated with erythrocytosis in 3% of patients and account for 15% to 20% of cases of inappropriate secretion of erythropoietin. A left flank mass of RCC may be mistaken for an enlarged spleen resulting from polycythemia vera. The differential diagnosis of erythrocytosis is discussed in Chapter 34, "Increased Blood Cell Counts," section I. Tumor production of erythropoietin may identify a subset of patients responsive to immunotherapy with interleukin-2 (IL-2) and interferon-α (IFN-α).

2. **Hypercalcemia,** which occurs in about 5% of patients, associated with parathyroid hormonelike proteins. Hypercalcemia may also be associated with widespread bony metastases.

3. **Fever** caused by tumor occurs in 10% to 20% of patients.
4. **Abnormal liver function (Stauffer syndrome)** occurs in 15% of patients. Leukopenia, fever, and areas of hepatic necrosis *without* liver metastases are noted. The resulting elevated serum levels of alkaline phosphatase and transaminase are reversed after nephrectomy.
5. **Hypertension** associated with renin production by the tumor occurs in up to 40% of patients and is alleviated by removal of the tumor.
6. **Hyperglobulinemia** can result in elevated erythrocyte sedimentation rate.
7. **Amyloidosis** occasionally occurs.

III. DIAGNOSIS
A. **Symptoms and signs.** Symptoms other than hematuria usually indicate large, advanced tumors. The classic triad of flank pain, a flank mass, and hematuria occurs in <10% of patients with RCC. The combined picture of anemia, hematuria, and fever is rare, but suggestive of renal cancer. The widespread use of ultrasound, CT, and MRI changed significantly the typical presentation of RCC. More than three-fourths of all locally confined tumors are found serendipitously (as an incidental finding), and thus a substantial proportion of patients are symptom free at the time of diagnosis. Therefore, symptoms and signs (as listed below) become rare and currently are more characteristic in cases presenting with advanced disease.

1. **Symptoms**
   a. Gross hematuria is rare.
   b. A steady, dull flank pain occurs in a few patients. Colicky pain may develop if blood clots are passed into the ureter.
   c. Weight loss may be a presenting feature in <15% of patients.
   d. Sudden onset of a left-sided or a right-sided varicocele is rare and usually suggests invasion into the renal vein or inferior vena cava, respectively.
   e. Leg edema is the result of locally advanced disease, which causes venous or lymphatic obstruction.
   f. Fever, plethora, or symptoms of hypercalcemia or anemia may be presenting features.
   g. Symptoms related to metastases, including bone pain or fracture, may occasionally be a presenting symptom.

2. **Physical findings**
   a. A palpable flank mass is rarely present.
   b. Fever occurs in about 15% of patients.
   c. Pallor from anemia may occur.

B. **Diagnostic studies**
   1. **Urinalysis** may reveal proteinuria and hematuria. *All patients with macroscopic or microscopic hematuria of any degree must have a thorough urologic evaluation.*
   2. **Routine studies**
      a. Complete blood count, LFT, and renal function studies
      b. Hyperglobulinemia may be present in patients with RCC because acute-phase reactant proteins are elevated.
      c. Chest radiographs may reveal multiple, large, round (cannonball-like) metastatic deposits that are characteristic of metastatic genitourinary neoplasms.
   3. **CT scanning of the kidneys** is most cost-effective method for evaluating a suspected renal mass and should be the first study for that purpose. Extension through the capsule is usually diagnosed correctly. CT does not detect minimal lymph node involvement.
   4. **MRI** may be as accurate as CT. MRI images demonstrate extension of tumor into the renal vein and vena cava more reliably in preparation for surgery.
   5. **Ultrasonography** with duplex Doppler may assist in imaging tumor thrombus in the inferior vena cava and in defining its extension. It cannot be used for local staging because regional lymph node involvement cannot be imaged.
   6. **Scans for staging** should be performed in the following situations:
      a. Bone scan, if there is bone pain or elevated serum alkaline phosphatase levels
      b. MRI of the brain, if there are signs of central nervous system abnormalities

7. **Percutaneous biopsy of a renal mass** has a controversial role and is also believed to be inaccurate in approximately 25% of the cases. This procedure should be restricted to patients with medical conditions that make surgery unduly hazardous and patients with metastatic disease for which a tissue diagnosis is necessary.

C. **Renal cysts** are usually classified using CT according to the chance of harboring malignancy (Bosniak's classification). The following approach is recommended to evaluate potential renal cysts:

1. If a renal cyst is suspected or demonstrated and the findings are not strongly suggestive of cancer, ultrasound is performed to determine whether the mass is cystic. If a simple cyst or a fatty tumor is demonstrated, no further follow-up is usually indicated. If a hyperdense cyst is imaged, the patient should have follow-up studies.

2. Rarely, all imaging modalities are not diagnostic, and surgical exploration is indicated.

3. Bosniak cyst types 3 and 4 are managed in the same fashion as renal cancers

IV. STAGING SYSTEM AND PROGNOSTIC FACTORS

A. **Staging system.** The reader is referred to a current American Joint Commission on Cancer (AJCC) manual for details of the TNM staging system.

B. **Prognostic factors**

1. **Pathologic stage** is the most important prognostic indicator.

   a. **Tumor size** > 10 cm is associated with poor prognosis in comparison to smaller lesions.

   b. **Venous extension.** Renal vein or vena caval involvement is not associated with a hopeless prognosis if managed properly; 25% to 50% of patients survive for 5 years.

2. **Histology.** Sarcomatous and unclassified patterns of RCC have a poor prognosis.

   a. **Nuclear grade** correlates with survival across all tumor stages. **Fuhrman's four-tiered system** is most commonly used; it takes into consideration nuclear size, nuclear shape, and nucleolar appearance.

   b. **Nuclear ploidy** was proposed as a potential prognostic marker for survival. Nondiploid tumors are thought to harbor a less favorable prognosis.

3. **Disease-free interval.** The length of time between nephrectomy and the development of metastases affects the survival of patients with metastatic disease.

   a. Nearly all patients who have metastases at the time of surgery or who develop metastases or local recurrence within 1 year of surgery die within 2 years if untreated.

   b. Patients who develop metastases >2 years after nephrectomy have a 20% 5-year survival rate from the time metastases are recognized.

4. **Integrated prognostic systems.** The TNM system can be augmented with more complex systems that take into account various prognostic factors, such as Fuhrman's nuclear-grading system and performance status to assess risk and the probability of survival with and without evidence of RCC. Such a system is shown in Figure 13.1.

V. PREVENTION AND EARLY DETECTION.
The incidence of renal cancer might be reduced if tobacco-smoking habits could be controlled. Early detection depends on prompt attention to hematuria and other symptoms suggestive of these cancers.

VI. MANAGEMENT

A. **Early disease**

1. **Surgery**

   a. **Nephrectomy** with removal of Gerota's fascia, the adrenal gland *in large or superior tumors,* and tumor in the renal vein or vena cava is the treatment of choice. Laparoscopic nephrectomy has become the standard procedure for stage T1 and T2 tumors.

   b. **Nephron-sparing surgery** (NSS, partial nephrectomy) is indicated for patients with localized RCC and a concomitant urologic or medical condition

Stage	N1M0	N2M0 or any M1						
Fuhrman's Grade	⇓	1		2		3		4
ECOG PS		0	≥ 1	0	≥ 1	0	≥ 1	0	≥ 1
RISK GROUP	Low		Int	Low	Intermediate (Int)			High

Survival	Years after neph	RISK GROUP		
		Low	Int	High
Disease-Specific, following neph (%)	1	87	63	21
	2	65	41	11
	3	56	31	0
	4	37	23	0
	5	32	20	0
Following immunotherapy (%)	1	85	62	25
	2	55	42	17
	3	47	32	0
	4	33	25	0
	5	26	23	0
Progression-Free, following immunotherapy (%)	1	45	30	0
	2	33	21	0
	3	25	19	0
	4	25	16	0
	5	25	12	0

Figure 13.1. UCLA Integrated Staging System: Risk group assignment for patients with metastatic renal cell carcinoma. To obtain a patient's risk group, begin at the top of the decision box and progress downward using the AJCC N and M stages, Fuhrman's grade, and ECOG performance status. ECOG PS, Eastern Cooperative Oncology Group performance status (see inside of back cover); Int, intermediate risk; Neph, nephrectomy. Modified from Zisman A, Pantuck A, Wieder J, et al. Risk group assessment and clinical outcome algorithm to predict the natural history of patients with surgically resected renal cell carcinoma. *J Clin Oncol* 2002;20:4559, with permission.

that jeopardizes overall renal function. NSS for patients with a normal contralateral kidney gives equivalent results to radical nephrectomy for small peripheral or polar lesions <4 cm in diameter. Patients with bilateral cancer or only one functional kidney may undergo NSS. Laparoscopic partial nephrectomy has gained popularity over the open NSS procedure. Less invasive approaches to the renal mass, such as cryoablation and radiofrequency ablation, are still being evaluated.

   c. **Preoperative occlusion of the renal artery** using angiographic techniques has been advocated by some urologists, but is seldom indicated. The hypervascular nature of renal cancer often results in hemorrhage during surgery, particularly with large, bulky tumors. Occlusion procedures make the operation technically easier, but the patient may suffer considerable discomfort from pain, fever, and nausea.

   d. **Contraindications to surgery** include high surgical risk because of unrelated medical diseases. Since the emergence of targeted therapies, the role of surgery ("adjunctive nephrectomy") in the presence of distant metastases is once again under investigation.

   2. **RT** has no established role in the management of early renal cancers.

   3. **Chemotherapy** has no established role in the management of early renal cancers.

B. **Advanced disease**

   1. **Surgery**

      a. **Nephrectomy.** The appearance of targeted oral therapy for systemically advanced RCC with sorafenib (Nexovar) and sunitinib (Sutent) has made immunotherapy a second-line treatment. The role of cytoreductive nephrectomy followed with targeted therapy will be revisited within the frame of large clinical trials, but it is generally accepted to perform cytoreductive nephrectomy before targeted therapy is instituted.

Spontaneous regression of metastases after nephrectomy occurs rarely (<1%) and is far exceeded by the associated surgical morbidity and mortality. The hope for spontaneous regression is never an indication for surgery. Palliative nephrectomy is indicated in patients with metastases to alleviate severe symptoms, such as pain, paraneoplastic syndrome, or severe hemorrhage, if all of the following criteria are met:

(1) The performance status of the patient is at least 30% on Karnofsky's scale (see inside back cover) or is expected to improve substantially if hemorrhage was controlled.

(2) The only symptoms are in the area of the primary tumor. Sites of metastatic disease must be asymptomatic.

(3) The tumor has a reasonable chance of being resectable.

b. Resection of metastases. RCC metastasectomy can be considered only if the following criteria are met:

(1) The interval from nephrectomy to the detection of metastases is at least 2 years.

(2) The metastasis is proved to be solitary by all of the following studies: physical examination, bone scan, chest CT scan, normal LFT (normal CT scan if LFT are abnormal), and brain CT scan (if the patient has neurologic symptoms).

2. RT is used to palliate symptoms from metastases to the central nervous system and bone. Generally, renal tumors are relatively radioresistant.

3. Drug therapy

a. Antiangiogenic agents sorafenib (Nexovar) and sunitinib (Sutent) have been approved for the treatment of advanced RCC. These compounds act primarily via the inhibition of VEGF receptor and platelet-derived growth factor receptor. Their use is associated with 60% to 70% clinical benefit (combined response rate and stable disease) and doubling of progression-free survival to approximately 20 months. These agents have dramatically changed the management of advanced RCC and have become first-line drugs of choice for patients presenting with metastatic disease as well as those whose disease progresses after immunotherapy.

The most frequent side effects of the current targeted agents are fatigue and gastrointestinal toxicity. A specific side effect is the hand-foot syndrome, which consists of a painful rush in the palms of hands and feet that mandates treatment discontinuation.

b. Immunotherapy. The role of immunotherapy for kidney cancer has decreased and is being supplanted by rapid progress with antiangiogenic agents. Nonetheless, IL-2 remains the only potentially curative treatment in selected patients with metastatic RCC.

(1) IL-2 administered alone in high-dose regimens produces a response rate of 15% to 20% in good-risk patients and durable remissions lasting for more than a decade in 10% of patients. Significant morbidity and 4% mortality associated with high-dose IL-2 make this therapy very difficult and applicable to only small minority of patients. IL-2 administered in lower dosages or in combination with IFN produces inferior response rates when compared with high-dose IL-2 in randomized trials. Ongoing efforts exist to establish reliable predictive factors to identify those patients who will benefit from high dose IL-2 therapy and justify the risk of significant morbidity.

(2) IFN-α as a single agent has modest antitumor activity in the setting of RCC, with a response rate of approximately 15%. With the emergence of effective targeted therapies, IFN-α is used primarily in clinical trials evaluating possible synergistic effects in combination with antiangiogenic agents.

c. Future developments in the treatment of RCC include redefining the role of nephrectomy in advanced cases, the development of other antiangiogenic agents, and inhibitors of m-TOR pathway (e.g., temsirolimus).

 URINARY BLADDER CANCER

I. EPIDEMIOLOGY AND ETIOLOGY

  A. Incidence (Table 13.1). Bladder cancers constitute 4.5% of all cancers in the United States. The disease is 2.5 times more frequent in men than in women and is most frequent in industrial northeastern cities. The average age of onset is the sixth to seventh decade. The incidence doubles in men >75 years of age versus younger men.

  B. Risk factors and carcinogens

    1. Occupational exposure is associated with 20% of cases. Historically, aniline dye workers were afflicted 30 times more than the general population. Aromatic amines and related compounds are the most abundant bladder carcinogens today. These are chemical intermediates of anilines, rather than the aniline dyes themselves. Leather, paint, and rubber industry workers also appear to have an increased risk for bladder cancer. Proven chemical carcinogens in these industries are 2-naphthylamine, benzidine, 4-aminobiphenyl, and 4-nitrobiphenyl.

    2. *Schistosomum haematobium* infection of the bladder is associated with bladder cancer, particularly with squamous cell histology, in endemic regions of Africa and the Middle East.

    3. Smoking increases the risk for bladder cancer fourfold in a dose-dependent fashion. Of men who die of bladder cancer, 85% have a history of smoking.

    4. Pelvic irradiation increases the risk for bladder cancer fourfold.

    5. Drugs. Cyclophosphamide unequivocally increases the risk for bladder cancer. Other drugs that have been implicated in animal studies but not proved in humans are phenacetin, sodium saccharin, and sodium cyclamate.

II. PATHOLOGY AND NATURAL HISTORY

  A. Pathology

    1. Histology. Of bladder cancers, 90% are transitional cell carcinoma (TCC), and 8% are squamous cell types. Adenocarcinomas, sarcomas, lymphomas, and carcinoid tumors are rare.

    2. Sites of involvement. Bladder tumors involve the posterior and lateral walls often and involve the superior wall least often. Patients with bladder carcinoma also frequently have carcinomas in other urinary tract sites.

    3. Types of bladder cancer

      a. Single papillary cancers are the most common type (70%) and the least likely to show infiltration.

      b. Diffuse papillary growths with minimal invasion

      c. Sessile cancers are often high grade and invasive.

      d. Carcinoma *in situ* (CIS; flat intraepithelial growth) appears either the same as normal mucosa or as a velvety red patch.

    4. The panurothelial abnormality or field defect. Bladder cancer appears to be associated with premalignant changes throughout the urothelial mucosa. This concept is suggested by the following observations:

      a. Up to 80% of patients treated for superficial tumors develop recurrences at different sites in the bladder.

      b. Multiple primary sites are present in 25% of all patients with bladder cancer.

      c. Random biopsies of apparently normal areas of mucosa in patients with bladder cancer frequently show CIS.

      d. Depending on the reported series, patients with bladder CIS also have ureteral CIS (10% to 60%) and urethral CIS (30%).

      e. About 40% of patients presenting with carcinoma of the renal pelvis or ureter develop tumors elsewhere in the urinary tract, usually in the bladder.

B. Natural history
1. **CIS of the bladder** is multifocal and can affect the entire urothelium. Up to 80% of patients with untreated CIS develop invasive bladder cancer within 10 years after diagnosis; the disease is lethal for most of these patients.
2. **Low-grade superficial carcinomas** have a better prognosis than CIS. Although the recurrence rate is 80%, 80% of patients with these tumors survive 5 years. Invasive cancer develops in only 10% of patients with superficial tumors, often in association with CIS. More than 80% of patients with both superficial cancers and CIS develop invasive malignancies.
3. **High-grade or invasive tumors** are associated with adjacent areas of CIS in 85% of cases. Squamous cell cancers and adenocarcinomas are usually high grade and have an aggressive clinical behavior. Other uncommon and very aggressive histologic variants include sarcomatoid cancer, small cell carcinoma, and micropapillary tumors.
4. **Mode of spread.** Bladder cancers spread both by lymphatic channels and by the bloodstream. High-grade lesions are more likely to metastasize. Of patients with distant metastases, 30% do not have involvement of the draining lymph nodes. Distant sites of metastases include bone, liver, lung, and, less commonly, skin and other organs. Uremia from ureteral compression by a large pelvic mass, inanition from advancing cancer, and liver failure are the usual causes of death.
5. **Iatrogenic tumor implantation.** High-grade bladder cancer cells exfoliated by cystoscopy, brushing, transurethral biopsy, or resection were reported to seed other areas of the bladder. Mucosal sites damaged by inflammation or instrumentation appear to be most receptive to such implants.
6. **Associated paraneoplastic syndromes**
   a. Systemic fibrinolysis
   b. Hypercalcemia
   c. Neuromuscular syndromes
   d. Leukemoid reaction

III. DIAGNOSIS
A. Symptoms and signs
1. **Symptoms**
   a. Hematuria occurs as a presenting feature in 90% of patients.
   b. Bladder irritability occurs in 25% of patients. Hesitancy, urgency, frequency, dysuria, and postvoiding pelvic discomfort may mimic prostatitis or cystitis. These symptoms occur in patients with CIS as well as in those with tumors that are large, extensive, or near the bladder neck.
   c. Pain in the pelvis or flank is associated with locally advanced disease.
   d. Edema of the lower extremities and genitalia develops from venous or lymphatic obstruction.
2. **Physical findings.** The patient is carefully examined for metastatic sites. It is mandatory that a bimanual examination is performed by the urologist through the rectum each time the patient is put under general anesthesia or having a cystoscopy done. The importance of the bimanual examination cannot be overemphasized. It supplies pertinent information concerning local extension of the disease not obtainable by current imaging modalities.

B. Diagnostic studies
1. **Routine studies**
   a. CBC, LFT, and renal function tests
   b. Urinalysis
   c. Chest radiograph
2. **Cystoscopy** is the cornerstone procedure for diagnosing bladder cancer. Biopsy is performed on abnormal areas. Biopsies of normal areas at random are performed to search for CIS. Cystoscopy is followed by bimanual pelvic examination under anesthesia in both men and women. Cystoscopy is indicated for patients with the following clinical features:

   a. Any gross or microscopic hematuria and a normal upper urinary tract imaging (except female patients with a single episode of acute bacterial cystitis who are <40 years of age and do not smoke)

   b. Unexplained or chronic lower urinary tract symptoms

   c. Urine cytology that is suspicious for cancer

   d. A history of bladder cancer

3. Urography. An intravenous pyelogram (IVP) is performed in all patients with unexplained hematuria or cystoscopic or cytologic evidence of tumor in an attempt to search for primary sites in the ureters or renal pelvis. It is advisable to perform an IVP before cystoscopy, because if a poorly visualized upper system or nonconclusive filling defect is imaged, retrograde pyelography may be performed using a ureteral catheter inserted during the same cystoscopy session.

4. CT urography (CTU). CT scanning of the abdomen and pelvis typically includes three phases: a noncontrast phase, an early postcontrast phase, and the pyelographic phase. During the noncontrast phase, abnormal calcifications (i.e., urinary stones) can be identified. The early postcontrast phase obtained minutes after IV administration of contrast serves to discern renal lesions and to differentiate between abnormal lymph nodes and normal anatomic structures. During the pyelographic phase, the contrast material is observed as it is excreted into the collecting system, allowing the identification of abnormal filling defects within the collecting system. Owing to its higher resolution and diagnostic accuracy, CTU has largely supplanted IVP as the imaging modality of choice for the upper urinary tract.

    It is important to obtain a CTU in any patient with hematuria, a history of bladder cancer, or positive cytology. CTU is also useful for staging invasive bladder cancer or upper tract TCC. Abnormally enlarged lymph nodes and visceral metastasis can be observed by CTU. Local invasion into pelvic organs or tumor infiltration into the perivesical fat can also be observed. CT is not reliable for the detection of local invasion, however.

5. Urine cytology detects about 70% of bladder cancers that are subsequently diagnosed by cystoscopy. Cytologic evaluation should not be the primary diagnostic method for patients suspected of having bladder cancer. Urine cytology is useful for the following purposes:

   a. Following patients with a history of bladder cancer

   b. Screening symptom-free patients who are exposed to environmental carcinogens

   c. Evaluating patients with chronic irritative bladder symptoms before cystoscopy is done

6. Bladder tumor markers. Bladder tumor antigen (BTA), nuclear matrix protein 22 (NMP-22), telomerase activity, fibrin degradation products assay, and others are being tested to replace or decrease the frequency of cystoscopy, to serve in follow-up of TCC patients, and to assist in screening and evaluation of hematuria. Some of these tests are promising, but the current standard care for a patient with hematuria or history of TCC remains cystoscopy.

7. Fluorescent *in situ* hybridization (FISH). Because bladder cancers are associated with typical chromosomal aberrations, their detection in the urine is an accurate and noninvasive modality of TCC detection. The current commercially available FISH test (Urovysion) uses four chromosomal probes to detect an abnormal number of chromosomal copies (CEP17, CEP3, and CEP7) and a single locus-specific indicator probe (9p21). FISH has a sensitivity of 81% and a specificity of 96%, far better than those of cytology.

8. Scans. Bone scans should be performed in patients with bone pain or elevated serum alkaline phosphatase or transaminase levels.

IV. STAGING SYSTEM AND PROGNOSTIC FACTORS

  A. Staging system. The reader is referred to a current AJCC manual for details of the TNM staging system.

B. **Prognostic factors.** The most important clinical prognostic factors are tumor stage, tumor grade, and the presence of CIS. Untreated patients have a 2-year survival rate <15% and a median survival of 16 months.

1. **Histology.** Squamous cancers and adenocarcinomas have poorer prognoses than TCC. Likewise, the other aggressive histologic subvariants confer a poor prognosis.

2. **Invasion** of muscle, lymphatics, or perivesical fat is associated with a poor prognosis. Invasive cancer is associated with a 50% mortality rate in the first 18 months after diagnosis. Delaying cystectomy >12 weeks following the diagnosis of muscle invasive disease (stage T2) may hamper patient survival.

3. **CIS** progresses to invasive carcinoma in 80% of patients within 10 years of diagnosis.

4. **Tumor grade**
   a. A close relationship exists between tumor grade and stage. Tumor grade alone affects survival in patients with superficial tumors. The 5-year survival rate is 85% with low-grade lesions and 30% with high-grade lesions. Virtually all high-grade superficial tumors become invasive if left untreated.
   b. Chromosome number correlates with tumor grade. Tetraploid and aneuploid cells, as opposed to diploid cells, are associated with invasive tumors.
   c. Several phenotypic properties that have been offered as markers for biologically more aggressive disease include enhanced expression of the Lewis x antigen; expression of defective p53, together with overexpression of the *Rb* gene and abnormal epidermal growth factor receptor; reduced expression of transforming growth factors β1, p27, and p15.

5. **Size of the primary tumor** does not correlate with the risk for dissemination. Large superficial lesions, however, are more likely to recur after therapy than are small lesions.

6. **Multifocality** is associated with an increased recurrence risk as compared with cases that have a solitary tumor.

V. PREVENTION AND EARLY DETECTION

A. **Prevention.** Protecting factory workers in certain industries from continuous exposure to bladder carcinogens (e.g., with protective clothing) may be beneficial. The benefit gained by reducing the intake of coffee or artificial sweetener has not been determined. All people should be discouraged from smoking. Folate-enriched diet has been associated with a decreased risk for bladder cancer.

B. **Early detection** depends on prompt evaluation of all patients with hematuria or chronic irritative bladder symptoms.

VI. MANAGEMENT

A. **Early disease: overview**

1. **Superficial low-grade tumors** not associated with CIS are managed by transurethral resection and, when indicated, intravesical chemotherapy. Although the recurrence rate is 80% with this management, the prognosis is good. Fulguration is added in cases of excessive numbers of small lesions.

2. **CIS** is usually multifocal, persistent, and recurrent; it is highly likely to evolve into invasive cancer, which often involves the urethra and ureters. Choice of therapy may be based on the degree of urothelial atypia; however, the pathologic distinction between severe dysplasia and CIS is often difficult to make.

   a. **Borderline cases.** Patients should have repeated urine cytology; cystoscopy and biopsy are repeated every 3 to 6 months. Some cases have an indolent course, with years passing before frank CIS is found.

   b. **True CIS.** Opinion is divided on the optimal therapeutic approach for apparently localized CIS. Localized, unifocal areas of CIS may be fulgurated. CIS localized to the bladder, without ureteral or urethral involvement, may be initially treated by intravesical therapy, provided there is no history of invasive tumor. Multifocal CIS (particularly if high grade, diffuse, or symptomatic) is treated with radical cystectomy; urethrectomy, ureterectomy, or both may also be necessary.

3. **Invasive tumors or superficial tumors with CIS** are best treated by pelvic lymph node dissection and radical cystectomy in women and radical cystoprostatectomy in men. Segmental resections of the bladder may be used in highly selected cases (see section VI.B.2). Radiotherapy and chemotherapy may be appropriate in some cases (see sections VI.C and D).

B. Early disease: surgery

1. **Transurethral resection of bladder tumor (TURBT)** is the cornerstone for treating and T staging newly diagnosed bladder neoplasia. One or more TURBT procedures and follow-up cystoscopy constitute sufficient treatment for most superficial tumors. Occasional patients with a small solitary invasive bladder cancer can be treated with TURBT alone with no need for radical cystectomy. Diligent patient selection and meticulous surveillance are absolute conditions for this approach.

2. **Segmental resection** (partial cystectomy) is associated with a high risk for recurrence. Of patients <50% are candidates for this procedure. Segmental resection can be considered for tumors with the following characteristics:

   a. Solitary

   b. Localized to the bladder dome

   c. Not associated with areas of CIS sought by multiple biopsies of urothelial mucosa

   d. Able to be removed with a 2-cm margin of healthy tissue

3. **Intravesical instillations.** Because the bladder is a storage organ with no absorptive capacity, cytotoxic agents can be safely instilled into the bladder with virtually no systemic effects. Chemotherapy or immunotherapy has been used for the treatment and prevention of recurrence of superficial bladder cancer. These agents have no role in the treatment of invasive bladder cancer. Chemotherapeutic agents include thiotepa, mitomycin C, valrubicin, and doxorubicin. Immunotherapy has consisted of bacillus Calmette-Guerin (BCG) with or without IFN-α.

   a. BCG is administered weekly for 6 weeks followed by maintenance administration of shorter courses. Maintenance BCG has been shown to augment the effects of a single 6-weekly course.

   b. Mitomycin C is also given weekly at a dose of 40 mg each time. A single instillation of mitomycin C immediately following TURBT has been shown to dramatically decrease the risk of tumor recurrence, most likely owing to the prevention of cancer cell seeding. No proof exists that maintenance intravesical chemotherapy has any benefit.

   c. BCG instillations are considered more effective in reducing the risks for recurrence and progression, as compared with chemotherapy. BCG is also curative for most patients with CIS. There is no proof, however, that any of these treatments can alter long-term disease-specific survival.

   d. Both chemotherapy and BCG are frequently associated with local side effects, such as bladder irritability, and both can rarely induce systemic adverse reactions. Of particular importance, systemic infection with BCG affects 5% of the cases and may lead to significant morbidity.

4. **Radical cystectomy,** the standard treatment for invasive bladder cancer, includes excision of the bladder, perivesical fat, and attached peritoneum. Men undergo removal of the entire prostate and seminal vesicles; women undergo *en bloc* removal of the uterus, adnexa, and cuff of the vagina. Lymphadenectomy is controversial; it probably does not improve survival but adds little morbidity and provides information for staging. Retrospective analysis of cystectomy series suggests that extensive lymphadenectomy (removal of >10 regional lymph nodes) is associated with improved survival. This concept is being evaluated prospectively in the large adjuvant chemotherapy trial in Europe.

   a. **Urinary diversion procedures.** The ureters are diverted into either a loop of ileum that functions as a conduit to an abdominal stoma (ileal conduit,

Bricker's procedure) or a reservoir. Generally, reservoirs are created by de-tubularizing and oversewing a bowel segment.

The reservoir may be implanted orthotopically as a neobladder draining through the urethra using the native sphincter mechanism or attached to a con-tinent conduit drained periodically by using intermittent self-catheterizations of the conduit stoma (*continent diversion*). Alternative urinary drainage pro-cedures, such as cutaneous implantation of the ureters and ureterosigmoidos-tomy, were largely abandoned because of a high rate of severe complications.

b. Indications for radical cystectomy

(1) Muscle invasive tumors

(2) True, severe CIS not responsive to intravesical therapy

(3) Superficial low-grade tumors that are diffuse, multiple, and frequently recurring and becoming difficult to control with recurrent TURBT and intravesical therapy

(4) High-grade tumors refractory to conservative measures

c. Complications of cystectomy

(1) Mortality rate of 1% to 3%

(2) Blood loss

(3) Rectal injury, ureterocutaneous fistulas, wound dehiscence or infection, or small bowel obstructions or fistulas may occur. Small bowel fistulas are associated with a substantial mortality rate.

(4) Thrombophlebitis, pulmonary embolism, and other cardiocirculatory complications

(5) Impotence in men; potency can be preserved in some men by sparing the corporal nerves.

d. Complications of urinary diversion

(1) Urinary tract infection

(2) Obstruction owing to stenosis (fibrosis or tumor growth)

(3) Urinary calculi occasionally occur. Calcium stones are the most common.

(4) Acid–base imbalance: Hyperchloremic metabolic acidosis is the most com-mon and results from the rapid reabsorption of ammonium followed by chloride from the urine-containing lumen through the intestinal epithe-lium into the plasma. The type of diversion (reservoir *vs.* conduit) and the specific type of bowel segment used determine the type, extent, and gravity of the accompanied electrolyte impairment. The most severe metabolic de-rangements reported were for diversions using sigmoid colon or jejunum.

C. Early disease: RT does not appear to alter the course of CIS favorably.

1. Indications for RT

a. RT is an alternative to surgery for highly motivated patients who desire to retain their bladder and potency within a bladder preservation protocol. These multiple modality treatment plans include aggressive TURBT, RT, and chemotherapy and are conducted in only a few dedicated institutions because such protocols mandate frequent follow-up visits and may end up in delayed cystectomy in up to 20% of cases.

b. Preoperative RT is seldom used. RT does not appear to improve expected sur-vival beyond that achieved by radical surgery alone, although local recurrence is reduced.

c. Postoperative radiation has no proved role in bladder cancer.

2. Complications of RT are discussed in Chapter 11, "General Aspects," section IV.A (radiation cystitis) and Chapter 30, section VI.D (radiation proctitis).

D. Early disease: chemotherapy

1. Adjuvant therapy with systemic cytotoxic agents for patients undergoing cystectomy has been associated with a delay in time to disease progression (8 to 12 months), but no conclusive evidence indicates the improvement of survival. Ongoing large clinical trials, it is hoped, will clarify the role of that strategy in the treatment of bladder cancer.

2. Neoadjuvant therapy is an attempt to provide the earliest possible treatment of micrometastatic disease and to facilitate definitive local therapy. Multiple single-institution trials of M-VAC (see section VI.E.3) indicate high response rates (60%) and complete responses (20% to 25%) on surgical resection. This approach remains experimental pending ongoing randomized trials.

E. Advanced disease

1. Surgery. An attempt to fulgurate large tumors that are bleeding uncontrollably or causing severe irritative symptoms is worthwhile. Often, these symptoms force the caregiver to perform palliative cystectomy and urinary diversion.

2. RT ameliorates hemorrhage in about half of patients and provides substantial local pain relief in areas of bone involvement. Tumor masses that threaten extension through the skin, particularly in the perineum, should be irradiated early. Bacterial cystitis should be treated effectively before the use of RT, if possible.

3. Chemotherapy. Cisplatin-based combination chemotherapy regimens have produced sustained complete responses in up to 45% of patients and represent the best current therapy for advanced bladder cancer, although toxicity can be substantial. Using gemcitabine plus cisplatin (GC) or taxanes seem to have comparable activity but reduced morbidity. The survival and median time to disease progression is similar for both regimens (7 to 8 months), but GC is believed to have a better safety and tolerability profile. Arterial infusion of these agents is experimental.

a. M-VAC is administered in 28-day cycles in the following dosages:

Methotrexate, 30 mg/m^2 IV on days 1, 15, and 22
Vinblastine, 3 mg/m^2 IV on days 2, 15, and 22
Doxorubicin (Adriamycin), 30 mg/m^2 IV on day 2
Cisplatin, 70 mg/m^2 IV on day 2

b. GC is administered in 28-day cycles for up to six cycles in the following dosages:

Gemcitabine, 1,000 mg/m^2 IV on days 1, 8, 15, and
Cisplatin, 70 mg/m^2 IV on day 2.

F. Patient follow-up

1. Patients with severe urothelial dysplasia should have urine cytology repeated every 2 to 3 months and cystoscopy with random biopsies every 3 to 6 months.

2. Patients with superficial low-grade cancer treated with intravesical chemotherapy should have cystoscopy performed at 3-month intervals.

3. Patients who have undergone cystectomy should be evaluated every 3 months for the first 2 years, every 6 months for the next 3 years, and yearly thereafter. Urinalysis and urine cytology should be performed at 6-month intervals to search for the development of new primary cancers in the upper urinary tract. Hematuria or a positive cytology should be evaluated with IV urography.

4. For patients having an ileal conduit or continent diversion, urethral washing for cytology is advisable periodically to diagnose local recurrence in the urethra. For the same purpose, patients having orthotopic diversions should have follow-up cystoscopy.

VII. SPECIAL CLINICAL PROBLEMS

A. Gross hematuria can complicate the course of locally advanced bladder cancer. Transurethral fulguration or RT may help. In some retractable cases, the bladder may be catheterized and filled with sterile water under pressure to attempt tamponade. Some physicians advocate instillation of 4% formaldehyde and 1% silver nitrate into the bladder under general anesthesia; the agent is retained for 15 minutes, then thoroughly rinsed out with 10% alcohol followed by normal saline. Irrigation of the bladder with dilute alum also may be effective in controlling hemorrhage.

B. Obstructive uropathy. Uremia can develop in patients with any type of urinary diversion. Obstruction caused by benign conditions, such as stones or stenosis, must be excluded. The urine should be examined for malignant cells, crystals, and blood. If the ureteral orifice can be located, a retrograde pyelogram is performed. Otherwise, IVP or renal radionuclide scan may show obstruction.

Endoscopy may be used to dilate stenotic lesions with some success. Exploratory surgery should be considered to solve the problem in patients who otherwise are clinically free of cancer. Patients with advanced disease commonly benefit from diverting externally with percutaneous nephrostomies or internally with ureteral stents.

C. Impotence. Despite nerve-sparing technique, impotence complicates radical cystectomy in men. Oral agents, intraurethral preparations, intracavernosal injection, and penile prostheses are the available solutions that usually permit restoration of potency and, often, orgasm in these patients.

D. Management of urinary symptoms is discussed in Chapter 5, section V.

URETHRAL CANCER

I. EPIDEMIOLOGY AND ETIOLOGY. Urethral cancer is extremely rare. Women are affected three times as often as men. The age of onset is usually >50 years. The etiology is not known, but urethral cancer may be associated with gonorrheal urethritis, strictures, or transitional cell carcinoma in the bladder.

II. PATHOLOGY AND NATURAL HISTORY.

A. Histology. Of cases, 80% are squamous cell carcinomas, usually arising from the stratified squamous epithelium of the posterior (proximal or bulbous) urethra (60%) or the anterior (distal or penile) urethra (30%). Fifteen percent are transitional cell carcinomas arising in the prostatic urethra. Adenocarcinomas possibly arise from Cowper's glands.

B. Clinical course. Urethral cancer is usually diagnosed late and involves inguinal nodes early on. It also spreads hematogenously to distant organs. Lesions of the anterior urethra are less likely to be associated with widespread metastases than are posterior lesions.

III. DIAGNOSIS. Patients have urinary hesitancy, hematuria, palpable mass, urethral discharge, perineal pain, or enlarged inguinal nodes. Transurethral biopsy establishes the diagnosis. The biopsy and imaging studies contribute to TNM staging.

IV. MANAGEMENT. In both female and male patients, the extensiveness of therapy is determined by the stage, location of the tumor (anterior *vs.* posterior urethra), and need for local palliation. In women, treatment varies between total urethrectomy and more extensive surgery, which includes cystectomy (with total or partial resection of the vagina), urethrectomy, and pelvic lymph node dissection. In men who have anterior urethral cancer, transurethral resection of the tumor followed by wide local excision is usually sufficient. If the corpora are infiltrated with tumor, partial or total penectomy is usually required. For posterior urethral disease, the combination of radical cystoprostatectomy, total penectomy, and pelvic lymphadenectomy offers improved results. RT has a limited role in urethral cancer therapy for selected cases. Combination chemotherapy regimens are used for patients with metastases.

PROSTATE CANCER

I. EPIDEMIOLOGY AND ETIOLOGY

A. Incidence (Table 13.1) of prostate cancer (CAP) rose continuously for >20 years. In 1987, it crossed the line of 100 cases per 100,000 (age adjusted, all male population). The peak incidence was seen in 1992 (191/100,000). The incidence declined from 1992 to 1995, and then leveled off. The rise in incidence is basically explained by improved detection capability, mainly using prostate-specific antigen (PSA) and transrectal ultrasound (TRUS) to aim prostate TrueCut biopsies.

The risk for prostate cancer increases steeply with age. One percent incidence is reached at 67 and 72 years of age for black and white men, respectively. A rise in death rate accompanies the rise in the incidence. An age-adjusted death rate peak of 27/100,000 was reported in 1991 in the United States. Thereafter, death rates declined slowly, perhaps because of treatment efforts.

B. Etiology. The cause of prostate cancer is unknown. Several factors are associated with an increased risk.

   1. Demography. The risk for developing prostate cancer is highest in Sweden, intermediate in the United States and Europe (and Japanese men who migrated to the United States), and lowest in Taiwan and Japan. Blacks are afflicted 30% more often than are whites. Corrected for stage, blacks also *may* have lower survival rates.

   2. Positive familial history of prostate cancer in the father or brother of a subject increases his risk sevenfold over the general population if the affected relative was diagnosed by 50 years of age. The relative risk declines to fourfold if the diagnosis of the first-degree relative was made after 70 years of age.

   3. Hormones. Altered estrogen and androgen metabolite levels have been suggested as a causative mechanism leading to prostate cancer occurrence.

   4. Other suggested risk factors, which are not fully established, are increased intake of vitamin A, decreased intake of vitamin D, and occupational exposure to cadmium.

II. PATHOLOGY AND NATURAL HISTORY

A. Histology. Almost all prostate cancers are adenocarcinomas. Transitional, small, and squamous cell carcinomas and sarcomas are rare. The prostate may be the site of metastases from bladder, colon, or lung cancer or from melanomas, lymphomas, or other malignancies.

B. Location. Prostate cancer tends to be multifocal and frequently (70%) arises from the peripheral zone of the prostate (the surgical capsule). Both of these characteristics make removal by transurethral resection of the prostate (TURP) unfeasible for curative intent.

C. Mode of spread. The biology of adenocarcinomas of the prostate is strongly influenced by tumor grade. Low-grade tumors may remain localized for long periods of time. The disease locally invades along nerve sheaths and metastasizes through lymphatic chains. Distant metastases can occur without evidence of nodal involvement. Distant metastases are nearly always present when lymph nodes are involved.

D. Metastatic sites. Bone is the most common site of prostate cancer metastases, almost always producing dense osteoblastic metastatic lesions. Occasionally, patients demonstrate uncharacteristic osteolytic lesions. Liver involvement also occurs, but metastases to the brain, lung, and other soft tissues are rare.

E. Associated paraneoplastic syndromes
   1. Systemic fibrinolysis
   2. Neuromuscular abnormalities

III. DIAGNOSIS

A. Symptoms and signs
   1. Symptoms. Currently, most patients with CAP are asymptomatic at diagnosis.
      a. Early prostatic cancer is usually asymptomatic and can be detected as a result of routine digital rectal examination (DRE). It is mainly discovered by serum PSA measurement or, rarely, during TURP for glandular hyperplasia. The presence of severe symptoms usually indicates advanced disease. Symptoms include hesitancy, urgency, nocturia, poor urine stream, dribbling, and terminal hematuria.
      b. The sudden onset and rapid progression of symptoms of urinary tract obstruction in men of the appropriate age is most likely to be caused by prostate cancer.
      c. Pain in the back, pelvis, or over multiple bony sites is the most common presenting complaint in patients with distant metastases.

    d. The sudden onset of neurologic deficiencies, such as paraplegia and incontinence resulting from extradural spinal metastases, may be a presenting feature or may develop during the course of the disease.

  2. Physical examination

    a. Check for induration or nodularity of the prostate, which often represents prostatic cancer. Nodules of prostatic cancer are typically stony hard and not tender.

    b. Examine lateral sulci and for palpable (abnormal) seminal vesicles.

    c. Evaluate inguinal nodes for metastatic disease.

    d. Evaluate for distant metastases by palpating the skeleton for tender foci and by performing an oriented neurologic examination looking for spinal cord compression.

B. Differential diagnosis of the enlarged prostate

  1. Acute prostatitis. Bacterial infection causes dysuria, pain, and often fever. The prostate is tender and enlarged but not hard. Examination and culture of prostatic fluid obtained by prostate massage may reveal the infectious agent.

  2. Chronic and granulomatous prostatitis caused by bacterial, tuberculous (including following intravesical BCG instillation), fungal, or protozoan infection may produce a mass that cannot be clinically distinguished from cancer. Biopsy may be necessary to make the diagnosis.

  3. Nodular hyperplasia (benign prostatic hypertrophy) is found in men >30 years of age and in 80% of men by 80 years of age. Urinary obstructive symptoms are common. Palpable nodules that are indistinguishable from cancer necessitate biopsy.

  4. Other possibilities. Rarely, calculi, amyloidosis, benign adenomas, or infarction of a hyperplastic nodule can cause obstruction or a mass suggestive of cancer.

C. Diagnostic studies

  1. Routine studies. Urinalysis, CBC, renal function tests, LFT, alkaline phosphatase, calcium, and chest radiographs

  2. PSA is a serine protease that serves as a marker unique to the prostate. Using PSA increases the number of biopsies performed and thus augments the number of patients diagnosed. It significantly augments the yield of DRE in diagnosing prostate cancer in general and organ-confined disease in particular.

    a. False-positive results. About 15% of patients with nodular hyperplasia have elevated PSA levels. PSA values can also be increased with prostatic inflammation, surgery, or endoscopy, but not with rectal examination. After a prostate biopsy, PSA is reported to be elevated for at least 6 to 8 weeks. Increased serum PSA concentration has been reported rarely in patients with cancers of the pancreas, parotid gland, and breast.

    b. Free PSA is the fraction of PSA that is not bound to the plasma antiproteases α_1-antichymotrypsin and α_2-macroglobulin. A *decreased ratio* of free PSA to total PSA is associated with increased probability of prostate cancer. For patients with elevated PSA and no suspect findings on palpation of the prostate, it is recommended to proceed with watchful waiting after one negative biopsy if the free-to-total PSA ratio >25%.

    c. Age-specific PSA. The normal range of PSA in patients without prostate cancer rises with age, mainly as a result of gland enlargement.

Age (years)	Age-specific serum PSA upper limit of normal (ng/mL)
40–50	2.5
50–60	3.5
60–70	4.5
70–80	6.5

    d. PSA density indices are mathematic modifications of PSA. The transitional zone (TZ) is located centrally; it is one of the PSA-producing parts of the prostate and is usually increased in size when benign prostate hyperplasia occurs. The indices adjust serum PSA levels for the prostate gland volume (*PSA density* = PSA/gland volume) or for the TZ volume (PSA TZ = PSA/TZ volume). These indices were found to improve positive-predictive and negative-predictive values in patients with total PSA levels of 4 to 10 ng/mL. PSA TZ is also reported to assist in staging, screening, and sparing prostate biopsies in some patients.

    e. Clinical utility of PSA. PSA can detect primary or recurrent tumors of very low volume and is useful for both diagnosis and follow-up. Although PSA is not sufficiently sensitive to be the sole screening method for prostate cancer, it is useful when combined with DRE. About 25% of patients with biopsy-proven prostate cancer have serum PSA levels <4 ng/mL. When PSA is combined with TRUS-guided prostatic biopsies, cancer is detected in 20% of patients with PSA values between 4 and 10 ng/mL and in 60% of patients with values >10 ng/mL.

        PSA values may show a progressive increase several years before metastatic disease becomes evident. Such a rise is an indication to look for local recurrence in previously treated patients using physical examination or TRUS. The search for metastatic disease in asymptomatic patients with PSA <10 ng/mL is not routinely indicated.

3. Acid phosphatase, previously the only marker for prostate cancer, is seldom used today.

4. Biopsy techniques

    a. TRUS-guided true-cut biopsy is the standard and most popular method to diagnose prostate cancer. A twelve-core set *is* taken by sampling the base, apex, and midgland on each side of the gland along two parallel lateral lines.

        Most cancers have a hypoechoic appearance in TRUS, although up to 30% of cancers may be isoechoic. When the indication for TRUS-guided biopsy is a PSA >4 ng/mL, the expected yield for diagnosing prostate cancer reaches 24%. When PSA is >4 ng/mL, the DRE is suspicious, and a hypoechoic lesion is imaged by TRUS, the yield rises to 45%.

    b. TURP. Prostate cancer may be found in approximately 5% of TURP performed for benign hyperplasia.

5. Bone scans. The probability of a positive scan is extremely low when the PSA is <10 ng/mL or symptoms are absent.

6. CT scans and MRI are used to assess tumor spread into lymph nodes or the pelvis. These studies are warranted only in high-risk patients who have a tumor that is confluent with the pelvic side wall on DRE, a high Gleason's score (see tumor grading in section IV.B.1), or PSA >20 ng/mL.

IV. STAGING AND PROGNOSTIC FACTORS

    A. Staging system. The TNM classification is used to stage prostate cancer is shown in Table 13.2.

    B. Prognostic factors

        1. Tumor grade strongly affects prognosis. Higher tumor grades are more frequently associated with lymph node and distant metastases. The **Gleason's scoring system** is most commonly used. This system is founded on the glandular appearance and architecture at relatively low-power magnification. Two scores of 1 to 5 points are given for a primary (predominant) site and a secondary (second most prevalent) site. Therefore, Gleason's score can sum from 2 to 10 points. Patients having Gleason's score of 7 and above have a worse prognosis than patients with lower scores.

        2. Involvement of seminal vesicles is associated with a poor prognosis, even in apparently early disease.

        3. Extension of tumor beyond the prostate capsule is associated with worse prognosis.

        4. High PSA values and elements of PSA kinetics, including rapid PSA rise (high PSA velocity) and short PSA doubling time, are associated with poor prognosis.

TABLE 13.2 TNM Staging System for Prostate Adenocarcinoma

Primary tumor (T)[a]		Regional lymph nodes (N)[a]	
TX	Primary tumor cannot be assessed	NX	Regional lymph nodes cannot be assessed
T0	No evidence of primary tumor		
T1	Subclinical tumor not evident by palpation or imaging	N0	No regional lymph node metastasis
		N1	Metastasis in regional lymph node(s)
T1a	≤5% cancerous tissue found incidentally on TURP	pNX	Regional lymph nodes not sampled
		pN0	No positive regional lymph nodes
T1b	>5% cancerous tissue found incidentally on TURP	pN1	Metastasis in regional lymph node(s)
T1c	Tumor found by needle biopsy (e.g., because of elevated PSA)	**Distant metastases (M)**	
		MX	Distant metastasis cannot be assessed
T2	Tumor confined to the prostate		
T2a	Tumor involves ≤$\frac{1}{2}$ of one lobe	M0	No distant metastasis
T2b	Tumor involves >$\frac{1}{2}$ of one lobe	M1	Distant metastasis is present
T2c	Tumor involves both lobes	M1a	Nonregional lymph node involvement (e.g., supraclavicular)
T3	Tumor extends through prostate capsule	M1b	Bony metastasis
T3a	Extracapsular extension (unilateral or bilateral)	M1c	Metastases to sites other than lymph nodes or bone (e.g., liver)
T3b	Seminal vesicle(s) involvement	**Histologic grade (G)**	
T4	Tumor is fixed or invades bladder neck, rectum, external sphincter, levator muscles, or pelvic wall	G1	Gleason 2–4 (well differentiated)
		G2	Gleason 5–6 (moderately differentiated)
		G3	Gleason 7–10 (poorly differentiated)

Stage groupings		
Stage	**TNM classification**	**Histologic grade (G)**
I	T1a N0 M0	G1
II	T1–2 N0 M0	G2, 3–4
III	T3 N0–1 M0	Any G
IV	T4 N0 M0; any T N1 M0; any T any N M1	Any G

[a]Pathologic substaging by biopsy or radical prostatectomy is designated by the "p" prefix for pT2–pT4 and pNX–pN1.
Adapted from the *AJCC Cancer Staging Manual.* 6th ed. New York: Springer-Verlag; 2002, with permission.

5. An array of Kattan nomograms is clinically useful for prognostication in a variety of clinical setups and treatment modalities using known prognostic factors (for reference: http://www.nomograms.org).

V. PREVENTION AND EARLY DETECTION. Screening for prostate cancer remains controversial. Early detection as a result of elevated PSA only (T1c disease) results, however, in the identification of more patients with organ-confined disease and perhaps contributes to a reduction in disease-specific mortality. American Cancer Society guidelines recommend that PSA screening and DRE begin at the age of 50 years. Screening at the age of 40 should be considered in men with positive familial or racial (blacks) risk factors.

VI. MANAGEMENT

A. Overview and philosophy.
The management of all stages of prostate cancer is controversial. This disease often has a long natural history; therefore, substantial numbers of patients survive 15 years or longer after the diagnosis (even without treatment). Furthermore, because the disease occurs in older men (who often have significant comorbid illnesses), many patients die from these conditions before they have symptoms or die from prostate cancer.

1. Investigators and clinicians vary widely in their use of surgery, RT, hormonal manipulation, and other measures for treating each stage of disease. Most clinicians agree, however, that treatment of early stage disease with either surgery or RT results in comparable survival. It is unclear at this time whether similar survival rates could be achieved with systemic therapies.

2. All options should be explored when it comes to treatment selection for a specific patient. No prospective head-to-head data are available to show an overall clear-cut advantage for radical retropubic prostatectomy (RRP) over RT, or vice versa. The long-term *survival* results of modern cryotherapy and modern brachytherapy are not yet ready for a critical comparison with the gold standard therapies. "Watchful waiting" is another option that should be considered.

A newer approach of **active surveillance** is replacing the "watchful waiting" approach. With active surveillance, patients are clinically monitored twice a year and tumor histology is re-evaluated with annual prostate biopsy to detect disease progression and allocate patients who deserve a curative effort at that point. Inclusion criteria are absence of palpable disease on DRE (T1c), Gleason score ≤6 in a single biopsy core, the absence of a large tumor (<10% of the core may be involved), and a low PSA (3.5 to 5.0 ng/mL) at diagnosis. It is plausible that a long PSA doubling time (i.e., >12 months) would also indicate an indolent disease.

These options should be carefully explained to the patient, exploring the advantages and disadvantages of each treatment modality. The treatment strategy should be tailored according to both the patient's clinical data and his expectations and lifestyle.

B. Surgery for early disease (stages T1 and T2)

1. Stage T1a. Prostate cancer is often discovered by histologic evaluation of specimens taken by TURP for hyperplasia. Management is controversial. Patients with stage T1a prostate cancer can usually be managed with watchful waiting. But, the clinical course of stage T1a is variable. If left untreated, a small but significant proportion of patients are at risk for disease progression and death. Thus, it is acceptable to offer treatment for cure in selected cases of T1a disease, such as with patients who are

a. 60 years of age or younger, and

b. Assumed to have a biologically significant disease:

  (1) High Gleason's score,

  (2) TURP weight <30 g, or

  (3) More than three chips containing adenocarcinoma

2. Stages T1b to T2b. These patients may be offered a treatment intended for cure (provided they do not have significant comorbid conditions), including radical RRP, RT, cryosurgery, or brachytherapy. Patients with PSA >10 ng/mL, Gleason Score =7, or palpable disease usually undergo pelvic lymphadenectomy during RRP or may undergo lymphadenectomy before definitive therapy other than RRP.

3. Stage T1c stands for CAP diagnosis driven by elevated serum PSA only. Currently, most CAP patients with organ-confined disease are diagnosed within the frame of clinical stage T1c. Most patients are offered treatment for cure. Recently, active surveillance is also offered to a selected subgroup of T1c patients (see inclusion criteria in section VI.A.2).

4. Complications of RRP and lymphadenectomy

a. RRP causes minor incontinence in 10% to 20% of patients. Severe incontinence is reported to occur in no more than 1% to 3%. Potency can be preserved by a skilled surgeon in up to 60% to 70% of younger patients who undergo nerve-sparing radical prostatectomy.

b. Complications of staging lymphadenectomy, which occur in about 20% of patients, include lymphocele, pulmonary embolus, wound infection, and lymphedema.

c. Persistent or recurrent disease following radical exterpiration of the prostate is rare provided that patients were carefully selected for surgery. It may occur in 10% to 40% of patients after RRP, depending on tumor stage, Gleason's score, and pretreatment PSA. Patients with higher risks for disease progression may benefit from multimodality treatment protocols.

5. Contraindications to RRP and lymphadenectomy. Generally speaking, RRP is reserved for men who are likely to be cured and who have a life expectancy of at least 10 years. Thus, the following constitute contraindications for radical prostatectomy:

a. Physiologic age >70 to 75 years

b. High-grade cancers (relative contraindication)

c. High serum PSA concentration (relative contraindication)

d. Invasion of the seminal vesicles (stage T3b)

e. Metastases to pelvic nodes

f. Disseminated cancer

C. RT for early disease (stages T1 to T3)

1. Indications. RT is widely used in the treatment of patients with stages T1 and T2 disease. Adjuvant androgen deprivation therapy for 6 months to 3 years has been shown to improve survival in this setting. The use of three-dimensional conformal technique and intensity-modulated RT (IMRT) allows improved results and with fewer side effects than standard RT.

RT for patients with stage T3 disease is also controversial, but most authorities would support the use of RT integrated with hormonal cytoreduction and radiobiologic sensitizers. For patients with locally advanced disease (stages T3 and T4), 3 years of adjuvant androgen deprivation therapy has been shown to prolonged survival in comparison with 6 months of androgen deprivation therapy in a randomized clinical trial. Increasing the radiation dose is advisable in this selected group. This may be achieved by using conformal external-beam irradiation, proton therapy, or brachytherapy. Other indications for RT include the following:

a. The patient's medical condition precludes surgery.

b. Node involvement is found at staging lymphadenectomy (RRP is not performed).

c. Residual malignant pelvic disease is found after prostate surgery (i.e., positive surgical margins and slowly rising PSA).

2. Complications after about 7,000 cGy given in 7 to 8 weeks and their approximate incidence rates in treated patients are as follows:

a. Impotence: 50% (may be less with conformal RT or brachytherapy)

b. Radiation proctitis with diarrhea, blood-streaked stools, and rectal urgency: <5% (see Chapter 30, section VI.D)

c. Dysuria, urinary urgency, and frequency: <5%

d. Perineal fistulas: <1%

e. Fecal and urinary incontinence: 1% to 2%

f. Urethral stricture: 1% to 5%

g. Persistent tumor or recurrent disease: 10% to 40%, depending on tumor stage, Gleason's score, and pretreatment PSA

3. Brachytherapy and cryotherapy are other therapies intended for cure. These modalities will be judged in the future when enough patients have been treated sufficiently long for ample follow-up data to become available.

4. Systemic therapy. Neither hormonal manipulation nor chemotherapy clearly improves the survival of patients with early prostate cancer.

D. Advanced disease

1. Surgery. TURP may be used to relieve bladder outlet obstruction even in the presence of advanced disease; however, orchiectomy alone is usually effective.

2. **RT** is useful in treating the following problems commonly encountered in prostate cancer patients:
    a. Isolated, painful bony metastatic sites, despite endocrine therapy
    b. Pelvic pain syndromes, urinary tract obstruction, and gross hematuria
    c. Metastases to retroperitoneal lymph nodes that produce back pain or scrotal and lower extremity edema
    d. Spinal cord compression from vertebral and extradural metastases is a common and rapidly progressive complication of prostate cancer. Cord compression is an emergency; MRI, administration of corticosteroids and definitive therapy must be undertaken within a few hours after onset of symptoms (see Chapter 32, section III).

3. **Androgen deprivation therapy** is the mainstay of treatment for symptomatic advanced prostate cancer because testosterone is the main growth factor for prostate cancer cells. The timing of androgen deprivation therapy is controversial because no conclusive evidence suggests that treatment of asymptomatic patients provides survival advantage. Prolonged androgen deprivation is associated with multiple side effects, including hot flushes, weight gain, erectile dysfunction, osteoporosis, and increased risk of diabetes and cardiovascular disease. Thus, treatment of patients with asymptomatic, advanced disease is not essential.

    Orchiectomy, luteinizing hormone-releasing hormone (LHRH) agonists, and antiandrogens are the available treatments. Each produces symptomatic relief in 80% of patients. Improvement is often dramatic; many bedridden patients crippled with bone pain return to a more functional status.

    a. **Orchiectomy** produces a rapid decline in testosterone level. It is an effective but irreversible procedure. Orchiectomy is advisable as primary treatment for advanced disease, particularly for patients who are noncompliant with androgen blockade or who require emergency blockade for spinal cord compression.
    b. **LHRH agonists,** such as leuprolide (Lupron) and goserelin (Zoladex), appear to be as effective as orchiectomy. These depot drugs are given every 3 months (22.5 mg for leuprolide and 10.8 mg for goserelin). The cost of ongoing treatment with LHRH agonists is substantially greater than with orchiectomy.
    c. **Antiandrogens combined with LHRH agonists** are believed by some investigators to be superior to LHRH agonists alone and to result in a small but significant survival benefit by "total androgen blockade." Flutamide (Eulexin, 250 mg PO given t.i.d.), bicalutamide (Casodex, 50 mg PO daily), or other antiandrogens are given along with the LHRH agonist.
    d. **Other agents** that may be helpful include the following:
        (1) **Progestins,** such as megestrol acetate, 40 mg PO q.i.d.
        (2) **Other drugs that inhibit androgen synthesis,** such as aminoglutethimide or ketoconazole (200 to 400 mg t.i.d.), have also been shown to be effective. These agents, however, are expensive and are often difficult to tolerate. The benefits of treatment with them are often difficult to separate from the benefits of corticosteroids, which are often given simultaneously.
        (3) **Corticosteroids,** such as prednisone and dexamethasone, often provide symptomatic improvement and may be associated with reductions in PSA levels.
        (4) **Zoledronic acid** (Zometa), 4 mg IV over 15 minutes monthly, is widely used for reduction in bone pain, in time to first skeletal-related events, and in the incidence of fractures and other complications of bone metastases.
        (5) **Strontium 89 infusion.** The beta emission of ^{89}Sr is used in selected hormone refractory patients to relieve skeletal pain. Responses last about 6 months. Hematologic toxicity is anticipated in the first 2 weeks after administration.
        (6) α_5**-Reductase inhibitors** (e.g., finasteride) are used for the treatment of benign prostatic hyperplasia. They are being evaluated in combination with other antiandrogens, for efficacy in treating patients with advanced prostate cancer, but so far no evidence indicates that they provide additional benefits to LHRH agonists and antiandrogens.

4. **Chemotherapy.** The first chemotherapy drug approved for the treatment of androgen-independent prostate cancer was mitoxantrone based on its palliative effects. Two large randomized clinical trials showed that chemotherapy with docetaxel (Taxotere) given every 3 weeks improves survival and provides superior palliation as compared with mitoxantrone. Second-line therapy after failure of docetaxel is usually not effective, but about 10% of patients may benefit from mitoxantrone or carboplatin. An oral platinum compound (satraplatin) is showing promise in the second-line setting and is currently undergoing clinical trials.

VII. SPECIAL CLINICAL PROBLEMS

A. **Cytopenias in prostate cancer** are usually part of the end-stage process caused by extensive tumor involvement of the bone marrow or by RT to major marrow-bearing sites. The anemia is typically normochromic and normocytic and sometimes a part of a leukoerythroblastic peripheral blood smear. Other causes must be considered.

B. **Obstructive uropathy and uremia** may be the fatal complication of prostate cancer. Orchiectomy or RT (followed by endocrine therapy or chemotherapy) may relieve the obstruction. Unlike uremic patients with other pelvic tumors, some patients with prostate cancer and ureteral obstruction may benefit from surgical intervention. Patients without pelvic pain syndromes and low-grade cancers should be considered for ureteral bypass by stent catheters or percutaneous nephrostomy.

C. **Dense-bone sclerosis on radiograph** in an adult man of the appropriate age who has bone pain usually is diagnostic of prostate cancer. Bone-containing prostate cancer is so densely sclerotic that attempts at marrow biopsy often result in "dry taps" and damaged biopsy needles. The radiologic appearance of Paget's disease is distinguished by the fluffy, cottonlike appearance of lesions, by thickening of the bone cortex, and by the dense sclerosis of the pelvic brim (*brim sign*).

D. **Extraosseous extension** of prostate cancer is common. Extension of skull or vertebral lesions can produce neurologic deficits. Extension of rib lesions can produce subcutaneous or pleuropulmonary masses. Retro-orbital and cavernous sinus masses can result in proptosis and visual loss. Extraosseous extension of bony lesions necessitates RT.

E. **Systemic fibrinolysis.** Activators of the fibrinolytic enzyme, plasmin, abound in prostatic tissue. Prostatic disease, especially carcinoma of the prostate, is among the few medical conditions that can produce both significant systemic fibrinolysis and disseminated intravascular coagulation (see Chapter 34, "Coagulopathy," section III, for diagnosis and management).

PENILE CANCER

I. EPIDEMIOLOGY AND ETIOLOGY

A. **Incidence.** Penile cancer constitutes about 0.5% of all cancers in men in the United States and Europe. The incidence is greatly increased in populations that do not uniformly practice circumcision. The average age of onset is about 60 years, peaking at about 80 years of age.

B. **Etiology.** The etiology of penile cancer is not known. Venereal disease is not a causative factor. The following data suggest that circumcision is preventative:

1. The disease is almost nonexistent in Jewish men, who are all circumcised shortly after birth.

2. In Africa and other countries where circumcision is not performed, penile cancer constitutes 20% of all cancers.

3. Muslims have an intermediate risk for penile cancer. Muslim boys are circumcised at puberty.

II. PATHOLOGY AND NATURAL HISTORY

A. **Premalignant lesions**

1. **Carcinoma *in situ***

a. **Erythroplasia of Queyrat** occurs on the glans and prepuce of uncircumcised men. The lesions are flat and reddened or are velvety plaques and may progress to invasive cancer in 10% of patients.

   b. Bowen's disease appears as a small eczematoid plaque anywhere on the penis. Squamous carcinoma *in situ* is demonstrated by histology. Bowen's disease of the penis, as with squamous carcinoma *in situ* in other areas of the skin not exposed to sun, is associated with a high incidence of carcinoma of the gastrointestinal tract and lungs.

2. Leukoplakia. Nonspecific plaques of leukoplakia on the glans are almost always associated with squamous carcinoma. Unlike leukoplakia lesions elsewhere, penile lesions are not white.

3. Giant penile condyloma (Buschke-Löwenstein tumor) grossly resembles a cauliflowerlike squamous cell cancer and may have foci of cancer. Surgical excision is mandatory.

B. Histology. Squamous cell carcinoma, usually well differentiated, constitutes nearly all penile cancers. Rare penile cancers include melanoma, sarcoma, and metastatic tumor. Squamous carcinoma of the penis may demonstrate variable degrees of keratin formation.

C. Clinical course. If left untreated, penile cancers usually cause death within 2 years.

1. Squamous penile cancer usually starts on the glans or coronal sulcus. As the disease progresses, the corpora cavernosa are invaded. The urethra is usually spared until late in the disease course.

2. The rich lymphatic drainage of this region results in metastases to the inguinal nodes (only one-third of palpable nodes are involved with tumor by histology). Lymphatic metastases are not common if the tumor is confined to the glans or prepuce.

3. The tumor disseminates through the lymphatic system and the bloodstream to distant organs in up to 10% of patients, most often to the lungs and, less frequently, to bone and other sites.

D. Paraneoplastic syndromes. Hypercalcemia may develop with no evidence of bony metastasis (20% of patients).

III. DIAGNOSIS is usually delayed substantially because of denial, personal neglect, shame, guilt, or lack of knowledge.

A. Symptoms and signs

1. The earliest lesion of penile carcinoma is described by patients as a nonhealing sore, often with an associated foul-smelling discharge. Phimosis may mask penile cancer until erosion through the prepuce occurs. Many patients have a long history of a mass. Urinary tract symptoms, such as pain and hematuria, are signs of locally advanced disease.

2. Physical examination usually reveals an exophytic mass. Infection of the tumor is usually present when the patient is examined for symptoms. In about 92% of patients, the tumor arises in the glans penis, prepuce, or both.

B. Laboratory studies

1. Routine blood tests, urinalysis, and chest radiographs are obtained.

2. Biopsy or imprint slides should be done for all patients with a penile mass or with any finding compatible with a precancerous lesion.

3. Liver and bone scans should be obtained only if abnormalities seen on physical examination or blood studies suggest liver or bone involvement.

4. MRI and ultrasound of the penis and pelvis are effective in the staging.

IV. STAGING SYSTEM AND PROGNOSTIC FACTORS

A. Staging system. The TNM classification is used for squamous cell carcinoma. The reader is referred to a current AJCC manual for details of the TNM system.

B. Prognostic factors. Poor prognostic features include endophytic and high-grade lesions, invasion of the shaft, and involvement of draining lymph nodes, especially at the iliac level or higher. Of patients with clinical stage Tis, Ta, or T1 (Jackson stage I or II) tumors, 10% have inguinal node involvement proved by surgery.

V. PREVENTION AND EARLY DETECTION. Prevention of penile cancer can be accomplished by routine early circumcision of male babies. Circumcision should be performed in patients with phimosis and penile discharge, inflammation, or induration. Early detection of penile cancer requires regular inspection of the prepuce and glans at physical examination and biopsy of suspected lesions.

VI. MANAGEMENT

A. Surgery is the principal modality of therapy for penile cancer in the United States. Partial penectomy is sufficient therapy if there is a 2-cm tumor-free margin.

1. Total penectomy is necessary for lesions that invade the body of the penis or are very large.

2. In younger patients with tumor confined to the prepuce, circumcision may be used if close follow-up can be assured; however, the recurrence rate is high.

3. Dissection or routine sampling of the superficial inguinal nodes for patients with low-stage (up to T2), but high-grade, lesions is recommended by some authorities; if the nodes contain tumor, a radical ilioinguinal lymphadenectomy is necessary. Radical lymphadenectomy is routinely performed in patients with stage T3 tumors. The extensiveness of the lymph node dissection (deep *vs.* superficial inguinal *vs.* pelvic node dissection; unilateral *vs.* bilateral; full *vs.* limited) varies according to local and regional disease extension.

B. RT. The primary role of RT is to avoid penectomy, especially in younger patients. This modality has been used for treating small primary stage I lesions (<3 cm in diameter); the results for RT alone (along with salvage surgery for failures) appear to be the same as those obtained when partial amputation is used as primary therapy.

C. Chemotherapy

1. **Premalignant lesions** may respond to topical therapy with fluorouracil or to laser therapy in selected cases.

2. **Penile cancer** appears to be responsive to combination chemotherapy: vincristine, bleomycin, and methotrexate (VBM regimen) or cisplatin and 5-fluorouracil. Some authorities use these drugs as an adjunct to surgery or RT for stage T3 and T4 tumors. Response rates of advanced cancer to these drugs may be as high as 50%.

Suggested Reading

Renal Cancer

Belldegrun A, et al. *Renal and Adrenal Tumors: Biology and Management.* Oxford, UK: Oxford University Press; 2003.

Escudier B, et al. Sorafenib in advanced clear-cell renal-cell carcinoma. *N Engl J Med* 2007; 356:25.

Motzer R, et al. Sunitinib versus interferon alfa in metastatic renal cell carcinoma. *N Engl J Med* 2007;356:115.

Pantuck A, et al. Changing the natural history of renal cell carcinoma. *J Urol* 2001;166:1611.

Rassweiler J, et al. Oncological safety of laparoscopic surgery for urological malignancy: experience with more than 1,000 operations. *J Urol* 2003;169:2072.

Twardowski P, Figlin R. Emerging targeted therapies for renal cell carcinoma. *Monographs in Renal Cell Carcinoma* 2006;1(2):10.

Whang YE, et al. Renal cell carcinoma. *Curr Opin Oncol* 2003;15:213.

Zisman A, et al. Improved prognostication of RCC using an integrated staging system (UISS). *J Clin Oncol* 2001;19:1649.

Zisman A, et al. Reevaluation of the 1997 TNM classification for RCC: T1 and T2 cutoff point at 4.5 cm rather then 7 cm better correlates with clinical outcome. *J Urol* 2001;166:54.

Zisman A, et al. Risk group assessment and clinical outcome algorithm to predict the natural history of patients with surgically resected renal cell carcinoma. *J Clin Oncol* 2002;20:4559.

Urothelial Cancers

Borden LS, et al. Bladder cancer. *Curr Opin Oncol* 2003;15:227.

Raghavan D. Molecular targeting and pharmacogenomics in the management of advanced bladder cancer. *Cancer* 2003;97:2083.

Sternberg CN, et al. Chemotherapy for bladder cancer: treatment guidelines for neoadjuvant chemotherapy, bladder preservation, adjuvant chemotherapy, and metastatic cancer. *Urology* 2007;69(1 Suppl):62.

Von der Maase H, et al. Gemcitabine and cisplatin versus methotrexate, vinblastin, doxorubicin and cisplatin in advanced or metastatic bladder cancer: results of a large randomized, multinational, multicenter, phase III study. *J Clin Oncol* 2000;17:3068.

Prostate Cancer

Akduman B, et al. The management of high risk prostate cancer. *J Urol* 2003;169:1993.

Axelson Bill, et al. Radical prostatectomy versus watchful waiting in early prostate cancer. *N Engl J Med* 2005;352(19):1977.

Graefen M, et al. International validation of a preoperative nomogram for prostate cancer recurrence after radical prostatectomy. *J Clin Oncol* 2002;20:3206.

Messing EM, et al. Immediate hormonal therapy compared with observation after radical prostatectomy and pelvic lymphadenectomy in men with node-positive prostate cancer. *N Engl J Med* 1999;341:1781.

Petrylak DP, et al. Docetaxel and estramustine compared with mitoxantrone and prednisone for advanced refractory prostate cancer. *N Engl J Med* 2004;351(15):1513.

Pisansky TM. External-beam radiotherapy for localized prostate cancer. *N Engl J Med* 2006;355(15):1583.

Tannock IF, et al. Docetaxel plus prednisone or mitoxantrone plus prednisone for advanced prostate cancer. *N Engl J Med* 2004;351(15):1502.

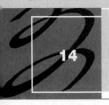

NEUROLOGICAL TUMORS

14

Lisa M. DeAngelis

I. EPIDEMIOLOGY AND ETIOLOGY

A. **Incidence.** Malignant primary brain tumors represent 2% (17,000 cases) of all cancers and 2.5% (10,000 cases) of cancer deaths annually in the United States (Table 14.1). The male-to-female ratio is 3:2. The incidence peaks at 5 to 10 years of age and again at 50 to 55 years of age. Brain cancers are the most common solid tumors in children; brain cancers occurring in childhood are discussed further in Chapter 18, "Brain Tumors."

B. **Etiology**

1. **Environmental factors,** such as tobacco, alcohol, and diet, have not been associated with primary central nervous system (CNS) tumors. Exposure to ionizing radiation, however, can induce the formation of meningiomas, nerve-sheath tumors, sarcomas, and astrocytomas. Exposure to electromagnetic radiation, including cell phones and computer terminals, does not cause brain tumors. Occupational exposure to vinyl chlorides may be a risk factor for astrocytomas; animal studies have shown that exposure to *N*-nitroso compounds, aromatic hydrocarbons, triazenes, and hydrazines increases the risk for astrocytoma formation, but it is not clear whether these compounds play a role in human tumor formation.

2. **Hereditary neurocutaneous syndromes**

   a. **Neurofibromatosis I** is a dominantly inherited condition of multiple neurofibromas, café-au-lait spots, axillary freckling, and Lisch nodules of the iris that confers an increased risk for optic glioma, intracranial astrocytoma, neurofibrosarcoma, neural crest–derived tumors (glomus tumor, pheochromocytoma), embryonal tumors, leukemia, and Wilms' tumor. The gene for this disorder is on chromosome 17q11, and its product, neurofibromin, is a tumor suppressor that regulates the Ras pathway, which transmits mitogenic signals to the nucleus.

   b. **Neurofibromatosis II** is a condition of multiple schwannomas, especially vestibular schwannomas, that is also associated with an increased risk for ependymoma and meningioma. The gene for this disorder is located on chromosome 22q12, and its product, merlin, encodes a member of the ezrin-radixin-moesin (ERM) family of membrane and cytoskeletal linker proteins thought to be important for cell motility and adhesion.

   c. **Tuberous sclerosis** (Bourneville disease) is a dominantly transmitted disorder characterized by the development of hamartomas, including subependymal nodules and cerebral cortical tubers that have abnormal cortical architecture and can be associated with mental retardation, epilepsy, and behavioral disturbances such as autism. Hamartomatous lesions of other organ systems include facial angiofibromas, forehead plaques, shagreen patches, cardiac rhabdomyomas, and renal angiomyolipomas and cysts. This disorder is associated with the formation of giant-cell astrocytomas. Two responsible tumor-suppressor genes, *TSC-1* (chromosome 9q34) and *TSC-2* (chromosome 16p13), have been identified.

   d. **Nevoid basal cell carcinoma syndrome** (Gorlin syndrome) is a dominantly inherited syndrome of multiple basal cell carcinomas that may be associated with the presence of medulloblastoma, meningioma, craniopharyngioma,

TABLE 14.1 Features of Common Central Nervous System Tumors

Tumor type	Age	Common location	Clinical features	Survival	RT	Chemotherapy
Astrocytoma	Adult > child	Supratentorial	Slow growing, may be present for years	5 yr MS	Yes	At recurrence
Anaplastic astrocytoma	Adult	Supratentorial	Rapidly growing	2.5 yr MS	Yes	Yes
Glioblastoma	Adult, elderly	Supratentorial	Rapidly growing, highly malignant	1 yr MS	Yes	Yes
Oligodendroglioma	Any	Supratentorial, often frontal	Seizures more common	5 yr MS	Yes	Yes
Brainstem glioma	Child > adult	Brainstem, especially pons	Marked morbidity from cranial nerve deficits	1 yr MS	Yes	Seldom
Pilocytic astrocytoma	Child > adult	Cerebellum and hypothalamus	Cure with total resection	80% 10 yr	Yes	Yes
Ependymoma	Child, adult	Fourth ventricle, cauda equina	Cure with total resection; can disseminate in CSF	70% 5 yr	Yes	Seldom
Medulloblastoma	Child > adult	Cerebellum	Likely to disseminate in CSF	70% to 80% 5 yr	Yes	Yes
Meningioma	Adult	Convexity, clival, thoracic	More common in women; cure with total resection	Long term	Yes	Rare
Primary CNS lymphoma	Adult	Multifocal, periventricular	CSF/ocular dissemination common	3–5 yr MS	Yes	Yes
Germinoma	Second and third decades	Pineal and suprasellar	Highly sensitive to chemotherapy and RT	80% 5 yr	Yes	Yes
Nongerminoma germ cell tumor	Second and third decades	Pineal and suprasellar	Mixed histologies, often marker positive	25% 5 yr	Yes	Yes

MS, median survival; CSF, cerebrospinal fluid; CNS, central nervous system; RT, radiation therapy.

and some systemic tumors (ovarian tumors, cardiac fibroma, maxillary fibrosarcoma, adrenal cortical adenoma, rhabdomyosarcoma, seminoma). Other features include jaw cysts, palmar and plantar pits, and spine and rib anomalies. The loss of a tumor-suppressor gene on chromosome 9q22 is responsible for this disorder. Its gene product, PTCH, is the human homologue of the *Drosophila patched* gene, part of the hedgehog signaling pathway, which is important in embryonic patterning and cell fate.

    e. Neurocutaneous melanosis is a developmental rather than inherited condition of large, hairy, pigmented benign nevi of the skin associated with infiltration of the meninges by melanin-containing cells. Although the pigmented lesions of the skin remain benign, the pigmented cells in the meninges often undergo malignant transformation with neural invasion, resulting in primary CNS melanoma.

3. Hereditary cancer syndromes

    a. von Hippel-Lindau disease is a dominantly transmitted disorder characterized by hemangioblastomas of the retina, cerebellum, and, less commonly, spinal cord. Other associated tumors include renal carcinoma, pheochromocytoma, islet cell tumors, endolymphatic sac tumors, and benign renal, pancreatic, and epididymal cysts. The disorder is due to the loss of a tumor-suppressor gene on chromosome 3p25-26. This loss results in the overexpression of vascular endothelial growth factor and erythropoietin, which are normally induced by hypoxia.

    b. Turcot syndrome is a rare autosomal dominant or recessive familial syndrome associated with colon cancer, glioblastoma, and medulloblastoma. It is due to a germ line mutation of the APC gene on chromosome 5q21, or the tumors can carry errors of the DNA replication mechanism with somatic mutations of either the hMLH-1 or the hPMS-2 gene, both of which encode proteins responsible for DNA mismatch repair.

    c. Li-Fraumeni syndrome is a clinical syndrome of familial breast cancer, sarcomas, leukemia, and primary brain tumors that is associated with germ line *p53* (chromosome 17) mutations.

4. Immune suppression. Transplant recipients and patients with acquired immunodeficiency syndrome (AIDS) have a markedly increased risk for primary CNS lymphoma.

II. DIAGNOSIS

  A. Clinical presentation depends on the location of the tumor and its rate of growth. In general, slow-growing tumors cause little in the way of focal deficits because the brain tissue is slowly compressed and compensatory mechanisms appear to occur. After they reach a certain size, the compensatory mechanisms fail or cerebrospinal fluid (CSF) pathways may be obstructed, causing increased intracranial pressure (ICP). Fast-growing tumors tend to be associated with considerable surrounding cerebral edema; the edema, in addition to the tumor mass, is more likely to cause focal deficits. Usually, the deficits caused by edema are reversible, whereas those caused by the tumor may not be reversible. Specific signs and symptoms associated with tumors of the CNS include the following:

    1. Headaches occur in about 50% of brain tumor patients. They are most likely to occur in younger patients with fast-growing tumors and are typically deep, dull, and not intense or throbbing. They are characteristically worse on arising in the morning and are exacerbated by straining or lifting. Lateralization of headaches occasionally facilitates tumor localization.

    2. Seizures. In 20% of patients >20 years of age, the onset of seizures is caused by a neoplasm. The seizures may be generalized or partial (focal). Simple partial seizures commonly consist of transient sensory or motor phenomena of a single limb or side. Complex partial seizures, often of frontal or temporal lobe origin, consist of changes in the level of consciousness or awareness of surroundings, frequently in conjunction with abnormal olfactory or gustatory phenomena.

Speech arrest may also occur. Generalized seizures result in loss of consciousness, bowel and bladder incontinence, and bilateral tonic–clonic movements. In patients with brain tumors, generalized seizures always have a focal origin even if the focal signature is not evident at seizure onset; evidence of focality is often found on postictal examination of the patient.

3. **Increased ICP** may result from a large mass or from obstructive hydrocephalus. Large supratentorial masses cause progressive obtundation and can lead to transtentorial herniation, which classically presents with an ipsilateral third-cranial-nerve palsy and contralateral hemiparesis. Hydrocephalus causes gait ataxia, nausea, vomiting, headache, and a decrease in level of alertness. If untreated, hydrocephalus can lead to central herniation, which is not heralded by a third-nerve palsy. Papilledema is a sign of increased ICP, but it is rarely seen in current brain tumor patients because of the availability of modern neuroimaging, which facilitates early diagnosis. Unusual signs and symptoms of increased ICP include visual obscurations, dizziness, and false localizing signs, the most common of which is sixth-cranial-nerve dysfunction owing to stretching of the nerve from downward pressure caused by a large supratentorial mass.

4. **Supratentorial tumors** usually present with focal signs and symptoms, including hemiparesis (frontal lobe), aphasia (left frontal and posterior temporal lobes), hemineglect (parietal lobe), and hemianopsia (occipital lobe).

5. **Hypothalamic tumors** may be associated with disturbance of body temperature regulation, diabetes insipidus, hyperphagia, and, if the optic chiasm is involved, visual-field deficits.

6. **Brainstem tumors,** such as brainstem gliomas, present with multiple cranial nerve deficits, hemiparesis, and ataxia.

7. **Nerve-sheath tumors,** such as acoustic neuromas, result in deficits of the involved cranial or spinal nerve. As the tumor enlarges, surrounding neural structures may also be compressed, leading to further symptoms.

8. **Cerebellar tumors** are associated with dysmetria, ataxia, vertigo, nystagmus, headache, and vomiting.

9. **Spinal cord tumors** present with spastic paraparesis and sensory loss below the level of the tumor as well as with disturbances of bowel and bladder function.

10. **Meningeal involvement** by primary CNS tumors is less common than with metastatic tumors (see Chapter 32) and is seen primarily with medulloblastomas, pineoblastomas, germinomas, primary CNS lymphomas, and, to a lesser degree, ependymomas. The hallmark for meningeal disease is neurological dysfunction at multiple levels of the neuraxis. Nonspecific features include seizures and changes in mentation.

B. **Evaluation.** Imaging studies must be performed to evaluate patients suspected of having CNS mass lesions.

1. **Computed tomography (CT) and magnetic resonance imaging (MRI)** are the primary imaging modalities for evaluating presumed CNS tumors. MRI is preferable because of its greater sensitivity, especially for mass lesions in the brainstem, posterior fossa, medial temporal lobes, and spinal cord. Contrast studies should always be performed because many tumors show contrast enhancement. CT should only be used for those patients unable to undergo MRI (e.g., pacemaker).

2. **Lumbar puncture** is almost never a part of the initial evaluation of a suspected CNS tumor and in fact is often contraindicated in this setting. It is used primarily to stage tumors known to disseminate along the neuraxis or to evaluate patients with clinical or radiographic evidence of meningeal dissemination (see section II.A.10). A notable exception is primary CNS lymphoma, which can be diagnosed in about 15% of patients by examination of CSF in lieu of biopsy.

3. **Angiography** is never required in the evaluation of suspected CNS tumors. It is useful in the preoperative evaluation of highly vascular tumors that require embolization to reduce the blood supply before surgical resection is performed. The need for angiography is determined by the neurosurgical consultant.

4. **Systemic evaluation.** After a mass lesion is demonstrated on CT or MRI scan, its specific etiology must be determined. The differential diagnosis includes primary tumors of the nervous system, metastatic tumors, stroke, and inflammatory or infectious processes (e.g., multiple sclerosis, cerebral abscess). Radiographic features can help differentiate among these diagnoses; combined with the patient's history and physical examination, they can lead to a presumptive diagnosis with reasonable certainty.

   A systemic evaluation is not necessary in the initial evaluation of a patient with a single lesion seen on MRI. Doing a comprehensive evaluation usually delays the diagnosis and is rarely informative. Such patients should immediately undergo surgical resection and any subsequent testing based on the pathology. If a primary brain tumor is found, no systemic evaluation is necessary. If a metastasis is identified, a systemic workup can proceed accordingly and be completed with a body positron emission tomography (PET) scan. This is a reasonable approach because resection is the optimal treatment for either a primary brain tumor or a single brain metastasis. If multiple lesions are identified on the initial MRI, a systemic evaluation is in order; body PET is largely replacing the individual organ imaging tests such as a chest CT scan.

5. **Surgery** is required for definitive diagnosis in most cases of suspected primary nervous system tumors and is usually a cornerstone of treatment as well. Exceptions include tumors not requiring surgical extirpation for therapy that can be diagnosed by other means, including imaging (e.g., neurofibroma, optic nerve glioma) or CSF examination (e.g., primary CNS lymphoma). In addition, when nonneoplastic processes (e.g., stroke, multiple sclerosis) are a consideration, clinical and radiographic observation may be appropriate.

III. ASTROCYTOMA AND GLIOBLASTOMA

A. **Pathology.** Astrocytomas are highly infiltrative tumors that are graded by their degree of anaplasia according to World Health Organization (WHO) definitions. Low-grade tumors are classified as astrocytoma (WHO grade II), those with more evidence of cytologic atypia and increased cellularity as anaplastic astrocytoma (WHO grade III), and those with highly malignant features as glioblastoma (GBM; WHO grade IV). Glioblastomas with sarcomatous features are gliosarcomas, and they behave in a fashion identical to GBMs. The very low grade pilocytic astrocytoma constitutes WHO grade I; it is almost exclusively seen in children. WHO grade III and IV tumors are malignant astrocytomas.

   The incidence of astrocytomas increases with age, and as the age of the patient increases, the astrocytoma is more likely to be of higher grade. Astrocytomas are most commonly supratentorial but may occur in the cerebellum, brainstem, and spinal cord.

   Immunohistochemical properties of neurological malignancies are shown in Appendix C-4.V.

B. **Radiology.** On CT or MRI scans, astrocytomas are usually solitary lesions primarily in the white matter. The astrocytoma (grade II) appears as a nonenhancing infiltrative mass best seen on T_2-weighted or fluid-attenuated inversion recovery (FLAIR) MRI sequences. The high-grade astrocytomas (grades III and IV) usually enhance after administration of contrast material and are surrounded by focal edema; occasionally, anaplastic gliomas do not enhance on MRI. GBMs often have central necrosis and may appear as *ring-enhancing lesions*. Uncommonly, cystic components may be associated with low- or high-grade astrocytomas.

C. **Treatment**

1. **Dexamethasone** reduces the cerebral edema associated with brain tumors by decreasing vascular permeability through its action on endothelial junctions. Neurological dysfunction from brain tumors is often due to the surrounding edema rather than to the tumor itself. Therefore, treatment with steroids usually results in considerable neurological improvement. Dosing schedules vary,

but the typical starting dose is 4 mg PO or IV every 6 hours. Doses should be reduced once definitive treatment has been undertaken (usually postoperatively or during RT), and most patients can be tapered off completely. Common steroid-related side effects in brain tumor patients include insomnia, weight gain, hyperglycemia, steroid myopathy, and affective disturbance.

2. **Surgical resection** should be performed whenever technically feasible. Not only is surgery necessary for adequate tissue sampling for pathological diagnosis, but it can also lead to neurological improvement from reduction of mass effect. The degree of surgical resection has been shown to correlate with survival, especially for higher-grade lesions. The term *gross total resection* refers to removal of all or nearly all tumor visualized radiographically. Based on the infiltrative nature of astrocytomas, however, residual tumor always remains. Postoperative MRI scans should be performed within 3 to 4 days of surgery to determine the extent of surgical resection. If resection is not possible, biopsy should be performed for histological diagnosis.

3. **Radiation therapy** (RT) substantially improves survival, and a dose–response relationship has been documented up to 6,000 cGy for high-grade tumors. Astrocytomas are treated with 5,000 to 5,400 cGy and anaplastic astrocytomas and GBMs with 6,000 cGy of radiation to the tumor and surrounding margins. Radiotherapy may be deferred in some patients with low-grade astrocytomas who have seizures controlled by antiepileptic drugs and no other neurological symptoms. Radiation sensitizers are not beneficial in the treatment of astrocytomas. Adjuvant (boost) RT, such as interstitial brachytherapy or radiosurgery, does not offer a survival advantage to patients with malignant gliomas. Complications of such therapies include steroid dependence and the need for further surgical debulking in one half of patients for control of radionecrosis.

4. **Chemotherapy** with temozolomide has become the standard of care for patients with GBM. It is given concurrently during RT at 75 mg/m^2/day continuously, and for at least six cycles as adjuvant therapy at a dose of 150 to 200 mg/m^2 for 5 consecutive days every 4 weeks. Treatment is usually well tolerated. Although efficacy has not been established for patients with anaplastic astrocytoma, many have adopted this regimen for all patients with malignant gliomas.

5. **Treatment at recurrence.** Astrocytomas, including GBM, may respond to treatment at recurrence, and treatment strategies usually parallel those given at diagnosis. The decision to treat at recurrence and the type of treatment to be administered depends on patient characteristics, such as age and performance status, and on tumor features, such as histological grade and surgical accessibility. Dexamethasone may be reinstituted to control neurological symptoms. Further surgical debulking should be performed if possible. Postoperatively, chemotherapy should be employed. Traditional agents include a nitrosourea, procarbazine, etoposide, or irinotecan. Alternatively, newer agents, such as the antiangiogenic drug bevacizumab (Avastin), have shown promise in this setting. Optimally, patients should be offered participation in a clinical trial if available. Further irradiation, such as stereotactic radiosurgery, rarely has a role in the treatment of these highly infiltrative neoplasms.

6. **Patient follow-up.** Patients with astrocytomas require lifelong follow-up. Low-grade astrocytomas can recur, often as higher-grade lesions, as long as 20 years after treatment. Tumor recurrence is usually at the primary site, but occasionally astrocytomas can become multifocal or recur at distal sites within the neuraxis. Metastasis to systemic tissues is exceedingly rare. Monitoring for tumor recurrence can best be achieved with serial neurological examinations and MRI scans. The rate of monitoring is individualized and depends on the grade of the tumor, the performance status of the patient, and the intention for further therapy.

D. **Survival.** Median survival is about 5 years for astrocytoma, 2.5 years for anaplastic astrocytoma, and 1 year for glioblastoma. About 5% of patients with GBM survive for 5 years or longer.

IV. OTHER GLIAL NEOPLASMS

A. Oligodendroglioma

1. **Pathology.** Oligodendrogliomas arise from the oligodendrocytes or myelin-producing cells of the CNS and may occur in conjunction with astrocytomas as a mixed tumor. Most are lower-grade lesions, but anaplastic tumors also occur. Oligodendrogliomas are characterized by loss of heterozygosity of chromosomes 1p and 19q, which may correlate with chemosensitivity and improved prognosis.

2. **Clinical features.** Compared with astrocytomas, oligodendrogliomas are more likely to cause seizures and have a higher tendency to hemorrhage (about 10% of patients). Oligodendrogliomas are most common in the frontal and temporal lobes, particularly in the insular cortex. Intratumoral calcifications are also a radiographic feature best appreciated on CT scan.

3. **Treatment** is similar to that for astrocytomas and includes dexamethasone for control of symptoms and aggressive surgical resection. Low-grade oligodendrogliomas may be followed, and many do not require immediate treatment. When therapy is required, oligodendrogliomas are chemosensitive and may be treated with temozolomide, deferring RT until necessary. High-grade oligodendrogliomas all require therapy at diagnosis. Adding chemotherapy to RT at the time of diagnosis significantly prolongs progression-free survival but has no effect on overall survival, suggesting that it may be administered at diagnosis or held until recurrence. Median survival of low-grade oligodendrogliomas exceeds 15 years and is about 5 years for the anaplastic oligodendroglioma.

B. Juvenile pilocytic astrocytoma (JPA)

1. **Pathology.** Pilocytic astrocytomas (grade I) differ in histology and clinical behavior from the astrocytomas discussed in section III. They are less invasive, more circumscribed, and much less likely to progress to a more anaplastic state.

2. **Clinical features.** Pilocytic astrocytomas tend to occur in children and young adults and have a predilection for the cerebellum, hypothalamus, optic chiasm, and thalamus. Radiographically, they are well-demarcated masses that enhance densely and homogeneously and may have cystic components.

3. **Treatment.** JPAs are not infiltrative or histologically progressive and, therefore, can be cured by surgical excision. Subtotally resected tumors may be observed or rarely require immediate focal irradiation. Nonresectable tumors (e.g., optic gliomas) may also be followed or can be treated with RT (5,400 cGy, focal fields) or, in very young patients, with chemotherapy if symptoms dictate the need for immediate treatment. JPAs respond to nitrosoureas, procarbazine, cyclophosphamide, vincristine, platinum compounds, and etoposide.

4. **Survival** depends on tumor location and extent of resection. The overall median survival rate is 80% at 10 years and 70% at 20 years.

C. Ependymoma

1. **Pathology.** Ependymomas arise from ependymal cells. Therefore, these tumors localize to the ventricular system and spinal canal, most often in the fourth ventricle and in the region of the cauda equina. They are more frequent in children but occur in adults as well. Most are histologically benign, but some types, including anaplastic ependymoma, ependymoblastoma, and myxopapillary ependymoma, can disseminate through the spinal fluid.

2. **Treatment.** Ependymomas can be cured by total resection, particularly the filum terminale myxopapillary ependymoma. Unfortunately, their location often prevents complete excision, and RT must often be administered postoperatively. Radiation is usually given to a focal field to a dose of 5,400 cGy. Chemotherapy plays less of a role in the treatment of ependymomas, but when used, platinum compounds are considered most effective. Temozolomide also has some activity.

D. Brainstem glioma

Brainstem gliomas are astrocytomas that arise in the brainstem, usually the pons, and are more common in children than adults. They can be any grade of astrocytoma, but their outcome is primarily determined by their location, so they are classified separately from the other astrocytomas. Patients present with multiple cranial nerve palsies and ataxia.

Surgical resection is not possible because of tumor location, and diagnosis is usually based on the typical radiographic and clinical findings. Biopsy is occasionally pursued, and only when an exophytic component is apparent on MRI. Treatment consists of focal RT, usually to 6,000 cGy. Chemotherapy is largely ineffective for brainstem gliomas. Median survival for patients with diffuse pontine gliomas is about 1 year. Patients with more localized, discrete tumors, particularly those in the midbrain or medulla, have a longer survival time of several years.

V. PRIMARY CNS LYMPHOMA

Primary CNS lymphoma (PCNSL) is discussed in Chapter 21, NonHodgkin Lymphoma, section VIII.C and Chapter 36, section II.G. Compared with gliomas, PCNSLs are more likely to cause cognitive and behavioral abnormalities and are less likely to cause seizures. These clinical features reflect the tendency of PCNSLs to localize to deep, periventricular structures and to be multiple in about 40% of patients. In addition, the eye is involved in about 25% of PCNSL cases at diagnosis, often producing visual symptoms suggestive of vitreitis. Radiographically, these tumors usually enhance homogeneously; rarely, they are nonenhancing lesions seen on FLAIR or T_2 MRI. Diagnosis is usually by stereotactic biopsy because resection does not improve survival. Chemotherapy with high-dose methotrexate-based regimens should be the first-line treatment in all patients.

VI. MEDULLOBLASTOMA

A. Pathology. Medulloblastomas are embryonal tumors arising from primitive germinal cells in the cerebellum; they most commonly localize to the vermis and fourth ventricle. They are more common in childhood but occur in young adults as well. Medulloblastoma is associated with isochromosome 17q and a unique microarray gene expression that is distinct from other CNS tumors.

B. Clinical features. Medulloblastomas often cause obstructive hydrocephalus from compression of the fourth ventricle. Therefore, patients often present with signs of increased ICP (e.g., gait ataxia, headache, nausea and vomiting) rather than with signs localizing to the site of their tumor.

C. Staging and treatment. Patients require full staging of the neuraxis, including contrast-enhanced MRI of the head and full spine and cytological examination of CSF, because medulloblastoma disseminates in the CSF. Spinal imaging can often be performed preoperatively. CSF should be obtained intraoperatively or not until 2 weeks after surgery to avoid false-positive results.

   1. Surgery. The extent of surgical resection correlates with survival in patients with medulloblastoma, and gross total resection should be attempted. Patients with persistent hydrocephalus may require placement of a ventriculoperitoneal shunt. Dexamethasone is used to control cerebral edema, especially in the perioperative period.

   2. Radiation Therapy, consisting of craniospinal irradiation, is required for all patients, including those with negative staging studies. The standard dose ranges from 3,000 to 3,600 cGy to the whole brain and spine with an additional boost to the tumor to 5,500 to 6,000 cGy and perhaps even less in patients with standard risk disease. However, data suggest that the craniospinal dose can be reduced to 2,400 cGy when adjuvant chemotherapy is used.

   3. Chemotherapy. Chemotherapy as part of initial treatment used to be reserved for patients with disseminated disease. However, increasingly it is being incorporated into the regimen of all patients because it may allow for reduction of the dose of craniospinal irradiation and subsequently a reduction in the long-term sequelae of treatment.

   The standard regimen incorporates lomustine, vincristine, and cisplatin or cyclophosphamide, vincristine, and cisplatin. In both regimens, weekly vincristine is given during radiotherapy at a dose of 1.5 mg/m^2 (to a maximum dose of 2 mg). After completion of RT, either lomustine at 75 mg/m^2 PO or cyclophosphamide at 1,000 mg/m^2 IV plus cisplatin at 75 mg/m^2 IV are given every 6 weeks; vincristine is given at 15 mg/m^2 for 3 weeks of each cycle. Eight 6-week cycles of chemotherapy are administered.

D. Prognosis. Patients with medulloblastomas who have had a gross total resection and who show no evidence of tumor dissemination (standard risk) have a 5-year survival rate of 70% to 80%. In cases of disseminated tumor (poor risk), the median survival is about 5 years.

VII. GERM CELL TUMORS

A. Pathology. Germ cell tumors arising in the nervous system are usually localized in the pineal and suprasellar regions. They are of two basic types: germinomas and nongerminomatous germ cell tumors. The former are highly sensitive to radiation and are analogous to systemic seminomas and dysgerminomas. The latter, including teratomas, choriocarcinomas, endodermal sinus tumors, and some tumors of mixed histology, are relatively resistant to radiation. All germ cell tumors except mature teratomas are malignant. They are more common in male patients and in those of Asian ancestry. They occur mostly in the first three decades of life.

B. Evaluation. Because germ cell tumors can readily disseminate in the neuraxis, all patients require complete staging, including contrast MRI of the brain and full spine, CSF cytological examination, and determination of serum and CSF α-fetoprotein and β-human chorionic gonadotropin levels.

C. Treatment. Surgical resection should be performed first with a goal of achieving a complete excision. If resection is not feasible, biopsy is necessary for histological diagnosis. Resection constitutes complete therapy for the rare mature teratomas. Germinomas without evidence of neuraxis dissemination are treated with irradiation of the tumor and surrounding ventricular system; even those with positive markers can be treated with irradiation alone. Nongerminomatous germ cell tumors and tumors with evidence of neuraxis dissemination are treated with craniospinal irradiation and chemotherapy. Regimens are similar to those used for systemic germ cell tumors. The 5-year survival rate is 90% for germinomas and may approach 50% for nongerminomas that are more resistant to therapy.

VIII. BENIGN NERVOUS SYSTEM TUMORS

A. Meningiomas are tumors arising from arachnoidal cells. Their incidence increases with age, and they are more common in women. Meningiomas may occur over the convexities, parasagittal along the falx, along the sphenoid wing, retroclival, or along the thoracic spine. Although most of these tumors are benign, some are histologically atypical or malignant. The tumors are recognized radiographically by their extra-axial location and their dense, homogeneous pattern of contrast enhancement. Patients with small asymptomatic meningiomas can be followed.

Treatment is surgical resection, which is often curative. Recurrent tumors may be treated with RT or stereotactic radiosurgery. These tumors are not responsive to chemotherapy. Receptors for estrogen, androgens, and especially progesterone have been demonstrated in meningiomas, but the tumors rarely respond to hormonal manipulation.

B. Craniopharyngiomas are congenital, cystic suprasellar tumors thought to arise from epithelial remnants of Rathke pouch. They present with dysfunction of the optic chiasm or hypothalamic–pituitary axis as a result of tumor compression. The tumor may contain calcifications and an oily, cellular debris that causes a severe chemical meningitis if a cyst ruptures into the spinal fluid. The tumor is histologically benign and can be cured by total resection. Unfortunately, this is often not possible, and RT may be required for tumor control.

C. Pituitary adenoma. Adenomas of the pituitary gland can be either secreting or nonsecreting tumors. Secretory tumors can cause acromegaly (growth hormone), infertility and galactorrhea (prolactin), or Cushing disease (adrenocorticotropic hormone, ACTH). These tumors are often microadenomas (<1 cm), but are usually visualized on MRI. Nonsecretory tumors are typically macroadenomas (>1 cm) and cause bitemporal hemianopsia because of optic chiasm compression, pituitary apoplexy resulting from hemorrhage into the tumor, or hypopituitarism. Treatment of either micro- or macroadenomas may consist of surgical resection, usually by the transsphenoidal route. However, secretory tumors may be treated pharmacologically: prolactinomas with cabergoline and growth hormone–secreting tumors with somatostatin or an analog such as octreotide. Recurrent tumors may require RT.

D. **Vestibular schwannoma (acoustic neuroma).** Vestibular schwannomas arise from the vestibular branch of the eighth cranial nerve. Initial symptoms are sensorineural hearing loss, tinnitus, and vertigo. Involvement of adjacent neural structures can cause facial weakness, facial numbness, dysphagia, and ataxia. On contrast-enhanced MRI scans, these tumors are seen as a homogeneous, densely enhancing mass that follows the eighth cranial nerve into the internal auditory canal; the diagnosis is usually clear on MRI. Management depends on the extent of hearing loss and whether bilateral tumors are present, but therapeutic options include surgical resection and focal irradiation with radiosurgery. Bilateral acoustic neuromas constitute a diagnosis of neurofibromatosis II. Spinal schwannomas cause a radiculomyelopathy and can be cured by total resection. Rarely, these tumors can have sarcomatous degeneration.

IX. SPECIAL CLINICAL PROBLEMS

A. **Seizures.** Seizures occur in about 25% to 30% of all brain tumor patients. Once a patient has had a seizure, they are maintained on anticonvulsants. The choice of agent usually depends on the common side effect profile and potential for drug interactions. Anticonvulsants that induce hepatic enzymes (e.g., phenytoin, carbamazepine) can enhance chemotherapy metabolism, resulting in subtherapeutic serum levels. Although frequently administered, *prophylactic anticonvulsants are ineffective in the prevention of seizures in brain tumor patients who have not had a seizure.* They should be avoided.

   1. **Phenytoin (Dilantin)**
      a. **Loading dose** is 18 mg/kg (usually 1 g for adults). Maintenance doses are 5 mg/kg per day (usually 300 mg/day for adults). Phenytoin given orally can be given once or twice a day because it has a half-life of about 24 hours. For intravenous administration, phenytoin is given in the form of fosphenytoin in *phenytoin-equivalent* (PE) doses (18 mg PE/kg loading; 5 mg PE/kg per day in divided doses maintenance) at a rate not to exceed 150 mg PE/minute. Parenteral loading of phenytoin should be performed with electrocardiogram, blood pressure, and respiratory monitoring.
      b. **Therapeutic levels** are 10 to 20 mcg/mL, but this is a general guide. Many patients have well-controlled seizures with a level <10 mcg/mL, and others do not experience toxicity with a level >20 mcg/mL. Dose adjustments should be made gradually, because phenytoin has zero-order kinetics, and small increases in the dose can sometimes result in large increases in serum levels.
      c. **Side effects** of phenytoin include cognitive impairment, hirsutism, megaloblastic anemia, leukopenia, and hepatic dysfunction. Allergic reactions manifesting as a rash occur in about 20% and can proceed to a Stevens-Johnson reaction. Toxicity is manifested by nystagmus, ataxia, and lethargy.
   2. **Phenobarbital** is rarely used because of its sedating effects. The loading dose is 20 mg/kg and may be administered up to a rate of 100 mg/minute. Maintenance doses are 1 to 5 mg/kg per day, usually 90 to 120 mg/day in adults, and may be given before bedtime as a single dose. Therapeutic levels are 15 to 40 mcg/mL. Sedation is the primary side effect.
   3. **Carbamazepine** is often a first-line agent in the treatment of seizures. It is available only in an oral form, and doses must be slowly increased to maintenance levels because rapid loading is not tolerated. Doses range from 7 to 15 mg/kg per day, divided into twice-daily or thrice-daily fractions, typically 600 to 1,000 mg/day for an adult. Therapeutic serum levels range from 6 to 12 mcg/mL. Side

effects include granulocytopenia, diplopia, nystagmus, fatigue, hepatic dysfunction, and allergic dermatitis. Monitoring of blood counts is required.

4. **Valproate (Depakote)** is administered orally at a dose of 15 mg/kg per day divided into thrice-daily doses and elevated by 5 mg/kg per day as needed to control seizures; the therapeutic level is 50 to 100 mcg/mL. Valproate is available as an IV preparation and is usually the second choice after phenytoin for a patient unable to take oral medication. Side effects include hepatic and pancreatic toxicity, thrombocytopenia, nausea, tremor, and alopecia. Monitoring of LFTs is required.

5. **Levetiracetam (Keppra)** is used with increasing frequency as a first-line antiepileptic. It is available in oral and IV preparations. Doses start at 500 mg b.i.d. and can be increased to 1,500 mg b.i.d. The dose is determined clinically as serum levels are unreliable.

6. **Newer anticonvulsants,** such as gabapentin, lamotrigine, topiramate, and vigabatrin, can be used at the discretion of the treating physician. Most of these agents do not induce the hepatic microsomal system.

B. **Hydrocephalus** can result from obstruction of CSF pathways, especially with intraventricular tumors or tumors in the upper brainstem. Patients with hydrocephalus present with headaches, nausea, vomiting, gait ataxia, urinary incontinence, and progressive lethargy. Large ventricles above the level of obstruction can be diagnosed with a noncontrast CT scan. Communicating hydrocephalus may also develop in patients treated for a brain tumor; one sees progressive ventricular enlargement on serial neuroimaging. Treatment of both forms of hydrocephalus consists of placement of a ventriculoperitoneal shunt.

C. **Radiation necrosis** can result from RT and is common after high-dose and interstitial irradiation. Clinically and radiographically, it is indistinguishable from tumor recurrence. Positron emission tomography (PET) or magnetic resonance spectroscopy (MRS) may be useful in distinguishing tumor recurrence from radiation necrosis. Radiation necrosis can be treated with dexamethasone, but surgical debulking is often required to relieve mass effect and to provide a definite tissue diagnosis.

D. **Deep-vein thrombosis (DVT)** occurs in about 20% of patients with high-grade gliomas and is optimally treated with anticoagulation. Although some physicians are concerned that anticoagulation poses increased risk for intracranial hemorrhage into a brain tumor, studies have not substantiated this risk. Therefore, anticoagulation is safe in this population. Inferior vena cava filters should be avoided because patients develop chronic venous stasis and edema and may develop pulmonary emboli from the filter. However, patients with DVT who are scheduled for craniotomy must be treated with a filter.

E. **Herniation** results from progressive mass effect in patients with large, edematous tumors. Herniation can be central in the case of midline tumors and hydrocephalus, uncal in the case of hemispheric lesions, or tonsillar in the case of posterior fossa tumors. Once recognized, herniation is an emergency that must be treated to decrease intracranial pressure. These interventions will reduce intracranial pressure, but they will only temporize until definitive treatment is initiated. The emergency methods include the following:

1. Elevation of the head of the bed
2. Hyperventilation to a P_{CO_2} of about 30 mm Hg
3. Creation of an osmotic gradient by administration of mannitol at 1 g/kg IV (usually 50 to 100 g in adults) or hypertonic saline
4. Dexamethasone, up to 100 mg IV

Suggested Reading

DeAngelis LM. Brain tumors. *N Engl J Med* 2001;344:114.

DeAngelis LM, Gutin PH, Leibel SA, et al. *Intracranial Tumors: Diagnosis and Treatment.* London: Martin Dunitz; 2001.

Forsyth PA, Weaver S, Fulton D, et al. Prophylactic anticonvulsants in patients with brain tumour. *Can J Neurol Sci* 2003;30:106.

Intergroup Radiation Therapy Oncology Group Trial 9402; Cairncross G, Berkey B, Shaw E, et al. Phase III trial of chemotherapy plus radiotherapy compared with radiotherapy alone for pure and mixed anaplastic oligodendroglioma: Intergroup Radiation Therapy Oncology Group Trial 9402. *J Clin Oncol* 2006;24(18):2707.

Packer RJ, Gajjar A, Vezina G, et al. Phase III study of craniospinal radiation therapy followed by adjuvant chemotherapy for newly diagnosed average-risk medulloblastoma. *J Clin Oncol* 2006;24(25):4202.

Padovani L, Sunyach MP, Perol D, et al. Common strategy for adult and pediatric medulloblastoma: a multicenter series of 253 adults. *Int J Radiat Oncol Biol Phys* 2007;68(2):433.

Stupp R, Mason WP, van den Bent MJ, et al. Radiotherapy plus concomitant and adjuvant temozolomide for glioblastoma. *N Engl J Med* 2005;352(10):987.

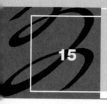

ENDOCRINE NEOPLASMS
Harold E. Carlson

15

I. **GENERAL CONSIDERATIONS.** Cancers of endocrine glands constitute <1% of all malignancies. Most malignant neoplasms derived from endocrine organs are not associated with clinical endocrinopathies, although several do produce unique syndromes and biochemical markers.

 A. **Steroid hormones** are usually produced by the tissue that normally produces them, such as the adrenal cortex and gonads, whether that tissue is healthy or cancerous. Occasionally, human chorionic gonadotropin (hCG)-producing tumors of the placenta or other organs (e.g., lung) have the capacity to transform androgens into estrogens. The mechanism of action for most steroid hormones depends on specific receptors in the target cell cytoplasm or nucleus.

 B. **Peptide hormones and catecholamines** appear to act at the cell surface, where they attach to specific receptors and modify intracellular concentrations of cyclic nucleotides, calcium, and kinases.

  1. **Amine precursor uptake and decarboxylation (APUD) cells** are theoretically derived from embryonic neuroectoderm (melanocytes, thyroid C cells, adrenal medulla, paraspinal ganglia, argentaffin cells of the intestine). These cells produce hormone mediators such as serotonin, catecholamines, histamine, and kinins. Neoplasia of these tissues gives rise to carcinoid tumors, pheochromocytoma, and medullary thyroid cancer; these tumors may also produce peptide hormones (e.g., adrenocorticotropic hormone [ACTH] and vasoactive intestinal polypeptide [VIP]) in addition to their natural products. Other peptide-producing endocrine tissues (e.g., parathyroid, pancreatic islet) demonstrate some APUD characteristics, even though they may not be derived from neuroectoderm.

  2. **Peptide hormones,** such as ACTH, hCG, and calcitonin, are produced by a wide variety of neoplastic tissues that may or may not normally synthesize detectable amounts of these hormones. Many of these peptides are synthesized as a *prehormone*. A segment of prehormone is enzymatically cleaved to form a storage molecule, a *prohormone*. The prohormone is further cleaved into the active hormone, which is secreted into the blood.

  3. **Gastrointestinal hormones,** such as insulin, glucagon, somatostatin, VIP, and gastrin, are normally produced by gut endocrine cells and the pancreatic islets. Neoplasms of these tissues commonly produce one or more of these hormones; gut hormones are also normally produced in the brain and may be products of a wide variety of other neoplasms.

 C. **Multiple endocrine neoplasias** (MEN) are inherited, Mendelian-dominant, endocrine tumor syndromes. Two categories of the syndrome are recognized.

  1. **MEN-1** (Wermer syndrome; menin tumor-suppressor gene located at chromosome 11q13)

   a. **Pituitary tumors** (acromegaly, nonfunctioning adenoma, prolactinoma, or ACTH-producing adenoma)

   b. **Pancreatic islet cell tumors,** including gastrinoma, VIPoma, glucagonoma, and insulinoma

   c. **Parathyroid hyperplasia**

  2. **MEN-2.** Medullary carcinoma of the thyroid is present in all patients with this syndrome. Cushing syndrome may develop as a consequence of ectopic ACTH production by medullary carcinoma or pheochromocytoma.

   a. MEN-2A (Sipple syndrome; *ret* oncogene located at chromosome 10q11)
      (1) Medullary carcinoma of the thyroid
      (2) Pheochromocytoma (bilateral)
      (3) Parathyroid hyperplasia
   b. MEN-2B (*ret* oncogene located at 10q11)
      (1) Medullary carcinoma of the thyroid
      (2) Pheochromocytoma (bilateral)
      (3) Multiple mucosal ganglioneuromas (lips, tongue, eyelids)
      (4) Marfanoid body habitus, high-arched palate, pes cavus, diverticulae, and sugar-loaf skull often accompany the endocrine abnormalities in MEN-2B.

II. CARCINOID TUMORS
   A. Epidemiology and etiology. Carcinoid cancers represent <1% of visceral malignancies. The cause of these tumors is unknown, but they may be associated with MEN-1.
   B. Pathology and natural history
      1. Primary tumor. Carcinoid tumors belong to the APUD system of tumors (see section I.B.1). The primary tumors are usually small and most commonly arise in the small intestine. They may also develop in the stomach, colorectum, lung, ovary, and rarely other organs. Appendiceal carcinoids are common but are usually of no clinical significance.
      2. Metastases tend to develop primarily in the liver. Bone metastases, which are often osteoblastic, also occur. Carcinoid metastases are indolent or slowly progressive and evolve over many years. Carcinoid tumors tend to produce desmoplastic responses, which can result in mesenteric fibrosis and bowel obstruction ("parachute intestine"). Hormonally inactive tumors usually cause death by replacing hepatic tissue, which leads to liver failure.
      3. Tumor products. Hormonally active tumors occur in 30% to 50% of patients and produce a variety of potentially lethal complications (*carcinoid syndrome*).
         a. Small intestine carcinoids never produce the carcinoid syndrome in the absence of liver metastases; the responsible hormonal mediators are degraded in their first pass through the liver.
         b. Benign and malignant lung carcinoids occur with about equal frequency; those that produce the carcinoid syndrome are malignant. Lung carcinoids can potentially produce hormonal effects without metastasizing; active tumor products pass directly into the circulation without being filtered by the liver. Most patients with endocrinologically active lung carcinoids, however, also have liver metastases. Bronchial carcinoids that produce ACTH or growth hormone–releasing hormone (GH-RH) may be benign, and Cushing syndrome or acromegaly may be the only endocrine manifestation.
         c. Symptomatic ovarian carcinoids are rarely associated with liver metastases.
         d. Humoral mediators of the carcinoid syndrome are serotonin, histamine, kinins, prostaglandins, and other hormonally active tumor products.
            (1) The major source of serotonin is dietary tryptophan, which normally is mostly metabolized to nicotinic acid. In carcinoid syndrome, tryptophan metabolism is directed to the production of serotonin (Fig. 15.1). Most patients with carcinoid syndrome develop chemical evidence of niacin deficiency, and some may develop clinically recognizable pellagra.
            (2) Other hormones and hormone metabolites that are found in some patients with carcinoid include calcitonin, gastrin, GH-RH, and ACTH. These substances may or may not produce clinical syndromes, but they should be searched for in patients with carcinoid and serum calcium abnormalities, peptic ulcer, acromegaly, or Cushing syndrome.

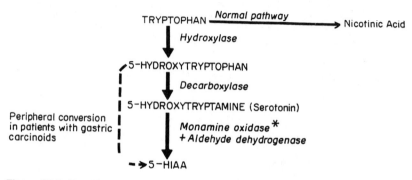

Figure 15.1. Hepatic metabolism of tryptophan and serotonin in carcinoid syndrome. The normal pathway (*thin arrow*) of tryptophan metabolism is impaired in carcinoid syndrome, resulting in excessive production of serotonin. *Monamine oxidase inhibitors interfere with the metabolism of serotonin and are contraindicated in patients with carcinoid syndrome. 5-HIAA, 5-hydroxyindoleacetic acid.

C. Diagnosis

1. **Symptoms: Endocrinologically inactive carcinoids.** Most carcinoid tumors are endocrinologically inactive. Patients who have these tumors may have appendicitis, bowel obstruction, or a painful, enlarged liver that results from metastases. Bronchial carcinoids may produce cough, hemoptysis, or frequent pulmonary infections.

2. **Symptoms: Endocrinologically active carcinoids**
   a. **Humoral mediators** produce attacks of flushing, diarrhea, hypotension, light-headedness, and bronchospasm in various combinations. Attacks may be spontaneous or precipitated by emotional stress, alcohol ingestion, exercise, eating, or vigorous palpation of a liver that contains metastatic deposits.
   b. **Heart failure** from valvular lesions commonly occurs in patients with long-standing carcinoid symptoms and appears to be related to serotonin excess. Ileal carcinoids produce tricuspid valve stenosis and insufficiency and pulmonary valve stenosis. Bronchial carcinoids with venous drainage into the left atrium can produce mitral valve disease.

3. **Physical findings**
   a. **The characteristic flush** differs somewhat according to the site of the primary tumor.
      (1) **Ileal carcinoid.** Purple flush involves the upper trunk and face and usually lasts <30 minutes.
      (2) **Bronchial carcinoid.** Deep, dusky purple flush over the entire body.
      (3) **Gastric carcinoid.** Generalized urticarialike, pruritic, and painful wheals, probably related to histamine production
   b. **Chronic skin changes** involve repeated episodes of flushing, especially with bronchial carcinoids, which cause thickening of the facial features, telangiectasis, enlargement of the salivary glands, and leonine facies. A pellagrous skin rash characterized by photosensitivity, atrophy of the lingual mucosa, and thickened skin may develop.
   c. Right heart failure with evidence of tricuspid valve disease
   d. Hepatomegaly
   e. Cushing syndrome and, occasionally, acromegaly

4. **Laboratory studies in all patients**
   a. Routine blood tests, particularly liver function tests (LFTs)
   b. Liver ultrasound or CT scan
   c. Chest CT scan to search for bronchial carcinoids
   d. Upper gastrointestinal barium series or endoscopy
   e. Nuclear scanning using a radiolabeled somatostatin analog

f. A histologic diagnosis is essential for management. Biopsy the site that is associated with the least morbidity and that has been determined by noninvasive tests to be probably affected.

5. **Laboratory studies** in patients with symptoms have traditionally consisted of 24-hour urine collections for 5-hydroxyindoleacic acid (5-HIAA), particularly in patients with midgut carcinoids. Serotonin is a product of tryptophan metabolism and is metabolized to 5-HIAA (Fig. 15.1). Fasting plasma 5-HIAA has been shown to be at least as sensitive and specific as urinary 5-HIAA. Platelet serotonin measurements may also be useful, particularly in foregut carcinoids, in which 5-HIAA production may be minimal.

   a. **Causes of elevated urine or plasma 5-HIAA** include the following:
      (1) Carcinoid syndrome
      (2) Other tumors that produce 5-HIAA include biliary, pancreatic islet, and medullary thyroid cancers.
      (3) Dietary intake of nuts, bananas, avocados, or pineapples within 48 hours of urine collection or 8 hours of plasma sampling.
      (4) Medications that must be stopped 1 day before 5-HIAA measurement include mephenesin and guaifenesin.
      (5) Malabsorption syndromes (celiac disease, Whipple disease, and tropical sprue) rarely increase 5-HIAA urine excretion above 20 mg per 24 hours.

   b. **Causes of falsely low 5-HIAA excretion.** Phenothiazines interfere with the color reaction of the urine test and must be stopped 2 to 3 days before the collection of urine.

   c. **Interpretation.** A urine level of 5-HIAA >9 mg per 24 hours in patients without malabsorption or >30 mg per 24 hours in patients with malabsorption is pathognomonic for carcinoid unless interfering foods or drugs have been ingested. The magnitude of 5-HIAA excretion in the urine roughly corresponds to the tumor volume; 5-HIAA excretion can also be used to monitor therapy. Normal values for plasma 5-HIAA are laboratory-dependent.

   d. **Chromogranin A (CgA)** is a soluble protein found in secretory granules in a variety of neuroendocrine cell types. Plasma CgA is elevated in nearly all patients with carcinoid tumors, but is nonspecific, since it is also elevated in patients with other neuroendocrine tumors such as pancreatic islet tumors, small cell lung cancer, medullary thyroid cancer, and pheochromocytoma. Serum CgA may also be elevated in patients receiving proton-pump inhibitors.

D. **Management.** The most important principle of management of metastatic carcinoid tumors is therapeutic restraint. These patients often survive for >10 years without antitumor treatment. Patients with endocrinologically active tumors are at especially high risk for complications from any procedure requiring anesthesia. Therapy should be focused on controlling the endocrine symptoms.

1. **Surgery** is useful for patients with localized primary carcinoids or metastatic tumors that produce obstruction. For patients with incidental appendiceal carcinoids that are ≤2 cm in diameter (which rarely metastasize), appendectomy is adequate treatment.

   Partial hepatectomy has been recommended by some physicians, particularly if the metastases are confined to one lobe of the liver. The mortality rate of hepatectomy and the long natural history of the disease, however, often dissuade the physician from recommending the procedure. Palliation of liver metastases may also be accomplished with cryosurgery or radiofrequency ablation.

2. **Hepatic artery occlusion** performed surgically or by catheterization and embolization of hepatic metastases has been successfully used to palliate endocrine symptoms or pain. Objective regression of manifestations occurs in 60% of patients for a median of 4 months. Side effects of arterial occlusion include fever, nausea, and LFT abnormalities. Both the response rate and the median duration of response appear to improve when occlusion is followed by sequenced chemotherapy (see section II.D.4).

3. **Radiation therapy (RT)** is used to palliate liver pain caused by far-advanced metastatic disease unresponsive to other treatments. However, carcinoid tumors are relatively radioresistant.

4. **Chemotherapy** is used late in the course of disease for treatment of symptomatic metastases and for patients with severe endocrine symptoms that do not respond satisfactorily to pharmacologic maneuvers (see section II.D.5). There is no general agreement on when (or even if) chemotherapy should be started in patients with malignant carcinoid. Single-agent therapy with 5-fluorouracil (5-FU), streptozocin, cyclophosphamide, doxorubicin (Adriamycin), dacarbazine, or interferon-α (IFN-α) has been associated with response rates of about 25%, with variable median durations of response. Endocrine symptoms may be palliated, but the effect of chemotherapy on survival is not known.

   a. **Combination chemotherapy regimens** have not clearly had a beneficial effect compared with single agents. The largest experience in the treatment of metastatic carcinoid tumors has been gained with the combination of 5-FU and streptozocin administered every 42 days (see section II.D.4.b for dosages). Cisplatin in combination with etoposide is useful for anaplastic forms of neuroendocrine carcinomas. Combinations of IFN-α (3 to 10 million units 3 times weekly) and octreotide have been more effective than monotherapy with either agent alone; however, autoimmune thyroid disease develops in some patients on long-term treatment with IFN, and its associated flulike syndrome may be problematic.

   b. **Sequenced chemotherapy after hepatic arterial occlusion** is initiated about 3 weeks after the procedure, which is performed for symptomatic hepatic metastases from carcinoid tumors or islet cell carcinomas. Substantial or complete relief from the endocrine syndromes is achieved in about 80% of selected patients, with a median duration of 18 months.

   The following two regimens are alternated every 4 to 5 weeks until the patient has stabilized with maximum tumor regression (usually about 6 months):

   (1) Doxorubicin (60 mg/m^2 IV on day 1) and dacarbazine (250 mg/m^2 IV daily for 5 days)

   (2) Streptozocin (500 mg/m^2) and 5-FU (400 mg/m^2), both given daily IV for 5 days

5. **Pharmacologic management.** It is probably not possible to control the symptoms of carcinoid syndrome completely with aggressive dietary tryptophan restriction and high-dose antiserotonin drugs alone.

   a. **Octreotide,** a somatostatin analog, reduces the production of 5-HIAA and ameliorates symptoms in about 90% of patients. The drug may have a tumoristatic effect as well. The dosage is usually 100 to 600 mcg SC daily in two to four divided doses. A long-acting depot form of octreotide is also available; the dose is 10 to 30 mg IM every 28 days, often supplemented by SC injections.

   b. **Hypotension,** the most life-threatening complication of carcinoid syndrome, is mediated by kinins (and perhaps prostaglandins) and can be precipitated by catecholamines. β-Adrenergic drugs (e.g., dopamine, epinephrine) must be strictly avoided because they may aggravate hypotension. Pure α-adrenergic (methoxamine, norepinephrine) and vasoconstrictive (angiotensin) agents are preferred for treating hypotension in carcinoid syndrome.

   (1) Methoxamine (Vasoxyl) is given IM at a dose of 0.5 mL (10 mg), or IV at a dose of 0.25 mL (5 mg) over 1 to 2 minutes (using a tuberculin syringe). The dose is repeated as necessary to maintain the blood pressure.

   (2) Angiotensin amide (Hypertensin), rather than methoxamine, is recommended by some anesthesiologists.

   (3) Corticosteroids may prevent episodes of hypotension.

   c. **Flushing** is mediated by kinins and histamine and may respond to several agents, including the following:

   (1) Prochlorperazine (Compazine), 10 mg PO 4 times daily

(2) Phenoxybenzamine (Dibenzyline), 10 to 20 mg PO twice daily

(3) Cyproheptadine (Periactin), 4 to 6 mg PO 4 times daily

(4) Prednisone, 20 to 40 mg PO daily, is useful for flushing as a result of bronchial carcinoids and occasionally for patients with other kinds of carcinoids.

(5) The combined use of H_1- and H_2-receptor antagonists has been effective in patients with carcinoid flush and documented hypersecretion of histamine. Diphenhydramine hydrochloride (Benadryl), 50 mg PO 4 times daily, plus cimetidine (Tagamet), 300 mg PO 4 times daily, have been used with success in some patients.

(6) Methyldopa (Aldomet) is useful in some patients.

(7) Monoamine oxidase inhibitors *are contraindicated* in carcinoid syndrome because they block serotonin catabolism and can aggravate symptoms (Fig. 15.1).

d. Bronchospasm is mediated by histamine and managed with aminophylline. Adrenergic agents, such as isoproterenol, do not appear to worsen bronchospasm for carcinoid and may also be used, although they may cause hypotension.

e. Diarrhea is mediated by serotonin and is often difficult to control. A recommended sequence for treatment before the use of octreotide is as follows:

(1) Belladonna alkaloids and phenobarbital combination (Donnagel-PG), 15 mL every 3 hours as needed

(2) Loperamide (Imodium) or diphenoxylate and atropine (Lomotil) as needed.

(3) Cyproheptadine (Periactin), 4 to 6 mg PO 4 times daily

(4) Methysergide maleate (Sansert), started at 8 to 12 mg/day and gradually increased to 20 to 22 mg/day if needed

(5) Ondansetron, 8 mg PO 3 times daily

f. Preparation for anesthesia. Patients with carcinoid syndrome are at high risk for the development of flushing and hypotensive episodes during surgery. Stimulation of adrenergic hormone release and use of drugs that induce hypotension (morphine, succinylcholine, and curare) must be minimized.

(1) Preoperative period. Patients should be premedicated with cyproheptadine, 4 to 8 mg PO. Methotrimeprazine, 10 mg IM, is given 1 hour before surgery. Methotrimeprazine is a phenothiazine with amnesic, analgesic, antihistaminic, and catechol blocker properties. This drug permits the use of lower doses of anesthetics and allows the avoidance of morphine.

(2) During surgery. Aminophylline can be used for bronchoconstriction, methotrimeprazine for flushing, and methoxamine for hypotension. Rapid, dramatic improvement has been reported after administration of intravenous somatostatin.

E. Special clinical problems associated with carcinoid syndrome

1. Bowel obstruction may result from dense fibrosis of the mesentery. Surgical relief is often impossible. Patients may improve with simple nasogastric decompression and fluid replacement.

2. Right ventricular failure results from tricuspid and pulmonic valve lesions. These lesions develop with far-advanced carcinoid syndrome, which has a poor prognosis independent of the heart lesions. Because of the high surgical risk in these patients, valve replacement may not be warranted. Heart failure should be medically managed with diuretics.

3. Pellagrous skin lesions may be treated with daily oral vitamin preparations containing 1 to 2 mg of niacin.

III. THYROID CANCER

A. Epidemiology and etiology

1. Incidence. Thyroid cancer accounts for about 2% of visceral malignancies; there are 33,000 new cases and 1,500 cancer deaths in the United States annually.

The risk increases with age. Women are affected more than men in a ratio of 3:2.

2. **Radiation exposure.** Radiation fallout and RT given over the neck region in intermediate doses (<2,000 cGy) for benign conditions (such as acne in teenagers, or enlarged tonsils or thymus glands in children) increase the risk for thyroid cancer, particularly the papillary type.

   a. The lag time between radiation exposure and the onset of thyroid cancer averages 25 years but ranges from 5 to 50 years. Most patients younger than 20 years of age with thyroid cancer have a history of neck irradiation.

   b. About 4% of patients with thyroid cancer have a history of radiation to the neck. Between 5% and 10% of patients who have a history of neck irradiation develop thyroid cancer; 25% have an abnormal thyroid by palpation.

   c. Thyroid cancers after neck irradiation are often multifocal but have an indolent course and a prognosis similar to that of spontaneous tumors.

   d. Neck irradiation also increases the risk for hyperparathyroidism and parotid gland tumors.

3. **Hereditary factors.** Medullary cancer of the thyroid may arise sporadically or as a dominantly inherited syndrome of MEN-2 (see section I.C.2). Thyroid tumors (including papillary and follicular carcinomas), as well as breast neoplasms, also occur frequently in Cowden multiple hamartoma syndrome and in familial adenomatous polyposis (including Gardner syndrome). Several oncogenes and tumor-suppressor genes have been implicated in the pathogenesis of thyroid neoplasms.

4. **Thyroid-stimulating hormone (TSH).** An increased risk for thyroid cancer may be present in patients with chronic TSH elevation, such as patients with congenital defects in thyroid hormone formation.

B. **Pathology and natural history.** The more aggressive histologic subtypes of thyroid cancer tend to affect older patients.

1. **Papillary cancers** (75% of thyroid cancers in adults) affect younger patients. Histologically, the tumor cells may be arranged in either papillary or follicular patterns; the diagnosis of papillary carcinoma is based on nuclear features, not on the presence or absence of follicles. Psammoma bodies may be present in histologic sections in about 40% of these tumors. Regional lymph nodes that drain the thyroid are involved in half of patients. Distant metastases to lungs, bone, skin, and other organs occur late, if at all.

2. **Follicular cancers** (15% of thyroid cancers) have a peak incidence at 40 to 50 years of age. They tend to invade blood vessels and to metastasize hematogenously to visceral sites, particularly bone. Lymph node metastases are relatively rare, especially compared with papillary cancers.

3. **Anaplastic giant and spindle cell cancers** (2% of thyroid cancers) occur most often in patients older than 60 years of age. Anaplastic thyroid cancers are aggressive cancers, which rapidly invade surrounding local tissues and metastasize to distant organs.

4. **Medullary thyroid cancers** (5% to 10% of thyroid cancers) secrete calcitonin. ACTH, histaminase, and an unidentified substance that produces diarrhea may also be secreted by these tumors. Amyloid may be seen on histologic examination. Metastases are mostly found in the neck and mediastinal lymph nodes and may calcify. Widespread visceral metastases occur late.

5. **Hürthle cell cancer** is a variant of follicular carcinoma and has a relatively aggressive metastatic course.

6. **Other tumors** found in the thyroid include lymphomas (3% to 5% of all thyroid cancers), a variety of soft tissue sarcomas, and metastatic cancers from kidney, colon and other primary sites. Small cell cancers of the thyroid are rare, are histologically similar to lymphoma, and spread both to lymph nodes and to distant sites.

C. **Diagnosis**

1. **Symptoms and signs**

   a. Symptoms. Some patients with thyroid cancer complain of an enlarging mass in the neck. Hoarseness may be the result of recurrent laryngeal nerve paralysis. Neck pain or dysphagia occasionally is a complaint. Patients without symptoms may have thyroid cancer discovered at thyroidectomy done for other reasons or as an incidental finding in the course of radiologic examinations of the neck (see section III.C.3.a).

   b. Physical findings. Thyroid cancer may be found on routine physical examination as a mass in the thyroid or in the midline up to the base of the tongue (thyroglossal duct remnant). Thyroid masses <1 cm in diameter often are not palpable. Most patients have a single palpable nodule; others have a normal, multinodular, or diffusely enlarged thyroid gland. Cervical lymph nodes are frequently palpable. Anaplastic cancer is often manifested by obvious masses infiltrating the skin and soft tissues of the neck or by respiratory distress.

2. Laboratory studies

   a. Routine studies. Chest radiographs and serum alkaline phosphatase levels should be obtained to look for evidence of metastatic disease in the lung, liver, or bone. Liver and bone scans and selected skeletal radiographs are indicated when the alkaline phosphatase level is elevated.

   b. Thyroid scans may be obtained in nonpregnant patients with palpable abnormalities of the thyroid who have a suppressed serum TSH, in order to document the existence of a "hot" nodule. Nonfunctional "cold" nodules are found in 90% of patients with palpable nodules, both benign and malignant, but only about 10% of cold nodules prove to be cancer. Routine isotope scanning of all thyroid nodules is therefore not indicated unless serum TSH is low.

   c. Thyroid ultrasonography is useful in determining the size and location of a nodule, diagnosing cystic lesions, detecting nonpalpable nodules or lymphadenopathy, and documenting the presence of features suggestive of malignancy (e.g., microcalcifications within the nodule). Purely cystic lesions, found in about 10% of patients with palpable nodules, are reported to be malignant in <1% of cases. Benign and malignant lesions cannot be confidently distinguished by ultrasonography if they contain mixed solid and cystic components or are entirely solid.

   d. Serum calcitonin assay. Patients with a family history of medullary thyroid cancer or other features of MEN-2 should have serum calcitonin measured. Normal basal values may require a calcitonin stimulation test using pentagastrin or calcium infusion. Patients with elevated serum calcitonin require neck exploration regardless of findings on physical examination or sonography.

3. Thyroid gland biopsy

   a. Needle aspiration biopsy is invaluable for cytologic diagnosis of thyroid nodules and for preventing unnecessary thyroidectomies. Many authorities recommend needle biopsy as the first step in evaluation of any thyroid lump. The accuracy of needle biopsy of the thyroid is >90% for benign lesions; the false-negative rate is 5% to 10%. Only about 10% of nodules are cancerous. Roughly, if 100 patients with nodules underwent needle biopsy rather than thyroidectomy, and if patients with clearly benign histopathology were excluded from surgery, one cancer would be missed, nine cancers would be appropriately resected, and 10 patients with benign lesions would have undergone unnecessary surgery. Therefore, the needle biopsy saves 80 of 100 patients from unnecessary surgery at the expense of missing one cancer, which is usually indolent and can be detected later. Patients with nonpalpable nodules >1.5 cm in diameter found on radiologic examinations should generally undergo sonogram-guided needle aspiration biopsy, as should those patients with smaller nodules that appear suspicious for malignancy on sonography.

   b. Open biopsy. Nodules interpreted as suspicious on needle biopsy should be removed.

D. Survival and prognostic factors

   1. Papillary adenocarcinomas. Decreased survival is not noted when compared with age-matched populations until 12 years after the diagnosis. Only 3% to 12% of patients die as a result of thyroid cancer. Even with distant metastases, patients often survive many years without therapy. The raw 10-year survival rate is 95% for patients <40 years of age and 75% for patients >40 years of age.

   a. Factors that have no adverse effect on prognosis

   (1) Gender

   (2) Radiation-related neoplasms

   (3) Regional lymph node metastases (increased recurrences, but normal survival)

   b. Factors that adversely affect prognosis, which both increase the recurrence rate and decrease the survival rate

   (1) Age >40 years

   (2) Size of nodule >5 cm (compared with <2.5 cm)

   (3) Tumor extends through the thyroid capsule

   (4) Presence of symptoms, such as hoarseness or dysphagia

   (5) Distant metastases

   (6) Residual tumor fails to take up [131]I

   (7) Subtotal thyroidectomy (compared with total or "near-total" thyroidectomy) for tumors >1.5 cm in diameter

   (8) Probably, postoperative therapy with thyroid hormone alone (compared with thyroid hormone and ^{131}I)

2. Follicular adenocarcinoma without vascular invasion has essentially the same survival rate as papillary carcinoma for age-matched populations. With significant vascular invasion, the 10-year survival rate drops to 35%.

3. Medullary carcinoma without lymph node involvement is nearly always cured with surgery. With lymph node involvement, the 5-year survival rate decreases to 45%.

4. Anaplastic carcinoma. Nearly all patients die within 6 to 8 months.

5. Thyroid lymphoma. Depending on the stage and histologic subtype, 5-year survival is 35% to 80%.

E. Management. No uniform opinion exists regarding the management of indolent varieties of thyroid cancer.

1. Surgery. Total or near-total thyroidectomy is the treatment of choice for all types of thyroid cancer. Overall, subtotal thyroidectomy is associated with double the recurrence rate and a lower survival rate than total thyroidectomy for papillary and follicular cancers. Subtotal thyroidectomy or lobectomy may be sufficient, however, for low-risk patients with small tumors (<1 cm). Medullary cancer of the thyroid is often bilateral, and total thyroidectomy is imperative.

   a. Neck nodes that appear to be involved clinically or on sonography should be removed. Routine radical or modified radical neck dissection, however, does not improve the rate of survival or recurrence, except in medullary carcinoma, and is responsible for increasing the rate of major complications. Selective neck dissection may be pursued, depending on the extent of disease.

   b. Complications. The major complications of thyroidectomy are hypoparathyroidism and vocal cord paralysis; death is rare. Combinations of these problems and other complications occur in 5% to 10% of patients subjected to total thyroidectomy; the incidence is doubled to tripled if neck dissection is added to the procedure.

2. Thyroxine. TSH suppression after thyroidectomy is essential because TSH stimulates the growth of most papillary and follicular tumors. Thyroxine is given in a dose sufficient to suppress serum TSH to low-normal or subnormal levels. Patients must be monitored for clinical signs of hyperthyroidism and the dose of thyroxine decreased to keep the patient clinically euthyroid. If ^{131}I is given, thyroxine is begun afterward.

3. Radioactive iodine. Fears of the leukemogenic potential of ^{131}I have abated because little increase in the incidence of acute leukemia has been found in many long-term studies. [131]I given postoperatively (usually about 30 to 100 mCi) to ablate thyroid remnants may improve survival in patients with papillary and follicular tumors. Thyroid tumors that do not take up ^{131}I are not ablated by the isotope. See Chapter 2, section IV.A.

a. Indications for ^{131}I. The true value of ^{131}I is not known and is difficult to determine because the isotope has been given to patients with thyroid cancer as part of standard practice for many years. Radioactive iodine may not be necessary in all postoperative patients, particularly those with localized, small tumors (<1 cm). Clear indications for postoperative ^{131}I in patients in whom the residual tissue demonstrates uptake include the presence of the following:

(1) Multiple tumors of the thyroid gland

(2) Tumors >2.5 cm

(3) Locally invasive tumors

(4) Remote metastases

b. Administration. ^{131}I may be given either when the patient demonstrates biochemical evidence of hypothyroidism or after treating the patient with recombinant human TSH. Both methods are based on the principle that TSH stimulates ^{131}I uptake in both residual thyroid tissue and residual carcinoma and that it permits ablation of both.

(1) Waiting for hypothyroidism means allowing the patient to become hypothyroid following thyroidectomy. In most cases, patients are given triiodothyronine (T3) in a dose of 25 mcg PO twice daily for about 3 weeks to avoid prolonged hypothyroidism. T3 is then discontinued and serum TSH is measured 7 to 10 days later. If serum TSH exceeds 30 μU/mL, serum thyroglobulin is measured and ^{131}I is given.

(2) Giving TSH. Recombinant human TSH (Thyrogen) is currently approved for diagnostic use and for stimulating^{131} uptake in normal thyroid remnants following thyroidectomy. The use of Thyrogen in the therapy of residual or recurrent cancer is being investigated.

4. Patient follow-up. In most patients with papillary or follicular cancer, serum levels of thyroglobulin (Tg) correlate with residual thyroid tissue (either normal or neoplastic) and can be used as a tumor marker after all normal thyroid remnants have been ablated. Current evidence suggests that serum thyroglobulin levels >1 to 2 ng/mL in patients receiving replacement thyroxine therapy indicate the presence of residual tumor.

Following initial therapy, most patients are monitored every year by assessing the serum Tg response to injected recombinant human TSH. Patients with residual tumor may demonstrate a Tg response even when the baseline serum Tg is <1 ng/mL. An ^{131}I scan may also be performed following the administration of recombinant human TSH, but the scan is less sensitive than the Tg response in documenting the presence of residual tumor, and often adds little useful information.

Localization of residual or recurrent tumor may also be achieved using sonography of the neck, MRI scans of the neck or other areas, or PET scans; of these, careful sonography is probably the most useful. The use of iodinated contrast agents (e.g., in CT scanning) should be avoided, if possible, because the large load of stable iodine will preclude the use of ^{131}I for 1 to 3 months.

If additional treatment with radioactive iodine is to be given, thyroxine therapy is stopped and the patient is given T3 as detailed in section III.E.3.b.1. T3 is then discontinued and serum TSH is allowed to rise; when serum TSH exceeds 30 μU/mL, serum Tg is measured and ^{131}I is given. Alternatively, thyroxine therapy may be continued, and recombinant human TSH given to stimulate ^{131}I uptake; this use of rhTSH is currently investigational.

5. Relapsing disease develops in about 12% of patients who have no evidence of disease after primary therapy. Tumors that are not treatable by the combination of surgery, thyroxine therapy, and repeat doses of ^{131}I respond poorly to external-beam RT and chemotherapy.

a. External-beam RT is probably indicated as adjuvant therapy after surgery for anaplastic thyroid cancer and for patients with progressing residual cancers that do not take up ^{131}I.

b. Chemotherapy for symptomatic, widespread metastatic thyroid cancer that is unresponsive to ^{131}I has not been particularly useful.

F. Special clinical problems associated with thyroid cancer

1. **Hypoparathyroidism** complicates total thyroidectomy in 5% to 10% of patients; it is rare after ^{131}I therapy. Hypoparathyroidism is transient in the majority of cases, and serum calcium levels normalize in 1 or 2 weeks.

   a. **Acute therapy.** Serum calcium levels and clinical evidence of hypocalcemia are checked daily following surgery for 1 to 2 days. If the serum calcium level is <8 mg/dL, oral calcium citrate (1 g 4 or 5 times daily) or calcium carbonate (2.5 g/day) is given; either preparation will provide about 1 g of elemental calcium per day. If the patient manifests tetany or the serum calcium is ≤6 mg/dL, intravenous calcium gluconate or lactate is given (1 g every 4 to 6 hours) and serum calcium levels are monitored more frequently.

   b. **Chronic therapy.** Patients with persistent hypocalcemia 1 week after thyroidectomy usually require chronic calcium supplements. If hypocalcemia recurs after 2 more weeks of therapy that has been followed by weaning off supplements, vitamin D therapy is necessary as well. Calcitriol is started at a dose of 0.25 mcg/day PO; calcium citrate or carbonate is continued. Serum calcium measurements are repeated weekly; if <8 mg/dL, the calcitriol is increased in 0.25-mcg increments weekly until the calcium level has normalized. Ergocalciferol may also be used; it is much less expensive than calcitriol but may cumulate and cause vitamin D intoxication. Serum calcium should be maintained in the low-normal range (8.5 to 9.5 mg/dL) to avoid hypercalciuria.

2. **History of neck irradiation.** Patients who have a history of neck radiation exposure and no palpable abnormalities should be followed by careful annual physical examination and sonography. Radiation-induced thyroid cancer typically has an indolent course and does not necessitate anxiety-provoking management.

IV. PHEOCHROMOCYTOMA

A. Epidemiology and etiology. Pheochromocytomas (PCCs) are rare tumors; they belong to the APUD system and produce symptoms by elaborating catecholamines. Extra-adrenal pheochromocytomas are called *paragangliomas*. Certain hereditary syndromes are associated with an increased risk for PCC or paraganglioma.

1. Dominantly inherited MEN-2 (see section I.C)
2. Dominantly transmitted PCC
3. Neurofibromatosis-type 1 (von Recklinghausen disease)
4. von Hippel-Lindau disease of central nervous system and retinal hemangioblastomas, renal cell carcinomas, and polycythemia
5. Familial paraganglioma syndromes due to mutations in succinic dehydrogenase subunits B and D

   Recent reports indicate that as many as 30% of patients with an apparently sporadic pheochromocytoma may, in fact, harbor a germ line mutation in one of these genes. Screening for these mutations should be performed in patients with bilateral, extra-adrenal or malignant pheochromocytomas, patients with a family history of one of the syndromes, patients diagnosed with a pheochromocytoma before the age of 20 years, or patients with other phenotypic features of one of the hereditary syndromes.

B. Pathology and natural history

1. **PCC originates** in the adrenal medulla (90% of patients) or in the paraganglia of the sympathetic nervous system. The paraganglia range from the organ of Zuckerkandl at the aortic bifurcation to the carotid bifurcation. Bilateral PCC frequently occurs in inherited syndromes and in 10% of noninherited cases.

2. **Metastases** to bone, liver, and lung occur in 10% of cases of PCC despite a histologically benign appearance. Metastases have an indolent growth pattern but are lethal because they often produce cardiovascular complications.

3. **Hyperglycemia** is common in patients with PCC. Patients also have an increased incidence of gallstones.
4. **Paraneoplastic complications of PCC**
   a. Polycythemia
   b. Hypercalcemia
   c. Cushing syndrome
C. **Diagnosis**
   1. **Symptoms and signs**
      a. **Symptoms.** The most common symptoms of PCC are episodes of various combinations of the following: headache, sweating, tachycardia, palpitations, pallor, nausea, and feeling of impending death. Episodes may be triggered by exercise, emotional upset, alcohol ingestion, physical examination in the area of the tumor, or micturition. Vague complaints of anxiety, tremulousness, fever, dyspnea, or angina are often mistaken for psychosomatic illness or thyrotoxicosis. Weight loss is common, but one-third of patients are overweight.
      b. **Hypertension** is present in 90% of patients. The hypertension is fixed (66% of patients) or paroxysmal (33%). Orthostatic hypotension occurs in 70% of patients.
      c. **Catechol cardiomyopathy.** Patients may have cardiovascular collapse after a vague history of arrhythmias and anxiety.
      d. **Patients with small tumors,** such as might be found when screening patients with a family history of a hereditary PCC syndrome or when evaluating patients with incidentally discovered adrenal masses, are often asymptomatic; the lack of symptoms does not exclude PCC.
   2. **Selection of patients for study.** All patients with an incidentally discovered adrenal mass should be screened for PCC. Young patients without hypertension but with documented atrial arrhythmia, evidence of an unexplained hypermetabolic state, or cardiomyopathy should be screened for PCC and thyrotoxicosis. The presence of PCC should be sought in patients with hypertension and any of the following:
      a. Age <45 years (PCC is a remediable, although rare, cause of hypertension)
      b. A family history of a hereditary PCC syndrome
      c. Episodic attacks typical of the syndrome
   3. **Chemical tests**
      a. **Catecholamine metabolites.** Measurement of plasma-free metanephrines appears to be the most sensitive technique to detect PCC. Ideally, the sample should be drawn following an overnight fast and after the patient has been at rest for 15 to 30 minutes. There is a 10% to 15% false-positive rate using this assay. Twenty-four-hour urine collections for measurement of fractionated metanephrines are somewhat less sensitive (10% to 30% false-negative rate), but are more specific than plasma-free metanephrines. Plasma catecholamine assays are also available but require meticulous technique in sample collection and handling. Elevated levels of catecholamines or their metabolites suggest the presence of PCC and mandate further studies. A large number of drugs affect either the metabolism or the assay of catecholamines. All drugs, except perhaps mild tranquilizers, sedatives, and analgesics, should be discontinued 72 hours before sample collection, if possible. To control hypertension during the evaluation, diuretics, angiotensin-converting enzyme inhibitors, or angiotensin-receptor blockers may be given.
         (1) **Misleading elevations in urinary catecholamine metabolites.** Phenothiazines and tricyclic antidepressants increase levels during acute therapy but may decrease catecholamine excretion during chronic therapy. Increased excretion of metabolites is commonly found with drugs that are catecholamines (e.g., isoproterenol) or catecholamine releasers (e.g., ephedrine, amphetamines, methylxanthines). Other agents include ʟ-dopa, nalidixic acid, or para-aminosalicylic acid (which affect the vanillylmandelic acid [VMA] level) and methyldopa, labetalol,

phenoxybenzamine, acetaminophen, buspirone, and monoamine oxidase inhibitors (which affect the total metanephrines [TMN] level).

    (2) Misleading low values may result from incomplete urine collections or the following drugs:

        (a) α-Methylparatyrosine, clonidine, reserpine, guanethidine, monoamine oxidase inhibitors, clofibrate, and methenamine mandelate (Mandelamine) affect the VMA level.

        (b) α-Methylparatyrosine, clonidine, reserpine, and guanethidine affect the TMN level.

  b. Fasting hyperglycemia is almost always present in patients with PCC; its absence makes the diagnosis doubtful.

  c. Pharmacologic tests (e.g., production of a vasodepressor response with phentolamine) are hazardous, have a poor predictive value, and no longer have a role in the diagnosis of PCC. Failure to suppress plasma catecholamines by clonidine, however, may be useful in diagnosis.

4. Radiographic techniques are used for localization of tumor in patients with a chemical diagnosis of PCC.

  a. Chest radiographs may reveal a paraganglionic tumor.

  b. CT scan may identify PCC.

  c. MRI scan shows a characteristic bright, hyperintense image on T2-weighted images in PCC.

  d. Selective venography. During this procedure, blood catecholamines can be sampled from several areas of the venous system to help locate small tumors. Venography is useful in the following circumstances:

    (1) When less invasive studies fail to show the tumor

    (2) To search for multiple primary sites, especially in patients with MEN syndromes

  e. Isotope scanning with ^{123}I-metaiodobenzylguanidine may be useful in demonstrating PCC, especially in extra-adrenal sites. Octreotide scanning appears to be less sensitive.

D. Management

1. Pharmacologic control of PCC is essential before invasive diagnostic tests or surgery are done.

  a. Phenoxybenzamine (Dibenzyline), 10 to 20 mg PO given twice daily, is a pure α-adrenergic blocker that controls both episodic and fixed hypertension. Other α-adrenergic blockers may also be used (e.g., doxazosin in doses up to 20 mg/day).

  b. Propranolol (Inderal), 10 to 40 mg PO given 4 times daily, is a β-adrenergic blocker that is useful for treating sweating, hypermetabolism, and arrhythmias. Propranolol should be used only after adequate α-adrenergic blockade is established to avoid worsening of hypertension.

  c. α-Methylparatyrosine metyrosine (Demser) blocks catecholamine synthesis in doses of 2 to 4 g/day PO.

  d. Labetalol, a combined α- and β-adrenergic blocker, can also be used in doses of 200 to 600 mg given twice daily.

2. Surgery

  a. Before surgery

    (1) Long-acting α- and β-adrenergic blockers should be continued preoperatively and throughout surgery.

    (2) Close attention should be paid to maintaining fluid and electrolyte balance. Preoperative volume expansion may be useful.

    (3) Central venous and arterial catheters should be placed to monitor blood volume and pressure changes closely.

  b. During surgery

    (1) Close ECG monitoring is necessary to manage arrhythmias.

    (2) Hypertensive episodes, which may occur while the tumor is being manipulated, are managed with nitroprusside infusion or rapid intravenous boluses of phentolamine (Regitine, 1 to 2 mg IV).

(3) Hypotensive episodes, which occur after the tumor's blood supply has been isolated, should be treated with intravenous fluids and norepinephrine.

(4) Obvious tumors and paraspinal ganglia should be carefully inspected. All visible tumor is removed. In patients with metastatic PCC, as much tumor as possible is removed to reduce catecholamine secretion.

c. After surgery

(1) Hypertension may develop as a result of fluid overload during surgery and is treated with intravenous furosemide and fluid restriction until the blood pressure is controlled.

(2) If hypertension persists for 2 or 3 days postoperatively, residual PCC must be suspected.

(3) All patients should have plasma-free metanephrines or 24-hour urine studies for VMA and TMN repeated about 1 week after surgery. Unsuspected residual tumors and tumor recurrences should be surgically removed.

3. Metastatic disease

a. RT is useful for palliating locally symptomatic metastases.

b. The usefulness of chemotherapy for unresectable disease is not established, although the combination of cyclophosphamide, vincristine, and dacarbazine produces objective responses in most patients. Symptoms of catecholamine excess are managed pharmacologically (see section IV.D.1).

c. Some patients may respond to therapeutic doses of ^{131}I-metaiodobenzylguanidine.

V. ADRENAL CORTICAL CARCINOMA

A. Epidemiology. Adrenal cancer causes 0.2% of cancer deaths. The average age at diagnosis is 40 years, but the tumor occurs at all ages. About 60% of the patients are women.

B. Pathology and natural history. Adrenal cancers are highly aggressive; they frequently metastasize to lungs, liver, and other organs and are large and bulky at the time of diagnosis. About half of these tumors produce functional corticosteroids, including cortisol, aldosterone, androgens, and estrogens.

C. Diagnosis

1. Symptoms and signs

a. Hormonally inactive tumors are discovered as large abdominal masses in patients with abdominal pain, weight loss, or evidence of metastases.

b. Hormonally active tumors present with the following:

(1) Rapid virilization (hirsutism, clitoromegaly, oligomenorrhea, or amenorrhea) in women

(2) Gynecomastia in men

(3) Precocious puberty

(4) Cushing syndrome with hypertension and glucose intolerance

2. Adrenal function tests. Patients with clinical or laboratory evidence (hypokalemic alkalosis) of hypercortisolism should have the dexamethasone suppression test and 24-hour urine collection for 17-ketosteroids or serum DHEA-sulfate performed. The differential diagnosis of causes of Cushing syndrome is shown in Table 15.1.

a. Dexamethasone suppression test. The 1-mg overnight dexamethasone suppression test is useful as an initial screening test in outpatients. Following the administration of 1 mg of dexamethasone at 11:00 p.m., serum cortisol is measured before 9:00 a.m. the next morning; serum cortisol is usually suppressed to <2 mcg/dL in normal individuals without Cushing syndrome.

Patients who do not suppress normally using the 1-mg dose should have a baseline measurement of serum cortisol and plasma ACTH at 7:00 to 8:00 a.m. on another day. An elevated serum cortisol level together with a suppressed plasma ACTH concentration suggests a primary adrenal cause of the patient's Cushing syndrome.

TABLE 15.1 **Differential Diagnosis of Causes of Cushing Syndrome**

Etiology	Pituitary Cushing syndrome	Ectopic ACTH secretion	Adrenal carcinoma	Adrenal adenoma
Serum potassium	N or ↓	↓↓	N or ↓	N or ↓
Urine 17-ketosteroids	↑	↑	↑ or ↑↑	↑ or ↑↑
Plasma ACTH	N or ↑	↑↑	↓	↓
Adrenal enlargement[a]	Bilateral	Bilateral	Unilateral	Unilateral

ACTH, adrenocorticotropic hormone; N, normal; ↓, decreased; ↓↓, markedly decreased; ↑, increased; ↑↑, markedly increased.
[a]Adrenal gland enlargement is determined by CT scan.

    b. Twenty-four-hour urine collection is obtained for urinary-free cortisol (upper limit of normal is <50 mcg per 24 hours in most laboratories) and 17-ketosteroids (upper normal limit is <14 to 26 mg per 24 hours, depending on the age and sex of the patient). The level of urinary-free cortisol is elevated in Cushing syndrome, no matter what the cause. Levels of 17-ketosteroids in excess of 50 mg in 24 hours make the diagnosis of adrenal carcinoma likely; levels >100 mg in 24 hours are diagnostic. Serum DHEA-sulfate can be measured as an alternative to urine 17-ketosteroids and is elevated in most cases of adrenal carcinoma.

3. Further studies

    a. Chest CT scan to search for metastases.

    b. Abdominal CT scan or MRI to look for abdominal masses not clinically evident. Small (<4 cm) benign adrenal masses are common incidental findings on CT examination; laboratory findings and follow-up CT scans may help in the differential diagnosis.

    c. Biopsy

        (1) In patients with metastatic disease, biopsy is performed on the most readily accessible site (e.g., superficial lymph nodes or liver with evidence of metastases).

        (2) If only intra-abdominal disease is evident, surgery is necessary for biopsy proof of the diagnosis.

D. Management. The median survival for untreated patients is 3 months. Treated patients may survive up to 5 years, depending on the extent of disease.

    1. Surgery should be used to resect as much tumor as possible. The contralateral adrenal gland should be inspected and removed if there is evidence of tumor.

    2. RT is used to palliate symptoms from local metastatic sites.

    3. Chemotherapy may be useful for reducing tumor bulk and controlling endocrine symptoms. Mitotane (o,p′-DDD) produces objective tumor regression or improvement of endocrine symptoms in 30% of cases. The combination of mitotane with etoposide, doxorubicin, and cisplatin has provided responses in 50% of patients. The use of mitotane as an adjuvant to surgery in localized disease may improve results. Pharmacologic management of hypercortisolism is discussed in Chapter 27, section VIII.C.

VI. ISLET CELL TUMORS

    A. General aspects. Islet cell tumors of the endocrine pancreas are uncommon. In addition to the specific endocrine manifestations associated with each kind of tumor, some have been associated with ectopic production of ACTH (Cushing syndrome) and other hormones. Many of these tumors are malignant and metastasize to the liver and regional lymph nodes.

1. **Diagnosis.** The diagnosis of islet cell tumor is usually suspected because of endocrine or biochemical abnormalities. Signs and symptoms of islet cell tumors are described according to the specific type. After abnormal hormonal products are detected, the following studies are done in all patients to determine the tumor's location and extent:
   a. LFTs and liver imaging
   b. Liver biopsy is the diagnostic method of choice if liver imaging suggests the presence of tumor.
   c. CT or MRI scans of the pancreas and duodenum may reveal isolated tumors. Selective angiograms have a yield of <50%. Endoscopic ultrasonography is useful in localizing tumors in the head of the pancreas or duodenal wall.
   d. Somatostatin receptor scanning using radioiodinated octreotide frequently demonstrates primary and metastatic islet cell tumors. More than 90% of PETs (pancreatic endocrine tumors) possess somatostatin receptors. Detection of somatostatin receptors by this method correlates well with response to treatment with octreotide.
   e. Selective arterial secretagogue injection is an extremely useful technique in which the desired pancreatic hormone (e.g., gastrin, insulin) is measured in the hepatic vein immediately following selective injection of pancreatic hormone stimulants such as calcium or secretin into individual branches of the celiac artery axis; although technically difficult, it is highly effective in localizing the source of hormonal hypersecretion.
   f. Exploratory laparotomy is indicated if there is clinical or laboratory evidence of an islet cell tumor, even if preoperative localization is unrevealing.

2. **Management**
   a. **Surgery.** Intraoperative pancreatic ultrasonography and intraoperative duodenoscopy are used to localize tumors. Benign tumors are excised. Cytoreductive surgery should be performed in all patients with malignant tumors when feasible. In patients with liver metastases, partial hepatectomy, cryotherapy, and radiofrequency ablation have all been used for palliation, with some increase in both survival and quality of life. Hepatic artery embolization is helpful in carefully selected patients, with or without postocclusion chemotherapy (see section II.D.2).
   b. **Chemotherapy** has been useful in half of patients with metastatic disease, by both decreasing tumor mass and ameliorating otherwise refractory endocrine symptoms. The presence of metastases to the liver or other sites does not justify instituting cytotoxic therapy in itself because such patients can still survive several years (e.g., a median of about 4 years for gastrinomas with liver metastases if gastric acid secretion is controlled). Chemotherapy is generally reserved for patients with documented progressive liver metastases or without control of symptoms by octreotide and other medical measures.
      (1) **Octreotide,** a somatostatin analog, inhibits hormone release in gastrinomas, insulinomas, VIPomas, glucagonomas, and GH-RHomas (tumors producing growth hormone–releasing hormone) and often relieves the symptoms of the associated clinical syndrome but usually has no effect on tumor mass. A sustained-release form can be given as a monthly intramuscular injection.
      (2) **Streptozocin** is the drug of choice for islet cell tumors and is associated with a 30% response rate. Other single chemotherapeutic agents are much less effective.
      (3) **Combination chemotherapy** with streptozocin and doxorubicin or 5-FU achieves a 40% to 60% response rate for an average duration of about 18 months. Alternatively, the combination of 5-FU and streptozocin can be sequenced with the combination of doxorubicin and dacarbazine after hepatic artery occlusion (see section II.D.4).
      (4) **IFN-**α in doses of about 5 million units 3 times weekly may control symptoms and biochemical abnormalities in some patients with little effect on tumor mass.

B. Gastrinoma (Zollinger-Ellison syndrome). About 60% of these tumors are malignant, 90% are multiple, and about 30% are associated with MEN syndromes; the majority are located in the duodenum, with smaller numbers in the pancreas. Duodenal gastrinomas have a 40% to 70% risk of spread to local lymph nodes, but a low (5%) risk of hepatic metastases, while pancreatic gastrinomas are more likely to spread to the liver. Prognosis is poorer in cases with hepatic metastases.

1. **Diagnosis**
   a. **Symptoms** include severe peptic ulcer disease and, often, severe diarrhea.
   b. **Laboratory studies**
      (1) **Upper gastrointestinal contrast radiographic studies and endoscopy** show severe ulceration and hypertrophic gastric folds.
      (2) **Fasting serum gastrin level** (normal value is <100 pg/mL) is usually elevated to >500 pg/mL. If gastrinoma is suspected but serum gastrin levels are not elevated, gastrin stimulation with calcium or secretin may be attempted. Calcium infusion (12 mg/kg of calcium gluconate over 3 hours) causes the gastrin level to more than double in patients with gastrinoma; the paradoxic increase in gastrin after secretin stimulation is used by some authorities to diagnose gastrinoma. Other causes of increased gastrin levels (use of proton-pump inhibitors, atrophic gastritis, vagotomy, retained antrum after Billroth II gastrojejunostomy, and G-cell hyperplasia) must be differentiated from gastrinoma. Atrophic gastritis is differentiated by gastric acid studies.
      (3) **Gastric secretory studies.** After an overnight fast, a nasogastric tube is placed, and four 15-minute aliquots are removed for analysis. Acid secretion of >10 mEq/h and a volume of >100 mL/h suggest gastrinoma. These studies clearly distinguish gastrinoma from atrophic gastritis.
   c. **Tumor location and extent.** See section VI.A.1.
2. **Management**
   a. Therapy with proton-pump inhibitors controls symptoms in most patients.
   b. Total gastrectomy is rarely necessary because ulcer symptoms can be controlled with proton-pump inhibitors. Curative tumor excision may be possible in patients without hepatic metastases, and tumor debulking may improve quality of life in those with limited spread to the liver.
   c. Chemotherapy is used for metastatic disease (see section VI.A.2.b).

C. Insulinomas are most likely to occur between the ages of 40 and 60 years. About 80% to 85% are benign, 5% to 10% are malignant, and 5% to 10% are multifocal; 80% are hormonally functional. Insulinomas are sometimes found in association with gastrinomas. A family history of diabetes mellitus is present in 25% of patients.

Insulinomas occur with equal frequency in the head, body, and tail of the pancreas; about 3% develop outside the pancreas. Malignant tumors are more frequent in male patients. When malignant, they metastasize to the liver primarily.

1. **Diagnosis.** The differential diagnosis of hypoglycemia is discussed in Chapter 27, section XII.A.
   a. **Symptoms.** Fasting hypoglycemia, often alleviated by meals, is usually the presenting feature of insulinoma. Symptoms include diaphoresis, nervousness, palpitations, hunger pangs, anxiety, asthenia, confusion, weakness, seizures, and coma. Many patients have personality or other psychiatric changes noticed by the family. Weight gain is occasionally reported. Weight loss and liver failure may develop with metastases to the liver.
   b. **Laboratory studies.** Measurements of fasting blood glucose and insulin levels are the cornerstone for diagnosis of insulinoma.
      (1) **Fasting hypoglycemia.** An overnight fast is begun at 10:00 p.m. Blood glucose and insulin measurements are then obtained at 6:00 a.m., noon, 6:00 p.m., and midnight. An inappropriately elevated plasma insulin level (>6 μU/mL) in the presence of hypoglycemia usually is diagnostic of insulinoma. If symptoms of hypoglycemia develop at any time, blood glucose and insulin levels should be measured; if the glucose concentration

is <40 mg/dL, the test should be terminated by giving the patient food or a 50-mL intravenous bolus of 50% dextrose.

(2) Other insulin assays. Proinsulin and C peptide are absent from commercial insulin preparations; their measurement by radioimmunoassay determines the role of exogenous insulin administration in the causation of hypoglycemia. In fasting patients, proinsulin levels are normally <20% of total insulin; a higher percentage of proinsulin is indicative of insulinoma.

c. Tumor location and extent. See section VI.A.1.

2. Management

a. Surgery. Surgical removal of the tumor is the treatment of choice for insulinoma.

b. RT as an adjuvant to surgery has not been shown to be helpful.

c. Chemotherapy may be used for advanced disease (see section VI.A.2.b).

d. Treatment of hypoglycemia

(1) Diazoxide, 150 to 600 mg PO daily, is effective in managing hypoglycemic symptoms. The drug can induce hyperglycemia, hyperosmolar coma, or ketoacidosis; urine sugar and ketones should be monitored daily. A mild diuretic, such as hydrochlorothiazide, 50 mg daily, should be given to counteract the sodium-retaining effect of diazoxide. Other complications of diazoxide therapy include cytopenias, lanugo hair growth, rashes, eosinophilia, and hyperuricemia.

(2) Corticosteroids (prednisone, 40 mg/day, or hydrocortisone, 100 mg/day) may be given to patients who do not respond to diazoxide.

(3) Subcutaneous injections of octreotide (or a monthly intramuscular injection of a sustained-release preparation) can be used to inhibit insulin secretion and restore euglycemia.

(4) Calcium channel blockers (e.g., verapamil, 80 mg t.i.d.) inhibit insulin secretion and have been successfully used to prevent hypoglycemic episodes.

(5) Patients with unresponsive hypoglycemia and unresectable insulinoma may be approached with several other, usually unsatisfactory, alternatives including continuous intravenous infusion of 10% dextrose solutions through a Broviac or Hickman catheter, hepatic irradiation, or infusion of 5-FU into the hepatic artery.

D. Glucagonomas are usually malignant, and most have metastasized at the time of discovery. The disease is suspected in patients who have diabetes mellitus that is moderately resistant to insulin and who have the following abnormalities:

1. Diagnosis

a. Symptoms and physical findings

(1) *D*ermatosis: A peculiar erythematous migratory skin rash that had waxed and waned over many years (often >6 years), especially involving perioral and perigenital regions (also the fingers, legs, and feet), occurs in 80% of patients.

(2) *D*epression or other personality changes reported by family members

(3) *D*iarrhea; abdominal pain

(4) *D*eep-vein thrombosis (half of patients)

(5) Oral cavity ulcerations and sore tongue are common.

(6) Weight loss

b. Laboratory studies

(1) Hyperglycemia (usually mild)

(2) Normocytic anemia

(3) Elevated fasting blood glucagon levels (normal is <100 pg/mL)

c. Tumor location and extent. See section VI.A.1.

2. Management. See section VI.A.2. Prophylactic measures to prevent venous thrombosis during the perioperative period are mandatory.

E. Pancreatic cholera syndrome (VIPoma). These islet cell tumors secrete VIP (vasoactive intestinal peptide); half are malignant.
   1. Diagnosis
      a. Symptoms include severe watery diarrhea, muscle weakness due to hypokalemia, flushing, psychosis, and hypotension.
      b. Laboratory studies
         (1) Serum chemistry studies show hypokalemia and, often, hypercalcemia.
         (2) Gastric secretory studies show achlorhydria or hypochlorhydria.
         (3) Serum levels of VIP are elevated (normal is <70 pmol/mL).
      c. Tumor location and extent. See section VI.A.1.
   2. Management
      a. Surgery. Removal of solitary tumors controls manifestations of the pancreatic cholera syndrome, including hypercalcemia. Debulking of extensive tumor may palliate the diarrhea.
      b. Chemotherapy (see section VI.A.2.b) is useful for controlling symptoms in patients with metastatic tumor. A long-acting somatostatin preparation (octreotide) usually lowers VIP levels and stops the diarrhea.
F. Other pancreatic endocrine tumors
   1. Somatostatinoma. Somatostatin (somatotropin-release inhibiting factor) inhibits numerous endocrine and exocrine secretory functions. Half of patients with somatostatinoma have other endocrinopathies as well. This rare tumor produces diabetes mellitus, diarrhea, steatorrhea, gastric achlorhydria, weight loss, and in many cases, gallstones. Metastases are present in most cases at presentation. Cases are discovered by accident; symptoms are investigated, the tumor is found, and then the assays to confirm the diagnosis of somatostatinoma are performed. No definite procedure for diagnosis has been established. Routine evaluation of diabetic patients for somatostatinoma is not worthwhile unless severe malabsorption is present. See section VI.A.2 for treatment recommendations.
   2. PPoma. Pancreatic polypeptide (PP) inhibits gallbladder contraction, and thus PPomas are usually silent biochemically. It appears that many cases of so-called nonfunctional islet cell tumors are actually PPomas. These tumors are usually found incidentally while evaluating the patient for abdominal symptoms. Caution must be exercised in interpreting elevated PP levels because they can occur in other conditions, such as the MEN-1 syndrome. Benign tumors should be excised. Malignant PPomas respond to octreotide and streptozocin.
   3. GH-RHomas are large tumors that excessively produce growth hormone–releasing hormone. About one-third of these rare tumors originate in the pancreas, and more than half originate in the lung. The diagnosis can be suspected in patients with acromegaly but without an imaged pituitary tumor or with an abdominal mass. The diagnosis can be confirmed with elevated plasma GH-RH levels. Surgical resection is performed if possible. Octreotide effectively lowers plasma GH-RH levels.

VII. OTHER ENDOCRINE CANCERS
A. Parathyroid carcinoma is rare. Patients usually present with a neck mass and severe hypercalcemia. Tumor growth is slow and tends to involve the neck and upper mediastinum; widespread metastases are uncommon. Many patients with parathyroid carcinoma have either somatic or germ line mutations in the *HRPT2* gene, located at chromosome 1q25; the gene product, parafibromin, appears to function as a tumor suppressor.
   1. Diagnosis
      a. Patients with parathyroid cancer usually have stigmata of hypercalcemia, including polyuria, polydipsia, constipation, mental status changes, hyperparathyroid bone disease, hypercalciuria, nephrocalcinosis, or renal stones.
      b. High serum calcium levels are typical (often >15 mg/dL). Patients appear to tolerate these high levels relatively well, although hypercalcemic nephropathy

and progressive bone disease ultimately complicate the course. Serum levels of parathyroid hormone are usually grossly elevated.

  c. The diagnosis is established by biopsy of obvious neck masses in patients with evidence of hyperparathyroidism.

  d. Patients with parathyroid carcinoma should be considered for DNA testing for germ line mutations in the *HPRT2* gene.

 2. Management

  a. Surgery. Surgical extirpation of as much tumor as possible is necessary. Periodic repeated surgical debulking is warranted to try to control both the local effects of the tumor and hypercalcemia.

  b. Hypercalcemia may be difficult to manage unless the tumor can be removed. Attempts should be made to normalize blood calcium levels; because this may be impossible, however, the alternative therapeutic goal is to reduce blood levels to the asymptomatic range. The management of patients with hypercalcemia is discussed in Chapter 27, section I. Chronic therapy with zoledronate (4 mg IV) or pamidronate (30 to 90 mg IV) every 7 to 30 days may be necessary. The calcimimetic agent, cinacalcet, may be used (30 to 60 mg/day PO) to suppress parathyroid hormone production and alleviate the hypercalcemia.

B. Pineal gland neoplasms are extremely rare and are usually found in boys and young men. Dysgerminoma is the most common tumor of the pineal gland, although gliomas, choriocarcinoma, and melanomas also occur. Most tumors are localized, but spread along the flow tract of cerebrospinal fluid often occurs. See Chapter 14, section VII, for diagnosis and management.

VIII. METASTASES TO ENDOCRINE ORGANS

A. Adrenal gland metastases. The adrenal gland is frequently the site of metastatic tumors, particularly from lung cancer, breast cancer, and melanomas. Adrenal insufficiency, although rare, can develop with bilateral adrenal metastases.

 1. Diagnosis

  a. Symptoms and signs. Patients with adrenal insufficiency develop malaise, asthenia, weakness, anorexia, decreased ability to taste salt, and salt craving. Hyperpigmentation of the skin and mucous membranes, particularly the gums, and orthostatic hypotension may occur.

  b. Laboratory findings include hyponatremia, hyperkalemia, and elevated blood urea nitrogen. Diagnosis is established by the following steps:

   (1) Obtaining a baseline serum cortisol level that is low (<5 mcg/dL)

   (2) Repeating the serum cortisol 1 hour after administering 0.25 mg of cosyntropin IV. Failure of the cortisol level to rise to a peak value of at least 19 to 20 mcg/dL is diagnostic of adrenal insufficiency.

 2. Management. Patients should be treated with fludrocortisone acetate (0.1 mg once or twice a day) and hydrocortisone (30 mg/day) or prednisone (5 to 7.5 mg daily). The correct dose of fludrocortisone is determined by measuring orthostatic blood pressure changes and blood electrolyte levels. If the orthostatic drop in blood pressure is >10 mm Hg, the fludrocortisone is increased by 0.05-mg increments every few days until orthostasis is corrected. If the patient develops hypertension, hypokalemia, or alkalosis, the fludrocortisone dose is decreased.

B. Thyroid gland metastases. The thyroid gland is occasionally involved with metastases but is rarely the presenting site for metastatic tumors. Non-Hodgkin lymphomas and carcinomas of the breast, ovary, cervix, kidney, esophagus, colon, and lung have been reported to produce thyroid metastases. Diagnosis is established, if necessary, by needle biopsy of the thyroid masses. Therapy depends on the presence of local symptoms, the nature of the primary tumor, and the presence of metastases elsewhere in the body.

C. Testicular metastases. Acute leukemia, melanoma, and carcinomas of the lung, prostate, bladder, and, occasionally, kidney can metastasize to the testes. A peritesticular mass, intratesticular mass, or stony-hard enlarged testis (particularly characteristic of leukemic infiltration) is found on physical examination. Biopsy is necessary to establish the diagnosis; a transinguinal approach is mandatory.

D. Ovarian metastases. Ovarian metastases may complicate melanomas and primary tumors of the breast, stomach, colon, lung, and, occasionally, other organs. Ovarian metastases are usually asymptomatic but occasionally are the presenting feature of the primary tumor. An ovarian mass is palpable on pelvic examination. Biopsy must be done to determine the diagnosis if no other sites of cancer are evident.

E. Pituitary metastases cannot be distinguished on clinical or biochemical grounds from pituitary adenomas. Patients with known cancers have about a 3% incidence of sellar or suprasellar metastases and a 1.5% incidence of pituitary adenomas. Radiologic discrimination is not possible. Primary cancers of the breast account for more than half of the cases and lung cancer for 20%; the remainder are caused by other carcinomas, melanomas, sarcomas, and leukemias. The triad of headache, extraocular nerve palsy, and diabetes insipidus is highly suggestive of sellar metastases whether or not the patient has a known cancer. Surgical exploration and decompression are essential unless precluded by progressive widespread metastases.

Suggested Reading

Carcinoid and Islet Cell Tumors
Arnold R, Rinke A, Schmidt Ch, et al. Chemotherapy. *Best Pract Res Clin Gastroenterol* 2005;19:649.
Mittendorf EA, Shifrin AL, Inabnet WB, et al. Islet cell tumors. *Curr Probl Surg* 2006;43:685.
Modlin IM, Kidd M, Latich I, et al. Current status of gastrointestinal carcinoids. *Gastroenterology* 2005;128:1717.
Modlin IM, Latich I, Zikusoka M, et al. Gastrointestinal carcinoids: the evolution of diagnostic strategies. *J Clin Gastroenterol* 2006;40:572.
Plöckinger U, Wiedenmann B. Management of metastatic endocrine tumors. *Best Pract Res Clin Gastroenterol* 2005;19:553.
Raut CP, Kulke MH, Glickman JN, et al. Carcinoid tumors. *Curr Probl Surg* 2006;43:391.
Zuetenhorst JM, Taal BG. Metastatic carcinoid tumors: a clinical review. *The Oncologist* 2005;10:123.

Thyroid Cancer
Fialkowski EA, Moley JF. Current approaches to medullary thyroid carcinoma, sporadic and familial. *J Surg Oncol* 2006;94:737.
Green LD, Mack L, Pasieka JL. Anaplastic thyroid cancer and primary thyroid lymphoma: a review of these rare thyroid malignancies. *J Surg Oncol* 2006;94:725.
Robbins RJ, Schlumberger MJ. The evolving role of ^{131}I for the treatment of differentiated thyroid carcinoma. *J Nucl Med* 2005;46:285.
Weber T, Schilling T, Büchler MW. Thyroid carcinoma. *Curr Opin Oncol* 2006;18:30.
Wein RO, Weber RS. Contemporary management of differentiated thyroid carcinoma. *Otolaryngol Clin N Am* 2005;38:161.
Woodrum DT, Gauger PG. Role of ^{131}I in the treatment of well differentiated thyroid cancer. *J Surg Oncol* 2005;89:114.

Pheochromocytoma
Eisenhofer G, Goldstein DS, Walther MM, et al. Biochemical diagnosis of pheochromocytoma: how to distinguish true- from false-positive test results. *J Clin Endocrinol Metab* 2003;88:2656.
Forssell-Aronsson E, Bernhardt P, Wängberg B, et al. Aspects of radionuclide therapy in malignant pheochromocytomas. *Ann NY Acad Sci* 2006;1073:498.

Jiménez C, Cote G, Arnold A, et al. Should patients with apparently sporadic pheochromocytomas or paragangliomas be screened for hereditary syndromes? *J Clin Endocrinol Metab* 2006;91:2851.

Lenders JWM, Eisenhofer G, Mannelli M, et al. Pheochromocytoma. *Lancet* 2005; 366:665.

Adrenal Cortical Carcinoma

Allolio B, Hahner S, Weismann D, et al. Management of adrenocortical carcinoma. *Clin Endocrinol* 2004;60:273.

Geller JL, Mertens RB, Weiss LM. Adrenocortical carcinoma. Many questions remain unanswered. *The Endocrinologist* 2005;15:309.

Roman S. Adrenocortical carcinoma. *Curr Opin Oncol* 2006;18:36.

Terzolo M, Angeli A, Fassnacht M, et al. Adjuvant mitotane treatment for adrenocortical carcinoma. *N Engl J Med* 2007;356:2372.

Young WF Jr. The incidentally discovered adrenal mass. *N Engl J Med* 2007;356:601.

Parathyroid Carcinoma

Rodgers SE, Perrier ND. Parathyroid carcinoma. *Curr Opin Oncol* 2006;18:16.

Metastases to Endocrine Glands

Komninos J, Vlassopoulou V, Protopapa D, et al. Tumors metastatic to the pituitary gland: case report and literature review. *J Clin Endocrinol Metab* 2004;89:574.

Papi G, Fadda G, Corselllo SM, et al. Metastases to the thyroid gland: prevalence, clinicopathological aspects and prognosis: a 10-year experience. *Clin Endocrinol* 2007;66:565.

Sebag F, Calzolari F, Harding J, et al. Isolated adrenal metastases: the role of laparoscopic surgery. *World J Surg* 2006;30:888.

Yada-Hashimoto N, Yamamoto T, Kamiura S, et al. Metastatic ovarian tumors: a review of 64 cases. *Gynecol Oncol* 2003;89:314.

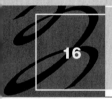

SKIN CANCERS
Bartosz Chmielowski, Antonio Ribas, and Richard F. Wagner, Jr.

MALIGNANT MELANOMA

I. EPIDEMIOLOGY AND ETIOLOGY

A. **Incidence.** Malignant melanoma is the sixth most common cancer among women and the fifth most common cancer among men in the United States. Malignant melanoma accounts for about 4% of all skin cancers, but it is responsible for 80% of deaths. The incidence of melanoma in the United States is 18.2 cases per 100,000/year, two-thirds in males and one-third in women. The median age at the time of diagnosis is 58 years, and only 0.9% of cases are diagnosed before the age of 20. The estimated number of new cases in the United States in 2007 is 59,940, and 8,110 patients would die of melanoma.

   The incidence of melanoma rose rapidly in the 1970s at about 6% per year; this rate decreased in the 1980s to about 3% per year. In the past decade the death rate from melanoma has decreased. White people have a 17 to 25 times higher risk for development of melanoma than blacks, but melanoma is diagnosed among all races.

B. **Risk factors.** The strongest risk factors for melanoma are a family history of melanoma, multiple benign or atypical nevi, and a previous melanoma. The list of additional risk factors includes immunosuppression, sun sensitivity, and exposure to ultraviolet radiation.

1. **Familial factors.** Approximately 10% of melanomas are familial. The higher risk of melanoma in these families may be attributed to both shared susceptibility genes and shared environment.

   a. **High-penetrance susceptibility genes.** Two genes, *CDKN2A* and *CDK4*, are associated with high-penetrance susceptibility. Mutated *CDKN2A* is the most prevalent gene in families with melanoma. It is located on chromosome 9p21 and it encodes cyclin-dependent kinase inhibitor 2A (p16INK4a). *CDK4* encodes cyclin-dependent kinase 4, which is one of the binding partners of p16INK4a. Mutations in *CDK4* are found much less frequently than *CDKN2A*. Also evidence exists for another, as yet unidentified, high-penetrance susceptibility gene at chromosome 1p22.

   The higher the number of family members with melanoma, the higher the probability of carrying a high penetrance gene. Mutated *CDKN2A* was found in 14% families with two cases of melanoma, in 67% families with six to seven cases, and 100% families with seven to ten cases. Overall, between 20% (in Australia) and 57% (in Europe) of the cases of familial melanoma are associated with *CDKN2A*.

   b. **Low-penetrance susceptibility genes.** Epidemiologic studies suggest that low-penetrance susceptibility genes are found frequently among families with melanoma. The *MC1R* gene, which encodes the melanocyte-stimulating hormone receptor, has been characterized best.

   c. **Familial atypical multiple mole-melanoma (FAMMM) syndrome,** also known as the familial dysplastic nevus syndrome, was described in 1978 in families whose members suffered from melanoma and had multiple (usually >100) large moles of variable size and color (reddish-brown to bright red) with pigmentary leakage. The median age of the development of melanoma in persons with this syndrome is 33 years, and 9% of affected people develop it before the age of 20. The syndrome is transmitted in autosomal dominant fashion, but there are sex differences in penetrance. Males develop melanoma less frequently and at an older age than women.

2. **Nevi.** Typical nevi are frequently precursors of melanoma, but more importantly they are markers of increased risk. One study showed that men who have at least 17 and women who have at least 12 small moles on the back are at 4.6 and 5.1 times higher risk of the development of melanoma, respectively. The lifetime risk for any mole to transform into melanoma by age 80 years is 0.03% for men and 0.009% for women.

   Congenital nevi are benign neoplasms that are present at birth and com-posed of nevomelanocytes. The malignant potential of giant congenital nevi varies between different types. Pigmented giant nevi have especially high risk for malignant transformation. Nevus sebaceous is associated with the develop-ment of basal cell carcinoma. Verrucous epidermal nevi and woolly hair nevi do not have malignant potential.

3. **Previous melanoma.** The rate of a second primary cutaneous melanoma is more than 10 times higher than the first one. The 1-year, 5-year, and 10-year probability of developing the second primary melanoma are 1% to 2%, 2.1% to 3.4%, and 3.2% to 5.3%, respectively. The greatest risk is within the first 2 years, but it remains elevated for at least 20 years. Males, elderly patients, and individuals with the first melanoma on the face, the neck, and the trunk are at especially high risk. The incidence of a third primary melanoma from the time of second primary melanoma is 16% at 1 year and 31% at 5 years.

4. **Immunosuppression.** Among organ allograft recipients, melanoma constituted 5% of skin cancers and was significantly higher than in the general population (2.7%). A sixfold to eightfold increase in melanoma rates has been observed among male kidney transplant recipients.

5. **Sun sensitivity.** Light-skinned and redheaded people frequently carry poly-morphism in the melanocortin receptor gene that results in a decreased melanin production after exposure to ultraviolet (UV) radiation and in an increased risk of melanoma.

6. **Exposure to sun and to UV radiation.** It is known that UV radiation causes genetic changes in the skin, impairs cutaneous immune function, increases the local production of growth factors, and induces the formation of DNA-damaging reactive oxygen species that affect keratinocytes and melanocytes. Epidemiologic studies revealed that mostly frequent but intermittent sun ex-posure and frequent sunburns, especially in the childhood, increase the risk of melanoma. Chronic low-grade sun exposure may be protective, although data also show that higher total exposure to the sun is associated with a higher risk of melanoma among non-Hispanic white individuals. In addition, exposure to UV light from recreational tanning salons is emerging as an important risk factor for melanoma.

7. **Occupational exposure.** Exposure to coal tar, pitch, creosote, arsenic com-pounds, or radium increases the risk of melanoma development.

II. **PREVENTION.** Avoidance of exposure to the sun during the midday hours, wearing skin-protecting clothing, sunglasses, use of sunscreens with a sun protective factor (SPF) of 15 or higher, and avoidance of sunburns and tanning beds are recommended as a primary prevention. Patients with a family or personal history of melanoma should undergo at least one annual skin examination performed by a dermatologist as a sec-ondary prevention. Suspicious lesions must be biopsied.

III. **PATHOLOGY AND NATURAL HISTORY**

   A. **Pathology.** Melanoma originates from melanocytes, the neural crest-derived cells that migrate into the epidermis during embryogenesis to reside in the basal layer of the epidermis. The overwhelming majority of melanomas originate in the skin, but some melanomas may arise from other primary sites. Potential extracutaneous sites include the choroidal layer of the eye and mucosal surfaces in the upper respiratory tract (most frequently, the nose and nasopharynx), gastrointestinal (GI) tract (most frequently, the anus), and genitourinary tract (most frequently, the vagina).

Several steps occur in the process of their malignant transformation. According to the Clark model, initially normal melanocytes proliferate and form a benign nevus. In the next phase, abnormal growth appears in the form of a dysplastic nevus. Melanoma may originate from a benign nevus, but it can also start from scattered melanocytes present in the normal skin. Next, in the radial growth phase, the cells acquire the ability to grow intraepidermally and have all the features of cancerous cells. Then, the lesion invades the dermis (vertical-growth phase) and finally spreads to other organs and other areas of the skin (metastasis). Not all melanomas pass through each of these individual phases, however.

B. Molecular events in the pathogenesis of melanoma. Several molecular alterations have known pathogenic effects in the transformation of melanocytes and the evolution of melanoma. In general, germline or somatic alterations in cell-cycle control, together with somatic activating mutations or amplifications of factors involved in signal transduction pathways, are required for melanoma development.

1. Alterations in signal transduction pathways. Mutually exclusive somatic activating point mutations in NRAS and BRAF, two members of the mitogen-activated protein kinase (MAPK) that provides proliferation signaling from surface receptors to the nucleus, are present in most melanomas. Paradoxically, BRAF mutation is also frequent in benign nevi, where its transforming effect may be counteracted by the phenomenon of oncogene-induced senescence. Somatic alterations in another signaling pathway important in cell growth, the phosphoinositide-3-OH kinase (PI3K) pathway, are also frequently found in melanoma, including loss of PTEN (phosphate and tensin homologue) and overexpression of protein kinase B (PKB, also known as Akt).

2. Aberrant cell cycle control. As described above, inherited mutations in the *CDKN2A* and *CDK4* genes are associated with high-penetrance susceptibility to melanoma. Somatic mutations in these and other cell-cycle control genes seem a requisite for the development of melanoma and escape from oncogene-induced senescence.

3. Other genetic events in melanoma pathogenesis. The microphthalmia-associated transcription factor (MITF) is required for melanocyte development. *MITF* gene amplifications are noted in a small subset of melanomas, and this gene has a complex relationship with melanoma oncogenesis. Several genetic alterations common in melanoma reduce sensitivity to apoptosis, including overexpression of Bcl-2 (B-cell leukemia/lymphoma-2), silencing of APAF-1 (apoptotic peptidase activating factor-1), and activation of NF-κB (nuclear factor kappa B).

C. Major clinical-histopathologic subtypes. Analysis of genome-wide alterations in DNA and sequencing of individual somatic mutations in key genes can be used to distinguish different melanoma subtypes with high accuracy, suggesting that these melanoma subtypes develop along distinct genetic pathways. Therefore, melanoma may soon be considered more than one disease based on improved knowledge of its molecular biology.

1. Superficial spreading melanoma compromises about 70% of all melanomas. It is most common in middle age and develops most frequently on the upper back of both sexes and on the legs of women, but it can occur in any anatomic location. Only 25% of lesions are associated with a pre-existing nevus. It spreads laterally (radial growth) for a period of time before it becomes invasive. The lesions appear as variably pigmented plaques or macules that have a bizarre shape with irregular borders. As the lesion progresses, the shape becomes more irregular and areas of regression can be noted. Progression correlates with the evolution of multiple shades of color from red (inflammation) through gray (regressed areas) to black (neoplastic melanocytes).

2. **Nodular melanoma** compromises about 15% to 20% of all melanomas. It is more common among elderly (the fifth and sixth decade of life), and it occurs twice as frequently in male than in female patients. The lesion appears as a darkly pigmented dome-shaped or polypoid nodule that can ulcerate and bleed early. Occasionally it can be amelanotic. These tumors grow rapidly and vertically from the onset.

3. **Lentigo maligna melanoma** (4% to 15% of melanomas) is most commonly seen in older individuals (in the sixth and seventh decade of life). It arises in sun-damaged areas of the skin, mainly on the face (90% cases). The lesion appears as a tan-brown macule, very often large in size (3 to 6 cm). The lesion grows slowly and the radial growth phase may last between 5 and 50 years before it starts growing vertically. Partial regression is not uncommon during evolution. The radial growth phase is called *lentigo maligna* (LM) or *Hutchinson's freckle*.

4. **Acral lentiginous melanoma** is the least common variant of radial growth phase melanomas. It compromises only 2% to 8% of melanomas in whites, but 30% to 75% cases in blacks, Hispanics, and Asians. It appears on the palms, soles, terminal phalanges, and mucous membranes as a dark brown to black, unevenly pigmented patch. Small elevation may suggest vertical growth.

5. **Rare types**
   a. **Nevoid melanoma** resembles benign nevi. It has verrucoid or dome-shaped appearance and can metastasize.
   b. **Desmoplastic melanomas** resemble a scar or fibroma and appear mainly on sun-exposed areas. Very often they are amelanotic. They tend to recur locally or as isolated metastasis.

D. **Mode of spread.** Melanoma first spreads through the lymphatic system forming satellite lesions and in-transit metastases and then it involves regional lymph nodes. *Satellite lesions* are skin or subcutaneous lesions within 2 cm of the primary tumor and represent intralymphatic extension of the tumor. *In transit metastases* are defined as lesions that are >2 cm from the primary tumor, but not beyond the regional lymph node basin. Finally, melanoma spreads hematogenously forming distant metastases in the skin, subcutaneous soft tissue, lungs, liver, brain, and other organs.

E. **Metastatic melanoma from an unknown primary site** accounts for approximately 2% to 6% of all melanoma cases. It is assumed that in most these cases the primary cutaneous melanoma regressed spontaneously. Metastases most often develop as cutaneous or subcutaneous nodules or as lymph node metastases. The survival of patients with unknown primary melanoma is similar to that of patients with known primary tumors when corresponding stages are compared.

F. **Paraneoplastic syndromes.** Most paraneoplastic syndromes occur in patients with widely metastatic melanoma, but some may precede the diagnosis (i.e., dermatomysositis, pemphigus, melanosis). A variety of paraneoplastic syndromes are associated with melanoma and can affect multiple organ systems, including

1. **Skin** (vitiligo, pemphipus, dermatomysositis, melanosis, acanthosis nigricans, systemic sclerosis). **Generalized melanosis** is a syndrome of progressive gray-blue skin discoloration frequently accompanied by melanuria, and sometimes also by melanoptysis or a dark brown blood serum. Melanosis is caused by the melanin (or its precursor) that is produced and secreted in an increased amount by malignant cells, and then deposited within macrophages throughout the body.

2. **Eyes.** Melanoma-associated retinopathy is a paraneoplastic syndrome characterized by frequent sudden onset of symptoms of night blindness, light sensations, visual loss, defect in visual fields, and reduced b-waves in the electroretinogram.

3. **Blood** (leukemoid reaction, eosinophilia, autoimmune neutropenia)

4. **Endocrine system** (hypercalcemia, Cushing syndrome, hypertrophic osteoarthropathy)

5. **Central and peripheral nervous system** (chronic inflammatory demyelinating polyneuropathy, opsoclonus-myoclonus)

IV. DIAGNOSIS

A. Symptoms

1. **The ABCDE rule.** Warning signs of melanoma are

   A: asymmetry
   B: irregular borders
   C: changes in color; pigmentation is not uniform
   D: diameter >6 mm
   E: enlargement of the lesion

   The changes in preexisting moles and appearance of a new mole with these features are highly suspicious for melanoma. More than 50% of the cases arise in apparently normal areas of the skin. Ulceration or bleeding usually represents deeper lesions.

2. **In-transit lesions and skin metastases** appear as skin or subcutaneous erythematous nodules between the primary tumor site and the regional nodal basin. The nodules do not have to be pigmented. As they grow, they can coalesce and ulcerate.

3. **Symptoms of the metastatic disease** are related to the involved site.

B. Physical examination.
A complete skin examination of the whole body should be performed, including scalp, axillae, genital area, interdigital webs, and mouth. Melanoma in men occurs more frequently on the trunk or head and neck, and in women on the extremities, but it can arise from any site on the skin surface. Although most primary lesions are pigmented, frequently skin metastases are not pigmented, and they may appear as red or subcutaneous nodules.

C. Differential diagnosis.
Compound nevi, halo nevi, dermal nevi, basal cell carcinoma, seborrheic keratosis, angiomas, and dermatofibromas may have features that suggest melanoma. Biopsy specimens of these lesions should be obtained. Precision of the diagnosis can be increased by use of a dermatoscope, an instrument that magnifies pigmented lesions about 10 times. The dermatoscope is especially invaluable for examination of flat to slightly raised pigmented lesions.

D. Biopsy.
All suspicious lesions should be biopsied and analyzed pathologically. A full-thickness excision with 1- to 3-mm margins should be performed if the tumor is highly suspected to be melanoma. Larger margins may interfere with planned sentinel lymph node biopsy. Incisional biopsies (punch biopsy or tangential), where part of the pigmented lesion is sampled for pathologic diagnosis, may be used for very large lesions or lesions on the face, palmar surfaces of the hand, sole of the foot, ear, distal digits, genitalia, or under nails. Incisional biopsies may fail, however, to diagnose melanoma or result in a more favorable early staging impression owing to sampling error, and if melanoma continues to be suspected or is diagnosed, the lesion should be rebiopsied or completely excised for pathologic re-evaluation and staging. Incisional biopsies do not increase the chance for melanoma metastases.

V. STAGING SYSTEM AND PROGNOSTIC FACTORS

A. Staging system.
The current staging system was developed by the American Joint Committee on Cancer (AJCC) in 2002 (Table 16.1).

B. Prognostic factors

1. **Primary lesion.** Tumor thickness and ulceration are the most powerful predictors of survival.

   a. **Tumor thickness** as a prognostic factor was first described by Alexander Breslow and it is traditionally reported as Breslow thickness in millimeters. The AJCC staging system uses 1-, 2-, and 4-mm cut-offs, but tumor thickness is really a continuous prognostic variable.

   b. **Ulceration** (the absence of intact epithelium over the tumor determined by pathologic analysis) indicates aggressive biology of melanoma.

   c. **Clark level** is an important prognostic factor for lesions thinner than 1 mm. Clark levels (Fig. 16.1), which specify the anatomic depth of invasion, are defined as follows:

| TABLE 16.1 | TNM Staging System for Cutaneous Melanoma |

Primary tumor (T)		Regional lymph nodes (N)[a]	
TX	Primary tumor cannot be assessed (inadequate or absent pathology)	NX	Regional lymph nodes cannot be assessed
T0	No evidence of primary tumor	N0	No regional lymph node metastasis
Tis	Melanoma *in situ*	N1	Metastasis in one node
T1a	≤1.0 mm thick and level II or III, no ulceration	N1a	Clinically occult (micrometastasis)
T1b	≤1.0 mm thick and level IV or V or with ulceration	N1b	Clinically apparent (macrometastasis)
T2a	1.01–2.0 mm thick without ulceration	N2	Metastasis in two to three regional lymph nodes or intralymphatic regional metastasis without nodal metastasis
T2b	1.01–2.0 mm thick with ulceration		
T3a	2.01–4.0 mm thick without ulceration	N2a	Clinically occult (micrometastasis)
		N2b	Clinically apparent (macrometastasis)
T3b	2.01–4.0 mm thick with ulceration	N2c	Satellite or in-transit metastasis without metastatic nodes
T4a	> 4.0 mm thick without ulceration		
T4b	>4.0 mm thick with ulceration	N3	Metastasis in four or more nodes, or matted nodes, or in-transit metastasis or satellite(s) with metastatic nodes

Distant metastases (M)

MX	Distant metastasis cannot be assessed
M0	No distant metastasis
M1	Distant metastasis is present
M1a	Metastasis to skin, subcutaneous tissue, or distant lymph nodes
M1b	Metastasis to lung
M1c	Metastasis to all other visceral sites; or distant metastasis with an elevated LDH

Pathologic stage grouping[a]

Stage	TNM classification
0	Tis N0 M0
IA	T1a N0 M0
IB	T1b,2a N0 M0
IIA	T2b,3a N0 M0
IIB	T3b,4a N0 M0
IIC	T4b N0 M0
IIIA	T1a–4a N1a,2a M0
IIIB	T1b–4b N1a,2a M0, T1a–4a N1b, 2b M0, T1a/b–4a/b N2c M0
IIIC	T1b–4b N1b,2b M0, Any T N3 M0
IV	Any T Any N M1

[a]Pathologic staging includes pathologic information about regional lymph nodes after complete or partial (sentinel) lymphadenectomy; pathologic stages 0 and IA do not require this information.
LDH, serum lactic dehydrogenase.
From the *AJCC Cancer Staging Manual*. 6th ed. New York: Springer-Verlag; 2002, with permission.

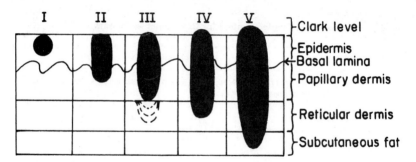

Figure 16.1. Clark levels of invasion for malignant melanoma.

Clark level I: Lesions confined to epidermis
Clark level II: Lesions extending beyond the basal lamina into the loose papillary dermis
Clark level III: Lesions forming a plaque within the papillary dermis
Clark level IV: Lesions invading reticular dermis.
Clark level V: Lesions invading the subcutaneous fat.

2. **Status of the regional lymph nodes.** The total number of nodal metastases is a significant predictor of outcome in patients with lymph node involvement. Moreover, patients in whom lymph node involvement was detected clinically have worse prognosis than those who required microscopic analysis. Satellite and in-transit lesions are considered an intralymphatic spread and they carry the same prognosis as the presence of lymph node metastases.

3. **Metastatic disease.** Patients who have nonvisceral metastases (skin, subcutaneous tissue, lymph nodes) carry a better prognosis than those who have visceral metastases. Elevated level of lactate dehydrogenase (LDH) is a poor prognostic factor.

4. **Survival according to the stage**

Stage	1-year survival	5-year survival
I	99% to 100%	94% to 99%
II	93% to 96%	56% (IIC) to 78% (IIA)
III	74% (N3 disease) to 95% (stage IIIA)	27% (N3 disease) to 68% (stage IIIB)
IV	42%	18%

C. **Staging work-up**
1. Breslow thickness, ulceration status, Clark level, margin status, and the presence of satellite lesions should be reported by the pathologist. Reporting of location, regression, mitotic rate, tumor infiltrating lymphocytes, vertical growth phase, angiolymphatic invasion, neurotropism, and histologic subtype is encouraged.
2. Physicians should obtain a complete history and physical examination, including the entire skin and locoregional lymph nodes.
3. Patients with stage 0 or IA melanoma do not require further studies. For deeper primary melanomas (stages II and III), further tests may be performed (LFT, LDH, and baseline whole body imaging).
4. All patients with surgically incurable locally advanced melanoma (stage IIIc) and metastatic melanoma (stage IV) should undergo complete blood work including LDH, and whole body imaging. Specific brain imaging is required, because approximately one-fifth of these cases will present with brain metastasis. Adequate brain imaging can be achieved with an MRI (preferable, because it has higher sensitivity for metastasis) or a CT scan of the brain with IV contrast.

Imaging of the rest of the body can be obtained by CT of the chest, abdomen, and pelvis with both oral and IV contrast, or a combined whole body fluorodeoxyglucose (FDG) positron emission tomography (PET) CT. The benefit of the FDG PET scan is that melanoma is associated with one with the highest accumulation rates of this PET tracer. If specific areas are involved that are not adequately imaged with CT scans (spinal, soft tissue or bone metastasis), dedicated MRI may be required.

VI. MANAGEMENT
A. Surgery
1. Management of the primary tumor
a. Cutaneous melanoma. The definitive surgical treatment for primary cutaneous melanoma is a wide excision. Some specialists recommend a 3-cm margin for lesions >2 mm. The usual recommended margin of the normal tissue depends on the depth of invasion of the primary tumor as follows:

Tumor thickness	Recommended surgical margin
In situ	0.5 cm
≤1 mm	1 cm
1.01 to 2 mm	1 to 2 cm
2.01 to 4 mm	2 cm
>4 mm	2 cm

Often, it is difficult to achieve a recommended excision margin in cases of melanoma located on the head or neck without skin grafting. Although some studies suggest that a narrower margin may result in better cosmetic results without influencing the overall survival, it is recommended that the tumor thickness—as opposed to cosmetic factors—guide the extent of the excisional surgery. Mohs' micrographic surgery may contribute to favorable outcomes, especially on the head and neck where extensive subclinical spread is relatively common.

b. Melanoma of the unusual sites
(1) Subungual melanoma is treated with partial digital amputation.
(2) The wide excision of a **plantar melanoma** frequently requires a variety of flap reconstructive procedures, especially when the lesion is located on a weight-bearing surface.
(3) Mucosal melanoma may arise from the epithelium lining the respiratory, GI, and genitourinary tracts. It often presents late with locally advanced or metastatic disease. If the disease is localized, it may require a major surgery (i.e., craniofacial resection for skull base tumors, radical vulvectomy for vulvar melanomas, or abdominal-perineal resection for anorectal melanomas).

2. Management of regional lymph nodes
a. Sentinel lymph node biopsy (SLNB). Randomized clinical trials in the 1980s demonstrated that elective lymph node dissection in patients without clinically involved lymph nodes did not increase survival in cases of melanoma. Conversely, data suggest that lymph node mapping and biopsy of the first draining lymph node (the so-called *sentinel lymph node*) can adequately detect lymph node metastasis with decreased morbidity. The SLN is identified by lymphoscintigraphy.

Patients who do not have clinically involved regional lymph nodes and whose primary tumor is >1 mm frequently undergo SLNB. SLNB should be done before a wide excision of the primary site, which obfuscates mapping of the SLN location.

Only 1% to 2% of patients who have an uninvolved SLN have metastases to non-SLN. For patients with positive SLNB, the recommendation is to have radical lymph node dissection (RLND). It is uncertain if patients with tumors <1 mm thick but presenting with high-risk features (ulceration, Clark level IV and V, histologic regression, or high mitotic rate) benefit from SLNB as well.

    b. Enlarged regional lymph nodes should be surgically removed. RLND allows 20% to 40% of patients with positive lymph nodes to be alive at 10 years. A thorough dissection of the involved nodal basin is required. It is recommended that at least 10 inguinal, 15 axillary, or 15 neck lymph nodes be dissected. The procedure can be complicated by delayed wound healing, wound infection, and the development of lymphedema or seromas. Complications occur more frequently after inguinal lymphadenectomy than after axillary lymphadenectomy.

3. Management of in-transit metastases

    a. If the patient does not have evidence of disseminated disease, in-transit metastases (single or multiple) could be resected with curative intent, but only 18% to 28% patients will remain free of disease at 5 years.

    b. Most patients are treated with either isolated limb perfusion (ILP) or systemic therapy. ILP is a procedure in which vasculature is separated surgically and chemotherapy (e.g., melphalan in high concentrations) can be perfused through the affected limb without exposing the rest of the body. Complete responses can be achieved in approximately 50% of cases, and about half of them are durable.

    c. Other patients can be treated with standard or experimental immunotherapies, such as interleukin-2 (IL-2), interferon (IFN), intralesional bacillus Calmette-Guérin (BCG), and anti-CTLA4 antibodies.

4. Surgical management of metastases. Patients with solitary metastases, oligometastatic melanoma (limited number of metastatic sites), or with residual lesions after successful immunotherapy may benefit from metastectomy.

B. Radiation therapy. In the adjuvant setting, hypofractionated RT to the primary side should be considered for patients with positive surgical margins and RT to the regional nodal basin for patients who had multiple positive lymph nodes (at least four), had a bulky disease (lymph nodes >3 cm), were found to have extranodal soft-tissue extension, or had recurrence. Patients with metastatic melanoma are rarely treated with RT. Radiation to pain-causing tumor or tumor invading vital structures can be used as palliation. Management of brain metastasis includes RT (see section VII.A).

C. Systemic therapy. Systemic therapy in patients with melanoma can be divided into two distinct groups: (*a*) chemotherapy, including cytotoxic agents with new small molecules and (*b*) immunotherapy. Chemotherapy targets dividing cells or their environment; it can lead to prolonged survival, but almost never results in cure. Immunotherapy stimulates the patient's own immune system to reject tumor. The rate of responses is frequently lower than with the use of chemotherapy, but it can result in cure in a small percentage of patients. Combination of chemotherapy and immunotherapy is called *biochemotherapy*. Current results of treatment with systemic therapy have been disappointing; therefore, all patients with melanoma should be encouraged to participate in clinical trials.

1. Adjuvant systemic therapy. Patients who present with involvement of regional lymph nodes (high-risk group) and patients with localized thick tumors (i.e., thickness >4 mm, or between 2 and 4 mm with ulceration, or thickness >4 mm with ulceration [intermediate-risk group]), may benefit from adjuvant therapy. Multiple agents have been tested in the adjuvant setting, but only interferon-alpha (IFN-α) has shown potential benefit.

    a. ECOG Trial 1648. Patients enrolled in the large, randomized ECOG 1648 trial were treated with high doses of IFN-α2b. The schedule consisted of IV therapy at maximal-tolerated doses of 20 MU/m^2 5 days/week for 4 weeks followed by 10 MU/m^2 subcutaneously three times a week for additional 48 weeks. After a median follow-up of 7 years, the treatment resulted in a prolonged relapse-free and overall survival of approximately 10%. Another large, randomized trial confirmed these results. Trials using low or intermediates doses of IFN have showed decreased or no benefit.

    b. Further analysis. When patients were followed for a longer time, and when the pooled analysis of three high dose IFN-α2b clinical trials was performed, the difference in overall survival was not statistically significant. Most patients required dose adjustment because of toxicity.

    c. Side effects of INF therapy included fatigue, nausea, fever, depression, neutropenia, and reversible elevation of liver enzymes.

    d. Autoimmunity as a complication of therapy with IFN-α can result in the development of clinical syndromes (hyperthyroidism, hypothyroidism, hypopituitarism, vitiligo, antiphospholipid syndrome) or of autoantibodies (antithyroid microsomal, antithyroglobulin, antinuclear, anti-DNA, antiplatelet, or anti–islet-cell antibodies). A prospective correlative analysis of 200 patients treated with high doses of IFN-α revealed that 25% of patients developed manifestations of autoimmunity (syndromes or autoantobodies). At a median follow-up of 46 months, a marked decrease in the rate of relapse (73% *vs.* 13%) and mortality (54% *vs.* 4%) was seen in patients treated with IFN-α who developed evidence of autoimmunity. Autoimmunity developed within the first month of treatment (induction phase with IV IFN-α) in 45% of patients, but in most, autoimmunity was not observed until months after the initiation of treatment. This study allows the identification of individuals who most likely have benefited from therapy, but does not help with selecting patients at the beginning of treatment.

    e. Recommendations. After discussion of side effects, adjuvant treatment with IFN-α should be offered to patients with completely resected skin melanoma of stages IIB, IIC, and III, who are <70 years of age and who are devoid of significant comorbid conditions. No evidence indicates that patients with less advanced melanoma benefit from adjuvant therapy.

2. Chemotherapy for metastatic melanoma. Metastatic melanoma is associated with median survival of 6 to 9 months. Only two agents have been approved by the U.S. Food and Drug Administration (FDA) for the use in metastatic melanoma, the chemotherapy agent DTIC and the immunotherapy agent IL-2.

    a. Dacarbazine (DTIC) is the only chemotherapeutic agent that has been approved by the FDA for treatment of patients with metastatic melanoma. It is a well-tolerated agent when 250 mg/m^2 is given IV daily for 5 days or 850 to 1,000 mg/m^2 once every 2 to 4 weeks. The response rates to DTIC are <20% (in newer trials, <12%), and most of these are partial responses with a median duration of response between 4 and 6 months. No randomized trials have been performed to show survival benefit for DTIC over placebo. Despite its low activity, DTIC remains the standard against which most new chemotherapy agents are compared.

    b. Temozolomide is an analog of dacarbazine that degrades to MTIC, the active metabolite of DTIC. It does penetrate the blood–brain barrier, so it can be used in patients with brain metastasis. When compared with DTIC, treatment with temozolomide resulted in no significant improvement in median survival. The drug is used at the doses of 200 mg/m^2 per day orally for 5 days every 28 days, or 75 mg/m^2/day for 6 weeks every 8 weeks. The extended dosing regimen of temozolomide may result in CD4 lymphocytopenia and opportunistic infections.

    c. Other single agents. Platinum-containing agents (cisplatin, carboplatin), nitrosoureas (carmustine, lomustine, fotemustine), microtubule toxins (vinblastine, vindesine), and taxanes (paclitaxel, docetaxel, abraxane) resulted in modest responses. None of these agents has been proved to be superior to DTIC in a randomized clinical trial.

    d. Combination chemotherapy. Multiple attempts have been made to improve treatment of metastatic melanoma by combining several cytotoxic agents. These regimens resulted in increased response rates, significant toxicity, and no prolongation in survival in randomized trials when compared with DTIC.

    e. Combination chemotherapy with targeted therapies. Several new agents have been studied in the treatment of melanoma.

(1) **Sorafenib,** a small molecule created initially as raf kinase inhibitor, but working most probably through blocking angiogenesis, had a very limited activity as a single agent. Two phase III trials of combination of chemotherapy with sorafenib are ongoing. Preliminary results showed no improvement in progression-free survival.

(2) **Oblimersen,** an antisense oligoneucleotide suppressing expression of bcl-2, in combination with dacarbazine improved response rate and progression-free survival, but not overall survival.

(3) **MEDI-522,** a humanized antibody against integrin αVβ3, in combination with DTIC, improved survival in an open label phase II trial.

3. **Immunotherapy for metastatic melanoma.**

a. **IL-2** given in high doses (600,000 to 720,000 U/kg every 8 hours for a maximum of 15 doses/cycle) resulted in a 16% response rates. Responses were higher in patients with stages M1a and M1b melanoma compared with patients with other visceral metastasis. Of responders, 44% were alive at 6-year follow-up. Because of these results, the FDA approved high-dose IL-2 for patients with metastatic melanoma. The treatment is associated with extensive toxicity and can be administered only in experienced centers.

b. **Interferon-α** produces responses in up to 16% of patients.

c. **Adoptive immunotherapy.** Adoptive transfer of *ex vivo* expanded tumor infiltrating lymphocytes (TIL) followed by treatment with high dose IL-2 to patients who received nonmyeloablative lymphodepleting conditioning regimen with fludarabine and cyclophosphamide resulted in 51% responses, including 9% complete responses. Adoptive transfer of lymphocytes that were *ex vivo* transduced with a retrovirus encoding a T-cell receptor for a melanoma-specific peptide led to response in 2 of 18 patients.

d. **Anti–CTLA-4 antibodies.** CTLA-4 is a molecule on the surface of activated T lymphocytes that is responsible for inhibiting immune responses. Blocking this molecule can potentially result in enhancement of antitumor responses. Two monoclonal antibodies against CTLA-4 (CP-675,206 and MDX-010) are being evaluated in advanced melanoma, with apparent overall response rates in the 15% range in phase I/II testing. Phase III clinical trials are underway.

e. **Vaccines.** A variety of therapeutic vaccination methods have been tested in patients with metastatic melanoma, including autologous dendritic cells pulsed with peptides, proteins, or tumor-derived RNA/DNA. Responses have been marginal.

4. **Biochemotherapy.** Combination of cisplatin-based chemotherapy with either high-dose IL-2 or IL-2 combined with IFN-α has been tested in multiple trials. Phase II trials reported promising response rates. These trials were followed by multiple phase III trials that consistently revealed that the addition of immunotherapy to combination chemotherapy increased toxicity significantly, but did not increase survival (in one study it decreased survival). The use of combination chemoimmunotherapy regimens is not recommended in the absence of well-designed, prospective, randomized protocols.

5. **Novel targeted therapies.** The improved understanding of the oncogenic events in melanoma provides novel targets for therapeutic intervention. Targeted agents are being developed that block the oncogenic signaling from mutations or genetic amplifications of members of the MAPK and PI3K signal transduction pathways. In addition, drugs that control kinases involved in cell-cycle control, promote apoptosis, and interfere with cell survival signals are in clinical development.

VII. SPECIAL CLINICAL PROBLEMS ASSOCIATED WITH MALIGNANT MELANOMA

A. **Brain metastases** are a common finding in patients with malignant melanoma. Male patients whose primary lesions were located on mucosal surfaces or on the skin of the trunk or head and neck, who had thick or ulcerated primary lesions, and who had acral lentiginous or nodular lesions are at especially high risk for the development of brain metastases. These metastases contribute to death in 95% of these patients. The median survival from the time of diagnosis of brain metastasis is 4 months, and only 14% to 19% patients survive 1 year.

Favorable prognostic factors include good performance status, younger age, absence of extracranial metastases, and the presence of a solitary brain metastasis. All patients with a new diagnosis of brain metastasis from melanoma should be evaluated for possible surgical resection or stereotactic irradiation utilizing convergent radiation beams. Control of progression in >90% of lesions can be achieved with these methods.

With multiple simultaneous metastasis (>6), whole brain radiation therapy may be the only feasible treatment approach. It is questionable whether chemotherapy with agents that can penetrate through the blood–brain barrier, such as temozolomide or fotemustine (not available in the United States), can enhance the response to radiation.

B. Cardiac metastases. Metastatic tumors to the heart are uncommon with the exception of melanoma. More than half of the patients with disseminated melanoma have cardiac involvement. Clinical findings are related to the location of the metastases and include heart failure symptoms caused by obstructive masses, syncope or arrhythmia caused by endomyocardial or conduction system involvement, and tamponade caused by pericardial involvement and effusion. Most patients remain asymptomatic.

C. Breast metastases. Melanoma is among the most commonly reported primary tumors to metastasize to the breast. Patients may have bilateral breast involvement. Breast involvement is usually associated with disseminated disease, but rare cases of the primary melanoma of the breast have been reported.

D. Gastrointestinal metastases. Malignant melanoma shows an unusual predilection to metastasize to the small intestine. Metastatic melanoma in the small bowel should be suspected in any patient with a history of malignant melanoma who develops GI symptoms or chronic blood loss. Uncontrolled bleeding, bowel obstruction, and intussusception may require palliative surgical resection of small bowel metastasis.

VIII. FOLLOW-UP
The goal of a follow-up is to identify potentially curable recurrence and to screen for secondary primary tumors. At least one annual skin examination by a dermatologist is recommended. Patients with high risk factors (including family history of melanoma, skin type, and presence of dysplastic nevi or nonmelanoma skin cancers) may require more frequent examination.

Patients with stage IA melanoma should be seen every 3 to 12 months, and the examination of regional lymph nodes should be emphasized. For patients with stage IB-III melanomas, history and physical should be performed every 3 to 6 months for 3 years, then every 4 to 12 months for 2 years, and annually thereafter. Patients with stage IV disease who are rendered disease free are followed as are patients with stage III disease. The regular follow-up should last between 5 and 10 years.

At clinician discretion, a chest x-ray study, LDH, LFT, and CBC may be obtained. Imaging studies (CT scan, PET scan) are ordered if clinically indicated. Abdominal or chest CT scans should be considered in patients with node-positive disease.

 BASAL CELL AND SQUAMOUS CELL CARCINOMAS

I. EPIDEMIOLOGY AND ETIOLOGY
A. Incidence. Nonmelanoma skin cancers (NMSC), mainly basal cell carcinoma (BCC) and squamous cell carcinoma (SCC), are the most common type of malignancy, but they account for <0.1% of cancer-related deaths. BCC is four to five times more common than SCC. The exact incidence is unknown, because these cancers are not reported to the registry; estimate is that there are 1.3 million cases a year.

B. Risk factors

1. **UV light exposure.** Excessive UV light exposure is the main risk factor. NMSC are >50 times less common in nonwhite population than in white persons. Of these cancers, 90% develop in sun-exposed areas of the body. Blue-eyed, fair-skinned, blond and red-haired people, and those who are easily sunburned are at increased risk.

2. **Exposure to ionizing radiation.** Individuals who were exposed to ionizing radiation (uranium miners, individuals treated with radiation, cancer survivors) have a higher risk of NMSC.

3. **Chronic immunosuppression and chronic use of glucocorticoids.** Organ transplant recipients have 60 to 250 higher risk of development of SCC than the general population. BCC occurs in this population only 10 times more commonly.

4. **Inorganic arsenic** exposure predisposes to the development of Bowen's disease, multiple BCC, and SCC, and is also associated with a higher incidence of intestinal carcinoma. Hard, yellowish hyperkeratotic plaques on the palms and soles provide a clue that the patient was exposed to arsenic.

5. **Other environmental risk factors** include smoking and phototherapy combined with psoralens.

6. **Infection**
   a. **Epidermodysplasia verruciformis,** which is primarily caused by human papillomaviruses (HPV) types 5 and 8, results in *in situ* and invasive SCC synergistically with other carcinogens, such as sunlight.
   b. **SCC** of the genitals and anal regions are strongly associated with HPV serotypes 16 and 18. Infection, usually through sexual transmission, increases the risk for regional SCC. **Verrucous carcinoma** (Buschke-Lowenstein tumor) is typically a slow-growing, HPV-associated (usually serotypes 6 and 11) neoplasm of the anogenital region that may deeply invade underlying structures.
   c. **Periungual SCC** is associated with HPV type 16.

7. **Chronic inflammation.** SCC can occasionally originate from the site of chronic ulcers or scars, sites of thermal burns, chronic draining osteomyelitis, and sinus tracts.

8. **Hereditary factors**
   a. **Basal cell nevus syndrome (Gorlin syndrome)** is a rare autosomal-dominant disorder caused by mutations in the human patched gene (PTCH). Multiple BCC lesions appear over the face, arms, and trunk during the late teenage years. Individuals also present with macrocephaly, bifid ribs, bone cysts, palmar and plantar pitting, kyphoscoliosis, spina bifida, short metacarpals, hyporesponsiveness to parathyroid hormone, medulloblastoma, and ovarian fibromata.
   b. **Xeroderma pigmentosum** is a multigenic, autosomal-recessive disorder in which DNA repair ability is impaired. Homozygotes have severe skin and eye sensitivity to sunshine. They develop SCC, BCC, and melanomas in the early childhood. Eye abnormalities include keratitis, iritis, opacification of the cornea, choroidal melanoma. Frequently, they also have from neurologic disorders (seizures, mental and speech disturbances). A severe form (De Sanctis-Cacchione syndrome) includes microcephaly, mental deficiency, dwarfism, and failure of gonadal development.
   c. **Oculocutanenous albinism** is a group of genetic disorders characterized by generalized decrease in pigmentation.

II. PATHOLOGY AND NATURAL HISTORY

A. **BCC** originates in the basal cell layer of the epidermis. Distant metastases from BCC are extremely rare. It has several recognized subtypes:

1. **Nodular BCC** is the most common type (~60% of cases). It arises predominantly on the head and neck as a well-circumscribed nodule with pearly or rolled borders and telangiectasias. Some lesions are pigmented and clinically indistinguishable from melanoma. They spread both over the surface and deeply into the tissues

to invade cartilage and bone. Larger tumors may develop central necrosis and ulcerate, forming a so called rodent ulcer.

2. **Superficial BCC** represents 30% of cases. Lesions usually arise on the trunk, are often multiple, and appear as red, scaly patches with areas of brown or black pigmentation. They spread over the skin surface and may have areas of nodularity.

3. **Sclerosing (morpheaform) BCC** represents 5% to 10% of cases. Lesions usually affect the face. The tumors resemble scars and may have an ivory-colored, ill-defined, indurated border. Histologically, the cancer cells are surrounded by a dense bed of fibrosis ("morphealike"). Considering all types of BCC, these have the highest recurrence rate after treatment.

4. **Cystic BCC** is uncommon. The tumor undergoes central degeneration to form a cystic lesion.

5. **Linear BCC** is a recently recognized morphologic clinical entity characterized by an increased risk for aggressive histopathologic pattern and increased subclinical tumor extension.

6. **Micronodular BCC** is defined histopathologically by small tumor nests and often exhibits covert subclinical growth.

B. **SCC** usually presents as a hyperkertotic papule, plaque or nodule. Hyperkartosis is an important feature of SCC. In 60% of cases, SCC arises from actinic keratoses.

1. **Cutaneous horns** usually represent a premalignant process of hyperkeratosis on an erythematous base, but occasionally may be a SCC.

2. **Bowen's disease** is a form of intraepithelial SCC *in situ*, but invasion may occur. It appears as a red-brown eczematoid plaque. It usually occurs on sun-damaged areas in older persons, but it may arise in mucous membranes. Although historically suspected, Bowen's disease is not associated with an increased risk for internal cancer. Bowenoid papulosis is an intraepithelial neoplasia of the genital area caused by HPV.

3. **Keratoacanthoma** is a hyperkeratotic nodule with a central keratin plug. It grows rapidly, distinguishing it from other forms of SCC. It may regress spontaneously, but it should be treated because it may further invade the dermis and involve deeper soft tissue.

4. **Basosquamous carcinoma** has features of both BCC and SCC, but it is usually grouped with SCC because of its more aggressive behavior and metastatic capacity.

5. **Metastases.** Tumors that metastasize are usually poorly differentiated. The incidence of metastasis is <3% for actinically induced SCC and 35% for nonactinically induced SCC. The draining lymph nodes are the most frequent sites of metastases, although distant organs are eventually involved.

III. DIAGNOSIS AND WORK-UP

Patients with suspicious lesions are offered a complete skin examination. If the lesion suggests SCC, examination of the regional lymph nodes should be performed. All suspicious lesions must be biopsied.

IV. STAGING SYSTEM AND PROGNOSTIC FACTORS

A. **TNM system** of staging has been developed by the American Joint Commission on Cancer (AJCC) for NMSC. More than 95% of BCC and SCC involve only local disease, and the staging system is rarely used. This system uses NX, N0, or N1 for unassessed, absent, or present regional lymph node metastasis, respectively, and MX, M0, or M1 for unassessed, absent, or present distant metastasis, respectively. Primary tumor stages are as follows:

TX	Primary tumor cannot be assessed
T0	No evidence of primary tumor
Tis	Carcinoma *in situ*
T1	Tumor ≤2 cm in greatest dimension
T2	Tumor 2 to 5 cm in greatest dimension
T3	Tumor >5 cm in greatest dimension

B. **Prognostic factors.** Several prognostic factors are associated with inadequate treatment of primary tumors.
   1. NMSC occurring on the head and neck and tumors >2 cm in diameter are more likely to recur.
   2. SCC in the genital area, on mucosal surfaces, or on the ear have a higher propensity to metastasize.
   3. Tumors that recur more frequently are those that are characterized by ill-defined clinical borders or perineural involvement, and those that present as recurrent disease or develop in chronically immunosuppressed individuals (especially, organ transplant recipients).
   4. BCC with micronodular, infiltrative, sclerosing, or morpheaform features and SCC with desmoplastic histologic features are also more likely to recur.
   5. Basosquamous carcinoma has a higher capacity to metastasize than BCC or SCC.
   6. Several risk factors also are applicable only to SCC. These factors include tumor at the site of chronic inflammation, rapidly growing tumors, symptomatic nerve involvement, depth of invasion, and moderately or poorly differentiated histology. Patients with any one high-risk feature belong to the high-risk group.

V. PREVENTION

Primary prevention is largely achieved by encouraging patients and other responsible parties to minimize sunlight exposure and other reducible risk factors. Early vaccination with Gardacil for females holds great potential to reduce the incidence of anogenital SCC. Skin erythema from solar exposure, even from UV light on cloudy days, represents skin damage that is cumulative over the years. The "healthy tan" represents the body's reaction to skin damage, and freckling should be recognized as an early sign of skin injury. Sunscreens with an SPF of ≥15 and protective clothing, including hats, are helpful. Those who fastidiously avoid sunlight exposure to decrease their risk for skin cancer should meet their vitamin D requirement through diet or dietary supplements.

Successful *secondary prevention* is dependent on a regular follow-up. About 40% of patients with NMSC will develop another NMSC within 5 years. These individuals are also at higher risk for development of melanoma.

VI. MANAGEMENT

A. **Actinic keratoses** (precancerous lesions for SCC) are treated with cryosurgery or topical treatment with 5-fluorouracil or imiquimod. Solaraze gel (diclofenac sodium, 3%) twice daily for 3 months is often effective topically if multiple lesions are present. Cryotherapy is associated with the risk of scarring, infection, and pigmentary changes; topical therapies are associated with application-site irritation. Topical methyl aminolevulinate photodynamic therapy is a new promising method.

B. **BCC and SCC** can be treated with surgical techniques, radiation therapy, and topical therapies. It is important to customize therapeutic approaches to the particular factors and the individual needs of patients.
   1. **Mohs' micrographic surgery** is the surgical method with the highest primary tumor cure rate (99% for BCC and 96% for SCC) and excellent cosmetic effects. Other techniques may require less training, be less costly, less invasive, or less time-consuming. Therefore, Mohs' surgery is recommended mainly for high-risk lesions and for recurrent tumors wherein the success rates are 95% for BCC and 93% for SCC.
   2. **Excision with postoperative margin evaluation.** The rate of cure is about 90% for primary tumors <2 cm in diameter when a 4- to 6-mm margin is applied. Larger or recurrent tumors require 10-mm margins, which may result in significant cosmetic or functional deficits; cure rates range from 50% to 85%.
   3. **Curettage and electrodessication** is effective for low-risk tumors. It should not be used for tumors in the hair-bearing areas, and it should be followed by surgical excision if the subcutaneous layer is reached.
   4. **Cryosurgery using liquid nitrogen** may be considered for patients with small, clinically well-defined primary tumors. It is especially useful for debilitated patients with medical conditions that preclude other types of surgery.

5. **Radiation therapy** is indicated in patients requiring extensive surgery or whose tumors are in surgically difficult locations. It should be avoided in young individuals, because of the risk of secondary malignancies. RT is also relatively contraindicated in patients with xeroderma pigmentosa, epidermodysplasia verruciformis, or the basal cell nevus syndrome, because RT may induce more tumors in the treated field. Adjuvant RT should be considered after surgery for SCC demonstrating perineural invasion, tumor thickness >4 mm, or invasion into muscle or periosteum owing to increased risk for local recurrence and nodal metastases.

6. **Superficial therapies** with topical 5-fluorouracil, imiquimod, or photodynamic therapy are used in patients with low-risk shallow cancers and in those who have contraindications for surgery and radiation therapy.

7. **Chemotherapy** has no adjuvant use for BCC or SCC. Experience in treating metastatic skin cancers is extremely limited. Fluorouracil, cisplatin, methotrexate, bleomycin, retinoids, and cyclophosphamide given singly and in combination have produced temporary tumor regression. Excellent response rates have been reported for advanced cases of SCC and BCC treated with cisplatin in combination with either a 5-day infusion of 5-fluorouracil (dosages similar to those used for head and neck cancers) or doxorubicin.

C. **Management of enlarged lymph nodes.** Occasionally, SCC can spread to the regional lymph nodes. Enlarged regional lymph nodes should undergo fine needle aspiration (FNA) or be biopsied. If lymph nodes are involved by tumor, a radical lymph node dissection followed by radiation therapy is recommended.

MERKEL CELL CARCINOMA

I. EPIDEMIOLOGY

Merkel cell carcinoma (MCC) is a rare type of skin cancer with the estimated incidence in the United States of 0.44 per 100,000 and 33% mortality, which is the highest mortality rate among cutaneous malignancies. The median age at presentation is 68 to 74 years.

A. **Risk factors.** Sun exposure, advanced age, and chronic immunosuppression are important risk factors. The tumor occurs mainly on sun-exposed areas and it is more common in patients treated with PUVA (psoralen [a light-sensitizing agent] is combined with controlled exposure to ultraviolet light A [UVA]). It also occurs more frequently in patients who are human immunodeficiency virus (HIV) positive, have had organ transplantation, or have been on chronic immunosuppression for rheumatoid arthritis. Transplant recipients develop MCC at a median age of 46 years.

B. **Prognostic factors.** Positive SLNB remain the worst prognostic factors. The 3-year recurrence rate is 60% in patients with positive SLNB and 20% when biopsy is negative. Contrary to melanoma, the depth of invasion is not a prognostic factor. Studies on other parameters for prognosis, such as tumor size, growth pattern, mitotic activity, necrosis, and inflammation, have revealed conflicting results.

II. PATHOLOGY AND NATURAL HISTORY

These cells, first discovered by Merkel in the snout skin of voles in 1875, are thought to originate from the neural crest and to act as mechanoreceptors. Tumors are assumed to be derived from the large, oval neuroendocrine Merkel cells that are located in the basal layer of the epidermis and are associated with terminal axons.

Initially, tumor cells spread from the primary site through the lymphatic system to local lymph nodes and then they can disseminate throughout the whole body. The most common sites of distant metastases are liver, brain, lungs, bones, and skin.

III. DIAGNOSIS

A. **Signs.** MCC manifests as a rapidly growing, painless, indurated, and erythematous to violaceous nodule. The lesions appear mainly in the sun-exposed areas. Head and neck (30% to 45%) and the extremities (35%) are the most common sites for the primary tumor, but the tumor can occur on the trunk, the buttocks, or genitalia. Most patients (75%) present with the disease localized to the primary skin site. Of cases, 25% are characterized by involvement of regional lymph nodes and 2% to 4% by distant metastases. Some patients (~2%) are diagnosed with the metastatic disease in the setting of the carcinoma of unknown primary site.

B. Diagnosis. Biopsy of the growing lesion is required for diagnosis. The three histologic types are trabecular, intermediate cell, and small cell, but histologic subtypes do not carry prognostic value. It is often difficult to differentiate MCC from other "small blue cell tumors."

C. Staging. Three-stage staging system has been most widely used.

Stage	Extent	5-Year survival (%)
Ia	Localized disease, tumor ≤2cm	81
Ib	Localized disease, tumor >2cm	67
II	Regional lymph nodes involved	52
III	Disease beyond the regional lymph nodes or distant metastases	11

Physical examination, concentrating especially on regional lymph nodes and computerized tomography scan of the chest, abdomen and pelvis, should be used as a part of staging investigations.

IV. MANAGEMENT

Merkel cell carcinoma is a rare disease, and no randomized trials have been performed to establish standard care.

A. Surgery. Patients who have no evidence of metastatic disease should be considered for primary RT or wide excision of the primary tumor with 2- to 3-cm margin. In some centers, primary RT is the treatment of choice because the malignancy is extremely radiosensitive. Some evidence from nonrandomized trials indicates that Mohs' micrographic surgery improves local tumor control when compared with standard surgical resection.

B. Assessment of the regional lymph nodes, Individuals who had negative lymph nodes on surgical assessment of their status by SNLB, elective lymph node dissection, or therapeutic nodal staging had a 97% 5-year disease-free survival (DFS) compared with a 75% 5-year DFS for individuals whose lymph nodes were assessed only clinically. Most of the centers recommend SNLB as the most appropriate method of lymph node status assessment. Patients who have a positive SNLB or have clinically or radiograpically demonstrable nodal involvement are treated with total lymphadenectomy.

C. Radiation therapy. Adjuvant RT to the primary site improves local tumor control. Patients treated with surgery alone are 3.7 times more likely to develop a local recurrence and 2.7 times more likely to develop a regional recurrence than patients who received combination surgery and RT. The rate of distant metastasis is similar between the groups. Adjuvant RT to nodes is recommended when SNLB has not been performed or when clinically or pathologically evident nodal disease is present. Efforts should be made to minimize potential delays before commencement of RT, because it may result in disease progression.

D. Chemotherapy. The role of adjuvant chemotherapy is controversial and most studies suggest that, although it may improve the locoregional control, it does not prolong survival. In a study performed by Trans-Tasman Radiation Oncology Group, patients with high-risk features (size of the primary tumor >1 cm, lymph node involvement, recurrence after primary therapy, or gross residual disease after resection) received synchronous RT and chemotherapy with carboplatin and etoposide; this approach resulted in an excellent overall survival at 3 years of 76%. In a subsequent follow-up study, a greater number of patients were compared with historical controls, and this comparison revealed no benefit in overall survival for individuals receiving chemotherapy.

Currently, chemotherapy is not recommended for patients with node-negative disease, but can be considered for high-risk patients. Individuals with metastatic disease should be treated with chemotherapy.

No standard chemotherapy regimen has been established, but regimens commonly used for the treatment of small cell lung cancer, such as CAV (cyclophosphamide, doxorubicin, vincristine), CEV (cyclophosphamide, etoposide, vincristine) with or without prednisone, and EP (etoposide, cisplatin) have been prescribed most frequently. Use of CAV or CEV resulted in 75% response rate, including 35% complete responses; EP resulted in 60% response rate and 35% complete responses. Median overall survival for patients treated with any type of chemotherapy is 22 months (ranging from 1 to 118 months) and at 2 years 36% individuals remain alive.

E. Treatment of recurrent disease. Locally and regionally recurrent disease is treated with surgery and RT or chemoradiation therapy. Systemic recurrence is treated with chemotherapy.

Suggested Reading

Malignant Melanoma

Balch CM, Soong SJ, Gershenwald JE, et al. Prognostic factors analysis of 17,600 melanoma patients: validation of the American Joint Committee on Cancer melanoma staging system. *J Clin Oncol* 2001;19(16):3622.

Kirkwood JM, Strawderman MH, Ernstoff MS, et al. Interferon alfa-2b adjuvant therapy of high-risk resected cutaneous melanoma: the Eastern Cooperative Oncology Group Trial EST 1684. *J Clin Oncol* 1996;14(1):7.

Miller AJ, Mihm MC Jr. Melanoma. *N Engl J Med* 2006;355(1):51.

Morton DL, Thompson JF, Cochran AJ, et al. Sentinel-node biopsy or nodal observation in melanoma. *N Engl J Med* 2006;355(13):1307.

Tsao H, Atkins MB, Sober AJ. Management of cutaneous melanoma. *N Engl J Med* 2004;351(10):998.

Basal Cell and Squamous Cell Carcinomas

Alam M, Ratner D. Cutaneous squamous-cell carcinoma. *N Engl J Med* 2001;344(13):975.

Clayman GL, Lee JJ, Holsinger FC, et al. Mortality risk from squamous cell skin cancer. *J Clin Oncol* 2005;23(4):759.

Rubin AI, Chen EH, Ratner D. Basal-cell carcinoma. *N Engl J Med* 2005;353(21):2262.

Merkel Cell Carcinoma

Gupta SG et al. Sentinel lymph node biopsy for evaluation and treatment of patients with Merkel cell carcinoma. The Dana-Farber experience and meta-analysis of the literature. *Arch Dermatol* 2006;142:685.

Krasagakis K, Tosca AD. Overview of Merkel cell carcinoma and recent advances in research. *Int J Dermatol* 2003;42(9):749.

Mojica P, Smith D, Ellenhorn JDI. Adjuvant radiation therapy is associated with improved survival in Merkel cell carcinoma of the skin. *J Clin Oncol* 2007;25:1043.

Swann M, Yoon J. Merkel cell carcinoma. *Semin Oncol* 2007;34(1):51.

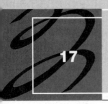

SARCOMAS

Charles A. Forscher and Dennis A. Casciato

I. EPIDEMIOLOGY AND ETIOLOGY. Primary mesenchymal tumors localized outside the skeleton, parenchymatous organs, or hollow viscera are generally designated as soft-tissue sarcomas (STSs). Sarcomas of the mediastinum, heart, and blood vessels are discussed in Chapter 19.

A. Incidence. Sarcomas constitute about 1% of all cancers and will account for an estimated 9,220 new cases of STS and 2,370 cases of bone sarcoma in the United States in 2007. These will be associated with 3,560 and 1,330 deaths, respectively.

    1. STSs outnumber bone sarcomas by a ratio of 3:1. In children, most STSs are rhabdomyosarcomas or undifferentiated tumors originating in the head and neck regions. In adults, STSs occur most frequently on the extremities or retroperitoneum and least frequently in the head and neck region.

    2. Bone sarcomas occur mostly between 10 and 20 years of age (osteogenic sarcoma) or between 40 and 60 years of age (chondrosarcoma).

    3. Most sarcomas show no sexual predilection. Incidence peaks during childhood and in the fifth decade.

B. Etiology. Certain kinds of sarcomas are associated with exposure to specific agents or with underlying medical conditions.

    1. Lymphangiosarcoma. Prolonged postmastectomy arm edema (Stewart-Treves syndrome)

    2. Angiosarcoma and other STSs. Polyvinyl chloride, thorium dioxide, dioxin, arsenic, and androgens

    3. Osteosarcoma. Radium (watch dials) exposure; postmastectomy irradiation; Paget disease of bone

    4. Fibrosarcoma. Postirradiation: Paget disease of bone

    5. Kaposi sarcoma. Cytomegalovirus and human immunodeficiency virus type 1 (HIV-1; discussed in Chapter 36, Section IV.)

    6. Leiomyosarcoma. HIV-1 in children

    7. Genetic diseases and syndromes

        a. Li-Fraumeni syndrome. Various sarcomas (especially rhabdomyosarcoma) and carcinomas of breast, lung, and adrenal cortex (*p53* gene)

        b. Neurofibromatosis. Schwannomas (*NF1* gene)

        c. Familial retinoblastoma. Osteosarcoma (*RB1* gene)

    8. Chromosomal aberrations are found in nearly all sarcomas. Characteristic translocations, particularly involving DNA transcription factors, are being defined (e.g., the X;18 translocation in synovial sarcoma and the 11;22 translocation in Ewing sarcoma).

II. PATHOLOGY AND NATURAL HISTORY

A. Histology and nomenclature. Sarcomas are given a bewildering variety of names that do not indicate biological behavior and usually do not influence therapeutic approach. The multipotential capacities of the mesenchymal tissue and the appearance of several histological elements in the same tumor often make clear-cut histological diagnosis difficult.

    1. Sarcomas are named for the tissue of origin (e.g., osteosarcoma, chondrosarcoma, schwannoma, liposarcoma). These names may be combined to describe multicomponent tumors (e.g., fibrous histiocytoma).

2. **Tumors are also named for special histological characteristics** or given a nondescriptive name because the tissue of origin is unknown (alveolar soft parts tumor, Kaposi sarcoma, Ewing sarcoma).

3. **Pathologists recognize several features in determining the grade of a sarcoma.** These include the degree of cellular differentiation, the presence (or absence) of mitotic activity, spontaneous necrosis, and vascular invasion. The other descriptive terms for the tumor are far less important. Expert pathological evaluation is crucial.

4. **The presence of osteoid formation** by the tumor cells suggests the diagnosis of osteogenic sarcoma. This must be distinguished from reactive or metaplastic bone formation by the pathologist.

5. **Immunohistochemistry** may be helpful in confirming the diagnosis of rhabdomyosarcoma and leiomyosarcoma. Expected immunophenotypes for the various sarcomas are shown in Appendix C-4.III and C-4.VIII.

6. **Cytogenetics** can be useful in the diagnosis of Ewing sarcoma, synovial sarcoma, and rhabdomyosarcoma. Newer techniques, such as fluorescent in situ hybridization (FISH) analysis, are also becoming increasingly useful.

B. **Natural history.** Generally, sarcomas arise *de novo* and not from pre-existing benign neoplasms. Tumors occasionally "dedifferentiate," however, from benign to malignant forms or from a lower grade to a higher grade. Sarcomas spread without interruption along tissue planes; they invade local nerve fibers, muscle bundles, and blood vessels. Histological sections usually show much greater local extension than is apparent on gross examination.

1. **Histological grade.** The biological behavior of sarcomas can usually be predicted by their histological grade. Low-grade tumors tend to remain localized; high-grade tumors (especially those with a marked degree of necrosis) metastasize early. Most osteogenic sarcomas, rhabdomyosarcomas, Ewing sarcomas, and synovial sarcomas are high-grade malignancies.

2. **Site of origin.** The site of origin of the sarcoma may suggest the cell type, as follows:

   a. **Head and neck**
      (1) Rhabdomyosarcoma (in a child)
      (2) Angiosarcoma (in an elderly person)
      (3) Osteogenic sarcoma (jaw)

   b. **Distal extremity**
      (1) Epithelioid sarcoma
      (2) Synovial sarcoma
      (3) Clear cell sarcoma
      (4) Osteogenic sarcoma (femur)

   c. **Proximal tibia or humerus.** Osteogenic sarcoma

   d. **Mesothelium.** Mesothelioma

   e. **Abdomen, retroperitoneum, and mesentery**
      (1) Leiomyosarcoma
      (2) Liposarcoma
      (3) Gastrointestinal stromal tumor (GIST; gastrointestinal sarcoma)
      (4) Desmoplastic small round cell tumor

   f. **Genitourinary tract**
      (1) Rhabdomyosarcoma (in a child)
      (2) Leiomyosarcoma (in an adult)

   g. **Skin**
      (1) Angiosarcoma, lymphangiosarcoma
      (2) Kaposi sarcoma
      (3) Epithelioid sarcoma
      (4) Dermatofibrosarcoma protuberans (on trunk)

3. **Metastases.** Sarcomas typically spread hematogenously. Lung metastases occur most commonly. Hepatic metastases can be seen from primary gastrointestinal or gynecologic sarcomas. The retroperitoneum can be a site of metastasis for extremity liposarcomas. Other sites, such as bone, subcutaneous tissue, and brain,

are less common and are often detected only after pulmonary metastases have developed (tertiary metastases).

a. Sarcomas that metastasize to lymph nodes

(1) Rhabdomyosarcoma

(2) Synovial sarcoma

(3) Epithelioid sarcoma

b. Sarcomas that rarely metastasize and are associated with a favorable survival

(1) Liposarcoma (myxoid and well-differentiated types)

(2) Fibrosarcoma (infantile and well-differentiated types)

(3) Malignant fibrous histiocytoma (superficial type)

(4) Dermatofibrosarcoma protuberans

(5) Parosteal osteosarcoma

(6) Kaposi sarcoma when not related to acquired immunodeficiency syndrome (AIDS)

4. Paraneoplastic syndromes associated with sarcomas

a. Hypoglycemia (particularly with retroperitoneal fibrosarcoma)

b. Hypertrophic osteoarthropathy (sarcoma of pleura or mediastinum)

c. Hypocalcemia

d. Oncogenic osteomalacia

C. Clinical aspects of specific STSs

1. Alveolar soft-part sarcoma

a. Tissue of origin (incidence). Unknown (rare)

b. Features. Unique histology with no benign counterpart; often indolent even with lung metastases, which are common. The sarcoma most associated with brain metastases. Commonly affects the thigh in adults and the head and neck in children. The 5-year survival rate exceeds 60%.

2. Angiosarcoma (hemangiosarcoma, lymphangiosarcoma)

a. Tissue of origin (incidence). Blood or lymph vessels (2% to 3%)

b. Features of hemangiosarcoma. Affects the elderly; aggressive. Arises in many organs, notably the head and neck region, breast, and liver; especially affects the skin and superficial soft tissues (whereas most STSs are deep). Dedifferentiation from a hemangioma is rare. The 5-year survival rate is <20%.

c. Features of lymphangiosarcoma. Affects older adults; aggressive. Arises in areas with chronic lymphatic stasis (especially postmastectomy). The 5-year survival rate is 10%.

3. Clear cell sarcoma

a. Tissue of origin (incidence). Now recognized as a form of malignant melanoma (rare)

b. Features. Affects adults <40 years of age; painless, firm, spherical masses on tendon sheaths and aponeurotic structures of distal extremities. The 5-year survival rate is about 50%.

4. Epithelioid sarcoma

a. Tissue of origin (incidence). Unknown (rare)

b. Features. Affects young adults; aggressive; typically appears on distal extremities. Epithelioid sarcoma and synovial sarcoma are the most common tumors of the hand and foot. Differs from other STSs by having a greater tendency to spread to noncontiguous areas of skin, subcutaneous tissue, fat, draining lymph nodes, and bone. The 5-year survival rate is about 30%.

5. Fibrosarcoma

a. Tissue of origin (incidence). Fibrous tissue (5% to 20%)

b. Features. Affects all age groups; arises in many mesenchymal sites; usually involves the abdominal wall or extremities. Ninety percent are well differentiated (desmoid). Dermatofibrosarcoma protuberans (rare) develops on the skin of the trunk and almost never metastasizes. Fibromyxosarcoma affects any soft-tissue site but usually develops on the extremities. Ten percent are poorly differentiated (high grade). Survival is directly related to tumor grade (also see section II.D.5).

6. **Malignant fibrous histiocytoma (MFH)/myxofibrosarcoma.** Many pathologists now prefer the term *myxofibrosarcoma* for these tumors. Some tumors previously felt to represent MFH are now classified as pleiomorphic liposarcomas or pleiomorphic sarcoma, not otherwise specified (NOS).
   a. **Tissue of origin (incidence).** Unknown (10% to 23%)
   b. **Features.** Age >40 years (<5% of affected patients are <20 years of age). MFH has become a common histological diagnosis. Develops in extremities (especially legs), trunk, and retroperitoneum. Superficial MFH develops close to the skin surface and is often low grade; the 5-year survival rate is 65%. Deep MFH usually is high grade; the 5-year survival rate is 30% to 60%.
7. **Hemangiopericytoma/solitary fibrous tumor**
   a. **Tissue of origin (incidence).** Blood vessels or fibrous tissue (<1%)
   b. **Features.** Affects all ages. Develops under finger tips (glomus tumors), on lower extremities or pelvis, in the retroperitoneum, and elsewhere. Benign and malignant versions. The 5-year survival rate is about 50%.
8. **Kaposi sarcoma (KS).** All varieties of KS are associated with human herpesvirus type 8 (HHV-8). KS typically presents as purplish blotches or nodules that may be painful or pruritic. Treatment of KS in patients with AIDS is discussed in Chapter 36.IV.
   a. **Tissue of origin (incidence).** Controversial (varied)
   b. **Features of classic KS.** Classically affects older adults with Mediterranean ancestry; extremely indolent lesions arise on lower extremities (occasionally on hands, ears, and nose) and rarely cause death.
   c. **Features of epidemic KS.** The epidemic and aggressive variety is associated with AIDS (see Chapter 36, IV), African children, renal transplant recipients, immunosuppressed nontransplantation patients, and Eskimos. These patients develop a widely disseminated, aggressive, and usually fatal form of the disease. Generalized cutaneous involvement, generalized lymphadenopathy, and visceral or gastrointestinal involvement are typical.
9. **Leiomyosarcoma, gastrointestinal stromal tumor (GIST), and metastasizing leiomyoma**
   a. **Tissue of origin (incidence).** Smooth muscle for leiomyoma and leiomyosarcoma; interstitial cell of Cajal for GIST (7% to 11%).
   b. **Features.** Affects all age groups. Develops in gastrointestinal tract, uterus, retroperitoneum, and other soft tissues. Generally refractory to chemotherapy and radiotherapy. The 5-year survival rate is 30%.
   c. **Gastrointestinal stromal tumors (GISTs)** are morphologically similar to leiomyosarcoma but have different immunohistochemical staining characteristics (see Appendix C-4.III). GISTs do not stain for actin (as leiomyosarcomas do), and most express CD117 (*c-kit* protein). Treatment of GIST is presented in section VII.C.7.
   d. **Leiomyoma peritonealis disseminata (LPD).** A condition in women, usually in reproductive years. Myriads of asymptomatic benign leiomyomas are usually scattered throughout the peritoneal cavity and range from 1 to 10 cm in size; they are stimulated by estrogen. LPD causes occasional mechanical problems with bowel or pain. Generally, no treatment is required; when symptomatic, treatment is with estrogens or antiestrogens.
   e. **Leiomyoma, benign metastasizing.** Histologically benign, these leiomyomas are typically discovered as persistent pulmonary nodules and possibly as a variant of LPD. Associated nodules in the pelvis are mostly in round ligaments of uterus and not as diffuse as in LPD. Treatment is surgical for symptomatic or progressive lesions.
10. **Liposarcoma**
    a. **Tissue of origin (incidence).** Fat tissue (15% to 18%)
    b. **Features.** Affects middle and older age groups, mostly men. Develops in thigh, groin, buttocks, shoulder girdle, and retroperitoneum. Does not arise from benign lipomas. Low-grade tumors in the extremity are now called *atypical lipomatous tumor*. The designation of well-differentiated liposarcoma

remains for tumors of the abdomen and retroperitoneum. The 5-year survival rate is 80% for low-grade liposarcomas and 20% for high-grade liposarcomas.

11. Mesothelioma
   a. Tissue of origin (incidence). Mesothelium
   b. Features. Age >50 years. Asbestos exposure is etiologic. Involves pleura and peritoneum; aggressively encases viscera. Highly lethal; the 5-year survival rate is <10% (see Chapter 8).

12. Myxoma
   a. Tissue of origin (incidence). Mesenchymal tissues
   b. Features. Usually found on extremities; has histological appearance of umbilical cord. The 5-year survival rate is about 80%.

13. Neurofibrosarcoma (schwannoma, neurilemoma)
   a. Tissue of origin (incidence). Nerve (5% to 7%)
   b. Features. Affects young and middle-aged adults and patients with neurofibromatosis type 1 (von Recklinghausen disease; about 10% develop sarcomatous changes during lifetime). Histologically resembles fibrosarcoma. Presents with thickening of nerves and without anatomic predilection. Superficial variety is low grade, spreads extensively along nerve sheaths without metastasizing, and has a 5-year survival rate of >90%. Penetrating variety is high grade with nodular growth, vascular invasion, and lung metastases and has a 5-year survival rate of <20%.

14. Rhabdomyosarcoma
   a. Tissue of origin (incidence). Striated muscle (5% to 19%)
   b. Features. By definition in the G-TNM staging system, all are grade 3. All types can occur in any age group, but the typical onset and distribution is noted below (see Chapter 18, "Rhabdomyosarcoma").
   c. Features of embryonal rhabdomyosarcoma. Affects infants and children; sites are head and neck (70%) and genitalia (15% to 20%). Includes sarcoma botryoid. The 5-year survival rate is about 70%.
   d. Features of alveolar rhabdomyosarcoma. Affects teenagers at any site; highly aggressive; histology resembles lung alveoli. The 5-year survival rate is about 50%.
   e. Features of pleomorphic rhabdomyosarcoma. Affects patients >30 years of age, is rare, and develops in extremities. Often is highly anaplastic; microscopically confused with MFH. The 5-year survival rate is about 25%.

15. Synovial sarcoma
   a. Tissue of origin (incidence). Unknown. Although these tumors can arise near joints, they are not composed of cells with synovial differentiation. The name is a misnomer that persists. They rarely arise within a joint space.
   b. Features. Affects young adults, but may occur from the second to fourth decade. Monophasic and biphasic subtypes are distinguished. Presents with hard masses, often painful, near tendons in the vicinity of joints of the hands, knees, or feet. Synovial and epithelioid sarcoma are the most common tumors of the hand and foot. Often calcified, with characteristic radiographic appearance. The majority of synovial sarcomas are high grade. Lymph node involvement may be seen in up to 20% of cases. The 5-year survival rate is from 30% to 50%.

D. Clinical aspects of specific bone sarcomas
   1. Adamantinoma
      a. Tissue of origin (incidence). Unknown; nonosseous (<1%)
      b. Features. Osteolytic tumor; often develops on upper tibia; resembles ameloblastoma of mandible. Indolent behavior; the 5-year survival rate is >90%.

   2. Chondrosarcoma
      a. Tissue of origin (incidence). Cartilage (30%)
      b. Features. Age, 40 to 60 years; <4% of patients are <20 years of age. Usually develops in shoulder girdle (15%), proximal femur (20%), or pelvis (30%).

Chondrosarcomas are the most common malignant tumors of the sternum and scapula. Most tumors are grade 1 or 2; higher-grade tumors metastasize frequently; however, tumor grade does not appear to affect prognosis. Local recurrence is a major problem in management. Usually refractory to both radiation therapy (RT) and chemotherapy. Dedifferentiated chondrosarcomas may, however, respond to chemotherapy. Complete surgical removal is the main determinant of recurrence and survival. The 5-year survival rate is about 50%.

(1) Central chondrosarcomas (75%) arise within a bone; peripheral chondrosarcomas (25%) arise from the surface of a bone. Peripheral lesions can become quite large without causing pain; central lesions present with a dull pain but rarely with a mass. Pain means that the apparently "benign" cartilage tumor on radiographs is probably a central chondrosarcoma.

(2) About 25% of chondrosarcomas represent malignant transformation of a pre-existing endochondroma or osteocartilaginous exostosis. The presentation of multiple benign cartilaginous tumors has a higher rate of malignant transformation than the corresponding solitary lesions.

3. Chordoma
  a. Tissue of origin (incidence). Primitive notochord cells (5%)
  b. Features. Develops in the midline of the neural axis at base of skull or sacrococcygeal area. The physaliferous cells are pathognomonic histologically. Indolent tumor with almost universal tendency for local recurrence. Low grade but eventually fatal after many years because of complications associated with invasion into neural tissues. Treated with surgery and RT. The 5-year survival rate is 50%.

4. Ewing sarcoma
  a. Tissue of origin (incidence). Unknown; nonmesenchymal elements of bone marrow (15%).
  b. Features. Affects children 10 to 15 years of age; rare in blacks; highly aggressive; arises in many bones, but especially the femoral diaphysis (see Chapter 18, "Ewing Sarcoma").

5. Fibrosarcoma of bone
  a. Tissue of origin (incidence). Fibrous tissue (2%)
  b. Features. Affects middle-aged patients in major long bones; develops occasionally in conjunction with an underlying disease (bone infarcts, osteomyelitis, benign giant cell tumor, Paget disease, after RT). Resembles fibrosarcoma, but osteoid is detected in parts of the lesion. Often high grade, which correlates with metastatic potential and survival (see section II.C.5).

6. Fibrous histiocytoma of bone
  a. Tissue of origin (incidence). Fibrous and primitive mesenchymal tissue (5%)
  b. Features. Affects older patients; arises *de novo* or as a complication of Paget disease. Most common sites are metaphyses of long bones, especially around the knee. In contrast to osteogenic sarcoma, serum alkaline phosphatase levels are normal. Pathological fracture is often the first manifestation. Aggressive with high rate of dissemination to lungs (also see section II.C.6).

7. Giant cell tumor of bone
  a. Tissue of origin (incidence). Unknown (<1%)
  b. Features. Patients usually >20. Most common sites are around the knee, radius, and sacrum. Tumor is usually benign but can be locally aggressive. Rare malignant transformation can occur.

8. Osteogenic sarcoma
  a. Tissue of origin (incidence). Bone (40% to 50%)
  b. Features of classic osteogenic sarcoma. Affects any age, but the onset is usually between 10 and 20 years; more common in boys and men. Most tumors originate in the metaphysis of long bones, the region of highest growth velocity. Tender, bony masses in the distal femur, proximal tibia, and proximal humerus account for 85% of cases. Nearly always high grade.
  c. Features of low-grade osteogenic sarcoma. Rare; central lesions can occur.

    d. Features of osteogenic sarcoma of the jaw. Affects patients between the ages of 20 and 40 years; men are more commonly affected; frequently detected during dental examinations. These tumors often have a cartilaginous component. High- and low-grade varieties are treated with hemimaxillectomy or hemimandibulectomy and reconstruction. Local control can often be a major problem if less than radical surgery is performed.

    e. Features of telangiectatic osteogenic sarcoma. Affects younger patients; a purely lytic tumor that can be confused with an aneurysmal bone cyst. Highly malignant; metastasizes early.

    f. Features of multifocal sclerosing osteogenic sarcoma. Rare; affects children <10 years of age. Develops multiple simultaneous primary sites in metaphyses; rapidly metastasizes to lung and soft tissues.

    g. Features of periosteal osteogenic sarcoma. Rare. Affects patients between the ages of 15 and 25 years; arises on external bone surface growing into the overlying soft tissues as an enlarging painless mass with minimal involvement of medullary canal. Histologically confused with chondrosarcomas. More than 50% metastasize (also see section II.D.9).

9. Parosteal (juxtacortical) sarcoma

    a. Tissue of origin (incidence). Bone surface (<2%)

    b. Features. A distinct clinical entity (see section II.D.8.g). Onset from 20 to 30 years of age. Characteristic exophytic lesion that is often on the posterior aspect of the distal femur or medial aspect of the proximal humerus. Presents as a fixed painless mass. Usually low grade with an indolent course; rarely involves medullary canal. Infrequently metastasizes; the 5-year survival rate is 80%.

10. Sarcomas of bone associated with other conditions

    a. Paget disease of the bone. Affects patients >60 years of age; the risk for sarcoma is 1,000-fold greater than in the general population at this age. Sarcomatous transformation occurs in 0.7% of patients with Paget disease and accounts for 5% to 14% of osteogenic sarcomas. The histological form varies among reported series but is usually osteogenic sarcoma, MFH, or fibrosarcoma; chondrosarcoma, giant cell tumor, and other forms occur infrequently. Tends to affect the pelvis and proximal femur; frequently presents as pathological fracture of the femur. Highly malignant.

    b. After high-dose RT. Sarcoma develops within the irradiated field (bone or adjacent soft-tissue structures) about 10 years after treatment. Highly malignant.

    c. Familial or bilateral retinoblastoma. A tumor-suppressor gene (*RB*) has been identified on the 13q chromosome in some patients with retinoblastoma. Patients who have a 13q deletion are at increased risk for later development of osteogenic sarcoma, not only in the irradiated field but also in long bones distant from irradiated sites about 10 to 20 years later. Highly malignant.

III. DIAGNOSIS

    A. Symptoms and signs are summarized in sections II.C and D. Patients with STS typically present with a painless, progressive swelling in an extremity; all such swellings are suspect for malignancy. Head and neck sarcomas manifest as proptosis, masses, or neurological abnormalities. Retroperitoneal sarcomas present with back pain, lower-extremity edema, and abdominal masses. Bone sarcomas usually result in visible enlargement of bone and pathological fractures.

    B. Biopsy. An accurate biopsy diagnosis is essential. Computed tomography (CT) or ultrasound-guided biopsies are increasingly employed at initial diagnosis and in the evaluation of possible recurrences. An open biopsy is still performed when the results of CT-guided biopsies are equivocal.

    C. Radiographic studies

        1. Plain radiographs of soft tissues may demonstrate bone involvement. Stippled calcification may be present within the mass. Patients with painful or enlarged bones should have radiographic study of these areas. The following findings are helpful for making the diagnosis of osteogenic sarcoma:

a. An osteoblastic appearance is often seen in osteosarcoma.
b. Periosteal reaction with elevated periosteum forming a triangle (*Codman's triangle*) with bone cortex. Any periosteal elevation in an apparent bone lesion is an indication for biopsy.
c. Sunraylike spiculation of bones
d. Onion-skin appearance (a common finding in Ewing sarcoma)

2. CT scans are most useful for evaluating retroperitoneal or head and neck regions. CT scanning of the extremities appears to be effective in delineating the extent of the tumor.

3. Magnetic resonance imaging (MRI) is comparable to CT scans in defining the relation of the tumor to neurovascular and skeletal structures, but MRI might be better for predicting resectability.

4. Arteriography may be useful in certain cases to plan surgical resection.

5. Radionuclide scans. Bone scan is performed in patients with bone sarcomas to search for multifocal disease. PET scanning is useful both for determining sites of disease and for assessing response to therapy.

6. CT of the thorax is necessary for all patients with sarcoma to detect lung metastases, which may be resected after the primary tumor is managed. An "old calcified granuloma" is an untenable radiological diagnosis in a young person with sarcoma.

7. Serum alkaline phosphatase levels are elevated in 60% of patients with osteogenic sarcoma and rarely in other bone sarcomas. When elevated at the time of diagnosis, this result is an important tumor marker to evaluate response to therapy.

IV. STAGING SYSTEM AND PROGNOSTIC FACTORS

A. Staging system. Tumor grade is the single most important prognostic factor in sarcomas and is incorporated into the G-TNM staging system.

1. Grade (G). All rhabdomyosarcomas, Ewing sarcomas, and synovial sarcomas are high grade. Three systems used for grading sarcomas and their relationships are as follows:

Two-tiered system	Three-tiered system	Four-tiered system
Low grade	G1: Low grade	G1: Well differentiated
		G2: Moderately differentiated
High grade	G2: Intermediate grade	G3: Poorly differentiated
	G3: High grade	G4: Undifferentiated

2. TNM staging classification for sarcomas is shown in Table 17.1.

B. Prognostic factors

1. Histological grade (the degree of differentiation, the amount of necrosis, and the number of mitoses per high-power microscopic field) is the single most important prognostic factor, especially for STS. The shortcoming of this system is less-than-ideal reproducibility.

2. Local recurrence predisposes to further recurrences. The absence of clear surgical margins, with or without postoperative RT, increases the rate of local recurrence in patients with STS but does not affect survival. The development of distant metastases after local recurrence may be either directly related to the recurrence or only a reflection of the more aggressive tumor biology.

3. Site of disease. Half of deaths in patients with STS occur in the 8% of patients with retroperitoneal lesions.

4. Tumor-suppressor gene *p53* is located on the short arm of chromosome 17. Nuclear accumulation of p53 protein appears to be a marker of tumor aggressiveness and may be a useful prognostic factor for STS.

C. Stage groupings and survival for STS are shown in Table 17.2.

D. Long-term survival. About 80% of all STSs that recur do so within 2 years. Patients with osteogenic sarcoma who survive 3 years without evidence of disease appear to be cured.

TABLE 17.1	TNM Staging of Sarcomas

Primary tumor (T)

Bone sarcomas

T1	Tumor ≤8 cm in greatest dimension
T2	Tumor >8 cm in greatest dimension
T3	Discontinuous tumors in the primary site

Soft-tissue sarcomas (adults)

T1	Tumor ≤5 cm in greatest dimension	
	T1a	superficial tumor
	T1b	deep tumor
T2	Tumor >5 cm in greatest dimension	
	T2a	superficial tumor
	T2b	deep tumor

Regional lymph nodes (N)

N0	No clinical regional lymph node metastases
N1	Regional lymph node metastases present

Distant metastases (M)

M0	No distant metastases
M1	Distant metastases present (for bones sarcomas, M1a has metastasis to the lung and M1b has metastasis to other distant sites)

V. PREVENTION AND EARLY DETECTION. The physician must suspect and biopsy all soft-tissue masses, *de novo* bony abnormalities, and periosteal elevations with an apparent bone lesion.

VI. MANAGEMENT OF BONE SARCOMAS

    A. Surgery. Treatment of osteogenic sarcomas results in a 65% to 80% 10-year, disease-free survival. Relapse after 3 years of disease-free survival is unusual.

        1. Limb-salvage surgery is now the standard treatment for most patients with osteogenic sarcomas of the extremities, where nearly 90% of these tumors originate. The historical fear of "skip metastases" (within the same bone of involvement) has proved excessive; the occurrence rate of skip metastases appears to be <10%. Only occasionally do patients require amputation. The widespread, successful use of limb-salvage therapy has been made possible by the following advances:

            a. Significant progress in the development of modern prostheses that are available immediately after surgery. For example, young children who would have had unacceptable leg-length discrepancy with limb-salvage procedures

TABLE 17.2	Stage Grouping and Survival for Soft-Tissue Sarcomas

	TNM stage	Grade	5-yr survival rate (%)
Stage I	T1a, 1b, 2a, 2b N0 M0	Low	85–90
Stage II	T1a, 1b, 2a N0 M0	High	70–80
Stage III	T2b N0 M0	High	45–55
Stage IV	Any T N1 M0	Any	0–20
	Any T N0 M1	Any	0–20

can now be given a prosthesis that can be lengthened as the patient grows (expandable prosthesis).

b. The use of preoperative (neoadjuvant) chemotherapy

(1) Preoperative chemotherapy can result in enough tumor shrinkage to permit the use of prosthesis and can allow time for fabrication of the prosthesis.

(2) Preoperative chemotherapy provides an *in vivo* drug trial to determine the drug sensitivity of an individual tumor and to customize postoperative chemotherapy regimens. Patients who have an excellent response to preoperative chemotherapy (>95% necrosis) have the most favorable long-term prognosis.

2. Amputation provides definitive surgical treatment in patients in whom a limb-sparing resection is not a prudent option. The procedures include hip disarticulation, hemipelvectomy, and forequarter resection. Although these procedures were once used for technically difficult resections and proximal tumors, most sarcomas of the shoulder girdle or knee can now be resected rather than amputated with the extremity.

B. Adjuvant RT is usually not necessary for osteogenic sarcomas of the extremities. Tumors of the jaw, facial bones, and axial skeleton require combined RT and limited surgery.

C. Chemotherapy

1. Preoperative (neoadjuvant) chemotherapy provides a response rate of 60% to 85% with combination regimens, including high-dose methotrexate (HDMTX) with leucovorin rescue. Response to preoperative chemotherapy is the single most important prognostic variable in predicting relapse-free survival.

2. Adjuvant chemotherapy is standard practice in the management of all patients with osteogenic sarcoma. Prospective, randomized, controlled studies demonstrated improvement in relapse-free survival for patients treated adjuvantly with chemotherapy compared with those treated with surgery alone (17% vs. 65% to 85% at 2 years). A steep dose–response curve has been repeatedly observed for chemotherapy of sarcomas: the higher the dose, the higher the response rate. Combination chemotherapy incorporating high-dose methotrexate, ifosfamide, doxorubicin, and cisplatin has produced the best responses.

D. Treatment of other bone sarcomas. Cryosurgery—using liquid nitrogen after curettage of a tumor cavity—can decrease local recurrence for aggressive benign bone tumors and low-grade sarcomas.

1. Chondrosarcoma. Complete surgical excision with limb-sparing procedures where applicable. Adjuvant RT or chemotherapy is not helpful, but may be tried in cases of dedifferentiated chondrosarcoma.

2. MFH of bone. Radical surgical resection. Because of the poor prognosis, adjuvant chemotherapy is justified, but its efficacy has not been proved.

3. Fibrosarcoma of bone. Surgery alone

4. Chordoma. The first surgical procedure has the best chance for cure. Inadequate surgery results in local recurrence and ultimate death. RT is also used adjuvantly with disappointing results. Heavy-particle irradiation appears promising for improving local control.

5. Ewing sarcoma is discussed in Chapter 18, "Ewing Sarcoma."

6. Giant cell tumor of bone. Surgical removal cures 90% of these tumors when benign. Amputation is reserved for massive recurrence or malignant transformation.

VII. MANAGEMENT OF STS

A. Surgery. Wide, adequate surgical resection with pathologically proven clear margins is the most effective therapeutic approach. Soft-part resection can be accomplished without amputation in at least 80% of patients.

1. Extent of resection. Surgical exploration of the tumor demonstrates apparent encapsulation; this is actually a *pseudocapsule*. Local recurrences develop in 80% of patients treated only by enucleation of the pseudocapsule. The surgeon must remove the localized sarcoma *within a complete envelope of normal tissue*; normal structures must be sacrificed if necessary to encompass the tumor. The biopsy site, skin, and most of the subcutaneous tissue, fibrous tissue, and (often) the adjacent muscle group should be included in the resection.

   2. Regional lymph node dissection. Node dissection is not done routinely for soft-tissue or bone sarcomas and is only performed if nodal involvement is suspected clinically.

   3. Amputation of painful extremities. Removal of a painful, functionless extremity that is the site of an eroding, necrotic tumor may be palliative, even in patients with metastatic disease. Surgery may be attempted after chemotherapy and RT have failed to control progressive disease.

   4. Resection of pulmonary metastasis is a reasonable measure in selected patients with resectable pulmonary metastasis and no other evidence of disease (see Chapter 29, section II). The best results of this approach are observed in patients with sarcomas or germ cell tumors, as compared with patients with carcinomas or melanomas.

B. RT is administered to the tumor bed before or after surgery (depending on the treatment center) for high-grade or large STSs to improve local control rates.

   1. Microscopically positive surgical margins increase the risk for local failure. The presence of microscopically positive surgical margins or the occurrence of local failure, however, does not affect overall survival. Adjuvant RT may be most important when achieving clear margins would require amputation or significant functional compromise of the extremity.

   2. For lesions distal to the elbow or knee, postoperative RT raised the ability rate to perform limb-salvage surgery to 95% and reduced the local recurrence rate to 10%. These results were the same as if radical amputation or muscle group excision were performed.

   3. Palliation. RT can provide palliation to sites of painful bony disease or to sites of unresectable local soft-tissue disease.

C. Treatment of STS for specific presentations

   1. Grade 1 and small grade 2 lesions are treated with surgery alone; the relapse rate is <10% with surgery alone. Adjuvant RT is not required.

   2. Grade 2 lesions that are proximal and large are treated with surgery and postoperative RT.

   3. Grade 3 or 4 lesions. RT is advisable before or after surgery.

   4. Head and neck STS. Appropriate therapy is not defined. Wide surgical excision and RT before or after surgery is advisable.

   5. Childhood rhabdomyosarcoma is treated intensively with chemotherapy, RT, and surgery (see Chapter 18, "Rhabdomyosarcoma").

   6. Retroperitoneal STS (mostly leiomyosarcomas and liposarcomas) must be radically extirpated. Complete resection is possible in about 65% of patients and strongly predicts outcome. Median survival with complete resection is 80 months for low-grade STS and 20 months for high-grade disease. Median survival with incomplete resection for all STSs is only 24 months. The survival rate is not affected by tumor type or size.

   7. GIST. Imatinib (Gleevec) has demonstrated activity in advanced GIST in up to 70% of cases with doses ranging from 400 to 800 mg/day. The durability of responses to imatinib is being evaluated. Trials in the adjuvant setting have shown an decreased rate of recurrence with the use of imatinib for 1 year following complete surgical resection. Sunitinib (Sutent) has demonstrated an improvement in time to progression and progression-free survival at a dose of 50 mg/day in those who have progressed after or were intolerant to imatinib.

   8. Kaposi sarcoma

      a. KS in AIDS. Highly active antiretroviral therapy (HAART) has markedly decreased the incidence of KS and is effective in the treatment of early KS. Management of KS in AIDS patients is discussed in Chapter 36, section IV.G.

      b. Classic KS. A topical treatment for cutaneous KS, 0.1% alitretinoin gel (Panretin), should be tried first for local control; however, local erythema and

TABLE 17.3	Combination Chemotherapy Regimens for Sarcoma		
Regimen (cycle: 21–28 days)	**Drug**	**Daily dose (mg/m^2)**	**Days given in cycle (route)**
Ifosfamide, high dose	Ifosfamide	Age $\geq$50 yr: 2,000 Age <50 yr: 2,250	For 7 days (CIV) For 8 days (CIV)
	Mesna	Age $\geq$50 yr: 2,000 Age <50 yr: 2,250	For 7 days (CIV) For 8 days (CIV)
Doxorubicin + cisplatin	Doxorubicin	75–100	Over 48–96 hr (CIV)
	Cisplatin	90–120	1 (IV)
Gemcitabine + docetaxel	Gemcitabine	900[b]	1 and 8 (IV)
	Docetaxel	100	8 (IV)[c]
CyVADic	Cyclophosphamide	500	1 (IV)
	Vincristine	1.4[a]	1 and 5 (IV)
	Doxorubicin	50	1 (IV)
	Dacarbazine	250	1 through 5 (IV)
MAID	Mesna	1,500–2,500	1, 2, and 3 (CIV)
	Doxorubicin	15–20	1, 2, and 3 (CIV)
	Ifosfamide	1,500–2,500	1, 2, and 3 (CIV)
	Dacarbazine	250	1, 2, 3, and 4 (CIV)

CIV, continuous intravenous infusion; IV, intravenously.
[a]Maximum, 2 mg.
[b]Gemcitabine dose reduced to 650 mg/m^2 if patient received prior pelvic RT.
[c]Support with granulocyte colony stimulating factor

dermatitis may limit its use. Liquid nitrogen can be used for the destruction of localized nodular lesions. RT, including electron beams, is useful for local disease; KS is very radiosensitive. Chemotherapy is inconsistently effective; vinca alkaloids appear to be the most active agents.

D. Chemotherapy for STS. Currently used combination chemotherapy regimens for sarcoma are shown in Table 17.3.

1. Single agents. The response rates of STS to doxorubicin, ifosfamide, or dacarbazine used as single agents are 30%, 30%, and 15%, respectively. Other drugs have response rates of <15%. Intra-arterial administration is not superior to intravenous administration.

2. Adjuvant chemotherapy is standard practice in the management of rhabdomyosarcoma in children. Adjuvant chemotherapy for STS in adults with high-grade tumors remains controversial.

a. A meta-analysis of randomized trials of adjuvant doxorubicin for STS demonstrated a reduction in local and distant recurrence rates and a trend toward improved overall survival; this survival benefit was most clear for those with extremity sarcomas. More recent trials using the combination of ifosfamide with an anthracycline (either epirubicin or doxorubicin) showed an advantage in both disease-free survival and overall survival for those receiving chemotherapy. Additionally, preoperative treatment with both RT and chemotherapy that includes ifosfamide has shown higher rates of complete pathological response at the time of surgery than prior preoperative regimens using either RT alone or RT with intravenous or intra-arterial doxorubicin.

b. At our institutions, patients with STS who are candidates for adjuvant chemotherapy typically are given two cycles of ifosfamide with mesna and one cycle of doxorubicin both before and after RT to the affected part. Dosages are shown in Table 17.3.

3. **Combination chemotherapy regimens** (e.g., CyVADic in Table 17.3) appear to provide no advantage over single agents for palliation or survival but are more toxic. Pulmonary and soft-tissue metastases are more responsive than liver and bone metastases.

   a. The combination of vincristine, actinomycin D, and cyclophosphamide (VAC) in children with rhabdomyosarcoma produces a response rate of 90% even with disseminated disease. Responses to these agents in other sarcomas are usually minimal and brief.

   b. The combination of gemcitabine and docetaxel (dosage and schedule are shown in Table 17.3) has shown promising activity in advanced leiomyosarcomas.

   c. Dose intensity probably correlates with response rates in the treatment of sarcomas. High-dose combinations of ifosfamide (with mesna uroprotection), doxorubicin, and dacarbazine (MAID regimen in Table 17.3) results in a higher response rate (45%) than single agents but at the expense of substantial myelosuppression. Ifosfamide as a single agent, when given in divided doses over several days at total doses of 10 to 14 g/m^2, can produce responses in patients previously treated with ifosfamide at lower doses. Comparison studies of lower doses of ifosfamide (6 g/m^2) versus higher doses ifosfamide (12 g/m^2), both given with doxorubicin at 60 mg/m^2, have not shown a clear benefit for the higher-dose regimens in terms of either disease-free or overall survival at 1 year.

Suggested Reading

Frustaci S, et al. Adjuvant chemotherapy for adult soft tissue sarcoma of the extremities and girdles: result of the Italian randomized cooperative trial. *J Clin Oncol* 2001;19:1235.

Goorin AM, et al. Presurgical chemotherapy compared with immediate surgery and adjuvant chemotherapy for nonmetastatic osteosarcoma: Pediatric Oncology Group Study POG-8651. *J Clin Oncol* 2003;21:1574.

Hensley ML, et al. Gemcitabine and docetaxel in patients with unresectable leiomyosarcoma: results of a phase II trial. *J Clin Oncol* 2002;20:2824.

Kattan MW, Leung DH, Brennan MF. Postoperative nomogram for 12-year sarcoma-specific death. *J Clin Oncol* 2002;20:627.

Lae ME, et al. Desmoplastic small round cell tumor: a clinicopathologic, immunohistochemical, and molecular study of 32 tumors. *Am J Surg Pathol* 2002;26:823.

Maki RG, et al. Randomized Phase II Study of gemcitabine and docetaxel compared with gemcitabine alone in patients with metastatic soft tissue sarcoma. *J Clin Oncol* 2007;19:2755

Meyers PA, et al. Osteosarcoma: a randomized, prospective trial of the addition of ifosfamide and/or muramyl tripeptide to cisplatin, doxorubicin and high dose methotrexate. *J Clin Oncol* 2005;223:2004.

Sarcoma Meta-analysis Collaboration. Adjuvant chemotherapy for localised resectable soft-tissue sarcoma of adults: meta-analysis of individual data. *Lancet* 1997;350:1647.

Van Oosterom AT, et al. Update of phase I study of imatinib (STI571) in advanced soft tissue sarcomas and gastrointestinal stromal tumors: a report of the EORTC Soft Tissue and Bone Sarcoma Group. *Eur J Cancer* 2002;38(Suppl 5):S83.

Worden FP, et al. Randomized phase II evaluation of 6 g/m^2 of ifosfamide plus doxorubicin and granulocyte colony-stimulating factor (G-CSF) with 12 g/m^2 of ifosfamide plus doxorubicin and G-CSF in the treatment of poor-prognosis soft tissue sarcoma. *J Clin Oncol* 2005;23(1):105.

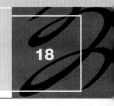

CANCERS IN CHILDHOOD
Theodore B. Moore and Carole G. H. Hurvitz

18

 INCIDENCE, LEUKEMIA, AND LYMPHOMA

I. **INCIDENCE AND OVERVIEW.** Although cancer is the second leading cause of death in children (12% of deaths), it is still relatively uncommon. The incidence of cancer is increasing, however. Fortunately, with modern aggressive multidisciplinary therapy, 5-year survival rates for children with cancer exceed 75%.

A. **Cooperative groups.** The treatment of children with cancer is highly specialized. Whenever possible, patients younger than 18 to 21 years of age should be treated in specialized centers related to one of the major pediatric cooperative groups, such as the Children's Oncology Group. More than 90% of children younger than 10 years of age are treated in such centers, and their mortality has decreased proportionally. Only about 30% of teenagers are enrolled in such centers, however, and the mortality rates in this group have not shown the same improvement.

B. **Incidence.** Leukemia and lymphoma make up almost half of the cases of malignancy in childhood, followed by central nervous system (CNS) tumors. The mortality rate for CNS cancers now exceeds that for acute lymphocytic leukemia.

There is no formal reporting system for malignant tumors in children in the United States. SEER (Surveillance, Epidemiology, and End Results) reports from the National Cancer Institute indicate that approximately 164 cases of cancer occur per 1 million population <20 years of age in the following incidences per million:

Leukemia—43	Neuroblastoma—8	Bone tumors—9
CNS tumors—29	Wilms' tumor—6	Retinoblastoma—3
Lymphomas—22	Soft tissue sarcomas—11	

II. **ACUTE LEUKEMIA** (see Chapter 25)

A. **Pathology.** Acute lymphoblastic leukemia (ALL) accounts for 80% to 85% of leukemias in childhood. Acute myelogenous leukemia (AML) accounts for 15% and chronic myelogenous leukemia accounts for 5% of cases.

In ALL, 15% to 25% of cases are T-cell, <5% are B-cell, and the remainder are precursor B-cell leukemias. Of the precursor B-cell leukemias, 70% possess the common acute lymphoblastic leukemia antigen (CALLA, CD-10). They are usually also terminal deoxynucleotidyl transferase–positive. Almost all are also CD-19–positive.

B. **Treatment** of acute leukemias in childhood involves induction of remission, prophylaxis to the CNS, and maintenance therapy. Standard treatment for ALL leads to long-term remission in >85% of cases. Induction therapy employs vincristine, prednisone, and L-asparaginase with the addition of daunomycin, depending on risk stratification. Intensification therapy includes CNS prophylaxis. During maintenance therapy, oral mercaptopurine is given daily and methotrexate weekly for 2 to 3 years. Many patients receive monthly pulses of vincristine plus prednisone or dexamethasone. One or two cycles of a reinduction regimen are often added in ALL.

Certain prognostic factors at diagnosis affect the outlook of children with ALL, and their treatment is modified accordingly. Children with poorer prognostic features require more intensive treatment than standard therapy.

397

1. **Favorable prognostic factors for ALL.** Average risk factors include initial white blood cell count (WBC) of <50,000/μL and age 1 to 9 years. Favorable features include pre-B subtype, L1 morphology, hyperploidy, lack of organomegaly, low bone marrow blasts on day 7 of induction therapy, trisomy of chromosomes 4 and 10, and t4:11 or Tel/AML1 translocations.

2. **Poor prognostic factors** include WBC >50,000/μL, age <1 year or >10 years, massive organomegaly, lymphomalike features, CNS involvement at diagnosis, mediastinal mass, failure to achieve remission by day 14 or 28, and certain chromosomal translocations, especially *MLL* gene rearrangements (11q23) in infants, and the Philadelphia chromosome.

3. **AML** requires intensive chemotherapy. It is often followed by allogeneic hematopoietic stem cell transplantation (HSCT) in first remission, which appears to provide the best survival if a suitably matched related donor is available. Otherwise, outcome with chemotherapy alone appears as good as with autologous or matched unrelated donor transplant as of this writing. HSCT (allogenic, autologous, or matched unrelated) is also often recommended for patients with ALL and AML who relapse.

C. **Survival.** The 5-year survival rate is >85% in children with "good-prognosis" ALL following standard therapy. Even children with poorer risk factors who receive intensive therapy have an overall long-term survival of at least 70%. Sites of relapse include the CNS, testes, and bone marrow. The risk for relapse after 2 years of therapy is very low. The 5-year survival rate with the best available regimens in children with AML is 65% in first remission when consolidated with a sibling donor HSCT and about 50% for those without.

III. LYMPHOMA

A. **Non-Hodgkin lymphoma** (see Chapter 21). In pediatrics, lymphomas can be considered to be lymphoblastic or nonlymphoblastic and localized or nonlocalized. Lymphoblastic lymphomas are usually T cell and, when nonlocalized, may be the same entity as T-cell leukemia; these illnesses are usually treated in the same way. Nonlymphoblastic lymphomas are usually B cell and are frequently Burkitt (or Burkitt-like) lymphoma.

Different combination chemotherapeutic regimens are necessary for the subtypes of lymphoma. Localized lymphomas respond very well to chemotherapy even when bulky, and have a cure rate of >90%. The prognosis for disseminated T-cell lymphomas is the same as for T-cell ALL. The outlook for disseminated nonlymphoblastic or B-cell lymphoma is about 50%.

B. **Hodgkin lymphoma** (see Chapter 21). There is no consensus on the treatment of Hodgkin lymphoma in children, with the exception of stage IV disease, which is primarily treated with chemotherapy. Chemotherapy is used for all stages of disease. Staging laparotomy is no longer recommended. Splenectomy is contraindicated in young children because of fatal infectious complications and increased risk for leukemia. The alternation of the COPP and ABVD regimens (defined in Appendix D-1) or a hybrid of them is frequently recommended rather than either regimen alone. In children, local-field rather than extended-field radiation is preferred in an effort to reduce long-term side effects, such as growth retardation and second cancers, especially breast cancer in girls. Second malignancies are a major problem with the risk approaching 40% by age 35 years for girls who have been irradiated. Current Children's Oncology Group (COG) treatment regimens are evaluating modulation of therapy based on initial response with a goal of minimizing toxicity while maintaining high cure rates.

BRAIN TUMORS

Neurologic malignancies are discussed in Chapter 14.

I. **EPIDEMIOLOGY.** Brain tumors in children may be associated with certain underlying diseases, including neurofibromatosis, tuberous sclerosis, and von Hippel-Lindau angiomatosis. Family clusters of CNS tumors have occasionally been reported.

II. PATHOLOGY AND NATURAL HISTORY

A. Pathology. Most CNS neoplasms in children are primary tumors of the brain; the single exception is meningeal metastases, which are common with leukemia and lymphoma. Astrocytomas are the most frequent type (about 50% of all cases). Medulloblastomas account for 25% of cases; ependymomas, 9%; and glioblastomas, 9%.

B. Sites of disease. Brain tumors in children tend to occur along the central neural axis (i.e., near the third or fourth ventricle or along the brain stem). Most brain tumors that occur during the first year of life are supratentorial. In patients between 2 and 12 years of age, 85% are infratentorial. In patients >12 years of age, the relative incidence of supratentorial tumors increases.

III. SYMPTOMS AND SIGNS

A. Symptoms. The most common symptoms include headaches, irritability, vomiting, and gait abnormalities. Morning headaches are most characteristic, but drowsiness and abnormal behavior are also common. Symptoms may be intermittent, particularly in very young children who have open fontanelles.

B. Physical findings include enlarged or bulging fontanelles in very young children and cerebellar abnormalities, papilledema, and sixth cranial nerve abnormalities in older children.

IV. TREATMENT AND SURVIVAL.
Survival rates for patients with low-grade astrocytomas are high if the tumor can be surgically removed (>90% at 5 years) and low if the tumor is high grade (<10% at 5 years). Survival for medulloblastoma depends on both local recurrence (<25% with surgery and radiotherapy) and spinal metastases (about 35% incidence without prophylactic spinal irradiation); this tumor is invariably recurrent when treated with surgery alone.

Chemotherapy is now being used more frequently in children with brain tumors in an attempt to improve survival and to reduce the use of radiation, which has devastating effects in young children. RT is deferred in children <3 years of age. Unlike childhood leukemia, relatively little improvement in survival has been obtained over the years. High-dose therapy with autologous HSCT support has shown some promise. In addition, experimental approaches using targeted therapies, novel chemotherapy and radiation delivery systems, and dendritic cell-based vaccine trials are currently under investigation.

NEUROBLASTOMA

I. EPIDEMIOLOGY AND ETIOLOGY.
Neuroblastoma is the most common congenital tumor and the most common tumor to occur during the first year of life. It rarely occurs in patients >14 years of age. About 40% occur in the first year of life, 35% from 1 to 2 years of age, and 25% after 2 years of age. Rarely, family clusters are reported.

II. PATHOLOGY AND NATURAL HISTORY.
Neuroblastoma has the highest incidence of spontaneous regression of any tumor in humans.

A. Histology. Neuroblastoma closely resembles embryonic sympathetic ganglia. The tumors partially differentiate into rosettes or pseudorosettes, mature ganglion cells, or immature chromaffin cells. Although histologically similar to ganglioneuromas and pheochromocytomas, neuroblastomas are clearly distinctive. Electron microscopy shows typical dendritic processes that contain granules with dense bodies, probably representing cytoplasmic catecholamines. The most primitive histologic type of neuroblastoma is composed of small round cells with scant cytoplasm. The ganglioneuroma is composed of larger, more mature ganglion cells with more abundant cytoplasm.

Homogeneously staining regions and double minute chromosomes seen in poor-prognosis neuroblastomas represent amplified *N-myc* segments. Amplification of *N-myc* is an intrinsic property of poor-prognosis tumors and can be rapidly detected by fluorescent *in situ* hybridization (FISH) concordant with Southern blot analysis.

B. Sites. The most common primary site is the adrenal gland (40% of cases); a tumor of the adrenal gland produces an abdominal mass. Involvement of posterior sympathetic ganglion cells results in both intrathoracic and intra-abdominal masses, the so-called *dumbbell tumor* that causes compression of the spinal cord.

C. Mode of spread. Most cases of neuroblastoma present with widespread metastatic disease. The most common metastatic sites include bone, bone marrow, liver, skin, and lymph nodes.

III. DIAGNOSIS

A. Symptoms. Abdominal pain and distention, bone pain, anorexia, malaise, fever, and diarrhea

B. Physical findings. Hepatomegaly, hypertension, orbital mass and ecchymosis, subcutaneous nodules (particularly in infancy), intra-abdominal mass, and Horner syndrome

C. Laboratory studies

1. Complete blood count (CBC), serum chemistry panel
2. Urine for total catecholamines and metabolites, including vanillylmandelic acid (VMA) and homovanillic acid (HVA)
3. Chest and abdominal radiographs
4. CT scan of the abdomen or thorax (possibly preceded by abdominal and renal ultrasound)
5. Bone scan
6. Bone marrow aspiration and biopsy to look for tumor cells
7. ^{131}I-MIBG (^{131}I-metaiodobenzylguanidine), which is specific for neuroblastoma and pheochromocytoma.
8. Examination of tumor for amplification of the *N-myc* gene

IV. STAGING SYSTEM AND PROGNOSTIC FACTORS

A. Staging system

Stage	Extent of disease
I	Localized disease surgically removed *in toto*
II	Regional disease, unilateral
III	Tumor crossing the midline
IV	Metastatic disease
IVS	Stage I or II primary tumor with metastases to liver, skin, and/or bone marrow without radiographic evidence of bony involvement (usually in very young infants)

B. Survival and prognostic factors. The prognosis for neuroblastoma is closely related to the age of the patient and stage of disease.

1. **Age.** Patients with congenital tumors have the most favorable prognosis, even with widespread disease, and they also have the highest rate of spontaneous regression without treatment. Patients who are between 1 and 5 years of age do worse than patients younger than 1 year or older than 5 years of age.

2. **Stage.** Patients with advanced disease, except for stage IVS, have a poor survival rate. The overall 2-year survival for neuroblastoma is >80% for stages I and II and <30% for stage IV. Stage IVS has a 90% survival rate. Patients with stage III and IV disease who have amplification of the *N-myc* gene do worse.

3. **The urinary VMA:HVA ratio** is an indirect measure of dopamine hydroxylase. Absence of this enzyme may convey a poorer prognosis (i.e., if the VMA:HVA ratio is <1.5) and may cast doubt on the diagnosis of neuroblastoma.

V. MANAGEMENT

A. Surgery. Localized disease is managed primarily by surgical resection. For metastatic disease, biopsy or excision of the primary tumor is important for *N-myc* gene assessment. Complete resection is usually delayed until after chemotherapy is administered but may be done at the time of diagnosis.

B. RT is used for bulky tumor in combination with chemotherapy.

C. **Chemotherapy**
1. **Residual localized or advanced disease.** Aggressive multimodal chemotherapy with doxorubicin, cyclophosphamide, etoposide, and cisplatin, combined with surgical resection and bone marrow transplantation, has improved survival in stage III and IV disease.
2. **Congenital disease.** In patients with congenital disease, specifically for stage IVS, chemotherapy is not used unless the tumor causes significant symptoms.
D. **HSCT** (usually autologous) after intensive radiation and chemotherapy appears to improve the outlook for patients with advanced disease, especially when used in conjunction with post transplant 13-*cis*-retinoic acid.
E. **Future directions.** Poor survival in the advanced stages of disease has spurred extensive research into targeted therapies. An especially promising target under evaluation is GD2 (disialoganglioside). Anti-GD2 has shown some efficacy, especially in patients with infiltrating marrow disease.

 WILMS' TUMOR (NEPHROBLASTOMA)

I. EPIDEMIOLOGY AND ETIOLOGY
A. **Incidence.** Wilms' tumor most frequently affects children between 1 and 5 years of age, and rarely those >8 years of age. The incidence is about 7 per 1 million in the childhood age group. Familial clusters have been described, particularly in patients with bilateral Wilms' tumors.
B. **Associated abnormalities.** Wilms' tumor has been associated with certain congenital anomalies, including genitourinary anomalies, aniridia (absence of an iris), and hemihypertrophy (Beckwith-Wiedemann syndrome). Deletion of the short arm of chromosome 11 has been associated with a syndrome of Wilms' tumor, mental retardation, microcephaly, bilateral aniridia, and ambiguous genitalia.

II. PATHOLOGY AND NATURAL HISTORY
A. **Histopathologic classification** is most accurate for determining the prognosis.
1. **Wilms' tumor.** Tumors that display mature elements and few anaplastic cells have the most favorable prognosis and are termed *favorable histology. Unfavorable histology* concerns tumors that have focal or diffuse anaplasia, rhabdoid sarcoma, or clear cell sarcoma. Unfavorable histology accounts for 12% of Wilms' tumors but almost 90% of deaths.
2. **Congenital mesoblastic nephroma** is a rare benign tumor that is common in infancy (the most common renal neoplasm during the first month of life) and can be histologically confused with Wilms' tumor. This tumor consists of spindle-shaped, immature connective tissue cells that have a distinctive fibroblastic appearance with only minimal nuclear pleomorphism and mitoses.
B. **Sites.** About 7% of Wilms' tumors are bilateral at the time of diagnosis.
C. **Mode of spread.** The lungs are the principal sites of metastases; liver and lymph nodes are the next most common sites. Bone marrow metastases are extremely rare and tend to be associated with clear cell subtypes of sarcomatous Wilms' tumor. CNS metastases are extremely rare.
D. **Paraneoplastic syndromes.** Wilms' tumors have been associated with increased erythropoietin (erythrocytosis) and with increased renin (hypertension).

III. DIAGNOSIS
A. **Symptoms.** The most common symptoms include enlarged abdomen, abdominal pain, and painless hematuria.
B. **Physical findings.** A palpable abdominal mass is the most common finding. Hypertension is sometimes present.
C. **Laboratory studies**
1. CBC, serum chemistries, urinalysis
2. Plain radiographs of the chest and abdomen
3. CT or, preferably, MRI scan of abdomen

IV. STAGING AND PROGNOSTIC FACTORS

A. Staging system

Stage	Extent of disease
I	Well-encapsulated tumor that is surgically removed in its entirety
II	Extension of tumor beyond renal capsule by local infiltration with extension along the renal vein, involvement of para-aortic nodes, and no residual macroscopic disease
III	Macroscopic residual disease or peritoneal metastases or contamination during nephrectomy
IV	Distant metastases, particularly to lung
V	Bilateral disease

B. Survival and prognostic factors.
The most important prognostic factors are the histopathologic classification and the clinical and surgical staging. Age at diagnosis is of minor importance, although younger patients appear to have a slightly better outcome. The overall 2-year survival rate is >95% for stage I, II, and III disease, with favorable histology, and about 50% for stage IV disease.

V. MANAGEMENT

A. Surgery. All patients must have surgery for both staging and removal of as much tumor as possible. A transabdominal incision is mandatory to examine the vessels of the renal pedicle and the noninvolved kidney. The tumor bed and any residual tumor should be outlined with metallic clips at the time of surgery.

B. RT is useful for treating stage III disease and metastatic disease to bone, liver, or lung.

C. Chemotherapy. Multiple courses of combination chemotherapy are the preferred treatment. The major active chemotherapeutic agents are actinomycin D, vincristine, and doxorubicin. Cyclophosphamide is an effective second-line drug. Cisplatin is active against Wilms' tumor and is being used in investigational protocols. The National Wilms Tumor Study is ongoing. The youngest patients are particularly susceptible to serious toxic effects from chemotherapy, particularly hematologic, and drug dosages should be reduced 50% for patients <15 months of age.

D. Treatment according to stage of disease. Surgery and chemotherapy are used for all stages of disease.

1. Stage I. RT is not necessary.

2. Stages II and III. RT is not needed for stage II with favorable histology but is used for unfavorable histology and stage III.

3. Stage IV or recurrent disease. If possible, surgery can be used. Chemotherapeutic agents can be restarted if they were discontinued or changed if relapse occurred during treatment. RT is useful for metastatic disease. Intensive chemotherapy with autologous HSCT may be beneficial in recurrent disease.

4. Stage V. Bilateral Wilms' tumor necessitates a special effort to preserve as much renal tissue as possible. Initially, biopsy is done, and then chemotherapy followed by judicious resection of the remaining tumor. Bilateral nephrectomy followed by chemotherapy, and renal transplantation is a last resort. The 3-year survival rate is 75% for these patients.

RHABDOMYOSARCOMA

I. EPIDEMIOLOGY AND ETIOLOGY.
Rhabdomyosarcoma (RMS) is the most common soft tissue sarcoma in children; there are about 8 cases per million population. Suggestive evidence of C-particle viruses in these tumors has been observed with electron microscopy, but the viruses have not been isolated.

II. PATHOLOGY AND NATURAL HISTORY

A. Histology. Four major histologic categories of this striated muscle neoplasm have been described: embryonal (including sarcoma botryoid), alveolar, pleomorphic, and mixed. Z bands can be seen with electron microscopy. Rhabdomyoblasts have acidophilic cytoplasm, which is often periodic acid–Schiff stain (PAS)–positive. There are characteristic genetic alterations that can be observed. Embryonal RMS may have a characteristic loss of heterozygosity at the 11p15 locus. The majority of alveolar RMS have a characteristic t(2;13) resulting in a chimeric *PAX3* and *FKHR* fusion gene product with a smaller percentage having t(1;13) involving *PAX7* and *FKHR*.

B. Sites. The head and neck are involved in 35% of cases, the trunk and extremities in 35%, and the genitourinary tract in 30%.

C. Mode of spread. These tumors have a great tendency to recur locally and to metastasize early through the venous and lymphatic systems. Any organ may be involved with metastases, but the lungs are most frequently affected.

III. DIAGNOSIS

A. Symptoms. The most common presenting symptom is a painless, enlarging mass. Hematuria and urinary tract obstruction is seen with primary tumors of the genitourinary tract. The painless swelling is often noticed after minor trauma that calls attention to the enlarging mass.

B. Physical findings include mass lesions, urinary tract obstruction, and a "cluster of grapes" protruding through the vaginal canal (sarcoma botryoid). Exophthalmos or proptosis occurs with head and neck primaries.

C. Laboratory studies
1. CBC, liver function tests
2. Plain radiographs and MRI or CT scans of involved areas
3. Bone marrow aspiration and biopsy
4. Gallium (and perhaps thallium) scans

IV. STAGING SYSTEM AND PROGNOSTIC FACTORS

A. Intergroup Rhabdomyosarcoma Study Staging System

Stage	Extent of disease
I	Localized disease, completely resected
II	Localized disease, microscopic residual tumor
IIA	Grossly resected disease with microscopic residual tumor and negative lymph nodes
IIB	Regional disease, completely resected, with no microscopic residual disease
IIC	Regional disease with positive lymph nodes, grossly resected
III	Incomplete resection or biopsy with residual gross disease
IV	Distant metastases

B. Survival and prognostic factors. Survival is closely correlated with stage. The 5-year survival rate with the standard VAC chemotherapy regimen (vincristine, actinomycin D, and cyclophosphamide) is almost 100% for stage I and II disease, >60% for stage III disease, and about 40% for stage IV disease. The overall survival rate is 70%.

V. MANAGEMENT. The treatment of RMS should be aggressive, even with localized disease. Surgery, RT, and chemotherapy should be used for all cases with any residual disease.

A. Surgery should include total excision, if possible, but radical surgery is unnecessary and unwarranted. Lymph node dissection is useful for staging in extremity or genitourinary tract tumors.

B. RT usually consists of 5,000 to 6,000 cGy given over 5 to 6 weeks to the primary tumor site with wide ports to include margins of all dissected tumors.

C. Chemotherapy. The VAC regimen is most commonly given. Studies that compared doxorubicin, etoposide, and ifosfamide with VAC for advanced disease showed no survival advantage, although the combination may be useful in recurrent or resistant disease. Chemotherapy is necessary for patients with the following indications:
1. Adjuvantly with stage I disease
2. With RT for stage II disease
3. To shrink the primary tumor either before or after surgery for stage III and IV disease, and continued as adjunctive therapy

EWING SARCOMA AND PRIMITIVE NEUROECTODERMAL TUMOR (EWING FAMILY TUMORS)

I. **EPIDEMIOLOGY AND ETIOLOGY.** The incidence of Ewing family tumors (EFT), Ewing sarcoma, and primitive neuroectodermal tumor (PNET) is about 1.5 cases per 1 million population. The disease is very rare among black children. Seventy percent of patients are <20 years of age. The peak incidence is at 11 to 12 years of age for girls and 15 to 16 years of age for boys. The male-to-female incidence ratio is 2:1. A reciprocal translocation between chromosomes 11 and 22 in about 85% of tumors creates a chimeric *ews-fli1* fusion gene.

II. **PATHOLOGY AND NATURAL HISTORY**
   A. **Histology.** EFT is a small cell tumor of bone or soft tissue characterized by islands of anaplastic, small, round blue cells (see Appendix C-4, section II, for immunophenotypes of small blue cell tumors). The spectrum of EFT includes Ewing sarcoma of bone, extraosseous Ewing sarcoma, and PNET. Ewing sarcoma and PNET carry the same chromosomal translocation.
   B. **Sites of disease.** These tumors occur predominantly in the midshaft of the humerus, femur, tibia, or fibula, but they also occur in the ribs, scapula, pelvis, or extraosseous sites. PNETs in the chest are called *Askin tumors*.
   C. **Mode of spread.** At the time of diagnosis, 20% to 30% of these tumors have metastasized. Most metastases are to the lung. Metastases to other bones or lymph nodes can also occur. CNS metastases, particularly meningeal, have been reported but are rare.

III. **DIAGNOSIS**
   A. **Symptoms.** Pain that is followed by localized swelling is the most frequent manifestation.
   B. **Physical findings** include tenderness and a palpable mass over the tumor site.
   C. **Preliminary laboratory studies** may show an elevated erythrocyte sedimentation rate and lytic bone lesions on radiograph (frequently, the lesions have an "onion-skin appearance"). A chest radiograph and CT should be obtained in all patients.
   D. **Special diagnostic studies**
      1. Bone scan
      2. MRI or CT scans of involved sites
      3. Gallium scan
      4. Positron emission tomography (PET)

IV. **STAGING AND PROGNOSTIC FACTORS**
   A. **Staging.** The two major stages for Ewing sarcoma and PNET are simply:
      1. Localized disease
      2. Metastatic disease
   B. **Survival and prognostic factors.** Patients with a primary tumor in a central location have a higher incidence of local recurrence and a generally poorer prognosis than do patients with tumors in other primary sites. The prognosis for patients with metastatic disease at the time of diagnosis remains grave; bone metastases have the worst prognosis. High WBC and fever at diagnosis also are associated with a poor prognosis. The disease-free survival depends on the response to chemotherapy.

V. **MANAGEMENT**
   A. **Treatment according to stage of disease**
      1. **Localized disease.** All patients with localized disease should receive intensive chemotherapy followed by complete surgical resection, if possible. If resection is not feasible or complete, RT is given. RT is not needed if the tumor can be removed with >1-cm margin.
      2. **Metastatic disease** is treated with intensive chemotherapy followed by surgical resection (if possible) or RT.
   B. **Chemotherapy** involves multiple drugs given in multiple cycles. The most active agents include vincristine, actinomycin D, high-dose cyclophosphamide, doxoru-

bicin, ifosfamide, and etoposide; combinations of these drugs are effective. Carmustine, methotrexate, and bleomycin also have activity against this disease and are useful in combination with the more active agents. The optimal combination of agents is controversial. High-dose chemotherapy with autologous HSCT is often used for consolidation in advanced stage disease with variable success.

C. Surgery. The initial procedure should be biopsy only. Open biopsy is preferred in children. Control of the primary tumor site is essential. Surgery is used in selected patients with localized disease and in patients with bulky metastatic disease. The total removal of tumor is not necessary in instances in which severe disabilities could result. Concerted efforts at limb preservation should be made.

D. RT is aimed at eradicating all disease while preserving limb function. The optimal volume of bone to be irradiated has not been determined.

    1. Nonbulky lesions. When combined with chemotherapy, delivering 4,000 to 5,000 cGy of RT to the entire bone with an additional 1,000 to 1,500 cGy coned down to the involved site yields good results.

    2. Leg-length discrepancies. In the past, when the probabilities for leg-length discrepancies were excessive (e.g., for younger children with lesions near the knee), patients underwent primary amputation plus chemotherapy. Expandable endoprosthetic reconstruction now makes surgical resection an option for younger children. This regimen usually results in better extremity function than limbs treated with orthovoltage irradiation. Limb-salvage procedures using chemotherapy are also frequently performed when appropriate.

    3. Pelvic primaries. Moderate doses of RT (4,000 cGy) with limited surgery are used for pelvic primary tumors because excessive morbidity is associated with large doses of radiation delivered to bowel and bladder. Chemotherapy must be used as well.

 RETINOBLASTOMA

I. EPIDEMIOLOGY AND ETIOLOGY

A. Incidence. Retinoblastoma occurs in about 3 per 1 million children annually. The average age of patients is 18 months, and >90% are <5 years old. The incidence in Asians is four times that in whites. Patients have a high risk for other neoplasms, particularly radiation-induced osteosarcomas that arise in treatment portals.

B. Familial retinoblastoma. About 40% of cases are hereditary. These have bilateral multifocal involvement, early age at diagnosis, secondary tumors, and a positive family history. Siblings have a 10% to 20% chance of developing retinoblastoma if the affected child has bilateral disease and about 1% if unilateral. The offspring of a patient who survived bilateral retinoblastoma have about a 50% chance of developing the disease.

II. PATHOLOGY AND NATURAL HISTORY

A. Histology. Retinoblastoma is a malignant neuroectodermal tumor. It appears histologically as undifferentiated small cells with deeply stained nuclei and scant cytoplasm. Large cells are sometimes seen forming pseudorosettes, particularly in bone marrow aspirates.

B. Mode of spread. Multiple foci of tumor in the retina are typical at the outset. Most patients die from CNS extension through the optic nerve or widespread hematogenous metastases.

III. DIAGNOSIS

A. Symptoms. The disease typically presents with a "cat's eye" (white pupil or leukokoria). A squint or strabismus is occasionally noted. Orbital inflammation or proptosis rarely occurs.

B. Physical findings are usually limited to the eye, but patients must have a complete neurologic examination. Ophthalmologic examination under anesthesia is essential for infants and small children, for both those with symptoms and those at high risk for developing the disease. Two pathognomonic features are as follows:

1. The typical pattern of fluffy calcifications in the retinas

2. The presence of vitreous seeding by tumor cells

C. Preliminary laboratory studies

1. CBC, liver function tests

2. MRI or CT scans of head and orbit (both scans performed with contrast)

D. Special diagnostic studies

1. Lumbar puncture with cerebrospinal fluid by cytocentrifuge

2. Bone marrow aspiration and biopsy

3. Serum levels of carcinoembryonic antigen and α-fetoprotein, which are frequently elevated in this disease

4. Urinary catecholamine levels, which are infrequently elevated

IV. STAGING SYSTEM AND PROGNOSTIC FACTORS

A. Staging system. The Reese-Ellsworth classification is most frequently used:

Group	Extent of disease
I	Solitary lesion or multiple tumors <4 disc diameters in size at or behind the midplane of the eye
II	Solitary lesions or multiple tumors 4 to 10 disc diameters at or behind the midplane of the eye
III	Any lesions anterior to the midplane, or solitary lesions larger than 10 disc diameters and behind the equator
IV	Multiple tumors, some larger than 10 disc diameters, or any lesion extending anteriorly to the ora serrata (junction of the retina and ciliary body)
V	Massive tumor that involves more than half the retina, or presence of vitreous seeding, or optic nerve involvement
VI	Residual orbital disease, optic nerve involvement and extrascleral extension

B. Survival and prognostic factors. The prognosis is related to both stage and the interval between discovery of clinical signs and the initiation of treatment. The survival rate is virtually 100% for groups I to IV and 83% to 87% for group V. After disease has invaded the orbit, the mortality rate exceeds 80% despite aggressive chemotherapy.

V. MANAGEMENT

A. Surgery is the primary modality of treatment. Prompt enucleation in unilateral disease and enucleation of the most extensively involved eye in bilateral disease are most commonly employed. Another approach has been to enucleate only those eyes with optic nerve involvement and to treat the remaining disease with RT. When enucleation is performed, as long a segment of the optic nerve as possible should be removed. Chemotherapy, photocoagulation, cryotherapy, and plaque radiotherapy may be used in selected cases.

B. RT is given, in most cases, to either the tumor bed or the nonremoved involved eye. Usually, the dose given is about 3,500 cGy in nine fractions over a 3-week period to the posterior retina. This technique, particularly when using megavoltage irradiation, is used to attempt to spare the anterior chamber and avoid cataract formation; it is unsuitable for tumors at or beyond the midpoint of the eye.

1. Radiocobalt applicators have been used for single lesions or discrete groups of small lesions.

2. RT without surgery is usually reserved for patients with advanced disease in both eyes, residual tumor after surgery, or tumors involving the optic nerve. Most patients should not have RT without surgery.

3. Light coagulation and cryotherapy have been used for discrete lesions, particularly for small recurrences.

C. Chemotherapy is useful for metastatic disease. Adjuvant therapy for localized disease has not been shown to increase longevity. Many chemotherapeutic agents are active (vincristine, actinomycin D, cyclophosphamide, and doxorubicin).

Suggested Reading

Arndt CA, Hawkins DS, Meyer WH, et al. Comparison of results of a pilot study of alternating vincristine/doxorubicin/cyclophosphamide and etoposide/ifosfamide with IRS-IV in intermediate risk rhabdomyosarcoma: a report from the Children's Oncology Group. *Pediatr Blood Cancer* 2008;50:33.

Bernstein M, Kovar H, Paulussen M, et al. Ewing's sarcoma family of tumors; current management. *Oncologist* 2006;11:503.

Matthay KK, Perez C, Seeger RC, et al. Successful treatment of stage III neuroblastoma based on prospective biologic staging: a Children's Cancer Group study. *J Clin Oncol* 1998;16:1256.

Nachman J, Sather HN, Cherlow JM, et al. Response of children with high-risk acute lymphoblastic leukemia treated with and without cranial irradiation: a report from the children's cancer group. *J Clin Oncol* 1998;16:920.

Pizzo PA, Poplack DG. *Pediatric Oncology, Principles and Practice.* 5th ed. Philadelphia: Lippincott Williams & Wilkins; 2006.

Pui CH, Evans WE. Treatment of acute lymphoblastic leukemia. *N Engl J Med* 2006; 354:166.

Rubnitz JE, Razzouk BI, Lensing S, et al. Prognostic factors and outcome of recurrence in childhood acute myeloid leukemia. *Cancer* 2007;109:157.

Siegel MJ, Finlay JL, Zacharoulis S, et al. State of the art chemotherapeutic management of pediatric brain tumors. *Expert Rev Neurother* 2006;6:765.

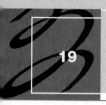

MISCELLANEOUS NEOPLASMS

Dennis A. Casciato

I. PRIMARY TUMORS OF THE MEDIASTINUM

A. General features

1. **Anatomy.** The mediastinum is bounded by the sternum anteriorly, the thoracic vertebral bodies posteriorly, the diaphragm inferiorly, and the first thoracic vertebrae superiorly. Its lateral boundaries are the parietal and pleural surfaces of the lungs. The mediastinum is arbitrarily divided into anterior, middle, and posterior segments by the heart and great vessels.

2. **Incidence.** The annual incidence of mediastinal tumors is 2/1 million population. Of mediastinal tumors, 75% are benign. Many are detected serendipitously in chest radiographs obtained for other reasons.

   a. **The most common mediastinal masses** are thymoma, teratoma, goiter, and lymphoma. Most mediastinal malignancies represent lymphomas or metastatic cancers from other sites.

   b. **Lymphomas** can involve the anterior, middle, or posterior mediastinum. Hodgkin lymphoma is the most common cause of isolated mediastinal disease among the lymphomas; the nodular sclerosing subtype has a predilection for the anterior mediastinum. Other lymphomas are infrequently limited to the mediastinum at the time of diagnosis. Lymphomas are discussed in Chapter 21.

   c. **Mediastinal goiters** without a cervical component are rare. They usually descend into the left anterosuperior mediastinum. Infrequently, they descend behind the trachea into the middle and posterior mediastinum. Mediastinal goiters contain foci of malignancy rarely.

3. **Age and sex.** Most of the tumors show no sexual predilection. Mediastinal teratomas usually arise after the age of 30 years. Benign thymomas may occur in any age group. Thymic carcinomas are more common in elderly men. Tumors of nerve tissue origin may occur at any age but are more common in children.

4. **Symptoms and signs.** Presenting symptoms depend on the tumor location, type, and rate of growth. Symptoms are more likely to be present with rapidly growing, malignant tumors. Hypertrophic osteoarthropathy can occur with any primary mediastinal tumor, particularly sarcomas.

   a. **Anterior mediastinal tumors** can present with retrosternal pain, dyspnea, upper airway obstruction, and development of collateral venous circulation over the chest. Dullness to percussion may be observed over the upper sternum.

   b. **Posterior mediastinal tumors** can cause tracheal compression (cough and dyspnea), phrenic nerve compression (hiccoughs or diaphragm paralysis), involvement of left recurrent laryngeal nerve (hoarseness), esophageal compression (dysphagia), vena cava obstruction, Horner's syndrome or pain, or palsies in the brachial or intercostal nerve distribution.

B. Tumors of the anterior and middle mediastinum

1. **Thymomas** represent 20% of all mediastinal tumors and are the most common cause of anterior mediastinal masses. They are composed of cells of both lymphocytic and epithelial origin. Thymomas are benign in 70% of cases and are locally invasive in 30%. Invasive thymomas involve the pericardium,

myocardium, lung, sternum, and large mediastinal vessels. Disseminated metastases are uncommon.

Histologic details have had little bearing on prognosis or evaluation of malignant potential; invasiveness of a thymoma at surgery is the best index of its malignancy. The World Health Organization classification, however, appears to reflect the invasiveness and prognosis of thymic epithelial tumors (see Okumura M, et al. in *Suggested Reading*). As a cautionary note, carcinoid tumors of the mediastinum may be misclassified as thymoma during cytologic interpretation of fine-needle aspirates.

a. Paraneoplastic immunologic syndromes associated with both benign and malignant thymomas occur frequently, do not affect prognosis, and may not reverse following thymectomy. These syndromes include the following:

(1) Myasthenia gravis occurs in more than half of patients with thymoma; manifestations are improved in about 70% of patients who undergo thymectomy. About 20% of patients with myasthenia gravis have thymomas. Patients suspected of having thymoma should have an assay of serum anti–acetylcholine-receptor antibody.

(2) Pure red-cell aplasia (PRCA, <5% of thymomas). About 10% of patients with PRCA have a thymoma in contemporary series. The pathophysiology of this complication is poorly understood. Thymectomy results in remission of PRCA in <20% of patients. Various immunosuppressive treatments have been attempted with variable success (cyclosporine, antithymocyte globulin), but can lead to significant morbidity, particularly with pulmonary infections.

(3) Immunodeficiency. Acquired hypogammaglobulinemia with low to absent levels of B-cells and CD4+ T lymphocytopenia (Good's syndrome) occurs in about 10% of patients with thymoma. Patients experience recurrent sinopulmonary infections secondary to encapsulated organisms, skin or urinary tract infections, and bacterial diarrheas. Therapy with intravenous immunoglobulins (IVIG) should be helpful in reducing the occurrence of infections.

(4) Rare paraneoplastic syndromes associated with thymoma
   (a) Ectopic Cushing's syndrome
   (b) Polymyositis, dermatomyositis, granulomatous myocarditis
   (c) Systemic lupus erythematosus
   (d) Churg-Strauss syndrome, microscopic polyangiitis, isolated pauci-immune necrotizing crescentic glomerulonephritis
   (e) Optic neuritis, limbic encephalitis
   (f) Hypertrophic osteoarthropathy

b. Therapy

(1) Surgical extirpation results in a cure rate that exceeds 95% for encapsulated, noninvasive thymomas. Less than 10% of resected encapsulated thymomas recur, sometimes years after excision. Surgery alone appears to be insufficient therapy for invasive thymomas.

(2) Radiation therapy, 3,000 to 5,000 cGy given postoperatively for locally invasive or incompletely excised thymomas, reduces the local recurrence rate from about 30% to 5% in 10 years. RT does not appear to be necessary for Masaoka stage II thymoma (microscopic transcapsular invasion or macroscopic invasion into the surrounding fatty tissue). The recurrence rate for locally invasive thymomas treated with RT alone is 20% to 30%.

(3) Combination chemotherapy regimens for locally advanced or metastatic disease usually involve cisplatin, doxorubicin, and cyclophosphamide. Corticosteroid therapy, including high doses, is also beneficial. Reports of chemotherapy efficacy are usually small phase II studies. These combinations consistently result in response rates that are >50%, less than half of those are complete responses. The median duration of complete responses in widespread disease is about 12 months. The 5-year survival rate for these patients is about 30%. For patients with locally advanced disease (for whom there is no standard therapy), it is reasonable to use induction chemotherapy first, followed by resection and RT.

(4) Somatostatin analogs, such as lanreotide (30 mg intramuscular [IM] every 14 days), combined with prednisone is effective therapy in thymic tumors refractory to standard chemotherapeutic agents. Of note, normal human thymus expresses messenger RNA (mRNA) and somatostatin receptor subsets.

2. Thymic carcinomas are obviously malignant histologically and are usually not associated with paraneoplastic syndromes. Neoplasms that are well circumscribed and low grade with a lobular growth pattern have a relatively favorable prognosis for survival (90% 5-year survival rate). High-grade thymic carcinomas are locally invasive; they are frequently associated with pleural or pericardial effusions and frequently metastasize to regional lymph nodes and distant sites. Cisplatin-based chemotherapy plus RT for high-grade tumors is associated with a 5-year survival rate of 15%. Carboplatin plus paclitaxel may also be helpful.

3. Thymic carcinoids are rare. About half have endocrine abnormalities, especially ectopic production of adrenocorticotropic hormone and multiple endocrine neoplasia syndrome, but carcinoid syndrome rarely occurs. Regional lymph node metastases and osteoblastic bone metastases develop in most patients. Metastases are often refractory to therapy.

4. Germ cell tumors (see Chapter 12). Teratomas (or dermoids) represent 10% of mediastinal neoplasms. About 10% of these are malignant, usually with a predominant epithelioid component, but occasionally with sarcomatous or endodermal elements. Malignant germ cell tumors of the mediastinum are usually large and solid.

a. Benign teratoma accounts for about 70% of mediastinal germ cell tumors, especially in children and young adults. They appear as a round, dense mass (often with a calcified capsular shell and occasionally with teeth). They are usually small with multilocular cysts and asymptomatic, but they can attain a large size. The serum of a patient with benign teratoma contains no α-fetoprotein (α-FP) or β-human chorionic gonadotropin (β-hCG). These characteristics often differentiate benign teratoma from germ cell malignancy. The treatment is surgical excision.

b. Seminoma, the most common malignant germ cell neoplasm of the mediastinum, occurs most frequently in men 20 to 40 years of age. The lesions are rarely calcified. Less than 10% of cases have an elevated β-hCG, and none has an elevated α-FP. Treatment of mediastinal seminoma is surgical excision if the tumor is small, followed by irradiation of the mediastinum and the supraclavicular nodes. For locally advanced disease, combination chemotherapy (see Chapter 12, section VI), followed by resection of residual disease, is preferred. The 5-year survival rate for these patients is >80%.

c. Mediastinal nonseminomatous germ cell tumors are malignant, aggressive, and usually symptomatic. They are usually associated with elevations of serum levels of β-hCG, α-FP, or lactate dehydrogenase (LDH). Choriocarcinoma in the mediastinum presents with gynecomastia and testicular atrophy in half of all male patients. Embryonal or yolk sac tumors of the mediastinum are highly aggressive cancers that are large and bulky at the time of diagnosis. Surgery may be required initially to establish the histologic diagnosis. Definitive treatment consists of aggressive chemotherapy as outlined for testicular cancer (see Chapter 12, section VI) followed by resection of residual masses. Mediastinal irradiation delays the initiation of chemotherapy, compromises bone marrow reserve (thus limiting the chemotherapy doses), and probably should not be used.

5. Other anterior mediastinal masses
   a. Goiter and thyroid cysts (10% of mediastinal masses)
   b. Lymphomas
   c. Parathyroid adenoma (10% are ectopic)

    d. Rare causes of anterior mediastinal masses
      (1) Thymic cysts
      (2) Thymolipoma
      (3) Lymphangioma (cystic hygroma)
      (4) Soft tissue sarcomas and their benign counterparts
      (5) Plasmacytoma
  6. Middle mediastinal masses
    a. Lymphomas
    b. Goiter
    c. Aortic aneurysm (10% of mediastinal masses in surgical series)
    d. Congenital foregut cysts (20% of mediastinal masses). About 50% of foregut cysts are bronchogenic, 10% are enterogenous (including esophageal duplication), and 5% are neuroenteric.
    e. Pericardial cysts
C. Tumors of the posterior mediastinum
  1. Neurogenic tumors are the most common cause of a posterior mediastinal mass and constitute 75% of neoplasms in the posterior mediastinum; about 15% are malignant, and half of these are symptomatic. Among mediastinal neoplasms, neurogenic tumors constitute 20% of cases in adults and 35% of cases in children.
    a. Neurofibromas and schwannomas are most common. *Malignant tumor of nerve sheath origin* is their malignant counterpart.
    b. Sympathetic ganglia tumors originate from nerve cells rather than nerve sheath. They are rare and range from benign ganglioneuroma to malignant ganglioneuroblastoma to highly malignant neuroblastoma. Some produce a syndrome identical to pheochromocytoma.
  2. Mesenchymal tumors, including lipomas, fibromas, myxomas, mesotheliomas, and their sarcomatous counterparts, are rare mediastinal tumors; more than half are malignant. Therapy necessitates surgical debulking. RT, chemotherapy, or both are used as a surgical adjuvant for treating sarcomas.
  3. Other posterior mediastinal masses
    a. Lymphomas
    b. Goiter
    c. Lateral thoracic meningocele

II. RETROPERITONEAL TUMORS
  A. Etiology. Excluding renal tumors, 85% of primary retroperitoneal neoplasms are malignant. About one-sixth of cases are Hodgkin lymphoma, and one-sixth are non-Hodgkin lymphoma. Sarcomas often appear in the retroperitoneum, particularly rhabdomyosarcoma (in children), leiomyosarcoma, and liposarcoma. Germ cell tumors, adenocarcinomas, and rare neuroblastomas account for most of the remainder of cases. Carcinomas of the breast, lung, and gastrointestinal tract can metastasize to retroperitoneal structures by way of the bloodstream or the spinal venous plexus.
  B. Evaluation
    1. Symptoms. Back pain, upper urinary tract obstruction, and leg edema caused by lymphatic or vena cava obstruction frequently are manifestations of retroperitoneal malignancies; arterial insufficiency does not appear to occur. Some patients develop fever or hypoglycemia as paraneoplastic syndromes.
    2. Laboratory studies. History, physical examination, chest radiographs, and routine blood studies are performed. Uremia can result from entrapment of the ureters. Intravenous pyelography, barium contrast study of the colon, and abdominal CT scanning are performed to evaluate the extent of tumor.
  C. Management. Exploratory surgery is necessary to establish the tissue diagnosis and to attempt resection of the tumor for potential cure, particularly for sarcomas. RT is used to treat residual disease. Chemotherapy is used for patients with lymphoreticular neoplasm or with tumors that are not responsive to RT. The specific chemotherapy selected depends on the tumor type.

III. CARDIOVASCULAR TUMORS

Primary cardiac tumors are exceedingly rare; cardiac metastases are more common (see Chapter 29, section V). Tumors of blood vessels are mostly sarcomas, which are discussed in Chapter 17. Some special types are discussed here.

A. Malignant heart tumors include fibrosarcoma, angiosarcoma, rhabdomyosarcoma, and endothelial sarcoma. Tumors usually arise in the right auricle and extend into the heart substance and valves. Their aggressive course is characterized by heart failure, angina, life-threatening arrhythmias, or cardiac rupture. The prognosis is hopeless.

B. Benign heart tumors

   1. Fibroma, myxoma, lipoma, and hemangioma typically arise in the atria. Presenting features include intermittent valvular obstruction with syncope or episodes of dyspnea and cyanosis.

   2. Atrial myxoma can cause a syndrome resembling microbial endocarditis with heart murmur, fever, joint pain, and systemic emboli. Patients with these findings and sterile blood cultures should have an echocardiogram, which is highly accurate for diagnosing myxoma of the heart. Occasionally, the diagnosis is established by the finding of myxomatous tissue in arterial embolectomy specimens.

C. Hemangiopericytomas are tumors of the capillaries, which look like very cellular fibrosarcomas but are rarely malignant. Histologic appearance and grade do not closely correlate with the metastatic potential; metastases occur in cases with apparently benign tumors. These highly vascular tumors are treated by resection after embolic therapy. Postoperative RT may reduce local recurrence. Metastatic tumors respond to doxorubicin.

D. Primary intravascular sarcomas are rare tumors that present with signs of focal vascular obstruction. Venous sarcomas, particularly leiomyosarcomas, are the most common IV sarcomas. Vena cava tumors can produce Budd-Chiari syndrome, renal failure, or pedal edema; patients may present with poorly defined back or abdominal pain. CT scan or venography suggests the diagnosis. Treatment is surgical resection, when technically feasible.

IV. CARCINOSARCOMAS

Carcinosarcomas are rare tumors, which have a histologic appearance of combined sarcomatous and epithelial elements. Conceptually, they represent carcinomas that develop sarcomatous elements via metaplasia of the epithelial element. Typically, they arise in the myometrium, prostate, or lung, but can occur elsewhere. Surgical resection is the treatment of choice. The role of postoperative irradiation is not clear. Recurrent or metastatic disease is associated with a dismal prognosis. Although ifosfamide has been advocated, the results of chemotherapy are anecdotal.

V. CYLINDROMA

Adenoid cystic carcinomas (or *cylindromas*) are rare tumors that most often arise in salivary glands or the large airways, but also can develop in the skin, breast, and other sites. Local recurrence after surgery is common. Pulmonary metastases are radiologically dramatic but often have an indolent course over several years. Primary tumors are treated surgically. Local recurrences may respond to RT. Symptom-free patients with lung metastases do not need specific treatment. Patients with symptomatic disease may respond to fluorouracil or doxorubicin.

VI. DENTAL TUMORS

A. Ameloblastomas appear to originate in odontogenic rests (remnants from the embryologic process of odontogenesis). Eighty percent occur in the mandible (70% in the molar areas). The remaining 20% of histologically similar tumors arise in other bones and, occasionally, soft tissues. Ameloblastomas are locally invasive and have a high risk for local recurrence after surgery. Distant metastases do not occur. Therapy is by surgical resection. Some surgeons use intraoperative cauterization or cryotherapy for better local control. RT has no role in managing the tumor or recurrences.

B. Cementoma is probably an area of calcified fibrous dysplasia and not a neoplasm.

C. Other dental tumors. Ameloblastic adenomatoid tumors, calcifying epithelial odontoma, ameloblastic fibroma, dentinoma, ameloblastic odontoma, and complex odontoma are all benign tumors of the embryologic precursors of teeth. Surgical removal is the therapy of choice. Transformation into malignancy may occur, but rarely.

VII. ESTHESIONEUROBLASTOMA

Olfactory neuroblastoma (ONB, or *esthesioneuroblastoma*) is an uncommon malignancy of the sensory epithelium of the nasal cavity close to the cribriform plate. This tumor is considered in the differential diagnosis of poorly differentiated, small, blue round cell neoplasms. The tumor's immunophenotype is that of a neuroendocrine tumor. Most patients present with Kadish stages B (within the paranasal cavity and paranasal sinuses) or C (extension beyond the paranasal cavity and paranasal sinuses). Aggressive biological behavior may represent a neuroendocrine carcinoma that is not ONB.

A. Presenting features are unilateral nasal obstruction, anosmia, epistaxis, rhinorrhea, sinus pain, headache, diplopia, or proptosis. It may be an incidental finding during polypectomy or nasal septoplasty. Metastases to neck nodes develop in about 30% of patients. Intracranial extension and orbital involvement are independent factors affecting outcome.

B. Multimodality therapy has improved survival for these patients. Disease-free survival at 10 years is about 85%. Aggressive surgical resection is the treatment of choice. Postoperative or neoadjuvant RT improves local control and survival. The results of salvage therapy on relapse are very good. The use of chemotherapy is anecdotal and is usually reserved for patients with high-grade tumors or advanced or relapsed disease.

VIII. PARAGANGLIOMAS (OR *CHEMODECTOMAS*)

These tumors have also been called *receptomas*, glomus tumors, carotid body tumors, and tympanic body tumors. These neoplasms originate in the neural crest and develop from paraganglia tissues, which are themselves chemoreceptor organs that are distributed throughout the body in association with the sympathetic chain. Nearly half originate in the head and neck region (particularly, at the carotid bifurcation and in the temporal bone), and the remainder develop in the mediastinum, retroperitoneum, abdomen, and pelvis. A conventional concept is that pheochromocytoma is simply a paraganglioma confined to the adrenal gland (see Chapter 15, section IV).

A. Occurrence. These uncommon neoplasms are either familial (predominantly men) or nonfamilial (predominantly women). They are multiple at several locations in 25% to 50% of the familial type and in 10% of the nonfamilial type.

B. Natural history. Paragangliomas, which are usually considered to be benign, are characterized by slow and inexorable growth from the site of origin. Clinical course and not histology is the indicator of tumor behavior. Manifestations depend on the cellular characteristics and tumor location. About 5% of tumors are functional, manifest excessive secretion of neuropeptides and catecholamines, and produce a syndrome identical to pheochromocytoma. Metastases, which are the exception rather than the rule, develop in organs that do not contain paraganglia tissue (lungs, lymph nodes, liver, spleen, and bone marrow).

C. Evaluation. Paragangliomas must always be considered as potentially multiple, especially in patients with a family history of such tumors. Patients should be screened for evidence of excessive catecholamine secretion.

Computed tomography or MRI is useful in delineating the tumors. Arteriography may be useful for tumor embolization done just before surgery or for evaluating contralateral crossover blood supply. Radionuclide scintigraphy using ^{131}I-meta-iodobenzylguanidine (MIBG) may be helpful in localizing both paragangliomas and pheochromocytomas. These tumors have a rich blood supply; caution must be exerted not to cause hemorrhage during biopsy. Fine-needle aspiration cytology is often useful if performed carefully.

D. Treatment. Surgical extirpation is the treatment of choice, particularly for small head and neck lesions, but technical expertise in vascular surgery is mandatory. RT is effective in local control and is probably the treatment of choice for lesions that are large or erode bone, particularly in older patients. Chemotherapy is generally ineffective for metastatic disease. To do nothing is an acceptable option in some patients because these lesions are often well tolerated for long periods.

IX. URACHAL CANCER

Urachal cancer arises in the primitive embryonic connection between the apex of the bladder and the umbilicus. Most of these tumors arise near the dome of the urinary bladder. The most common histologic type is adenocarcinoma. Adenocarcinomas evolve slowly and are asymptomatic until late in the course of disease. Presenting symptoms are painless hematuria, suprapubic mass, or passage of mucus in the urine. The presence of stippled calcification of a lower midline abdominal wall mass is almost pathognomonic for urachal carcinoma. Surgical resection is the therapy of choice.

Suggested Reading

Esthesioneuroblastoma

Argiris A, et al. Esthesioneuroblastoma: the Northwestern experience. *Laryngoscope* 2003;113:155.

Diaz EM, et al. Olfactory neuroblastoma: the 22-year experience at one comprehensive cancer center. *Head Neck* 2005;27:138.

Jethanamest D, et al. Esthesioneuroblastoma: a population-based analysis of survival and prognostic factors. *Arch Otolaryngol Head Neck Surg* 2007;133:276.

Loy AH, et al. Esthesioneuroblastoma: continued follow-up of a single institution's experience. *Arch Otolaryngol Head Neck Surg* 2006;132:134.

Paraganglioma

Al-Mefty O, Teixeira A. Complex tumors of the glomus jugulare: criteria, treatment, and outcome. *J Neurosurg* 2002;97:1356.

Fitoussi O, et al. Advanced paraganglioma: a role for chemotherapy? *Med Pediatr Oncol* 1999;33:129.

Thymoma

Agarwal S, Cunningham-Rundles C. Thymoma and immunodeficiency (Good syndrome): a report of 2 unusual cases and review of the literature. *Ann Allergy Asthma Immunol* 2007;98:185.

Ogawa K, et al. Postoperative radiotherapy for patients with completely resected thymoma. A multi-institutional, retrospective review of 103 patients. *Cancer* 2002;94:1405.

Okumura M, et al. The World Health Organization histologic classification system reflects the oncologic behavior of thymoma: a clinical study of 273 patients. *Cancer* 2002;94:624.

Palmieri G, et al. Somatostatin analogs and prednisone in advanced refractory thymic tumors. *Cancer* 2002;94:1414.

Rena O, et al. Does adjuvant radiation therapy improve disease-free survival in completely resected Masaoka stage II thymoma? *Eur J Cardio Thoracic Surg* 2007;31:109.

Thompson CA, Steensma DP. Pure red cell aplasia associated with thymoma: clinical insights from a 50-year single-institution experience. *Br J Haematol* 2006;135:405.

Other Neoplasms

DeLair D, et al. Ameloblastic carcinosarcoma of the mandible arising in ameloblastic fibroma: a case report and review of the literature. *Oral Surg Oral Med Oral Pathol Oral Radiol Endod* 2007;103:516.

Hansel D, Epstein JI. Sarcomatoid carcinoma of the prostate: a study of 42 cases. *Am J Surg Pathol* 2006;30:1316.

Macchiarini P, Ostertag H. Uncommon primary mediastinal tumours. *Lancet Oncology* 2004;5:107.

Perchinsky MJ, Lichtenstein SV, Tyers GFO. Primary cardiac tumors: forty years' experience with 71 patients. *Cancer* 1997;79:1809.

Spitz FR, et al. Hemangiopericytoma: a 20-year single-institution experience. *Ann Surg Oncol* 1998;5:350.

Strollo DC, Rosado-de-Christenson ML, Jett JR. Primary mediastinal tumors. *Chest* 1997;112:511 (Part I); 1344 (Part II).

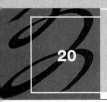

20 METASTASES OF UNKNOWN ORIGIN
Dennis A. Casciato

$\mathcal{T}$**he definition of metastases of unknown origin (MUOs).** MUOs are metastatic solid tumors (hematopoietic malignancies and lymphomas are excluded) for which the site of origin is not suggested by thorough history, physical examination, chest radiograph, routine blood and urine studies, and thorough histological evaluation.

$\mathcal{T}$**he predicament of MUO.** The detection of MUO usually represents the discovery of a far-advanced malignancy that is rarely curable and that is usually refractory even to palliative chemotherapy. Tumors that are potentially responsive to systemic treatment are found in only about 20% of all patients with MUO. The diagnostic evaluations inflicted on these patients in pursuit of the primary site are typically excessive and futile. The primary site is found in <15% of cases, and that discovery rarely affects the prognosis or treatment. All efforts to manage patients who meet the criteria defined above should be guided by the understanding that there are two basic categories of MUOs: (1) those that are treatable and (2) those that are not.

I. EPIDEMIOLOGY AND BIOLOGY
  A. Incidence. About 6% of patients with cancer present with MUO. MUO is the seventh most frequent malignancy, ranking below only cancers of the lung, prostate, breast, cervix, colon, and stomach.
  B. Age. The average age at onset is 58 years. Patients who present with a midline distribution of poorly differentiated carcinoma (10% of all MUO patients) have a median age of 39 years.
  C. Manifestations. Symptoms of metastasis, which are present in nearly all patients with MUO syndrome, are multiple in 30% of patients. The most frequent presenting features are the following:
   1. Pain (60%)
   2. Liver mass or other abdominal manifestations (40%)
   3. Lymphadenopathy (20%)
   4. Bone pain or pathological fracture (15%)
   5. Respiratory symptoms (15%)
   6. Central nervous system abnormalities (5%)
   7. Weight loss (5%)
   8. Skin nodules (2%)
  D. Aberrant natural history of tumors in the MUO syndrome compromises the ability to predict the primary site of disease. Carcinomas that occur commonly in the general population (namely, carcinoma of the breast, prostate, and bowel) make up only a small percentage of cases with MUO. About 75% of tumors in the MUO syndrome originate below the diaphragm. Importantly, patterns of dissemination by tumors do not follow typical pathways in the MUO syndrome. Examples are shown in Table 20.1. This observation represents the distinct biology of these malignancies wherein the metastatic behavior predominates unpredictably while the primary tumor remains occult.
  E. Mechanisms that could explain the presence of occult primary neoplasms include the following:
   1. Excision or electrocautery may have removed unrecognized primary lesions years before the appearance of metastatic lesions.

| **TABLE 20.1** | **Patterns of Dissemination by Tumors** | | |

		Metastatic site involved (% of cases)	
Type of carcinoma	Metastatic site	With primary site known	With MUO
Lung	Bone	30–50	5
Pancreas	Bone	5–10	30
Prostate	Liver or lung	15	>50

MUO, metastases of unknown origin.

2. The primary cancer may have shed metastases and then undergone spontaneous regression.

3. The primary tumor may be too small to be detected, even at autopsy.

4. The site of origin may be obscured by the extensiveness of metastases or by the atypical pattern of dissemination.

II. DIAGNOSIS AND HISTOPATHOLOGY

A. Performing a biopsy should be the first order of business. The pathologist should be informed before the biopsy that the primary site is not evident so that special studies can be planned.

1. Patients with metastases to neck lymph nodes only. Suspicious cervical nodes should *not undergo excisional biopsy* until a complete diagnostic evaluation of the head and neck has been performed (see Chapter 7, section X). About 35% of these patients have potentially curable cancers of the upper aerodigestive tract. This is not the case for patients with supraclavicular lymph nodes, which may be directly excised for histological examination.

2. Other patients who have suspected metastatic cancer. Biopsy of *the most accessible site* should be performed *before* specialized blood or radiological studies are done; the histological findings provide an invaluable guide for a rational diagnostic workup. Biopsy proof of metastatic cancer is necessary *at only one site*. If several areas of tumor involvement are suggested by the findings from the screening evaluation, the preferred biopsy site is that associated with the least morbidity (e.g., peripheral lymph nodes when palpable, bone marrow when a leukoerythroblastic blood picture is present, cytology of sampled effusions, or suspect skin lesions). The biopsy specimen should be placed in a fixative that allows immunoperoxidase analysis.

B. Role of the pathologist. Close communication between the clinician and the pathologist is especially important in cases of MUO. Morphological clues may make certain anatomic sites more likely and direct the sequence of investigation.

1. Histological problems

a. Poorly differentiated tumors, including adenocarcinomas, carcinomas, and small cell neoplasms, may be indistinguishable by light microscopy.

b. Squamous metaplasia overlying adenocarcinoma may be misread as squamous cell cancer.

c. Extensive fibrosis, a common sequela of squamous cell carcinoma and breast adenocarcinoma, may mask the underlying tumor.

d. Limitations of pathology. Pathologists are able to identify the primary site based on review of the biopsy alone in about 20% of cases of MUO. If they are given clinical information (especially the site of metastasis), the accuracy improves, but these tumors usually defy categorization for the origin of the tumor.

2. **Histological and histochemical clues for origin** are shown in Appendix C-1.
3. **Poorly differentiated, undifferentiated, or anaplastic carcinomas** should be further evaluated with immunoperoxidase stains and, in special circumstances, electron microscopy or molecular genetic analysis (if possible).
4. **Immunoperoxidase stains** are useful for poorly differentiated neoplasms to confirm the diagnosis of carcinoma, to identify patients with other neoplasms (e.g., lymphoma or melanoma), and occasionally to identify a site of recognized cancer. The predominant tumors identified by specific antigens delineated by immunohistochemistry are shown in Appendix C-2. A word of caution: These markers are stains attached to antibodies that must be *interpreted* for positivity, negativity, and relevance; none of these results is perfect.
   a. **Immunohistochemistry diagnostic algorithms**
      (1) An immunohistochemistry diagnostic algorithm based on microscopic findings (spindle cell, epithelioid, small cell, or undifferentiated morphologies) is diagrammed in Appendix C-3.I.
      (2) An immunohistochemistry diagnostic algorithm for carcinoma of unknown origin is diagrammed in Appendix C-3.II.
      (3) Expected immunophenotypes for specific tumors are shown in Appendix C-4.
   b. **The most useful immunoperoxidase stains** in the evaluation of patients with MUO syndrome are cytokeratins (CK) and those for lymphoma (CD45, leukocyte common antigen) and for melanoma (S100 protein, HMB45, Melan-A/Mart-1).
      The CK phenotypes (relative patterns of positivity and negativity for CK 7 and CK 20) have been employed in attempts to identify primary tumor sites with variable success (see Appendix C-3.I.). More discriminatory immunostains can then be selected based on these phenotypes; examples of such are shown in Appendix C-4.IX.
   c. Immunoperoxidase stains for neuron-specific enolase, synaptophysin, chromogranin, CD56, and CD57 are helpful in patients who could have primitive neuroendocrine tumors (PNETs).
   d. Immunoperoxidase stains for β-human chorionic gonadotropin (β-hCG) and α-fetoprotein (α-FP) are frequently performed for the possibility of a germ cell neoplasm but have not been helpful in these patients unless the clinical presentation suggests this entity.
   e. A few immunohistochemical markers have enough tissue-type specificity that allows for their use in trying to establish a primary tumor. These include:
      (1) PSA (prostatic adenocarcinoma and benign prostatic epithelium)
      (2) Thyroglobulin (thyroid follicular epithelium and nonmedullary thyroid carcinomas)
      (3) Thyroid transcription factor-1 (TTF-1; thyroid and lung cancers and carcinoid tumors)
      (4) Gross cystic disease fluid protein-15 (breast carcinoma and tumors of apocrine sweat glands or salivary glands)
      (5) RCC (renal cell carcinoma) and HepPar-1 (hepatocellular carcinoma) may prove to be helpful as well.
5. **Molecular diagnostics** continue to rapidly expand. Interphase cytogenetic analysis with fluorescent *in situ* hybridization (FISH) and genetic expression profiling can be performed on paraffin tissue. These techniques may provide anatomic pathologists with the tools to improve their ability to correctly predict the primary site for MUO in the future.

C. **Histological types of metastases**
   1. **Adenocarcinomas and undifferentiated carcinomas** account for >75% of cases of MUO. The natural history, prognosis, and poor responsiveness to therapy are similar for both of these histopathologies.
      a. **The primary site** is determined antemortem in only 15% of cases, even with exhaustive diagnostic efforts. When a primary site is determined, the sites of origin and relative frequencies are as follows:

(1) Pancreas (25%)

(2) Lung (20%)

(3) Stomach, colorectum, hepatobiliary tract (8% to 12% each)

(4) Kidney (5%)

(5) Breast, ovary, prostate (2% to 3% each)

b. **Undifferentiated and poorly differentiated large cell neoplasms** may represent carcinoma, extragonadal germ cell tumors, malignant melanoma, or large cell lymphoma. Lymphomas rarely are mistaken for adenocarcinomas, but the chance of confusion is increased if the tissue obtained is small or of poor quality. For example, gastric lymphoma and anaplastic large cell lymphoma are frequently misdiagnosed as carcinoma. These patients, in particular, require special study with immunoperoxidase techniques. Many patients with MUO who have been reported to achieve good results with chemotherapy ultimately were proved to have lymphomas.

2. **Squamous cell carcinomas** account for 10% to 15% of all MUO cases, and <5% if patients with metastases to cervical lymph nodes alone are excluded. Most squamous cancers that appear as MUO originate in the head and neck or lung. Other squamous cell cancer primary sites include the uterine cervix, penis, anus, rectum, esophagus, and occasionally, urinary bladder. Acanthocarcinomas (squamoid tumors) may develop in the gastrointestinal (GI) tract, notably in the pancreas and stomach. Squamous skin cancer that arises in a chronic osteomyelitis fistula may not be apparent until regional draining lymph nodes become involved.

3. **Melanoma** constitutes 4% of all cases of MUO, and about 4% of malignant melanoma cases present as MUO. It is important to distinguish melanoma from other histologies because metastases frequently involve lymph nodes alone, and these patients may be cured with appropriate therapy (see section V.A).

   a. Amelanotic melanoma may be mistaken as undifferentiated carcinoma. Malignant melanoma may be distinguished from tumors having obscure histology by use of immunohistochemical reagents that are specific for melanocytic lineage (HMB45, Melan-A/Mart1, PNL2). or for S100 protein (a cytoplasmic protein that is specific for nervous system tissue and is also present on human melanoma cell lines).

   b. Explanations of how melanoma can present as MUO:

      (1) The primary lesion may have been destroyed (e.g., by prior excision or cautery).

      (2) The primary lesion may have regressed spontaneously.

      (3) The tumor may have arisen *de novo* within a lymph node.

4. **Clear cell tumors.** Polygonal cells with clear cytoplasm can represent artifactual changes, benign neoplasms, or malignancies. Seminomas, nonseminomatous germ cell carcinomas, lymphomas, and benign tumors can be clear cell tumors with a virtually identical clear cell appearance. Differentiation requires detailed analysis of clinical, histological, immunohistochemical, and, occasionally, electron microscopic features.

5. **Small cell neoplasms, including PNETs or "oat cell" carcinomas,** develop in the entire alimentary canal, upper aerodigestive tract, thymus, breast, prostate, urinary bladder, uterine cervix, endometrium, and skin as well as in the lung. About 2% of small cell carcinomas originate in extrapulmonary sites. Although this subtype comprises only a small percentage of the patients who present with MUO, it represents one of the treatable varieties.

   a. **PNETs.** Low-grade PNETs are usually recognizable by light microscopy, have features of islet cell or carcinoid tumors, and often have an indolent behavior. Anaplastic small cell carcinomas and poorly differentiated PNETs behave aggressively and require immunohistochemical analysis of biopsies for synaptophysin and chromogranin.

   b. **Undifferentiated small cell neoplasms** may also represent a number of cancers that can be simply recalled with the mnemonic *MR. MOLSEN* [*m*yeloma, *r*habdomyoblastoma, *m*elanoma (amelanotic), *o*at cell carcinoma, *l*ymphoma, *s*eminoma (anaplastic), *E*wing sarcoma, *n*euroblastoma].

III. SITES OF METASTASES AND PROGNOSIS. *The prognosis in patients with MUO syndrome is unaffected by whether the primary lesion is ever found.*

A. Survival according to sites of metastases

1. **Patients with metastases to lymph nodes alone** have 5-year survival rates according to sites of involvement, which are as follows:

   a. Upper or middle cervical nodes alone (30% to 50%)

   b. Axillary nodes alone in women (25%)

   c. Groin nodes alone (50%, perhaps)

   d. Midline lymph node distribution with poorly differentiated adenocarcinoma, particularly in young men (30%)

   e. Melanoma to single peripheral lymph node region (30% to 45%)

2. **Patients with metastases to sites other than peripheral lymph nodes alone.** The median survival time for all patients ranges between <1 month and 5 months. More than 75% of patients die within 1 year of diagnosis. Subcutaneous metastases have a more favorable prognosis if the primary site is not the lung; bone marrow and epidural metastases have the worst prognosis (median survival time of <1 month).

3. **Particularly unfavorable prognostic features** in patients with MUO include the following:

   a. Multiple metastatic sites

   b. Supraclavicular lymph node involvement

   c. Well-differentiated or moderately differentiated adenocarcinoma histology

   d. Elevated serum alkaline phosphatase level

   e. Older age

   f. Lower performance status

B. Neck lymph node metastasis. Neck masses in adults, other than thyroid nodules, are malignant in 80% of cases. After 50 years of age, 90% of neck masses are malignant. About 35% of patients with MUO to upper and middle cervical lymph nodes can potentially be cured. However, MUO to lower cervical or supraclavicular lymph nodes is associated with an ominous prognosis. MUO to neck nodes is discussed in detail in Chapter 7, section X.

C. Axillary lymph node metastasis. Axillary lymphadenopathy that is excised for diagnosis is found to have benign disease in 75% of cases, lymphoma in 15%, and solid tumors (particularly adenocarcinoma) in 10%.

1. **The most likely sites of origin** of a solid tumor metastasizing to the axilla are the breast, lung, arm, and regional trunk. In patients with isolated malignant axillary lymphadenopathy, the primary site is detected in only half of the cases.

2. **Breast cancer.** Breast cancer accounts for 70% of cases of MUO involving axillary lymph nodes in women when the primary site is eventually diagnosed. About 0.5% of all breast cancer patients present with masses palpable in the axilla and not in the breast.

D. Groin lymph node metastasis. The primary tumor is detectable in 99% of patients having malignant groin lymphadenopathy. Metastases are most likely to arise from the skin (especially the lower extremities and lower half of the trunk), genital and reproductive organs, rectum, anus, or urinary bladder.

E. Midline lymphadenopathy (anterior mediastinal or retroperitoneal with or without peripheral lymphadenopathy) represents a highly treatable presentation of MUO when it is associated with *poorly differentiated carcinomas* (undifferentiated carcinoma, poorly differentiated carcinoma, or poorly differentiated adenocarcinoma). The cell lineage with this form of MUO is uncertain, but some are extragonadal germ cell tumors. Most patients are men, with a median age of 39 years and rapidly growing tumor masses. Many patients have achieved excellent responses to cisplatin-based combination chemotherapy (see section V.E).

F. Other sites of metastases

1. **Bone and bone marrow metastases**

   a. Bone cortex. When a primary site is found, carcinoma of the lung accounts for most patients with MUO who have bone metastases. When presenting as an MUO, pancreatic carcinoma frequently involves the skeleton (in contrast to its usual behavior). The median survival time of patients presenting with MUO and predominantly bone metastases is 3 months.

   b. Bone marrow is shown to be involved by aspiration or biopsy techniques in 10% to 15% of MUO cases during life, particularly in patients who prove to have lung, breast, or prostate cancer. Leukoerythroblastic peripheral blood smears are the most accurate barometers of bone marrow involvement in patients with solid tumors. The median survival time of patients presenting with MUO as marrow metastases is <1 month.

2. **Intrathoracic metastases**
   a. Pulmonary metastases may be solitary, and primary lung cancer lesions may be multiple. MUO presenting as a solitary pulmonary nodule is rare; when it does occur, it is most frequently associated with colorectal carcinoma or sarcoma.
   b. Effusions. Pleural effusions, when caused by malignant disease, are associated with an unknown primary tumor in 20% of cases. Pericardial effusions rarely occur as the predominant manifestation of MUO.

3. **Intra-abdominal metastases** most frequently involve the liver and originate in the GI tract, but the primary site is determined during life in only about 30% of cases.
   a. Liver metastases. Differentiating between primary hepatocellular carcinoma and metastatic carcinoma of unknown origin in the liver may be difficult. Carcinomas of the prostate or ovary metastasize to the liver more frequently when they present as MUO than when they occur as known primaries. The median survival time of patients presenting with MUO and predominantly liver metastases is <4 months.
   b. Ascites, when caused by malignant disease, is associated with MUO in 10% of cases. The median survival time of patients presenting with MUO and predominantly malignant ascites is <1 month, except for women with peritoneal carcinomatosis, which is considered to be a variant of ovarian carcinoma (see section V.F). Approximately 55% of women who present with malignant ascites have a primary site identified in the ovary. Histologic features that suggest ovarian carcinoma include papillary configuration, psammoma bodies, and poorly differentiated carcinoma.

4. **Central nervous system metastases**
   a. Brain metastases are most frequently associated with bronchogenic carcinoma and second most frequently with MUO syndrome. The primary site eventually becomes evident during life in 40% of cases, and 90% of these are lung carcinoma. Excision of single metastatic brain lesions does not improve survival beyond that experienced by other patients with MUO syndrome, but occasional patients experience prolonged survival without evidence of further recurrence. The median survival time of patients presenting with MUO and single brain metastasis that is resected is 3 to 6 months.
   b. Spinal cord compression is occasionally a manifestation of MUO syndrome. In these cases, laminectomy has been traditionally recommended as the first step to establish the histopathological diagnosis. However, the median survival time of patients presenting with MUO and epidural metastasis is <2 months, and such an aggressive approach is often not justified.

5. **Cutaneous metastases** are associated with carcinomas of the breast and lung in most cases. When skin metastases represent the initial manifestation of cancer, renal adenocarcinoma or bronchogenic carcinoma is the most likely possibility. The region of the skin near the primary tumor is most often involved. **Umbilical nodules** (*Sister Joseph nodules*) represent intra-abdominal carcinomatosis. The median survival time of patients presenting with MUO and predominantly skin metastases is 7 months if the primary site does not prove to be the lung.

IV. SEARCHING FOR THE PRIMARY TUMOR SITE. When the primary site of cancer is evident, the biopsy is performed 1 week earlier and the number of diagnostic tests ordered is significantly fewer than when patients present with MUO. Unfortunately, the usual behavior of physicians is to pursue the occult primary site through a prolonged investigative pathway with a bewildering scope of expensive, time-consuming, and potentially dangerous tests.

Even if all patients undergo exhaustive evaluation with barium enema (BE), upper GI series, intravenous pyelogram (IVP), skeletal survey, lung tomography, mammography (women), abdominal and pelvic CT scans, endoscopy, and a variety of radionuclide scans, <15% *of patients* with MUO syndrome (excluding those who have disease only in cervical nodes) have the primary site established before death. Part of the 15% includes patients in whom the primary tumor becomes clinically evident on follow-up.

Searching for the primary tumor site should be guided by the following questions:

A. **What is the effect on outcome of finding the primary site? None!** To reiterate: The prognosis in patients with MUO syndrome is unaffected by whether the primary lesion is ever found. This observation applies not only to metastases involving visceral or skeletal sites but also to metastases involving lymph nodes alone at any site (including the neck) with any histology (carcinoma or melanoma).

B. **What are the clinical clues?**
   1. **Histology.** The finding of squamous carcinoma obviates the need to investigate organs in which adenocarcinomas develop. If the pathologist is not certain of the diagnosis because of the morphology or quality of the specimen, special studies or another biopsy may be in order.
   2. **Presentation.** The history, physical examination, and screening studies should be reviewed with awareness of the natural histories of the potentially causal malignancies. The atypical behavior patterns of certain malignancies when presenting as MUO should also be remembered (see section I.D).

C. **Which advanced malignancies are treatable?** They are:
   1. **Metastases to unilateral lymph nodes alone**
      a. Melanoma to peripheral lymph nodes in a single region
      b. Squamous cell or undifferentiated carcinoma in the upper two-thirds of the cervical chain
      c. Adenocarcinoma in the axillary chain in women
      d. Carcinoma in unilateral groin nodes
   2. **Metastases that are sensitive to systemic therapy**
      a. Small cell carcinomas or PNETs
      b. Peritoneal carcinomatosis in women
      c. Poorly differentiated carcinoma metastatic to retroperitoneum and/or mediastinum, with or without involvement of peripheral lymph nodes, particularly in younger men
      d. Adenocarcinomas that are treatable in advanced stages (breast, ovary, prostate, and thyroid). Together these constitute <15% of cases of MUO, but they should be considered in patients with appropriate constellations of findings.
      e. Lymphomas should be considered in any patient with a poorly differentiated or undifferentiated neoplasm or with tumors that respond exquisitely to chemotherapy.

D. **What are the limitations of diagnostic studies?** Despite subjection to an alarming battery of tests, >85% of patients with MUO do not have the primary site determined while they are alive. Furthermore, many of the diagnostic tests are *just as frequently misleading as they are helpful.*
   1. **Pathology.** Review of the initial biopsy does not contribute to the origin of the malignant neoplasm in 80% of cases of MUO. Histopathological classification of tumors can vary by >50% among different reviewers of the same specimen.
   2. **Chest radiographs.** No chest radiographic pattern, including the number of lesions, can distinguish a metastasis from a primary lung cancer.
   3. **Upper GI series, BE, and IVP.** Fewer than 5% of patients with MUO who undergo these studies have abnormal results in the absence of abdominal symptoms, occult blood in the stools, or hematuria. Abnormal results usually consist of findings that provide no useful information (e.g., organ displacement by tumor). Upper GI series, BE, and IVP each suggests a primary malignant lesion in

5% to 10% of cases of MUO; the numbers of true-positive and false-positive results and the minimum number of false-negative results are about equal, however.

4. **Mammography** is usually performed in women with MUO but has not been helpful in identifying the primary site, even in women with axillary lymph node metastases alone. MRI of the breasts may increase the yield of detecting primary lesions in the latter group of patients.

5. **CT scans.** Some reported series have detected the primary site in about 30% of patients with MUO. However, other series reported that CT scans have not improved the frequency of detecting occult primary sites except in patients with squamous cell MUO to cervical lymph nodes. These scans often detect other sites of metastases. However, it is unusual for the information resulting from CT scans to result in improved outcome.

6. **Radionuclide scans.** Staging disease in asymptomatic sites is a dubious practice for patients with disease that is already considered lethal.

    a. **Thyroid scans** are associated with equal frequencies of true-positive, false-positive, and false-negative results. Thus, these scans are nearly useless in MUO.

    b. **Positron emission tomography** (PET) with ^{18}F-fluoro-2-deoxy-D-glucose (FDG) still needs to be adequately investigated to determine its true usefulness for patients with MUO. FDG PET has not been helpful in evaluating MUO patients with the exceptions of patients with squamous cell carcinoma metastasis to cervical lymph nodes alone and possibly of women with metastatic adenocarcinoma in axillary lymph nodes alone.

    c. **Bone scans** may be abnormal in the absence of symptoms related to the skeleton and may be useful for determining the extent of disease if that information is believed to be helpful.

    d. **Gallium scans** are useless in MUO.

7. **Ultrasonograms** have a high rate of false positivity in the evaluation of MUO, giving particularly erroneous results in retroperitoneal areas.

8. **Arteriography and screening endoscopy,** including bronchoscopy, upper GI endoscopy, sigmoidoscopy, and colonoscopy, are overly invasive and of no value in patients with the MUO syndrome and no other clinical indication to invoke these procedures.

9. **Serum tumor markers,** including CEA, CA 125, CA 15-3, CA 19-9, and β-hCG, are generally of little use in determining the primary site because of their lack of specificity. All five of these markers are commonly elevated in patients with MUO. Even PSA determinations are associated with false-positive and false-negative results.

10. **Estrogen receptor** determination has not been helpful in identifying the primary site or in prescribing therapy for patients with MUO.

11. **Postmortem examination,** the ultimate diagnostic test, fails to detect the primary site in 25% of MUO cases.

V. **MANAGEMENT.** My recommendations for the management of patients with MUO syndrome are diagrammed in Figure 20.1.

A. **Malignant melanoma involving peripheral lymph nodes only**

1. **Evaluation**

    a. Inquire about skin lesions that may have been removed previously.

    b. Search the skin carefully for a possible primary lesion; biopsy any suspect lesion.

    c. Exclude visceral disease with history and physical examination (especially ophthalmoscopy), chest radiographs, LFTs, and CT scans of the liver and brain.

2. **Recommended treatment** for malignant melanoma involving lymph nodes alone is radical lymphadenectomy of the affected nodal region. The procedure is repeated if the tumor recurs and the patient has no other evidence of disease. The use of interferon for melanoma is discussed in Chapter 16, in the section "Malignant Melanoma."

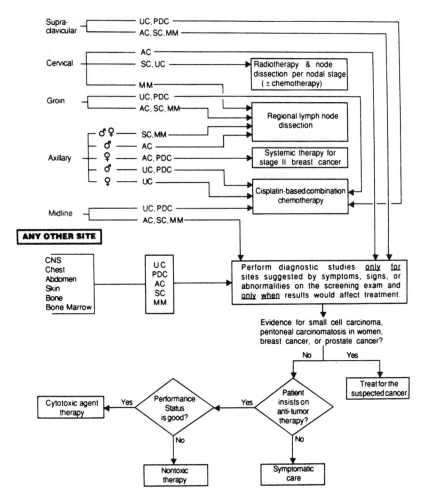

Figure 20.1. An approach to the treatment of patients with metastases of unknown origin. AC, adenocarcinoma; PDC, poorly differentiated carcinoma; SC, squamous cell carcinoma; UC, undifferentiated carcinoma; MM, malignant melanoma; CNS, central nervous system.

    3. Results of treatment. Both the 5- and 10-year survival rates using radical lymphadenectomy are 30% to 45%. The prognosis with lymphatic metastasis is affected neither by knowing the primary site nor by having a history of a pre-existing lesion. The prognosis is best if the metastasis involves only one node, and not the cervical chain, and if surgical intervention is prompt and aggressive.

B. Metastatic disease in neck lymph nodes only, particularly in the upper and middle cervical nodes, is potentially curable with radiation therapy (RT) or node dissection under appropriate circumstances. Excisional biopsy of these nodes should not be performed because it distorts surgical planes and may result in poor outcomes if it proves to be a primary squamous cell carcinoma originating in an occult site in the head and neck. Fine-needle aspiration for cytology is preferable. Supraclavicular lymphadenopathy, on the other hand, rarely represents curable disease; these nodes may be excised directly for histological examination. The evaluation and management of MUO to neck lymph nodes are discussed in detail in Chapter 7, section X.

C. Metastatic disease in unilateral axillary lymph nodes only. The major treatable malignancies presenting as MUO in axillary lymph nodes are occult breast carcinoma, amelanotic melanoma mistaken as undifferentiated carcinoma, and malignant lymphoma mistaken as carcinomas. Axillary metastases from breast cancer without an evident breast mass are most likely to emanate from the upper outer quadrant of the ipsilateral breast.

  1. Evaluation
    a. Search for a primary site in the breasts, lungs, and regional skin.
    b. If no primary lesion is found, perform an excisional biopsy.
    c. In women with adenocarcinoma or poorly differentiated carcinoma, perform mammography (although the diagnostic yield is poor) and assess hormone-receptor activity and HER2 status.
    d. MRI of the breasts and positron emission tomography (PET) scanning have aided the identification of primary tumors, even after normal physical examination and mammography.

  2. Occult breast cancer (axillary nodal metastasis without a clinically detectable primary tumor in the breast) accounts for 0.5% of all breast cancer patients. Ultimately, 30% to 50% of female patients develop evidence of a primary breast cancer. The primary tumor becomes evident in <20% of these patients if the breast is treated with RT.

  3. Recommended treatment
    a. Lymphoma. See Chapter 21.
    b. Malignant melanoma. See section V.A.
    c. Women with adenocarcinoma or poorly differentiated carcinoma. Treat for stage II breast cancer. Mastectomy had been traditionally performed but is not justifiable in these patients.
    d. Other patients. Axillary node dissection is performed, attempting to achieve local control and long-term survival.
    e. RT to the axilla is frequently given, but there is no evidence to indicate that survival is improved over that achieved with resection of the involved nodes alone.

  4. Results of treatment. Patients who have MUO and prove to have breast cancer can be expected to have the same survival as patients with stage II disease. The 5- and 10-year survival rates are identical with and without mastectomy and with and without the primary tumor ever becoming manifest. All other patients who are treated with excision of clinically involved nodes or axillary dissection have a 20% to 25% long-term survival rate (2 to 10 years).

D. Metastatic disease in unilateral groin lymph nodes only
  1. Evaluation
    a. Search for a primary site on the skin, anus, rectum, vulva, vagina, cervix, penis, and scrotum.
    b. If no primary lesion is found, perform an excisional biopsy.

  2. Recommended treatment
    a. Lymphoma. See Chapter 21.
    b. Melanoma. See section V.A.
    c. Carcinoma. Perform a superficial groin node dissection (affords local control with less morbidity than radical dissection). Simple excision of the involved node may be sufficient treatment, however.
    d. RT does not appear to be necessary.
    e. Chemotherapy has been useful for carcinomas of the anus and cervix. Although combined chemoradiotherapy has not been extensively used in this

relatively small patient population, the empiric addition of platinum-based chemotherapy may be useful.

3. Results of treatment. Half of patients treated with excisional biopsy or superficial groin dissection alone appear to survive >2 years. A significant proportion of these patients had unclassifiable carcinomas that may have been amelanotic melanoma.

E. Poorly differentiated carcinoma with midline lymphadenopathy (especially in young men) are managed as extragonadal germ cell tumors.

  1. Evaluation

    a. Perform CT scans of the chest, abdomen, and pelvis.

    b. Measure serum levels of β-hCG and α-FP. Elevated levels support the diagnosis of extragonadal germ cell tumor, but the results do not affect the probability of response to treatment.

  2. Recommended treatment. Administer four cycles of cisplatin-based combination chemotherapy using regimens recommended for testicular cancer in patients with acceptable performance status.

  3. Results of treatment. The response rate with disease confined to the mediastinum, retroperitoneum, or peripheral lymph nodes is 60% to 75%, with complete remissions observed in 50% of patients. In some series, the median survival time for patients achieving a complete remission is >4 years; the 5-year survival rate is 35% for patients with disease confined to the retroperitoneum and peripheral lymph nodes and 15% for those with disease affecting predominantly the mediastinum. For patients with this histology and metastases to other sites, the response rate to cisplatin-based chemotherapy is 20%, and the 5-year survival rate is about 5%.

F. Peritoneal carcinomatosis in women

  1. Evaluation

    a. Perform pelvic examination and paracentesis with cytological and biochemical analysis of the ascitic fluid.

    b. Perform CT scans of the abdomen and pelvis.

    c. Evaluate for other causes of malignant ascites clinically.

  2. Recommended treatment. If no extraovarian primary site is evident, perform exploratory laparotomy. If peritoneal carcinomatosis is confirmed without an extraovarian primary site, treat the patient as if she had ovarian carcinoma by performing total abdominal hysterectomy, bilateral salpingo-oophorectomy, omentectomy, and cytoreductive debulking of metastases. Thereafter, treat with a platinum-based combination chemotherapy regimen for 6 to 8 months. Second-look laparotomy is not a consideration in these patients.

  3. Results of treatment. The median survival rates are 1.5 to 2 years for all patients, 2.5 years for patients with limited residual disease after surgery, and 1 year for patients with extensive residual disease after surgery. About 10% to 25% of patients survive 3 years. Most long-term remissions have been observed in patients who had successful cytoreduction before receiving chemotherapy.

G. Small cell carcinoma (PNET) MUO

  1. Evaluation

    a. Evaluate the biopsy with neuroendocrine markers (e.g., chromogranin, synaptophysin, neuron-specific enolase).

    b. Perform CT scans of the chest and abdomen.

    c. Perform bone marrow biopsy if the patient has a leukoerythroblastic anemia or increased serum alkaline phosphatase.

  2. Recommended treatment

    a. Low-grade PNETs are relatively resistant to chemotherapy. Aggressive regimens should be avoided. For patients with small cell carcinoma MUO to cervical lymph nodes alone, some authorities recommend treatment with RT or neck dissection alone.

    b. Poorly differentiated PNETs are often highly sensitive to chemotherapy. Use cisplatin and etoposide combination chemotherapy. If a complete remission is obtained, consider administering RT to the known previous sites of disease.

3. **Results of treatment.** The response rate of poorly differentiated PNETs to chemotherapy is 35% to 70%, and the 2-year survival rate is about 40%. Long-term survival can be seen in patients who achieve a complete response after treatment for limited disease. Prolonged survival also occurs in patients presenting with cervical node metastases from occult primary small cell tumors of the minor salivary glands or paranasal sinuses after treatment with RT or neck dissection alone.

H. All other patients with MUO syndrome

1. **Evaluation.** All patients should receive a complete history and physical examination (including the breasts, rectum, and pelvis), chest radiograph, and routine laboratory tests. Because of the low frequency of detecting the primary site in patients with MUO and the frequently misleading results of radiological studies, radiological or radionuclide studies are justified only in the presence of either specific abnormalities in the screening evaluation or possibilities suggested by review of histopathology.

   When the initial database does not suggest a primary organ site, further evaluation is usually fruitless and is not indicated. It is important to recognize that these patients have incurable cancer that is usually refractory to treatment. With the exception of treatable malignancies, documenting a site is more important to the patient (or physician) psychologically than therapeutically.

2. **For possible breast or prostate cancer:** Treat according to the principles established for those malignancies, especially considering hormonal manipulations. Breast cancer could be suspected in women with bone or upper torso soft-tissue metastases, even with negative mammography results. Prostate cancer could be suspected in men with metastases only to bones of the pelvis or lumbar spine, particularly if the PSA level is elevated.

3. **For all other patients with adenocarcinoma MUO to viscera:** Nearly 80% of these patients have MUO metastases from cancers of the pancreas, GI tract, lung, and other or never-to-be-known sites that are usually refractory to chemotherapy. When patients with malignancies that are poorly differentiated or metastases that are restricted to lymph nodes are excluded, <20% of patients experience partial tumor regression after treatment with cytotoxic agents (used singly or in combination). Responses are associated with only a minimal (if any) improvement in survival. Median survival is reported to be improved by 4 to 6 months in patients who respond to therapy compared with those who do not, but this form of reporting data is largely discredited. One must be very cautious when reading about chemotherapy results in this heterogeneous group of patients, because differences may be due to patient selection factors.

   The most optimistic reports of response to therapy were with the combination of carboplatin and paclitaxel (with or without etoposide or gemcitabine). Response rates to carboplatin–taxane combinations are 25% to 35%, with median survivals being 6 to 9 months. These combinations appear to yield superior survival (20% at 2 years) in phase II clinical trials when compared with previous regimens that used doxorubicin-based or cisplatin-based combinations.

4. **Recommended treatment.** For most patients with disseminated MUO, particularly those with low performance status, we do not recommend chemotherapy. My recommendations are based on performance status and are as follows for patients who request therapy:

   a. **Patients with good performance status**

      (1) **Adenocarcinoma presenting as a single metastatic lesion.** Most patients who present with a single metastatic lesion manifest other metastatic sites within a relatively short period of time. However, definitive local treatment (surgical excision or RT) sometimes produces long disease-free intervals.

      (2) **Multiple metastatic sites.** An empiric trial of combination chemotherapy with carboplatin and paclitaxel may be considered. Alternative choices include gemcitabine plus either docetaxel or cisplatin, or cisplatin or carboplatin plus irinotecan or etoposide.

     b. Patients with poor performance status. Best supportive care without chemotherapy. If the patient demands treatment, nontoxic drugs or dosages can be offered.

Suggested Reading

Abbruzzese JL, et al. Analysis of a diagnostic strategy for patients with suspected tumors of unknown origin. *J Clin Oncol* 1995;13:2094.

Berry W, et al. Results of a phase II study of weekly paclitaxel plus carboplatin in advanced carcinoma of unknown primary origin: a reasonable regimen for the community-based clinic? *Cancer Invest* 2007;25:27.

Casciato DA. Metastases of unknown origin. In: Haskell CM, ed. *Cancer Treatment.* 5th ed. Philadelphia: WB Saunders; 2001:1556–1578.

Fizazi K, ed. *Carcinoma of an Unknown Primary Site.* New York: Taylor & Francis; 2006.

Giordano TJ, et al. Organ-specific molecular classification of primary lung, colon, and ovarian adenocarcinomas using gene expression profiles. *Am J Pathol* 2001;159:1231.

Greco FA, et al. Taxane-based chemotherapy for patients with carcinoma of unknown primary site. *Cancer J* 2001;7:203.

Greco FA, et al. Gemcitabine, carboplatin, and paclitaxel for patients with carcinoma of unknown primary site: a Minnie Pearl Cancer Research Network study. *J Clin Oncol* 2002;20:1651.

Kemeny MM. Mastectomy: is it necessary for occult breast cancer? *N Y State J Med* 1992; 92:516.

Le Chevalier T, et al. Early metastatic cancer of unknown primary presentation: a clinical study of 302 consecutive autopsied patients. *Arch Intern Med* 1988;148:2035.

Nystrom JS, et al. Identifying the primary site in metastatic cancer of unknown origin. *JAMA* 1979;241:381.

Pavlidis N, et al. Evaluation of six tumor markers in patients with carcinoma of unknown primary. *Med Pediatr Oncol* 1994;22:162.

Hematopoietic Malignancies

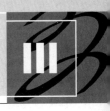

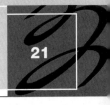

HODGKIN AND NON-HODGKIN LYMPHOMA

21

Lauren C. Pinter-Brown and Dennis A. Casciato

 EVALUATION OF SUSPECTED LYMPHOMA

I. SYMPTOMS AND SIGNS

A. History

1. **Painless lymphadenopathy,** involving any of the superficial lymph nodes, is the most common chief complaint of patients with Hodgkin lymphoma (HL) and non-Hodgkin lymphoma (NHL).

2. **Systemic symptoms.** Fevers, night sweats, and weight loss are characteristic in advanced presentations of HL and aggressive NHL but may be encountered in all stages and pathologic types of lymphoma. Marked fatigue and general weakness may also be reported, not always correlating with the degree of anemia.

   a. **Pruritus,** often intense, may be the presenting symptom in HL, particularly the nodular sclerosis subtype, and may antedate diagnosis by months or years.

   b. **Pel-Ebstein fever** is periodic and uncommon, but characteristic of HL.

3. **Pain**

   a. **Alcohol-induced pain** in areas of involvement is infrequent but is pathognomonic of HL.

   b. **Abdominal pain** or discomfort may be due to splenomegaly, bowel dysfunction due to adenopathy, or hydronephrosis.

   c. **Bone pain** may reflect localized areas of bone destruction or diffuse marrow infiltration.

   d. **Neurogenic pain** is caused by spinal cord compression, plexopathies, nerve root infiltration, meningeal involvement, and complicating varicella zoster.

   e. **Back pain** suggests massive retroperitoneal nodal involvement, often with psoas muscle invasion.

B. Physical examination
should evaluate for hepatosplenomegaly, the presence of effusions, evidence of neuropathy, and signs of obstruction (e.g., extremity edema, superior vena cava syndrome, spinal cord compression, hollow viscera dysfunction). Lymph node chains must be carefully examined, including the submental, supraclavicular, infraclavicular, epitrochlear, iliac, femoral, and popliteal nodes.

1. **The lymph nodes** are examined for size, multiplicity, consistency, and tenderness. Lymphomatous involvement typically imparts a rubbery consistency, not the rock-hard quality of carcinoma.

2. **The tonsils and oropharynx** are thoroughly examined. Waldeyer's ring involvement mandates complete evaluation of the nasopharynx, oropharynx, and hypopharynx by endoscopy.

II. DIFFERENTIAL DIAGNOSIS (Table 21.1) compares clinical features of HL and NHL.

A. Lymphadenopathy

1. **Infections.** Patients, particularly young children with apparent viral or other infections, may develop striking lymphadenopathy. Such patients should be evaluated for infectious processes and observed for clear-cut resolution. Microorganisms associated with prominent lymphadenopathy include Epstein-Barr virus (EBV; infectious mononucleosis), cytomegalovirus (CMV), human immunodeficiency virus (HIV), hepatitis virus, secondary syphilis, mycobacteria, some

TABLE 21.1   Comparison of Hodgkin and Non-Hodgkin Lymphomas

Characteristic	In Hodgkin lymphoma	In non-Hodgkin lymphoma	
		Low-grade	Others
Site of origin	Nodal	Extranodal (∼10%)	Extranodal (∼35%)
Nodal distribution	Centripetal (axial)	Centrifugal	Centrifugal
Nodal spread	Contiguous	Noncontiguous	Noncontiguous
CNS involvement	Rare (<1%)	Rare (<1%)	Uncommon (<10%)
Hepatic involvement	Uncommon	Common (>50%)	Uncommon
Bone marrow involvement	Uncommon (<10%)	Common (>50%)	Uncommon (<20%)
Marrow involvement adversely affects prognosis	Yes	No	Yes
Curable by chemotherapy	Yes	No	Yes

fungi, and *Toxoplasma, Brucella,* and *Rochalimaea* species infection. In some cases, biopsy is required for diagnosis of specific infectious diseases.

2. Systemic immune disorders, such as rheumatoid arthritis, Sjögren syndrome, and systemic lupus erythematosus, are associated with both benign lymphadenopathy and lymphoma. Progressive or asymmetric lymphadenopathy mandate biopsy.

3. Patients at risk for HIV infection present problems requiring individualization in management. Persistent generalized lymphadenopathy is a part of the acquired immunodeficiency syndrome (AIDS) spectrum, but lymphadenopathy can also be caused by opportunistic infections, Kaposi sarcoma, or lymphoma.

4. Lymph nodes that are usually benign
   a. Occipital. Consider scalp infection.
   b. Posterior auricular. Usually viral or scalp infection
   c. Shotty inguinal nodes. Often present with no obvious cause, but may suggest external genital or lower extremity infections.

5. Cervical nodes. Patients with isolated enlargement of high or middle cervical lymph nodes often harbor occult primary carcinoma of the head and neck. The special approach required for these patients is discussed in Chapter 7, section X.

B. Midline masses
   1. Retroperitoneal masses (see Chapter 19, section II)
   2. Mediastinal masses may occur in a variety of nonneoplastic and neoplastic (both primary and metastatic) conditions (see Chapter 19, section I).
   3. Hilar masses. Isolated symmetric bilateral hilar lymphadenopathy (without mediastinal mass) is strongly suggestive of sarcoidosis, and many experts believe that observation alone could suffice in this clinical setting. Unilateral hilar masses are frequently secondary to lung cancer; metastatic disease must also be considered. Coccidioidomycosis and histoplasmosis enter the differential diagnosis in the appropriate clinical and geographic milieu.

C. Splenomegaly. The diagnosis can usually be made with careful history taking and physical examination, laboratory evaluation, CT scans of abdomen, bone marrow biopsy or aspiration with flow cytometric analysis, and, occasionally, liver biopsy. When a diagnosis cannot be established by these means, careful follow-up of the patient is warranted. Splenectomy should be considered for diagnosis in patients with massive or progressive isolated splenomegaly.

   1. Normal. A palpable spleen is occasionally seen in otherwise healthy young adults of thin body habitus.
   2. Infections include most pathogens listed in section II.A.1, bacterial endocarditis, malaria, and abscess.

3. **Secondary to portal hypertension** (congestive splenomegaly). Patients with chronic liver disease or portal or splenic vein thrombosis may have no other findings to direct the diagnostic search. Portal hypertension may be documented by ultrasound of the abdomen with Doppler or by liver–spleen scanning, which reveals redistribution of the radionuclide to the spleen and marrow.

4. **Storage diseases,** particularly Gaucher disease, may produce prominent splenomegaly; characteristic cells are seen in the bone marrow in most cases.

5. **Tumors** are predominantly hematologic, including lymphomas and leukemias. Metastases, particularly from melanoma and breast cancer, and primary splenic sarcomas may also occur.

6. **Myeloproliferative disorders** such as polycythemia vera, agnogenic myeloid metaplasia (myelofibrosis), and chronic myelogenous leukemia may cause marked splenomegaly.

7. **Autoimmune disorders.** Rheumatoid arthritis (Felty syndrome), systemic lupus erythematosus, and autoimmune hemolytic anemia may produce splenomegaly (not isolated autoimmune thrombocytopenia) and can usually be diagnosed by history and associated laboratory findings.

8. **Miscellaneous.** Splenic cysts, thyrotoxicosis, sarcoidosis, chronic nonimmune hemolysis, and amyloidosis are unusual causes of splenomegaly.

III. BIOPSY PROCEDURES

A. **Sites and methods of diagnostic biopsy.** Tissues or organs that are suspected of involvement are subjected to generous open biopsy for primary diagnosis wherever possible. Fine-needle aspiration cytology is mainly used for staging evaluation or for proving recurrence but may sometimes allow cytologic diagnosis *if expertise in interpretation is available.*

1. **Peripheral node biopsy.** One of the largest accessible lymph nodes is excised whenever peripheral lymphadenopathy is present. Small lymph nodes may be more readily removed but may be uninvolved.

2. **Inguinal lymph nodes** are frequently enlarged because of chronic inflammatory processes in the lower extremities. These nodes should be excised only when other sites are not suspect or when pathologic involvement is clearly anticipated.

3. **Bone marrow biopsy** combined with aspiration is used for staging and may lead to diagnosis, particularly in the presence of abnormal circulating cells or cytopenias.

4. **Mediastinoscopy or limited thoracotomy** (e.g., Chamberlain procedure) for definitive diagnosis is required for a substantial proportion of patients with mediastinal masses.

5. **Laparotomy** is used to diagnose some cases of lymphoma restricted to the abdomen and may include biopsies of the liver and random lymph nodes as well as the primary area in question. If HL is suspected, splenectomy may be performed as part of a staging procedure.

6. **Laparoscopy** assesses the liver and peritoneum and allows extensive biopsy, obviating the need for laparotomy in some patients.

7. **Endoscopic gastric biopsy** with staining for *Helicobacter pylori* may be helpful in the diagnosis of gastric MALToma. Repeated attempts with deeper biopsies and immunoperoxidase staining for leukocyte common antigen and keratin intermediate filaments may be helpful in the differential diagnosis between lymphoma and carcinoma. Small bowel involvement beyond the duodenum usually requires open biopsy, although capsule biopsies may be suggestive of lymphoma in some cases.

8. **Retroperitoneal and mesenteric masses** may be evaluated by imaging-guided Trucut biopsy or fine-needle aspiration with immunologic analysis of the specimens, obviating the need for laparotomy.

B. **Handling the biopsy material.** The procured biopsy specimen is submitted to the pathologist directly and *not placed in a fixative* by the operating surgeon to ensure the best use of the available tissue. Prior communication with the pathologist is advantageous. Maintaining frozen sections is preferable for subsequent analysis. Pathology tissue processing includes the following procedures:

1. **Touch preparations** (imprints), which provide cytologic detail and material for immunologic phenotyping

2. **Immunologic phenotyping** with monoclonal antibodies can be crucial to diagnosis. Lymphoid cells are characterized immunologically using flow cytometry. Discriminatory immunophenotypes in lymphoma are shown in Appendix C-5. A common NHL panel should include assessment of expression of CD2 or CD3, CD5, CD19 or CD20, and CD23 in blood, bone marrow, or biopsy specimens. Classic Reed-Sternberg (RS) cells are usually CD15-positive and CD30-positive. More surface markers may need to be analyzed if this screening is inconclusive or if rare entities (such as natural killer [NK] cell or hairy cell leukemia) are considered.

3. **Special handling of tissues** for procedures that may occasionally be used in difficult diagnostic problems or research such as cytogenetics, molecular genetic analysis, and electron microscopy

4. **Microbial culture** of submitted material when the clinical picture or tissue suggests infection

IV. CLINICAL EVALUATION. The extent of the staging evaluation is determined by the individual case presentation, the histopathologic diagnosis, and the effect of the stage on treatment planning.

A. Evaluation of blood tests

1. **Hematologic manifestations** are discussed in Chapter 34.

2. **Diagnostically abnormal circulating lymphoid cells or lymphocytosis** are seen in some patients with either indolent or aggressive forms of NHL. Lymphoid cells are characterized immunologically using flow cytometry, and monoclonality may be established by κ:λ ratios (B cell) or gene rearrangement technology (T and B cell); these techniques are capable of detecting minute clones of circulating lymphoma cells not detectable by inspection of the blood smears.

3. **Acute-phase reactants,** such as the erythrocyte sedimentation rate (ESR), fibrinogen, haptoglobin, and serum copper levels, may parallel disease activity, especially in HL.

4. **Liver function tests** are unreliable in predicting lymphomatous involvement of the liver. Marked elevation of alkaline phosphatase and occasionally frank cholestatic jaundice may complicate HL as a paraneoplastic event without direct liver involvement. Extrahepatic biliary obstruction may also occur with lymphoma caused by enlarged nodes in the porta hepatis.

5. **Renal function tests.** Elevated creatinine and blood urea nitrogen levels suggest ureteral obstruction and, less commonly, direct renal involvement. Uric acid nephropathy or hypercalcemia may contribute to renal insufficiency. Frank nephrotic syndrome as a paraneoplastic phenomenon may complicate HL and other lymphomas (see Chapter 31).

6. **Serum uric acid.** Hyperuricemia is a common manifestation of high-turnover-rate (aggressive) NHL and may also be seen with extensive lower grade lymphomas. Treatment of high-grade NHL or treatment of sensitive bulky low-grade lymphoma may provoke brisk tumor lysis, leading to further elevation of uric acid and renal shutdown (see Chapter 27, section XIII). Hypouricemia may be seen in HL.

7. **Hypercalcemia** has been noted in some cases of lymphoma and may be secondary to production of parathyroid hormone-related peptide, or activation of vitamin D by lymphoma tissue.

8. **Serum lactate dehydrogenase (LDH)** levels reflect tumor bulk and turnover, particularly in the aggressive NHL, and are considered an independent prognostic factor.

9. **Serum immunoglobulins.** Polyclonal hypergammaglobulinemia is commonly seen in HL and NHL. Hypogammaglobulinemia is particularly common in the

small lymphocytic lymphomas and late in the disease. Monoclonal spikes are seen occasionally in NHL patients.

B. Evaluation of the chest

1. **Chest radiographs** may demonstrate mediastinal and hilar lymphadenopathy, pleural effusions, and parenchymal lesions. A cavitating lesion is more typical of infection than lymphomas.

2. **CT scans** tend to replace chest x-rays because they can demonstrate parenchymal and mediastinal abnormalities in more detail.

3. **Thoracentesis and pleural biopsy** may demonstrate direct lymphomatous involvement of the pleura. Obstruction of mediastinal lymphatic–venous drainage may result in cytologically negative or chylous effusions.

C. Evaluation of the abdomen and retroperitoneum

1. **CT scans** are useful in delineating abnormal enlargement of nodes in retroperitoneal, mesenteric, portal, and other lymph node sites. The CT scan also detects splenomegaly and, with constant enhancement, may define space-occupying lesions in the liver, spleen, and kidneys.

2. **Bipedal lymphangiography** has been abandoned because of improvements and availability of alternative imaging techniques and because expertise in performance and evaluation is frequently unavailable.

3. **Abdominal ultrasonography** is too insensitive to be useful in routinely assessing abdominal lymphadenopathy. It is occasionally helpful in distinguishing hepatic or splenic lesions (cystic vs. solid) and in excluding an obstructive basis for renal insufficiency and jaundice.

D. Evaluation of the gastrointestinal (GI) tract. Direct involvement of the GI tract is uncommon in HL but is common in NHL. Patients with Waldeyer's ring lymphoma, suggestive GI symptoms, extensive abdominal nodal involvement, unexplained iron deficiency, or GI bleeding are evaluated with upper GI series and complete small bowel follow-through. Barium enema may be necessary. Endoscopic examination and biopsy of accessible abnormalities are performed. Routine GI tract evaluation for patients with mantle cell lymphoma is performed in some centers.

E. Evaluation of the central nervous system (CNS). Spinal fluid examination is routinely used to exclude occult lymphomatous involvement of the meninges in patients with Burkitt lymphoma (BL) or lymphoblastic lymphoma and is often performed in patients with intermediate-grade or high-grade lymphoma involving testes, paranasal sinuses (B-cell histology), or with extensive bone marrow involvement. In these cases, the incidence of CNS disease is in the 5% range. Patients with AIDS-related lymphoma may require CT or MRI scans of the brain and spinal fluid analysis. Symptoms suggestive of intracranial, spinal cord, or peripheral nerve involvement require immediate diagnostic evaluation.

F. Nuclear scans

1. **Positron emission tomography (PET)** using ^{18}F-fluorodeoxyglucose scans tends to replace gallium scans. It seems to be more sensitive in detecting unsuspected metastasis or in differentiating active versus uninvolved nodes with accuracy approaching 95% depending on nodal histology. Similar to gallium scans, PET is somewhat less reliable in indolent lymphoma. False-positive results can be produced by any inflammation, whereas faint normal uptake of muscles, the bowel, and bone marrow recovering from chemotherapy should be differentiated from involvement. The advent of combined PET/CT scan is thought to increase the accuracy of the procedure and may eventually become the gold standard for staging and following patients.

2. **Gallium scans.** [67]Ga scans are primarily used in assessing residual radiographic mediastinal and, less often, retroperitoneal abnormalities after therapy. Persistent ^{67}Ga uptake in these areas strongly suggests residual tumor instead of fibrosis or necrosis. To be useful in such follow-up, a ^{67}Ga body scan is recommended before therapy. [67]Ga scans can be unreliable below the diaphragm because of competing uptake in the GI tract, liver, and spleen.

HODGKIN LYMPHOMA

I. EPIDEMIOLOGY AND ETIOLOGY

A. Incidence. HL accounts for about 1% of new cancer cases annually in the United States, or 7,000 cases per year.

1. Age. HL demonstrates a bimodal age–incidence curve in the United States and some industrialized European nations. The first peak, constituting predominantly the nodular sclerosis subtype, occurs in the 20s and the second peak occurs after 50 years of age. In third-world countries, the first peak is absent, but there is a significant incidence of mixed cellularity and lymphocyte-depleted HL in men.

2. Sex. About 85% of children with HL are boys. In adults, the nodular sclerosing subtype of HL shows a slight female predominance, whereas the other histologic subtypes are more common in men.

B. Risk factors. In Western countries, the first peak of HL is associated with a higher social class, advanced education, and small family size; a delayed exposure to a common infectious or other environmental agent has been suggested. HL may be associated with EBV infection, but the significance of this association is unclear. A slightly increased incidence of HL has been demonstrated with HIV infection; HIV-associated HL (see Chapter 36, section III) often presents with constitutional symptoms, advanced stage, and unusual sites of involvement (e.g., marrow, skin, leptomeninges).

II. PATHOLOGY AND NATURAL HISTORY

A. Histology. The pathologic diagnosis of HL depends on the presence of RS cells and their variants in *an appropriate pathologic milieu*. The bulk of lymphatic tissue involved by HL is not composed of neoplastic cells but rather a variety of normal-appearing lymphocytes, plasma cells, eosinophils, neutrophils, and histiocytes existing in different proportions in the various histologic subtypes. Important variants of RS cells include L&H (lymphocyte and histiocyte) cells, lacunar cells, and RS-like cells. (See Appendix C-5. Discriminatory Immunophenotypes for Lymphocytic Neoplasms).

1. The Rye classification for HL relates the histopathologic subtypes to clinical behavior and prognosis. This older classification system comprises lymphocyte-predominant (LP), nodular sclerosing (NS), mixed-cellularity (MC), and the uncommon lymphocyte-depleted (LD) varieties of HL. The LP subtype was further divided into nodular LP and diffuse LP subtypes. Immunohistochemistry, however, has resulted in deletion of the diffuse LP subtype and redefinition of the nodular LP subtype (see section II.A.2).

2. The World Health Organization (WHO) classification divides HL into *nodular LP HL* and *classical HL*. Classical HL in this newer classification system comprises the lymphocyte-rich, NS, MC, and LD varieties.

a. Nodular LP HL with its L&H cells, which are not classical RS cells, is now clearly recognized to be most like an indolent B-cell NHL and not true HL. For that reason, nodular LP HL is distinguished from classical HL in the new WHO classification. Table 21.2 shows this classification system with distinguishing histopathologic features, clinical correlates, and immunophenotypes.

b. Diffuse LP HL in the Rye classification has disappeared as an entity. In the new WHO classification of lymphocytic neoplasms (see Appendix C-6.I.), what was thought to be diffuse LP HL is now classified as lymphocyte-rich classical HL (with true RS cells that are CD30-positive), Laennert lymphoma (lymphoepithelioid peripheral T-cell lymphoma), T-cell–rich B-cell lymphoma, or other entities.

3. RS cells and their variants

a. RS cells are giant cells that have more than one nucleus and large, eosinophilic, inclusion-like nuclei. Single-cell polymerase chain reaction analysis has shown that the RS cells are B cells that originate in the germinal centers of lymph nodes. RS cells and the accompanying mononuclear *Hodgkin cells*

Histologic subtype	Frequency (%)	Histopathology	Clinical characteristics	Common stages
Nodular lymphocyte predominant HL[b]	5	L&H ("popcorn cells") intermingled with polymorphous infiltrate; nodular or nodular and diffuse patterns	Males; usually localized to peripheral nodes; frequent relapses; excellent prognosis	I–IIA
Lymphocyte-rich CHL[c]	5	RS scattered in background of small lymphocytes; nodular and diffuse patterns; absent eosinophils and neutrophils	Older males; localized to peripheral nodes; fewer relapses; excellent prognosis	I–IIA
Nodular-sclerosing CHL[c]	70	RS variable; nodular growth pattern with collagen bands and "lacunar cells"; heterogeneous cellularity with numerous eosinophils and neutrophils	Females; mediastinal masses and peripheral nodes	I–IIIA or B
Mixed-cellularity CHL[c]	20–25	RS more frequent in a mixed inflammatory background without nodular sclerosing fibrosis	Frequently retroperitoneal; often symptomatic	II–IVA or B
Lymphocyte-depleted CHL[c]	<5	RS predominant in variable patterns, including diffuse fibrosis; depleted of nonneoplastic lymphocytes	Aggressive course; liver and marrow involved with relative sparing of peripheral nodes	III–IVB

HL, Hodgkin lymphoma; L&H, lymphocytic and histiocytic cells; CHL, classical HL; RS, Reed-Sternberg cells; EMA, epithelial membrane antigen; ALK-1, anaplastic lymphoma kinase.
[a]World Health Organization classification system.
[b]L&H cells immunophenotype: CD15$^-$, CD30$^-$, CD20$^+$, CD45$^+$, EMA$^\pm$, CD79a$^+$.
[c]Classical HL—RS immunophenotype: CD15$^+$, CD30$^+$, CD20$^\pm$, CD45$^-$, EMA$^-$, ALK-1$^-$.

variants are the neoplastic cells in HL and are surrounded by a reactive cellular infiltrate. Classic RS cells usually express CD15 and CD30. CD30 (Ki-1) is an antigen that is also expressed in anaplastic large cell lymphoma and occasionally in other forms of NHL (e.g., large B-cell lymphoma [LBCL]). RS cells express CD20 infrequently, but not CD 45 (leukocyte common antigen).

   b. The lacunar cell is a variant of the RS cell and has the *same immunophenotype*. It characterizes NS HL and is often far more plentiful than classic RS cells in that subtype.

   c. L&H cells are RS-like but have a *different immunophenotype*. L&H cells manifest B-cell markers (CD20, CD45, and CD79a), but not CD15 or CD30. Although the L&H cells are believed to be of monoclonal origin, the surrounding B-cell infiltrates may be polyclonal. L&H cells were identified in nodular LP HL, which is now considered a separate entity because of its distinct immunophenotype.

   d. RS-like cells are found in a variety of infectious, inflammatory, and neoplastic disorders, including infectious mononucleosis, lymphoid hyperplasia associated with phenytoin therapy, and immunoblastic lymphomas.

B. Mode of spread (see Table 21.1). HL almost always originates in a lymph node. Whenever a primary diagnosis of HL is made in an extranodal site without contiguous nodal involvement, the diagnosis should be highly suspect. For much of its natural history, HL appears to spread in an orderly fashion through the lymphatic system by contiguity. Histologic types other than NS, however, often skip the mediastinum, and disease appears in the neck and upper abdomen. The axial lymphatic system is almost always affected in HL, whereas distal sites (e.g., epitrochlear and popliteal nodes) are rarely involved. Hematogenous dissemination occurs late in the course of disease and is characteristic of the LD subtype.

C. Sites of involvement
   1. Peripheral lymph nodes. Cervical or supraclavicular lymphadenopathy occurs in >70% of cases. Axillary and inguinal lymph nodes are less frequently involved. Generalized lymphadenopathy is atypical of HL. Left supraclavicular lymphadenopathy is more strongly associated with abdominal involvement (specifically, splenic involvement) than is right-sided disease.

   2. Thorax
      a. The anterior mediastinum is a prime location for NS HL. Mediastinal precedes hilar lymph node involvement.

      b. Lung involvement may occur by direct contiguity with hilar involvement in HL as well as by hematogenous dissemination. Pulmonary involvement by HL may produce discrete nodules and irregular, interstitial, or even lobar infiltrates.

      c. Pleural effusion may occur secondary to mediastinal compression of vascular–lymphatic drainage and by direct pleural involvement. Chylous effusions occasionally occur.

      d. Pericardial involvement may be found on CT scans, but overt cardiac tamponade is uncommon.

      e. Superior vena cava syndrome is more frequent in NHL than in HL.

   3. Spleen, liver, and upper abdomen
      a. The spleen, splenic hilar nodes, and celiac nodes are the earliest abdominal sites of involvement in infradiaphragmatic HL. Mesenteric lymph nodes are rarely involved in HL.

      b. At least 25% of spleens not clinically enlarged harbor occult HL at laparotomy, and as many as half of spleens believed to be enlarged on physical examination or radiologic assessment are histologically normal.

      c. Liver involvement is uncommon at diagnosis and is almost always associated with infiltration of the spleen.

   4. Retroperitoneal lymph node involvement tends to occur relatively late in the course of supradiaphragmatic HL and after spleen, splenic hilar, and celiac nodal involvement. Periaortic involvement without splenic involvement is uncommon.

The retroperitoneal nodes are, however, affected early in the course of inguinal presentations of HL.

5. **The bone marrow** is rarely involved at the time of diagnosis of HL. Patients with advanced-stage disease, systemic symptoms, and MC or LD histologies have a higher risk for bone marrow involvement. Biopsy is mandatory to evaluate the bone marrow because HL is difficult to diagnose on marrow aspirates.

6. **Bone.** Osseous involvement of HL usually produces an osteoblastic reaction mimicking prostatic carcinoma. Extradural masses may result in spinal cord compression. Sternal erosion by mediastinal NS HL may occur.

7. **Other extranodal sites** are rarely involved in HL. Liver or skin involvement is rare and usually a late manifestation of disease. CNS involvement is very uncommon with the exception of extrinsic spinal cord compression. Clinical involvement of meninges, brain, Waldeyer's ring, GI tract, kidney, and other extranodal sites usually suggests an alternative diagnosis.

III. STAGING SYSTEM AND PROGNOSTIC FACTORS

A. **Staging** is the most crucial determinant of prognosis and treatment in HL. The *Ann Arbor Staging System* had previously been universally used but has been modified to take into account important prognostic factors, particularly mediastinal bulk. The modified system is called the *Cotswolds Staging Classification* and is shown in Table 21.3.

B. **Prognostic factors**

1. **Stage** is clearly the single most important prognostic factor in HL. Within each stage, the presence of B symptoms confers a poorer prognosis. About 60% of patients with HL in the United States have stage I or II disease at the time of diagnosis. The percentage of patients with stage III or IV disease is generally higher in third-world countries and in lower socioeconomic enclaves.

TABLE 21.3   **Cotswolds Staging Classification of Hodgkin Lymphoma**

Stage	Description
I	Involvement of a single lymph node region or lymphoid structure
II	Involvement of two or more lymph node regions on the same side of the diaphragm (the mediastinum is considered as a single site, whereas hilar lymph nodes are lateralized). The number of anatomic sites should be indicated by a subscript (e.g., II_3)D.
III	Involvement of lymph node regions or structures on both sides of the diaphragm
	III_1 With involvement of splenic hilar, celiac, or portal nodes
	III_2 With involvement of para-aortic, iliac, and mesenteric nodes
IV	Involvement of one or more extranodal sites in addition to a site for which the designation "E" has been used

Designations applicable to any disease stage

A	No symptoms
B	Fever (temperature higher than 38°C), drenching night sweats, or unexplained loss of >10% of body weight within the preceding 6 months
X	Bulky disease (a mediastinal mass exceeding one-third the maximum transverse diameter of the chest or the presence of a nodal mass with a maximal dimension >10 cm)
E	Involvement of a single extranodal site that is contiguous or proximal to a known nodal site
CS	Clinical stage
PS	Pathologic state (as determined by laparotomy or biopsy)

2. **Histopathology.** With advances in therapy, the value of histopathologic subtype as an independent prognostic variable (apart from stage) is less clearly defined than it was in the past.
3. **Adverse prognostic factors** were evaluated by an international group in a multivariate retrospective analysis of 4,695 patients, mostly with extensive disease (see Hasenclever, et al. in "Suggested Reading"). Patients with no adverse factors had an 84% freedom from progression, whereas the presence of *each factor* depressed the freedom from progression curve plateau by about 8%. Interestingly, neither tumor bulk nor histology emerged as independent factors. The seven independent prognostic factors identified were as follows:

Adverse factor	Relative risk of relapse
Male sex	1.35
Age ≥45 years	1.39
Stage IV disease	1.26
Hemoglobin <10.5 g/dL	1.35
White blood cell (WBC) count >15,000/μL	1.41
Lymphocyte count <600/μL or <8% of WBC	1.38
Serum albumin <4 g/dL	1.49

4. **Independent adverse prognostic factors for NS HL** include eosinophilia, lymphocyte depletion, and RS cell atypia.
5. **Adverse prognostic factors in early stage HL** include ESR ≥50 mm/hour, four or more separate sites of nodal involvement, bulky mediastinal mass (defined as >33% of the maximum intrathoracic diameter) or any mass ≥10 cm, or extranodal sites of disease.

IV. DIAGNOSIS

A. **Clinical evaluation.** See "Evaluation of Suspected Lymphoma," sections I through IV.
B. **Staging evaluation**
1. Adequate surgical biopsy reviewed by experienced hematopathologist. Fine-needle aspiration is not an adequate means of initial diagnosis.
2. Thorough history and physical examination
3. Laboratory tests: CBC with differential and platelet count, serum chemistries including LDH, ESR, urinalysis
4. CT scan of the neck, chest, abdomen, and pelvis with contrast
5. Bone marrow aspiration and biopsy (bilateral iliac crest) unless clinical stage IA to IIA with no anemia or other blood count depression
6. Bone scan in presence of bone pain, or elevated serum alkaline phosphatase or calcium level
7. PET scans are optional but are useful in follow-up of residual masses on chest radiograph or CT scan after therapy, given the propensity of treated HL nodes to remain visible on CT scans.
8. HIV testing should be considered in patients whose disease presentation is primarily extranodal.
9. Pregnancy test and fertility counseling in patients of childbearing age should be performed with staging evaluation.
C. **Staging laparotomy.** Systematic evaluation by staging laparotomy revealed that at least 25% of patients with supradiaphragmatic presentations and negative clinical subdiaphragmatic evaluations had occult HL discovered at laparotomy (predominantly in the spleen, splenic hilar nodes, or celiac lymph nodes). Liver involvement was extremely uncommon in the absence of extensive splenic involvement.

The main purpose of staging laparotomy and splenectomy was to save patients with truly supradiaphragmatic or stage III$_1$A disease from the long-term complications of alkylator-based chemotherapy (MOPP regimen in Appendix D-1 and equivalents). Patients with a negative laparotomy or limited upper abdominal disease would be treated with radiation alone. The advent of improved diagnostic modalities, less toxic curative chemotherapy (ABVD regimen in Appendix D-1 and equivalents), and the success of combined-modality approaches have eliminated the need for surgical staging.

V. MANAGEMENT: PRIMARY THERAPY

- **A. Treatment philosophy.** More than one treatment approach may be used in the management of cases of HL. The challenge is to determine a course of therapy that preserves cure while minimizing long-term complications.
- **B. Surgery** is limited to diagnosis, possibly laparotomy, and laminectomy for spinal cord compression.
- **C. RT alone** is still used in the United States to treat many patients with stage IA or possibly IIA disease nonclassical HL. However, it is increasingly replaced in the treatment of classical HL with combined-modality treatment.
  - **1. Radiation dose.** HL may be locally sterilized in almost all cases with 3,000 to 4,400 cGy given at a rate of about 1,000 cGy per week. Lesser doses may be adequate as consolidation after chemotherapy.
  - **2. Radiation fields** (Fig. 21.1)
    - **a. Mantle field** encompasses the cervical, supraclavicular, infraclavicular, axillary, hilar, and mediastinal lymph nodes to the level of the diaphragm. Preauricular fields are added for patients with high cervical lymphadenopathy. The lungs and much of the heart are shielded by lead blocks, although many radiotherapists administer some radiation ($\leq$1,500 cGy) to the lung on the involved side, if hilar lymph nodes are enlarged. The whole heart may be treated if the pericardium is involved. A small gap must be left between the inferior border of the mantle field and the superior border of the periaortic field to obviate potential severe spinal cord injury caused by overlap.
    - **b. Inverted-Y field** includes the spleen or splenic pedicle and the celiac, periaortic, iliac, inguinal, and femoral lymph nodes. The kidneys, much of the pelvic marrow, and the testes are shielded.

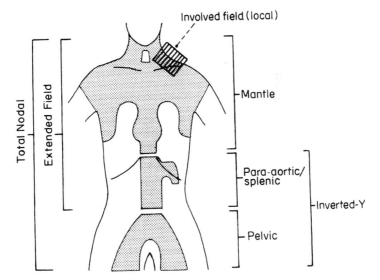

Figure 21.1. Radiation fields used in Hodgkin lymphoma. Stippled area is the area irradiated. See text for descriptions.

    c. Spade and pelvic fields. The inverted-Y field may be divided into a *spade field,* encompassing the splenic pedicle (or spleen) and periaortic nodes, and a *pelvic field,* including the iliac, inguinal, and femoral lymph nodes.

    d. Subtotal nodal or subtotal lymphoid irradiation consists of mantle and spade fields.

    e. Total nodal or total lymphoid irradiation is uncommonly used and consists of mantle and inverted-Y fields.

    f. Involved-field radiation therapy (IFRT) consists of sites of known disease only and is used with curative intent only in combination with chemotherapy. It has become the most common use of RT in HL with other fields previously described of mostly historical interest. Doses given in combined-modality therapy range from 2,000 to 3,600 cGy.

D. Combination chemotherapy is the mainstay modality for all stages of classical HL and advanced stages of nonclassical HL. Chemotherapy, often in combination with RT, is also preferable for patients with early-stage disease and/or bulky disease. The selection among the available regimens is often guided by the desire to avoid long-term toxicities associated with specific treatments. The advent of the nonleukemogenic, gonadal-sparing ABVD chemotherapy regimen expanded the use of chemotherapy to patients with earlier stages and obviated the need for laparotomy; it has replaced the historic MOPP. More aggressive regimens such as BEACOPP (Appendix D-1, section II) may improve on ABVD (see section V.D.3), especially in patients with advanced disease. Maintenance therapy is not recommended.

    1. Useful chemotherapy regimens for HL are shown in Appendix D-1. These regimens must be strictly followed because delays in therapy or reduction in dosages not indicated by the protocol can clearly compromise results. The total dose and dose rate (dose intensity) are important in achieving cure. Regimens used as salvage therapy in HL are shown in Appendix D-3.

    2. MOPP or COPP regimen (Appendix D-1, section I). The National Cancer Institute (NCI) recommends that vincristine should not be limited to a 2-mg maximum dosage in this regimen, but most clinicians sustain the 2-mg limit. Treatment is administered in 28-day cycles for two additional cycles beyond the attainment of a restaged complete response (CR) and a minimum of six cycles (6 months).

        a. The CR rate using the MOPP regimen is between 70% and 80% for stages III and IV HL. About 60% to 70% of CR cases are durable, with relapses rare after 42 months. More than 80% of patients with stage IIIA or IVA disease survive 10 years without recurrence of disease. Histologic subtype appears to have little effect on results with MOPP.

        b. The MOPP regimen is particularly emetogenic, and it is associated with myelosuppression neuropathy, leukemogenesis, and infertility. It is believed that COPP (replacing mechlorethamine with cyclophosphamide) may be better tolerated.

    3. ABVD regimen (Appendix D-1, section I) is superior to the MOPP regimen and causes much less leukemia and infertility. Potential cardiac toxicity caused by doxorubicin and pulmonary toxicity caused by bleomycin (particulary with the concomitant use of granulocyte growth factors) have been occasional problems using this schedule. The concern is heightened when combined with mediastinal RT. ABVD-based treatment has replaced MOPP as the standard regimen for HL.

        a. Generally, the same therapeutic rules as with the MOPP regimen apply: 6 to 8 monthly cycles are usually administered, and at least two cycles beyond maximum response.

        b. Pulmonary function should be monitored. If dyspnea, pneumonitis, or significant reduction to <40% of predicted lung diffusion capacity is noted, bleomycin should be discontinued. Bleomycin pneumonitis usually responds to corticosteroids and mandates discontinuation of bleomycin.

        c. Cardiac function should be monitored in patients with pre-existing heart disease and in those receiving high cumulative doses of doxorubicin. A baseline measurement of left ventricular ejection fraction is suggested before beginning doxorubicin administration.

4. **MOPP and ABVD in alternating cycles and the MOPP/ABV hybrid** have both been found to be less satisfactory than ABVD alone. While MOPP/ABV and ABVD were equally efficacious, the hybrid regimen was associated with increased acute toxicity, myelodysplastic syndrome, and leukemia in a randomized trial. While MOPP/ABVD and ABVD were both superior regimens to MOPP alone, ABVD was less myelotoxic than the combined regimen.

5. **Dose-intense regimens** have been developed with the hope of improving outcome, especially in patients with high-risk HL. The value of these regimens remains unclear.

   a. **BEACOPP.** This 3-week cycle regimen has been compared favorably to COPP–ABVD in randomized prospective and mature studies. Higher response rates are reported with dose escalation and mandatory use of growth factors, possibly with a higher risk for secondary leukemia. The effect on sterility is not fully evaluated.

   b. **Stanford-V** (Appendix D-1, section II). Excellent results achieved with this weekly regimen in phase II studies have not yet been confirmed in randomized studies.

   c. **High-dose chemotherapy** followed by autologous stem cell transplantation (SCT) for patients in first remission has been proposed but not satisfactorily tested.

6. **Compared effectiveness**

   a. A large, randomized trial conducted by a cooperative group showed that ABVD alone may be as effective as MOPP plus ABVD and more effective than MOPP alone in the management of most patients with advanced HL. ABVD is considered the standard first-line treatment for most patients and is superior to MOPP in efficacy and toxicity profile.

   b. A three-arm randomized clinical study compared COPP–ABVD with standard-dose BEACOPP and escalated-dose BEACOPP (see Diehl, et al., 2003, in "Suggested Reading"). The 5-year relapse-free rates were 69% for COPP–ABVD, 76% for standard BEACOPP, and 87% for escalated BEA-COPP. The 5-year survival rate was 83% for the COPP–ABVD arm, 88% for the standard-dose BEACOPP arm, and 91% for the escalated-dose BEACOPP arm. Patients with advanced HL and adverse prognostic factors appear to derive benefit from dose escalation. BEACOPP in one of its forms can clearly be considered the treatment of choice for selected patients with high-risk HL.

7. **Combined-modality treatment** is becoming popular in the management of early-stage disease. The advantage of this approach is the limitation of radiation to the involved area only (and thus the reduction of the total dose), reducing long-term radiation-related complications.

   a. IFRT can complement an abbreviated course of chemotherapy in patients with clinical stage I or II and nonbulky disease.

   b. IFRT may be prescribed after a full course of chemotherapy to consolidate previously bulky areas of disease that respond only partially to chemotherapy. IFRT to prior sites of disease, however, may not be helpful for patients who achieve a CR with chemotherapy.

E. **Treatment controversies and recommendations in classical HL** (Table 21.4)

   1. **Stages IA and IIA**

      a. **Supradiaphragmatic disease.** Traditionally, most patients used to undergo staging laparotomy and, if found to have pathologic stage I or II disease, would receive subtotal nodal irradiation. This approach resulted in an 80% probability of disease-free survival. Overall survival, on the other hand, may not be affected because most patients who relapse after RT can be salvaged by chemotherapy.

      Excellent disease-free survival, however, has been documented after treatment with an abbreviated course of chemotherapy (two to four cycles) followed by IFRT. ABVD regimen or the Stanford V regimen (Appendix D-1, sections I and II) is often used. In a randomized study using four cycles of ABVD, there was no difference in outcome between groups irradiated

TABLE 21.4	Hodgkin Lymphoma: Recommended Treatment According to Clinical Presentation

Presentation	Recommended treatment
Early stages	
Classical HL IA–IIA	ABVD × 4 cycles with IFRT or Stanford V for 2 cycles with IFRT
NLP HL IA-IIA	IFRT alone; observation (if patient cannot tolerate RT); chemotherapy followed by IFRT can be used in CS IIA
IB, IIB	Full-course chemotherapy
Advanced stages	
Bulky disease stage I–II	ABVD × 6 cycles or Stanford V for 3 cycles with RT to bulky site
Clinical stage III–IV and/or presence of B symptoms	ABVD × 6–8 cycles (or Stanford V or BEACOPP)

HL, Hodgkin lymphoma; IFRT, involved field radiation therapy; NLP, nodular lymphocyte-predominant; RT, radiation therapy; CS, clinical stage.

with 2,000 or 4,000 cGy, suggesting that the dose of radiation can also be reduced.

b. Infradiaphragmatic disease. Generally, similar principles apply for early disease. Most patients could be treated with a combined-modality approach or full course combination chemotherapy.

c. Current studies intend to assess the minimum number of cycles of a first-line regimen, such as ABVD, that can be given without compromising outcome. Less aggressive chemotherapy may suffice for patients with no risk factors, such as anemia, elevation of ESR, or bulky disease.

2. **Stages IB and IIB** management is somewhat controversial. Early-stage B disease has a nearly 50% relapse rate when treated with radiation monotherapy. It is preferable to treat such patients with a full course of chemotherapy, although a combined-modality approach may be considered.

3. **Bulky mediastinal presentations.** About 60% of patients with stage IA to IIB disease and bulky mediastinal masses fail treatment with RT alone; relapses occur predominantly in the mediastinum and lungs. Full-course combination chemotherapy and IFRT are recommended for these patients. Patients with bulky mediastinal disease and more advanced stages (IIIA to IVB) may also receive mediastinal RT at the end of chemotherapy. Using both modalities, results approaching the cure rate for patients without large mediastinal masses may be attained.

4. **Stage IIIA.** The 10-year disease-free survival rate using chemotherapy alone is 80%. Such results are superior to RT alone and probably cannot be improved by combined-modality therapy.

5. **Stage IIIB or IV.** The ABVD regimen is probably adequate management for most patients, although medically fit patients with adverse features may benefit from BEACOPP. Results of randomized studies to assess the efficacy of Stanford V regimen are awaited.

6. **E (extranodal) presentations.** Patients with contiguous limited extranodal disease (such as a single bone involved adjacent to an involved lymph node) can sometimes be managed by radiation alone or more frequently in combination with chemotherapy. Multiple E lesions and extensive E disease (such as a large pulmonary lesion) are best managed with chemotherapy or a combined approach.

7. **HIV and HL.** Patients with HIV usually present with stage IV disease involving the bone marrow. The desired intensity of the treatment should be weighed against the patient's tolerance. Full-course chemotherapy should be tried with

curative intent in patients with good performance status and controlled viremia (see Chapter 36, section III).

VI. MANAGEMENT AFTER PRIMARY THERAPY

A. Restaging. All CRs resulting from either irradiation or chemotherapy must be verified by a restaging evaluation that consists of the repetition of all examinations that were initially abnormal.

1. The initial restaging occurs 2 to 3 months after completion of radiation and traditionally after three or four cycles of chemotherapy, provided that all palpable and radiographic disease has disappeared.

2. Restaging mandates repeat biopsy of previously involved and accessible stage IV sites, such as liver or bone marrow.

3. Persistent and stable abnormalities on chest radiograph or CT scan in the mediastinum are not uncommon (particularly in patients treated for NS). Occasionally, persistent stable abdominal masses or palpable nodal masses may also occur. These abnormalities demand close follow-up. In most cases, however, these findings represent only fibrosis and do not require biopsy. PET scanning is useful in distinguishing viable HL from fibrosis.

B. Follow-up. Most relapses after therapy occur within the first 2 to 5 years, although later recurrences have been observed.

1. Follow-up should occur every 2 to 4 months the first 2 years, every 3 to 6 months for the next 3 to 5 years. Follow-up examinations include:

  a. History and physical examination

  b. CBC, chemistry panel, ESR, chest radiographs

  c. CT scans every 3 to 6 months for the first 3 years

  d. Thyroxine and thyroid-stimulating hormone (TSH) levels at least annually (see section VII.A.1) if radiation to the neck has been administered.

2. Health maintenance counseling and cancer screening are imperative for long-term survivors of HL. Smoking cessation and avoidance of additional practices associated with increased risk for cancer should be encouraged. If irradiation above the diaphragm was administered, women should be encouraged to start annual mammograms 5 to 8 years after treatment, or earlier if 40 years of age (whichever comes first). Some groups have suggested the addition of breast MRI for screening in this high-risk population.

3. PET scanning is not recommended for surveillance due to the high false-positive rate. Any management decisions should not be based on PET scanning alone but require clinical or pathologic correlation.

C. Salvage therapies

1. RT failures are generally treated with combination chemotherapy with results at least as successful as with *de novo* chemotherapy.

2. Chemotherapy failures

  a. Failure to achieve a CR with effective combination chemotherapy is associated with a poor prognosis. Although alternate combinations may be temporarily useful, long-term disease control is unlikely. Such patients should be referred for autologous stem cell transplant (ASCT) or less likely for allogeneic bone marrow transplantation (BMT). The decision depends on the age of the patient, the availability of a donor, bone marrow status, and responsiveness to a salvage chemotherapy regimen.

  b. Relapses after chemotherapy-achieved CR. The initial combination can be used again (provided there is no cardiotoxicity risk) if the unmaintained CR lasts >1 year, but it should not be used again if the CR lasts <1 year. No known available regimen is capable of producing long-term disease-free survival in >10% to 20% of chemotherapy relapsed cases. Patients who respond to salvage chemotherapy should be referred for consideration of ASCT.

  c. Patients who are resistant to MOPP and ABVD may experience brief (although occasionally long) responses to alternate chemotherapy. Single-agent therapy with a nitrosourea, vinca alkaloid, etoposide (possibly the oral form), or combinations of these and other agents may be helpful. Gemcitabine is emerging as an active agent, particularly in combination with vinorelbine or platinum. Second-line and third-line combination chemotherapy regimens are shown in Appendix D-3. Chemotherapy failures with predominantly nodal relapses may benefit from extended-field irradiation, which results in some long-term disease-free survival. Allogeneic BMT can be considered for young patients. Experimental trials would also be appropriate to consider for the treatment of this patient population.

3. **Intensive chemoradiotherapy with ASCT** has undergone extensive study. High doses of chemotherapy (potentially myeloablative), often combined with total-body irradiation, are administered ("conditioning regimen"), and either autologous bone marrow or peripheral stem cells (mobilized by growth factors) are used to rescue the patient from prolonged myelosuppression. This procedure is performed in most centers with a mortality rate of <5%; the hospital stay averages 3 weeks. Candidates include patients who have either relapsed after a CR or never achieved a CR with adequate combination chemotherapy. About 60% of chemosensitive candidates and 40% of patients failing induction chemotherapy achieve prolonged disease-free survival.

4. **Other therapies.** Immunoconjugates, such as anti-CD30 immunotoxins, and radioimmunotherapy have been tested in patients with HL in phase I studies, with inconclusive results so far. Rituximab is being used for nodular LP HL.

VII. SPECIAL CLINICAL PROBLEMS IN HL

A. Sequelae and complications of therapy

1. **Hypothyroidism.** Overt hypothyroidism can be expected in 10% to 20% of patients and elevation of serum TSH in up to 50% of patients treated with mantle-field RT or neck irradiation. Replacement therapy corrects the problem.

2. **Sterility.** RT poses problems for female patients who receive pelvic irradiation without oophoropexy and appropriate gonadal shielding. The testes are shielded during irradiation. MOPP and similar therapies produce near-universal sterility in male patients and can be anticipated to produce sterility in women in their late 20s or older. ABVD is not associated with sterility. BEACOPP is expected to cause sterility in many patients, although the incidence is unknown. Sperm banking is encouraged in male patients about to receive MOPP, BEACOPP, ASCT, or similar therapies.

3. **Lung damage**

   a. **Radiation pneumonitis.** Mantle-field irradiation routinely produces a paramediastinal fibrosis that is usually not clinically significant. When large ports are necessitated by large mediastinal-hilar masses, the potential for more severe reaction exists. In addition, patients given MOPP who have a prior history of mantle-field irradiation may experience an abrupt episode of pneumonitis, presumably secondary to steroid withdrawal. Therefore, prednisone is avoided after mantle-field irradiation, even if the radiation was administered years earlier.

   b. **Bleomycin pulmonary toxicity.** Almost all patients treated with bleomycin (in ABVD and the like) experience a reduction in their lung diffusion capacity. This reduction is usually asymptomatic and slowly improves after treatment. Severe idiopathic pulmonary toxicity is occasionally seen at bleomycin doses of >50 mg, although it usually does not occur until cumulative doses exceed 200 mg/m^2.

   Even more severe pulmonary toxicity (pulmonary infiltrates, restrictive defects, exertional dyspnea) is reported when bleomycin is given in combination with mediastinal RT. These adverse effects depend partly on the total dose of bleomycin and the radiation field. Caution is needed in patients who already have compromised lung function.

4. **Cardiac damage**

   a. **Radiation.** The risk for radiation pericarditis is relatively small when modern anteroposterior weighted radiation ports are used and when large portions of the heart are not radiated. Radiation pericarditis with or without pericardial effusion or tamponade can develop, however. Constrictive pericarditis is a rare complication of RT.

b. **Chemotherapy.** Doxorubicin, which is a component of ABVD and related regimens, is a well-known cardiotoxic agent. The incidence of cardiotoxicity is related to the cumulative dose and probably to peak serum levels. The cumulative dose of doxorubicin in ABVD is usually 300 mg/m^2, below the clinically significant cardiotoxic level when given without radiation. Administration of mediastinal and/or neck RT, however, increases the chance of cardiomyopathy, pericarditis, or coronary artery disease and other accelerated atherosclerotic disease and valvular disorders as well as the potential for delayed cardiomyopathy.

5. **Aseptic necrosis of the femoral heads** has been reported and is probably secondary to prednisone therapy in MOPP.

6. **Depressed cellular immunity.** Progressive loss of cell-mediated immunity with the development of cutaneous anergy, lymphocytopenia, and increased susceptibility to a variety of organisms is associated with advancing HL, even in the absence of therapy. Treatment with chemotherapy, corticosteroids, and RT accentuates these abnormalities. Late in the course of HL, hypogammaglobulinemia may also develop.

   a. **Infections associated with depressed cell-mediated immunity and therapy** (particularly corticosteroids) include *Listeria, Toxoplasma*, and *Mycobacterium* spp, fungi, and slow viruses (such as progressive multifocal leukoencephalopathy). Patients treated with corticosteroids are at particularly increased risk for infections with *Pneumocystis carinii* and CMV.

   b. **Herpes zoster** appears in >25% of patients, particularly in patients with irradiated dermatomes and in those undergoing splenectomy. Generalized cutaneous involvement is not uncommon, but visceral involvement is rare.

   c. **Splenectomy-related infections** involve encapsulated micro-organisms, particularly pneumococci, and less commonly *Haemophilus influenzae* and *Salmonella* sp, especially in children. Pneumococcal infection in an asplenic host can be rapidly fatal. Vaccination with polyvalent pneumococcal vaccine, hemophilus, and meningococcus is recommended before splenectomy, although its effectiveness in this population is not certain. Early, aggressive treatment with antibiotics of all febrile patients after splenectomy is mandatory.

7. **Secondary neoplasms**

   a. **Acute myelogenous leukemia,** often preceded by a prodrome of myelodysplastic syndrome, develops in 2% to 10% of patients treated with MOPP or similar combined-modality therapy containing alkylating agents. The problem appears to be greatest in patients older than 40 years of age and may be increased in patients undergoing splenectomy. The leukemia generally occurs between 3 and 10 years after treatment, is often associated with total or partial deletion of chromosomes 5 and 7, and has an extremely poor prognosis. Acute leukemia is extremely uncommon in patients treated with RT alone and appears to be rare in patients treated with ABVD.

   b. **NHL** may occur during the course of HL and may represent an evolution of the natural history of disease rather than a treatment complication. Most reported cases are high-grade B-cell tumors, with a particularly high incidence in cases of nodular LP HL. As previously noted, LP HL may be a B-cell lymphoma (see section II.A.2). High-grade peripheral T-cell lymphomas and mycosis fungoides have also complicated HL, particularly the NS type.

   c. **Epithelial tumors and sarcomas** are being increasingly reported as complications of RT and possibly of combined-modality therapy, and actuarial statistics suggest a rate of second neoplasms exceeding 20% with prolonged follow-up. Tumors may include breast cancer, sarcoma, melanoma, lung cancer, and other solid tumors. The relative risk for cancer appears to be higher for younger patients and synergistic to other predisposing factors. This significant risk applies to a patient population treated in the 1960s and 1970s; modern strategies limiting radiation exposure may reduce this risk.

8. Neurologic complications

a. Lhermitte's sign, which follows thoracic irradiation for HL, is an innocuous but worrisome finding for the patient. It consists of shocklike sensations down the back and legs, often precipitated by flexing the neck, and it gradually disappears.

b. Transverse myelopathy is a rare but serious complication of RT that is usually caused by failure to leave an appropriate gap between the mantle and abdominal ports.

9. Retroperitoneal fibrosis has been described as a complication of HL treatment.

B. Synchronous neoplasms. HL is said to be associated with an increased risk for simultaneous Kaposi sarcoma, leukemia, NHL, and myeloma.

C. Nephrotic syndrome, as a remote effect of malignancy, occurs most often in patients with HL. Lipoid nephrosis is typical (see Chapter 31, section IV). **Other paraneoplastic phenomena** that have been described in the setting of HL include autoimmune hemolysis, immune thrombopenia, neurologic deficits, and jaundice.

D. Pregnancy in HL. See Chapter 26.

E. Ichthyosis. Adult-onset ichthyosis is associated with HL in 75% of cases (see Chapter 28, section II.I).

NON-HODGKIN LYMPHOMA

I. EPIDEMIOLOGY AND ETIOLOGY

A. Incidence. NHL occurs with increasing frequency, with about 60,000 new cases annually in the United States. The incidence is rising dramatically for unknown reasons.

B. Age and sex. Small lymphocytic lymphomas occur in the elderly. Lymphoblastic lymphoma has a predilection for male adolescents and young adults. Follicular lymphomas occur mainly in middle-adult life. BL occurs in children and young adults.

C. Etiology. Viral etiology and abnormal immune regulation have been implicated in the development of lymphomas. The two mechanisms may be interrelated. An etiologic agent, however, can be identified in only a minority of cases.

1. Pathogens

a. RNA viruses. The human T-cell lymphotrophic virus type 1 (HTLV-1) is associated with adult T-cell leukemia-lymphoma (ATLL). HIV produces AIDS, and the resultant immune deficiency is associated with high-grade B-cell lymphomas. Chronic hepatitis C virus infection has been associated with indolent B-cell lymphoma.

b. DNA viruses. EBV has been found in the genome of African BL cells. EBV is also detected in biopsies of nasal T-cell and NK-cell lymphoma. This virus has also been associated with lymphomas in situations characterized by reduced immune surveillance, such as in patients with the X-linked lymphoproliferative syndrome, organ transplantation, and, in many instances, HIV-associated lymphoma.

c. Chronic _H. pylori_ infection of the gastric mucosa is clearly associated with gastric lymphoma. Eradication of the infection produces remission in more than two-thirds of patients.

2. Immunodeficiency or immune dysregulation states associated with development of lymphomas include the following:

a. AIDS

b. Organ transplant recipients

c. Congenital immunodeficiency syndromes (e.g., agammaglobulinemia, ataxia-telangiectasia, Wiskott-Aldrich syndrome)

d. Autoimmune disorders (e.g., Sjögren syndrome, rheumatoid disease, lupus erythematosus, Hashimoto thyroiditis).

e. Phenytoin may cause a spectrum from benign lymphoproliferation to frank lymphoma.

3. **Treatment-related.** The potential role of chemotherapy or RT in the development of NHL after HL and myeloproliferative disorders remains uncertain.

II. PATHOLOGY AND NATURAL HISTORY

A. **Two complementary classification systems for NHL** have been used: the Working Formulation (WF) and the WHO classification, which was based on the Revised European American Lymphoma (REAL) classification. The WF captures and describes the most common lymphomas in terms of biologic behavior or "grades." The REAL/WHO classifications intend to distinguish lymphoma entities based on their unique clinical, pathologic, immunologic, and/or genetic characteristics and includes the uncommon lymphomas. Because of its dependence on immunophenotypic and cell lineage analysis, the REAL/WHO system is more reproducible.

B. **The WF** was previously the most commonly used system for the classification of NHL in the United States. This scheme was developed in 1982 as the result of a consensus panel made up of distinguished hematopathologists, each previously espousing his or her own classification. The WF attempts to associate clinical behavior with descriptive histopathologic features of NHL. However, it does not incorporate accepted information regarding B-cell or T-cell origin of lymphomas and does not recognize a large variety of newly described clinicopathologic entities. Table 21.5 shows the WF with the frequencies, some clinical correlates, and median survival rates for the various types of NHL using pre-rituximab chemotherapeutic regimens.

TABLE 21.5 The Working Formulation Classification of Non-Hodgkin Lymphoma[a]

Type of lymphoma	Frequency (%)	Median age (yr)	Stage III or IV (%)	Marrow involved (%)	Median survival (yr)
Low grade					
A—Small lymphocytic; plasmacytoid	3.6	60	89	71	5.0
B—Follicular, small cleaved cell	22.5	54	82	51	7.2
C—Follicular, mixed (small cleaved and large cell)	7.7	56	73	30	5.1
Intermediate grade					
D—Follicular, large cell	3.8	55	73	34	3.0
E—Diffuse, small cleaved cell	6.9	58	72	32	3.4
F—Diffuse, mixed (small cleaved and large cell)	6.7	58	55	14	2.7
G—Diffuse, large cell	19.7	57	54	10	1.5
High grade					
H—Immunoblastic (large cell)	7.9	51	49	12	1.3
I—Lymphoblastic	4.2	17	73	50	2.0
J—Small, noncleaved (Burkitt, non-Burkitt)	5.0	30	66	14	0.7
Total[a]	88.0				

Extracted from Rosenberg SA, Berard CW, Braun BW Jr, et al. National Cancer Institute sponsored study of classifications of non-Hodgkin's lymphomas. Summary and description of a working formulation for clinical usage. *Cancer* 1982;49:2112.
[a]The Working Formulation was based on a study of 1,014 patients. It does not include cutaneous T-cell lymphomas, adult T-cell leukemia-lymphoma, diffuse intermediately-differentiated lymphocytic lymphoma, and malignant histiocytosis, which constitute 12% of cases.

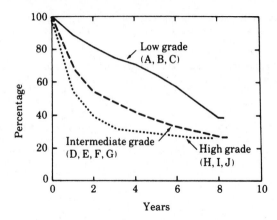

Figure 21.2. Actuarial survival curves for the National Cancer Institute's Working Formulation subtypes of lymphomas. Each of the three major prognostic categories (grades) is significantly different from the other (*p* <0.0001). Table 21.5 defines the histopathologic subtypes A through J for the grades. (From Rosenberg SA, et al. National Cancer Institute sponsored study of classifications of non-Hodgkin's lymphomas. Summary and description of a working formulation for clinical usage. *Cancer* 1982;49:2112, with permission.)

1. **Grades.** The WF divides NHLs into low, intermediate, and high grades that reflect their biological aggressiveness. The dividing lines between these categories are sometimes arbitrary.

    a. In general, small cell size, round or cleaved nuclei, and a low mitotic rate characterize low-grade NHLs. The intermediate/high-grade NHLs usually manifest larger cell size, prominent nucleoli, and a higher mitotic rate.

    b. Clinically, it is useful to consider low-grade NHLs as being indolent or nonaggressive, whereas the intermediate-grade and high-grade NHLs are aggressive diseases with a short, untreated natural history. Many clinicians approach immunoblastic lymphomas in a similar fashion to the intermediate-grade NHLs and consider lymphoblastic lymphomas and the small noncleaved NHLs, particularly the Burkitt variant, as high-grade NHLs requiring special management.

2. **Survival curves** based on the WF are shown in Figure 21.2.

C. **The WHO/REAL classification** was established after a consensus of hematopathologists in 1993. It incorporates immunophenotypic characteristics to determine cell lineage and to define subtypes by a more scientific method. It recognizes several less common entities that were unclassifiable by the WF. The WHO accepted the REAL proposal with some additions and should be the current classification standard. The WHO classification, which serves as a common language among hematologists, is shown in Appendix C-6, section I.

    1. WHO/REAL entities may include lymphomas of various clinical behaviors, provided that they originate from the same cell type. Leukemias are considered to be an extreme of the spectrum of certain lymphoproliferative disorders.

    2. Acute lymphocytic leukemias and lymphoblastic lymphomas are grouped together.

    3. Chronic lymphocytic leukemia (CLL) is classified together with small lymphocytic lymphoma because they both consist of small, round, B lymphocytes that are positive for CD5 and CD23.

    4. All follicular lymphomas constitute one group with grade designation (grades 1 to 3).

    5. Mantle cell lymphoma (MCL) is recognized as a separate entity with its distinct features and clinical aggressiveness. MCL was previously described as small

lymphocytic lymphoma, diffuse small cleaved cell lymphoma, or at times follicular lymphoma in the WF.

6. Immunoblastic lymphoma is classified as diffuse large cell lymphoma and is no longer recognized as a separate entity.

7. Detailed classification of T-cell and NK-cell malignancies is attempted in this system. Such lymphomas were not recognized by the WF.

8. Because about two-thirds of the NHL histologies are follicular or diffuse large cell, clinical decisions often rely on WF principles.

D. Pathogenesis

1. **Monoclonal antibodies** can identify epitopes on lymphoid cells characteristic of developmental stages of B-cell and T-cell ontogeny. The antibodies are used with flow cytometry in cell suspensions and with indirect immunoperoxidase labeling in frozen sections. Some of the most useful antibodies are shown in Appendix C-5. Monoclonality of B-cell lymphomas is usually established by showing marked dominance of a single light-chain (κ or λ) type.

2. **Gene rearrangements.** B cells and T cells must rearrange DNA to assemble antigen-specific receptors. Each clone rearranges its genes in a unique way that can be differentiated from the germ line pattern by Southern blot techniques. Identification of gene rearrangements for immunoglobulin and T-cell receptor loci can establish cellular lineage, monoclonality, and sometimes stage of differentiation for lymphoid neoplasms. The application of the polymerase chain reaction method may enable detection of down to one clonal cell in one million using amplification of breakpoint regions by specific primers.

3. **Specific chromosomal translocations** (Table 21.6) have been associated with histologically distinct lymphoma types. The genetic material found at or near the breakpoint of each translocated chromosome is frequently highly informative and provides clues regarding pathogenesis. For example, in BL, the transforming c-*myc* cellular oncogene found on chromosome 8 is involved in a translocation

TABLE 21.6 **Chromosomal Translocations in Lymphoma**

Lymphoma type	Translocation	Genes at breakpoint
B-cell lymphoma		
Small lymphocytic	t(14;19)(q32;q13)	Heavy chain; *BCL-3*
Plasmacytoid	t(9;14)(p13;q32)	Heavy chain;—
Mantle cell	t(11;14)(q13;q32)	*BCL-1*; heavy chain
Follicular	t(14;18)(q32;q21)	Heavy chain; *BCL-2*
Small noncleaved	t(8;14)(q24;q32)	*MYC*; heavy chain
(including Burkitt)	t(2;8)(p12;q24)	kappa; *MYC*
	t(8;22)(q24;q11)	*MYC*; lambda
Large cell	t(3;14)(q27;q32)	*BCL-6*
	t(3;22)(q27;q11)	
	t(2;3)(p12;q27)	
T-cell lymphoma		
Lymphoblastic	Variable involvement of T-cell receptor genes	—
Anaplastic large cell (Ki-1)	t(2;5)(p23;q35)	—

Key: CD5, Leu-1 or T-101; CD10, common acute lymphocytic leukemia antigen (CALLA); Sig, surface immunoglobulin; Cig, cytoplasmic immunoglobulin; TdT, terminal deoxynucleotidyl transferase.
See Appendix C-4 for leukocyte differentiation antigens and Appendix A for glossary of cytogenetic nomenclature.

within or adjacent to the heavy-chain gene on chromosome 14 or to one of the light-chain genes (κ on chromosome 2 or λ on chromosome 22).

In the follicular lymphomas, the translocation also involves the heavy-chain gene on chromosome 14, which is this time juxtaposed with the so-called *BCL-2* gene on chromosome 18. The *BCL-2* gene appears to be significantly involved in the abrogation of *apoptosis* (programmed cell death). Thus, the activation of the *BCL-2* gene by translocation in follicular lymphomas may result in the excessive longevity or accumulation of lymphoma cells, implying a defect in cell death rather than a pure problem of proliferation in that disease. In MCL, the heavy-chain gene on chromosome 14 and the *BCL-1* gene on chromosome 11 are brought into proximity. The *BCL-1* gene encodes cyclin-D1, which is involved in the cell cycle.

Such cytogenetic abnormalities can be demonstrated with the use of florescence *in situ* hybridization techniques to analyze specific genetic abnormalities that a tumor may possess.

4. **Production of lymphokines** by tumor cells may be related to the symptoms or manifestations of specific lymphomas. For example, production of interleukin (IL)-4 by T cells in Lennert lymphoma may explain the exuberant proliferation of histiocytes in that disease, whereas in angioimmunoblastic lymphomas, IL-6 production may result in plasmacytosis and hypergammaglobulinemia.

5. **The pattern of surface antigens** (Appendix C-5) found on lymphoma cells when flow cytometry or immunohistochemical staining is used may help identify or corroborate certain lymphoma types. For example, the CD5 antigen, a pan T-cell antigen expressed by a small minority of B lymphocytes, is found on the neoplastic cells of patients with small cell lymphocytic lymphoma and MCL but is absent from the cells of follicular lymphomas and monocytoid B-cell lymphoma.

III. **NATURAL HISTORY.** NHL exhibits a remarkable range of natural histories, with doubling times varying between days (e.g., BL) and years (some low-grade NHLs). Treatment tends to have a much more dramatic effect on intermediate/high-grade NHLs (collectively also called *aggressive*) than on low-grade NHLs. Early bone marrow involvement and hematogenous and noncontiguous dissemination characterizes NHL, particularly the low-grade types, in sharp contrast to the distribution in HL. Extra-axial nodes, including epitrochlear and mesenteric nodes, are often involved, again in distinction to HL (Table 21.1). Intermediate- and high-grade NHLs often present in extranodal sites, including Waldeyer's ring, GI tract, skin, bone, and CNS.

A. **B-cell lymphomas: low grade** (see Appendixes C-5 and C-6)

1. **Small lymphocytic lymphoma** is the tissue or nodal counterpart of CLL and classically presents with diffuse lymphadenopathy and marrow involvement. Cells are positive for CD5, CD20, and CD23. CLL and chronic B-cell prolymphocytic leukemia are discussed in Chapter 23, in "Chronic Lymphocytic Leukemia."

2. **Lymphoplasmacytic lymphomas** include Waldenström's macroglobulinemia may manifest monoclonal IgM spikes in the serum. The cellular composition of plasmacytoid lymphocytic lymphoma is made up of lymphocytes, plasma cells, and hybridized forms with features of both. Cells are usually CD20-positive, in contrast to frank plasma cells. Hyperviscosity syndrome caused by the IgM protein that forms asymmetric pentamers or neuropathy may dominate the clinical picture in Waldenström's macroglobulinemia, which is discussed in detail in Chapter 22.

3. **Follicular lymphoma.** The follicular lymphomas include lymphocytic infiltrates that are composed mostly of small cleaved cells with increasing numbers of large cells with increasing grade. Cells are positive for CD10 and CD20 and negative for CD5.

   a. **Cytogenetics.** Follicular lymphomas bear the t(14;18) translocation that results in upregulation of *BCL-2* expression. The *BCL-2* gene product is considered a potent inhibitor of apoptosis.

    b. Follicular lymphoma subtype, according to the WHO classification, is defined by the average number of large cells (centroblasts) in a high-power field (hpf):

> Grade 1, if <5 large cells/hpf,
> Grade 2, if 5–15 large cells/hpf,
> Grade 3, if >15 large cells/hpf.

    c. Aggressiveness. Follicular lymphomas grades 1 and 2 are generally considered to be low grade. The rarer follicular large cell type, or grade 3, is considered by most as intermediate grade, although it is not clear that the natural history is distinct. Cytologic transformation to intermediate-grade or high-grade NHL may occur at any point in the disease and is often characterized by *p53* mutation. A similar transformation may take place in other forms of low-grade NHL.

    d. Behavior. The follicular lymphomas tend to present as nodal disease. About 85% of cases are stage III or IV at presentation, with frequent bone marrow involvement (>50% of cases). The liver, spleen, and mesenteric nodes are often involved. Follicular lymphomas often progress slowly and may not require immediate therapy. Temporary spontaneous regressions are observed in up to 30% of cases. Follicular lymphomas are highly responsive to therapy, but the effect of any specific treatment on survival is modest, and few patients are cured. Average survival times vary between 6 and 10 years in the past, with possible increases in median survival times in the "rituximab era."

4. Marginal-zone lymphoma is believed to be derived from parafollicular or marginal-zone cells that surround the mantle zone. Cells are negative for CD10 and CD5 and positive for CD20.

    a. MALTomas (MALT: mucosa-associated lymphoid tissue) are a group of extranodal lymphomas that frequently present as localized tumors in the stomach, lung, breast, thyroid, and other extranodal sites.

      (1) In some cases, a pre-existing organ-associated autoimmune disease is noted (e.g., Sjögren syndrome or Hashimoto thyroiditis). Many of these were designated *pseudolymphomas* in the past.

      (2) The natural history includes prolonged survival without widespread dissemination and suggests a role for RT or surgery in management.

      (3) Gastric MALToma is clearly associated with *H. pylori* infection and regresses in two-thirds of the patients after its eradication.

    b. Splenic lymphomas are an uncommon form of marginal-zone lymphomas. These are characterized by pronounced splenic enlargement, often without systemic disease, and with blood and/or bone marrow involvement. Cells often have villi (splenic lymphoma with villous lymphocytes).

    c. Nodal marginal zone lymphomas may also be called **monocytoid lymphomas** because of their appearance.

5. Hairy cell leukemia is characterized by an indolent course, hypersplenism, and neutropenia. Characteristic lymphocytes may be seen with the tartrate-resistant acid phosphatase (TRAP) stain. Cells are characteristically positive for CD103, CD22, CD11c, and often CD25. This disease is discussed in Chapter 23, in "Hairy Cell Leukemia."

B. B-cell lymphomas: intermediate grade and high grade (see Appendix C-5 and Appendix C-6)

1. Mantle cell lymphoma (MCL) is a unique B-cell lymphoma with an adverse prognosis. It is derived from CD5-positive, CD20-positive, CD23-negative lymphocytes surrounding the germinal center. It is associated with the t(11;14) translocation, which results in up-regulation of cyclin D1, a promoter of cell cycling.

    a. MCL may present with a variety of histologic variations ranging from a pseudofollicular pattern to a blastic form. The most common appearance is a diffuse, small cell, slightly irregular infiltrate.

    b. MCL usually presents at advanced stage with B symptoms and involvement of the GI tract and bone marrow. Conventional chemotherapy usually produces disappointingly short remissions and a median survival of about 2.5 years.

c. **Mantle-zone lymphoma** with a "mantle zone pattern" is an uncommon indolent variety of MCL without invasion of the follicular center of the involved lymph nodes.

2. **Diffuse large B-cell lymphomas (DLBCL).** About 30% of cases originate in extranodal sites, such as the GI tract and Waldeyer's ring, sinuses, bone, or CNS. In contrast to most low-grade NHLs, localized presentations (stage I and II disease) are common, and bone marrow involvement is less frequent (<25% of cases). Localized presentations (stage I and II disease) may be curable in up to 80% of cases, whereas disseminated disease (stage III and IV disease) is curable 50% of the time.

a. **AIDS-related NHLs** are almost universally intermediate-grade or high-grade B-cell lymphomas (see Chapter 36, section II). Most patients present with extranodal disease, often including the GI tract, bone, jaw, and CNS (as parenchymal involvement), but almost any organ can be involved. Dissemination to bone marrow and meninges is characteristic.

b. **Posttransplantation lymphoproliferative disorders** describe a spectrum of oligoclonal lymphoproliferation following intense, often iatrogenic, immunosuppression in organ transplant recipients and also occurring in other immunocompromised patients. It is believed that polyclonal or oligoclonal B-cell proliferation is initially driven by EBV infection escaping immune surveillance. Ongoing proliferation results in true malignant transformation and development of monoclonal aggressive NHL.

The disease typically manifests with hectic fever, malaise, and cytopenias. Nodal involvement may or may not be noted at presentation. These lymphomas share similar histology and a proclivity for extranodal involvement with AIDS lymphomas. This disorder may respond to withdrawal of immunosuppression in early stages, but systemic chemotherapy and/or monoclonal antibody therapy may be required. The prognosis depends largely on comorbid conditions and the length of the time from transplant to diagnosis of the lymphoma.

c. **Primary effusion lymphoma** is an aggressive lymphoma originating in serosa and presenting with effusions. Dissemination of disease is the rule. It has been strongly associated with presence of the human herpes virus type 8 (HHV-8) and HIV infection.

3. **The "high-grade" B-cell lymphomas** are rapidly proliferating lesions with an extremely high mitotic rate and doubling times as brief as 24 hours. Many lymphomas associated with AIDS or organ transplantation are this type.

a. **Burkitt lymphoma** has a distinctive morphology, natural history, and behavior and is divided into African (endemic), sporadic, and immunosuppressive types. The cells are all nearly equal in size and contain prominent small nucleoli and cytoplasmic lipid vacuoles. In the non-Burkitt type of small noncleaved lymphoma, the cells have a less homogeneous cellular size and composition. BL is discussed later in section VIII.E.

b. **B-cell lymphoblastic lymphoma** is classified with B-lineage acute lymphoblastic leukemia (ALL) and is approached similarly (see Chapter 25, "Acute Leukemia" section).

C. **T-cell NHLs** constitute about 20% of NHLs in Western societies. T-cell lymphomas have been analyzed in detail by the REAL/WHO classifications (see Appendix C-6), despite the difficulty arising from the rarity of certain categories.

1. **Precursor T-cell lymphoblastic leukemia/lymphomas** (including T-cell ALL) are malignancies of immature T cells that occur predominantly in male adolescents and young adults. The nuclei are often convoluted in appearance, and the mitotic rate is high.

a. **Terminal deoxynucleotidyl transferase (TdT)** activity is characteristically positive in these patients. TdT positivity is generally restricted to lymphoblastic lymphoma, ALL (pre-B, T, and null subtypes), and the lymphoid blast crisis of chronic myelogenous leukemia; it is not seen in other NHLs.

    b. Clinical aspects. Patients usually present with anterior mediastinal masses and often manifest pleural effusion, pericardial effusion, or superior vena cava syndrome. Bone marrow and peripheral blood involvement are frequent, and the syndrome then merges with T-cell ALL. Meningeal involvement is anticipated unless CNS prophylaxis is used. Therapy that is similar to that used for ALL may cure half of the cases of lymphoblastic lymphoma.

  2. Peripheral T-cell and NK-cell neoplasms refer to all NHLs of T-cell or NK-cell origin except precursor T-cell lymphoblastic leukemia/lymphoma. The spectrum includes low-grade disorders, such as mycosis fungoides (MF), the most common cutaneous T-cell lymphoma, and a variety of other more aggressive clinicopathologic syndromes. With the exception of MF and large granular lymphocytic leukemia, T-cell lymphomas tend to be clinically aggressive even if the morphology suggests a low-grade behavior. It appears that the noncutaneous peripheral T-cell lymphomas (PTCLs) have a poorer prognosis than intermediate/high-grade B-cell NHLs stage for stage. Occasionally, hemophagocytic syndrome can occur.

    a. The pathologic manifestations of PTCL often include infiltration of T-cell lymph node regions (paracortical) and increased atypical epithelioid venules. The pleomorphic tumor cells often exhibit clear cytoplasm and occasionally resemble RS cells. These tumors frequently contain an admixture of interdigitating cells, epithelioid cells, eosinophils, and plasma cells. Many peripheral T-cell lymphomas would be placed in the *diffuse mixed* category of the WF.

    b. Clinical aspects of PTCL. PTCLs often develop in middle-aged to elderly patients, who present with constitutional symptoms (B symptoms). Most patients have nodal-based stage III or IV disease with frequent hepatosplenomegaly. Pulmonary and skin involvement are not uncommon. Eosinophilia and polyclonal hypergammaglobulinemia develop in some cases.

D. Peripheral T-cell and NK-cell entities (see Appendixes C-5 and C-6)

  1. Adult T-cell leukemia-lymphoma (ATLL) was initially described in southwestern Japan but has been subsequently seen throughout the world, including the United States. The HTLV-1 virus apparently causes the disease. Cutaneous involvement, lymphadenopathy, organomegaly, a leukemic blood picture, hypercalcemia with osteolytic bone lesions, and pulmonary involvement characterize ATLL. The cells frequently show a remarkable "knobby" configuration of the nuclei. Immunologically, the cells are CD4-positive. The response to treatment has been poor; combinations of zidovudine and interferon (IFN) may be useful. A prodromal, less aggressive chronic and smoldering phase is also recognized, which may clinically appear indistinguishable from MF, but with positive serology for the causative agent, HTLV-1.

  2. Aggressive NK-cell leukemia-lymphoma is a rare and rapidly fatal NK-cell malignancy. It is more prevalent among Asians than whites. The immunophenotype is identical to extranodal nasal-type NK-/T-cell lymphomas.

  3. T-cell prolymphocytic leukemia is discussed in Chapter 23, section VI.B of "Chronic Lymphocytic Leukemia".

  4. T-cell or NK-cell large granular lymphocytic leukemia is an indolent disease with subtle lymphocytosis of the blood or bone marrow and paraneoplastic neutropenia. It usually does not require treatment. Responses to cyclosporine have been reported. This is also discussed in Chapter 23, section III.D.6 of "Chronic Lymphocytic Leukemia".

  5. Anaplastic large cell lymphoma (ALCL) is usually of T-cell origin. Occasional cases appear to be of undefined lineage (null cell). The large anaplastic cells are positive for Ki-1 (CD30), an antigen initially described in HL but later found to be present in some neoplastic cells in a variety of aggressive NHLs. It is often associated with t(2;5), which results in fusion of the nucleophosmin gene *NPM* to a tyrosine kinase, ALK (anaplastic lymphoma kinase). The presence of t(2;5) is believed to confer a better prognosis.

    Pathologically, the cases are frequently confused with epithelial tumors (carcinomas) or melanoma. The confusion is sometimes compounded by positive staining for epithelial membrane antigen and by a sinusoidal distribution, which is characteristic of carcinomas or melanomas. Pathologically, it can be confused with HL, with lymphomatoid papulosis (a relatively benign cutaneous condition with similar histology and spontaneous regressions), or with cutaneous anaplastic lymphoma, which has an excellent prognosis with local treatment despite almost always being ALK-negative. Treatment of ALCL is similar to that of large cell B-cell lymphoma and is believed to have a slightly better outcome.

6. **Angioimmunoblastic T-cell lymphoma.** Immunoblastic lymphadenopathy and angioimmunoblastic lymphadenopathy with dysproteinemia (AILD) were originally described as abnormal immune reactions clinically characterized by fever, skin rash, autoimmune hemolytic anemia, polyclonal hypergammaglobulinemia, and generalized lymphadenopathy. Pathology revealed diffuse effacement of lymph node architecture, involvement by immunoblasts and plasma cells, and often an abnormal vascular network. Immunohistochemistry and gene rearrangement studies have indicated that many of these patients have underlying T-cell lymphomas from the onset. The course may vary in aggressiveness, with occasional spontaneous remissions. Satisfactory and prolonged responses to corticosteroids or cyclosporine can be seen. More often, patients require treatments similar to aggressive NHL.

7. **Nasal-type NK-cell and T-cell lymphomas** include the former angiocentric lymphoma and lethal midline granuloma (malignant midline reticulosis). The neoplastic cells in these disorders involve vessels and lead to an angiodestructive necrotizing process. Nasal NK-/T-cell lymphoma involves the palate and sinuses, but metastasis can occur. The course can be indolent but is more commonly aggressive, particularly if disseminated. It is uncommon in the United States and more common in Asia. In contrast to aggressive diffuse large cell B-cell lymphoma of the nasal cavity, nasal NK-/T-cell lymphoma does not usually extend to the CNS. Cells usually are positive for T-cell markers and CD56. Chemotherapy and RT can be curative for localized disease.

8. **Hepatosplenic T-cell lymphoma** is characterized by sinusoidal infiltration of the liver by cytotoxic T cells expressing the γ–δ rather than the most common α–β T-cell receptor complex. The bone marrow is nearly always involved and lymph nodes are rarely involved. This rare form of NHL is often associated with a hemophagocytic syndrome. Despite the bland appearance of the cells, the clinical course is usually relentless.

9. **Enteropathy-type T-cell lymphoma** presents with ulcerative intestinal lesions in patients with gluten-sensitive (celiac disease) or other enteropathy most commonly. Patients present with abdominal pain, often associated with perforation. It is uncommon in the United States.

10. **Subcutaneous panniculitislike T-cell lymphoma** is rare and is characterized by infiltration of the subcutaneous tissue with cytotoxic T-cells, expressing the α–β T-cell receptor complex. Patients present with multiple subcutaneous nodules, usually in the absence of other sites of disease. A hemophagocytic syndrome is a possible complication and often the harbinger of an aggressive clinical course.

11. **Mycosis fungoides and the Sézary syndrome** are described separately (see section VIII.B).

E. **Histiocytic and dendritic cell neoplasms** represent a rather confusing category of ill-defined very rare diseases. The cells of origin, histiocytes and accessory cells, have a major role in the processing and presentation of antigen to both T and B cells.

1. **Malignant histiocytosis-hemophagocytic syndrome** (fever, jaundice, hepatosplenomegaly, coagulopathy, and hemophagocytosis) has been described and most often represents a complication of T-cell lymphoma. Etoposide and sometimes cyclosporine have been reported to control this syndrome.

2. **Langerhans cell histiocytosis** is a condition caused by clonal proliferation of Langerhans cells. Most cases occur in childhood. Langerhans cell histiocytosis is associated with both HL and NHL. It may be localized or generalized with variable aggressiveness. Unifocal disease occurs in a majority of cases

(eosinophilic granuloma), usually involving bone. Multifocal, unisystem disease (Hand-Schüller-Christian disease) involves several sites in one organ system (usually the bone). Combination chemotherapy may be necessary for multiple system involvement.

F. Immunological abnormalities

1. Hypogammaglobulinemia is typically seen in small lymphocytic lymphoma but may develop in other lymphomas, particularly after treatment.

2. Paraprotein spikes, often IgM, are seen particularly in lymphoplasmacytic lymphomas but are also noted in other B-cell malignancies and in AILD.

3. Warm or cold antibody immune hemolytic anemias may be seen with any B-cell malignancy, particularly in the small lymphocytic type.

4. Additional autoimmune phenomena, such as circulating anticoagulants (e.g., acquired von Willebrand disease) or angioedema (associated with C′1 esterase deficiency), may occur, especially in the small lymphocytic lymphomas.

5. Polyclonal hypergammaglobulinemia is commonly observed in patients with AIDS or PTCL.

6. Defects in T-cell function are prominent in ATLL even before treatment, and in other lymphomas after treatment.

IV. STAGING SYSTEM AND PROGNOSTIC FACTORS

A. The Ann Arbor Staging System was used for HL and is applied to NHL, but histopathologic subtype is the prime determinant of survival in NHL. MF has a different staging system (see section VIII.B).

B. Survival (see Fig. 21.2 and Table 21.5)

1. **Low-grade lymphomas** are rarely curable and appear to cause a steady percentage of deaths annually. It is possible that the rare, early stages of low-grade NHL (stage I or II) may be curable in some cases, but even this is uncertain. Survival time averaged between 6 and 10 years for follicular lymphomas in the pre-rituximab era.

2. **Intermediate-grade and high-grade lymphoma** survival curves generally display two components: a rapid falloff in the first 1 to 2 years followed by an eventual plateau representing a presumptively cured population. About 80% to 90% of patients with stage I or early stage II disease and 50% with stage III or IV intermediate/high-grade lymphomas may be curable.

3. **MCL** survival curve shows a rapid and steady decline, with no survival plateau, and a median survival time of 2 to 2.5 years with conventional chemotherapy.

C. Prognostic factors. Extent of disease at presentation and survival rates are shown in Table 21.5.

1. **Low-grade lymphomas**

   a. **Sensitivity to therapy** is a prognostic sign in that the attainment of a CR or an excellent partial response (PR) with duration of over 1 year identifies patients who are likely to do well.

   b. **Early stage.** Stage I and II cases constitute <15% of all patients with low-grade lymphoma. In one small series, 80% of stage I and II patients younger than 40 years of age who were treated with RT were disease-free 10 years after diagnosis.

   c. **Follicular mixed (grade 2) lymphomas.** It is unclear whether there is a difference in long-term outcome based on grade.

   d. **The FLIPI scale** (Follicular Lymphoma International Prognostic Index) may be helpful to determine prognosis of patients with follicular lymphoma. Variables (score one point per variable) included in this score are (mnemonic: *NOLASH*):

   > Greater than 4 **No**dal areas of involvement
   > Abnormal **L**DH
   > **A**ge >60 years
   > **S**tage III or IV
   > **H**emoglobin <12 g/dL

Those with a low FLIPI score (0 to 1) have a 5-year survival of 90%, and those with a high score (3 or greater) have a 53% 5-year survival in the pre-rituximab era.

   e. The international prognostic index (IPI) described in section IV.C.2.a is also useful in stratifying patients with indolent lymphoma.

2. **Intermediate/high-grade lymphomas.** Stage I or II presentations, constituting 30% to 40% of these lymphomas, are highly curable (about 80%), although tumor bulk (>10 cm in largest diameter) adversely affects outcome.

   a. The IPI has established *five independently important prognostic factors.* The 5-year survival rate was 73% for patients manifesting none or one of the adverse risk factors and 26% for patients with four or five risk factors in the pre-rituximab era. In the post-rituximab era, even those with 3 to 5 points have a 4-year progression-free survival of 55%. These important **adverse risk factors** are as follows (mnemonic: *APLES*):

   (1) Age older than 60 years
   (2) Performance status (ECOG >1; see inside back cover)
   (3) LDH abnormal
   (4) Extranodal sites more than one
   (5) Stage III or IV

   b. Gene profiling. Retrospective microarray analysis of gene expression has identified subgroups of DLBCL with distinct gene cluster expression patterns. Recognized subgroups may resemble the expression profile of the follicular center cells, which confers better prognosis, or the expression pattern of activated lymphocytes, which confers a worse outcome in the pre-rituximab era. This association is independent of the IPI and may explain why treatment fails in certain patients who have a favorable IPI score. In addition to prognostic information, the evolution of gene profiling is expected to offer significant insight into the pathophysiology of the disease and in the identification of putative therapeutic targets.

V. STAGING EVALUATION

   A. Clinical evaluation. See "Evaluation of Suspected Lymphoma," sections I through IV.

   B. Initial staging evaluation

   1. The staging evaluation as outlined in "Hodgkin Lymphoma" section IV.B is generally applicable in NHL. Laboratory evaluation should also include uric acid, serum protein electrophoresis, hepatitis B testing, and HIV if diagnosis is high-grade B-cell malignancy. β_2-Microglobulin may be substituted for ESR.

   2. Flow cytometry on the peripheral blood and bone marrow in low-grade lymphomas may define a clonal excess and suggest hematogenous involvement, even when circulating lymphoma cells are not seen.

   3. Diagnostic spinal tap is indicated in lymphoblastic lymphoma, lymphomas occurring in AIDS, BL, and probably in intermediate/high-grade lymphomas with extensive marrow, sinus, or testicular involvement or with any parameningeal focus.

   4. Upper GI and small bowel series should be performed in patients with GI symptoms, unexplained iron deficiency, and/or Waldeyer's ring involvement. Endoscopic evaluation is performed as indicated, particularly in MCL.

   C. Restaging evaluation is performed to verify CR (all lymph nodes that were ≥1.5 cm). All abnormal studies are repeated, including biopsies of accessible previously involved sites, particularly with potentially curable histologies.

   Patients with intermediate-grade or high-grade lymphomas and residual masses on CT scans or radiographs should be followed closely with serial studies; stable residual masses usually do not contain lymphoma. PET is often used to ensure negativity of the presumed inert residual mass. The frequent presence of residual masses has resulted in the definition of "unconfirmed CR" (CRu), whereby all the requirements for CR exist except that a residual lymph node may be >1.5 cm, provided it has been reduced by >75% in the bidimensional product. This designation has been largely eradicated by the use of PET scanning in staging.

VI. THERAPY FOR INDOLENT LYMPHOMAS

A. True stage I and II disease (15% cases): RT to a dose of 2,400 to 3,600 cGy may be administered to all known sites of disease (including draining lymph nodes in E presentation). Large RT fields do not increase the cure rate and may decrease tolerance to chemotherapy later. Prolonged disease-free survival has been reported in some patients.

B. Stage III and IV disease

1. No treatment. Most patients with advanced indolent disease may be observed with no therapy and without adverse influence on survival. Spontaneous remissions may occur during the period of no therapy. Therapy is instituted in the presence of any systemic symptoms, rapid nodal growth, or imminent complications of the disease, such as significant cytopenias, obstructive phenomena, or effusions. The median times for "requiring therapy" vary from 16 months for the follicular mixed group, to 48 months for the follicular small cleaved group, and to 72 months for the small lymphocytic group.

2. Single-agent chemotherapy with chlorambucil or cyclophosphamide gives good responses in indolent NHL. Cyclophosphamide has the disadvantages of alopecia and hemorrhagic cystitis. The purine analogs, fludarabine and cladribine, exhibit activity rivaling the alkylating agents; up to 50% of patients with previously treated low-grade lymphomas respond to these purine analogs. Dosages are as follows:

a. Chlorambucil, 2 to 6 mg/m^2 PO daily

b. Fludarabine, 25 mg/m^2 IV daily for 5 days every 4 weeks

c. Cladribine, 0.14 mg/kg per day IV over 2 hours for 5 days every 4 weeks, or 0.1 mg/kg/day by continuous IV infusion for 7 days every 4 weeks

3. Combination chemotherapy. Multiagent therapy may be used if a more rapid response is required. Chlorambucil or cyclophosphamide plus corticosteroids in pulse doses, and fludarabine plus mitoxantrone combinations are commonly used regimens (see Chl & P, CVP, and FMD in Appendix D-2, section I for regimens and dosages).

Single-agent or combination chemotherapy produces CRs or excellent PRs in 60% to 80% of patients. Doxorubicin-containing regimens have no clear advantages for low-grade NHL and are often reserved for later stages of the disease or adverse presentations. Treatment is generally continued until a maximum response is achieved. Maintenance chemotherapy does not prolong survival, may compromise further treatment, and is potentially leukemogenic.

4. Rituximab (Rituxan, MabThera) is a chimeric humanized anti-CD20 monoclonal antibody approved for the treatment of refractory or relapsed indolent B-cell lymphoma, and the first-line therapy of follicular lymphoma when combined with CVP. It is believed to mediate cytotoxicity through activation of antibody-dependent cytotoxic T cells, possibly by activation of complement, and by mediating direct intracellular signaling.

a. An overall 50% response rate with a median duration of about 1 year is expected for indolent B-cell lymphomas with rituximab monotherapy. Small lymphocytic lymphoma may be less responsive than follicular NHL because of lower expression of CD20 antigen. Responses of about 30% have been reported in large cell lymphoma that is relapsed or refractory to treatment or occurs in patients that have not been treated but are over age 60. Combinations of rituximab with a variety of chemotherapy regimens are feasible and are believed to be synergistic, with documented increased disease-free survival. Rituximab allows for flexibility in its coadministration with chemotherapy, with no particular schedule known to be more advantageous.

b. The established dose of rituximab is 375 mg/m^2 IV weekly for 4 or 8 weeks. The maximum tolerated dose has not been defined, but it is doubtful that higher doses improve outcome. There are no criteria for choosing the 4- or 8-week dosing.

Retreatment on progression is feasible with an expected response rate of 40%. Given its lack of cytotoxicity, maintenance regimens have been investigated and usually demonstrate considerable delay of progression; however, given the frequently successful retreatment on progression, it is unclear whether maintenance with rituximab really delays the time to refractoriness to this agent.

c. Mild infusion-related fever or rigors are common, particularly during the first infusion. Cytopenias develop occasionally. Reactions resulting in death (anaphylaxis, tumor lysis syndrome, adult respiratory distress syndrome) have also been seen, mainly in patients with circulating lymphoma cells or the elderly; slow escalation of the dose as tolerated is recommended for such patients. Reactivation of latent viruses has been reported, as well as immune phenomena such as serum sickness and lupus-like syndromes. The resulting B-cell depletion for 6 months or more seems to be well tolerated but may contribute to ongoing hypogammaglobulinemia. Precipitation of hyperviscosity on lymphoplasmacytoid lymphomas has been seen.

5. Radioactive monoclonal antibodies offer the advantage of targeted radioimmunotherapy. Responses rates of 50% to 80% have been reported in previously treated patients. ^{131}I-labeled anti-CD20 (tositumomab [Bexxar]) and ^{90}Y-labeled anti-CD20 (ibritumomab tiuxetan [Zevalin]) are available.

a. A randomized study of Zevalin versus rituximab demonstrated a higher response rate (80% vs. 55%) and a higher CR rate (30% vs. 15%) for the radioimmunoconjugate.

b. The treatment is given once and is well tolerated with the exception of cytopenias. Grade IV cytopenia occurs in one-third of the patients. Nadirs occur during the sixth and seventh weeks following therapy. Patients are excluded from this treatment with >25% involvement or hypocellularity in the bone marrow, with platelets <100,000/μL, or with neutrophil counts <1,500/μL.

c. Radiation hazard with Zevalin is negligible, whereas lead shielding and more stringent release instructions are needed for Bexxar.

6. IFN-α has been used in several randomized studies as part of either induction or maintenance therapy for previously untreated patients. No clear-cut dose schedule is superior, and doses as low as two to three million units 3 times weekly may produce responses in up to 40% to 60% of patients.

The place of IFN-α in the routine management of follicular lymphoma is not clear. Results of some series suggest a potentiation of response rates, a prolongation of remission duration, and possibly an effect of IFN-α on survival.

7. Palliative RT is used for sites of bulky disease and to relieve obstruction or pain. RT alone may be used when most of the disease sites do not require treatment but one or two areas are troublesome. However, multiple courses of RT exhaust the marrow and are discouraged when chemotherapy is an effective alternative.

C. Histologic conversion. Indolent lymphomas that transform to an aggressive cell type usually have a poor prognosis. Limited, relatively asymptomatic presentations, however, may respond well to treatment used for intermediate/high-grade NHL. The CNS can be involved (particularly the meninges) in transformed NHL and is rarely affected in low-grade NHL. High-dose chemotherapy and stem cell support for cases of transformed chemosensitive low-grade NHL should be considered.

D. Primary cutaneous B-cell lymphoma (CBCL) is defined as having no extracutaneous dissemination at presentation and for 6 months thereafter. See Appendix C-6, section II for classification of cutaneous lymphomas. They are most commonly follicular and indolent with a good prognosis. Localized CBCL is treated with RT, even for multifocal disease. Polychemotherapy or monoclonal antibody therapy is reserved for noncontiguous anatomic sites or extracutaneous spread. The diagnosis of primary cutaneous LBCL, leg type, confers a poorer prognosis and may mandate a different treatment approach.

E. Experimental therapies
  1. **Monoclonal antibodies** of several types, in addition to rituximab, have been used in the treatment of low-grade (and some aggressive) NHL. Targets include B-cell antigens (e.g., CD23, CD19, CD20, CD22) or more generalized common antigens (CD5, CD25, CD80, CD40).
      a. **Alemtuzumab** (Campath-1H) is a humanized antibody against CD52 (present in B cells, T cells, and monocytes) and is believed to have satisfactory activity in CLL, prolymphocytic leukemia, and certain T-cell lymphomas but modest action against indolent NHL.
      b. **Immunotoxins** have been under investigation but remain of unclear benefit.
  2. **Idiotype vaccines** have been used in a limited fashion to stimulate cellular and humoral immune response against the idiotype of the lymphoma cells. Generation of idiotype vaccines is labor-intensive. Infusion of autologous dendritic cells pulsed with idiotype have been used for the same purpose. Although an immune response is produced in most patients with minimal disease, the magnitude of clinical benefit is unclear.
  3. **Antisense oligonucleotide** treatment against *BCL-2* or other targets is undergoing investigation.
  4. **Selective inhibitors.** Several agents targeting selected processes, such as angiogenesis, proteasomes, signal transduction, cyclins, and histone deacetylase enzymes, are under investigation.
  5. **Autologous bone marrow or peripheral stem cell support** following high-dose chemotherapy is undergoing extensive study in patients with relapsed or newly diagnosed low-grade NHL. Although no convincing data support high-dose therapy in the routine management of low-grade NHL, it can be used in relatively young patients with adverse presentations in an effort to prolong remissions.
  6. **Allogeneic BMT or SCT** is proposed by certain centers for the treatment of refractory young patients with related donors and should probably be reserved as a last resort. The use of nonmyeloablative, less toxic preparative regimens has been shown to be a particularly useful allogeneic transplant approach in patients with indolent lymphoma with excellent early disease-free survival.

VII. **THERAPY FOR AGGRESSIVE NHL.** Therapy for special lymphoma subtypes is discussed in section VIII. Therapy for AIDS-associated lymphoma is discussed in Chapter 36, section II. Useful combination chemotherapy regimens for these malignancies are shown in Appendixes D-2 and D-3.
  A. **Localized presentations of intermediate/high-grade NHL.** Nonbulky (<10 cm) stages IA and IIA cases, including extranodal (E) presentations, can be successfully managed by three cycles of a doxorubicin-containing regimen (i.e., CHOP) followed by IFRT (equivalent to 3,000 cGy in 10 fractions). Virtually all patients achieve CR, and the actuarial relapse-free survival exceeds 80%. Another approach is full-course chemotherapy with or without subsequent RT.
  B. **Stage I–II (bulky), III, and IV disease** is treated with full-course CHOP chemotherapy (Appendix D-2, section II). For areas of bulky disease, IFRT may benefit the patient if all bulky disease that was present before giving chemotherapy can be safely encompassed by the radiation ports.
      Pursuant to the results of the randomized Groupe d'Etude des Lymphomes de l'Adulte (GELA) study in which elderly patients with aggressive NHL demonstrated a survival advantage (see Coiffier, et al. in "Suggested Reading"), rituximab is added to each cycle of CHOP. The addition of rituximab to CHOP increased the overall survival at 3 years from 49% to 62% when compared with treatment with CHOP alone. One can expect long-term disease control ("cure") in roughly 50% of patients with advanced-stage, intermediate/high-grade NHL treated with R-CHOP and similar programs. Results from randomized trials comparing standard R-CHOP with dose-dense R-CHOP given every 2 weeks with growth factors are awaited.
      Despite claims to the contrary, there is no proof that any of the more complex and more toxic regimens are superior to CHOP. Some of these alternative

regimens (m-BACOD, M-BACOD, MACOP-B, ProMACE/CytaBOM) are shown in Appendix D-2, section II. The results of an intergroup trial comparing CHOP with three of the purportedly more effective combinations showed CHOP to be equally active and less toxic. The claims for improved outcome reported in single-institution trials using other regimens are likely the result of incomplete follow-up and selection bias.

1. **Complete restaging** to assess completeness of response is mandatory. Restaging is usually done after three to four cycles of CHOP and again after six cycles. Patients are generally given at least two additional cycles of therapy after attainment of CR (usually a total of six to eight cycles). Ideally, patients should be in CR after the fourth cycle.

2. **CNS prophylaxis** using intrathecal chemotherapy, sometimes complemented by cranial irradiation, appears to be indicated in situations associated with a high risk for meningeal relapse. This strategy is particularly advised in cases of involvement of the paranasal sinuses, when there is contiguous spread to the CNS, and in the small noncleaved lymphomas (especially the Burkitt type). Other indications may include lymphoblastic lymphoma, primary testicular lymphoma with metastases, and intermediate/high-grade lymphomas that involve the bone marrow extensively, although the latter indication is more controversial.

3. **Autologous SCT** has been proposed as consolidation during first remission for high-risk patients but is of no proven efficacy in multiple randomized trials.

4. **Maintenance therapy** does not enhance survival and thus is not advised.

C. **Refractory or relapsed intermediate/high-grade lymphomas**

1. **Refractory patients** failing to achieve a CR may be salvaged with consolidation RT if the involved area is not extensive. Salvage chemotherapy, followed by autologous SCT, is the preferred approach, if feasible. Patients achieving a PR may have a 20% to 40% chance of cure, but the long-term survival rate of truly refractory patients is in the 10% range, so that high-dose chemotherapy is not generally recommended. Allogeneic BMT can be considered for these patients.

2. **Salvage chemotherapy regimens** often employ high-dose cytosine arabinoside, corticosteroids, and cisplatin with or without etoposide (see ESHAP in Appendix D-3). Combinations employing ifosfamide (ICE, MINE) and other potentially helpful regimens (CEPP-B, EVA, mini-BEAM, VAPEC-B, and infusional EPOCH) are also shown in Appendix D-3. Any of these regimens could be combined with rituximab, but the impact of this practice is unclear. These programs generally produce significant but short-lasting remissions in 40% to 50% of patients. A small proportion of patients, probably fewer than 10%, have prolonged responses.

3. **High-dose chemotherapy plus RT with autologous bone marrow or stem cell support.** A similar strategy to that employed in HL has been adopted for intermediate-grade NHL after relapse from standard CHOP-like chemotherapy. A conditioning regimen based on high-dose chemotherapy, sometimes combined with total-body irradiation, is used and followed by reinfusion of cryopreserved peripheral blood progenitor cells (stem cells) mobilized by growth factors. The results of this strategy are best in chemosensitive recurrences, in which about 40% of patients may derive long-term, disease-free survival. The results are far less optimistic in patients whose disease is chemoresistant or in patients who have never achieved remission. The relative merits of salvage chemotherapy followed by autologous BMT have been convincingly proved in a multicenter randomized European study (the PARMA study).

4. **Allogeneic BMT** differs from autologous BMT or SCT in that a potential graft-versus-lymphoma immune reaction may complement the effects of the conditioning regimen. The degree to which this effect exists in lymphoma is subject to debate and may vary with the type of lymphoma. Allogeneic BMT may be most reasonable in young patients who have a suitable donor match and who do not fall into the favorable categories for benefit from autologous transplantation.

5. **Experimental therapies.** Monoclonal antibody approaches similar to those employed in low-grade NHL are under investigation.

D. Therapy for MCL with standard chemotherapy regimens has generally been ineffective at achieving long-term remissions. The hyper-CVAD regimen (see Appendix D2, section III) alternated with high-dose methotrexate plus high-dose cytarabine has been proposed for treatment of MCL by the M.D. Anderson Cancer Center. Rituximab has been supplemented to the regimen. Allogeneic or autologous transplantation after two or four rounds of chemotherapy is considered for patients younger than 65 years of age. Aggressive approaches to MCL such as this may have shifted the survival curve to the right, but it still remains unclear if long-term remission is possible. Patients who relapse may receive palliative treatment with agents such as rituximab, bortezomib, and/or radioimmunotherapy.

E. Therapy for lymphoblastic lymphoma is patterned after therapy for the closely related ALL. Overall results of therapy indicate a 40% long-term, disease-free survival, with the best prognosis seen in patients who have minimal or no marrow involvement, no CNS involvement, and normal serum LDH levels. Patients with poor prognostic presentations of lymphoblastic lymphoma are being considered for early allogeneic BMT or more intensive primary chemotherapy programs.

Stanford University researchers reported a 94% freedom-from-relapse rate at 5 years for patients without the previously named adverse prognostic factors with a regimen that involves 1 month of induction therapy, 1 month of CNS prophylaxis, 3 months of consolidation, and, finally, 7 months of maintenance therapy, as follows:

Cyclophosphamide, 400 mg/m^2 PO for 3 days, on weeks 1, 4, 9, 12, 15, and 18
Doxorubicin, 50 mg/m^2 IV, on weeks 1, 4, 9, 12, 15, and 18
Vincristine, 2 mg IV, on weeks 1, 2, 3, 4, 5, 6, 9, 12, 15, and 18
Prednisone, 40 mg/m^2 daily for 6 weeks (tapered off); then for 5 days on weeks 9, 12, 15, and 18
CNS prophylaxis consists of whole-brain RT (2,400 cGy in 12 fractions) and intrathecal methotrexate (12 mg for each of six doses) given between weeks 4 and 9
L-Asparaginase, 6,000 U/m^2 IM (maximum, 10,000 U) for five doses at the beginning of CNS prophylaxis
Maintenance therapy consists of methotrexate (30 mg/m^2 PO weekly) and 6-mercaptopurine (75 mg/m^2 PO daily) during weeks 23 to 52.

F. Therapy for ATLL with polychemotherapy has been largely ineffective. A combination of zidovudine (AZT) and IFN-α has been stated to show promise. Occasionally, patients may benefit briefly from combination chemotherapy programs used in intermediate/high-grade NHL or from 2-deoxycoformycin, a purine analog. Investigational agents are attractive treatment options for this group of patients.

G. Therapy of peripheral T-cell lymphomas. Patients with non-B-cell aggressive lymphomas usually relapse after aggressive chemotherapy and fare worse than patients with B-cell NHL. Often the remissions may last only for a few weeks (kinetic failure). Aggressive approaches with autologous or allogeneic SCT are justified. Participation in clinical trials is highly recommended for this group of patients.

1. **Angioimmunoblastic lymphoma (AILD)** has been managed with generally poor results by conventional chemotherapy or corticosteroids, although occasional long-term responses or spontaneous regressions have occurred. More recently, responses to IFN-α, cyclosporine, or high-dose chemotherapy with stem cell support have been described in small series or case reports.

2. **Angiocentric lymphoma** with localized involvement of the palate and sinuses (lethal midline granuloma) may benefit from RT followed by chemotherapy.

3. **Primary cutaneous CD30 (Ki-1)-positive T-cell disorders** comprise a spectrum of closely related skin lesions that, although they may look identical microscopically, can be distinguished on physical examination of the patient's skin.

   a. **Lymphomatoid papulosis** has the best prognosis and is often a self-limited disease. It appears as crops of <2-cm nodules that may have central ulceration and leave scars, but spontaneously resolve within 6 to 8 weeks.

b. **Cutaneous anaplastic large cell lymphoma** (C-ALCL), which appears as single >2-cm skin lesions often with ulcerative centers, can be treated with local irradiation or surgery or if multiple, single-agent chemotherapy (cyclophosphamide or weekly low-dose methotrexate) with or without corticosteroids or RT. Spontaneous remission can occur in up to 30% of cases within 6 to 8 weeks. It can often be confused with ALCL, which is treated as a common aggressive lymphoma.

VIII. SPECIAL LYMPHOMA SYNDROMES

A. **Systemic Castleman disease.** Initially, Castleman disease referred to *localized giant lymph node hyperplasia,* usually involving the mediastinum or abdomen. The disease is associated with infection with HHV-8 and probably promoted by viral IL-6 production. A disorder exhibiting the histopathologic features of the plasma cell type of Castleman disease but with a generalized presentation has been described.

1. **Clinical features**
   a. Fever, malaise, and weakness
   b. Lymphadenopathy, usually generalized
   c. Organomegaly
   d. Edema, anasarca, and effusions
   e. Pulmonary and CNS involvement
   f. Anemia, thrombocytopenia, polyclonal hypergammaglobulinemia, and elevated ESR
2. **Histopathology** shows preservation of lymph node architecture, but with prominent germinal centers, either hyperplastic or hyalinized, and diffuse marked plasma cell infiltration.
3. **Clinical course** is either persistent or episodic with remissions and exacerbations. Lymphoma or Kaposi sarcoma occasionally develops. The median survival time is 30 months.
4. **Treatment.** Corticosteroids and antitumor agents used in NHL have met with occasional responses. IL-6 has been implicated in the pathogenesis of this disorder, with a reported clinical response to treatment with an anti–IL-6 antibody.

B. **Mycosis fungoides (MF) and Sézary syndrome (SS)** are CTCLs (see Appendix C-6 section II for classification of CTCL). Both are malignant cutaneous lymphoproliferative disorders of helper T cells (CD4-positive). Approximately 15% to 20% transform to CD30-positive or CD 30-negative large cell lymphoma.

1. **Dermatologic presentation** is in localized patches or plaques evolving into tumor nodules in MF and diffuse exfoliative erythroderma associated with abnormal circulating cells in SS.
2. **Histopathology** shows atypical T cells with irregular cerebriform nuclei (MF cells) infiltrating the epidermis and the upper dermis, forming characteristic Pautrier's microabscesses. Enlarged lymph nodes do not always show overt lymphomatous infiltration, but techniques such as T-cell–receptor gene arrangement may be positive.
3. **Natural history.** A long history of undiagnosed skin disease often precedes the specific diagnosis.
   a. **Cutaneous stages of MF**
      (1) Patch stage
      (2) Plaque stage
      (3) Tumor stage
   b. **Lymph node involvement** occurs with increasing skin involvement. Histologically confirmed lymph node involvement with complete lymph node effacement on microscopic examination conveys a poor prognosis.
   c. **Visceral involvement.** Almost any organ can be involved late in the disease, particularly the liver, spleen, lung, and GI tract, but the marrow is relatively spared. A peculiar epitheliotropic pattern of dissemination may be observed.
4. **Staging system.** A variety of systems have been proposed, including a TNM system. One example is the following:

Stage I
    Stage IA   Limited patches/plaques (<10% body surface area)
    Stage IB   Generalized patches/plaques (>10% body surface area)
Stage II
    Stage IIA   Limited or generalized patches/plaques with palpable
                 lymphadenopathy, not pathologically involved
    Stage IIB   Cutaneous tumors
Stage III   Generalized erythroderma with or without adenopathy but
                 without histologic involvement of lymph nodes or viscera
Stage IV   Histologic involvement of lymph nodes, blood, or viscera at
                 any cutaneous stage

5. **Prognosis.** About 90% of patients with stage IA survive >15 years with treatment; median survival is not different from age-matched controls. Median survival time is 2 to 4 years from onset of tumor stage or lymph node involvement and <2 years from visceral involvement.

6. **Topical treatment**
   a. **Topical corticosteroids** frequently achieve good responses.
   b. **Topical nitrogen mustard** is useful in the patches or plaque stages. It can be used for involved skin only or in a total body application. Cutaneous allergic reactions may develop.
   c. **Psoralen with ultraviolet light A (PUVA) or narrow band UVB** repeated 2 to 3 times a week is effective for the patch or plaque phase. Long-term benefits and side effects are poorly defined.
   d. **Bexarotene** (Targretin) gel is a retinoid that selectively binds to the retinoid X-receptor (RXR) family of retinoid receptors. The response rate of localized patch or plaque disease to the gel is >60%. Bexarotene is the only retinoid that has been approved for this indication.
   e. **Electron-beam RT** to the total skin is technically demanding but has produced durable remissions, particularly in early stages of disease. Local electron-beam RT can be used in the treatment of tumors, especially if they are few in number.

7. **Systemic chemotherapy and investigational approaches** have resulted in short-term responses without an effect on survival.
   a. **Systemic chemotherapy** is recommended only for patients with advanced disease. A variety of single agents (e.g., methotrexate, corticosteroids, alkylating agents, gemcitabine, etoposide, doxorubicin, pegylated liposomal doxorubicin) achieve temporary responses in 30% of patients. The purine analogs 2-deoxycoformycin (pentostatin), cladribine, and fludarabine have all also shown response rates of about 30%. Combination chemotherapy is advocated for those with disease transformation to large cell lymphoma.
   b. **Bexarotene** (Targretin) is an oral rexinoid that is approved in the treatment of CTCL. The most common side effects are hypertriglyceridemia, central hypothyroidism, and myelosuppression.
   c. **IFN-α** has response rates of 15% to 50% in MF/SS.
   d. **Denileukin diftitox** (DAB_{389}-IL-2, Ontak) is a fusion protein between IL-2 and diphtheria toxin that was approved for the treatment of CTCLs failing other treatments. Most common side effects include vascular capillary leak syndrome, abnormal liver function tests, and infusion reactions.
   e. **Antibody therapy.** Transient responses to monoclonal T-cell antibodies, such as alemtuzumab (Campath), have been observed in CTCL.
   f. **Extracorporeal photophoresis (ECP),** a systemic form of PUVA therapy, is an effective immunoadjuvant therapy for CTCL. The procedure involves exposure of leukapheresed mononuclear cells to a psoralen photoactivating agent and UVA *ex vivo* followed by reinfusion of the treated cells. ECP induces an anti-idiotype cytotoxic T-cell response against circulating tumor cells. ECP is most effective with the erythrodermic phase (SS) of CTCL.

g. **Vorinostat (Zolinza)** is an oral histone deacetylase inhibitor that has been approved for the treatment of the skin manifestations of CTCL. The most common sides effects are GI, thrombopenia, and constitutional.

C. **Primary CNS lymphoma (PCNSL)** is essentially always of high histologic grade (large cell, immunoblastic) and of B-cell origin. Lesions are primarily parenchymal and involve deep periventricular structures. Multiple lesions occur in 20% to 40% of cases. The leptomeninges are involved in 30% of cases at diagnosis and in most cases at autopsy.

1. **Etiology and epidemiology**
   a. PCNSL accounts for about 1% of brain tumors and 1% of extranodal lymphomas. The disease is associated with advanced age (>60 years), AIDS, drug-induced immunosuppression (e.g., for transplantation), and congenital immunodeficiency syndromes.
   b. PCNSL accounts for roughly 50% of all lymphomas seen in transplant recipients and occurs at a somewhat lower frequency in AIDS. In AIDS cases, PCNSL appears in a setting of severe CD4 depression, with counts frequently $<50/\mu L$.
   c. Relationship to EBV infection is suggested by discovery of the *EBV* genome in some cases of PCNSL arising in transplant recipients and AIDS patients.

2. **Clinical presentations** include headache, personality changes, and hemiparesis. Symptoms of meningeal infiltration or spinal cord compression are less common. Associated systemic lymphoma is rare. Ocular lymphoma (appearing as uveitis) may precede or follow the diagnosis of CNS lymphoma. PCNSL complicating AIDS is associated with a median survival time of <3 months.

3. **Evaluation.** The diagnosis can usually be made with stereotactic biopsy and without formal surgical exploration.
   a. **Brain CT scan.** Deep periventricular lesions often involve the corpus callosum, basal ganglia, or thalamus and often appear hyperdense before contrast dye injection. Contrast often produces generalized intense enhancement, unlike the picture of gliomas and metastases. In AIDS patients, the precontrast scan may be hypodense.
   b. **Brain MRI** may reveal additional lesions not seen by CT scan.
   c. **Lumbar puncture.** Nonspecific elevation of cerebrospinal fluid (CSF) protein is common. Abnormal cells may be found in 25% to 35% of patients undergoing lumbar puncture at diagnosis. Identification of malignant cells may be enhanced by immunofluorescent techniques with monoclonal antibodies.
   d. Ophthalmologic examination, including slit-lamp examination
   e. HIV antibody; HIV titer if positive
   f. Enumeration of the CD4 count
   g. Abdominal CT scan, chest radiograph
   h. Bone marrow biopsy

4. **Therapy**
   a. **Corticosteroids** are extremely effective in PCNSL. Lesions may disappear on steroids alone and preclude histologic diagnosis after steroids are given.
   b. **Whole-brain RT (WBRT)** was previously the preferred treatment for PCNSL. Doses of 4,000 to 5,000 cGy appear necessary, with 1,000 to 1,500 cGy focal boost to the tumor bed. However, WBRT is associated with severe delayed neurotoxicity. Up to 90% of patients over 60 years of age develop totally debilitating dementia, gait ataxia, and urinary dysfunction within 1 year of treatment, if they survive. Delayed treatment-related cerebrovascular disease, alone or in combination with progressive leukoencephalopathy, has been observed in younger patients 7 to 10 years after WBRT.
   c. **Chemotherapy** with high doses of methotrexate (>3 g/m^2) has become the preferred treatment because it improves disease-free survival significantly and because it is not associated with the high rate of neurotoxicity from combined-modality treatment. The response rate to high doses of methotrexate is 70% to 95%, with an expected 2-year survival rate of 60% and median survival of 32 months. Relapses are treated with WBRT and/or salvage

chemotherapy. Intrathecal chemotherapy is not given unless CSF cytology is positive.

D. Primary gastrointestinal lymphoma (PGL) is the most common form of solitary extranodal disease and may occur in the stomach, small bowel, and large bowel.

1. **Associated diseases.** The incidence of enteropathy-type T-cell lymphoma is increased in patients with ulcerative colitis, regional enteritis, or celiac disease. α-Heavy-chain disease is present in some patients with the Mediterranean type of PGL. MALToma of the stomach is associated with *H. pylori* infection.

2. **Histopathology.** PGL may originate from either T cells or B cells. MALToma, follicular lymphoma, MCL, or other aggressive lymphomas may be found anywhere along the GI tract. B-cell PGL tends to present at lower stages, have fewer complications, and have a better prognosis than T-cell PGL.

3. **Symptoms and physical findings.** Anorexia, nausea, vomiting, weight loss, GI bleeding, or abdominal pain is present in most patients. An abdominal mass may be present, but peripheral lymphadenopathy is not common.

4. **Complications.** Obstruction may complicate the course of PGL. Perforation or hemorrhage may be either a presenting sign or a complication of treatment for PGL. Therapy can cause perforation by the lysis of the lymphoma's involvement of the full thickness of the wall of the organ involved.

5. **Diagnosis.** Endoscopy or barium contrast radiographs usually show large mucosal folds, ulceration, masses, lumen narrowing, or annular strictures. Gastric lymphomas may be indistinguishable from peptic ulcer by both radiologic and endoscopic criteria. Undifferentiated carcinoma or adenocarcinoma of the GI tract may be confused with intermediate/high-grade lymphoma even after expert histologic evaluation; immunohistochemical verification of diagnosis is mandatory. Multiple sites of involvement should be excluded by barium follow-through or endoscopy.

6. **Management of PGL**

   a. **Surgical management.** Laparotomy may be needed to establish the diagnosis or treat complications. Resection of bowel should be considered in cases with solitary lesions, intractable bleeding, or high risk of perforation. Subtotal gastrectomy for gastric lymphoma is rarely performed.

   b. **Medical management** should be based on histologic subtype and extent of disease. Intermediate/high-grade lesions are treated primarily with combination chemotherapy, such as CHOP. The 2-year survival after CHOP is better than 90% for B-cell PGL and 25% to 35% for T-cell PGL.

7. **Gastric MALToma.** *H. pylori*–associated MALToma of the stomach usually has low-grade histology. Occasionally, transformation to a large-cell lymphoma may occur. Significant mucosal thickening may be present before spread to regional or distant nodes. *H. pylori* can usually be found in endoscopic biopsies.

   a. **Treatment of *H. pylori*.** MALToma usually regresses after eradication of *H. pylori*. At least a 70% CR is expected but may be observed up to 6 months after treatment. A t(11;18) translocation is a predictor for no response to antibiotic therapy. The following 2-week regimen can be used for *H. pylori* (amoxicillin may be used instead of metronidazole in case of intolerance):

   Clarithromycin (Biaxin), 500 mg b.i.d.
   Metronidazole (Flagyl), 500 mg b.i.d.
   Omeprazole (Prilosec), 20 mg b.i.d.

   b. **Antineoplastic therapy.** Patients with a large-cell component, deeply penetrating disease, or with metastatic disease are not expected to respond to antimicrobial therapy. IFRT is used for disease localized to the stomach (3,000 to 3,300 cGy). Gastrectomy is probably not superior to RT for local control and has been abandoned. Rituximab can also be used if RT is contraindicated. Systemic chemotherapy is used for more advanced disease that is symptomatic or bulky.

E. Burkitt lymphoma (BL) is a specific subtype of the small, noncleaved cell, high-grade NHL. The cells in BL are very uniform with round or oval nuclei, two to

TABLE 21.7 Clinical Features of Burkitt Lymphoma

Feature	Endemic (Africa)	Sporadic
Association with Epstein-Barr virus	Yes	Rarely
Chromosomal translocation	t(8;14), common	t(8;14), common
Sites of involvement	Jaw, orbit	Abdomen, gastrointestinal tract, marrow
Lymph node involvement	Rarely	Not infrequently
Therapy	50% prolonged survival rate with cyclophosphamide	Requires multiple agents
Relapse	Survival possible	Guarded prognosis

five prominent nucleoli, and cytoplasm rich in RNA. The cells are of B lineage, expressing monoclonal surface IgM with *c-myc* overexpression. A consistent series of cytogenetic translocations (Table 21.6) and explosive growth characterizes BL.

1. **Epidemiology and etiology**
   a. BL is endemic in certain regions of equatorial Africa and other tropical locations. A sporadic form of BL occurs in the United States and throughout the world. The disease occurs predominantly in childhood but can be seen in young adults, particularly in the sporadic form.
   b. EBV has been found in the genome of endemic BL but rarely in the sporadic form. Very high EBV antibody titers are seen in the endemic form.
2. **Clinical features** of BL are shown in Table 21.7.
3. **Staging system.** A variety of systems have been proposed. The NCI system is as follows:

Stage	Disease distribution
A	Single solitary extra-abdominal site
AR	Intra-abdominal: >90% of tumor resected
B	Multiple extra-abdominal sites
C	Intra-abdominal tumor
D	Intra-abdominal plus one or more extra-abdominal sites

4. **Prognosis.** Before effective treatment, only 30% of sporadic cases survived. Using combination chemotherapy and CNS prophylaxis, the survival rate is at least 60%. Children and young adults with limited stage (A, AR, B) disease have an excellent prognosis with a 90% survival rate. Bone marrow and CNS involvement carry a poor prognosis. Adult cases of BL, particularly those of advanced stage, do more poorly than childhood cases.
5. **Treatment**
   a. Cyclophosphamide therapy alone has been curative for many localized presentations in Africa.
   b. Multiagent, aggressive regimens are necessary for the sporadic form as well as for Burkitt-like NHL. One such program would be hyper-CVAD with or without rituximab. Another appropriate treatment alternates two cycles of CODOX-M with two cycles of IVAC (see Appendix D-2, section III) in patients with Burkitt-like NHL, with excellent results. Low-risk patients (those with normal LDH and complete resection of an abdominal tumor or single extraabdominal mass) may be treated with CODOX-M alone combined with intrathecal prophylaxis. *CHOP is not adequate therapy for this group of patients.*
   c. Because of the extremely rapid growth rate, massive acute destruction of tumor with initial chemotherapy usually results in tumor lysis syndrome and mandates prophylaxis for tumor lysis syndrome when the patient is initially treated (see Chapter 27, section XIII).

Suggested Reading

Hodgkin Lymphoma

Aleman BMP, et al. Involved-field radiotherapy for advanced Hodgkin's lymphoma. *N Engl J Med* 2003;348:2396.

Bonnadonna G, et al. ABVD plus subtotal nodal versus involved–field radiotherapy in early-stage Hodgkins disease: long-term results. *J Clin Oncol* 2004;22:2285.

Canellos GP, et al. Chemotherapy of advanced Hodgkin's disease with MOPP, ABVD, or MOPP alternating with ABVD. *N Engl J Med* 1992;327:1478.

Diehl V, et al. HD10: Investigating reduction of combined modality treatment intensity in early stage Hodgkin's lymphoma. Interim analysis of a randomized trial of the German Hodgkin Study Group. *J Clin Oncol* 2005;23:561S.

Diehl V, et al. Standard and increased-dose BEACOPP chemotherapy compared with COPP–ABVD for advanced Hodgkin's disease. *N Engl J Med* 2003;348:2386.

Dores GM, et al. Second malignant neoplasms among long-term survivors of Hodgkin's disease: a population-based evaluation over 25 years. *J Clin Oncol* 2002;20:3484.

Hasenclever D, et al. A prognostic score for advanced Hodgkin's disease. *N Engl J Med* 1998;339:1506.

Loeffler M, et al. Dose response relationship of complementary radiotherapy following 4 cycles of combination chemotherapy in intermediate stage Hodgkin's disease. *J Clin Oncol* 1997;15:2275.

Meyer RM, et al. Randomized comparison of ABVD chemotherapy with a strategy that includes radiation therapy in patients with limited-stage Hodgkin's lymphoma: National Cancer Institute of Canada Clinical Trials Group and the Eastern Cooperative Oncology Group. *J Clin Oncol* 2005;23:4634.

Non-Hodgkin Lymphoma

Armitage JO, et al. New approaches to classifying non-Hodgkin lymphomas: clinical features of the major histologic subtypes. *J Clin Oncol* 1998;16:2780.

Browne WB, et al. The management of unicentric and multicentric Castleman's disease: a report of 16 cases and a review of the literature. *Cancer* 1999;85:706.

Coiffier B, et al. CHOP chemotherapy plus rituximab compared with CHOP alone in elderly patients with diffuse large-B-cell lymphoma. *N Engl J Med* 2002;346:235.

Daum S, et al. Intestinal non-Hodgkin's lymphoma: a multicenter prospective clinical study from the German Study Group on intestinal non-Hodgkin's lymphoma. *J Clin Oncol* 2003;21:2740.

DeAngelis LM. Primary central nervous system lymphoma: a curable brain tumor. *J Clin Oncol* 2003;21:4471.

DeAngelis LM, Iwamoto FM. An update on therapy of primary central nervous system lymphoma. *Hematology (Am Soc Hematol Educ Program)* 2006;311.

Feugier P, et al. BCL2 expression is a prognostic factor for the activated B-cell like type of diffuse large B-cell lymphoma: a study by the Groupe d'Etude des Lymphomes de l'Adulte. *J Clin Oncol* 2005;23:4117.

Fisher RI, et al. New treatment options have changed the survival of patients with follicular lymphoma. *J Clin Oncol* 2005;23:8447.

Habermann TM, et al. Rituximab-CHOP with or without maintenance rituximab in patients 60 years of age or older with diffuse large B-cell lymphoma (DLBCL). An update. *J Clin Oncol* 2006;24:3121.

Iqbel J, et al. BCL2 expression is a prognostic factor for the activated B-cell-like type of diffuse large B-cell lymphoma. *J Clin Oncol* 2006;24:961.

Jaffe ES, Harris NL, Stein H, et al. World Health Organization Classification of Tumors. Pathology and genetics of tumors of hematopoietic and lymphoid tissue. Lyon, France: IARC; 2001.

Khouri IF, et al. Hyper-CVAD and high-dose methotrexate/cytarabine followed by stem-cell transplantation: an active regimen for aggressive mantle-cell lymphoma. *J Clin Oncol* 1998;16:3803.

Liu Q, et al. Improvement of overall and failure-free survival in stage IV follicular lymphoma: 25 years of treatment experience at the University of Texas M.D. Anderson Cancer Center. *J Clin Oncol* 2006;24:1582.

Marcus R, et al. CVP chemotherapy plus rituximab compared with CVP as first-line treatment for advanced follicular lymphoma. *Blood* 2005;105:1417.

McClain KL, Natkunam Y, Swerdlow SH. Atypical cellular disorders. *Hematology (Am Soc Hematol Educ Program)* 2004;283.

Montoto S, et al. Risk and clinical implications of transformation of follicular lymphoma to diffuse large B-cell lymphoma. *J Clin Oncol* 2007;25:2426.

Rosenwald A, et al. The use of molecular profiling to predict survival after chemotherapy for diffuse large-B-cell lymphoma. *N Engl J Med* 2002;346:1937.

Sehn LH, et al. The revised International Prognostic Index (R-IPI) is a better predictor of outcome than the standard IPI for patients with diffuse large B-cell lymphoma treated with R-CHOP. *Blood* 2007;109:1857.

Solal-Celigny P, et al. Follicular lymphoma international prognostic index. *Blood* 2004;104:1258.

Van Oers MHJ, et al. Chimeric antii-CD20 monoclonal antibody (rituximab; mabthera) in remission induction and maintenance treatment of relapsed/resistant follicular non-Hodgkin's lymphoma. Final analysis of a Phase III randomized Intergroup clinical trial. *Blood* 2005;106:107a.

Willemze R, et al. WHO-EORTC classification for cutaneous lymphomas. *Blood* 2005; 105:3768.

Wilson WH, et al. The role of rituximab and chemotherapy in aggressive B-cell lymphoma: a preliminary report of dose-adjusted EPOCH-R. *Semin Oncol* 2002;1(Suppl 2):41.

Winter JN, et al. Prognostic significance of Bcl-6 protein expression in DLBCL treated with CHOP or R-CHOP: a prospective correlative study. *Blood* 2006;107:4207.

Witzig TE, et al. Randomized controlled trial of Yttrium-90-labeled ibritumomab tiuxetan radioimmunotherapy versus rituximab immunotherapy for patients with relapsed or refractory low-grade, follicular, or transformed B-cell non-Hodgkin's lymphoma. *J Clin Oncol* 2002;20:2453.

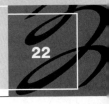

PLASMA CELL DYSCRASIAS AND WALDENSTRÖM'S MACROGLOBULINEMIA

James R. Berenson and Dennis A. Casciato

22

Immunoglobulins are produced by B lymphocytes and plasma cells. Properties of normal serum immunoglobulins are shown in Table 22.1. A clone of cells producing immunoglobulins may proliferate to sufficient mass that a monoclonal protein (M-protein or paraprotein) is detectable as a peak or "spike" on serum protein electrophoresis (PEP). The "M" in M-protein can stand for monoclonal, myeloma, macroglobulinemia, or the M-like appearance of the serum PEP graph. These disorders are included in the World Health Organization's classification of neoplastic diseases of lymphoid tissues (Appendix C-6). Their immunohistochemistry phenotypes are shown in Appendix C-5.

I. EPIDEMIOLOGY AND ETIOLOGY

- **A. Classification** of diseases associated with monoclonal paraproteinemia
  1. **Plasma cell neoplasms**
     a. Multiple myeloma (MM)
     b. Amyloidosis
     c. Heavy-chain disease
     d. Papular mucinosis
  2. **Other neoplastic diseases**
     a. Waldenström's macroglobulinemia (WM)
     b. Malignant B-cell non-Hodgkin lymphoma, chronic lymphocytic leukemia (CLL)
     c. Neoplasms of cell types not known to synthesize immunoglobulins (solid tumors, monocytic leukemia, myelodysplastic syndromes)
  3. **Non-neoplastic disorders**
     a. Monoclonal gammopathy of undetermined significance (MGUS)
     b. Autoimmune diseases (e.g., systemic lupus erythematosus)
     c. Hepatobiliary disease
     d. Chronic inflammatory diseases
     e. Immunodeficiency syndromes
     f. Miscellaneous diseases (e.g., Gaucher's disease)
     g. Pseudoparaproteinemia (see section IX.C)
- **B. Incidence.** MGUS, MM, and WM are the most common disorders associated with M-proteins. The average age at the time of diagnosis is 60 years, and the incidence increases with age.
  1. **MGUS** (formerly *benign monoclonal gammopathy*). The approximate incidence of MGUS is 0.2% for patients 25 to 49 years of age, 2% for those 50 to 79 years of age, and 10% for those 80 to 90 years of age.
  2. **MM** develops in 3/100,000 population and constitutes 1% of new cancer cases in the United States. The average age is 62 years and >75% of patients are >70 years of age. Men and women are affected about equally. MM is the most common lymphohematopoietic malignancy in blacks.
  3. **WM** has an incidence that is about 5% to 10% of that of MM. Two-thirds of cases occur in men.
  4. **Lymphomas.** Excluding MGUS, MM, and WM, about half of the patients with monoclonal gammopathies have lymphocytic lymphoma or CLL. The M-protein is nearly always either IgM or IgG and usually causes no symptoms. Patients

| **TABLE 22.1** | Normal Human Serum Immunoglobulins |

Ig (heavy chain)	MW (×1,000)	t₁/₂ (days)	Portion of Ig (%)	IV (%)
IgG[a] (γ)	150	20	75	52
IgA (α)	160	6	15	55
IgM (μ)	900	5	10	75
IgD (δ)	180	3	0.2	75
IgE (ε)	190	3	0.005	40

Ig, immunoglobulin; IV, proportion of Ig distributed intravascularly; MW, molecular weight; $t_{1/2}$, half-life.
[a]Four subclasses comprise IgG. About 70% of IgG is IgG₁, 17% is IgG₂, 8% is IgG₃, and 5% is IgG₄. The data shown apply to all subtypes except IgG₃. IgG₃ differs from the other subclasses in that 65% is distributed intravascularly, its serum half-life is 7 days and is not affected by high serum concentrations, it most avidly binds complement (other subclasses do so weakly, if at all), and it is most likely to produce hyperviscosity.

with other types of lymphoma do not have an increased incidence of monoclonal proteins.

C. Etiology. No specific etiologic agent for the plasma cell dyscrasias has been found. Predisposing factors in humans appear to be the following:

1. **Radiation exposure,** which slightly increases the risk for MM
2. **Chronic antigen stimulation.** Many M-proteins have been shown to be antibodies directed against specific antigens, such as microbial antigens, red blood cell antigens, neural antigens, lipoproteins, rheumatoid factors, and coagulation factors. Chronic antigenic stimulation (e.g., chronic osteomyelitis or cholecystitis) may predispose to the development of MM or MGUS. Patients with autoimmune disease may be at high risk for MM. A recent case-controlled study suggests that female patients who have had silicone gel breast implants also may be at high risk for MM.
3. **Environmental exposure.** Exposure to benzene in the workplace and the use of hair dye are associated with an increased incidence of MM. Farmworkers have been shown to be at high risk for MM in several epidemiologic studies. The role of pesticides as a possible etiologic factor has not been determined, however.
4. **Human herpesvirus 8 (HHV-8)** has been found in the nonmalignant bone marrow dendritic cells of patients with myeloma. It remains to be determined if HHV-8 contributes to the growth of the malignant plasma cells in these patients.

D. Cytogenetics

1. **MM.** Multiple, complex karyotypic changes are observed in the malignant plasma cells of most patients. Fluorescent *in situ* hybridization (FISH) analysis has shown that most patients with MM have malignant cells with translocations involving chromosome 14 at the site of the immunoglobulin heavy-chain gene locus and a limited number of nonimmunoglobulin partner chromosomes. Unlike the site of translocation in other B-cell malignancies that involves the joining region JH, the location of the breakpoint in myeloma usually occurs in the switch regions that are involved in heavy-chain class switching from Cμ to another heavy-chain class.

   a. The most common sites of the nonimmunoglobulin breakpoints include chromosomes 11 at the site of cyclin D, chromosome 16 at the site of the c-*MAF* proto-oncogene, and chromosome 4 at the site of the fibroblastic growth factor receptor 3. Loss of material on the long arm of chromosome 13 occurs in nearly 20% of patients. The presence of specific chromosomal abnormalities has prognostic value in MM.

   b. Mutations of *ras* genes occur in about 20% of myelomas and are associated with a poor prognosis. Similarly, mutations of *p53* are found in 15% to

20% of cases and are associated with more advanced and clinically aggressive disease. Abnormalities in c-*MYC* proto-oncogene may occur much more commonly than was previously suggested.

   c. Gene-expression profiling has identified specific subgroups of patients with MM. These studies have suggested a markedly different outcome depending on the expression of specific genes. These profiles also may predict responsiveness to specific therapies.

   d. Telomerase activity and telomere length, indicators of the aging of specific cells, are directly related to the type of myeloma as well as to the outcome among patients. Patients with higher telomerase activity and shorter telomere length tend to have a poor prognosis.

   2. MGUS. Studies have shown that patients with MGUS have similar karyotypic abnormalities to patients with MM.

   3. WM. Complex karyotypes are also commonly observed in WM. Occasional patients have translocations involving the immunoglobulin heavy-chain locus on chromosome 14 and either c-*MYC* on chromosome 8 or *BCL-2* on chromosome 18.

II. PATHOLOGY AND NATURAL HISTORY

   A. Bone marrow pathology is usually distinctive in MM and WM. Plasma cells that constitute >20% of the nucleated marrow cells (*excluding erythroblasts*) are characteristic but not diagnostic of MM.

   1. MGUS. Normal plasma cells rarely exceed 10% of bone marrow cells.

   2. MM. Plasma cells usually constitute 20% to 95% of the marrow cells; they have abundant basophilic cytoplasm and eccentric nuclei with paranuclear clear zones. Immaturity of the plasma cells is evident with the presence of prominent nucleoli ("myeloma cells"). Bone marrow biopsy showing monotonous infiltration with plasma cells is the only diagnostic criterion for MM accepted by many authorities. The presence of large, homogeneous infiltrates or nodules of plasma cells is highly suggestive of MM. Early in its course, however, marrow involvement is patchy, and normal marrow particles may be obtained.

   3. WM may closely resemble CLL. Bone marrow in WM contains 10% to 90% plasmacytoid lymphocytes or small mature lymphocytes; mast cells are often prominent.

   4. Reactive plasmacytosis. Peripheral blood plasmacytosis occurs in many viral illnesses (including human immunodeficiency virus [HIV] infection), serum sickness, and plasma cell leukemia (which is rare). Bone marrow plasmacytosis, when not caused by myeloma, is characterized by a diffuse distribution (not infiltrative) and alignment of mature plasma cells along blood vessels or near marrow reticulum cells. Reactive bone marrow plasmacytosis is commonly seen in many disorders, including the following:

   a. Viral infections
   b. Serum sickness
   c. Collagen vascular disease
   d. Granulomatous disease
   e. Liver cirrhosis
   f. Neoplastic disease
   g. Marrow hypoplasia

   B. Natural history of MGUS. MGUS occurs in nearly 5% of individuals over the age of 70. Although these individuals are symptom-free at diagnosis, nearly 25% of cases progress to a malignant disorder (usually MM) over 8 to 10 years. Importantly, the risk for malignancy remains constant over time (~1%/year). The risk of developing MM from MGUS is directly related to the size of the monoclonal peak. The number of circulating monoclonal plasma cells may also predict for a higher risk of developing MM. Some studies suggest that patients with MGUS are at higher risk of developing accelerated bone loss and fractures, especially of the vertebral bodies.

1. **Karyotypic abnormalities** in these patients are similar to those seen with MM.
2. **The presence of depressed normal immunoglobulin levels** occurs in many patients with MGUS, but is not associated with a higher risk for infection and does not predict a higher risk for malignancy.
3. **Peripheral neuropathy** is not uncommon and may be associated with a monoclonal antibody with reactivity to a myelin-associated glycoprotein (see section IX.B).

C. **Natural history of WM.** The natural history of WM resembles lymphocytic lymphoma much more than MM. Indeed, separating WM from MGUS, CLL, or lymphocytic lymphoma with IgM spikes may be more arbitrary than real. WM originates from clones of lymphocytes or plasma cells that synthesize μ chains.

Lymphadenopathy, splenomegaly, and hyperviscosity are hallmarks of WM; skeletal lesions and impaired renal function are unusual. Concomitant macroglobulinemia and osteolytic lesions usually signify malignant lymphoma or solid tumor rather than primary WM. Glomerular lesions are frequent in WM, but renal failure is uncommon. Low levels of light chains in the urine occur in about 25% of patients.

D. **Natural history of MM.** Three to 20 years of clonal growth may pass before MM becomes clinically evident. The disease may be localized (7% of cases), indolent (3%), or disseminated and progressive (90%). Manifestations of disease progression arise from bone marrow and skeletal involvement, plasma protein abnormalities, and the development of renal disease.

1. **Hematopoiesis** is often impaired. At the time of diagnosis, 60% of patients have anemia; 15%, leukopenia; and 15%, thrombocytopenia. Nucleated red blood cells and immature granulocytes may be present in the peripheral blood (leukoerythroblastic reaction).

2. **Plasmacytomas** (plasma cell tumors) may develop anywhere in the skeleton or, rarely, in extraskeletal sites, such as the nasopharynx or paranasal sinuses. Localized plasmacytomas produce a monoclonal spike in the serum or urine protein electrophoresis in only half of the cases. The median survival is >8 years. Most plasmacytomas that appear to be solitary become generalized in about 3 years, particularly those involving the skeleton. Extraskeletal plasmacytomas have a better prognosis than those of skeletal origin and less frequently progress to multiple myeloma.

3. **Skeletal disease in MM**

   a. **Osteolytic lesions.** Multiple osteolytic lesions are present in about 70% of patients, single osteolytic lesions or diffuse osteoporosis in 15%, and normal skeletal radiographs in 15%. Lesions are most commonly seen in the skull, vertebrae, ribs, pelvis, and proximal long bones. The use of MRI indicates that skeletal abnormalities exist in nearly all patients with myeloma.

   Previously it was thought that the demineralization and lytic lesions occur as a result of osteoclastic-activating factors and osteoblastic-inhibitory factors produced by neoplastic plasma cells and activated by inflammatory cytokines. The loss of bone in these patients, however, now appears to be a complex interplay involving the tumor cells, stromal cells in the bone marrow, and both the osteoblasts and osteoclasts. The factors responsible involve other important molecules, including macrophage colony-stimulating factor, vascular endothelial growth factor, specific matrix metalloproteinases, and the receptor for activation of nuclear factor-κB (NF-κB). The latter receptor is designated as "*RANK*" and is coupled with RANK ligand (RANKL) to comprise the RANKL-RANK signaling pathway.

   (1) **RANK–RANKL proteins** play a key role in the development of myeloma bone disease. Increased levels of RANKL have been found in myeloma bone marrow and are associated with enhanced bone loss.

   (2) **Osteoprotegerin (OPG),** the natural soluble decoy inhibitor of RANKL–RANK signaling, is decreased in MM bone marrow and blood. Blockade of RANKL prevents skeletal lesions in animal models of MM.

(3) **The chemokine macrophage inflammatory protein (MIP1-α)** also appears to play a key role in myeloma bone disease. MIP1-α is elevated in myeloma bone marrow; it is associated with increased bone loss and may stimulate myeloma cell growth.

(4) **Dickkopf1 (DKK1),** an inhibitor of osteoblast development and function, also has an important role in myeloma bone disease. Levels of DKK1 are elevated in the blood and bone marrow from patients with myeloma compared with normal subjects. The inhibition of osteoblast function ultimately leads to a loss of bone formation and enhanced bone loss.

b. **Osteoblastic lesions** occur in <2% of patients, often in association with neuropathy and the POEMS syndrome. Because of their rarity, the diagnosis of MM should be doubted in the presence of osteoblastic lesions.

c. **POEMS syndrome** is a multisystem disorder usually associated with osteo-sclerotic myeloma. It is characterized by the combination of **p**olyneuropathy (chronic inflammatory demyelinating neuropathy), **o**rganomegaly, **e**ndocrinopathy, **M**-protein (mainly IgG-γ or IgA-γ), and **s**kin changes (hyperpigmentation, thickening, hypertrichosis). Various other signs, such as cachexia, fever, edema, clubbing, and telangiectasia, can also occur. Autoantibodies to peripheral nerve components are absent. The syndrome appears to be the result of marked activation of the proinflammatory cytokines. Patients with POEMS syndrome, particularly those associated with Castleman's disease, have been found to contain HHV-8.

d. **Hypercalcemia.** About 10% of patients with MM present with hypercalcemia, and 10% develop it during the course of their disease. This complication results from enhanced bone resorption, resulting in the release of calcium into the circulation. Hypercalcemia is a major cause of renal failure among patients with MM, and normalization of the serum calcium often reverses the renal dysfunction. It is important to avoid bedrest and immobilization because these factors can contribute to both the development and worsening of hypercalcemia. Serum alkaline phosphatase levels are usually normal, but may be increased with recalcification of fractures.

4. **Protein abnormalities**
   a. **Frequency.** The incidence of monoclonal immunoglobulins in MM and in comparison to MGUS is shown in Table 22.2.
   b. **Increased excretion of κ or λ light chains in the urine** depends on the rate of unbalanced synthesis of excess light chains, plasma volume, degradation rate, renal catabolism, and urine volume. Monoclonal light chains in the urine are present in two-thirds of all patients with MM and present without an M-protein in the serum in 25%.
   c. **Serum free light chains** are identified among many patients with so-called nonsecretory disease.
   d. **Normal immunoglobulins** are usually decreased in the serum of patients with MM and are occasionally decreased in patients with MGUS. The

TABLE 22.2 **Frequency of Monoclongal Immunoglobulins in MM and MGUS**

M-protein	MM	MGUS
IgG	52%	65%
IgA	22%	25%
IgM	Very rare	10%
Light chains only	25%	Nil
Nonsecretory	<1 %	—

MM, multiple myeloma; MGUS, monoclonal gammopathy of undetermined significance.

mechanism of inhibition of their synthesis is unknown. Older series showed a high rate of infection with encapsulated organisms that was thought related to patients' marked decrease in normal serum immunoglobulins. The risk for infection, however, largely occurs during chemotherapy-induced neutropenia or at the terminal stages of the disease.

e. Other plasma alterations (see section IX.A). Hyperviscosity is unusual in MM (<5% of patients).

5. **Renal dysfunction,** both acute and chronic, occurs at diagnosis in 15% to 20% of cases and develops during their course in most patients with MM. Patients with MM secreting only light chains commonly present with renal failure. The most important causes of renal dysfunction in these patients are hypercalcemia and myeloma kidney.

a. Myeloma kidney is generally attributed to the deposition of κ and λ chains in the distal and collecting tubules, which is where the light chains are catabolized. The tubules dilate, apparently obstructed by casts surrounded by multinucleated giant cells, and undergo cellular atrophy. Glomerular basement membrane disease also occurs in most patients with myeloma kidney. In most instances, proteinuria contains monoclonal light chains only. These abnormalities occur slightly more commonly in MM associated with λ-chain production.

Malignant myeloma is the most common cause of the **adult Fanconi's syndrome** (aminoaciduria, glycosuria, phosphaturia, and electrolyte loss in the urine). Fanconi's syndrome may precede the recognition of MM by many years.

b. Amyloidosis also develops commonly in MM. It affects the glomeruli and results in nonselective proteinuria.

c. Inconstant findings that may aggravate renal function include pyelonephritis, metabolic abnormalities in addition to hypercalcemia (nephrocalcinosis and hyperuricemia), glomerulosclerosis, and focal myeloma cell infiltration. Renal tubular acidosis occasionally occurs. Nephrotic syndrome is rare in MM unless amyloidosis supervenes. Recent studies suggest, however, that chronic administration of IV pamidronate may also be associated with nephrotic syndrome (see below).

d. Intravenous contrast-dye studies should be done with caution (if at all) because patients with MM are more susceptible to renal dysfunction after such studies, particularly if they are dehydrated.

6. **Neurologic dysfunction** often develops in MM and is the result of several pathogenetic mechanisms.

a. Central nervous system (CNS). Spinal cord and nerve root compression develops in about 15% of patients and is usually caused by epidural plasmacytoma. Amyloidosis is a rare cause of epidural masses. Collapse of vertebral bodies can also cause spinal cord compression but, more likely, produces radicular symptoms secondary to nerve root compression. Cranial nerve palsies can develop from tumor occlusion of calvarial foramina. Intracerebral and meningeal plasmacytomas are rare. With the longer survival of myeloma patients, meningeal myeloma, however, seems to be occurring more frequently than had been previously observed.

b. Peripheral neuropathy. The carpal tunnel syndrome, which is usually the result of amyloid infiltration of the flexor retinaculum of the wrist (causing entrapment of the median nerve), is a common peripheral neuropathy in MM. Infiltration of nerve fibers and vasa nervorum with amyloid can also produce peripheral neuropathy. Additionally, peripheral neuropathy may be associated with monoclonal immunoglobulins to myelin-associated glycoproteins (see section IX.B). Rarely, patients with MM and POEMS syndrome develop a characteristic peripheral neuropathy. The most common cause of peripheral neuropathy in patients with MM is from treatment with drugs such as thalidomide, bortezomib, or arsenic trioxide.

c. Neurologic paraneoplastic syndromes (see Chapter 32, section V).

III. DIAGNOSIS

A. **Symptoms.** Fatigue, weakness, and weight loss are common in both MM and WM.

  1. **Skeletal pain** occurs in 70% of patients with MM at the time of diagnosis but is rare in patients with WM.

  2. **Symptoms of hypercalcemia** (see Chapter 27, section I) are present in about 10% of patients with MM at the time of diagnosis and develop in another 10% later in the course of the disease.

  3. **Hyperviscosity syndrome symptoms** (bleeding, neurologic dysfunction, visual disturbances, or congestive heart failure) are present in about 50% of patients with WM and in less <5% of patients with MM (see section IX.A.1).

  4. **Cold sensitivity** may occur in patients with cryoglobulins, especially in WM (see section IX.A.2).

B. **Physical findings**

  1. **Hepatosplenomegaly** is present in 40% of patients with WM at the time of diagnosis and is uncommon in MM except with the POEMS variant.

  2. **Lymphadenopathy** occurs in 30% of patients with WM but is rare in patients with MM except late in the disease.

  3. **Bone tenderness** in patients with MM often signifies recent fracture or subperiosteal infiltration with malignant cells.

  4. **Neurologic abnormalities** are frequent in MM; neurologic abnormalities in WM are caused by hyperviscosity or demyelination.

  5. **Purpura** signifies thrombocytopenia in MM and hyperviscosity syndrome in WM. Occasionally, patients with MM will develop coagulopathies associated with purpura.

C. **Laboratory studies.** The following studies should be obtained in the investigation of patients with suspected plasma cell neoplasms:

  1. **Routine studies:** CBC, blood urea nitrogen, creatinine, electrolytes; calcium, albumin, and total protein

  2. **Serum proteins** evaluated with PEP, immunoelectrophoresis (IEP), and quantitative immunoglobulins (QIG). Because of the inherent variability of results of these tests, it is critical to perform both of these tests in diagnosing and following response to therapy. The following assays are also useful:

     a. **Serum β_2-microglobulin ($\beta2m$)** reflects tumor mass and is a standard measure of tumor burden in MM.

     b. **C-reactive protein (CRP)** is a surrogate marker for interleukin-6 (IL-6), which is a prime stimulator of myeloma growth.

     c. **Lactic dehydrogenase (LDH),** which may be a measure of tumor burden in lymphomalike or plasmablastic myeloma

     d. **Serum viscosity,** if hyperviscosity is suspected.

     e. **Free light chains** may be measured in the serum, especially among patients with "nonsecretory disease" or with changing renal function among patients with only the presence of urinary paraprotein (see below).

  3. **Urine light chains.** Twenty-four–hour excretion of protein and PEP and IEP of a specimen concentrated 100- to 200-fold (urine dipsticks are usually not sufficiently sensitive to detect light chains, and Bence-Jones protein assays are unreliable). About 20% of patients with MM have urinary M-proteins only, and 20% to 30% of patients will show the presence of both serum and urine M-protein. It is important to measure both the urine and the serum M-proteins on an ongoing basis to determine the patient's response to treatment.

     Approximately 1% to 2% of patients with myeloma do not show the presence of serum or urine M-protein. This occurrence appears to result largely from aberrant rearrangements of the immunoglobulin genes that normally produce antibodies in the malignant plasma cells.

  4. **Bone marrow aspiration and biopsy** are necessary to establish the diagnosis. Bone marrow findings are discussed in section II.A. Flow cytometry may help confirm the diagnosis. Cytogenetic studies may detect abnormalities. Biopsy of

a solitary osteolytic lesion, masses, skin nodules, or enlarged lymph nodes may be necessary in selected cases.

Because myeloma can be a "patchy disease" in the bone marrow, there is marked heterogeneity in different parts of the bone marrow in terms of the percentage of tumor involvement. It is important to recognize that the use of the bone marrow aspirate and biopsy to establish the severity or progression of the patient's MM is of limited use.

5. Evaluation of the skeleton

    a. Complete skeletal radiographic survey, including skull and long bones, is required in all patients suspected of having MM.

    b. MRI of the spine may be necessary in some patients if there is a paraspinal mass or signs of cord or nerve root compression or solitary plasmacytoma of bone. This will determine if there is spinal cord involvement and can help to determine the extent of myeloma involvement in the spine. It has become more important to evaluate the spine accurately with the development of several surgical techniques that help immensely in controlling back pain caused by compression fractures from bone loss in patients with MM.

    c. Computed tomography scan (avoiding the use of contrast dyes) for evaluation of suspected extradural extraosseous plasmacytoma

    d. Positron emission tomography (PET) scans occasionally may be helpful to evaluate extent of disease. The routine use of PET scans cannot yet be recommended to follow patients with MM.

    e. Bone scans are of limited usefulness in MM because most lesions are osteolytic, and bone scans require perilesional osteoblastic activity to be positive. Positive bone scans in MM usually indicate regions of fracture or arthritis, except in the rare event of osteoblastic myeloma.

    f. Bone densitometry studies may be useful in following patients with MM. This study may help predict the risk for skeletal complications as well as the response to bisphosphonates among these patients.

    g. Bone formation and resorption markers may predict risk of skeletal complications but should not be performed routinely.

6. Special studies. Serum viscosity, cryoglobulins, and rectal biopsy or analysis of joint effusions for amyloid are obtained when indicated.

D. Protein studies. Some serum immunoglobulin properties that have clinical relevance are listed in Table 22.1. Kinetic studies of protein synthesis in animals and humans show tumor burden to be closely correlated with the quantity of M-protein in the blood ($\sim$1 g/dL corresponds to 100 g of tumor and 1×10^{11} plasma cells).

    1. Protein electrophoresis is extremely valuable for recognizing cases of monoclonal gammopathies and for following quantitative changes in spikes. PEP, however, is only a presumptive screening test; IEP must be done to establish the diagnosis of monoclonal gammopathy. Examples of serum and urine PEP patterns are shown in Figure 22.1.

        a. M-proteins appear as tall, narrow, sharply defined peaks (spikes) that reflect their structural homogeneity. They are usually located in the γ or γ–β region. Monoclonal peaks in the α or α–β region are usually not caused by M-proteins but by reactant proteins (see section IX.C).

        b. IgG spikes are usually tall, narrow, and located in the β region. **IgA spikes** are usually broader because the molecule tends to form polymers of different sizes; they are located in the β region. **IgM spikes** are usually located near the point of origin. **IgD spikes** usually cause only slight deflections in the pattern because the protein is present in a relatively small concentration.

        c. Light chains are not ordinarily found in the serum because light chains are rapidly catabolized by the kidney or excreted in the urine. Light chain spikes may be found in the serum of patients with renal insufficiency or in instances in which polymerization of light chains has occurred.

           (1) The normal ratio of κ-to-γ chains in humans is 2:1. This normal ratio is usually maintained when excretion of light chains is owing to renal disease

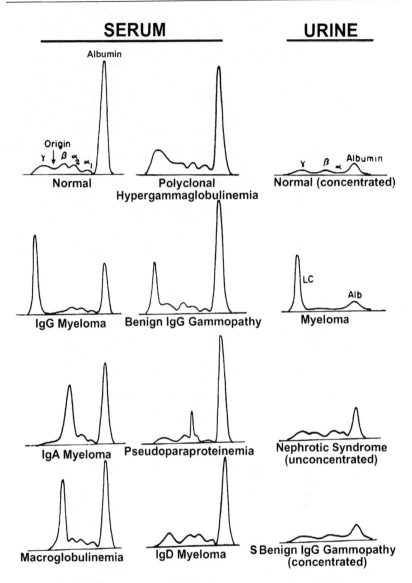

Figure 22.1. Electrophoresis patterns. Alb, albumin.

  SERUM. Normal: the point of application of serum is indicated. Polyclonal hypergammaglobulinemia: occurs in many conditions. Benign immunoglobulin G (IgG) gammopathy: normal levels of albumin and gamma globulins plus a peak in the γ region. Pseudoparaproteinemia: small peaks in β or α regions (see section IX.C).

  URINE. Myeloma: typical homogeneous peak of light chains (LC) in γ region. Nephrotic syndrome: panproteinuria. Benign IgG gammopathy: normal pattern in urine.

but is significantly altered when the excretion is caused by malignant gammopathies.

(2) Urinary excretion of monoclonal light chains is found in 50% to 60% of patients with MM and in 10% to 20% of patients with WM. Patients with MGUS may also show light chains in the urine, but the amount of monoclonal urinary protein is usually <1 g/24 hours.

(3) A recently developed assay, the *free lite assay,* is able to assess free light chains in the serum of a patient with myeloma. This assay can be important for following patients who have deteriorating renal function (more accurately than 24-hour urine paraprotein levels, which may be unreliable for patients with kidney dysfunction and oliguria) or who have nonsecretory myeloma (a serum light chain may be detected and followed). The usefulness of this assay in following patients long term has not yet been clearly demonstrated, however.

2. IEP determines the exact heavy chain class (γ, α, μ, δ, ϵ) and light chain type (κ, λ) of the M-protein and distinguishes polyclonal and monoclonal increases in gammaglobulins. IEP is more sensitive than PEP for low-concentration or heterogeneous globulin mixtures.

3. QIG estimations are excellent for measuring normal or decreased immunoglobulin levels and are useful for distinguishing MGUS from MM. QIG are unreliable, however, if levels are markedly increased or if protein aggregation has occurred. The variability in QIG estimation with assays measured in the same laboratory over time makes it imperative that both QIG and serum PEP be done to assess the response of patients to therapy.

4. Serum viscosity. The rate of descent of serum at 37°C through a calibrated capillary tube is compared with that of distilled water. Plasma is not used because elevated levels of fibrinogen can markedly affect the results. Normal values for serum viscosity ratios range from 1.4 to 1.9. Symptoms usually do not develop unless the serum viscosity >4.

E. Differentiation of plasma cell dyscrasias. In the absence of biopsy proof of malignant disease, differentiating MGUS from early malignant disease may be impossible at the initial examination. To establish the diagnosis, serial evaluations of the patient and M-protein level must be done for several months or years. Table 22.3 indicates the important data that need repeated observation. These data

TABLE 22.3 **Protein Variables for Predicting Benign Versus Malignant Monoclonal Gammopathy**

Variable	Monoclonal gammopathy of undetermined significance (MGUS)	Malignant monoclonal gammopathy (MM, WM, B-cell lymphomas)
Serum M-protein concentration		
IgG	<2.0 g/dL	>2.0 g/dL
IgM	<2.0 g/dL	>2.0 g/dL
IgA	<1.0 g/dL	>1.0 g/dL
Other serum immunoglobulins	Normal or decreased	Decreased
Change in M-protein concentration over time	Stable or transient	Increases
Serum albumin	Normal	Decreased
Urine light chains	Absent or normal κ:λ ratio (2:1) and <300 mg/day	Present with abnormal κ:λ ratio and/or >30 mg/dL or >300 mg/day

MM, multiple myeloma; WM, Waldenström's macroglobulinemia.

predict benign or malignant monoclonal gammopathy, but none is diagnostic by itself; patients with MGUS may slowly progress to MM. About 25% of patients with MGUS progress to MM or a related B-cell malignancy (WM, lymphoma, or amyloidosis). The most important findings that suggest malignant disease are significant and progressive increases in the serum M-protein or urinary light chain concentration.

1. **IgM monoclonal gammopathies** may be benign or owing to WM, lymphoproliferative disorders, or epithelial tumors that can present with a serum abnormality years before the neoplasm becomes evident. Thus, the division of IgM gammopathies into MGUS, primary or Waldenström's macroglobulinemia, and secondary macroglobulinemia is at times arbitrary. A very small percentage of patients with myeloma present with an IgM monoclonal gammopathy; these patients have typical features of myeloma with osteolytic bone disease, renal dysfunction, or both.

2. **IgG, IgA, and IgD monoclonal gammopathies: diagnostic criteria for MM.** To establish the diagnosis of MM, invasion or destruction of normal tissues by the uncontrolled growth of plasma cells must be proved by biopsy. High concentrations of monoclonal serum immunoglobulins (>3.5 g/dL for IgG, >2 mg/dL for IgA) or urinary light chains (>1 g/day) are nearly diagnostic of MM. MM, however, often remains subclinical or indolent (so-called *smoldering myeloma*) for many years. If the diagnosis of MM cannot be proved, the working diagnosis becomes MGUS, and the patient is examined at regular intervals to detect changes in clinical or laboratory findings.

IV. STAGING SYSTEMS AND PROGNOSTIC FACTORS

A. **Staging systems for MM.** Distinguishing patients with low, intermediate, and high volumes of tumor mass before institution of therapy is useful for prognosis: 1×10^{12} cells correspond to 1 kg of tumor, and 3 to 5×10^{12} cells are usually incompatible with life in the average-sized patient.

1. **The classic Salmon-Drurie staging system** for MM is shown in Table 22.4.

2. **The International Staging System** (ISS) has replaced the Salmon-Drurie system. The ISS involves measurement of serum β2m and albumin. The ISS consists of the following stages in the order of worsening prognosis:

Stage I: serum β2m <3.5 mg/L and serum albumin ≥3.5 g/L
Stage II: neither stage I nor III
Stage III, serum β2m ≥5.5 mg/L

3. **Serum β2m** is the light chain moiety of classic human leukocyte antigens (HLA) and is found on the surface membranes of most nucleolated cells. Patients with MM and higher initial values of β2m appear to have a worse prognosis. Despite the high correlation of β2m levels with renal function, β2m has emerged as an important independent prognostic factor.

a. Elevated β2m levels are also found in patients with acute or chronic myelocytic leukemia, lymphoproliferative disorders, myeloproliferative disorders, myelodysplastic syndromes, benign or malignant liver diseases, and autoimmune diseases.

b. Serum albumin also is decreased among patients with poor outcome and represents an assessment of nutritional status as well as pro-MM cytokine activity.

B. **Prognostic factors**

1. **MGUS.** If a patient with the presumptive diagnosis of MGUS remains stable for 2 years, the chance for malignant disease is about 20%.

2. **WM.** Median survival is about 3 to 4 years for patients who are unresponsive to treatment and about 5 to 7 years for responsive patients. Survival for 10 to 20 years, however, is not rare. The development of complications, such as hyperviscosity, hemorrhage, or infection, contributes to death. Age >60 years, male gender, and hemoglobin <10 g/dL are associated with shortened survival time.

TABLE 22.4	Salmon-Durie Staging System for Multiple Myeloma

Stage	Extent of disease

I	**Low tumor mass** ($<0.6 \times 10^{12}$ plasma cells/m^2). Patients must have *all* of the following:
	 Hemoglobin >10 g/dL
	 Serum calcium: normal or $\leq$12 mg/dL
	 Low M-component production rates
	    IgG <5 g/dL
	    IgA <3 g/dL
	    UPEP M-component light chain <4 g/24 hrs
	 Skeletal x-ray: normal or with a solitary plasmacytoma

II	**Intermediate tumor mass** (0.6–1.2×10^{12} plasma cells/m^2). Patients who qualify for neither stage I nor III

III	**High tumor mass** ($>1.2 \times 10^{12}$ plasma cells/m^2). Patients having *any one* of the following:
	 Hemoglobin <8.5 g/dL
	 Serum calcium >12 mg/dL
	 High M-component production rates
	    IgG >7 g/dL
	    IgA >5 g/dL
	    UPEP M-component light chain >12 g/24 hrs
	 Extensive lytic bone lesions

Substage A	Serum creatinine <2 mg/dL
Substage B	Serum creatinine $\geq$2 mg/dL

UPEP, urine protein electrophoresis.

3. **MM.** The overall median survival time of patients with MM is about 4 to 5 years. The prognosis in MM is improving with the wide array of new agents available to treat patients.
   a. **Tumor mass.** Patients with a low tumor mass have a median survival time of 3.5 to 10 years. Patients with a high tumor mass have a median survival time of 0.5 to 3 years.
   b. **C-reactive protein and IL-6.** Elevated IL-6 levels may possibly portend a poor prognosis. CRP levels appear to reflect IL-6 serum levels, but most patients with MM do not have elevated CRP levels.
   c. **Labeling index (LI).** The LI is indicative of the percentage of cells undergoing mitosis. A high LI (>3%) is associated with a poor prognosis in MM.
   d. **Cytogenetic abnormalities**
      (1) **Abnormalities associated with a poor prognosis**
         (a) The absence of chromosome 13 portends a poor prognosis when identified by conventional cytogenetics but not by FISH.
         (b) Abnormalities involving chromosome 4 or 16 also correlate with a poor prognosis and may better predict outcome than chromosome 13 loss alone.
         (c) Abnormality of chromosome 14
         (d) Gains on the long arm of chromosome 1
      (2) **Abnormalities associated with a good prognosis.** Translocations involving chromosome 11 portend an improved survival.
   e. **Renal function** previously was thought to be an important prognostic factor. Increasing degrees of azotemia were associated with progressively shorter life expectancies. Advances in plasmapheresis, dialysis, and supportive care have made this a less important prognostic factor. The outcome for patients whose

renal function normalizes with therapy is not different from that for patients who present with normal renal function.

f. Response to therapy. The response to therapy has been shown to be related to outcome. Only patients who show progressive disease during initial therapy definitely have a worse outcome, however. The extent of response from initial therapy, as long as the patient does not show disease progression, is not a very good prognostic factor. Paradoxically, patients who respond too rapidly to therapy with melphalan and prednisone (>50% reduction in <3 months) have a poor prognosis.

g. Immunoglobulin class. Although earlier studies suggested that patients with IgD or λ-light chain disease had a worse prognosis, analyses of prognostic factors in large MM trials have not shown the paraprotein type to be a prognostic factor.

h. Other prognostic factors. The presence of a *p53* deletion, plasmablastic morphology, higher numbers of circulating monoclonal plasma cells, or higher serum levels of LDH, soluble IL-6 receptor, or syndecan-1 also predict a poor outcome. In early stage disease, the pattern and number of MRI abnormalities predict both progression to symptomatic disease and overall survival. The gene-expression profiling pattern may predict outcome as well.

V. PREVENTION AND EARLY DETECTION

The availability of PEP and of screening chemistry panels has probably resulted in earlier detection of monoclonal gammopathies. If IEP were used for screening populations, the incidence of MGUS might well double, but survival would not be affected.

VI. MANAGEMENT OF WM

A. Diagnosis

1. Diagnostic criteria for WM

a. IgM monoclonal gammopathy of any concentration

b. Bone marrow infiltration by small lymphocytes, plasmacytoid lymphocytes, and plasma cells in a diffuse, interstitial, or nodular pattern

c. The immunophenotype is positive for surface immunoglobulin, CD19, and CD20, and is negative for CD5, CD10, and CD23.

2. Additional workup at presentation

a. Chest x-ray study, CT scan of chest, abdomen, and pelvis

b. Serum viscosity, cold agglutinins, and cryocrit

c. Hepatitis serology

B. Treatment. Patients with asymptomatic disease, without anemia, hyperviscosity, renal insufficiency, or neurologic abnormalities, should be monitored for clinical status and by PEP until disease progression is confirmed.

1. Indications for treatment

a. Anemia, pancytopenia

b. Symptomatic hyperviscosity, cryoglobulinemia, or neuropathy

c. Bulky lymphadenopathy or symptomatic organomegaly

d. Amyloidosis

e. Cryoglobulinemia

f. Cold agglutinin disease

g. Transformation to another aggressive B-cell malignancy

2. Treatment alternatives. Patients are treated similarly to low-grade lymphomas (see Chapter 21). Hyperviscosity is relieved by plasmapheresis because >70% of the protein is in the plasma rather than the tissues (see section IX.A), but it is required only in a few patients with high IgM levels. Several options can be considered.

a. Alkylating agents (usually chlorambucil), nucleoside analogs (fludarabine or cladribine), or rituximab alone or in combinations are usually tried first. Patients with WM should be treated with only several courses of these agents because decreases in M-protein can occur for many months after discontinuing the drug. In addition, treatment with rituximab may be associated with an initial rise in IgM, the so-called "flare" response, followed by a drop in serum IgM levels and tumor burden. Plasmapheresis should be considered for patients showing a significant increase in IgM during the first 2 months of anti-CD20 treatment.

b. If progressive disease develops >6 months following treatment, the same therapy can be repeated. If progressive disease develops <6 months, the alternative class of drugs should be tried.

c. With disease progression following failure of treatment with the above agents, an IMID (thalidomide or lenalidomide) with or without dexamethasone, or a clinical trial involving stem cell transplantation can be considered. Bortezomib combined with steroids also may be an option for these patients. It is important to note that patients failing one bortezomib- or IMID-containing regimen may respond to another.

VII. MANAGEMENT OF MGUS AND SOLITARY, SMOLDERING, OR STAGE I MM

A. MGUS. Patients should have PEP studies every 3 months for the first year, every 6 months for the next 2 years, and then yearly thereafter. Patients with MGUS should not be treated with cytotoxic agents. Only patients showing significant rises in M-protein levels should have additional diagnostic studies (bone marrow aspirate and biopsy, skeletal survey). It may be useful to obtain periodic bone density studies on these patients because of their higher risk to develop bone loss and fractures. Intermittent treatment with IV zoledronic acid may improve bone density, although its impact on fracture risk remains unknown.

B. Solitary osseous plasmacytoma is potentially curable and is treated with at least 4,500 cGy of RT to the involved field. It is important to recognize that many patients treated for a solitary osseous plasmacytoma actually have systemic disease. In fact, the presence of additional lesions on MRI among these patients suggests that they are at high risk to develop MM. This should be taken into consideration before an attempt is made at curative local RT. The M-protein is measured every 3 to 6 months as indicated. Radiologic skeletal survey is performed annually or when symptoms develop. Disease that is refractory to RT (<50% reduction in the M-protein) or that progresses is treated as for stage II or III MM.

C. Solitary extraosseous plasmacytoma is also potentially curable and is treated with surgery, at least 4,500 cGy of RT to the involved field, or both. The M-protein is followed and measured every 3 months for 1 year, then annually. CT scans should be repeated every 6 months for the first year and thereafter as indicated clinically. Disease that is refractory to RT (<50% reduction in the M-protein) or that progresses is treated as for stage II or III MM.

D. Systemic smoldering or stage I myeloma

1. Definition of smoldering MM

a. M-protein component:

IgG >3.5 g/dL and <5.0 g/dL
IgA >2.0 g/dL and <3.0 g/dL
Urinary light chains <1.0 g/24 hours

b. Plasma cell infiltration of bone marrow is >10% but <20%

c. No anemia, renal failure, or hypercalcemia

d. No bone lesions on skeletal survey

2. Clinical course. The disease progresses in most patients, but patients may do well for many months or years before progression occurs. The risk is highest (5%/year) during the first 5 years. Significant risk factors for more rapid progression to symptomatic disease include a level of paraprotein >3 g/dL, the IgA subtype, and bone marrow showing >10% plasma cells.

3. Treatment. Patients are observed without treatment until the disease progresses to symptomatic or active disease (anemia, hypercalcemia, renal insufficiency, bone lesions) or associated amyloidosis. Several clinical trials, however, are underway attempting to slow the progression of disease with the use of single-agent thalidomide. In addition, clinical trials are investigating the use of cyclo-oxygenase 2 (COX-2) inhibitors and IL-1 antagonists to treat this small group of patients with myeloma. Whether bisphosphonates should be used routinely in these patients has not been clearly established. Among patients with severe bone loss demonstrated on bone densitometry, however, it is certainly reasonable to consider this option.

VIII. MANAGEMENT OF STAGE II OR III MM
Maximizing ambulation, administration of chemotherapy, glucocorticoids, bisphosphonates, stem cell transplantation (SCT), and RT have been the mainstays of treatment. Newer agents, such as bortezomib, thalidomide, and lenalidomide, have shown efficacy in the treatment of these patients in both first-line and relapsed or refractory disease settings. Notably, the newer agents show higher response rates when combined with glucocorticoids or cytotoxic agents.

A. Older chemotherapy regimens for MM. Several alkylating agents (melphalan, cyclophosphamide, chlorambucil, and nitrosoureas) are equally effective in producing responses. Refractoriness to one alkylating agent is often associated with responsiveness to another alkylating agent. Exposure to myelotoxic agents (particularly alkylating agents) should, however, be limited to avoid compromising stem cell reserve before stem cell harvest in patients who may be candidates for SCT.

Treatment should continue for two cycles beyond maximal response; continued therapy does not prolong the duration of the plateau phase. Traditional regimens for MM are as follows:

1. Dexamethasone alone: 40 mg PO daily for 4 days every other week

2. M&P (cycle frequency is 4 to 6 weeks)

Melphalan: 10 mg/m^2 PO on days 1 through 4
Prednisone: 60 mg/m^2 PO on days 1 through 4

3. VAD (cycle frequency is 4 weeks)

Vincristine: 0.4 mg/day for 4 days by continuous IV infusion
Doxorubicin (Adriamycin): 9 mg/m^2/day for 4 days by continuous IV infusion
Dexamethasone: 40 mg PO on days 1 through 4, 9 through 13, and 17 through 21

4. EC (cycle frequency is every 4 weeks)

Etoposide: 100 mg/m^2 IV on days 1 through 3
Cyclophosphamide: 1,000 mg/m^2 IV on day 1

5. DVD (cycle frequency every 4 weeks)

Doxil (liposomal doxorubicin): 30 to 40 mg/m^2 IV on day 1
Vincristine: 2 mg IV on day 1
Dexamethasone: 40 mg PO on days 1 through 4

6. Other regimens

a. M-2 protocol (cycle frequency is 5 to 6 weeks)

Melphalan: 0.25 mg/kg PO on days 1 through 4
Prednisone: 1 mg/kg PO on days 1 through 7
Vincristine: 0.03 mg/kg IV on day 1
BCNU (carmustine): 1 mg/kg IV on day 1
Cyclophosphamide: 10 mg/kg IV on day 1

b. VBAP (cycle frequency is 3 weeks)

Vincristine: 1 mg IV on day 1
BCNU (carmustine): 30 mg/m^2 IV on day 1
Doxorubicin (Adriamycin): 30 mg/m^2 IV on day 1
Prednisone: 100 mg PO on days 1 through 4

7. Response rates to older regimens

   a. Response rates to daily low-dose, single alkylating-agent therapy is about 30% and appear to be equivalent to pulse therapy given every 4 to 6 weeks. The addition of prednisone to an alkylating-agent regimen (e.g., M&P) increases the response rate to 50% to 60%.

   b. Responses to VAD occur more rapidly and are somewhat more frequent than to M&P. The duration of response to up-front VAD chemotherapy is approximately 15 to 18 months and of similar duration for other up-front regimens.

   c. Corticosteroids alone (dexamethasone) may produce response and survival rates nearly equivalent to those achieved with infusional VAD or M&P.

   d. Other combination chemotherapy regimens have not been shown to improve survival when compared with M&P. Durable complete responses to these regimens are rare.

B. Newer regimens for the treatment of MM

   1. IMID-regimens. The mechanisms of action of the IMID (thalidomide [Thalomid] and lenalidomide [Revlamid]) are incompletely understood but are thought to be immunomodulatory and antiangiogenic. Both agents are very active in MM but differ in their toxicity profile. The dose-limiting side effects are neurologic (somnolence, peripheral neuropathy) for thalidomide and hematosuppression (mainly thrombocytopenia) for lenalidomide. Both agents are teratogenic and thrombophilic.

   a. Thalidomide (with or without dexamethasone or other steroids): a dose of 100 mg PO daily at night is as effective, but with fewer neuropathic effects, than higher doses.

   b. MPT (cycle frequency is every 4 weeks)

   Melphalan: 4 mg/m^2 daily on days 1 through 7
   Prednisone: 40 mg/m^2 daily on days 1 through 7
   Thalidomide: 100 mg daily at night

   c. Rev/Dex (cycle frequency is every 4 weeks)

   Revlimid (lenalidomide): 25 mg PO daily for 21 days followed by a 7-day rest period
   Dexamethasone: 40 mg PO weekly

   d. BLT-D (daily)

   Biaxin (clarithromycin): 500 mg PO twice daily
   Thalidomide: 100 to 200 mg PO at bedtime
   Dexamethasone: 40 mg PO weekly

   e. Response rates

   (1) Thalidomide leads to durable responses in one-third of relapsing patients. The response rate to thalidomide plus dexamethasone is 60% with a 15% complete response rate. Thalidomide alone is associated with a 30% response rate even after progression of disease following autologous SCT. Although this agent used up front with dexamethasone improves response rate and progression-free survival compared with dexamethasone alone, no improvement is seen in overall survival, an observation that may reflect patients failing steroids alone receive thalidomide at the time of progressive disease.

   (2) Lenalidomide with dexamethasone is also associated with a 60% response rate and approximately 20% complete response.

   2. Velcade (bortezomib) regimens. Dose-limiting side effects of bortezomib are peripheral neuropathy (predominantly sensory) and hematosuppression (especially thrombocytopenia). Fatigue, fever, and gastrointestinal (GI) side effects are also common.

   a. Velcade: 1 or 1.3 mg/m^2 IV bolus (IVB) on days 1, 4, 8, and 11; cycle frequency is every 3 weeks

b. Velcade/Dex (cycle frequency is every 3 weeks)

Velcade: 1.3 mg/m^2 IVB days 1, 4, 8, and 11
Dexamethasone: 40 mg PO weekly

c. BAM (cycle frequency is every 4 weeks)

Bortezomib: 1 mg/m^2 IVB on days 1,4, 8 and 11
Ascorbic acid: 1 g PO daily on days 1 through 4
Melphalan: 0.1 mg/kg daily days 1 through 4

d. VMP (cycle frequency is every 6 weeks)

Velcade: 1.3 mg/m^2 IVB on days 1, 4, 8, 11, 22, 25, 29, and 32
Melphalan: 9 mg/m^2 daily on days 1 through 4
Prednisone: 60 mg/m^2 daily on days 1 through 4

e. Doxil/Velcade (cycle frequency every 3 weeks)

Doxil (liposomal doxorubicin): 30 mg/m^2 IV on day 4
Velcade (bortezomib): 1.3 mg/m^2 IVB on days 1, 4, 8, and 11

f. Response rates. Although bortezomib as a single agent shows a 30% response rate, adding steroids increases the response rate to >50%. Adding melphalan to bortezomib increases the response rate to nearly 70%.

C. Duration of therapy. Patients should be treated until a plateau phase (stabilization of M-protein levels for several months) is achieved. Continuation of chemotherapy beyond plateau phase has not been demonstrated to prolong survival but does increase the risk for secondary malignancies, especially acute leukemia. Few data exist on how long to continue the newer agents such as bortezomib and the IMID once a maximal response is achieved, but most patients remain on these agents albeit at often a reduced or less frequent dosing schedule until disease progression occurs.

1. **For patients with disease that responds or stabilizes following therapy,** choices are observation without further therapy until disease progression occurs, maintenance therapy, or high-dose regimens with SCT. No treatment while watching disease parameters is a justifiable option.

2. **Maintenance therapy** is controversial. Some studies have reported that maintenance therapy with prednisone (50 mg PO every other day) or recombinant interferon-α (IFN-α) prolongs the response to conventional therapy in patients who have a near complete response or in those with IgA or light chain myeloma. The use of prednisone (50 mg PO every other day) as maintenance therapy after even a minor response to VAD was shown to improve significantly both progression-free and overall survival without significant toxicity.

Although remissions are sustained longer with the addition of IFN to prednisone, a significant survival benefit for maintenance therapy with this cytokine after conventional therapy has not been demonstrated. Maintenance therapy with IFN alone has yielded inconsistent results. Although one recent study suggests the combination of thalidomide and pamidronate following tandem transplant may improve overall survival, no other studies have been done to help guide the use of thalidomide or bortezomib as maintenance therapy.

D. High-dose regimens have generally contained myeloablative doses of alkylating agents with or without total-body irradiation (TBI). TBI is generally not given to patients who received prior local RT and is associated with a higher degree of treatment-related morbidity and mortality. Most institutions currently use high-dose IV melphalan as the sole treatment for patients having myeloablation for their MM. With high-dose regimens, the response rates are higher, and a significant proportion of patients show elimination of the M-protein. All candidates for this intensive therapy must have sufficient cardiac, pulmonary, hepatic, and renal function.

1. **High-dose therapy with autologous peripheral blood SCT** in some studies is associated with increased rates of complete remission, improved

event-free survival, and increased overall survival when compared with conventional chemotherapy, particularly in patients <60 years of age. Other studies, however, have not shown a difference in overall survival despite the higher complete remission rate among patients who have high-dose therapy.

Stem cells are harvested from the blood of patients at the time of maximal response to conventional chemotherapy. Autologous peripheral blood SCT is not curative, but improvements in supportive care have reduced the treatment-related mortality rate to 1% to 2% in most centers.

A study in France suggests that patients having a **tandem transplant** approach (two sequential autologous SCT) may have an improved outcome compared with those having a single transplant. The intensity of chemotherapy in that study was suboptimal, however; thus, the superiority of double compared with single SCT is questionable. Other studies have not confirmed the benefit of double transplant for this patient population.

2. **Allogeneic SCT** is associated with high treatment-related mortality rates (nearly 40%); thus, the use of this procedure has been reduced to primarily clinical trials for younger patients who have a compatible donor. Studies have used **donor leukocyte infusions** with some reduction in M-protein levels but also with significant graft-versus-host disease toxicity. Some centers are now performing **tandem (double) transplantations** for these patients (autologous SCT followed by allogeneic SCT). A study suggests a high complete remission rate when patients have this latter approach, but the long-term outcome of these patients is yet to be determined and the risk of chronic graft-versus-host disease is high and associated with a significant treatment-related mortality.

3. **Autologous bone marrow transplantation.** Because many tumor cells are found in the autograft, attempts have been made to *purge* autografts of tumor using stem cell selection. Although this procedure successfully eliminates tumor cells in the autograft, it does not improve overall survival, probably because of the relatively high tumor burden remaining in the patient even after myeloablative chemotherapy.

E. **Considerations for choices of treatment for MM**
   1. **Treatment choices for initial therapy** of MM have greatly increased recently as a result of the introduction of bortezomib, thalidomide, and lenalidomide in the first-line setting. Because these regimens have not been evaluated against each other and response rates and progression-free survival are similar between the different regimens, choice of initial therapy must take into account the severity of the myeloma and the patient's work- and life-style and comorbid conditions.

      a. Although long-term use of alkylating agents is associated with permanent stem-cell toxicity, short courses with lower doses in the newer regimens are unlikely to have an impact on stem cell function.

      b. Thalidomide-containing regimens, including thalidomide and dexamethasone or MPT, are oral and convenient, but they are associated with irreversible neuropathy and a high risk of thromboembolic events, requiring many patients to receive long-term anticoagulation prophylaxis. Similarly, Rev/Dex is also associated with significant risk of thromboembolic effects and also marrow suppression.

      c. Bortezomib-containing regimens, including Velcade/Dex, BAM, and VMP, are also associated with neurotoxicity but the effects are generally reversible.

   2. **SCT.** Patients who are considering high-dose chemotherapy with hematopoietic support may receive these up-front regimens for several months and then have stem cell collection, high-dose chemotherapy, and stem cell infusion.

   3. **Patients who relapse** may be considered for another treatment with the same new agent (bortezomib, thalidomide, or lenalidomide) with a different chemotherapeutic agent or for another new agent alone or in combination with steroids or chemotherapy. In addition, although arsenic trioxide shows only modest activity as a single agent, it is very active in combination with melphalan and IV ascorbic acid. The EC combination and single-agent therapy with

topotecan or vinorelbine show moderate activity in relapsing patients; however, the duration of responses with these combinations is extremely brief.

4. **Patients with disease progression following therapy** can be treated with ESHAP (see Appendix D-3), cyclophosphamide with VAD, thalidomide, lenalidomide, bortezomib, or arsenic trioxide. As a single agent in these circumstances, bortezomib is associated with a 35% response rate, about 5% of which are complete responses. The addition of bortezomib or arsenic trioxide to small doses of melphalan, cyclophosphamide, or anthracyclines can produce responses even among patients who were previously resistant to these chemotherapeutic agents. The combination of thalidomide and bortezomib has also been associated with a high response rate. It is important to recognize these observations in planning therapy for relapsing patients who have been previously treated with chemotherapeutic agents.

F. **Supportive care** is extremely important in MM. Bedrest is often necessary because of the painful bony lesions or fractures. Bedrest, however, further promotes bone demineralization, which may lead to hypercalcemia.

1. **Bisphosphonates** (pamidronate, 90 mg IV over >2 hours, or zoledronic acid, 4 mg IV over 15 minutes) given monthly are indicated for all patients with stage II or III MM (and perhaps stage I as well). These agents have significantly decreased the incidence of skeletal complications in this disease. Bisphosphonates reduce pain and analgesic usage and prevent the deterioration of quality of life compared with placebo.

It is important to recognize that these agents occasionally are associated with **renal dysfunction**. The type of renal lesion is different, however, between the two bisphosphonates. Pamidronate more often will cause a glomerular lesion initially associated with proteinuria, which may be at nephrotic levels. By contrast, zoledronic acid more often causes tubular dysfunction and, thus, is not often associated with albuminuria.

Recent reports suggest that bisphosphonates are associated with an increased risk of **osteonecrosis of the jaw** (ONJ). This complication occurs more frequently among patients who have had recent dental surgery or trauma, poor dental hygiene, or who abuse alcohol or use tobacco. Before initiating bisphosphonate treatment, patients should have a complete dental examination and any dental extractions or removal of jawbone(s) should be completed several months before initiating these drugs to reduce the risk of ONJ. The course of ONJ is variable and many patients do not show worsening of the condition, although this can occur. No studies have evaluated whether discontinuing these drugs among patients with this complication affects the course of ONJ. It is clear that surgical intervention to treat this problem should be kept to a minimum and undertaken only by dental professionals experienced with this problem.

2. **Skeletal complications**

   a. **Surgery** for MM is restricted to orthopedic procedures. Fractures of long bones usually require fixation with a medullary pin and postoperative irradiation. Sometimes, impending fractures with large osteolytic lesions of the femoral head are internally fixed prophylactically. If the diagnosis of the underlying disease is in doubt, acute spinal cord compression or vertebral fracture may make laminectomy necessary. Either vertebroplasty or kyphoplasty should be considered for symptomatic vertebral compression fractures. Kyphoplasty may reverse the compression fracture and can lead to immediate and sustained pain relief for patients with symptomatic vertebral compression fractures, especially when they occur in either the thoracic or the lumbar spine. The risk of leakage of the cement appears to be lower with this procedure than with veretebroplasty, although these procedures have not been evaluated in any randomized studies.

   b. **RT** in low doses is useful for palliation of lesions that are localized or that cause spinal cord or nerve root compression. Small subcutaneous tumors or small painful lesions in bone may be treated with only a single dose of 800 cGy. Large osteolytic lesions in long bones should be irradiated before a fracture occurs. Large lytic lesions or paraspinous masses rarely need >2,000 cGy given over 5 days. Many patients, however, will have significant pain relief with effective treatment of their underlying myeloma. In some patients, it may be prudent to wait before initiating RT to relieve pain.

   c. Back pain is relieved by RT unless the pain is caused by compression fracture. Because spinal cord compression is a common complication in MM, the physician should not hesitate to order an MRI or CT myelogram in patients with MM who have new or changing back pain. This should be treated emergently if it occurs (see Chapter 32, section III). The use of RT to the spine should be done judiciously. The spine represents a large reservoir for the production of normal bone marrow and, thus, its compromise with RT must be taken into consideration among patients who will require myelotoxic treatment for their underlying disease.

   d. Pain relief may be achieved with focal RT. Analgesics should be prescribed in a regimen that gives the most consistent pain relief. Nonsteroidal anti-inflammatory drugs (NSAID) should be avoided to decrease the chances of renal dysfunction.

   e. Ambulation should be maximized as early as possible after the onset of fractures or pain. Corsets and braces are often effective in relieving back pain by stabilizing the spine until chemotherapy or RT becomes effective.

   f. Calcium and vitamin D deficiencies occur in many patients with myeloma and serum calcium levels may also be reduced with bisphosphonate treatment. Thus, oral calcium (1,000 mg daily) and vitamin D (800 IU daily) is recommended. Monitoring of serum calcium is necessary, however, because occasionally patients may develop hypercalcemia.

   g. Fluoride is not effective in increasing bone remineralization in patients with MM; fluoride treatment results only in increased bone density because of fluorosis.

3. Hydration. Patients must be repeatedly reminded to drink 2 to 3 L of liquids daily to promote urinary excretion of light chains, calcium, and uric acid. This simple reminder has been shown to improve survival greatly in some studies.

4. Infections are the foremost cause of death in patients with MM. Infections must be investigated and treated urgently. These patients have similar infections to other cancer patients treated with chemotherapy. In fact, the risk for infection is primarily during periods of chemotherapy-induced neutropenia or in the terminal stages of the disease. Although the use of prophylactic antibiotics and IVIG may be attempted in patients with recurrent infections, most patients do not require these interventions. IVIG therapy should be considered in cases of recurrent, life-threatening infections. Pneumococcal and influenza vaccine should also be considered.

5. Renal failure is best prevented by hydration, treatment of hyperuricemia and hypercalcemia, and avoidance of both IV contrast media and NSAID. Recent randomized studies have not demonstrated the benefit of plasmapheresis. When renal failure becomes severe, some patients may be candidates for hemodialysis treatment, especially if they have a reasonable prognosis and have not failed initial therapy. Azotemia may improve slowly in these patients; it may take several months for these patients to discontinue dialysis treatment.

IX. SPECIAL CLINICAL PROBLEMS IN PATIENTS WITH PLASMA CELL DISORDERS

A. Plasma alterations in patients with M-proteins

   1. Hyperviscosity syndrome. The blood cells normally contribute more to the whole-blood viscosity than do plasma proteins. The development of hyperviscosity with M-proteins depends on their concentration and their ability to aggregate or polymerize. WM is typically associated with hyperviscosity. Symptoms usually do not occur unless the serum M-protein concentration exceeds 3 to 4 g/dL and the serum viscosity index exceeds 4.

a. **Complications** of hyperviscosity include the following:
   (1) **Bleeding diathesis** is manifested by spontaneous bruising, purpura, retinal hemorrhages, epistaxis, or mucosal bleeding. The hemorrhagic diathesis is compounded by thrombocytopenia. Bleeding in the hyperviscosity syndrome appears to be a result of the following:
      (a) **Interference with coagulation,** especially the third stage of coagulation (polymerization of fibrin monomer), resulting in prolongation of clotting times
      (b) **Impaired platelet function** resulting in abnormalities of bleeding times, clot retraction, and other platelet functions
   (2) **Retinopathy** is manifested by venous dilation and segmentation ("link-sausage" appearance), retinal hemorrhages, and papilledema.
   (3) **Neurologic symptoms,** which develop in about 25% of patients, include malaise, focal neurologic defects, stroke, and coma.
   (4) **Hypervolemia** develops with an increase of M-protein concentration, resulting in distention of peripheral blood vessels and increased vascular resistance. Plasma volume expansion may actually lessen the viscosity, but may also precipitate congestive heart failure (which occurs in about 10% of patients who have hyperviscosity).
b. **Management.** Hyperviscosity syndrome is treated by reducing the quantity of M-protein in the serum. Reduction of M-protein concentrations with cytotoxic-agent therapy takes several weeks or months. Symptomatic patients should be treated with plasmapheresis, 4 to 6 units daily, until the viscosity index is <3. Patients with hyperviscosity caused by monoclonal IgM usually respond to plasmapheresis more rapidly than those with IgG or IgA gammopathies because IgM has a predominantly intravascular distribution (Table 22.1). Additionally, an exponential relationship exists between serum viscosity and IgM level, so that, for example, a 20% decrease in IgM concentration results in a 100% decrease in serum viscosity. Improvement should be monitored by noting changes in clinical findings, coagulation tests, and serum viscosity determinations.
2. **Cold sensitivity** may afflict patients with M-proteins (especially IgM) that have physicochemical properties that permit cold precipitation. The cryoglobulins in plasma cell dyscrasias and lymphoproliferative disorders are monoclonal. The cryoglobulins in other disorders (e.g., collagen vascular diseases and viral infections) are circulating soluble immune complexes (IgM–IgG, IgA–IgG, IgG–IgG). Manifestations include cold urticaria, Raynaud's phenomenon, and vascular purpura in the absence of severe thrombocytopenia.
3. **Cold agglutinins** are IgM with a specificity for specific red blood cell antigens (usually Ia) at temperatures <37°C. These proteins may be responsible for a mild extravascular complement-dependent hemolysis and acrocyanosis but not for other symptoms of cold sensitivity unless cryoglobulins are also present.
4. **Pseudohyponatremia** may be observed with high levels of M-proteins (plasma water is displaced by the M-protein).
5. **Anion gaps,** noted with measurement of serum electrolytes (serum concentration of sodium chloride bicarbonate), may be decreased in patients with cationic monoclonal proteins. The decreased gap is produced by the increase of chloride and bicarbonate anions.
B. **Peripheral neuropathy (PN)**
   1. **PN associated with gammopathy** occurs especially in patients with IgM monoclonal gammopathies. About 5% of patients with a sensorimotor neuropathy have an associated monoclonal gammopathy. Nearly 10% of patients with WM or with MGUS and an IgM paraprotein develop a demyelinating peripheral neuropathy. Sural nerve biopsies demonstrate monoclonal IgM deposition on the outer myelin sheath. The antibody can be shown to react with myelin-associated glycoprotein (MAG) in half of the cases. These patients usually have a mostly sensory or ataxic polyneuropathy, whereas patients with non–MAG-reactive antibodies usually have both a sensory and a motor component to their

neuropathy. Treatment with plasmapheresis may be effective in some cases. Other forms of treatment have included high doses of glucocorticosteroids, IVIG, and rituximab.

2. PN associated with treatment. PN more often results from treatment of plasma cell disorders with agents such as thalidomide or bortezomib. Most patients receiving thalidomide will develop irreversible neuropathy after 6 months of treatment. Approximately one-third of patients treated with bortezomib develop treatment-related neuropathy, which may be painful but is reversible in most cases. The risk of neuropathy with these two agents is directly related to the dose used. Drugs such as gabapentin (Neurontin), pregabalin (Lyrica), duloxetine (Cymbalta), doxipen, and over-the-counter alpha lipoic acid may be helpful to reduce the severity of this complication.

C. Pseudoparaproteinemia. The PEP can detect serum proteins when the concentration >200 mg/dL. In certain situations, a nonimmunoglobulin homogeneous protein concentration may >300 mg/dL and appear as a spike on PEP. The location of these spikes usually are in the α and β regions but may be in the β–γ region. The differential diagnosis is clarified by review of the clinical picture, the location of the PEP spike, and IEP. Conditions that may produce pseudoparaproteinemia include the following:

1. Hyper-α_1-globulinemia (acute-phase reactant in many inflammatory and neoplastic diseases)

2. Hyper-α_2-globulinemia (nephrotic syndrome or hemolysis)

3. Hemoglobin–haptoglobin complexes (intravascular hemolysis)

4. Hyperlipidemia

5. Hypertransferrinemia (iron deficiency)

6. Bacterial products

7. Desiccated serum

8. Fibrinogen (if plasma is measured)

D. Pseudomyeloma. Several malignancies, including lymphoma and cancer of the breast, bowel, or biliary tract, can be associated with the production of an M-protein. These same malignancies may produce lytic lesions in the skeleton and induce marrow plasmacytosis. Pseudomyeloma must be distinguished from true myeloma.

E. Therapy-linked acute leukemia is discussed in Chapter 34, section I.D in "Cytopenia."

F. Heavy chain diseases (HCD) are rare plasma cell lymphocytic neoplasms characterized by secretion of abnormal heavy chains (γ, α, or μ) without light chains (κ, λ). α-HCD is the most common, and μ-HCD is the rarest. The heavy chains may also be excreted in the urine and detected by urine PEP. Normal immunoglobulin levels are usually suppressed. Diagnosis of these disorders necessitates detailed immunochemical investigation. IEP is the crucial test; it should demonstrate reaction of antisera with the appropriate heavy chain but not with light chains.

1. α-HCD nearly always involves only the α_1 subtype of heavy chain and is associated with GI lymphomas.

2. γ-HCD usually affects elderly patients. Generalized lymphadenopathy, hepatosplenomegaly, involvement of Waldeyer's ring, fever, pancytopenia, and eosinophilia are common features of the disease. The illness initially resembles granulomatous disease or Hodgkin's disease. Biopsies of lymph nodes and bone marrow are rarely diagnostic. The disease has a variable course, developing over a few months to several years. A satisfactory treatment plan has not been established.

3. μ-HCD nearly always occurs in patients with CLL, and the two disorders are treated in the same manner. In μ-HCD, however, lymphadenopathy is infrequent and, in contrast to other HCDs, large amounts of κ–light chains are excreted in the urine. The rare disease may be suspected when a patient with CLL has unusual vacuolated plasma cells (characteristic of μ-HCD) in the bone marrow.

G. Amyloidosis may be primary (with or without associated plasma cell or lymphoid neoplasms), secondary to a variety of chronic inflammatory diseases or hereditary disorders (familial Mediterranean fever), or associated with the aging process. The disease is characterized by organ deposition of fibrillar substances of many different types. The fibrils are mostly or exclusively composed of immunoglobulin light chains (especially the λ type) in amyloidosis associated with primary amyloidosis and myeloma, but the fibrils are composed of substances other than light chains in secondary amyloidosis.

1. **Organ distribution of amyloid.** The various forms of amyloidosis overlap considerably. **Secondary amyloidosis** affects the kidneys, spleen, liver, or adrenal glands and rarely involves the heart, GI tract, or musculoskeletal system. **Primary amyloidosis and amyloidosis associated with MM** mostly affect the heart, GI tract, skeletal muscle, ligaments (carpal tunnel syndrome), and peri-articular and synovial tissue (articular manifestations) as well as the tongue (macroglossia) and skin. Skin involvement most commonly is located in the periorbital and skin-fold regions and is manifested by spontaneous purpura and ecchymoses, which may be aggravated by coagulation factor X deficiency, which occasionally accompanies amyloidosis; postproctoscopic eyelid ecchymoses are characteristic. Involvement of the respiratory tract, endocrine glands, and peripheral and autonomic nervous systems also occurs.

2. **Diagnosis**
   a. **Biopsy** of an involved organ (especially the carpal ligament, sural nerve, rectum, or gingivae) must be performed to establish the diagnosis of amyloidosis; liver or renal biopsy may result in hemorrhage. Amyloid deposits have a homogenous eosinophilic appearance on light microscopy. Confirmation is made by the demonstration of specific birefringence by polarized microscopy of specimens stained with Congo red.
   b. **Monoclonal light chains** in the urine are found in both the primary type and in amyloidosis associated with MM. Many patients with primary amyloidosis are found to have developed plasma cell disease if they survive sufficiently long.

3. **Prognosis.** Patients with amyloidosis live a median of about 2 years, although the prognosis varies greatly depending on the type of amyloid and sites as well as extent of organ involvement. Patients with primary amyloidosis generally have the worst outcome. Those with cardiac involvement have the worst prognosis, whereas patients with renal disease have a better outcome.

4. **Treatment** of amyloidosis is directed at both the affected organs and the underlying process producing the amyloid deposits. Data are insufficient to identify optimal therapy for this plasma cell disorder. Treatment options include M&P, VAD, moderately high-dose melphalan, and high-dose melphalan with autologous SCT. Recent results of a randomized study, however, show no overall survival advantage with high-dose therapy compared with conventional treatment despite the increase in progression-free survival with the more intensive treatment. Studies also suggest that thalidomide and lenalidomide, with or without the addition of glucocorticoids and bortezomib, may be effective for patients with amyloidosis and may lead to long-term remissions. The significant neurotoxic side effects of both thalidomide and bortezomib must be considered in choosing these agents for patients with amyloidosis with neuropathy.

H. Papular mucinosis (lichen myxedematosus) is a dermatologic condition characterized by cutaneous papules and plaques that result from the deposition of a mucinous material. The disease is often preceded by chronic pyoderma. It demonstrates an M-protein, usually IgG-λ, with a characteristic mobility (slower than any other gammaglobulin component), and a strong affinity for normal dermis. Other manifestations of MM (plasmacytosis, osteolysis, and excretion of light chains) are rare. Treatment with melphalan is often beneficial.

Suggested Reading

Multiple Myeloma

Attal M, et al. Single versus double autologous stem-cell transplantation for multiple myeloma. *N Engl J Med* 2003;349:2495.

Barlogie B, et al. Treatment of multiple myeloma. *Blood* 2004;103:20.

Berenson JR, Crowley JJ, Grogan TM. Maintenance therapy with alternate-day prednisone improves survival in multiple myeloma patients. *Blood* 2002;99:3163.

Bergsagel PL, Kuehl WM. Molecular pathogenesis and a consequent classification of multiple myeloma. *J Clin Oncol* 2005;23:6333.

Child JA, et al. Medical *Research* Council Adult Leukaemia Working Party. High-dose chemotherapy with hematopoietic stem-cell rescue for multiple myeloma. *N Engl J Med* 2003;348:1875.

Fonseca R, et al. Clinical and biologic implications of recurrent genomic aberrations in myeloma. *Blood* 2003;101:4569.

Greipp PR, et al. International staging system for multiple myeloma. *J Clin Oncol* 2005;23:3412.

Kyle RA, et al. Review of 1027 patients with newly diagnosed multiple myeloma. *Mayo Clin Proc* 2003;78:21.

Kyle RA, et al. Clinical course and prognosis of smoldering (asymptomatic) multiple myeloma. *N Engl J Med* 2007;356:2582.

Lauta VM. A review of the cytokine network in multiple myeloma. *Cancer* 2003;97:2440.

Magrangeas F, et al. Gene expression profiling of multiple myeloma reveals molecular portraits in relation to the pathogenesis of the disease. *Blood* 2003;101:4998.

Maloney DG, et al. Allografting with nonmyeloablative conditioning following cytoreductive autografts for the treatment of patients with multiple myeloma. *Blood* 2003;102:3447.

Rajkumar SV, et al. Thalidomide as initial therapy for early-stage myeloma. *Leukemia* 2003;17:775.

Richardson PG, et al. A phase 2 study of bortezomib in relapsed, refractory myeloma. *N Engl J Med* 2003;348:2609.

Sezer O, et al. RANK ligand and osteoprotegerin in myeloma bone disease. *Blood* 2003;101:2094.

Terpos E, et al. Clinical implications of chromosomal abnormalities in multiple myeloma. *Leuk Lymph* 2006;47:803.

Weber D, et al. Thalidomide alone or with dexamethasone for previously untreated multiple myeloma. *J Clin Oncol* 2003;21:16.

Wu K-D, et al. Telomerase and telomere length in multiple myeloma: correlations with disease heterogeneity, cytogenetic status, and overall survival. *Blood* 2003;101:4982.

Yeh HS, Berenson JR. Treatment of myeloma bone disease. *Clin Cancer Res* 2006;12:6279s.

Other Topics

Berenson JR, et al. Zoledronic acid is superior to pamidronate in the treatment of hypercalcemia of malignancy: a pooled analysis of two randomized, controlled clinical trials. *J Clin Oncol* 2001;91:1191.

Dimopoulos MA, et al. Treatment of plasma cell dyscrasias with thalidomide and its derivatives. *J Clin Oncol* 2003;21:4444.

Merlini G, Stone MJ. Dangerous small B-cell clones. *Blood* 2006;108:2520.

Rajkumar SV, et al. Monoclonal gammopathy of undetermined significance, Waldenstrom macroglobulinemia, AL amyloidosis, and related plasma cell disorders: diagnosis and treatment. *Mayo Clin Proc* 2006;81:693.

Seldin DC, et al. Tolerability and efficacy of thalidomide for the treatment of patients with light chain-associated (AL) amyloidosis. *Clin Lymphoma* 2003;3:241.

Treon SP, et al. CD20-directed antibody-mediated immunotherapy induces responses and facilitates hematologic recovery in patients with Waldenstrom's macroglobulinemia. *J Immunother* 2001;24:272.

Vijay A, Gertz MA. Waldenstrom macroglobulinemia. *Blood* 2007;109:5096.

CHRONIC LEUKEMIAS

Gary Schiller, Dennis A. Casciato, and Ronald L. Paquette

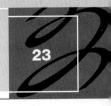

23

 CHRONIC LYMPHOCYTIC LEUKEMIA

I. EPIDEMIOLOGY AND ETIOLOGY

A. Incidence. Chronic lymphocytic leukemia (CLL) is the most common type of leukemia in Western countries, accounting for one-third of cases. The incidence in the United States is 3.5 cases per 100,000. The disease is rare in Asians. Ninety percent of patients are >50 years of age, and the median age at diagnosis is approximately 65 years. Men are affected more often than women by a ratio of 2:1.

B. Etiology

1. **Genetic factors.** The vast majority of cases are sporadic, but familial clusters of CLL have been described. The incidence in relatives of patients with leukemia is two- to threefold greater than that of the general population. The etiology in the majority of cases is unknown.

2. **Immunological factors.** Inherited and acquired immune deficiency is often associated with CLL and other lymphoproliferative neoplasms. This observation supports a concept that defective immune surveillance may result in proliferation of malignant cell clones and increased susceptibility to potential leukemogenic transduction, such as by viruses.

3. **Molecular and cytogenetic aberrations.** Somatic mutations of the immunoglobulin gene take place in the germinal center of secondary lymphoid follicles after antigen exposure. IgV_H hypermutations are detected in approximately half of the cases of CLL, indicating that the cells are derived from postgerminal center or memory B cells and do not express ZAP-70, a molecule usually required for selective activation of T cells but aberrantly expressed in some cases of (B-cell) CLL. Some cases of CLL show characteristics of naive B cells with unmutated antigen receptors and are ZAP-70 positive.

   Chromosomal abnormalities are detected in >80% of cases of CLL by use of interphase fluorescence *in situ* hybridization (FISH). CLL is characterized by loss or gain of chromosomal genetic material rather than by translocations. Conventional cytogenetics typically miss these abnormalities. Incidence, genes involved, and clinical features of the most common chromosome abnormalities are shown in Table 23.1.

4. **Radiation and cytotoxic agents.** Populations exposed to ionizing radiation or cytotoxic chemotherapy do not have an increased incidence of CLL.

II. PATHOLOGY AND NATURAL HISTORY

A. Pathology. CLL is characterized by suppression of programmed cell death (apoptosis) of mature B cells. Increased levels of Bcl-2 protein have been identified in cells taken from patients with CLL. Two other *BCL-2* family gene products may prevent apoptosis of CLL cells. *BCL-xL*, which is expressed at high levels in CLL, enhances the efforts of *Bcl-2*, whereas *BCL-xS*, which is expressed at low levels in CLL cells, is a *Bcl-2* antagonist. Furthermore, nonclonal CD4+ T cells and cells of the bone marrow stroma may support and sustain survival of the neoplastic B cell clone.

1. The leukemia cells have low levels of surface immunoglobulin and display a single heavy-chain class, typically μ; some cells display both μ and δ; less commonly, γ,

TABLE 23.1	Chromosomal Abnormalities In Chronic Lymphocytic Leukemia		
Chromosome	**Frequency (%)**	**Involved genes**	**Clinical characteristics**
Del 13q14.3	>50	Telomeric to *RB1*	Good prognosis, low CD38, mutated V_H genes
Del 11q22–q23	19	*ATM*	Poor prognosis, extensive lymphadenopathy
Trisomy 12	15	*MDM-2*	Intermediate prognosis, high CD38, unmutated V_H genes, atypical morphology
Del 17p13.3	15	*p53* (deleted)	Poor prognosis, >10% prolymphocytosis, Richter transformation

α, or no heavy-chain determinant is found. The leukemia cells display either κ or λ light chains, but never both.

2. Surface membrane antigens include the B-cell antigens CD19, CD20, and CD23; CD22 and CD79b are weak or negative. The CD11c and CD25 antigens are found on the cells in half of the cases. CD5 is always present on CLL cells. Expression of CD38 has been associated with an unfavorable prognosis (see Appendix C-5, "Discriminatory Immunophenotypes for Lymphocytic Neoplasms").

3. CLL is associated with a defect in the B-cell receptor (BCR), which is faintly expressed.

B. Natural history

1. Immunological abnormalities in CLL

  a. Advanced disease is associated with hypogammaglobulinemia and an increased risk of infection with encapsulated bacterial organisms.

  b. A variety of *in vitro* lymphocyte function tests are abnormal. Many studies have suggested decreased helper T-cell functions, and patients may have an inversion of the normal helper T-cell–to–suppressor T-cell ratios.

  c. Monoclonal paraproteins are not routinely identified; however, when one uses more sensitive techniques, it appears that most patients with CLL secrete small amounts of paraproteins [usually immunoglobulin M (IgM)]. These paraproteins rarely produce symptoms of hyperviscosity.

  d. Coombs-positive warm antibody hemolytic anemia occurs in about 10% of patients and immune thrombocytopenia in about 5%. Immune neutropenia and pure red blood cell aplasia are rare.

  e. Compared with the general population, the incidence of skin carcinoma is increased eightfold and visceral epithelial cancers twofold in patients with CLL.

2. Clinical course. The natural history of CLL is highly variable. Survival is closely correlated with the stage of disease at the time of diagnosis. Because most patients are elderly, >30% die of diseases unrelated to leukemia.

  a. Manifestations. In 25% of patients, CLL is first recognized at routine physical examination or by a routine CBC. Clinical manifestations develop as the leukemia cells accumulate in the lymph nodes, spleen, liver, and bone marrow.

   (1) Pulmonary infiltrates and pleural effusions are common late in the course of disease.

   (2) Renal involvement is common in CLL, but functional impairment is unusual in the absence of obstructive uropathy, pyelonephritis, or hyperuricemia secondary to tumor lysis from therapy.

   (3) Transformation into a diffuse large cell lymphoma (Richter syndrome) or prolymphocytic leukemia occurs in <5% of patients.

   (4) Skin involvement is rare.

(5) Osteolytic lesions and isolated mediastinal involvement are unusual and suggest a diagnosis other than CLL.
  b. **Progressive disease** is accompanied by deterioration of both humoral and cell-mediated immunity. As the disease progresses, patients develop progressive pancytopenia, persistent fever, and inanition. During the latter stages of disease, cytotoxic chemotherapy is generally ineffective, and dosages are restricted because of pancytopenia. Death is usually caused by infection, bleeding, or other complications of the disease.
    (1) Herpes zoster is the cause of 10% of infections in CLL patients.
    (2) Bacterial pathogens associated with hypogammaglobulinemia include *Streptococcus pneumoniae, Haemophilus influenzae,* and *Legionella sp.*
    (3) *Pneumocystis jiroveci* may be the causative infectious agent in patients with pulmonary infiltrates.

III. DIAGNOSIS

  A. **Symptoms and signs.** Patients with CLL that was discovered incidentally are usually asymptomatic. Chronic fatigue and reduced exercise tolerance are the first symptoms to develop. Advanced and progressive disease are manifested by severe fatigue out of proportion to the degree of the patient's anemia, fever, bruising, and weight loss.

   Lymphadenopathy, splenomegaly, and hepatomegaly should be carefully assessed. Edema or thrombophlebitis may result from obstruction of lymphatic or venous channels by enlarged lymph nodes.
  B. **Laboratory studies**
    1. **Hemogram**
      a. **Erythrocytes.** Anemia may be caused by lymphocyte infiltration of the bone marrow, hypersplenism, autoimmune hemolysis, and other factors. Red blood cells are usually normocytic and normochromic in the absence of prominent hemolysis.
      b. **Lymphocytes.** The absolute lymphocyte count typically ranges from 10,000 to 200,000/μL but may exceed 500,000/μL. Lymphocytes are usually mature appearing with scanty cytoplasm and clumped nuclear chromatin. When blood smears are made, the cells are easily ruptured, producing typical "basket" or "smudge" cells.
      c. **Granulocytes.** Absolute granulocyte counts are normal until late in the disease.
      d. **Platelets.** Thrombocytopenia may be produced by bone marrow infiltration, hypersplenism, or immune thrombocytopenia.
    2. **Other useful studies** that should be obtained in patients with CLL include the following:
      a. Biologic markers of the disease, including FISH, ZAP-70 expression, and perhaps IgV$_H$ gene rearrangement
      b. Flow cytometry of the peripheral blood lymphocytes
      c. Renal and liver function tests
      d. Direct antiglobulin (Coombs) test
      e. Serum protein electrophoresis
      f. Chest radiographs
      g. Computed tomography (CT) scans, which can be used to evaluate mediastinal, retroperitoneal, abdominal, and pelvic lymph nodes
    3. **Bone marrow examination** is usually not necessary to establish the diagnosis in patients with persistent lymphocytosis. The bone marrow of all patients with CLL contains at least 30% lymphocytes. The pattern of bone marrow infiltration is an important prognostic factor (see section IV.A.2). The indications for bone marrow aspiration and biopsy include the following:
      a. Borderline cases of lymphocytosis when the diagnosis is in doubt
      b. Thrombocytopenia, to distinguish immune thrombocytopenia from severe bone marrow infiltration
      c. Coombs-negative, unexplained anemia

    4. Lymph node biopsy in patients with CLL shows malignant lymphoma of the small lymphocytic type. A lymph node biopsy is not indicated in CLL unless the cause of the lymph node involvement is in doubt, particularly when Richter transformation is suspected.

C. Establishing the diagnosis of CLL. The National Cancer Institute (NCI) Working Group on CLL has established useful guidelines for the minimum diagnostic requirements for this disease, which are as follows:

    1. Absolute lymphocytosis (5,000/μL or more) with mature-appearing lymphocytes that is sustained

    2. Characteristic immunophenotype of monoclonal B cells

        a. Expression of pan–B-cell antigens (CD19, CD20, and CD23)

        b. Coexpression of CD5 on the leukemic B cells

        c. Surface immunoglobulin of low intensity (most often IgM)

D. Differential diagnosis

    1. Benign causes of lymphocytosis in adults

        a. Viral infections, especially hepatitis, cytomegalovirus, and Epstein-Barr virus (EBV). Lymphadenopathy and hepatosplenomegaly are absent or mild in elderly patients with infectious mononucleosis. The presence of fever, LFTs compatible with hepatitis, and positive EBV serologies should distinguish mononucleosis from CLL.

        b. Brucellosis, typhoid fever, paratyphoid, and chronic infections

        c. Autoimmune diseases; drug and allergic reactions

        d. Thyrotoxicosis and adrenal insufficiency

        e. Postsplenectomy

    2. Hairy cell leukemia must be differentiated from CLL because management of the two disorders is different. Diagnosis depends on recognizing the pathognomonic hairy cells by immunophenotyping.

    3. Cutaneous T-cell lymphomas are suspected if skin involvement is extensive. Differentiation from CLL is made by identifying the convoluted nuclei and helper T cells (with immunohistochemistry and flow cytometry) that are characteristic of this disease.

    4. Leukemic phase of non-Hodgkin lymphoma (NHL) is usually distinguished from CLL morphologically and immunologically. NHL cells are often cleaved, whereas CLL cells are never cleaved. In addition, NHL cells demonstrate intense surface immunoglobulins without the CD5 and CD23 antigens, and the opposite is generally true for CLL cells.

    5. Prolymphocytic leukemia has large lymphocytes with prominent nucleoli. Lymphadenopathy is minimal; splenomegaly is massive (see section VI.B).

    6. Large granular lymphocytic leukemia/lymphoma (LGLL) has a characteristic morphology with abundant pale to clear, sharply defined cytoplasm and multiple distinct azurophilic granules of varying size. The cells are either T cells or NK cells, and most correspond to natural killer cells. The immunophenotype is positive for CD3, CD8, CD16, and CD57. LGLL is indolent and almost uniformly associated with neutropenia. Rheumatoid arthritis is present in about one third of patients.

IV. STAGING SYSTEM AND PROGNOSTIC FACTORS

A. Prognostic factors. Routine CBCs may detect asymptomatic cases of CLL, but this has no bearing on the overall survival of these patients. If survival has been improved (and it is not clear that it has), effective treatment of complicating infections in CLL probably has been more responsible for the improvement than cytotoxic agents.

    1. Clinical staging is helpful for determining prognosis and deciding when to initiate treatment. Anemia and thrombocytopenia adversely affect prognosis when they are due to leukemic infiltration ("packing") of the bone marrow but not when they are due to autoimmune destruction of red blood cells or platelets.

    2. The pattern of bone marrow infiltration also appears to affect prognosis. Patients with nodular or interstitial patterns of bone marrow involvement have longer survival times than patients with diffuse ("packed") involvement.

TABLE 23.2 The Modified Rai Classification of Chronic Lymphocytic Leukemia

Stage	Extent of disease	Risk	Median survival (yr)
0	Lymphocytosis of bone marrow ($\geq$40% lymphocytes) and blood (>5,000/μL)	Low	10
I	Stage 0 plus lymphadenopathy	Intermediate	7
II	Stage 0 or I plus splenomegaly and/or hepatomegaly	Intermediate	7
III	Stage 0, I, or II plus anemia (hemoglobin <11.0 g/dL)[a]	High	2
IV	Stage 0, I, or II plus thrombocytopenia (platelets <100,000/μL)[a]	High	2

[a]Excluding anemia or thrombocytopenia caused by immunologic destruction of cells.

3. **V genes.** Two subsets of CLL are defined by the IgV$_H$ mutational status. Patients with somatic mutations of the V genes generally have a better prognosis than those with unmutated V genes.
4. **CD38 expression** on CLL cells generally is associated with a poorer prognosis than absent or low-level expression of CD38.
5. **Chromosome abnormalities** as described in Table 23.1 may predict outcome.
6. **Other adverse prognostic factors** appear to be a lymphocyte doubling time of <12 months and an elevated serum β_2-microglobulin level.
B. **Staging system.** The *modified Rai classification* of CLL with median survivals is shown in Table 23.2 (see section III.C for differences with the NCI Working Group criteria).

V. MANAGEMENT
A. **Indications for treatment.** CLL is usually indolent. Treatment of asymptomatic stable disease is not warranted. The magnitude of the blood lymphocyte count does not indicate the need to start therapy. The initiation of therapy should be timed according to the clinically assessed pace of disease. Complete remission is not a necessary goal. The indications for instituting therapy in CLL are as follows:
1. Persistent or progressive systemic symptoms (fever, sweats, weight loss)
2. Lymphadenopathy that causes mechanical obstruction or bothersome cosmetic deformities
3. Progressive enlargement of the lymph nodes, liver, or spleen
4. Stage III or IV (high-risk) disease that results from the replacement of bone marrow with lymphocytes
5. Immune hemolysis or immune thrombocytopenia, which are treated with prednisone alone
6. Rapid lymphocyte doubling time
B. **Chemotherapy.** Fludarabine is superior to alkylating agents in its associated complete response rate and duration of response but not in overall survival. Drug dosage schedules for CLL are as follows.
1. **Nucleosides.** Fludarabine may be the initial treatment of choice for patients who would benefit from a rapid and sustained remission, such as those designated for further aggressive therapy. Prolonged treatment with fludarabine and other nucleoside analogs, such as cladribine or pentostatin, however, are also associated with marked immunosuppression and an increased risk of opportunistic infections and autoimmune hemolysis.
   a. **Fludarabine,** 25 to 30 mg/m^2 IV daily for 5 consecutive days every 4 weeks
   b. **Cladribine** (2-chlorodeoxyadenosine, 2-CdA), either 0.10 mg/kg daily by continuous IV infusion for 7 days, or 0.14 mg/kg daily IV over 2 hours for 5 consecutive days every 4 to 5 weeks

    c. Pentostatin at 4 mg/m² IV every 2 weeks. Typically this drug, and the others mentioned above, are combined with an alkylating agent and/or rituximab.

2. Alkylating agents remain useful and effective for palliative therapy.

    a. Chlorambucil, 0.1 mg/kg PO daily for 3 to 6 weeks as tolerated; the dose is usually tapered to 2 mg daily until the desired effect is achieved. Alternatively, 15 to 30 mg/m² PO may be given for 1 day (or divided over 4 days) every 14 to 21 days; the dose is adjusted to tolerance.

    b. Cyclophosphamide, 2 to 4 mg/kg PO daily for 10 days; the dose is then adjusted downward for continued therapy until the desired effect is achieved.

3. Monoclonal antibodies can be useful for problematic CLL.

    a. Rituximab (Rituxan) is an anti-CD20 chimeric monoclonal antibody (see Chapter 4, section VII.G). The dose of 375 mg/m² weekly for 4 weeks, as used for non-Hodgkin lymphoma, has minimal activity in previously treated patients with CLL but is quite useful as part of combination therapy in untreated patients. Dose escalation with the weekly schedule or thrice-weekly administration increases the clinical response significantly with minimal toxicity. Similar to alemtuzumab, the complete remission rate is low. However, rituximab has less myelosuppression and is a better candidate to combine with chemotherapy than alemtuzumab. The primary toxicity associated with rituximab is an infusion-related cytokine release syndrome that is typically associated with the first infusion.

    b. Alemtuzumab (Campath-1H) is a humanized anti-CD52 monoclonal antibody whose antigen is expressed on more than 95% of mature B and T lymphocytes and may be used for the treatment of fludarabine-refractory CLL. Alemtuzumab preferentially eliminates CLL cells from the blood, bone marrow, and spleen but is less effective in nodal sites of disease. Approximately one-third of the patients will have a partial response to alemtuzumab; complete responses are rare. Dosing is discussed in Chapter 4, section VII.B.

        Side effects of alemtuzumab include cytokine release syndrome, immunosuppression, and neutropenia. The acute infusion reactions following intravenous administration are markedly reduced with subcutaneous injection. The immunosuppression has resulted opportunistic infections; trimethoprim/sulfamethoxazole (Bactrim) and acyclovir are recommended for prophylaxis.

4. Modern combination therapies have resulted in high response rates (70% to 95%) and high complete response rates (20% to 65%) in previously untreated patients. Variations in the following regimens are in active clinical trials. **Prophylaxis** with fluconazole, acyclovir, and Bactrim are recommended for all of these therapies.

    a. Fludarabine and cyclophosphamide. Fludarabine (25 mg/m² IV on Days 1 to 3) and cyclophosphamide (250 mg/m² IV on Days 1 to 3) are given every 4 weeks for six cycles (30% to 50% achieve a complete remission, CR).

    b. Fludarabine and rituximab. Fludarabine (25 mg/m² IV on Days 1 to 5) is given every 4 weeks for six cycles. Rituximab (375 mg/m²) is given on Days 1 and 4 of the first cycle and on Day 1 of cycles 2 to 6 (50% CR rate).

    c. Fludarabine, cyclophosphamide, and rituximab. Fludarabine (25 mg/m² IV on Days 1 to 3) and cyclophosphamide (250 mg/m² IV on Days 1 to 3) are given every 4 weeks for six cycles. Rituximab is given at a dose of 375 mg/m² 1 day before the first course and increased to 500 mg/m² on Day 1 for cycles 2 to 6 (65% CR rate).

    d. Pentostatin and cyclophosphamide. Pentostatin (4 mg/m² IV) and cyclophosphamide (600 to 900 mg/m² IV) are given every 3 weeks for six cycles (17% CR in previously treated patients). A newer regimen with Rituximab uses lower doses of pentostatin (4 mg/m²) and cyclophosphamide (600 mg/m²).

5. Treatment of resistant disease is controversial. Clearly, if patients were initially treated with an alkylating agent, then fludarabine or a fludarabine combination (see above) should be initiated. If a patient is resistant to fludarabine, then single-agent alkylators, alemtuzumab, or pentostatin plus cyclophosphamide should be considered. However, if patients have previously responded to fludarabine, then one of the fludarabine combinations should be considered. The role of autologous and allogeneic stem-cell transplants is limited in CLL patients, who are typically elderly and poor candidates for transplantation. However, in selected patients, stem-cell transplants can be considered.

C. Radiation therapy (RT). Local irradiation is recommended only for reduction of lymph node masses that threaten vital organ function and that respond poorly to chemotherapy. Splenic irradiation may result in improvement of disease elsewhere and may temporarily improve signs of hypersplenism; however, the clinical usefulness of splenic irradiation has not been established. Total-body irradiation remains investigational and potentially dangerous.

D. Surgery. Splenectomy is indicated in CLL patients who have immune hemolytic anemia or immune thrombocytopenia that either fails to respond to corticosteroid therapy or must be treated with corticosteroids chronically. Splenectomy may also be helpful in patients with problematic hypersplenism.

VI. SPECIAL CLINICAL PROBLEMS IN CLL

A. Richter syndrome. About 5% of patients with CLL develop a diffuse large-cell lymphoma with rapid clinical deterioration and death occurring within 1 to 6 months. The clinical features include fever, weight loss, increasing localized or generalized lymphadenopathy, lymphocytopenia (as well as other cytopenias), and dysglobulinemia. Combination chemotherapy with CHOP (see Appendix D-2, section II) is usually tried but is rarely effective.

B. Prolymphocytic leukemia is a rare variant of CLL. The main clinical feature is massive splenomegaly without substantial lymph node enlargement. Leukocytosis usually exceeds $100,000/\mu L$ and is characterized by large lymphoid cells with single prominent nucleoli. Tissue sections show almost no mitotic figures despite the immature appearance of the leukemic cells.

1. Eighty percent of cases involve B cells that have different surface markers than typical CLL (the B cells of prolymphocytic leukemia show intense surface immunoglobulin, the CD19 and CD20 B-cell antigens, but typically not the CD5 antigen). Twenty percent of cases are T cell, usually with a T-helper phenotype (CD3 and CD4 positive).

2. A small percentage of CLL patients develop a "prolymphocytoid" transformation, whereby more than 30% of the peripheral blood cells are prolymphocytic. This differs from *de novo* prolymphocytic leukemia in that the cells maintain the immune features of CLL and the clinical course resembles typical CLL, albeit in a late stage of the disease.

3. Single-agent therapy with fludarabine, cladribine, or alemtuzumab or combination therapy with CHOP may be useful.

 HAIRY CELL LEUKEMIA

I. EPIDEMIOLOGY AND ETIOLOGY. Hairy cell leukemia (HCL; leukemic reticuloendotheliosis, lymphoid myelofibrosis) accounts for about 2% of all leukemias. The disease occurs more frequently in men than women by a ratio of 5:1. The median age of patients is 55 years; patients <30 years of age are unusual. The etiology is unknown.

II. PATHOLOGY AND NATURAL HISTORY

A. Pathology. The pathognomonic cells with irregular cytoplasmic projections can be identified in the peripheral blood, bone marrow, liver, and spleen of affected patients. Hairy cells are B lymphocytes in virtually every case (rare T-cell variants have been reported).

B. Natural history. The natural history is characterized by neutropenia. The time course can be variable, ranging from a relatively fulminant course to a waxing and waning course of exacerbations and spontaneous improvements, and to prolonged survival measured in decades. Most patients are able to function normally throughout most of their illness.

Patients with HCL usually present with an insidious development of nonspecific symptoms, splenomegaly, neutropenia, and sometimes pancytopenia. Progression of disease is manifested by bleeding because of thrombocytopenia, anemia requiring transfusions, and recurrent infections.

III. DIAGNOSIS

A. Symptoms and signs. Weakness and fatigue are the presenting symptoms in about 40% of cases. Bleeding, recent infection, or abdominal discomfort is present in about 20% of patients.

Splenomegaly occurs in 95% of patients. Hepatomegaly is seen in about 40% of patients. Peripheral lymphadenopathy is rarely present in patients with HCL; however, CT scans of the abdomen may reveal retroperitoneal lymphadenopathy.

B. Preliminary laboratory studies

1. CBC. Anemia and thrombocytopenia occur in 85% of patients. About 60% of patients have granulocytopenia; 20% have increased hairy cells with leukocytosis and absolute granulocytopenia.

2. Blood chemistries. Only 10% to 20% of patients have abnormal liver or renal function tests. Polyclonal hyperglobulinemia or decreased normal immunoglobulin concentrations occurs in 20% of patients.

C. Special diagnostic studies. The diagnosis of HCL is made by identifying the pathognomonic mononuclear cells in the peripheral blood or bone marrow, but an immunophenotype characteristic of HCL is required. The cells have irregular and serrated borders with characteristic slender, hairlike cytoplasmic projections and round, eccentric nuclei with spongy chromatin. The cytoplasm is sky blue without granules.

1. Immune flow cytometry demonstrates a characteristic pattern of CD19, CD20, CD22, CD11c, CD25, and CD103 positivity. Hairy cell variants may be CD25 or CD103 negative and typically do not have a favorable prognosis.

2. Phase-contrast microscopy with supravital staining of fresh preparations is valuable for demonstrating the cellular characteristics because the cytoplasm of hairy cells is often poorly preserved in films mixed with Wright's stain.

3. Tartrate-resistant acid phosphatase (TRAP). HCL cells have a strong acid phosphatase activity, which is resistant to inhibition by 0.05 molar tartaric acid (due to the presence of isoenzyme 5 of acid phosphatase); the acid phosphatase in leukocytes from most patients with lymphomas and CLL is sensitive to tartrate. A strongly positive TRAP study is present in most patients with HCL but is not required for the diagnosis and can be detected in patients with other lymphoid malignancies. Cytochemical staining for TRAP is often omitted.

4. Bone marrow aspiration frequently is unsuccessful ("dry tap"). Marrow biopsy shows a characteristic loose and spongy arrangement of cells, even with extensive infiltration with hairy cells. Fibrosis of the marrow with reticulin fibers is also characteristic in areas of HCL infiltration and accounts for the high frequency of dry taps.

5. Splenic morphology. The spleen is the most densely infiltrated organ in HCL. The red pulp may contain a unique vascular lesion: pseudosinuses lined by hairy cells.

D. Differential diagnosis. It is important to distinguish HCL from other diseases because management is substantially different. HCL is most often confused with CLL, malignant lymphoma, histiocytic medullary reticulosis, myelofibrosis, or monocytic leukemia. Differentiation is made by identifying the pathognomonic cell, the characteristic immune profile, TRAP test, and pathological findings of the bone marrow biopsy.

IV. STAGING SYSTEM AND PROGNOSTIC FACTORS.
The median survival in the natural history of HCL appears to be 5 to 10 years, but this has been dramatically altered by current therapies.

V. MANAGEMENT

A. The decision to treat. Many cases tend to have an indolent course, and these patients have excellent survival without therapy. Therapy may be deferred for asymptomatic patients until the patient develops symptomatic anemia or clinically worrisome granulocytopenia and/or thrombocytopenia.

B. Cladribine is the treatment of choice for HCL. The drug is given by continuous intravenous infusion *once only* at a dose of 0.1 mg/kg per day for 7 days. Other regimens have been published, including a 5-day bolus IV treatment. Virtually all patients respond, and 95% achieve complete response. Relapse occurs in 35% of patients, usually after 3 years, and most respond to an additional course of cladribine. Toxicity has been limited to transient fever, usually associated with neutropenia. Survival at 9 years exceeds 95% in patients treated with cladribine.

C. Pentostatin (Nipent) is also highly effective therapy for HCL. Most patients not only have normalization of their CBC but also have a complete response with disappearance of hairy cells from their bone marrow (rarely seen with IFN-α). Complications include skin rash and neurotoxicity. The dosage is 4 mg/m^2 IV every 2 weeks for 3 to 6 months.

D. Interferon-α (IFN-α) is a highly effective agent in reversing the pancytopenia and splenomegaly in HCL. Dosages of IFN ranging from 2 to 4 million U daily or three times weekly for 1 year achieve responses in 90% of patients with HCL. Complete response with disappearance of hairy cells from the bone marrow, however, are unusual.

E. Splenectomy has achieved at least a partial response in 75% of patients and historically had been the standard therapy for HCL but, like interferon therapy, is no longer used as primary therapy.

F. Other therapy. Rituximab has been effective for treatment of HCL in case reports. Immunotoxin therapy, such as that studied with an anti-CD22 immunoconjugate, may be useful in the future.

 CHRONIC MYELOGENOUS LEUKEMIA

I. EPIDEMIOLOGY AND ETIOLOGY. Chronic myelogenous leukemia (CML) is a myeloproliferative disorder with a characteristic cytogenetic abnormality and a propensity to evolve from a chronic phase into a blast phase with features similar to acute leukemia.

A. Incidence. CML has an incidence of approximately 1 case in 100,000 population and composes 20% of adult leukemias in Western countries. The median age at onset is in the mid-50s, although children are also affected.

B. Etiology. The cause of most cases of CML is unknown, although radiation exposure is a known risk factor.

II. PATHOGENESIS AND NATURAL HISTORY

A. Clonality. CML is a clonal disease of an abnormal stem cell. Myeloid, erythroid, megakaryocytic, and B lymphoid cells are involved in the malignant clone.

B. The Philadelphia chromosome (Ph^1) is the diminutive chromosome produced by an unbalanced translocation between chromosomes 9 and 22. This translocation, designated t(9;22), fuses the 3' portion of the *c-ABL* gene on the long arm of chromosome 9 (band q34) to the 5' end of the breakpoint cluster (*BCR*) gene on the long arm of chromosome 22 (band q11). The resultant fusion gene encodes a chimeric protein of 210 kilodaltons (p210) with constitutive tyrosine kinase activity. The *BCR-ABL* protein stimulates the proliferation and enhances the survival of CML hematopoietic progenitor cells.

1. Atypical (Ph^1-negative) CML. Approximately 1% to 2% of cases that appear clinically to be CML are Ph^1-negative by bone marrow cytogenetics, FISH, and polymerase chain reaction (PCR) amplification for the *BCR-ABL* fusion gene. Some cases may have a translocation involving chromosome 5q31–35, which encodes the *PDGFRB* gene. The clinical course is poorly characterized as many case series were published before availability of FISH and PCR assays, and probably included a majority of cases with occult *BCR-ABL* translocations. Nevertheless, anemia, thrombocytopenia, and splenomegaly appear to be clinical consequences of this disorder.

Therapy with imatinib may benefit patients with the *PDGFRB* gene rearrangement. In the absence of this specific abnormality, hydroxyurea would be the myelosuppressive therapy of choice, if required for management of leukocytosis or splenomegaly.

2. **Ph^1 chromosome in acute leukemia.** The Ph^1 chromosome can be found in *de novo* acute leukemia. Approximately 30% of adults with acute lymphoblastic leukemia (ALL) and 2% of adults with acute myelogenous leukemia (AML) present with the Ph^1 chromosome. Some of these cases represent CML in blast crisis that was never diagnosed in the chronic phase; effective treatment may reverse some cases to a chronic phase.

C. **Clinical course.** Three stages of CML are recognized: chronic phase (CP), accelerated phase (AP), and blast phase (or blast crisis, BP). Approximately 85% of patients are diagnosed while in chronic phase. All stages of disease can present with fatigue, low-grade fevers, night sweats, and early satiety or abdominal pain from splenomegaly. Symptoms tend to be more severe when advanced disease is present. Evolution of accelerated or blast phase from the chronic phase can be suggested by the development of anemia, thrombocytopenia, leukocytosis with immature myeloid cells or basophilia, increasing splenomegaly, or recurrent constitutional symptoms while on therapy. The disease status should be reevaluated in this setting.

Cytogenetic changes other than the Ph^1 abnormality are commonly observed in association with blast crisis evolution. Approximately 70% of blast crises are myeloid, in which the blasts display a phenotype indistinguishable from acute myeloid leukemia. The remaining cases of blast crisis are lymphoid, in which the blasts are B lymphoblasts similar to acute lymphoid leukemia.

III. CLINICAL MANIFESTATIONS
A. Symptoms and signs
1. CML is asymptomatic in approximately 20% of patients and is discovered incidentally by routine blood counts.
2. The excessive numbers of metabolically active myeloid cells can cause fevers and sweats. Fatigue and malaise are also commonly present.
3. Bone pain and tenderness can result from the expanding leukemic mass in the marrow.
4. Splenomegaly is present in the majority of cases, and it may be massive. It can be manifested as early satiety, abdominal fullness, or pain. Hepatomegaly is less common and is usually asymptomatic.
5. Marked leukocytosis (particularly white blood cell counts [WBC] exceeding 100,000/μL) can be associated with symptoms of leukostasis. Manifestations may include visual changes, seizures, and cerebral or myocardial infarctions. Similar complications can result from severe thrombocytosis.
6. **Progression to accelerated phase or blast crisis** is suggested by the recurrence of constitutional symptoms, including fevers, sweats, anorexia, and bone pain while on therapy. Recurrent or worsening splenomegaly also suggests disease progression. The development of blast crisis may be accompanied by infection or bleeding due to neutropenia or thrombocytopenia, respectively. Lymphadenopathy can develop in lymphoid blast crisis.

B. Laboratory studies
1. **Leukocytes.** The WBC usually exceeds 30,000/μL and usually ranges from 100,000 to 300,000/μL at the time of diagnosis. The peripheral blood smear in the chronic phase is often described as appearing like a bone marrow aspirate smear due to presence of all stages of myeloid cell maturation. Myeloblasts

constitute <15% of the leukocytes in the peripheral blood, and promyelocytes plus blasts combined compose <30% in the chronic phase. Eosinophil and basophil counts are often elevated, but basophils constitute <20% of the peripheral blood leukocytes in the chronic phase.

2. **Platelets.** Thrombocytosis is common, and the platelet count may exceed 1,000,000/μL at presentation. Thrombocytopenia is unusual in the chronic phase. Platelet aggregation tests are commonly abnormal.

3. **Erythrocytes.** The hemoglobin level is usually normal, but a mild normocytic, normochromic anemia can be present. A few nucleated red blood cells can be seen on the peripheral blood smear.

4. **Bone marrow aspiration and biopsy** should be performed on all patients as part of the diagnostic evaluation. This is necessary to evaluate the stage of disease at presentation. In all cases, the marrow is markedly hypercellular as a result of massive myeloid hyperplasia, resulting in a markedly increased myeloid-to-erythroid ratio. Megakaryocyte numbers are frequently increased. Fibrosis may also be present in variable amounts but is rarely profound.

5. **Cytogenetic analysis** should be performed at the time of bone marrow examination on all patients. The characteristic t(9;22) is identified in the majority of patients. However, complex translocations infrequently occur that can mask the *BCR-ABL* translocation. In this situation, FISH or PCR for *BCR-ABL* can identify the characteristic abnormality. Cytogenetics are particularly important to determine if additional chromosomal abnormalities associated with advanced disease are present.

6. **Fluorescence *in situ* hybridization (FISH)** for the *BCR-ABL* gene rearrangement can be performed on peripheral blood or bone marrow. This assay does not require dividing cells and is slightly more sensitive than cytogenetics at detecting minimal residual disease during therapy. It can be useful if complex chromosomal translocations are present.

7. **Polymerase chain reaction (PCR)** is a molecular assay performed on the peripheral blood that identifies the *BCR-ABL* translocation. The **quantitative PCR (Q-PCR)** assay is the most sensitive method to follow residual disease during the treatment of CML. A baseline Q-PCR assay should be obtained on all patients so that subsequent measurements during therapy will permit an accurate assessment of response in relation to the pretreatment level of disease. Like the FISH test, the PCR assay is capable of detecting the *BCR-ABL* rearrangement if complex chromosomal translocations occur.

8. **Leukocyte alkaline phosphatase** activity in circulating granulocytes is decreased or absent in CML and was previously helpful diagnostically. This test has been supplanted by FISH and PCR assays for *BCR-ABL*.

9. **Uric acid.** Hyperuricemia and hyperuricosuria are typically present.

IV. DIAGNOSTIC CRITERIA AND PROGNOSTIC VARIABLES

A. **World Health Organization (WHO) diagnostic criteria for chronic phase (CP) CML** include:
1. Peripheral blood leukocytosis due to increased numbers of mature and immature neutrophils
2. Prominent dysgranulopoiesis
3. Promyelocytes, myelocytes, and metamyelocytes >10% of WBCs
4. Basophils <2% of WBCs
5. Monocytes <10% of WBCs
6. Bone marrow hypercellular with granulocytic proliferation and dysplasia, with or without erythroid or megakaryocytic dysplasia
7. <20% blasts in the blood or bone marrow

B. **WHO criteria for diagnosis of accelerated phase (AP) CML** requires one or more of the following:
1. Blasts 10% to 19% in the blood or bone marrow, or
2. Basophils ≥20% of peripheral blood leukocytes, or

3. Platelets $\geq 1,000,000/\mu L$ unresponsive to therapy or $\leq 100,000/\mu L$ unrelated to therapy, or

4. Increasing spleen size and/or increasing WBC count unresponsive to therapy, or

5. Cytogenetic evidence of clonal evolution (cytogenetic abnormalities in addition to the Ph^1 chromosome)

C. WHO criteria for diagnosis of blast phase CML (blast crisis, BP)

    1. Blasts $\geq 20\%$ of bone marrow cells or peripheral WBC, or

    2. Extramedullary blast formation (e.g., osteolytic bone lesions, lymphadenopathy), or

    3. Large foci or clusters of blasts in bone marrow

D. Differential diagnosis

    1. Leukemoid reactions rarely show the full spectrum of myeloid cells (especially myelocytes, promyelocytes, or blasts) in the peripheral blood and lack the *BCR-ABL* Translocation.

    2. Other myeloproliferative disorders may present with leukocytosis and thrombocytosis but will not have the *BCR-ABL* translocation.

    3. Chronic neutrophilic leukemia is an exceedingly rare disorder (if it is a real disease) that can be considered when no other cause for persistent, mature neutrophilia is found. Cytogenetics are normal.

E. Prognostic variables. Although a variety of prognostic variables were identified that predicted the outcome of CML to interferon therapy, the remarkable efficacy of imatinib in the treatment of newly diagnosed CML has rendered these predictors useless. Ongoing assessment of response during therapy has emerged as a much more important predictor of progression-free survival. Stage of disease, however, remains a critical determinant of outcome. Chronic phase is defined as absence of accelerated or blast phase.

V. MANAGEMENT

A. Imatinib (Gleevec) is an inhibitor of *BCR-ABL* tyrosine kinase activity that has remarkable activity in CML. Long-term progression-free survival of CML patients on imatinib therapy correlates with the depth of response.

    1. Imatinib dosing. The standard dose of imatinib is 400 mg/day. Suboptimal cytogenetic response may warrant a dose increase to 600 mg/day, or 800 mg/day administered in divided doses as 400 mg b.i.d. Potential side effects include fluid retention, nausea, diarrhea, muscle cramps, skin rashes, fatigue, and myelosuppression. If moderate toxicity warrants dose reduction, re-escalation to a standard dose should be attempted once side effects abate. It is important to be aware that **the minimum dose capable of inducing a cytogenetic response is 300 mg/day.** Failure of a patient to tolerate this dose warrants a change in therapy.

    2. Acquired imatinib resistance is defined as loss of a previous hematologic or cytogenetic response. The best understood mechanism of resistance is the development of point mutations in *BCR-ABL* that decrease sensitivity of the protein to the inhibitory effects of imatinib. *BCR-ABL* mutation analysis is commercially available and should be sent if acquired resistance develops. CML with most of the common *BCR-ABL* mutations can be effectively treated by the second-generation kinase inhibitors dasatinib or nilotinib. However, *BCR-ABL* harboring the T315I mutation is resistant to both second-line agents. Patients with this mutation should be referred to a center that is evaluating investigational agents for this mutation. Another mechanism of resistance is amplification of *BCR-ABL* copy number, as detected by FISH.

B. Close monitoring of response is essential to optimize patient outcomes. Patients who do not achieve response end points within appropriate time frames should be considered for imatinib dose escalation, therapy with an alternative tyrosine kinase inhibitor, or allogeneic bone marrow transplantation.

    1. Complete hematologic response (CHR) is defined as a normalization of the peripheral blood counts and can be expected in >95% of chronic-phase patients. Failure to achieve this end point by 3 months warrants a reassessment of the treatment approach.

2. **Major cytogenetic response** (MCR) is defined as a reduction of the percentage of Ph[1] chromosomes to <35% of bone marrow metaphases. **Complete cytogenetic response** (CCR) is defined as normalization of the bone marrow cytogenetics. Ideally, an MCR should be observed by 6 months and a CCR by 1 year. The absence of any cytogenetic response at 6 months, less than an MCR at 12 months, or less than a CCR at 18 months should prompt consideration of a change in treatment.

3. **Major molecular response** (MMR) is defined as at least a 3-log (1,000-fold) reduction in the level of disease measured by Q-PCR. Patients who achieve this end point by 1 year have a 0% risk of disease progression to AP or BP at 5 years.

4. **Response monitoring** should include a bone marrow aspiration and biopsy at baseline and every 6 months until a complete cytogenetic response is achieved. A Q-PCR should be performed every 3 months. A bone marrow biopsy should be repeated if unexplained peripheral blood abnormalities occur or there is progressive increase in the Q-PCR assay. A 10-fold increase in Q-PCR is considered clinically significant.

C. **Second-generation *BCR-ABL* kinase inhibitors** have been developed to treat CML patients who are resistant to or intolerant of imatinib. **Dasatinib** (Sprycel) is a novel SRC and ABL kinase inhibitor that has been FDA approved for this indication. **Nilotinib** (Tasigna) is an imatinib analog that has also been approved by the FDA. Both agents are active against *BCR-ABL* mutations (other than T315I) that confer imatinib resistance, and they appear to be well tolerated by patients who experience intolerable side effects to imatinib. Both agents are more potent inhibitors of the *BCR-ABL* kinase than imatinib, but they have not yet been compared with imatinib or with each other in clinical trials.

1. **Dasatinib** can induce a CHR in approximately 90% of chronic phase patients who lose their response to imatinib or are intolerant of it. Approximately 50% of such patients will develop an MCR. Although follow-up is relatively short, these responses appear to be durable. The FDA-approved dose is 70 mg PO b.i.d., but a subsequent clinical study demonstrated that 100 mg PO daily is equally effective and better tolerated. Side effects include peripheral blood cytopenias and pleural effusions.

2. **Nilotinib** 400 mg PO b.i.d. can produce CHR rates of 80% in CP patients with acquired resistance or intolerance to imatinib. MCRs occur in approximately 50% of these patients. Common side effects include peripheral blood cytopenias, skin rash, and liver function abnormalities.

D. **Bone marrow transplantation (BMT)** is the only therapy that is known to be curative for CML, but its role in the management of this disease has become difficult to define due to the marked success of imatinib and the second-generation kinase inhibitors. The tyrosine kinase inhibitors are not currently believed to be capable of curing CML. The disadvantage of transplantation is that there is a 15% to 20% risk of morality at 1 year in young patients, and the risk increases with the age of the patient. In comparison, the risk of death during the first year on tyrosine kinase therapy is approximately 2% in patients with a median age of >50 years, and use of imatinib before transplantation does not appear to adversely affect outcome. Therefore, BMT is primarily reserved as a salvage therapy for patients who are at high risk (AP or BP at diagnosis) or who are having suboptimal response to medical therapy.

Careful monitoring of response to imatinib using cytogenetics and Q-PCR should permit the prediction of long-term benefit from medical therapy and identification of patients who should be considered for transplantation due to inadequate response. The risks and benefits of ongoing medical therapy versus transplantation must be highly individualized and should be discussed in detail with patients as therapy proceeds. The risk of relapse is unacceptably high if BMT is performed in BP and therefore is not routinely performed. AP disease is also associated with an increased risk of relapse, so when there are clinical indications that medical therapy will be inadequate, transplantation should be considered while the patient is still in chronic phase.

The expected outcomes of BMT for CML include:

1. Disappearance of the Ph^1 chromosome
2. Long-term (5 to 10 years) disease-free survival is reported in 60% to 80% of patients in chronic phase CML who are treated with BMT using related donors. Allogeneic transplants using 10/10 matched unrelated donors produce survival results approximately 5% points lower than for patients receiving transplants from matched related donors. Survival rates after BMT appear to plateau after 3 to 7 years.
3. Young patients undergoing BMT face a 15% to 20% probability of transplant-related death within 1 year of the procedure. Significant graft-versus-host disease (GVHD) occurs in 10% to 60% of cases and is the cause of death in 5% to 15% of patients. The risk of severe GVHD and mortality increases with age and with degree of HLA disparity between the donor and recipient.
4. Survival rates decrease by half when using BMT in the accelerated phase and by half again when used in the blast phase.
5. Relapses of CP disease can be effectively treated with lymphocyte infusions from the original donor (donor lymphocyte infusions, or DLI) without additional chemotherapy. CCR can be expected in approximately 60% of patients with chronic phase CML treated with DLI. The predominant risk of this therapy is worsening GVHD. Patients who relapse with AP or BP disease should ideally be returned to CP before the use of DLI.

E. **Younger patients who are considered good candidates for an allotransplantation** should be referred to a transplant center to discuss this option. Human leukocyte antigen (HLA) typing of the patient and siblings should be performed to determine the potential availability of a related donor. Because the therapeutic landscape for CML is still evolving, candid discussions about the risks and benefits of transplantation and tyrosine kinase inhibitors should be undertaken. Close monitoring of response to imatinib is essential, as discussed previously. Failure to achieve a CHR at 3 months, any degree of cytogenetic response at 6 months, less than an MCR at 12 months, or less than a CCR at 18 months should prompt consideration of switching to a second-generation tyrosine kinase inhibitor or reconsideration of the transplant option. Similar considerations apply should there be loss of hematologic, cytogenetic, or molecular response at any time, suggestive of acquired imatinib resistance.

F. **Management of the accelerated phase (AP) or blast crisis (BP).** Patients who present in AP or BP should be started on imatinib 600 mg/day. Long-term outcome data for newly diagnosed AP and BP patients treated with imatinib are lacking. However, AP patients who achieve an excellent reduction in disease burden, such as a MMR, are likely to have a very low rate of disease progression. As in CP, lesser degrees of response convey a higher risk of relapse or progression to BP.

1. For any patient, the choice between ongoing imatinib therapy and transplantation must take into consideration the depth of response and the individualized risks of the transplant procedure.
2. BP patients, regardless of the depth of response, will all ultimately relapse with recurrent disease, usually within a few months. Therefore, definitive therapy with allogeneic BMT should be expeditiously undertaken if a BP patient can be returned to AP or CP with imatinib.
3. All side effects of imatinib are potentially more severe in patients who present with advanced disease. Patients who experience severe cytopenias (neutrophils <500/μL or platelets <20,000/μL) on imatinib should have a bone marrow biopsy to determine if the low counts are due to the drug or the disease. If the bone marrow is hypocellular without increased blasts, then the imatinib should be held until the neutrophils are $\geq$1,000/μL and the platelets are $\geq$50,000/μL. If increased numbers of blasts persist in the bone marrow, imatinib should be continued, and the bone marrow biopsy should be repeated in 2 to 4 weeks if the cytopenias persist.

G. **Other treatment modalities**

1. **Allopurinol,** 300 mg/day PO, is given to all patients at diagnosis and is continued until the WBC normalizes.

2. **Leukapheresis** rapidly decreases the granulocyte count for short periods of time but is time-consuming and expensive. This procedure is useful in the following circumstances:
   a. Patients with central nervous system or pulmonary symptoms from leukostasis, which usually develops when the WBC count exceeds 100,000/μL, especially with significant proportions of blasts. Leukapheresis is implemented emergently in combination with imatinib.
   b. Patients with priapism
   c. Pregnant patients, in whom imatinib and cytotoxic agents are contraindicated
3. **Interferon-alpha (IFN-α)** can induce hematologic and cytogenetic responses in CML patients and was the standard therapy for many years. However, a landmark randomized clinical trial of imatinib versus IFN-α plus cytarabine demonstrated a markedly higher cytogenetic response rate and much greater tolerability for imatinib than IFN-α–based therapy. There does not currently appear to be any role for IFN-α in the management of CML, as it is appears to be less effective and more toxic than second-generation tyrosine kinase inhibitors in patients who do not respond well to imatinib.
4. **Hydroxyurea** (1 to 3 g per day PO) has been used for many years to rapidly reduce the blood counts of CML patients. It is well tolerated, but it does not induce cytogenetic responses. The rapid effectiveness of the tyrosine kinase inhibitors has relegated hydroxyurea to a minor role in therapy. It can be used as a bridge between kinase inhibitors to control blood counts, when necessary.
5. **Chemotherapy** does not have an established role in the management of CML. Historically, lymphoid blast crisis has had a 20% to 40% response rate to ALL-type chemotherapy regimens, whereas myeloid blast crisis has a response rate of <20% to AML induction. The use of chemotherapy plus tyrosine kinase inhibitors may be useful in lymphoid blast crisis, as it has been in Ph[1] positive ALL. Because most CML patients currently develop blast crisis while on imatinib, the results of ongoing trials of second-generation kinase inhibitors plus chemotherapy may provide guidance for this patient population.
6. **Splenic irradiation** is not indicated for splenomegaly in CML.
7. **Splenectomy** is not indicated for splenomegaly in CML.

VI. SPECIAL CLINICAL PROBLEMS IN CML
A. **False platelet counts.** Patients with AP or BP CML may develop severe, refractory thrombocytopenia. Platelet counts that incorrectly show improvement may be found in patients with marked leukocytosis and advancing disease. The false platelet count happens because the granulocytes become disrupted in the test tube, and automatic platelet counting machines enumerate the larger leukocyte granules as platelets. The paradox is resolved by reviewing the peripheral blood smear and estimating platelet numbers.
B. **Other false laboratory results.** Pseudohyperkalemia, pseudohypoglycemia, and pseudohypoxemia are discussed in Chapter 24, section II.G, "Comparable Aspects."

CHRONIC MYELOMONOCYTIC LEUKEMIA

I. **TERMINOLOGY.** Chronic myelomonocytic leukemia (CMML) is classified as a "myelodysplastic/myeloproliferative syndrome" in the WHO system (Table 25.2). It is divided into two subtypes (CMML-1 and CMML-2), depending on the percentage of blasts in the bone marrow.

II. DIAGNOSIS
A. **Clinical features.** CMML most commonly affects the elderly. Splenomegaly is commonly present and tends to increase as the disease progresses. Hepatomegaly is uncommon, and lymphadenopathy is rare.
B. **Diagnosis** according to the WHO classification requires all of the following:

1. A persistent, unexplained monocytosis (>1,000/μL) must be present.
2. The Ph[1] chromosome or *BCR-ABL* fusion gene must be absent.
3. Fewer than 20% blasts (myeloblasts, monoblasts, and promonocytes) must be present in the bone marrow, and dysplasia must involve one or more myeloid lineages.
4. If dysplasia is not evident, there must be a clonal cytogenetic abnormality, the monocytosis must have been present for at least 3 months, and other potential causes of the monocytosis must have been excluded.

C. **Additional laboratory abnormalities** are commonly observed.
   1. **Leukocytosis** in the range of 11,000 to 50,000/μL (because of increased numbers of both granulocytes and monocytes) is present in most patients, but leukopenia occasionally occurs. The morphology of the leukocytes is characteristically abnormal. Cells with nucleoli in the peripheral blood are uncommon.
   2. **Mild anemia,** often macrocytic
   3. **Thrombocytopenia** is mild in most patients and severe in 15%. Some patients have normal platelet counts. Rarely, thrombocytosis is observed.
   4. **Serum lysozyme** levels are usually elevated.
   5. **Leukocyte alkaline phosphatase** values are variable but rarely as low as those in CML.

D. **Bone marrow aspirates** in CMML are very hypercellular. Granulocytic hyperplasia with increased numbers of promyelocytes and myeloblasts is prominent. The myeloid series in the marrow often has monocytoid features, but pure monocytic hyperplasia is unusual. Blasts account for <10% of the nucleated cells in CMML-1 and for 10% to 19% in CMML-2. Myelodysplasia is typically present in one or more cell lines.

E. **Cytogenetic abnormalities** occur in approximately 40% of cases, but the Ph[1] chromosome is absent. It is important to evaluate whether there is rearrangement of the *PDGFRB* gene on chromosome 5q33 by FISH or PCR. It can partner with ETV6 on chromosome 12p13, HIP1 on chromosome 7q11, RAB5 on chromosome 17p13, and others. The fusion gene created by these translocations encodes a protein in which the tyrosine kinase activity of *PDGFRB* is constitutively active. Treatment of patients with *PDGFRB* gene rearrangements with imatinib has induced hematologic and cytogenetic remissions due to the ability of the drug to inhibit the kinase activity of *PDGFRB*.

F. **Molecular abnormalities** include point mutations of the *KRAS* gene, predominantly in patients without cytogenetic abnormalities. These mutations enhance the intrinsic activity of the encoded proteins.

III. **CLINICAL COURSE.** Distinguishing CMML from acute myelomonocytic leukemia is essential. CMML-1 often has an insidious onset and an indolent course. Most of these patients live ≥2 years, and many survive >5 years. Patients with CMML-2 have a high risk of AML evolution.

IV. **MANAGEMENT**
   A. **Imatinib** should be administered to patients with rearrangement of the *PDGFRB* gene on chromosome 5q33. Complete remissions have been observed with imatinib 400 mg/day in this uncommon subset of CMML patients.
   B. **Hypomethylating agents,** including azacytidine or decitabine, have been reported to induce remissions in the majority of CMML patients. The randomized trials of these drugs versus supportive care in MDS patients included small numbers of CMML patients. These studies demonstrated a superior response rate and progression-free survival for study patients treated with hypomethylating agents versus best supportive care. The drugs should be dosed as for MDS, and at least three to four cycles should be given before assessing response, unless there is evidence of progressive disease.
   C. **Hydroxyurea** can be used to reduce the leukocytosis or splenomegaly in CMML, but it does not induce remissions.

D. Induction chemotherapy, as for acute myeloid leukemia, should be deferred until acute leukemia or life-threatening cytopenias develop.

E. Erythropoiesis-stimulating agents may be considered for patients with low-risk disease (bone marrow blasts <5%) and symptomatic anemia.

F. Blood product transfusions are standard supportive care measures in CMML patients with symptomatic anemia and/or thrombocytopenia.

Suggested Reading

Chronic Lymphocytic Leukemia

Chiorazzi N, Rai KR, Ferranini M. Chronic lymphocytic leukemia. *N Engl J Med* 2005;352:804.

Damle RN, et al. B-cell chronic lymphocytic leukemia cells express a surface membrane phenotype of activated, antigen-experienced B lymphocytes. *Blood* 2002;99:4087.

Dighiero G, et al. Chlorambucil in indolent chronic lymphocytic leukemia. French Cooperative Group on Chronic Lymphocytic Leukemia. *N Engl J Med* 1998;338:1506.

Dohner H, et al. Genomic observations and survival in chronic lymphocytic leukemia. *N Engl J Med* 2000;343:1910.

Hamblin TJ, et al. Unmutated Ig V(H) genes are associated with a more aggressive form of chronic lymphocytic leukemia. *Blood* 1999;94:1848.

Mavromatis B, Cheson BD. Monoclonal antibody therapy of chronic lymphocytic leukemia. *J Clin Oncol* 2003;21:1874.

O'Brien SM, et al. Rituximab dose-escalation trial in chronic lymphocytic leukemia. *J Clin Oncol* 2001;19:2165.

Rai KR, et al. Fludarabine compared with chlorambucil as primary therapy to chronic lymphocytic leukemia. *N Engl J Med* 2000;343:1750.

Shanafelt TD, et al. Pentostatin, cyclophosphamide, and rituximab regimen in older patients with chronic lymphocytic leukemia. *Cancer* 2007;109:2291.

Van Den Neste E, et al. Chromosomal translocations independently predict treatment failure, treatment-free survival and overall survival in B-cell chronic lymphocytic leukemia patients treated with cladribine. *Leukemia* 2007;21:1715.

Weiss MA, et al. Pentostatin and cyclophosphamide: an effective new regimen in previously treated patients with chronic lymphocytic leukemia. *J Clin Oncol* 2003;21:1278.

Hairy Cell Leukemia

Chadha P, et al. Treatment of hairy cell leukemia with 2-chlorodeoxyadenosine (2-CdA): long-term follow-up of the Northwestern University experience. *Blood* 2005;106:241.

Cheson BD, et al. Treatment of hairy cell leukemia with 2-chlorodeoxyadenosine via the group C protocol mechanism of the National Cancer Institute: a report of 979 patients. *J Clin Oncol* 1998;16:3007.

Goodman GR, et al. Extended follow-up of patients with hairy cell leukemia after treatment with cladribine. *J Clin Oncol* 2003;21:891.

Kreitman RJ, et al. Efficacy of the anti-CD22 recombinant immunotoxin BL22 in chemotherapy-resistant hairy-cell leukemia. *N Engl J Med* 2001;345:241.

Chronic Myelogenous Leukemia

Druker BJ, et al. Efficacy and safety of a specific inhibitor of the Bcr-Abl tyrosine kinase in chronic myeloid leukemia. *N Engl J Med* 2001;344:1031.

Goldman JM, Druker BJ. Chronic myeloid leukemia: current treatment options. *Blood* 2001;98:2039.

Hehlmann R, Hochhaus A, Baccarani M. European Leukemia Net. Chronic myeloid leukaemia. *Lancet* 2007;370(9584):342.

Kantarjian H, et al. Hematologic and cytogenetic responses to imatinib mesylate in chronic myelogenous leukemia. *N Engl J Med* 2002;346:645.

Kantarjian HM, et al. Nilotinib (formerly AMN107), a highly selective Bcr-Abl tyrosine kinase inhibitor, is effective in patients with Philadelphia chromosome-positive chronic myelogenous leukemia in chronic phase following imatinib resistance and intolerance. *Blood* 2007;110(10):3540.

Weisdorf DJ, et al. Allogeneic bone marrow transplantation for chronic myelogenous leukemia: comparative analysis of unrelated versus matched sibling donors. *Blood* 2002;99:1971.

Chronic Myelomonocytic Leukemia
Aribi A, et al. Activity of decitabine, a hypomethylating agent, in chronic myelomonocytic leukemia. *Cancer* 2007;109:713.

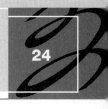

MYELOPROLIFERATIVE DISORDERS

24

Ronald L. Paquette and Dennis A. Casciato

 COMPARABLE ASPECTS

The World Health Organization (WHO) classification of the chronic myeloproliferative disorders (MPDs) includes polycythemia vera (PV), chronic idiopathic myelofibrosis (MF), essential thrombocythemia (ET), chronic eosinophilic leukemia (CEL)/hypereosinophilic syndrome (HES), chronic myelogenous leukemia (CML), chronic neutrophilic leukemia, and unclassifiable chronic MPD. Chronic myelomonocytic leukemia (CMML) has features of both an MPD and a myelodysplastic syndrome (MDS). Details on CML and CMML are presented in Chapter 23. This chapter will focus on PV, ET, MF, CEL/HES, and systemic mastocytosis (SM).

The MPDs each result from a genetic alteration within a pluripotent hematopoietic progenitor cell that induces the excessive production of one or more cell lineages. The individual diseases are distinguished by the predominant lineage that is overproduced. Table 24.1 compares important clinical and distinguishing features of the MPDs. There is considerable overlap between several of the MPDs. Long-term observation may be required to clarify the diagnosis. Unclassifiable MPDs is the best designation for patients who have leukoerythroblastic blood smears, normal red blood cell mass, and a hypercellular marrow that shows only mild fibrosis.

Erythrocytosis, granulocytosis, eosinophilia, basophilia, and thrombocytosis may be due to disorders other than MPDs, as discussed in Chapter 34 sections I to V in "Increased Blood Cell Counts". Similarly, bone marrow fibrosis may be secondary to a variety of other etiologies, as discussed in Chapter 34, section I.B in "Cytopenia".

I. PATHOGENESIS. The MPDs are clonal neoplastic disorders that arise from a single pluripotential hematopoietic stem cell. The molecular abnormalities underlying many of the MPDs are rapidly becoming elucidated.

A. Molecular and cytogenetic abnormalities. A mutation of the Janus kinase 2 (*JAK2*) gene has been identified in PV, ET, and MF. The JAK2 protein is a tyrosine kinase that is phosphorylated by the receptors for erythropoietin (EPO), thrombopoietin, granulocyte colony-stimulating factor, granulocyte-macrophage colony-stimulating factor, and interleukin-3 in response to ligand binding. Activation of *JAK2* in this way initiates a signalling cascade that induces cell proliferation in response to these growth factors.

1. The most commonly observed mutation results in the replacement of valine by phenylalanine at position 617 (V617F) of *JAK2*. The mutated protein enables hematopoietic cells to survive in the absence of growth factors and to have enhanced proliferation when exposed to low growth factor concentrations. The *JAK2* V617F mutation occurs in approximately 95% of PV, 50% of ET or MF, 20% of unclassifiable MPD, and 2% of HES. The mutation is homozygous in approximately 40% of PV due to mitotic recombination. Mutations involving exon 12 of *JAK2* have been identified in some PV patients without the V617F mutation. In addition, a point mutation of the gene encoding the thrombopoietin receptor (MPL) has been identified in a small number of patients with MF or ET. The mutated MPL receptor activates the *JAK* signalling pathway in the absence of thrombopoietin.

2. Chromosome analyses have established that a clonal cytogenetic abnormality is present in erythroblasts, neutrophils, basophils, macrophages, megakaryocytes,

TABLE 24.1 Clinical Features of the Myeloproliferative Disorders and Chronic Myelogenous Leukemia

Feature	PV	ET	MF	U-MPD	CML
Degree of cellular proliferation[a]					
Erythrocytosis	2+	N	N or D	N	N
Thrombocytosis	1+ → 2+	4+	2+ → 4+	1+	1+ → 2+
Granulocytosis	1+ → 2+	N → 2+	D → 2+	1+ → 2+	4+
Marrow fibrosis	1+	N → 1+	3+ → 4+	N → 1+	N → 1+
Extramedullary hematopoiesis	Late	A → 1+	2+ → 4+	A → 1+	N → 1+
Proportion of patients with:					
Splenomegaly	75%	30%	95%	Variable	95%
Hepatomegaly	40%	A	75%	A	50%
Cytogenetics					
Ph[1] chromosome	A	A	A	A	80%
Abnormal karyotypes	10%–20%	A	35%	Unknown	Ph[1], *bcr/abl*
Preeminent clinical features	Hyperviscosity, thrombosis	Thrombosis, hemorrhage	Pcikilocytosis, splenomegaly	Leukoerythroblastosis	Leukemic infiltration
Transition to acute leukemia	Uncommon	Rare	5%–10% at 10 yrs	Unknown	6% at 5 yrs

PV, polycythemia vera; ET, essential thrombocythemia; MF, myelofibrosis with myeloid metaplasia; U-MPD, unclassifiable myeloproliferative disorder; CML, chronic myelogenous leukemia; N, normal; D, decreased; A, absent.
[a]The designations 1+ → 4+ indicate relative degrees of prominence.

and subsets of B lymphocytes, but *not* in fibroblasts. Abnormal karyotypes are found in about 20% of PV cases at the time of diagnosis, with deletions of 20q or 13q or trisomies of 8 or 9 being most common.

3. In MF, abnormal karyotypes are found in 35% of cases; deletions of 20q or 13q and partial trisomy 1q account for 70% of the abnormal karyotypes found. The frequency of chromosomal abnormalities increases over time, particularly if patients are treated with chemotherapeutic agents. In some cases of CEL, a very small interstitial deletion on chromosome 4q12 fuses the *FIP1L1* and platelet-derived growth factor receptor *(PDGFR)-A* genes, producing a novel transforming fusion gene. The t(5;12)(q33;p13) occurs in other CEL cases and fuses the *PDGFR-B* gene to the *ETV6* gene.

B. **Hematopoiesis in the MPDs** is generally characterized by autonomous growth of progenitor cells in the absence of growth factors and hypersensitivity to the proliferative effects of growth factors.

1. **Erythropoiesis** *in vitro* in semisolid media normally requires exogenous EPO. Bone marrow progenitor cells from patients with PV form colonies *in vitro* without exogenous EPO and proliferate in response to very low EPO concentrations. Serum EPO levels are usually low in PV and are normal or elevated in most cases of secondary polycythemia.

2. **Granulocytopoiesis** is frequently increased in all MPDs to varying degrees and is manifested by neutrophilia and myeloid hyperplasia in the marrow.

3. **Megakaryocytopoiesis.** Megakaryocyte progenitors from ET patients are able to grow autonomously *in vitro* without added thrombopoietin.

4. **Extramedullary hematopoiesis** occurs in the liver and spleen in patients with MF and contributes to organ enlargement. However, the degree of organomegaly does not correlate well with the level of extramedullary hematopoiesis.

C. **Bone marrows in MPDs** demonstrate hypercellularity that is often trilineage but are diagnostic of a specific disorder only in MF. Megakaryocytes are greatly increased in number and size in ET and MF at all stages of disease and to a lesser degree in PV. Reticulin also can be increased in all MPDs, but collagen fibrosis occurs only in MF and in PV that has converted to MF.

1. **Fibrosis of the marrow** develops in all patients with MF and in some patients with PV or ET over time. The fibrosis is caused by the release of cytokines, including transforming growth factor-β and basic fibroblast growth factor, from clonal megakaryocytes or monocytes. The growth factors act on nonclonal fibroblasts and stromal cells and induce increased deposition of various interstitial and basement membrane glycoproteins, including collagen types I, III, IV, and V. Type III collagen is uniformly and preferentially increased. The fine reticulin fibers that are visible with silver stains are principally type III collagen and do not stain with trichrome dyes.

2. **MF.** Marrow fibrosis is prominent in MF. Megakaryocytes are increased in number, and they are atypical, enlarged, and immature. Neutrophilic granulopoiesis is hyperplastic. A marked neovascularization is also present, even in the early proliferative phase of the disease.

3. **PV.** Trilineage hyperplasia in the marrow is the hallmark of PV. Erythroid hyperplasia is prominent. Megakaryocytes are enlarged, clustered, mature, and pleomorphic with multilobulated nuclei. Iron stores are absent or decreased in most untreated patients. In secondary erythrocytosis, erythroid hyperplasia may be present, but megakaryocytes remain small and normal with no tendency to cluster.

4. **ET.** Increased numbers of enlarged megakaryocytes with mature cytoplasm and multilobulated nuclei and a tendency to cluster in a bone marrow with normal or slightly increased cellularity constitute the hallmarks of ET. In reactive thrombocytosis, increased numbers of megakaryocytes may be present, but they have normal size and morphology and no tendency to cluster.

II. COMPLICATIONS OF THE MPDs

A. **Thrombotic phenomena,** both venous and arterial, can complicate untreated PV and ET. Myocardial and cerebrovascular ischemia are the most serious events, but thrombosis can occur anywhere in the venous or arterial system. For example, PV is the most common cause of hepatic vein thrombosis (Budd-Chiari syndrome). In PV, two-thirds of thrombotic events occur either at presentation or before diagnosis, and one-third occur during follow-up.

1. **Risk factors** for thrombosis in PV and ET include age >60 years, history of a prior thrombotic incident, and elevated white blood cell (WBC) count at presentation.

2. **In PV,** the risk of thrombosis increases with the hematocrit, so phlebotomy is performed to keep the hematocrit <45% in male patients and <42% in female patients. Low-dose aspirin reduces the risk of thrombotic complications in PV without increasing the risk of major bleeding.

3. **In ET,** the level of the platelet count does *not* correlate with the risk of thrombosis. However, reducing the platelet count and WBC to normal levels reduces the risk of thrombotic events. Normalization of the platelet count using hydroxyurea (HU) is more effective than using anagrelide in preventing arterial thrombotic events in patients at high risk for thrombosis. Low-dose aspirin is used in ET patients with high risk of thrombosis, but its benefit has not been evaluated in randomized, controlled trials.

B. **Microvascular arterial thrombosis** is easily and best controlled by low-dose aspirin or by reduction of platelet count to normal levels.

1. **Erythromelalgia** is the most characteristic vaso-occlusive manifestation in MPDs and is most often associated with PV or ET. It is caused by the toxic effects of platelet arachidonic acid on arterioles. Localized painful erythema and warmth occur in the distal portions of the extremities and may progress to cyanosis or necrosis of toes or fingers.

2. **Microvascular arterial thrombosis** in PV or ET is usually transient and not progressive. Manifestations can include ocular disturbances, amaurosis fugax, diplopia, headache, vertigo, hypaesthesia, paraesthesia, dysarthria, aphasia, and syncope. If superimposed on a previously compromised vasculature, these events could result in stroke, myocardial infarction, or digital gangrene.

C. **Hemorrhagic phenomena** occur in PV, ET, and late MF, but they occur far less commonly than thrombotic events. Easy bruisability and purpura are the usual manifestations. Bleeding can be reversed by reducing the platelet count, platelet transfusion, or administering desmopressin (DDAVP).

1. **Bleeding** can occur spontaneously without relationship to the platelet count, but it occurs especially when the count exceeds 1,000,000/μL in uncontrolled myeloproliferation.

2. **Acquired von Willebrand disease** develops occasionally in the MPDs. This coagulopathy is characterized by a *very high platelet count*, a normal or prolonged bleeding time, normal factor VIII and normal von Willebrand factor (vWF) antigen levels, but with decreased vWF–ristocetin cofactor activity, decreased collagen-binding activity, and a decrease or absence of large vWF multimers. This condition simulates type II vWF deficiency. The increased number of platelets appears to be directly responsible for the observed decrease of large vWF multimers in plasma that leads to the tendency for spontaneous bleeding at very high platelet counts.

D. **Hypercatabolism.** Hyperuricemia and hyperuricosuria are present in nearly all patients with active MPD. Treatment with allopurinol can prevent gouty arthritis, uric acid nephropathy, and nephrolithiasis, but its necessity is unproven. Pruritus is a frequent problem, particularly in PV. Fever, heat tolerance, and weight loss ensue when the disease becomes rapidly progressive.

E. **Interconversions of the MPDs** are uncommon. The only consistent transformation is the conversion of PV into MF (approximately 5% of PV cases).

F. **Transformation to acute myelogenous leukemia (AML).** The risk of progressing to AML is approximately 2% for ET, 5% for PV, and 10% for MF within 10 years of diagnosis. The risk for AML transformation is higher in patients with MF who have undergone splenectomy. Prior treatment with alkylating agents or radioactive phosphorus (^{32}P) also increases the risk.

G. Misleading laboratory results

1. **Normal hematocrits in patients with PV** can represent erythrocytosis masked by hemorrhage, iron deficiency, increased plasma volume, or splenomegaly with sequestration.

2. **Pseudocoagulopathy.** Prolonged clotting times in patients with marked erythrocytosis are usually the result of excessive amounts of anticoagulant relative to the small plasma volume in the test tube. Accurate determinations can be made if the volume of anticoagulant is adjusted for the hematocrit.

3. **Pseudohyperkalemia.** Marked thrombocytosis may result in elevated serum potassium concentrations because platelets release potassium during the clotting reaction. The true level is determined by measuring the potassium concentration in plasma rather than in serum.

4. **Pseudo–hyper-acid-phosphatemia.** Platelets are rich in acid phosphatase. Marked thrombocytosis may result in spurious elevations of enzyme levels measured in serum and plasma.

5. **Pseudohypoglycemia.** Leukocytes metabolize glucose from serum in test tubes. Dramatically low blood glucose concentrations may result from marked granulocytosis. More accurate glucose levels can be measured if the sample is analyzed immediately after the sample is drawn.

6. **Pseudohypoxemia.** Oxidative respiration is used by monocytes and immature leukocytes to a greater extent than by mature leukocytes and platelets and is not used by mature erythrocytes. Falsely low oxygen tensions may be seen in patients with severe thrombocytosis or granulocytosis because of oxygen consumption within the test tubes. The presence of hypoxemia may be clarified if specimens are collected in test tubes containing fluoride and are immediately placed in ice.

 POLYCYTHEMIA VERA

See "Comparable Aspects" at the beginning of this chapter for pathogenesis, bone marrow findings, complications, and misleading laboratory results of the MPDs. Familial cases occur occasionally in PV.

I. DIAGNOSIS. PV is a clonal MPD that harbors a *JAK2* mutation (most commonly V617F) in approximately 95% of cases. Therefore, mutation analysis of the *JAK2* gene will help to segregate PV from secondary causes of erythrocytosis. The WHO has not yet incorporated this specific assay into its diagnostic criteria. Although the erythroid series is the predominant proliferating cell lineage in PV, panmyelosis is common.

A. WHO diagnostic criteria for PV

1. **Category A criteria**

A1   Increased red blood cell mass >25% above mean normal predicted value, or hemoglobin >18.5 g/dL in men, >16.5 g/dL in women, or >99th percentile of method-specific reference range for age, sex, and altitude of residence

A2   No cause of secondary polycythemia, including:
a. Absence of familial erythrocytosis
b. No elevation of serum EPO level due to hypoxemia (Po_2 ≥92%), high oxygen affinity hemoglobin, truncated EPO receptor, or inappropriate EPO production by tumor

A3   Splenomegaly

A4   Clonal genetic abnormality other than the Philadelphia chromosome or *BCR-ABL* fusion gene in marrow cells

A5   Endogenous erythroid colony formation *in vitro*

2. **Category B criteria**

B1   Thrombocytosis >400,000/µL
B2   Granulocytosis >12,000/µL

B3   Bone marrow biopsy showing panmyelosis with prominent erythroid and megakaryocytic proliferation

B4   Low serum EPO levels

3. **The diagnosis of PV** is established by the presence of the following:

A1 and A2 plus any other category A item, or
A1 and A2 plus any two from category B

B. Laboratory studies

1. **Red blood cell mass (RBCM).** Autologous RBCs are ^{51}Cr-labeled, injected intravenously, then a blood sample is drawn to quantitate the dilution of the labeled cells and calculate the circulating RBCM. Unfortunately, the radionuclide assessment of RBCM using ^{51}Cr is rarely available today.

2. **Clonal genetic abnormality.** The presence of the *JAK2 V617F* mutation in the blood or bone marrow cells is adequate to demonstrate a clonal etiology for the erythrocytosis. It is present in approximately 95% of PV. Absence of a *JAK2* mutation suggests a secondary cause for the erythrocytosis. (See Comparable Aspects, Section IA.)

3. **Erythroid colony-forming assay.** PV bone marrow demonstrates EPO independency in culture. However, this assay is cumbersome and not routinely performed by clinical laboratories and it has been supplanted by the *JAK2* mutation analysis.

4. **Supportive studies**
   a. **CBC.** Erythrocytes are usually normocytic and normochromic unless iron deficiency is present. Poikilocytosis and anisocytosis accompany the transition into MF late in the disease course. Granulocytosis in the range of 12,000 to 25,000/µL occurs in two-thirds of patients at presentation. Early forms may be present but are not frequent. Two-thirds of patients have basophilia. Platelet counts usually are in the range of 450,000 to 800,000/µL, occasionally with abnormal morphology.
   b. **Serum EPO levels** can be normal or reduced in PV. Although autonomous expansion of the RBCM would be expected to suppress EPO production, this assay cannot reliably distinguish between PV and EPO-driven erythrocytosis. EPO production is depressed and circulating EPO catabolism is increased as the RBCM expands from any cause. Furthermore, a normal serum EPO level is common in hypoxic erythrocytosis unless the hypoxemia is extreme.
   c. **Abdominal ultrasonography or CT scanning** can rule out renal or hepatic causes of erythrocytosis and quantitate spleen size.
   d. **Bone marrow examinations** can be used to demonstrate panmyelosis and abnormal megakaryocyte morphology consistent with PV, quantitate the extent of reticulin fibrosis if transition to MF is suspected, or evaluate the percentage of blasts if transformation to AML is a concern.

C. Differential diagnosis

includes the other MPDs and relative or secondary erythrocytosis (see Chapter 34, section I in "Increased Blood Cell Counts"). Reduced plasma volume, hypoxemia, renal cysts or carcinoma, hepatic neoplasms, or uterine myomata can cause secondary erythrocytosis.

II. CLINICAL COURSE.

The survival of patients with PV approaches that of a matched otherwise healthy population with modern therapy. The median survival exceeds 12 years.

A. Predominant signs and symptoms

early in the disease are secondary to increased red blood cell mass that results in plethora and hyperviscosity. Modest splenomegaly is present in 75% of cases and hepatomegaly in 40%. Splenomegaly is caused by an increased splenic red blood cell pool and not by extramedullary hematopoiesis, which is absent early in the disease. Pruritus develops in 15% to 50% of cases, urticaria in 10%, and gout in 5% to 10%.

1. **Hyperviscosity** results in decreased blood flow and, consequently, in tissue hypoxia. Manifestations include headache, dizziness, vertigo, tinnitus, visual disturbances, stroke, angina pectoris, claudication, and myocardial infarction.

2. **Thrombotic manifestations** can result from hyperviscosity associated with the increased RBCM.

a. **Types of events.** Both arterial and venous thrombosis occur in PV, more commonly in women than in men. Approximately two-thirds of the thrombotic events are severe and life-threatening. including cerebrovascular accidents, myocardial infarctions, pulmonary infarctions, and axillary, hepatic, portal, splenic or mesenteric vein thromboses. The remaining one-third of events are uncomplicated deep vein or other thromboses.

b. **Thrombosis-related risk factors.** High risk is conveyed by age >65 years or a history of prior thrombosis. The risk of thrombosis, especially myocardial infarction, is increased by a WBC >15,000/μL. A history of smoking, hypertension, hypercholesterolemia, congestive heart failure, or diabetes mellitus increases the risk to a lesser degree. *Thrombocytosis does not increase the risk of thrombosis.*

3. **Hemorrhagic manifestations** (10% to 20% of patients) include epistaxis, ecchymosis, and gastrointestinal (GI) bleeding. Minor mucosal bleeding is most common. Acquired abnormalities of vWF can occur with marked thrombocytosis (see "Comparable Aspects," section II.C).

B. **Phases of disease**

1. **Erythrocytic phase.** The phase of persistent erythrocytosis that necessitates regular phlebotomies lasts from 5 to 25 years. The manifestations of erythrocytosis and severity of complications depend on comorbid conditions and sufficient use of phlebotomy.

2. **Spent phase.** Eventually, the patient enters a "spent" or "burned-out" phase; the need for phlebotomies is greatly reduced, or the patient enters a long period of apparent remission. Anemia eventually supervenes, but thrombocytosis and leukocytosis usually persist. The spleen increases in size, but little marrow fibrosis is present.

3. **Myelofibrotic phase.** Myelofibrosis develops in 5% to 10% of patients with PV, particularly in those who were exposed to chemotherapy or radiotherapy. The development of increased marrow reticulin or osteosclerosis, however, is not synonymous with the "spent phase." When myelofibrosis does develop, it is not necessarily a progressive or destructive process, does not affect survival, and is potentially reversible. When cytopenias and progressive splenomegaly develop, the clinical manifestations and course become similar to that of MF.

4. **Terminal phase.** In patients who die from PV, death results from thrombotic or hemorrhagic complications. Death is attributed to myelofibrosis in <10% of cases. Historically, patients treated with radioactive phosphorus or alkylating agents had an increased risk of developing acute myeloid leukemia compared to those treated by phlebotomy or HU.

C. **Pregnancy and PV.** Pregnant patients with PV have an increased incidence of premature births, fetal wastage, pre-eclampsia, and postpartum hemorrhage. Pregnancy does not affect the course of PV.

III. **MANAGEMENT.** The therapeutic challenge in PV is balancing the control of manifestations with the risks for thrombosis, hemorrhage, and leukemic transformation.

A. **Principles of treatment**

1. Reduce the hematocrit with phlebotomy

2. Administer low-dose aspirin to reduce thrombotic risk

3. Avoid overtreatment or elective surgery

4. Control panmyelosis with HU in patients who have one of the following characteristics:

a. A high risk for thrombotic complications (age >60 or prior thrombosis) or a high requirement for phlebotomy (more frequently than every 2 months)

b. Symptomatic splenomegaly

c. Uncontrolled systemic symptoms (e.g., intractable pruritus, weight loss) or poor venous access

d. Pathologic bleeding in the presence of thrombocytosis

e. Progressive granulocytosis (often a harbinger of extramedullary hematopoiesis or disease acceleration) or progressive thrombocytosis

5. Avoid potentially leukemogenic myelosuppressive agents, especially in young patients.

B. Medical management

1. **Phlebotomy** alone prevents thrombosis and may be adequate treatment for many years. The hematocrit is maintained at <45% for men, 42% in women, and 36% in pregnancy. No additional treatment may be needed in stable patients who are at low risk for thrombosis (<60 years of age and no history of thrombosis).

   a. Initially, 500 mL of blood may be removed every other day (only 250 mL of blood should be removed in patients with serious vascular disease).

   b. About 200 mg of iron is removed with each 500 mL of blood (the normal total-body iron content is about 5 g). Iron deficiency is a goal of chronic phlebotomy treatment. Symptomatic iron deficiency (glossitis, cheilosis, dysphagia, asthenia, pruritus) resolves rapidly with iron administration.

2. **Myelosuppressive therapy** controls the blood counts, minimizes complications from increased circulating elements, reduces symptomatic organomegaly, improves pruritus, and may delay myelofibrosis.

   a. **HU,** 10 to 30 mg/kg daily PO, is arguably the drug of choice for treating panmyelosis. It is effective in most patients within 12 weeks and reduces the incidence of thrombotic events by 50%. The leukemogenic risk of this drug appears to be low. Occasional side effects of HU include fever, rash, stomatitis, leg ulcers, gastric discomfort, and possible renal dysfunction.

   b. **Interferon-α (IFN-α)** suppresses the proliferation of hematopoietic progenitors, inhibits bone marrow fibroblast progenitor cells, and antagonizes the action of platelet-derived growth factor (PDGF). IFN-α, given at a dose of 500,000 to three million units SQ 3 times weekly, can control myeloproliferation, reduce splenomegaly, ameliorate pruritus, and possibly delay myelofibrosis. IFN-α, however, is associated with significant side effects including flulike symptoms, fatigue, weight loss, altered mental status, depression, and exacerbation or development of autoimmune disease. Peripheral neuropathy is a common side effect associated with chronic IFN-α administration, can be severe, and does not improve with discontinuation of the drug. IFN-α is not leukemogenic and it does not damage the bone marrow. Nevertheless, its potentially severe toxicities relegate it to second-line therapy.

   c. **Radioactive phosphorus** (^{32}P), 2 to 5 mCi, controls panmyelosis in 80% of patients within 2 months and may be effective for 2 years or longer. However, it increases the incidence of acute myeloid leukemia (approximately fivefold), lymphomas, and cancers of the skin and GI tract. Therefore, its use is rarely warranted.

   d. **Alkylating agents** (chlorambucil, busulfan, and melphalan) can successfully control panmyelosis and reduce the incidence of thrombosis but unacceptably increase the incidence of acute myeloid leukemia (13-fold).

3. **Low-dose aspirin** (81 to 100 mg/day) reduces the risk of major thrombotic events in PV, including myocardial infarction, stroke, pulmonary embolism, and major venous thrombosis. Aspirin also ameliorates erythromelalgia or other microvasculature problems. Aspirin may be contraindicated in patients with a history of prior GI hemorrhage.

4. **Supportive care**

   a. **Hyperuricemia,** if associated with complications, is treated with allopurinol, 100 to 600 mg/day PO. Other measures are discussed in Chapter 27, section IX.

   b. **Platelet transfusions** are given for important bleeding, even if the platelet count is normal or elevated, because platelet function abnormalities may be present.

   c. **Anticoagulation** for acute thrombotic complications is managed as for patients without PV.

   d. **Pruritus** is multifactorial and may be resistant to therapy. The following may be helpful:

      (1) Histamine blockers, such as hydroxyzine 25 mg PO q.i.d., cyproheptadine (4 mg PO t.i.d.), or cimetidine (300 mg PO t.i.d.) should be tried initially.

(2) Selective serotonin reuptake inhibitors, including paroxetine 20 mg/day or fluoxetine 10 mg/day, have been helpful in some patients.

(3) Low-dose ferrous sulfate supplementation to treat pruritus that may be caused by iron deficiency may be considered. If iron is given, the hematocrit must be closely monitored for the expected increase in phlebotomy requirements.

(4) Cholestyramine or psoralen-activated ultraviolet light therapy may be helpful in some cases.

(5) If the above measures fail, HU or IFN-α may be necessary.

e. Symptomatic splenomegaly may be addressed with HU or IFN-α.

C. Surgery

1. Elective surgery should be avoided in patients with PV. More than 75% of patients with uncontrolled PV who undergo surgery develop hemorrhagic or thrombotic complications, and about one-third of patients die as a result. The longer the disease is controlled, the fewer the complications that will occur. The following approach is recommended:

   a. Phlebotomy. The hematocrit should be reduced to 45%. If there is evidence of clinically significant arterial disease, reducing the hematocrit to 35% to 40% may be justified. The blood obtained by phlebotomy can be saved for autologous transfusion.

   b. Prevention of perioperative thromboembolism. Elastic stockings or pulsating boots should be used to speed blood flow through the calf. Low-dose heparin or low-molecular-weight heparin can be given until the patient returns to normal activity, if there are no contraindications.

2. Emergency surgery. Aggressive phlebotomy should be performed prior to surgery, if possible. Consider reinfusing the patient's plasma to prevent depletion of clotting factors.

3. Splenectomy is occasionally performed for massive splenomegaly in the myelofibrotic phase of PV. Unfortunately, progressive hepatomegaly from extramedullary hematopoiesis or transformation to AML can follow this procedure. A high rate of perioperative mortality may be expected for elderly or frail patients.

 ESSENTIAL THROMBOCYTHEMIA

See "Comparable Aspects" at the beginning of this chapter for pathogenesis, bone marrow findings, complications, and misleading laboratory results of the MPDs.

I. DIAGNOSIS. The megakaryocyte is the predominant proliferating cell line in the panmyelosis of ET.

A. Diagnostic criteria for ET. The diagnosis of ET is based largely on the exclusion of other MPDs or MDS associated with increased platelet counts, and reactive thrombocytosis.

1. JAK2 mutation is present in approximately 50% of ET and, if present, excludes secondary causes of thrombocytosis

2. Platelet counts: WHO criteria require sustained platelet counts exceeding 600,000/μL, although some patients may present with lower counts.

3. Absence of other causes of thrombocytosis

   a. No prior splenectomy

   b. No iron deficiency as assessed by the serum ferritin or bone marrow hemosiderin.

   c. No evidence of malignancy, infection, inflammation, GI bleeding, or other causes of reactive thrombocytosis

4. Bone marrow examination shows hypercellularity, markedly increased numbers of megakaryocytes, and clumps of platelets and megakaryocytes (see "Comparable Aspects," section I.C). Cytogenetic studies show no Philadelphia chromosome or *BCR/ABL* gene rearrangement (observed in CML), and no 5q⁻ or 3q chromosome abnormality (observed in MDS).

B. Laboratory studies
1. **Erythrocytes.** Hypochromic, microcytic anemia is present in >60% of patients. Howell-Jolly bodies are found in 20% of patients and indicate splenic atrophy from repeated infarctions.
2. **Granulocytosis** is present in half of cases, usually in the range of 15,000 to 30,000/μL. Myelocytes and earlier forms are rare, and basophilia is mild, if present.
3. **Platelet counts** always exceed 600,000/μL and are often present as clumps or megakaryocytic fragments. Counts may reach 15,000,000/μL.

C. Differential diagnosis of ET includes reactive thrombocytosis, familial thrombocytosis related to increased levels of thrombopoietin, the other MPDs, CML, and MDS. The MDS subtypes that are most frequently associated with thrombocytosis include refractory anemia with the 5q⁻ chromosomal abnormality or refractory anemia with ringed sideroblasts. Reactive thrombocytosis is discussed in Chapter 34, section III of "Increased Blood Cell Counts."

II. CLINICAL COURSE
A. Predominant signs and symptoms. Two-thirds of patients do not have symptoms when ET is discovered. The spleen may be enlarged (one-third of cases), normal, or atrophic. Hepatomegaly is absent. Extramedullary hematopoiesis is not a major feature of ET. Pruritus develops in 10% to 15% of patients.

B. Thrombotic, embolic, or hemorrhagic episodes of varying severity are the most common spontaneous manifestations of ET (see "Comparable Aspects," section II). Neither the level of the platelet count nor platelet function tests correlate with thrombotic risk, except that platelet counts above 1,500,000/μL are associated with an increased bleeding risk. Homozygosity for the *JAK2* mutation increases the risk for complications compared with heterozygosity or absence of the mutation.
1. **Thrombotic episodes** are most frequently venous, with deep vein thrombosis and pulmonary emboli as the most frequent manifestations. Splenic, hepatic, portal, and cerebral veins are also often affected. Arterial thromboses primarily affect small and medium-sized vessels, and most frequently cause digital ischemia or infarction.
2. **Hemorrhage episodes** occur most frequently in the mucous membranes or skin. Life-threatening hemorrhage rarely occurs except after trauma or surgery or in the presence of antiplatelet drugs.
3. **Pregnancy** is associated with increased occurrence of spontaneous abortions due to thrombosis of placental vessels, particularly in the presence of the *JAK2* mutation. Cardiovascular events are not increased in patients with ET during pregnancy.

C. Survival approaches that of matched, otherwise healthy controls. The median survival exceeds 10 years, and the 5-year survival rate is >80%. Transformation of ET into acute leukemia is rare if leukemogenic agents have not been used.

III. MANAGEMENT
A. Principles. The mainstay of treatment for ET is observation without treatment for low-risk patients, or low-dose aspirin and myelosuppression for high-risk patients. Patients with either hemorrhagic or vaso-occlusive complications should be treated promptly to lower the platelet count.

B. Medical management
1. **Low-risk disease** is present in patients with age <60 years and no prior history of thrombosis. The level of the platelet count alone does not dictate a need for therapy. Low-dose aspirin (81 to 100 mg/day) may be considered for patients with low-risk disease by extrapolation from data involving PV patients.
2. **High-risk disease** warrants the use of cytoreductive therapy in addition to low-dose aspirin and is characterized by any of the following:
   a. Age >60 years
   b. History of thrombotic complications
   c. Cardiovascular risk factors (e.g., tobacco use, hypertension, obesity, diabetes mellitus)

3. **Myelosuppressive therapy.** Drugs are administered to achieve platelet counts <450,000/μL. If thrombotic events still occur, dosages are adjusted to maintain platelet counts well within the normal range.

   a. **HU** is the most commonly employed myelosuppressive treatment for ET (see "Polycythemia Vera," section III.B.2.a). It is effective in controlling thrombocytosis, leukocytosis, and in reducing thrombotic complications for patients who are at high risk. HU is more effective than anagrelide in preventing arterial thromboses in patients with high-risk ET, and it is better tolerated.

   b. **Anagrelide** controls thrombocytosis in >80% of patients, usually within 1 to 2 weeks. It is a selective inhibitor of platelet production. The maintenance dosage is usually 2 to 2.5 mg/day in two to four divided doses. The main side effects of anagrelide are headaches, palpitations, fluid retention, and other neurologic, GI, and cardiac manifestations. It should be used with caution in patients with heart disease. Chronic administration cause progressive anemia. It is more likely than HU to be associated with progressive marrow fibrosis.

   c. **IFN-α** is effective in controlling thrombocytosis and pruritus. Its ability to prevent thromboembolic complications is unknown. It causes more frequent and severe side effects than either HU or anagrelide (see "Polycythemia Vera," section III.B.2.b) but may be useful if treatment is required during pregnancy.

   d. **Radioactive phosphorus** can induce prolonged suppression of platelet counts, but it is leukemogenic. Its use should be avoided, with the possible exception of elderly high-risk patients who are not compliant with oral medications (see "Polycythemia Vera," section III.B.2.c).

   e. **Alkylating agents** (melphalan, busulfan, or chlorambucil) effectively reduce platelet counts but are leukemogenic and carcinogenic. Avoid their use in ET, particularly in younger patients (see "Polycythemia Vera," section III.B.2.d).

4. **Antiplatelet drugs.** Manifestations of microvascular arterial thrombosis (erythromelalgia, transient ischemic attacks, and ocular disturbances) in ET can be eliminated by reducing the platelet count into normal levels. Low-dose aspirin should be used in patients who have had thrombotic manifestations, but its efficacy in the primary prevention of thrombosis in ET is unproven. The use of aspirin and other antiplatelet drugs may increase the risk of bleeding, particularly when the platelet count exceeds 1,000,000/μL. Aspirin may be contraindicated in patients with a history of peptic ulcer disease.

5. **Plateletpheresis** is indicated for emergency treatment of life-threatening complications of severe thrombocytosis and is nearly always associated with improvement in hemorrhagic and thrombotic symptoms.

6. **Cardiovascular risk factors** should be modified when possible.

C. **Splenectomy** greatly aggravates thrombocytosis, can be life-threatening, and is contraindicated in patients with ET.

D. **Pregnancy with ET** is successful in 55% of cases and is most frequently complicated by spontaneous abortion during the first trimester (35% of pregnancies). Maternal complications occur in about 5% of pregnancies. Abortion cannot be predicted by history or therapy or platelet counts, although a decline in the platelet count has been observed in some patients with successful pregnancies. Specific therapies for ET during pregnancy, including plateletpheresis, do not appear to modify the clinical outcome. The ideal management for women with ET during pregnancy is speculative, but IFN-α is often recommended for those who require platelet count reduction because it is not considered to be teratogenic.

 CHRONIC IDIOPATHIC MYELOFIBROSIS

See "Comparable Aspects" at the beginning of this chapter for pathogenesis, bone marrow findings, complications, and misleading laboratory results of the MPDs. Chronic idiopathic MF is also known as *myelofibrosis with myeloid metaplasia* and *agnogenic myeloid metaplasia*. Familial cases occur occasionally in MF. Radiation exposure is associated with an increased incidence of MF but accounts for only a small percentage of cases. No other etiologic factors have been determined.

I. DIAGNOSIS. Monoclonal megakaryocytes and polyclonal fibroblasts are the predominant proliferating cell lines in the panmyelosis of MF.

  A. Diagnostic criteria for MF (according to the PV Study Group) consist of the following:

  1. Splenomegaly
  2. Leukoerythroblastic blood smears (nucleated red blood cells and granulocytosis) with prominent anisocytosis and poikilocytosis
  3. Normal ^{51}Cr red blood cell mass (should be measured, if possible, if the hematocrit is >40%)
  4. Bone marrow examination that demonstrates fibrosis involving more than one-third of the cross-sectional area, and the fibrosis is not secondary to some identifiable cause (see Chapter 34, section I.B in "Cytopenia").
  5. Absence of Ph^1 chromosome
  6. **Osteosclerosis** appears as patchy sclerotic lesions on radiographs of the pelvis, spine, or long bones in approximately half of the MF patients. These lesions may resemble metastases from carcinoma.

  B. Laboratory studies

  1. **JAK2 mutation analysis** is positive in approximately 50% of MF patients. Presence of the mutation excludes secondary causes of fibrosis but does not exclude other MPDs.
  2. **Erythrocytes.** Anemia is moderate in two-thirds of patients at presentation. Dacrocytes ("teardrop" cells), ovalocytes, pronounced anisocytosis, polychromasia, and nucleated red blood cells make up the characteristic and nearly pathognomonic blood picture of MF. The anemia is usually due to ineffective erythropoiesis.
  3. **Granulocytes** usually range from 10,000 to 30,000/µL. Blasts and promyelocytes constitute <10% of the granulocytes. Granulocytopenia occurs in 15% of patients. Basophils are only slightly increased.
  4. **Platelets** are increased in one-third, normal in one-third, and decreased in one-third of patients with MF, depending on the stage of disease. Platelets usually have abnormal morphology.
  5. **Bone marrow examination** shows hypercellularity, granulocytic hyperplasia, and markedly increased numbers of atypical megakaryocytes. Fibrosis is patchy and variable in distribution; reticulin is always increased and is striking in half of the patients. The extent of fibrosis *is not correlated* with the duration of disease, splenic size, or degree of splenic myeloid metaplasia. See "Comparable Aspects," section I.C.
  6. **Immunologic abnormalities,** such as monoclonal antibodies (10%), positive direct Coombs' tests (20%), polyclonal hyperglobulinemia, rheumatoid factor, antinuclear antibodies, antiphospholipid antibodies, or circulating immune complexes are found in more than half of the patients with MF.

  C. Differential diagnosis of MF includes the other MPDs, CML, MDS, AML of the M7 subtype, hairy cell leukemia, Hodgkin lymphoma, metastatic carcinoma associated with marrow fibrosis (desmoplastic reaction), autoimmune diseases (especially systemic lupus erythematosus), and disseminated mycobacterial infection. A long list of other disorders associated with secondary myelofibrosis are discussed in Chapter 33, section I.B in "Cytopenia."

II. CLINICAL COURSE

  A. Symptoms are proportional to the severity of anemia and splenomegaly. Virtually all patients have splenomegaly, which may be massive, and three-fourths of patients have hepatomegaly. One-fourth of patients do not have symptoms at the time of diagnosis. Progression to AML is commonly manifested by fever, weight loss, and debilitating bone pain.

  B. Chronic MF. The clinical course of MF is extremely variable. Some patients are symptom-free for long periods without treatment. Hemorrhagic manifestations rarely develop until late in the disease when severe thrombocytopenia develops. Death is due to heart failure, infection, hemorrhage, postsplenectomy mortality, or transformation to AML. Development of AML occurs in approximately 10% of MF patients.

The median survival in patients with MF is 4 to 5 years, but survival can range from <2 years to >10 years (20 years, in some reports) for patients, depending on risk factors. Splenic size and bone marrow findings have not been found to be significant prognostic factors. The expected survival is inversely related to the number major risk factors that a patient demonstrates.

1. Accepted risk factors in MF

Hemoglobin <10 g/dL
WBC count <4,000/μL or >30,000/μL
Presence of >10% circulating precursors (blasts, promyelocytes, myelocytes)

2. Probable risk factors in MF

Abnormal karyotype
Age >65 years
Presence of constitutional symptoms

C. Associated syndromes
   1. Portal hypertension and varices in MF are caused by massive increases in splenoportal blood flow and decreased hepatic vascular compliance. The decreased compliance is due to extramedullary hematopoiesis and its secondary collagen deposition.
   2. Extramedullary hematopoietic tumors can develop in any location. Foci of these tumors on serosal surfaces can cause effusions containing immature hematopoietic cells.
   3. Neutrophilic dermatoses are skin lesions with intense polymorphonuclear neutrophil infiltration. These raised tender plaques can progress to bullae or pyoderma gangrenosum.

III. MANAGEMENT
   A. Medical management. Available therapies for MF have not been shown to impact survival. Treatment is therefore directed toward amelioration of symptoms.
   1. Packed red blood cells are transfused to alleviate symptoms of anemia.
   2. Androgens, such as fluoxymesterone (Halotestin; 10 mg PO b.i.d.) or danazol (200 to 400 mg PO b.i.d.), improve anemia in approximately one-third of MF patients. Several months of treatment are necessary before improvement is evident. Combination of androgens with glucocorticoids may improve the response rate.
   3. Glucocorticoids, such as prednisone (20 to 30 mg/day), can ameliorate systemic symptoms and anemia in a minority of MF patients.
   4. Erythropoiesis stimulating agents in doses of 10,000 to 20,000 units 3 times per week can improve the anemia in some MF patients. Lower pretreatment serum EPO levels (<125 U/L) are associated with an increased likelihood of response.
   5. Thalidomide in low doses (50 to 100 mg/day) in combination with prednisone can improve anemia and thrombocytopenia associated with MF. Higher doses of thalidomide increase toxicity without additional therapeutic benefit. Sedation, fluid retention, peripheral neuropathy, and venous thromboembolism can complicate its use in this patient population.
   6. Lenalidomide is a thalidomide analog that has myelosuppression as its principal toxicity. In doses of 10 mg PO daily it can improve anemia, thrombocytopenia, and splenomegaly in some MF patients.
   7. Chemotherapy with low doses of HU (15 to 20 mg/kg/day) can reduce leukocyte and platelet counts, symptomatic splenomegaly, or symptoms of hypercatabolism (fever, sweats, or weight loss). The response to treatment is unpredictable and careful monitoring is recommended to avoid excessive bone marrow suppression. 2-Chlorodeoxyadenosine (2-CdA) can also reduce leukocyte and platelet counts in MF patients. It may also decrease marrow fibrosis and reverse

hepatomegaly developing after splenectomy. Alkylating agents such as busulfan, cyclophosphamide, and melphalan can also be effective cytoreducing agents in MF, but their use should be avoided because of potent leukemogenic effects.

8. **IFN-α** can be cytoreductive in some patients with MF. However, its use is often complicated by intolerable side effects and peripheral blood cytopenias (see "Polycythemia Vera," section III.B.2.b).

9. **Anagrelide** can reduce the platelet count, but no other clinical manifestation of MF.

B. **Bone marrow or peripheral blood stem cell transplantation** is potentially curative for MF but it is associated with a high rate of morbidity and mortality. Therefore, standard allogeneic transplantation should be considered primarily for younger patients who have high-risk disease. The use of nonmyeloablative conditioning therapy may reduce the risks of this procedure and extend the use of transplantation to older patients.

C. **Splenectomy** should be approached cautiously but it may beneficial in patients who have painful splenomegaly, serious cytopenias, or hypercatabolism. The mortality rate is <10% if the procedure is performed by experienced surgeons, but postoperative morbidity exceeds 30%. Peripheral blood cytopenias may persist or worsen if a significant amount of extramedullary hematopoiesis was carried out in the spleen prior to splenectomy. There is no reliable preoperative test to predict the contribution of splenic hematopoiesis. Progressive hepatomegaly and an increased risk for blast transformation after splenectomy are also major concerns. Splenectomy in medically suitable patients with MF can be considered in the following situations:

1. Persistent discomfort because of a grossly enlarged or infarcted spleen unresponsive to less aggressive measures

2. Refractory anemia accompanied by increasingly more frequent transfusions

3. Refractory, severe thrombocytopenia in the absence of evidence of disseminated intravascular coagulation

4. Hypercatabolic symptoms that are not responsive to myelosuppression

5. Portal hypertension associated with bleeding varices. Based on circulatory dynamic studies performed at the time of surgery, the following procedures should be performed:

   a. Splenectomy alone for portal hypertension secondary to markedly increased blood flow from the liver to the spleen

   b. Portosystemic shunt may be considered for portal hypertension secondary to intrahepatic obstruction to blood flow

D. **Radiation therapy (RT)**

1. Small doses (20 to 300 cGy per course given in daily fractions of 20 cGy) of RT to the spleen can relieve pain and early satiety secondary to massive splenomegaly in MF, usually for a few months. RT can be considered when splenectomy is contraindicated. Blood counts must be monitored carefully during splenic RT because severe cytopenias can develop rapidly.

2. RT may also palliate focal areas of periostitis, extramedullary hematopoietic tumors, and ascites secondary to myeloid metaplasia of the peritoneum.

CHRONIC EOSINOPHILIC LEUKEMIA AND HYPEREOSINOPHILIC SYNDROME

I. DEFINITION AND MANIFESTATIONS

A. **CEL and HES** are characterized by blood and bone marrow eosinophilia, and by tissue infiltration with relatively mature eosinophils resulting in multisystem organ dysfunction. The WHO distinguishes CEL from HES by the former having evidence of clonality, such as a cytogenetic abnormality or increased numbers of blasts in the blood or bone marrow. HES, on the other hand, is considered idiopathic but not necessarily clonal. CEL and HES occur predominantly in men, usually between the ages of 20 and 50 years.

B. **Etiology and pathogenesis.** CEL is associated most commonly with a small interstitial deletion on chromosome 4q12 that fuses the platelet-derived growth factor A

(*PDGFRA*) gene to the *FIP1L1* gene, producing a novel transforming fusion gene. This deletion is too small to be detected by routine cytogenetics but it can be identified by fluorescence *in situ* hybridization (FISH) or reverse transcriptase polymerase chain reaction (PCR) for the *FIP1L1-PDGFRA* fusion. Rarely, CEL can be associated with a translocation involving the *PDGFRB* gene on chromosome 5q31-33 and the *ETV6* gene on chromosome 12p12-13, resulting in the formation of another novel fusion gene.

The etiology of HES is idiopathic by definition. In some cases there may be overproduction of cytokines that stimulate eosinophil production, such as granulocyte-macrophage colony-stimulating factor, interleukin-3, or interleukin-5. Other cases may be CEL with occult translocations of *PDGFRA* or *PDGFRB* and therefore be misdiagnosed as HES.

C. Organ system involvement

1. **Hematopoietic system involvement.** The absolute eosinophil count must be >1,500/μL for longer than 6 months in the absence of other causes of eosinophilia to entertain the diagnosis, and usually ranges from 3,000 to 25,000/μL. The eosinophils are usually mature but often contain decreased numbers of granules that are small in size. Half of the patients have a normocytic, normochromic anemia. Bone marrow cytology shows myeloid hyperplasia with 25% to 75% of these cells being eosinophils, which are shifted to the left in maturation. Increased numbers of myeloblasts and cytogenetic abnormalities are absent.

2. **Cardiac involvement** (55% to 75% of cases). Myocardial necrosis is associated with the presence of increased numbers of eosinophils seen on endomyocardial biopsy. Thrombi develop in the ventricles or atria and can embolize. Mitral or tricuspid valvular regurgitation and restrictive cardiomyopathy due to endomyocardial fibrosis develop after about 2 years of eosinophilia.

3. **Neurologic involvement** (40% to 70%). Clinical syndromes include cerebral thromboembolism originating in the heart, encephalopathy, and peripheral sensory polyneuropathy. Biopsy findings are inconsistent.

4. **Lung involvement** (40% to 50%) usually manifests as a chronic nonproductive cough. The chest radiograph is usually clear. Pulmonary function test abnormalities are rare in the absence of congestive heart failure or pulmonary emboli arising from the right ventricle. Diffuse or focal infiltrations develop in 20% of patients. Bronchial asthma is a rare occurrence in CEL or HES.

5. **Cutaneous involvement.** Skin rashes develop in >50% of cases. Urticarial or angioedematous lesions, erythematous papules and nodules, or mucosal ulcers may develop.

6. **Involvement of other organs.** Splenomegaly develops in 40% of cases. Rheumatologic manifestations include arthralgias, effusions, and Raynaud's phenomenon. Eosinophilic gastritis, enterocolitis, chronic active hepatitis, and Budd-Chiari syndrome have been observed in CEL and HES. Visual blurring caused by microemboli or microscopic hematuria may occur.

II. **DIFFERENTIAL DIAGNOSIS.** See Chapter 34, section IV in "Increased Blood Cell Counts" for eosinophilia.

A. **Other chronic MPDs.** Patients with CEL or HES rarely have expansions of other cell lines besides eosinophils to the extent seen in the other chronic MPDs and do not develop severe myelofibrosis.

B. **Other hematopoietic malignancies,** especially acute myelomonocytic leukemia with inv(16) cytogenetics, T-cell lymphoma, and Hodgkin lymphoma.

C. **Eosinophilic syndromes limited to specific organs** lack the multiplicity of organ involvement often found in CEL or HES.

D. **Churg-Strauss syndrome** is the major vasculitis associated with eosinophilia. It is characterized by asthma, pulmonary infiltrates, eosinophilia, paranasal sinus abnormalities, neuropathy, and blood vessels showing extravascular eosinophils. Asthma is usually absent in HES and may be the only feature that distinguishes it from Churg-Strauss syndrome.

III. DIAGNOSIS

A. Diagnostic criteria for HES

1. Persistently increased absolute eosinophil count >1,500/μL for longer than 6 months
2. Absence of parasites, allergies, or other causes of eosinophilia
3. Evidence of organ system involvement
4. Absence of chromosome abnormalities, which would justify the diagnosis of CEL

B. Helpful studies

1. Complete history and physical examination, CBC, liver and renal function tests, and urinalysis
2. Immunoglobulin E levels and serologic tests for collagen vascular disorders
3. Chest radiograph
4. Electrocardiogram, echocardiogram, and serum troponin T assay to assess cardiac involvement
5. Bone marrow aspirate and biopsy with chromosome analysis
6. FISH and PCR assays for *PDGFRA* and *PDGFRB* gene rearrangement
7. T-cell receptor gene rearrangement assay to rule out clonal T-cell disorder
8. Biopsy of skin lesions
9. Serum tryptase level and *c-KIT* mutation analysis to rule out systemic mastocytosis
10. Several stool samples for ova and parasites
11. Duodenal aspirates and blood serology to exclude *Strongyloides* sp infection

IV. PROGNOSIS.
Historically, >75% of patients survived for at least 5 years and 40% survived at least 10 years, depending on the ability to manage the effects of end-organ damage. Congestive heart failure or a WBC count >90,000/μL at presentation is associated with a poor prognosis. The impact of imatinib therapy on survival has not yet been assessed.

V. MANAGEMENT.
All patients with CEL or HES should be given a trial of imatinib 400 mg daily because even patients without identifiable *PDGFRA* or *PDGFRB* gene rearrangement have been reported to respond to this therapy. Doses as low as 100 mg/day are effective to treat some patients. When *PDGFRA* and *PDGFRB* translocations are present, monitoring of disease status every 3 months while on therapy by quantitative PCR (if available) or FISH should be performed. In patients with baseline cardiac abnormalities, serial monitoring of troponin T levels should be performed after initiating imatinib therapy to monitor for exacerbation of cardiac dysfunction. This potential complication of therapy may be reduced by pretreatment with glucocorticoids of at-risk patients.

Patients not responding to imatinib may benefit from glucocorticoid therapy, although treatment is usually reserved for symptomatic disease. Cytoreductive therapy with HU or INF-α can sometimes be beneficial for symptomatic patients. These agents are discontinued if organ dysfunction improves and the eosinophil count is reduced to or near the normal range.

MASTOCYTOSIS

I. PATHOGENESIS

Mastocytosis includes a heterogeneous group of diseases characterized by abnormal growth and accumulation of mast cells (MCs) in one or more organ systems. Although not classically listed as a myeloproliferative syndrome, MCs are myeloid cells and are derived from CD34-positive progenitors; thus, mastocytosis is included in this chapter.

MCs express stem cell factor receptor, CD2, and CD25. c-*KIT* is the proto-oncogene that encodes the tyrosine kinase receptor for stem cell growth. Cutaneous mastocytosis typically presents as urticaria pigmentosa or diffuse cutaneous mastocytosis, accounts for >85% of cases, and usually has a benign course. Malignant mastocytosis is an uncommon disease; it is most frequently reported in Israelis and light-skinned whites. The *c-KIT* proto-oncogene plays an important role in hematopoiesis in general, in MC growth in particular, and in all categories of MC disease. The mutation seen in MC disorders is located in the tyrosine kinase domain of the *c-KIT* receptor. Mutations are associated with autonomous phosphorylation and activation of the receptor. More than 80% of patients with systemic mastocytosis (SM) have the point mutation of *c-KIT* at codon 816 (mostly D816V) detected by PCR or other technologies. The histopathologic diagnosis may be difficult but is facilitated using basic dyes and immunostaining against tryptase.

II. WHO CLASSIFICATION OF MC DISEASE is as follows (note that the D816V mutation has been found in all of these categories):

Cutaneous mastocytosis (CM)
Indolent systemic mastocytosis (ISM)
Aggressive systemic mastocytosis (ASM)
Systemic mastocytosis with associated clonal, hematologic non-MC lineage disease (SM-AHNMD; e.g., AML, chronic myelomonocytic leukemia, MDSs, MPDs, and CEL/HES)
MC leukemia
MC sarcoma and extracutaneous mastocytoma (very rare localized phenomena)

MCs infiltrate any organ that contains mesenchymal tissue (particularly the lymph nodes, liver, spleen, and bone marrow) and produce local destructive or fibrotic changes. Organ infiltration often indicates acceleration of the disease.

III. CLINICAL FEATURES. CM typically affects children, presents as urticaria pigmentosa or diffuse cutaneous mastocytosis, accounts for >85% of cases of MC disease, and usually has a benign course that resolves before puberty. SM is an uncommon disease, affects mostly adults, and is most frequently reported in Israelis and light-skinned whites.

A. Skin changes. Urticaria pigmentosa is the most common early manifestation of systemic disease. Brownish skin nodules diffusely infiltrated with MCs may be localized or diffuse, flat or raised, bullous or erythematous. Mild skin trauma may produce urticaria or dermatographia.

B. Organ infiltration may develop years after skin lesions have appeared and is manifested by hepatomegaly, lymphadenopathy, bone pain (osteosclerotic lesions on radiographs are common), bone marrow fibrosis, and, occasionally, MC leukemia. MCs infiltrate any organ that contains mesenchymal tissue (particularly the lymph nodes, liver, spleen, and bone marrow) and can produce local destructive or fibrotic changes. Osteosclerotic lesions on radiographs are common. Extracutaneous organ infiltration often indicates acceleration of the disease. Hyperchlorhydria occasionally occurs and can result in peptic ulcer and malabsorption.

C. Hyperhistaminemia symptoms may be precipitated by exposure to cold, alcohol, narcotics, fever, or hot baths, and include the following:
   1. Erythematous flushing, urticaria, edema, pruritus
   2. Abdominal pain, nausea, vomiting (occasionally diarrhea), flatulence, steatorrhea
   3. Sudden hypotension

IV. DIAGNOSIS. The histopathologic diagnosis of SM may be difficult but is facilitated using basic dyes and immunostaining against **tryptase.** The source of cells assayed for the *c-KIT* D816V mutation should be the bone marrow since use of peripheral blood led to falsely negative assays in 80% of cases.

A. CM is confirmed by skin biopsy; bone marrow biopsy is not needed. Serum tryptase levels are normal.

B. SM is diagnosed by biopsies of both skin and bone marrow. Because of its implications regarding treatment, the *c-KIT* mutation variant should be determined. The diagnosis of SM is established with the major criterion plus one minor criterion or three minor criteria.

   1. Major criterion for diagnosis: multifocal dense MC infiltrates ($\geq$15 MCs per infiltrate) in the bone marrow or other extracutaneous organ

  2. Minor criteria
   a. Less than 25% of MCs are spindle-shaped or atypical in infiltrates or marrow smears
   b. Expression of CD2 and/or CD25 on marrow MC
   c. *c-KIT* point mutation at codon 816 (mostly D816V) in marrow or extracutaneous organ
   d. Serum tryptase level >20 ng/mL (except in cases of SM-AHNMD, where this criterion does not apply)

V. MANAGEMENT. In the vast majority of patients with ISM, the condition is very stable over many years. Results of various treatments have been unsatisfactory.
A. Histamine antagonism by H_1- and H_2-receptor blockade may help flushing, itching, and gastric distress. Cyclo-oxygenase inhibition may prevent prostaglandin D_2-induced hypotension when indicated. Oral cromolyn (200 mg PO q.i.d.) may prevent GI symptoms and bone pain.
B. Cytoreduction is considered when the patient develops evidence of decreased organ function such as anemia (hemoglobin <10g/dL), neutropenia (<1000/μL), thrombocytopenia (<100,000/μL), abnormal liver function tests, ascites, hypersplenism, malabsorption with weight loss, or large osteolytic lesions and/or severe osteoporosis.
   1. Cladribine (2-CdA) is associated with a major response rate of about 50%. The dosing schedule is 0.1 to 0.15 mg/kg/day given IV over 2 to 3 hours for 5 consecutive days every 2 to 6 months for one to six cycles.
   2. INF-α2b is associated with a major response rate of about 20%, as well as significant morbidity from the drug. Doses have ranged from 9 to 42 million units per week, usually given with glucocorticoids. Alkylating agents, cyclosporine, INF, and corticosteroids occasionally help.
   3. Imatinib (Gleevec) targets are detectable in SM. However, the D816V mutation, which is present in the vast majority of patients, confers relative resistance to imatinib.

   Imatinib is very effective in patients with SM and eosinophilia who harbor the *FIP1L1-PDGRFA* fusion, but not the D816V mutation. The responsive patients tended to have a high serum tryptase level (>150 ng/mL) and be females with skin lesions. Patients with SM and eosinophilia who do express the D816V mutation, however, are not responsive to imatinib. Dasatinib, however, is active *in vitro* in patients with the D816V *KIT* mutation; clinical trials with dasatinib for SM are ongoing.
   a. For ASM associated with eosinophilia, the starting dose for imatinib is 100 mg/day.
   b. For ASM without the D816V *c-KIT* mutation or with unknown c-*KIT* mutational status, the starting dose of imatinib is 400 mg/day.
C. Treatment approach
   1. CM and ISM. Patients are treated with drugs targeting only histamine mediators unless they have severe osteopenia or recurrent shocklike episodes. Patients with smoldering SM are observed expectantly; cytoreduction can be considered with progression.
   2. ASM with slow progression can be treated with 2-CdA or INF-α. In the absence of D816V, consider imatinib.
   3. ASM with rapid progression or MC leukemia is treated with polychemotherapy, with or without 2-CdA or INF. In the absence of D816V, consider imatinib. Stem cell transplantation can also be considered.
   4. SM-AHNMD components are treated independently.

Suggested Reading

Myeloproliferative Disorders

Campbell PJ, Green AR. The myeloproliferative disorders. *N Engl J Med* 2006;355:2452.
Jones AV, et al. Widespread occurrence of the JAK2 V617F mutation in chronic myeloproliferative disorders. *Blood* 2005;106:2162.

Kralovics RK, et al. A gain-of-function mutation of JAK2 in myeloproliferative disorders. *N Engl J Med* 2005;352:1779.

Pardanani AD, et al. MPL515 mutations in myeloproliferative and other myeloid disorders: a study of 1182 patients. *Blood* 2006;108:3472.

Thiele J, Kvasnicka HM. A critical reappraisal of the WHO classification of the chronic myeloproliferative disorders. *Leuk Lymphoma* 2006;47:381.

Vardiman JW, Harris NL, Brunning RD. The World Health Organization (WHO) classification of the myeloid neoplasms. *Blood* 2002;100:2292.

Wadleigh M, et al. After chronic myelogenous leukemia: tyrosine kinase inhibitors in other hematologic malignancies. *Blood* 2005;105:22.

Polycythemia Vera

Fruchtman SM, et al. A PVSG report on hydroxyurea in patients with polycythemia vera. *Semin Hematol* 1997;34:17.

Landolfi R, et al. Efficacy and safety of low-dose aspirin in polycythemia vera. *N Engl J Med* 2004;350:114.

Landolfi R, et al. Leukocytosis as a major thrombotic risk factor in patients with polycythemia vera. *Blood* 2007;109:2446.

Schafer AI. Molecular basis of the diagnosis and treatment of polycythemia vera and essential thrombocythemia. *Blood* 2006;107:4214.

Scott LM, et al. JAK2 exon 12 mutations in polycythemia vera and idiopathic erythrocytosis. *N Engl J Med* 2007;356:459.

Spivak JL. Polycythemia vera: myths, mechanisms, and management. *Blood* 2002;100:4272.

Vannucchi AM, et al. Clinical profile of homozygous *JAK2* 617V>F mutation in patients with polychythemia vera or essential thrombocythemia. *Blood* 2007;110:840.

Essential Thrombocythemia

Carobbio A, et al. Leukocytosis is a risk factor for thrombosis in essential thrombocythemia: interaction with treatment, standard risk factors, and Jak2 mutation status. *Blood* 2007;109:2310.

Griesshammer M, Heimpel H, Pearson TC. Essential thrombocythemia and pregnancy. *Leuk Lymphoma* 1996;22(suppl 1):57.

Harrison CN, et al. Hydroxyurea compared to anagrelide in high-risk essential thrombocytopenia. *N Engl J Med* 2005;353:33.

Murphy S, et al. Experience of the Polycythemia Vera Study Group with essential thrombocythemia: a final report of diagnostic criteria, survival and leukemic transition by treatment. *Semin Hematol* 1997;34:29.

Passamonti F, et al. Increased risk of pregnancy complications in patients with essential thrombocythemia carrying the *JAK2 (617V>F)* mutation. *Blood* 2007;110:485.

Myelofibrosis

Barosi G. Myelofibrosis with myeloid metaplasia: diagnostic definition and prognostic classification for clinical studies and treatment guidelines. *J Clin Oncol* 1999;17:2954.

Cervantes F, et al. Identification of "short-lived" and "long-lived" patients at presentation of idiopathic myelofibrosis. *Br J Haematol* 1997;97:635.

Mesa RA, et al. A phase 2 trial of combination low-dose thalidomide and prednisone for the treatment of myelofibrosis with myeloid metaplasia. *Blood* 2003;101:2534.

Pullarkat V, et al. Primary autoimmune myelofibrosis: definition of a distinct clinicopathologic syndrome. *Am J Hematol* 2003;72:8.

Tefferi A. Myelofibrosis with myeloid metaplasia. *N Engl J Med* 2000;342:1255.

Tefferi A, et al. Lenalidomide therapy in myelofibrosis with myeloid metaplasia. *Blood* 2006;108:1158.

Hypereosinophilic Syndrome

Cools J, et al. A tyrosine kinase created by fusion of the PDGFRA and FIP1L1 genes as a therapeutic target of imatinib in idiopathic hypereosinophilic syndrome. *N Engl J Med* 2003;348:13.

Fletcher S, Bain B. Diagnosis and treatment of hypereosinophilic syndromes. *Curr Opin Hematol* 2007;14:37.

Gotlib J, et al. The FIP1L1-PDGFRα fusion tyrosine kinase in hypereosinophilic syndrome and chronic eosinophilic leukemia: implications for diagnosis, classification, and management. *Blood* 2004;103:2879.

Klion AD, et al. Elevated serum tryptase levels identify a subset of patients with a myeloproliferative variant of idiopathic hypereosinophilic syndrome associated with tissue fibrosis, poor prognosis and imatinib responsiveness. *Blood* 2003;101:4660.

Mastocytosis

Garcia-Montero AC, et al. KIT mutation in mast cells and other bone marrow hematopoietic cell lineages in systemic mast cell disorders: a prospective study of the Spanish Network on mastocytosis (REMA) in a series of 113 patients. *Blood* 2006;108:2366.

Kluin-Nelemans HC, et al. Cladribine therapy for systemic mastocytosis. *Blood* 2003;102:4270.

Orfao A, et al. Recent advances in the understanding of mastocytosis: the role of KIT mutations. *Br J Haematol* 2007;138:12.

Pardanani A, et al. Imatinib for systemic mast-cell disease. *Lancet* 2003;362:535.

Pauls JD, et al. Mastocytosis: diverse presentations and outcomes. *Arch Intern Med* 1999;159:401.

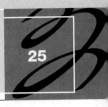

ACUTE LEUKEMIA AND MYELODYSPLASTIC SYNDROMES   25

Gary Schiller, Mary C. Territo, and Dennis A. Casciato

 ACUTE LEUKEMIA

I. EPIDEMIOLOGY AND ETIOLOGY

A. Incidence. Acute leukemia afflicts 3 to 4/100,000 population annually (11,000 new cases/year) in the United States. Children account for 25% of cases. Acute leukemia is the most common malignant disease of childhood.

1. Cell type. Of cases of acute lymphoblastic leukemia (ALL), 80% occur in children, and 90% of cases of acute myelogenous leukemia (AML) occur in adults.

2. Age. In adults, AML rates begin to rise exponentially after 50 years of age; the age-specific incidence rates are 3.5/100,000 in adults 50 years of age, increases significantly to 15 at age 70 and 35 at age 90. The mean age for AML in the United States is 63 years. A peak incidence of ALL occurs at 3 to 4 years of age; the incidence steadily decreases after 9 years of age and rises in incidence after 40 years of age. Despite being considered a childhood cancer, the age-related increase in incidence of most cancers also pertains to ALL.

3. Sex. Acute leukemia shows a male predilection only in very young and elderly patients.

B. Etiology

1. Hereditary

a. Hereditary syndromes that are associated with chromosomal abnormalities, a high risk of acute leukemia, and excessive chemosensitivity include the following:

(1) Bloom syndrome is a recessively transmitted disease occurring predominantly in people of Jewish ancestry. Chromosome breaks are readily found in cytogenetic studies. The syndrome is characterized by short and thin stature, delicate features, telangiectatic lesions over the malar eminences of the face, photosensitivity, and a variety of other cutaneous abnormalities (acanthosis nigricans, hypertrichosis, ichthyosis, and café-au-lait spots). AML is the type of leukemia that develops in these patients.

(2) Fanconi's congenital pancytopenia (Fanconi's aplasia) is an autosomal recessive disease often associated with multiple chromosomal abnormalities. Clinical features include skeletal abnormalities (absence of radii, hypoplasia of the thumbs), squinting, microcephaly, small stature, and hypogonadism. AML, as well as skin carcinoma, often complicates this syndrome.

(3) Down's syndrome (mongolism, trisomy 21) is associated with an increased risk for both AML and ALL.

(4) Ataxia telangiectasia is associated with an increased incidence of lymphoid malignancies, including ALL.

b. Siblings of younger patients with acute leukemia have a fivefold increased risk of developing leukemia. If one member of a monozygotic twinship develops acute leukemia, the risk that the other twin will also be affected is 1:4, especially if the patient is <8 years of age and it is within 1 year of the first diagnosis of leukemia.

2. Radiation is a well-documented leukemogenic factor in humans. Increased incidence of leukemia proportional to the cumulative radiation dose has been demonstrated in populations exposed to atomic bombs, in patients irradiated for ankylosing spondylitis, and in radiologists (before current protective precautions). Doses <100 cGy are not believed to be associated with the development of leukemia. The types of leukemia induced by radiation are ALL, AML, and chronic myelogenous leukemia (CML), but not chronic lymphocytic leukemia.

3. **Viruses** have not been shown to be etiologic for acute leukemias in humans, although an association is seen with Epstein-Barr virus with ALL-L3 (Burkitt leukemia). HTLV-1 is discussed in Chapter 21, in "Non-Hodgin Lymphoma".

4. **Chemicals.** The ability of chemicals to produce acute leukemia and pancytopenia is likely related to their ability to mutate or ablate the bone marrow stem cells.

   a. **Benzene and toluene** were identified as carcinogens associated with acute leukemia a century ago. Acute leukemia develops 1 to 5 years after exposure and is often preceded by bone marrow hypoplasia, dysplasia, and pancytopenia.

   b. **Drugs.** Drug-induced acute leukemia is usually preceded by myelodysplasia. Alkylating agents and topoisomerase II inhibitors given for prolonged periods are associated with a markedly increased risk of AML when compared with the general age-matched population. Exposure to arsenicals has also been implicated as an increased risk factor for leukemia development. Secondary AML currently accounts for 10% to 20% of all AML cases.

5. **Hematologic diseases.** Transformation into acute leukemia ("blast crisis") is seen in >80% of cases of CML, and is part of its natural history. Patients with myelodysplastic syndromes (MDS) clearly have an increased likelihood for evolution to AML. The incidence of AML in myeloproliferative disorders (MPD), myeloma, and certain solid tumors is increased by the use of chemotherapy.

6. **Smoking.** Cigarette smoking is associated with approximately 50% increase in leukemia risk. Cigarette smoking has a deleterious effect on survival in AML by shortening complete remission duration and subsequent survival. It has been associated with severe infections during aplasia. Leukemogenic compounds favoring complex karyotypic abnormalities could also be involved.

II. PATHOLOGY, CLASSIFICATION, AND NATURAL HISTORY OF ACUTE LEUKEMIA

A. Classification

1. **Morphologic features of acute leukemias**

   a. **The French–American–British (FAB) histopathologic classification** of acute leukemia was originally proposed in 1976. This system has been supplanted by the World Health Organization (WHO) classification below. The FAB defined the M1–M7 and L1–L3 subtypes of acute leukemia as follows:

FAB Subtype	Acute leukemia type
M0:	Myeloblastic without maturation
M1:	Myeloblastic with minimal maturation
M2:	Myeloblastic with maturation
M3:	Promyelocytic; M3v: Promyelocytic ("microgranular")
M4:	Myelomonocytic; M4 Eos: Myeloblastic with abnormal eosinophils (Eos)
M5:	Monocytic: poorly (M5a) or well differentiated (M5b)
M6:	Erythroleukemia
M7:	Megakaryoblastic
L1:	ALL, childhood form
L2:	ALL, adult form
L3:	ALL, Burkitt-type

   b. **Auer rods** are abnormal condensations of cytoplasmic granules. Their presence in the immature cells distinguishes AML from ALL; their absence is not diagnostically helpful.

   c. **Cytologic features** of the acute leukemia subtypes, particularly the nuclear configurations, cytoplasm granularity, and prevalence of Auer rods, are shown in Appendix C-7, section I.

   d. **Cytochemistry.** Identifying the type of early cell may be difficult, but it is facilitated by readily available and traditionally used histochemical techniques, particularly for myeloperoxidase and nonspecific esterase (see Appendix C-7, section II). Myeloperoxidase activity can be assessed by both cytochemistry and flow cytometry.

   e. **Immunologic markers assessed by flow cytometry** usually distinguish ALL from AML as well as identify their subtypes. These markers are summarized in Appendix C-7, section II. Antibodies against platelet glycoproteins (CD41 or CD61) are useful in distinguishing megakaryocytic (M7) leukemia. Flow cytometry has largely replaced cytochemistry for classification of acute leukemias in most centers. Flow cytometry is most useful when using antibodies against panmyeloid antigens (CD13 and CD33), monocyte antigens (especially CD11b and CD14), and hematopoetic progenitor cell antigens (CD34 and HLA-DR).

2. **The WHO classification** has replaced the FAB classification. The FAB classification, which provided a consistent morphologic and cytochemical framework, did not reflect the cytogenetic or clinical diversity of the disease. The WHO classification system takes into account the developing knowledge of the biology of AML, its distinct subtypes divided into diseases characterized by proliferative biology and diseases characterized by disorders of maturation. The WHO classification of AML is as follows (with corresponding FAB designations and approximate proportions of AML cases in brackets):

   a. **AML with recurrent cytogenetic abnormalities** (Table 25.1)

      AML with abnormal bone marrow eosinophils and inv(16)(p13;q22) or t(16;16)(p13;q22) [M4 Eo, 10% to 12%]

      Acute promyelocytic leukemia and variants; t(15;17)(q21;q11) and its variants [M3, M3v; 5% to 8%]

      AML with t(8;21)(q22;q22); (AML1/ETO) [M2, 5% to 12%]

      AML with 11q23 (MLL) abnormalities [M5 or M1, 5% to 6%]

   b. **AML with multilineage dysplasia [M2 or M6]**

      Following MDS or MDS/MPD

      Without antecedent MDS

   c. **AML and MDS, therapy-related** (alkylating agents, topoisomerase inhibitors, other types)

   d. **AML not otherwise categorized**

      AML minimally differentiated [M0, 5%]

      AML without maturation [M1, 10%]

      AML with maturation [M2, 30% to 45%]

      Acute myelomonocytic leukemia [M4, 15% to 25%]

      Acute monoblastic and monocytic leukemia [M5a, M5b; 5% to 8%]

      Acute erythroid leukemia [M6, 5% to 6%]

      Acute megakaryoblastic leukemia [M7, 3% to 5%]

      Acute panmyelosis with myelofibrosis [M7, rare; "acute myelofibrosis"]

      Acute basophilic leukemia (very rare)

   e. **Myeloid sarcoma** ("chloroma," "granulocytic sarcoma"; extramedullary masses of monoblasts or myeloblasts)

   f. **Acute lymphocytic leukemias** are now included in the WHO classification of lymphoid tissues as "precursor B cell lymphoblastic leukemia/lymphoma" and "precursor T cell lymphoblastic leukemia/lymphoma" (see Appendix C-6, section I). These were designated as ALL- L1, L2, or L3 in the FAB system.

3. **The two most significant differences between the FAB and the WHO classifications** are

| TABLE 25.1 | Cytogenetic Abnormalities and Prognosis of Acute Myelogenous Leukemia in Adults | | |

Cytogenetic abnormalities	Fusion genes	Frequency in adults (%)			Frequency of FLT3ITD[a] (%)
		<45 yrs	All	>45 yrs	
Favorable prognosis					
t(8;21)(q22;q22)	AML1/ETO	5–8 (<55 yrs)		Rare	9
inv(16)(p13;q22)	CBFβ/MYH11	10		Rare	7
t(16;16)(p13;q22)					
t(15;17)(q21;q11)	APL-RARα	15		Rare	37
Variants:					
t(11;17)(q23;q11)	PLZF-RARα				
t(5;17)(q32;q11)	NPM-RAR-α				
t(11;17)(q13;q11)	NuMA-RARα				
Intermediate prognosis					
Normal karyotype		5–20			34
+8		10			28
Others: −Y, +6					
All other karyotypes not considered favorable or unfavorable		—			20–30
Unfavorable prognosis					
Abnormal 11q23[b]	MLL	5–7			0
Common variants:					
t(4;11)(q21;q23)	MLL/AF4				
t(9;11)(p22;q23)	MLL/AF9				
t(11;19)(q23;p13.1)	MLL/ELL				
t(11;19)(q23;p13.3)	MLL/ENL				
t(6;9)(p23;q34)	DEK/CAN	<10			—
t(3;3)(q21;q26)	Ribophorin/EV11	3–5			17
−5/del(5q)		<10		>10	0
−7/del(7q)		<10		>10	7

[a]FLT (a tyrosine kinase growth factor receptor) mediates hematopoietic stem cell proliferation and differentiation. *FTL3* mutations (internal tandem duplication of exon 11 and 12 termed FLT3ITD) are common in AML and could be an important prognostic indicator.
[b]>50% of AML cases in infants.

    a. A lower blast threshold for the diagnosis of AML: The WHO defines AML when the blast percentage reaches **20%** in the bone marrow (rather than 30% as defined by FAB).

    b. Patients with recurring clonal cytogenetic abnormalities should be considered to have AML regardless of the blast percentage: t(8;21)(q22;q22), t(16;16)(p13;q22), inv(16)(p13;q22), or t(15;17) (q22;q12).

4. A more clinically relevant classification of AML can be achieved if two distinct subgroups with different biological features are recognized.

    a. AML that evolves from MDS is associated with multilineage dysplasia, poor risk cytogenetics, and a poor response to therapy. The incidence of this type increases with age and is consistent with the hypothesis that MDS and MDS-related leukemia results through multiple insults to the molecular constitution of the hematopoietic stem cell.

b. AML that arises *de novo* usually lacks significant multilineage dysplasia. It is often associated with favorable-risk cytogenetic findings and has a better response to therapy with a higher likelihood of failure-free and overall survival. This type of leukemia has a relatively constant incidence throughout life and is the type most likely to be observed in children and young adults. Some types are clearly related to disorders of differentiation such as AML characterized by core-binding-factor abnormalities, t(8;21) or inv 16 or t(15;17). Others are characterized more by proliferative defects such as AML with normal cytogenetics (often with FLT3 mutations).

B. Pathology. Bone marrow examination in acute leukemia demonstrates hypercellularity with a monotonous infiltration of immature cells. Normal marrow elements are markedly decreased. Erythroblast maturation is commonly megaloblastoid in all types of AML, especially subtype M6. Cytologic features of the AML subtypes are shown in Appendix C-7, section I.

At the time of diagnosis, the kidneys are clinically involved in about 25% of cases; the lungs, joints, or gastrointestinal (GI) tract in 5% of cases; and the heart in 2% of cases. At postmortem examination, virtually all organs are infiltrated with leukemia cells.

C. Natural history. Leukemic cells generally replicate more slowly than their normal counterparts. Hematopoiesis is disturbed even before the proportion of blast cells in the marrow is conspicuously increased. Immature and malfunctioning leukocyte progenitors progressively replace the normal bone marrow and infiltrate other tissues. Relapse is inevitable in most patients unless complete remission after induction and consolidation therapy lasts at least 4 years. Relapse is associated with progressively poorer response to therapy and, if second or subsequent remission is achieved, progressively shorter duration of remission. Unsuccessful therapy is usually followed by death within 2 months. Death in acute leukemia is usually caused by either infection or hemorrhage.

D. Biology of acute promyelocytic leukemia (APL)

  1. Morphology. Classified as M3 in the FAB classification, APL is characterized morphologically by the presence of blasts cells with heavy azurophilic granules, bundles of Auer rods ("faggot cells"), and a bilobed or reniform nucleus. Although most acute APL cases fit the description of hypergranular blasts, a cytologic microgranular variant (M3v) has been identified. The blasts in M3v have a bilobed, multilobed, or reniform nucleus and, under the usual staining, are devoid of granules or contain only a few fine azurophilic granules. The apparent paucity of granules is owing to their submicroscopic size. M3v is commonly associated with hyperleukocytosis and accounts for 15% to 20% of APL cases.

  2. Immunophenotyping. APL blasts are positive for CD33 and CD13 but negative for HLA-DR and usually have a low-level expression of CD34. M3v blasts tend to be positive for CD34, CD2, and CD19.

  3. Cytogenetics. Both the classic and the M3v forms of APL are associated with a specific cytogenetic abnormality, t(15;17)(q22;q21). This translocation disrupts the APL gene on chromosome 15 and the retinoic acid receptor α (RARA) on chromosome 17, resulting in a fusion gene (APL/RARA). The protein product of APL/RARA retains the retinoic acid (RA) ligand-binding domain and plays a key role in leukemogenesis, as well as in mediating the response to retinoids. Expression profiling by microarray is likely to be used in the future as an adjunct to cytogenetics or as a replacement.

  a. Three other alternative translocations associated with APL have been characterized:

  t(11;17)(q23;q21) involving the *PLZF* gene on chromosome 11
  t(5;17)(q35;q21) involving the *NPM* gene on chromosome 5
  t(11;17)(q13;q21) involving the *NuMA* gene on chromosome 11

b. APL/RARA-mediated APL is sensitive to retinoids, as are the variants *NPM*/RARA- and *NuMA*/RARA-mediated APL. In contrast, *PLZF*/RARA-associated APL is considered resistant to retinoids as well as arsenic trioxide.

III. DIAGNOSIS
A. Symptoms
1. **Nonspecific fatigue and weakness** are the most common symptoms. Bruising, fever, and weight loss are frequent.
2. **Central nervous system (CNS) involvement** may be manifested by headaches, nausea, vomiting, blurred vision, or cranial nerve dysfunction.
3. **Abdominal fullness** usually reflects hepatosplenomegaly, which is more frequent in ALL or the monocytic subtype of AML.
4. **Oliguria** may result from dehydration, uric acid nephropathy, or disseminated intravascular coagulation (DIC).
5. **Obstipation** may signify disorders of hypocalcemia or hypokalemia; potassium wasting may occur in monocytic leukemia.

B. Physical findings
1. **General examination**
   a. Pallor, petechiae, and purpura are the most frequent findings in acute leukemia.
   b. Sternal tenderness to palpation, lymphadenopathy, and hepatosplenomegaly are much more common in ALL than in AML.
   c. Meningismus may indicate CNS involvement. CNS leukemia is most common in ALL. When seen in patients with AML, M4 (particularly with abnormal bone marrow eosinophils) and M5 subtypes are commonly involved. It is far less common in the remaining AML subtypes but can be seen at relapse.
   d. Leukemic infiltrates in the optic fundus appear like Roth's spots with flame hemorrhages.
2. **Extramedullary infiltration or masses of blasts,** especially involving the skin, orbits, breasts, gingivae, or testes, are most likely to occur in acute monocytic leukemias (M5) and ALL.
3. **Bleeding** out of proportion to the degree of thrombocytopenia suggests the presence of DIC, particularly common in M3 acute leukemia.
4. **Signs of infection** should be carefully elicited.

C. Laboratory studies.
Evaluation of the peripheral blood smear should be done in every case where leukemia is in the differential diagnosis. Finding circulating leukemic blasts establishes the diagnosis, but this should be confirmed by the evaluation of the bone marrow from which successful cytogenetic analysis is more likely. Fluorescent *in situ* hybridization (FISH) for common, recurring molecular abnormalities, may identify distinct clonal abnormalities not easily elicited by conventional cytogenetics.
1. **Hemogram**
   a. **Leukocytes.** The WBC count is elevated in about 60% of cases, normal in 15%, and decreased in 25%, depending on the referral base of the treatment center. Circulating blasts are demonstrated in virtually every case of acute leukemia; however, some patients present with a very low percentage of circulating blasts.
   b. **Erythrocytes.** 90% of patients have a normocytic, normochromic anemia, which is usually severe. Reticulocytes are nearly always decreased. Macrocytosis usually reflects megaloblastic maturation and suggests a history of prior MDS. Circulating nucleated red blood cells should always prompt further evaluation of the bone marrow.
   c. **Platelets** are decreased in 90% of cases and are <50,000/μL in about 40%.
2. **Biochemical tests** that should be obtained include the following:
   a. Serum uric acid, ionized calcium, phosphorus, magnesium, and lactic dehydrogenase (LDH) levels

   b. Serum renal and liver function tests.

   c. Coagulation tests for DIC (see Chapter 34, section II in "Coagulopathy")

3. Bone marrow findings are discussed earlier, in section II. Blasts in excess of 20% establish the diagnosis of acute leukemia.

4. Flow cytometry results for AML are shown in Appendix C-7, section II. Results for ALL are shown in Appendix C-5.

5. Cytogenetic testing is essential in every new patient because of its prognostic significance. Cytogenetic abnormalities distinguish unique types of AML and are the single most predictive factor for response to treatment, duration of response, and relapse. The abnormalities are categorized as "favorable-," "standard- or intermediate-," and "unfavorable or poor"-risk cytogenetics (Table 25.1).

6. Radiographic studies that should be obtained include the following:

   a. Chest radiograph to look for leukemic or infectious infiltrates

   b. Bone radiographs of painful or tender areas to look for periosteal elevation or bony destruction from extramedullary bone masses

7. Cerebrospinal fluid (CSF) examination should be performed at some time in all patients with ALL, where it is usually part of the induction therapy. CSF evaluation should be done in patients with acute monocytic leukemia and in those patients with AML who have meningismus or CNS abnormalities. Cytarabine or methotrexate may be instilled into the CSF at the completion of the examination because of the possibility of leukemic contamination from the blood (see section IX.B).

   The fluid should be cultured for acid-fast bacilli, fungi, and bacteria. Meningeal involvement with leukemia is associated with decreased sugar and increased protein concentrations, pleocytosis, and leukemic cells identified by cytologic examination.

8. Surveillance bacterial cultures of the nose, pharynx, axillae, and perianal regions identify organisms that may have colonized the patient. These cultures, however, are not commonly helpful in determining the etiologic agents responsible for serious infection in the patient with neutropenia. Cultures of the blood, urine, sputum, and any symptomatic areas should be obtained in all febrile leukemic patients.

IV. PROGNOSTIC FACTORS AND SURVIVAL

Complete remission (CR) is the paramount prognostic factor in all forms of acute leukemia. A CR is defined as all of the following:

- Bone marrow contains <2% blasts
- Granulocyte and platelet counts have recovered
- Resolution of organomegaly may be required in a clinical-trial setting

A. AML prognostic factors. The most important factors portending a **poor prognosis** in AML are

   1. Advanced age (typically described as age >60)

   2. Antecedent myelodysplasia

   3. Therapy-related AML

   4. High WBC count at presentation

   5. Unfavorable cytogenetics

B. ALL prognostic factors. ALL is not a uniform disease but consists of subtypes with distinct biological, clinical, and prognostic features. The most important prognostic factors are age, initial WBC count, and immunophenotype, as well as cytogenetic features.

   1. Favorable prognostic factors in adult ALL. The Cancer and Leukemia Group B (CALGB) identified the following clinical and biological features that correlate with favorable long-term outcome:

      a. Younger age

      b. WBC count ($\leq$30,000/μL)

      c. Absence of the Philadelphia chromosome (Ph[1])

2. Adverse prognostic factors in ALL

a. Clinical characteristics
  (1) Older age
  (2) WBC count >30,000/μL
  (3) Late achievement of CR (occurring after >3 to 4 weeks)

b. Immunophenotype
  (1) Pre–B-cell ALL
  (2) Pro–T-cell, pre–T-cell
  (3) Mature T-cell ALL

c. Cytogenetics and molecular genetics
  (1) t(9;22)(p34;q11) [Ph^1]; *BCR/ABL* fusion gene: occurs in 25% of adults with ALL
  (2) t(1;19)(q23;p13); *PBX/E2A*: occurs in 25% of children with ALL
  (3) Abnormal 11q23; *MLL* gene rearranged: poor prognosis in infants <1 year of age and adults
  (4) t(4;11)/ALL1-AF4; common clinical features of this subtype include:
    (a) High WBC count (median 180,000/μL)
    (b) L1 or L2 morphology with B-cell lineage
    (c) Unfavorable immunophenotype (CD10−, CD19+, HLA-DR+) with frequent coexpression of myeloid markers (CD15+, CDw65+)
  (5) Expression of multidrug resistance (rarely assayed)

3. Response rates and survival

a. AML.
About two-thirds of patients achieve a CR to standard induction chemotherapy. The median survival is 12 to 24 months for patients who achieve CR; the median duration of first remission is 10 to 12 months. About 20% of patients who achieve CR (5% to 15% of all patients) survive ≥5 years, and many of these patients may be cured. Most relapses occur within 3 years.

Approximately 50% of patients with "favorable" cytogenetics who achieve CR survive. Only 10% to 15% of patients in CR achieve long-term survival if they are >60 years or develop AML following primary or secondary MDS.

b. ALL (also see Acute Leukemia in Chapter 18, Cancers in Childhood)
  (1) **"Standard-risk" children** (1 to 9 years of age, WBC count <50,000/μL, precursor B-cell subtype, and without adverse prognostic factors). Of cases, <20% relapse if properly treated, and >80% have a 5-year disease-free survival. Relapse or death is unusual in these patients after 4 years of continuous CR.
  (2) **"High-risk" children** (those with adverse prognostic factors) have remission duration and survival similar to those of adults, yet some series report 70% of patients surviving disease-free for 4 years. The survival time for infants is <2 years.
  (3) **Adolescents and adults** have a median first CR duration of 12 to 24 months and a median survival time of 24 to 30 months. Late adolescents (17 to 21 years of age) appear to have a substantially improved survival time if treated with aggressive pediatric protocols. The median survival time is <18 months for patients >60 years of age with an elevated WBC count at presentation.

V. MANAGEMENT OF EVERY PATIENT WITH ACUTE LEUKEMIA WHO MAY UNDERGO ALLOGENEIC HEMATOPOIETIC STEM CELL TRANSPLANTATION (HSCT)
The following precautions are very important in all patients (generally, <65 years of age) who are eligible for allogeneic HSCT:

- **Leukocyte reduction and irradiation of all administered blood products**
- **Obtain HLA typing** of the patient for both class I and class II antigens on admission and before giving any treatment that will suppress blood counts.

■ **Assess cytomegalovirus (CMV)** antibody titers on admission. All blood products should be screened and negative for CMV until titers become available. CMV-seronegative patients should probably receive CMV-negative products if allotransplant is ever contemplated, whereas CMV-positive patients can receive CMV-safe products (positive but leukofiltered).

VI. MANAGEMENT OF AML

A. Remission induction. Intensive chemotherapy, nearly always to the point of severe myelosuppression (which generally occurs about 7 to 12 days after treatment is begun), is presently required to achieve CR in patients with AML. Cytarabine and an anthracycline are usually administered. Cytarabine has been given in doses ranging from 100 mg/m^2 to 6,000 mg/m^2, but it is not clear that higher dosages in induction give better results. Daunorubicin, idarubicin, and mitoxantrone at equipotent doses also appear to give similar results. Idarubicin, however, appears to induce higher remission rate in patients with an elevated WBC count at presentation. A typical regimen is as follows:

Cytarabine 200 mg/m^2/day by continuous IV infusion for 7 days, and
Idarubicin, 12 mg/m^2 (or daunorubicin, 45 mg/m^2, or mitoxantrone, 12 mg/m^2)
IV push on days 1, 2, and 3

If the blasts are not cleared from the blood and bone marrow after the first course of treatment, and if the patient can tolerate another such intensive treatment, the combination therapy is repeated again. A CR is achieved in 60% to 75% of patients with good medical support, usually about 1 month after initiating treatment. More than 95% of CR are achieved with one or two courses of induction chemotherapy.

1. Toxicity of induction therapy

a. Tumor lysis syndrome can occur with its associated hyperuricemia, hyperphosphatemia, hypocalcemia, and hyperkalemia. Patients with acute leukemia should be given allopurinol (300 to 600 mg daily), if possible beginning 12 to 48 hours before starting chemotherapy.

b. Cardiac abnormalities. Anthracyclines may be associated with electrocardiographic changes, arrhythmias, or congestive heart failure. All patients must have a nuclear heart scan or an echocardiogram to assess the left ventricular ejection fraction before starting an anthracycline.

c. Tissue necrosis. Anthracyclines are vesicants and, if infiltrated out of the veins into the tissues, will cause severe tissue necrosis. A safer approach would be to use a well-secured central venous access catheter (i.e., Hickman catheter), which should be checked for position and good blood return before infusing the anthracycline.

d. Pancytopenia secondary to bone marrow suppression is both caused by the disease and a goal of therapy. This results in infectious and hemorrhagic complications. Patients will also become dependent on transfusions until remission is achieved and normal hematopoiesis is restored.

e. Nausea and vomiting tend to be minimal with an effective antiemetics regimen. The emetic potential of cytarabine is low, but patients need effective antiemetics during the anthracycline administration. A typical regimen involves serotonin antagonist (ondansetron, dolasetron, or granisetron) and dexamethasone (10 mg PO daily) for the 3 days of anthracycline administration.

f. Alopecia is the rule and is usually reversible.

g. Toxicity of high-dose cytarabine. When used at high dose (2 to 3 g/m^2 over 1 to 3 hours), cytarabine can be associated with cerebellar, ophthalmologic, and GI toxicity, particularly in patients > 60 years of age. These toxicities occur in much lower frequency when given in lower dosages (1.5 g/m^2) or when a much lower dose of drug is infused over longer periods of time (100 to 400 mg/m^2 by continuous IV infusion).

2. **Elderly patients.** The treatment of patients ≥65 years of age is controversial. Elderly patients often cannot tolerate the toxic effects of intensive induction therapy as well as can younger patients; the treatment-related mortality during induction is between 10% and 30% with intensive regimens. Furthermore, elderly patients often develop AML with adverse disease features, often following antecedent MDS or with high-risk cytogenetics.

   a. Less intensive treatment using attenuated dosages of drugs, oral agents (hydroxyurea or etoposide), or "low-dose cytarabine" (10 mg/m^2 SC daily) have been shown to be associated with less myelosuppression, fewer early deaths, and longer outpatient survival than standard intensive induction therapy. The use of supportive care alone is a reasonable option for some elderly patients with AML, particularly for those who are not in good general medical condition, although survival is typically measured in weeks to months.

   b. Other, less intensive regimens for elderly patients who are in good general medical condition under investigation include

      (1) Cytarabine, 100 mg/m^2/day for 5 days given by continuous IV infusion; and idarubicin, 12 mg/m^2 IV for one dose only

      (2) Gemtuzumab ozogamicin as a single-agent induction treatment

      (3) Various doses and schedules of drugs approved for myelodysplasia, such as decitabine and azacytidine

      (4) Investigational agents (e.g., tipifarnib, a farnesyltransferase inhibitor)

B. **Postremission therapy.** After CR is achieved, the most important goal is to prevent recurrence. Leukemic cells that are not clinically apparent are nearly always present in the bone marrow. Therapy to eradicate residual leukemia is required, or recurrence is inevitable. The best form of postremission therapy, however, remains controversial. Patients <60 years of age are usually presented three potential postremission options.

   1. **Intensive chemotherapy.** Relatively high doses of drugs are given shortly after the patient has achieved CR, has regained normal hematologic function, and has recovered clinically from any complications of prior therapy. Cytarabine alone, or with an anthracycline, is commonly used.

      A randomized study treated patients <60 years of age with four cycles of consolidation cytarabine using three different dosages (100 mg/m^2, 400 mg/m^2, and 3 g/m^2). Cytarabine was given over 3 hours every 12 hours on days 1, 3, and 5 for a total of six doses. The higher dose of cytarabine achieved a 45% disease-free survival at 4 years, whereas lower doses were associated with poor survival (25% in the 100 mg/m^2 group). Older patients, however, did not benefit from any dosage and had a 15% disease-free survival at 4 years.

   2. **Autologous HSCT** may offer a lower risk of relapse compared with intensive chemotherapy, but relapse remains higher than that associated with allogeneic transplantation. The major cause of death remains disease recurrence.

      Three prospective randomized trials comparing intensive chemotherapy with autologous HSCT demonstrated a lower relapse rate in the transplant arm (40% *vs.* 57%), but no overall survival advantage (56% *vs.* 46%). The high transplant-related mortality rate in these cooperative-group studies (12%) offset the antileukemic advantage provided with the autograft. With transplant mortality now decreasing to <5%, this may translate into improved overall survival for the autografted patients.

   3. **Allogeneic HSCT.** Most prospective studies have failed to show a survival advantage for allogeneic transplantation in good-risk patients (those with favorable cytogenetics) in first remission. On the other hand, reduced relapse and improved disease-free survival was demonstrated in standard-risk patients. Poor-risk patients with unfavorable cytogenetics seem to derive the maximal benefit from allogeneic HSCT.

C. **Treatment of relapses.** Relapses in AML are typically systemic (i.e., in the marrow and elsewhere). Occasionally, extramedullary relapse (e.g., chloromas in skin or lymph nodes) may precede systemic relapse. Up to half of those with recurrent AML achieve a second CR using either the same drugs that induced first remission or investigational drugs. A variety of investigational drugs have been developed to supplant high-dose cytarabine in the relapsed setting. Eligible patients with an available histocompatible stem cell donor should be strongly considered for allogeneic HSCT.

D. Gemtuzumab ozogamicin (Mylotarg). More than 80% of patients with AML have myeloid blast cells that express the CD33 surface antigen. Calicheamicin, a highly potent antitumor antibiotic that cleaves double-stranded DNA at specific sequences, was conjugated to a humanized anti-CD33 monoclonal antibody to produce Mylotarg. The drug was used to treat patients with AML who were in first relapse and who had no history of an antecedent hematologic disorder; their median age was 61 years. Of patients treated with Mylotarg, 30% obtained remission. The most frequent toxicities were myelosuppression and infusion-related symptoms; after licensing, hepatic veno-occlusive disease (hyperbilirubinemia, elevated hepatic transaminase levels) was identified in patients who had previously been heavily treated, especially in those who had had a stem-cell transplant. (See Chapter 4, section VII.E. for dosage.)

VII. MANAGEMENT OF ACUTE PROMYELOCYTIC LEUKEMIA (APL)

A. Induction. All-*trans*-retinoic acid (ATRA, 45 mg/m^2/day in two divided doses) is given daily throughout the induction period. Either idarubicin is given in conventional doses (12 mg/m^2) but with increased number of doses (on days 2, 4, 6, and 8 of the induction course) or daunorubicin is given for 3 consecutive days in doses higher than the normal 45 mg/m^2. The role of cytarabine is not established for APL. CR rates were in the range of 70% to 95% in the Italian cooperative group (GIMEMA) and the Spanish cooperative group (PETHEMA) studies. Both ATRA and arsenic trioxide act as differentiative agents in APL.

B. Consolidation. Following CR in APL, it is mandatory to administer consolidation therapy to avoid relapse. Although the optimal regimen is not clearly defined, most protocols utilize an anthracycline with or without cytarabine.

C. Maintenance. The North American Intergroup APL study, randomized patients who achieved CR after two courses of consolidation chemotherapy to either a year of daily maintenance ATRA at standard doses or to observation. Patients who received ATRA during both induction and as maintenance had a 5-year disease-free survival of 75%, whereas patients who received no ATRA maintenance had an inferior 5-year disease-free survival of 55%. Other regimens use ATRA maintenance for 2 weeks every 3 months for 2 years with oral chemotherapy (6-mercaptopurine and methotrexate) on a quarterly basis.

D. APL differentiation syndrome (APLDS) is a cardiorespiratory syndrome manifested by fever, weight gain, respiratory distress, interstitial pulmonary infiltrates, pleural and pericardial effusion, episodic hypotension, and acute renal failure. The disorder is attributed to rapid differentiation of blasts to (clonal) neutrophils with subsequent vascular complications and can be induced by either ATRA or arsenic trioxide. The incidence is 25% when ATRA is used alone. The concurrent administration of chemotherapy and ATRA may reduce the incidence to below 10%, but this has not been clearly established. Corticosteroids can be effective as prophylaxis and therapy of the differentiation syndrome. The mortality rate with APLDS has declined from 30% to 5%, likely reflecting earlier recognition and earlier institution of dexamethasone therapy. No factors are clearly predictive of APLDS.

E. DIC. Coagulopathy exacerbated by cytotoxic chemotherapy was previously seen in >90% of patients with APL and resulted in severe hemorrhagic manifestations in excess of that expected for the degree of thrombocytopenia. Both the incidence and severity of DIC have substantially decreased with differentiation therapy. Laboratory abnormalities include not only features associated with DIC (decreased fibrinogen and increased fibrin and fibrinogen degradation products), but also evidence of increased fibrinolysis (acquired deficiency of the fibrinolysis inhibitor, α_2-antitrypsin).

Patients should be monitored closely for the development of DIC and treated at its first sign. Transfusions with platelets and cryoprecipitate (to sustain fibrinogen levels) are the mainstays of therapy. Heparin is now rarely used. Antifibrinolytic agents, such as epsilon-aminocaproic acid, may be useful in the setting of excess fibrinolysis.

VIII. MANAGEMENT OF ACUTE LYMPHOBLASTIC LEUKEMIA (ALL)

A. Remission induction

1. **Children** (also see Chapter 18). The combination of vincristine and prednisone (V + P) produces CR in 85% to 90% of cases of childhood ALL. L-asparaginase is typically added. Most children achieve CR within 4 weeks of therapy; if CR is not achieved within 6 weeks, no value is found in continuing the drugs unless under unusual circumstances such as in ataxia telangiectasias. Children often achieved CR without prolonged myelosuppression.

    a. **Standard-risk patients** are treated with V + P plus L-asparaginase for 4 to 6 weeks.

    Vincristine, 1.5 mg/m^2 (maximum 2 mg) IV push weekly
    Prednisone, 40 mg/m^2 PO daily
    L-asparaginase, 6,000 U/m^2 (maximum 10,000 U) IM three times weekly for a total of nine doses

    b. **High-risk patients** are treated with V + P, L-asparaginase, and daunorubicin (25 mg/m^2) IV weekly for two doses.

2. **Adults.** The V + P regimen results in CR in 45% to 65% of adults with ALL. The addition of an anthracycline (with or without L-asparaginase) increases the CR rate to 75%. Regimens with five drugs may further increase the CR rate to 85%; an example regimen is the following (see Larson RA, et al. in *Suggested Reading*):

    Cyclophosphamide, 1,200 mg/m^2 IV on day 1
    Daunorubicin, 45 mg/m^2 IV on days 1, 2, and 3
    Vincristine, 2 mg IV on days 1, 8, 15, and 22
    Prednisone, 80/m^2 IV or PO on days 1 through 21
    L-asparaginase, 6,000 U/m^2 SC on days 5, 8, 11, 15, 18, and 22

3. **Toxicity of induction therapy**

    a. **V + P**

    (1) Intestinal colic and constipation (bulk laxatives should be used prophylactically)

    (2) Peripheral neuropathy (usually reversible)

    (3) Bone marrow suppression

    (4) Alopecia (uncommon)

    b. **V + P plus an anthracycline.** Same as above, in section VIII.A.3.a, along with nausea, vomiting, stomatitis, alopecia, myelosuppression, and possibly cardiac toxicity.

    c. **V + P and L-asparaginase.** Same as above, in section VIII.A.3.a, with the addition of coagulation defects with decreased fibrinogen level, allergic reactions, and encephalopathy, hyperbilirubinemia, elevated hepatic transaminases, pancreatitis, phlebitis, or thrombosis.

B. CNS prophylaxis after induction chemotherapy prevents early CNS relapse and is mandatory in ALL. The CNS is the initial site of relapse in more than half of children unless prophylaxis is given and it is also a frequent site of relapse in adults.

1. **Regimens.** The form of CNS prophylaxis is controversial. Many authorities recommend intrathecal methotrexate (6 to 12 mg/m^2 of preservative-free methotrexate up to a maximum of 15 mg/dose is given twice weekly for five to eight doses). Intrathecal methotrexate is often combined with craniospinal irradiation (~2,400 cGy in 12 fractions over 2.5 weeks) for patients >1 year of age. Intrathecal methotrexate alone is recommended by some authorities for patients at low risk for relapse (age 2 to 9 years, WBC count <10,000/µL, and CD10+). For adults, prophylactic intrathecal chemotherapy alone is considered sufficient.

2. **Toxicity of CNS prophylaxis**
   a. **Transient encephalopathy,** which can be fatal, may develop in about 70% of children in 4 to 8 weeks after completion of cranial irradiation, especially if methotrexate is given in the maintenance program. Symptoms of encephalopathy include somnolence, headache, vomiting, and low-grade fever. Spinal fluid examination shows pleocytosis with neutrophils and mononuclear cells. The differential diagnosis includes CNS infection, cerebrovascular accidents, and leukemic meningitis, which should be distinguishable by MRI scans and by spinal fluid culture and cytology.
   b. **Alopecia** after cranial irradiation
   c. **Headache** after intrathecal drug administration
   d. **Chemical arachnoiditis** with meningismus and back pain related to epidural extravasation of methotrexate
   e. **Leukoencephalopathy** may develop in patients given large doses of IV methotrexate after brain irradiation.
   f. **Neuropsychological effects** of treatment are common, especially in children <6 years of age. Memory, mathematic, and motor skills may be impaired. CNS prophylaxis and the systemic drugs that have activity in the CNS (methotrexate, prednisone, vincristine, and L-asparaginase) are thought to cause these problems; however, the disease itself may also contribute.
C. **Intensive postremission therapy**
   1. **Consolidation treatment** with an intensive multidrug regimen has been shown to improve survival in children and is considered standard treatment. A retrospective analysis in adults showed a superior outcome among trials implementing multidrug intensive consolidation, but randomized trials are inconclusive. High-dose cytarabine may be beneficial for T-cell ALL and some high-risk subgroups. High-dose methotrexate may be useful in B-cell lineage ALL.
   2. **Allogeneic HSCT** in first CR has been demonstrated to improve survival for adults with ALL in all age categories. It is not recommended for first CR for children with standard-risk ALL, but HSCT may be important for specific subgroups of ALL (patients with the Philadelphia chromosome) or for those who relapse after initial remission.
D. **Maintenance therapy** for 2 to 3 years is mandatory in childhood ALL and is typically used in adults as well.
   1. **Effective drugs.** Methotrexate (20 mg/m^2 PO to a maximum of 35 mg weekly) plus mercaptopurine (50 to 75 mg/m^2 PO daily) are the cornerstones of maintenance therapy in ALL. It is important that the drugs be given in dosages sufficient to produce myelosuppression to produce an impact on disease-free survival. Monthly pulses of V + P are also given. Intrathecal chemotherapy is typically administered every 90 days.
   2. **Toxicity of maintenance therapy**
      a. Therapy is interrupted if any of the following occurs:
         (1) Significant myelosuppression (which is dose-limiting but a necessary goal)
         (2) Abnormal LFT
         (3) Stomatitis, diarrhea
         (4) Renal tubular necrosis secondary to the methotrexate (renal function is closely monitored)
      b. Immunosuppression (increased susceptibility to infection, particularly varicella and *Pneumocystis jiroveci*)
      c. Growth inhibition
      d. Skin disorders
      e. Osteoporosis with long-term methotrexate treatment
   3. **When to stop maintenance therapy**
      a. **Children.** Prolonged chemotherapy is of greatest consequence in children because adverse late, side effects may develop. Most children in remission are treated for 30 to 36 months; 20% of children taken off treatment relapse, most within the first year. Elective testicular biopsy of boys before stopping maintenance therapy has been shown to be of no clinical value.

   b. Adults. Most adults with ALL relapse despite maintenance therapy. The question of how long adults with ALL should continue maintenance is yet to be answered but it seems that prolonged and more dose-intensive regimens lead to better results. We recommend maintenance therapy for at least 2 years in adults with ALL based on the experience with children.
E. Treatment of relapses. ALL may relapse systemically or in sanctuary sites (testicle or CNS).
   1. Extramedullary relapse. Without CNS prophylaxis, relapse only in the CNS is common. Relapse in the testis occurs, but less commonly. Patients who have solitary extramedullary relapse and normal bone marrow may be treated with local therapy alone (i.e., CNS irradiation plus intrathecal chemotherapy for CNS relapse or irradiation of the testicle for testicular relapse). Frequently, relapse in these sites predict for systemic relapse.
   2. Systemic relapse may be successfully treated with the agents used to induce the original remission in half of the cases but any relapse should prompt consideration of allogeneic transplantation.
   3. Subsequent remissions. Each subsequent remission becomes progressively shorter, and drugs available for maintenance therapy are progressively limited. Patients who relapse after cessation of maintenance therapy have a better prognosis than those who relapse during therapy.

IX. MANAGEMENT OF ACUTE LEUKEMIAS: OTHER ISSUES
A. Supportive care
   1. Indwelling tunneled central venous catheters are used during the induction phase to facilitate the administration of IV therapies and the sampling of blood for laboratory tests.
   2. Blood component therapy
      a. Platelet transfusions are clearly indicated for patients with severe thrombocytopenia when there is active bleeding, fever, or infection. Without petechiae or bleeding, platelets are transfused prophylactically when counts are 10,000/μL to 20,000/μL unless the patient is febrile, at which point platelets should be kept at a slightly higher level of 20,000/μL owing to enhanced platelet consumption.
      b. Packed red blood cell transfusions are used to treat symptomatic anemia and active hemorrhage. The hemoglobin concentration is generally kept ≥ 8 g/dL because these patients have aregenerative bone marrows. If the patient is actively bleeding or has a medical history, transfusion is given to target a higher hemoglobin level.
      c. Granulocyte transfusions are not generally recommended. They can be used, however, in certain settings such as an overwhelming fungal sepsis, when the patient is past the induction phase and has no evidence of leukemia on bone marrow evaluation and is expected to recover within a short period of time. In the absence of a reasonable chance of recovery, granulocyte transfusions should not be used.
      d. Growth factors (G-CSF and granulocyte macrophage-CSF [GM-CSF]) may be given on completion of administration of the induction chemotherapy after a repeat bone marrow biopsy on days 10 to 14 is proven to be devoid of leukemic elements. Their use may shorten the duration of neutropenia by 2 to 4 days and appears to decrease morbidity. Studies do not indicate that these factors impair the efficacy of chemotherapy.
   3. Infections. It is critical to initiate prompt empiric IV antibiotics in the event of fever. The choice of antibiotics is institution dependent, but should always contain adequate coverage of gram-negative bacteria and also *Staphylococcus aureus* in patients suspected of having a catheter-related infection. For persistently febrile patients, empiric coverage with antifungal agents has been demonstrated to improve survival.
      a. Management of neutropenic fever is thoroughly discussed in section II of Chapter 35.

        b. Prophylaxis against infection (see Chapter 35, section II.A.2.c).
    4. Tumor lysis syndrome (see Chapter 27, section XIII).
B. Treatment of meningeal leukemia
    1. Manifestations. Meningeal leukemia should be considered in the setting of cranial neuropathy, other neurologic signs, or altered mental status. Blast cells identified by cytologic evaluation of the CSF is diagnostic but evaluation of the CSF is not sensitive.
    2. Treatment. Optimal treatment has not been determined. Most patients are given cranial or craniospinal irradiation over a 3-week period plus intrathecal chemotherapy. Intrathecal therapy alone may be insufficient.
        a. Drugs. Preservative-free methotrexate (6 to 12 mg/m^2 to a maximum of 15 mg) or cytarabine (50 to 100 mg) is used for intrathecal therapy. Methotrexate should be avoided in the setting of renal failure. Toxic effects of methotrexate in the periphery may be prevented by giving IV or oral leucovorin.
        b. Diluents. Artificial spinal fluid (Elliott's B solution) is available at some institutions to dilute the cytotoxic agents.
        c. Technique. Intrathecal chemotherapy is given isovolumetrically and gradually by serial withdrawal and injection of spinal fluid with a syringe containing the chemotherapeutic agents. The drugs can be administered by lumbar or cisternal puncture, or through an inserted intraventricular (Ommaya) reservoir.
        d. Duration. Intrathecal chemotherapy is given at 2- to 7-day intervals until abnormal cells and excess protein are cleared from the spinal fluid. Therapy is often continued at 1- to 2-month intervals for a period thereafter.
C. Special clinical problems
    1. Leukostasis is more common in AML than in ALL and frequently occurs in patients with WBC count >100,000/µL. Sludging impairs circulation and results in organ dysfunction. The circulating blast count can be rapidly reduced with leukapheresis, thereby reducing the risks of leukostasis, DIC, and metabolic abnormalities associated with tumor lysis. Hydroxyurea (3 g/day) or alternative chemotherapy should be instituted with leukapheresis.
    2. Ocular and gingival involvement. Irradiating eyes involved with leukemic infiltrates may prevent blindness. Gingival enlargement in patients with monocytic leukemia does not require special treatment because it should resolve with induction chemotherapy.
    3. Patients exposed to varicella zoster infections should be given acyclovir and zoster immune globulin (see section V.B. in Chapter 35).
    4. Acute leukemia during pregnancy (see Chapter 26, section IV).

 MYELODYSPLASTIC SYNDROMES

Patients who have MDS are at a high risk for developing AML. Theoretically, defects in stem cells account for ineffective hematopoiesis and for a wide variety of abnormalities. The diagnosis of a primary MDS may be made only in the absence of conditions that produce secondary myelodysplasia, namely, exposure to radiation and cytotoxic therapy. Folic acid and vitamin B$_{12}$ deficiencies produce a reversible picture similar to myelodysplasia.

I. CLINICAL FEATURES
    MDS usually affects patients >65 years of age, particularly men. Symptoms are nonspecific and usually reflect the degree of anemia. Physical examination is usually normal. Various cytopenias, usually including macrocytic anemia, may persist for months to years. The bone marrow is usually abnormal.

II. DYSHEMATOPOIESIS
    Dyshematopoiesis is manifested by cytopenias in the presence of a normocellular or hypercellular bone marrow. Components and features of dyshematopoiesis, which occur in various combinations for each syndrome, are as follows:

A. Dyserythropoiesis

1. **Peripheral blood.** Anemia and reticulocytopenia from ineffective erythropoiesis; anisocytosis, poikilocytosis, basophilic stippling; macrocytosis (when megaloblastoid maturation is present); and dimorphic (normocytic, normochromic, and microcytic, hypochromic) red blood cell populations

2. **Bone marrow.** Erythroid hyperplasia or hypoplasia; ringed sideroblasts; megaloblastoid maturation (multinucleation, nuclear fragments, karyorrhexis, or cytoplasmic vacuoles)

3. **Other assays.** Decreased CD55 and CD59 expression on granulocytes or erythrocytes defines paroxysmal nocturnal hemoglobinuria. Periodic acid Schiff (PAS)-positive cytochemistry, and increased fetal hemoglobin levels may be detected in some cases of myelodysplasia.

B. Dysgranulocytopoiesis

1. **Peripheral blood.** Neutropenia; decreased or abnormal neutrophil granules; neutrophil hyposegmentation (pseudo-Pelger-Huët anomaly), hypersegmentation, or bizarre nuclei

2. **Bone marrow.** Granulocytic hyperplasia; abnormal or decreased granules in neutrophil precursors; increased numbers of blast cells

3. **Other assays.** Decreased neutrophil alkaline phosphatase score and myeloperoxidase activity

C. Dysmegakaryopoiesis

1. **Peripheral blood.** Thrombocytopenia; large platelets with abnormal and decreased granularity

2. **Bone marrow.** Reduced numbers of megakaryocytes; micromegakaryocytes; megakaryocytes with large, single nuclei or multiple, small separated nuclei

3. **Other assays.** Abnormal platelet function tests

III. CLASSIFICATION

A. The French–American–British classification of MDS initially categorized patients based entirely on morphology and dysplastic changes in at least two of the three hematopoietic cell lines into six subtypes:

1. Refractory anemia (RA): <5% marrow blasts
2. RA with ringed sideroblasts (RARS): <5% blasts plus ≥15% ringed sideroblasts
3. RA with excess blasts in transformation (RAEB): 5% to 20% marrow blasts
4. RAEB in transformation (RAEB-T): 21% to 30% marrow blasts
5. Chronic myelomonocytic leukemia (CMML): ≤20% marrow blasts plus peripheral blood monocytosis > 1,000/μL
6. AML: >30% marrow blasts

B. The WHO revised and restructured the traditional FAB classifications of AML, MDS, and MPD. The presence or absence of the Philadelphia (Ph[1]) chromosome [t(9;22)(q34;q11)] and *BCR/ABL* fusion gene was taken into account (Table 25.2).

1. **WHO classification of MDS** lowered the blast percentage threshold for the definition of AML from 30% to 20%. The category of RAEB-T was eliminated. The WHO classification for MDS is shown in Table 25.2.

2. **WHO classification of MPD** is as follows:

   Polycythemia vera
   Chronic idiopathic myelofibrosis (with extramedullary hematopoiesis)
   Essential thrombocythemia
   Chronic myelogenous leukemia (CML)
   Chronic neutrophilic leukemia
   Chronic eosinophilic leukemia
   Chronic MPD, unclassified

3. **WHO classification of myelodysplastic/myeloproliferative disease (MDS/ MPD)** acknowledges the overlap between MDS and MPD entities. This category includes myeloid disorders that have both myelodysplastic and myeloproliferative features at the time of initial presentation. The MDS/MPD diseases are:

TABLE 25.2	World Health Organization (WHO) Classification of Myelodysplastic Syndromes and Myeloid Leukemias

Diseases	Peripheral blood	Bone marrow[a]
Myelodysplastic syndromes		
MDS, unclassified (MDS-U)	Cytopenias: ≥ 1 Blasts: None or rare Auer rods: None	Dysplasia in granulocytes or megakaryocytes only Blasts: <5% Auer rods: None
Refractory anemia (RA)	Cytopenia: Anemia Blasts: None or rare	Erythroid dysplasia only Blasts: <5% RS: <15%
RA with RS (RARS)	Same as RA	Same as RA except RS: ≥ 15%
Refractory cytopenia with multilineage dysplasia (RCMD)	Cytopenias: ≥ 2 Blasts: None or rare Auer rods: None Monocytes <1,000/μL	Dysplasia in ≥ 10% of cells in ≥ 2 MCL Blasts: <5% Auer rods: None RS: <15%
RCMD with RS (RCMD-RS)	Same as RCMD	Same as RCMD except RS: ≥ 15%
Refractory cytopenia with excess blasts-1 (RAEB-1)	Cytopenias Blasts: <5% Auer rods: None Monocytes <1,000/μL	Dysplasia in ≥ 1 MCL Blasts: 5% to 9% Auer rods: None
RAEB-2	Cytopenias Blasts: 5% to 19% Auer rods: $\pm$ Monocytes <1,000/μL	Dysplasia in ≥ 1 MCL Blasts: 10% to 19% Auer rods: $\pm$
Myeloid leukemias		
Chronic myelomonocytic leukemia (CMML)[b]	Persistent monocytosis $\geq 1,000/\mu$L, unexplained	Dysplasia in ≥ 1 MCL and/orcytogenetic abnormalities; no Ph[1]
CMML-1	Blasts: <5%	Blasts: <10%
CMML-2	Blasts: 5% to 19%	Blasts: 10% to 19%
Chronic myelogenous leukemia (CML)[b]		Presence of Ph[1] in the appropriate milieu; see Chapter 23. *CML*
Acute myelogenous leukemia (AML)		Blasts: ≥ 20% or specific recurrent cytogenetic abnormalities; see Appendix C-7

MCL, Myeloid cell line; MDS, myelodysplastic syndrome; Ph[1], Philadelphia chromosome or *BCR/ABL* fusion gene; RS, ringed sideroblasts
[a]See section II for definitions of the various dysplasias.
[b]CML in the WHO classification is defined as a myeloproliferative disease (MPD), although this contention is debatable. Myelodysplastic/myeloproliferative disease (MDS/MPD) is a category in the WHO system that includes myeloid disorders that have both dysplastic and proliferative features at the time of initial presentation and that are difficult to assign to either the MDS or MPD group of diseases. MDS/MPD includes CMML and is presented in section III.B.3.

Chronic myelomonocytic leukemia (CMML, CMML-1, CMML-2)
Atypical chronic myeloid leukemia
Juvenile myelomonocytic leukemia
MDS/MPD, unclassified

a. Diagnostic criteria for CMML and its subtypes are shown in Table 25.2.

b. Atypical CML is a very aggressive disorder. It is characterized by marked granulocytic and often multilineage dysplasia (which is not seen in chronic-phase CML) and the absence of the Ph^1 chromosome and *BCR/ABL* fusion gene.

c. Juvenile myelomonocytic leukemia affects infants and young children, manifests neutrophilic and monocytic proliferation, and lacks the Ph^1 chromosome and *BCR/ABL* fusion gene.

IV. GENE ABNORMALITIES

A. Cytogenetic abnormalities are nonrandom and occur in 40% to 60% of patients with MDS. Cytogenetics abnormalities traditionally associated with MDS (involving chromosomes 3q, 5q, 7q, 12p, and 20q11–12, and trisomy 8) are "secondary" genetic events. The unbalanced translocation between chromosomes 1 and 7 [t(1;7)(p11;p11)] results in trisomy for the long arm of chromosome 1 and monosomy for the long arm of chromosome 7 and may be causally related to therapy-related MDS.

B. Molecular mutation and gene methylation. In adults with MDS, disease progression has been associated with mutations in genes such as *p53*, and *FLT3* (see Table 25.1 for the frequency of *FLT* mutations in AML). *FTL3* mutations are now considered one of the most common mutations in AML (35% in older adults) and an important predictor of poor outcome.

Disease progression is also associated with progressive methylation and transcriptional inactivation of critical cell cycle regulatory genes, such as *p15 INK4b* that normally function to inhibit cyclin-dependent kinase activity at the G_1 phase of the cell cycle. Patients with MDS have also been shown to have defective activation of signal transduction pathways, particularly involving STAT5, in response to erythropoietin, which may account in part for defective erythropoiesis and persistent anemia.

C. The 5q–syndrome is recognized as a distinct clinical entity that predominantly affects females and has a favorable prognosis with a low risk of transformation to AML. This entity is to be distinguished from AML characterized by a deletion of chromosome 5 or 5q. Patients have macrocytic anemia, modest leukopenia, normal or high platelet counts, bone marrow erythroid hypoplasia, hypolobulated megakaryocytes, and bone marrow blast counts <20%.

The breakpoint most frequently cited is 5q12–14 (proximal breakpoint) and 5q31–33 (distal breakpoint). Many hematopoietic growth factors and growth factor receptor genes, including interleukins (IL) and colony-stimulating factors (CSF), have been localized to chromosome 5q. Those localized to 5q13–33 include IL-3, IL-4, IL-5, IL-9, CSF-1R, ras p21 activator protein, and interleukin regulatory factor-1 (IRF-1). The deletion of these genes seems to contribute to the clinical development of the 5q–syndrome.

V. PROGNOSIS

Life expectancy in MDS ranges from several months to 10 years, depending on the initial presentation, cytopenia, cytogenetics, and age. Age >45 to 50 years is a major unfavorable prognostic factor. The **IPSS** is a weighted prognostic grouping based on cytopenias, cytogenetics, and blast percentage in the bone marrow. The IPSS classifies patients into low-, intermediate-, or high-risk groups by scoring for initial bone marrow blasts, cytogenetics (favorable *vs.* unfavorable), and lineage cytopenia. The IPSS and associated median survivals are shown in Table 25.3.

VI. MANAGEMENT OF MDS

Because treatment for MDS is unsuccessful in most patients, patients should be encouraged to enroll into clinical trials. Treatment selection should be based on the patient's

TABLE 25.3	International Prognostic Scoring System (IPSS) for Myelodysplastic Syndromes				

	IPSS score				
Covariates	**0**	**0.5**	**1.0**	**1.5**	**2.0**
Bone marrow blasts	<5%	5% to 10%	—	11% to 20%	21% to 30%
Cytogenetics	Normal −Y del (5q) del (20)	Other	−7 del (7q) ≥3 abnormalities	—	—
Cytopenias Hg <10 g/dL Neutrophil count <1,500/μL Platelet count <100,000/μL	0 or 1 cytopenias	2 or 3 cytopenias	—	—	—

		Median survival (Yr)	
Total score	**Risk group**	**Age ≤70 yrs**	**Age ≥70 yrs**
0 = IPSS Low		>9.4	>5.8
0.5–1.0 = IPSS Intermediate 1		5.5	2.2
1.5–2.0 = IPSS Intermediate 2		1.0	1.4
2.5 = IPSS High		0.2	0.4

age, performance status, and IPSS subgroup categorization. Following are some of the therapeutic options available to patients, either through standard care or through available clinical trials.

A. Supportive therapies: treatment of anemia. Erythropoietin (EPO) increases hemoglobin levels in approximately 15% of patients; 5% to 10% of patients may have a decrease in red cell transfusion requirements. Responses usually occur within 2 to 3 months, if they are to occur. Pretreatment serum EPO concentrations are inversely correlated with probability of response.

   1. High doses of EPO (40,000 to 60,000 U weekly) may be helpful. Dosage is adjusted if the drug is effective. Response is more likely if the patient has ringed sideroblasts and serum EPO levels <500 mU/mL.

   2. The combination of EPO and G-CSF (1 μg/kg/day) may increase the response rate of the anemia, producing synergistic erythropoietic activity in patients who fail to respond to erythropoietin alone.

B. Remittive therapies

   1. Immunomodulatory agents: thalidomide, at low doses, has been shown in some trials to improve the degree of anemia and decrease red cell transfusion requirements. **Lenalidomide** (10 mg/m²/day for 21 days monthly) has also been shown to improve hemoglobin and transfusion dependence in some patients with MDS. Lenalidomide is most effective in patients with 5q deletions where 80% of patients achieve an erythroid response; transient cytogenetic responses can also be seen. Responses are less common (~40%) in patients with MDS with normal or other cytogenetic findings.

   2. DNA hypomethylating agents. A randomized phase III trial of azacitidine (75 mg/m²/day SC for 7 days every 28 days) compared with supportive care alone identified the value of azacitidine to improve blood cell counts, decrease or eliminate transfusion requirements, and improve both survival and quality of life. Decitabine produced a similar spectrum of improvement in a randomized phase III trial leading to U.S. Food and Drug Administration (FDA) approval.

3. **Immunosuppressive therapy.** Low marrow cellularity and absence of blasts increase the likelihood of response of MDS to immunosuppressive agents such as prednisone, antithymocyte globulin (ATG), and cyclosporine.

C. **Curative therapies for high-risk MDS.** Induction chemotherapy followed by allogeneic HSCT may lead to complete resolution of myelodysplasia. Although commonly believed that HSCT is the only curative option for MDS, the projected 3-year disease-free survival for patients <60 years of age is dependent on the risk category of disease. Allogeneic HSCT should only be offered in intermediate- or advanced-disease settings.

Standard chemotherapy for MDS or MDS-related AML is associated with lower response rates than in *de novo* AML. This disparity is owing to advanced age in patients with MDS, poor risk cytogenetics, and increased expression of multidrug resistance.

D. **Management of CMML** is discussed in Chapter 23, Chronic Myelomonocytic Leukemia.

Suggested Reading

Acute Leukemia

Bullinger L, Dohner K, Bair, E, et al. Use of gene-expression profiling to identify prognostic subclasses in adult acute myeloid leukemia. *N Engl J Med* 2004;350:1605.

Fielding AK, et al. Medical Research Council of the United Kingdom Adult ALL Working Party; Eastern Cooperative Oncology Group. Outcome of 609 adults after relapse of acute lymphoblastic leukemia (ALL); an MRC UKALL12/ECOG 2993 study. *Blood* 2007;109:944.

Gandhi V, Plunkett W. Clofarabine and nelarabine: two new purine nucleoside analogs. *Curr Opin Oncol* 2006;18:584.

Kottaridis PD, et al. The presence of a FLT3 internal tandem duplication in patients with acute myeloid leukemia (AML) adds important prognostic information to cytogenetic risk group and response to the first cycle of chemotherapy: analysis of 854 patients from the United Kingdom Medical Research Council AML 10 and 12 trials. *Blood* 2001;98:1752.

Larson RA, et al. A five-drug remission induction regimen with intensive consolidation for adults with acute lymphoblastic leukemia: cancer and leukemia group B study 8811. *Blood* 1995;85:2025.

Marks DI, Aversa F, Lazarus HM. Alternative donor transplants for adult acute lymphoblastic leukaemia: a comparison of the three major options. *Bone Marrow Transplant* 2006;38:467.

Oliansky DM, et al. The role of cytotoxic therapy with hematopoietic stem cell transplantation in the therapy of acute myeloid leukemia in children: an evidence-based review. *Biol Blood Marrow Transplant* 2007;13:1.

Rowe JM, et al. ECOG; MRC/NCRI Adult Leukemia Working Party. Induction therapy for adults with acute lymphoblastic leukemia: results of more than 1500 patients from the international ALL trial: MRC UKALL XII/ECOG E2993. *Blood* 2005;106:3760.

Sievers SL, et al. Efficacy and safety of gemtuzumab ozogamicin in patients with CD33-positive acute myeloid leukemia in first relapse. *J Clin Oncol* 2001;19:3244.

Stone RM. Induction and postremisson therapy: new agents. *Leukemia* 2003;17:496.

Stone RM. Novel therapeutic agents in acute myeloid leukemia [Review]. *Exp Hematol* 2007;35(4 Suppl 1):163.

Tallman MS, et al. Acute promyelocytic leukemia: evolving therapeutic strategies [review]. *Blood* 2002;99:759.

Tallman MS, et al. Clinical description of 44 patients with acute promyelocytic leukemia who developed the retinoic acid syndrome. *Blood* 2000;95:90.

Vardiman JW, et al. The World Health Organization (WHO) classification of the myeloid neoplasms. *Blood* 2002;100:2292.

Myelodysplastic Syndromes

Borthakur G, Estey AE. Therapy-related acute myelogenous leukemia and myelodysplastic syndrome. *Curr Oncol Rep* 2007;9:373.

Catenacci D V-T, Schiller GJ. Myelodysplasic syndromes: a comprehensive review. *Blood Rev* 2005;6:301.

Estey EH. Current challenges in therapy of myelodysplastic syndromes. *Curr Opin Hematol* 2003;10:60.

Greenberg P, et al. International scoring system for evaluating prognosis in myelodysplastic syndromes. *Blood* 1997;89:2079.

Kornblith AB, et al. Impact of azacytidine on the quality of life of patients with myelodysplastic syndrome treated in a randomized phase III trial: a CALGB study. *J Clin Oncol* 2002;20:2441.

Kurzrock R, et al. Pilot study of low-dose interleukin-11 in patients with bone marrow failure. *J Clin Oncol* 2001;19:4165.

Melchert M, Kale V, List A. The role of lenalidomide in the treatment of patients with chromosome 5q deletion and other myelodysplastic syndromes. *Curr Opinion Hematol* 2007;14:123.

Sanz G, Sanz M, Greenberg P. Prognostic factors and scoring systems in myelodysplastic syndromes. *Haematologica* 1998;83:358.

Web Sites

MDS Foundation Web site: www.mds-foundation.org

Aplastic Anemia–MDS Web site: www.aamds.org

Complications IV

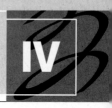

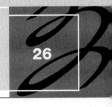

SEXUAL FUNCTION AND PREGNANCY
Eric E. Prommer

I. SEXUAL FUNCTION IN PATIENTS WITH CANCER

A. Background. Sexuality is a complex and subjective concept that changes over time as a person ages and gains experience. Sexuality as a concept can include body image (how someone sees oneself physically and perceives one's overall health and sexuality), sexual response (interest, function, and satisfaction), sexual roles, and relationships. Sexuality is a personal expression of one's self and one's relationship with others.

The effects of cancer and its treatment on sexuality are not usually included in assessments and plans of care for patients, nor are they often addressed in patient education. The disease and its treatments may cause patients to doubt their humanness and their passion for living; at the same time, their body image and their ability to express themselves sexually may become altered. Consequently, closeness, sharing, and other aspects of sexual expression may be avoided or neglected at a time in life when these experiences can be most beneficial. Factors affecting sexual function in cancer patients include the following:

1. **Psychological factors.** In the early stages of cancer diagnosis and treatment, patients may confront feelings of depression, fear of death or of treatment consequences, apprehension of functional loss, deterioration of self-esteem, or impairment of a long-lasting emotional and sexual balance with their spouse. Both patient and spouse may experience difficulties in discussing sexual relationship issues, feeling that it is not appropriate when confronting cancer. Libido is adversely affected from the initial steps of diagnosis and treatment planning, and sexually oriented thoughts and desire, if they exist, may result in feelings of guilt and further suppression of sexuality. Patients may experience fears—often unrealistic—of potential harm to themselves or their partner during sexual activity, especially when cancer treatment is ongoing. Patients must be evaluated and treated for depression.

2. **Body-image alterations.** Body-image changes for men and women are related to perceived losses and influences. The term *influences* relates to the quality of relationships before the diagnosis of cancer and the amount of control and information the patient had at the time of diagnosis. For women, losses include missing body parts (mastectomy), loss of menses, loss of sexual sensation, and, ultimately, loss of womanhood. For men, body-image changes as a result of treatment include loss of ejaculatory function, incontinence, penile deformities, and skin changes.

3. **Physical symptoms.** Uncontrolled symptoms impair all aspects of sexual function, including sexual interest and sexual desire. Fatigue, gastrointestinal symptoms (nausea, diarrhea), urinary tract symptoms, sleep disorders, and pain can alter sexual function. Surgical treatment, chemotherapy, radiation therapy, combined-modality treatment, and biologic and hormonal therapies may all exacerbate physical symptoms.

4. **Drug effects.** Chronic opioid consumption to control pain in cancer patients has been demonstrated to induce hypogonadism in men and further exacerbate depression, fatigue, and sexual ill health. In men, hypogonadism is also due to androgen-deprivation therapies or bilateral orchiectomy. Treatment of depression and anxiety in cancer patients with psychotropic drugs may further impair sexual

557

function by adverse effects on libido, erection ejaculation, and orgasmic function. Selective serotonin-reuptake inhibitors (SSRIs) also have been reported to decrease libido in up to 40% of patients. SSRIs and tricyclic antidepressants (TCAs) have been shown to impair orgasmic function; indeed, they are used in clinical practice to treat premature ejaculation.

5. **Impaired sexual response.** Even before a diagnosis of cancer, women may have problems with sexual function. More than 40% of healthy women have been reported to have one or more sexual problems, such as vaginal dryness, lack of sexual interest, dyspareunia (pain with intercourse), difficulty reaching orgasm, or lack of pleasure with sexual activity. Cancer and its treatment can compound these difficulties.

6. **Sexual roles and relationships.** Research from cancer survivors suggests that survivors who had a good sexual relationship before therapy continued to have a satisfying relationship after surgery for breast cancer. Understanding and support from the partner were critical for the survivor to be able to obtain and maintain healthy sexual roles and relationships. The partner's overall sexual health and function may also influence a survivor's sexual roles.

7. **Cultural differences.** Research from breast cancer patients suggests that culture may affect body image. There are no data on cultural effects when it comes to male sexuality and cancer.

B. **Sexual problems specific to women**

1. **Germ cell depletion** is discussed in section III. Indirect indicators of menopause are amenorrhea, increased serum follicle-stimulating hormone (FSH) and luteinizing hormone (LH) levels, and symptoms of estrogen deficiency. Symptoms include hot flashes, loss of vaginal lubrication, atrophy of genital structures, and discomfort with intercourse.

2. **Hormonal therapy for breast cancer.** Tamoxifen, which is commonly used in women with breast cancer, may have a positive estrogenic effect on the vaginal mucosa or may contribute to vaginal atrophy and dyspareunia. Patients who are taking tamoxifen often experience hot flashes or vaginal discharge. Tamoxifen does appear to have a somewhat proestrogenic effect on serum lipids and bone density. Aromatase inhibitors may have a lower incidence of estrogen deficiency symptoms compared with tamoxifen, with an as yet unknown effect on general sexual function.

3. **Chemotherapy** may cause ovarian failure (see section III.B). Emotional and physical changes can also adversely affect sexual function. The effect of chemotherapy on ovarian androgen output is unknown. Diminished androgen production affects libido.

4. **Radiation therapy (RT).** Effects of ionizing radiation on sexual function depend on age, field, and dose (see section III.A). RT for cervical cancer leads to vaginal fibrosis, dyspareunia, and ovarian failure. Symptoms may not become apparent until 1 year after treatment.

5. **Pelvic surgery**

   a. **Cervical conization** does not impair desire, arousal, or orgasm.

   b. **Radical hysterectomy** has been shown to have no negative impact on sexual satisfaction after abdominal hysterectomy, whether subtotal or total. The only predictor of negative sexual experience of partners after hysterectomy was negative sexual experience before hysterectomy. Women may need to experiment with different positions to experience comfortable penetration.

   c. **Radical cystectomy** can lead to decreased vaginal lubrication and dyspareunia. Newer techniques, such as a quality-of-life (QOL) measurements, have shown that newer surgical procedures can maintain sexual function compared with traditional techniques. These newer approaches with cystectomy involve (a) bilateral nerve-sparing (NS) surgical technique; (g) preservation of the anterior vaginal wall (to enhance lubrication) and anterior vaginal tubularization (to preserve the depth of the vagina); and (c) avoidance of routine hysterectomy.

d. Abdominal-perineal resection (APR). Sexual and bladder functions are quite often sacrificed when a conventional low anterior resection and APR with an extended lymph node dissection (LND) are performed in patients with advanced lower rectal carcinoma. These complications are due to injury of the pelvic plexus. APR commonly causes dyspareunia but orgasmic function is preserved.

The consensus is that the iatrogenic genitourinary dysfunctions are mostly caused by either a non–sphincter-sparing procedure or a non–nerve-sparing surgical approach. The practice of total mesorectal excision (TME) in rectal cancer treatment has substantially improved autonomous pelvic nerve preservation with reduction of sexual dysfunction rates.

e. Total pelvic exenteration with vaginal reconstruction results in loss of vaginal lubrication, loss of some erotic zones, dyspareunia, decreased intensity of orgasm, and the need to relearn how to achieve orgasm.

6. Mastectomy. There are consistent benefits of breast conservation or lumpectomy over mastectomy alone in preserving women's body image and comfort with sexuality. It is clear that the type of primary surgery a woman receives for her breast cancer continues to play an important role in her body image and feelings of attractiveness, with women undergoing lumpectomy experiencing more positive outcomes than women undergoing mastectomy, with or without reconstruction. Women often feel less feminine and less physically attractive after mastectomy. About one-third experience significant anxiety or depression and are unable to enjoy or tolerate making love. A similar percentage of patients' partners reported decreased sexual activity after mastectomy and fears of causing pain during intercourse. Men's reactions to seeing their partner's incision and chest wall area appear to have prognostic value: if the reaction is primarily empathic rather than negative, the prognosis for good sexual adjustment appears favorable. Women treated with lumpectomy and breast irradiation have improved self-image compared with those treated with mastectomy. Women who undergo breast reconstruction have a better body image than those who do not.

C. Sexual problems specific to men. Men treated for testicular cancer, prostate cancer, and Hodgkin lymphoma (HL) are particularly at risk for sexual dysfunction (see section II.A). Twenty percent of surviving testicular cancer patients have reported that they have been sexually inactive; many have reported decreased sense of pleasure with orgasm, anxiety, and marital unhappiness.

1. Germ-cell depletion. Clinical indicators of germ-cell depletion include decreased testicular size, severe oligospermia or azoospermia, infertility with elevated serum LH and FSH levels, and decreased testosterone level.

2. Impotence. The reported incidence of impotence in the general population is about 10%: 8% at 50 years of age, 20% at 60 years of age, and 80% at 80 years of age. The incidence of impotence in men treated for cancer is increased, particularly for men with tumors involving the pelvis and genital tract. Often, men emotionally relate impotence to a loss of masculinity, with attendant fear, anxiety, depression, and feelings of diminished self-worth.

Temporary or permanent erectile impotence is the most common symptom of sexual dysfunction in men with cancer. Recovery of erectile function is more likely in men <60 years of age and may take months to years. Pre-existing conditions, such as diabetes, cardiovascular disease, and antihypertensive medication, exacerbate the risk for erectile dysfunction. Ejaculatory dysfunction occurs less frequently and may be due to retrograde ejaculation or dry orgasm. The presence of nocturnal tumescence is helpful in differentiating nonorganic from organic causes of impotence.

3. Systemic therapy. Fatigue, nausea, alopecia, anxiety, and other general effects of chemotherapy interact to diminish libido during treatment.

a. Chemotherapy is thought to suppress Leydig cell function, resulting in decreased serum testosterone, increased serum LH levels, and resultant loss of desire and erectile function. Chemotherapeutic agents associated with neuropathy (e.g., vinca alkaloids) can cause dry orgasm with preservation of pleasurable sensation. The effect of chemotherapy on spermatogenesis is discussed in section II.C.

b. Hormonal therapy for prostate cancer can impair all phases of the sexual response cycle. Gonadotropin-releasing hormone (GnRH) agonists (e.g., leuprolide, goserelin) reduce serum testosterone to prepubertal levels and lead to loss of libido, difficulty with arousal, and diminished intensity of orgasm. Hot flashes may occur. In addition, flutamide and similar agents can cause gynecomastia.

4. RT

   a. Prostate cancer. RT can result in loss of erectile function in 20% to 80% of patients treated for prostate cancer. Younger men with intact sexual function before RT are most likely to regain adequate erectile function. Semen volume is also reduced with RT, leading to little or no ejaculatory fluid.

   b. Testicular cancer. Patients who receive radiation to the pelvis and retroperitoneum have an increased incidence of erectile dysfunction. The effects of RT on sperm count are discussed in section II.B.

   c. Testicular shielding should be used if the distance between the testes and the radiation field boundary is <30 cm. Radiation dose to the testes is reduced to <10% of the total dose if this method is used.

5. Surgery. After the recovery period from pelvic surgery itself, the desire phase generally remains intact. Orgasmic function may be normal or reduced.

   a. Radical prostatectomy causes impotence or impaired erection in most patients, although partial recovery of erectile function is possible. Parasympathetic stimulation causes tumescence; sympathetic stimulation causes detumescence. One or both of these autonomic bundles are at risk during radical prostatectomy.

   b. Nerve-sparing techniques during radical prostatectomy allow a greater percentage of men to recover erectile function (reportedly up to 85%). Closer analysis, however, has disclosed that many men do not have erections firm enough for vaginal penetration.

   c. Radical cystectomy results in erectile dysfunction and dry orgasm. With nerve-sparing procedures, up to 67% may recover erectile function.

   d. APR leads to problems with erection (55%) and dry orgasm as a result of nerve damage.

   e. Total pelvic exenteration results in permanent impotence and dry orgasm.

   f. Retroperitoneal lymph node dissection (RPLND) leads to retrograde ejaculation. With *modified* RPLND in clinical stage I nonseminomatous germ-cell tumor patients, ejaculatory function can be preserved in about 90% of cases.

D. Guidelines for treatment of sexual problems

1. Initial history should include information about the patient's sexual function before diagnosis. Patients at particular risk for dysfunction include those in relationships characterized by conflict and poor emotional adjustment, younger patients, those who want more children, and those with a history of rape or incest.

2. Brief counseling can alleviate most problems. Physicians should include the sex partner in discussions and recognize and deal with feelings and fears. In addition, clinicians should specifically tell patients that it is all right to resume sexual activity and that cancer is not contagious.

3. Refer for expert assistance if needed: occasionally, patients need the services of a sex therapist or marital counselor or a referral to a urologist. An invaluable resource is the pamphlet "Sexuality and Cancer" (separate pamphlets for women and men), available from the American Cancer Society; it can be downloaded from their Web site (www.cancer.org).

4. Control pain and treat depression.

5. For men with erectile dysfunction

   a. Oral therapy with sildenafil (Viagra), vardenafil (Levitra), and tadalafil (Cialis) is efficacious in half of patients or more regardless of the underlying cause. These drugs are contraindicated in patients taking nitrates. Efficacy improves when there is preservation of neurovascular bundles. Oral therapy is considered first-line therapy.

b. Second-line therapy involves intraurethral or intracavernosal administration of vasoactive agents such as alprostadil (MUSE).

c. Vacuum erection device (VED) provides a well-tolerated, cost-effective, non-invasive, nonmedical alternative to intracavernosal injection therapy in the population with erectile dysfunction following prostatectomy. Proper instruction and reinforcement in the use of the VED are crucial to its overall efficacy. Patient satisfaction with VED varies significantly, compared with the placement of a penile prosthesis. Penile prosthetic devices include rod implants and inflatable cylinders (pump in scrotum). Implants are usually placed via coronal incision.

d. Small studies suggest combinations of the above may be helpful.

6. For men with testicular cancer

a. Depo-Testosterone, 200 to 300 mg IM every 3 weeks, for hypotestosteronism (check serum testosterone levels)

b. Imipramine, 25 to 50 mg daily PO, may induce antegrade ejaculation in those who have undergone RPLND.

7. For women with dyspareunia and vaginal fibrosis

a. Vaginal dilators of graduated sizes can help women learn to relax voluntary muscles progressively until penetration can be achieved without pain.

b. Water-based lubricants and vaginal moisturizers can be used.

8. For women with dyspareunia and vaginal dryness. Vaginal dryness is one of the most important predictors of sexual health. Vaginal moisturizers can be used on a regular basis to decrease dryness and subsequent associated irritation. Polycarbophil-based vaginal moisturizers (such as Replens, Hill Dermaceutical, Sanford, FL) can be used. For women whose symptoms are not controlled by nonhormonal preparations, using low-dose estrogen creams or tablets applied intravaginally are options. With these agents, systemic absorption is probably minimal. Conjugated estrogens, such as Premarin in the form of vaginal creams, can be used at a very small dose of 0.3 mg (one-eighth of the applicator dose) daily for 3 weeks, followed by maintenance with the same dose administered only twice weekly. This dose is associated with a low incidence of endometrial proliferation. Estradiol vaginal tablets (Vagifem, Novo Nordisk, Princeton, NJ) are also available and have been shown to have even less systemic absorption when compared with estrogen vaginal creams.

9. Vasomotor symptoms are traditionally treated with antidepressants. This treatment is justified due to increases in monoamine oxidase activity, as well as lower serum serotonin levels compared with premenopausal women. Estrogen enhances serotoninergic transmission by decreasing the levels of monoamine oxidase, increasing the availability of free tryptophan to the brain and enhancing serotonin transport. SSRIs, such as venlafaxine (Effexor) at 75 mg/day, are recommended. One concern associated with the use of SSRIs to treat hot flashes in women with breast cancer is the interaction of these drugs with tamoxifen. There are no long-term data on survival and recurrence rates of breast cancer in women taking tamoxifen and SSRIs concomitantly

Hot flashes and vaginal dryness remain legitimate indications for hormone replacement therapy (HRT), which must be individualized and done with informed consent. The Women's Health Initiative study showed increased rates of stroke, pulmonary embolism, and breast cancer in women taking HRT.

10. For women with breast cancer

a. The dictum that estrogen replacement therapy is contraindicated is being challenged. A decision for such replacement therapy must be individualized.

b. Early discussion of the option of breast reconstruction may alleviate feelings of loss and poor self-image. A prosthesis should be fitted as soon as feasible for a normal silhouette in clothing. The Reach to Recovery program of the American Cancer Society exposes the patient to women with breast cancer who have made successful adjustments.

II. REPRODUCTIVE FUNCTION IN MEN WITH CANCER

A. Pretreatment hypogonadism in cancer patients

1. **Testicular cancer.** More than 80% of men with disseminated germ-cell tumors are oligospermic or azoospermic before therapy, probably owing to effects of the disease itself and abnormalities of the malignancy-prone testis.

2. **Hodgkin lymphoma (HL).** More than half of the men with HL have low sperm counts and poor motility before treatment.

3. **Metastatic cancer** of any type may be associated with low levels of testosterone in up to two-thirds of male patients. Malnutrition is believed to play a significant role.

B. Effects of RT in men.
The testes are exquisitely sensitive to radiation. Doses as low as 15 cGy result in transient suppression of spermatogenesis. The duration of azoospermia is proportional to the magnitude of the RT dose. At 200 to 300 cGy, recovery takes 3 years, and at 400 to 500 cGy, azoospermia can persist for 5 years. A dose of >600 cGy results in permanent sterility.

C. Effects of chemotherapy in men.
Spermatogenesis is highly susceptible to toxic effects of certain chemotherapeutic agents, depending on age and total dose per m^2, particularly when administered in combinations.

1. **Alkylating agents** cause germ-cell depletion in a dose-related fashion. Drugs reported to be definitely associated with azoospermia include chlorambucil (possibly reversible if total dose is <400 mg), cyclophosphamide (possibly reversible if total dose is <6 to 10 g), nitrogen mustard, busulfan, procarbazine, and nitrosoureas.

2. **Other drugs** probably associated with germ-cell depletion include doxorubicin, vinblastine, cytosine arabinoside, and cisplatin. Effects of methotrexate, 5-fluorouracil, 6-mercaptopurine, vincristine, and bleomycin are either unknown or unlikely to cause damage.

3. **Combination regimens.** Therapy with MOPP (nitrogen mustard, vincristine, procarbazine, and prednisone) for HL leads to testicular atrophy in 80% of patients and 100% sterility. The ABVD regimen (doxorubicin, bleomycin, vinblastine, and dacarbazine) is an alternative to MOPP, with a reported 35% occurrence of azoospermia during therapy but an eventual return of spermatogenesis in nearly 100% of cases; similar regimens based on mitoxantrone show similar results. About half of the patients treated with cisplatin, vinblastine, and bleomycin for nonseminomatous testicular cancer regain spermatogenesis within 2 to 3 years.

D. Measures to protect reproductive function in men

1. **Sperm banking** can be offered to men who are likely to suffer prolonged or permanent sterility. Between 50% and 80% of patients with HL or testicular cancer, however, have low sperm counts (<20 million/mL) with poor motility (<50%) before treatment. Sperm banking should be offered to all patients at risk for treatment-related infertility. Surveillance in lieu of chemotherapy or RT may be offered to men with good-prognosis testicular cancer, which optimizes fertility.

2. **Artificial insemination** may be tried in women whose partner's posttreatment sperm quality is good despite low sperm count.

3. **In vitro fertilization (IVF)** techniques in men with very low sperm counts can result in successful production of an embryo with relatively few sperm. In addition, IVF can be carried out before cancer therapy with cryopreservation of embryos. Intracytoplasmic sperm injection enables even apparently azoospermic men to achieve fertilization. Only a single viable sperm is needed for micropipette insertion into an ovum. Consultation with fertility specialists should be considered due to the rapidly changing knowledge and practice in this field.

4. Nerve-sparing procedures for prostatectomy, modified RPLND to reduce retrograde ejaculation, and testicular shielding for RT are discussed in sections I.C.4.c and I.C.5.b.

III. REPRODUCTIVE FUNCTION IN WOMEN WITH CANCER

A. Effects of RT in women.
The effects of radiation on fertility are strongly influenced by age as well as by RT field and total dose. Cessation of menses for variable periods

of time occurs at doses >150 cGy. A dose of 500 to 600 cGy to the ovaries usually results in permanent ovarian failure. After total nodal irradiation, 70% of women <20 years of age resume normal menses, whereas 80% of women >30 years of age do not.

Oophoropexy, or sequestering the ovaries surgically in midline behind the uterus, reduces the risk for infertility in half of women undergoing inverted-Y field irradiation. Sparing one ovary in women <40 years of age prevents premature menopause.

B. Effects of chemotherapy in women. The likelihood of permanent ovarian failure after chemotherapy increases with age. Menses rarely return after age 35 to 40 years. Use of GnRH agonists before and during chemotherapy may prove useful in preventing premature ovarian failure.

1. Alkylating agents. Cyclophosphamide, nitrogen mustard, Alkeran, busulfan, and procarbazine are clearly associated with ovarian failure.

2. Other drugs. Methotrexate, 5-fluorouracil, and 6-mercaptopurine are unlikely to cause ovarian dysfunction. Agents with unknown effects on the ovary include doxorubicin, bleomycin, vinca alkaloids, cisplatin, nitrosoureas, cytosine arabinoside, etoposide, vinorelbine, paclitaxel, and interferon.

3. Combination regimens. MOPP leads to ovarian dysfunction in 40% to 50% of women treated for HL. Nearly all patients <25 years of age experience a return of normal menses, but these patients may experience very early menopause (before 30 years of age). ABVD is associated with a much lower incidence of infertility than is MOPP.

Ten years after receiving combination regimens for malignant ovarian germ-cell tumors (with drugs including cisplatin, vincristine, doxorubicin, etoposide, dactinomycin, bleomycin, methotrexate, and cyclophosphamide), two-thirds of women aged 14 to 40 years had regular menses, whereas about 10% had amenorrhea or premature ovarian failure.

IV. PREGNANCY AND CANCER
A. Background

1. Incidence. Cervical cancer is the most common malignancy complicating pregnancy, occurring in 1 in 1,000 pregnancies, followed by breast cancer (1 in 3,000), melanoma and ovarian cancer (1 in 10,000), and colon cancer, leukemia, and lymphoma (1 in 50,000 to 1 in 100,000).

2. Natural history. The incidence of malignancy is not increased in pregnancy. Pregnancy neither alters the biological behavior or prognosis of cancer nor reactivates cancer in remission. Metastasis to the placenta or fetus is very rare but can occur with malignant melanoma.

3. Teratogenesis. The definition of *teratogenesis* has been broadened to encompass not merely morphological abnormalities readily apparent at birth but also other types of malformation, growth retardation, fetal death, and developmental disability. The incidence of major malformations apparent at birth in the general population is about 3% to 4%. Damage from chemotherapeutic agents in the first trimester is more likely to cause morphological abnormalities and spontaneous abortion. Exposure during the second and third trimesters is more likely to cause intrauterine growth retardation, microcephaly, and developmental delay with attendant risks for mental retardation and learning problems.

B. Diagnostic studies during pregnancy

1. Biopsies under local anesthesia carry essentially no risk to the fetus. Biopsy procedures using general anesthesia present minimal risk to the fetus.

2. Studies to avoid: radionuclide scans, contrast studies of the gastrointestinal and urinary tracts, abdominal and chest CT scans, and pelvic and lumbosacral spine films. Studies should only be done if results would have a significant effect on treatment decisions.

3. Mammograms lack sensitivity in pregnancy because of breast engorgement and histological changes. Up to half of pregnant women with a breast mass have a negative mammogram.

4. **Chest radiographs** can be done safely with proper abdominal shielding. The dose of ionizing radiation to the fetus is about 0.008 cGy.
5. **Bone scans** are relatively contraindicated in pregnancy. The fetus receives a dose of about 0.1 cGy. Because of low yield, bone scans are not justified in asymptomatic stage I and II breast cancer patients and can be deferred until postpartum. MRI is preferred in place of bone scans.
6. **Ultrasonography** does not involve ionizing radiation and is safe.
7. **Other permissible radiological studies.** Brain CT scans and radiographs of the cervical spine or long bones are probably associated with radiation doses to the fetus of <0.5 cGy if the abdomen and uterus are properly shielded.
8. **MRI.** Although no risks to the fetus from MRI have been demonstrated, first-trimester use should be avoided if possible. MRI has proven useful in pregnancy as an alternative to ionizing radiation in many instances, including studies of the brain, liver, and skeleton, and in staging cervical cancer.
9. **Sentinel node imaging** can safely be performed as the ^{99m}Tc dose to the fetus is negligible.

C. **Principles of cancer therapy during pregnancy**
1. Pregnancy prevention should be emphasized in all women of childbearing age with cancer and in the context of the patient's personal goals. All options, including pregnancy termination, should be discussed.
2. Accurate determination of gestational age should be made before commencing diagnostic studies or therapy.
3. When maternal cure is possible and delay would compromise this goal, therapy should be instituted as soon as possible. If feasible, chemotherapy should be delayed until the second or third trimester or after delivery.
4. Therapeutic abortion (TAB) may be performed up to the 24th week of gestation. TAB should be offered to the patient if her fetus has received a dose of ionizing radiation in excess of 10 cGy during the first trimester.
5. Breast-feeding is usually contraindicated because chemotherapeutic agents are excreted into human milk and have caused neutropenia in infants.

D. **Surgery during pregnancy.** Surgical treatment is far less likely to affect pregnancy adversely than is chemotherapy or RT. General anesthesia is an uncommon cause of teratogenesis. The fetus is exquisitely sensitive to hypoxia; the anesthesiologist and surgeon must take special precautions to ensure adequate oxygenation.

E. **RT during pregnancy**
1. A dose of 10 cGy to the fetus during the first trimester carries a substantial risk for fetal damage. No increase in the incidence of spontaneous abortion, growth retardation, or congenital malformations has been noted when the dose of radiation is <5 cGy at any time during pregnancy.
2. Defects most commonly seen with radiation damage include microcephaly, growth retardation, and ocular abnormalities. Late effects of radiation in early pregnancy include an increased incidence of thyroid cancer and leukemia.

F. **Chemotherapy during pregnancy**
1. **Pharmacokinetics.** Absorption, distribution, and metabolism of chemotherapeutic agents are undoubtedly altered by the multiplicity of physiological changes accompanying pregnancy. Because the effects of pregnancy on pharmacokinetics are unknown, standard drug dosages are used. It can be assumed that most antineoplastic drugs cross the placenta.
2. **First-trimester exposure.** When folic acid antagonists and concomitant RT are excluded, single agents lead to congenital defects in 6% of infants exposed in the first trimester.
   a. **Antimetabolites.** Folic acid antagonists are the agents most frequently associated with teratogenesis and should not be used in the first trimester. Methotrexate is an abortifacient and is teratogenic. Methotrexate has caused facial anomalies, bone and limb deformities, and variable intellectual impairment (aminopterin syndrome). Although other antimetabolites, including cytarabine and 5-fluorouracil, have been associated with fetal malformation, 6-mercaptopurine has not.

b. Alkylating agents are less frequently associated with fetal malformation than are antimetabolites. A 14% overall occurrence rate has been reported in one series; cyclophosphamide was associated with congenital defects in three of seven exposed infants.

c. Vinca alkaloids. Vinblastine resulted in malformation in 1 of 14 exposed infants. No data are available for vincristine.

d. Others. Procarbazine is associated with fetal malformation. Diethylstilbestrol (DES) has been linked to clear-cell vaginal cancer in offspring.

e. Combination chemotherapy regimens are associated with a 25% rate of fetal malformation. MOPP was linked to congenital defects in four of seven exposed infants.

3. Second- and third-trimester exposure. Forty percent of fetuses exposed to a variety of antineoplastic agents in the second and third trimesters have exhibited low birth weight, with its attendant risk for developmental delay. Other potential adverse effects include prematurity, spontaneous abortion, and major organ toxicity.

G. Recommendations concerning therapeutic abortion (TAB)

1. TAB not recommended

a. Treatment does not jeopardize the pregnancy (e.g., surgery for breast cancer)

b. Refractory malignancies for which treatment has no significant impact

2. TAB considered, but not strongly recommended

a. Treatment may be delayed with reasonable safety until fetal maturity allows delivery.

b. Treatment may be delayed into the second or third trimester, when the fetus is relatively resistant to the effects of chemotherapy (e.g., acute leukemia) or RT.

3. TAB strongly recommended

a. Cancers in which curative therapy cannot be delayed or accomplished during pregnancy (e.g., most gynecologic malignancies).

b. Treatment that is likely to cause abortion or fetal malformation is required in the first trimester (e.g., MOPP, methotrexate, pelvic RT).

V. MANAGEMENT OF SPECIFIC CANCERS AND PREGNANCY

A. Cervical cancer

1. Screening. Papanicolaou (Pap) smears should be done on all prenatal patients.

2. Evaluation of cervical dysplasia. Colposcopy can be done. Endocervical curettage biopsy is contraindicated. In the absence of invasive disease, there is no urgency to treat cervical dysplasia during pregnancy. Cervical conization should be avoided, but it may need to be done to exclude invasive disease. In pregnancy, conization is associated with cervical hemorrhage and a high incidence of incomplete resection.

3. Staging and treatment. The extent of invasive disease is often underestimated because of limitations of physical examination and diagnostic procedures. Treatment of invasive cervical cancer, using either surgery or RT, is incompatible with fetal survival. Consideration may be given to expectant management of early-stage cervical cancer (stage IA with <3 mm invasion) until delivery. Radical trachelectomy may be considered for early-stage cervical cancer to preserve future reproductive function.

B. Breast cancer

1. Screening. A delay in diagnosis of 5 months or more has been observed in gravid patients with breast cancer, resulting in node-positive disease in 74% of patients, as compared with 37% in nonpregnant patients. Physiological changes in the breasts during pregnancy hamper adequate physical examination. Serial breast examinations should be done throughout pregnancy, and masses should be investigated promptly. Clinicians have tended to observe breast masses 2 months longer in pregnant than in nonpregnant patients.

2. Diagnosis. Mammograms are not helpful during pregnancy. Fine-needle aspiration may be inaccurate, and excisional biopsy is the procedure of choice. Estrogen and progesterone receptor studies may be falsely negative or difficult to interpret.

3. **Treatment.** Modified radical mastectomy is the procedure of choice. Lumpectomy with radiation results in unacceptable radiation exposure to the fetus. Tamoxifen is contraindicated during gestation. Adjuvant chemotherapy should be delayed until at least the second or third trimester, or, if possible, until after delivery.

C. **Hodgkin lymphoma**
   1. Limit staging procedures that may expose the fetus to radiation.
   2. If the disease is diagnosed during the first trimester, either perform a TAB and proceed as usual or delay chemotherapy or RT until later in the pregnancy.
   3. If the disease is diagnosed during the second or third trimester:
      a. Try to delay therapy until delivery if the mother's outcome will not be adversely affected.
      b. If therapy is necessary, proceed with proper counseling regarding possible growth and developmental abnormalities.
      c. Very-limited-field RT has been largely successful. Internal scatter from standard mantle field RT can result in fetal exposure of 50 to 250 cGy.

D. **Non-Hodgkin lymphoma** is generally a more virulent disease and poses a greater risk to the mother and secondarily to the fetus than does HL. Therapeutic recommendations parallel HL, except for the possibility of protracted delay of treatment with indolent lymphomas.

E. **Genetic counseling.** Retrospective studies and case reports of patients who were treated for malignancy in childhood or adolescence and bore children later show a 4% rate of major malformations in offspring. This rate is similar to the risk borne by the general population. The late effects of cancer treatment on infants exposed *in utero* are unknown. Female survivors of cancer who later become pregnant, particularly those who have had abdominal radiation, have an increased rate of preterm delivery and low-birth-weight infants.

Suggested Reading

Boice JD, Miller RW. Childhood and adult cancer after intrauterine exposure to ionizing radiation. *Teratology* 1999;59:227.

Incrocci L, Slob AK, Levendag PC. Sexual dysfunction after radiotherapy for prostate cancer: a review. *Int J Radiat Oncol* 2002;52:681.

Kendirci M, Bejma J, Hellstrom WJ. Update on erectile dysfunction in prostate cancer patients. *Curr Opin Urol* 2006;16(3):186.

Kuczyk M, et al. Sexual function and fertility after treatment of testicular cancer. *Curr Opin Urol* 2000;10:473.

Nguyen C, Montz FJ, Bristow RE. Management of stage I cervical cancer in pregnancy. *Obstet Gynecol Surv* 2000;56:633.

Nicklas AH, Baker ME. Imaging strategies in the pregnant cancer patient. *Semin Oncol* 2000;27:623.

Partridge AH, Garber JE. Long-term outcomes of children exposed to antineoplastic agents in utero. *Semin Oncol* 2000;27:712.

Pelusi J. Sexuality and body image. *Cancer Nurs* 2006;29(2 Suppl):32.

Salonia A, Briganti A, Deho F, et al. Women's sexual dysfunction: a review of the "surgical landscape." *Eur Urol* 2006;50(1):44.

Schover LR. Counseling cancer patients about changes in sexual function. *Oncology* 1999;13:1585.

Tal R, Mulhall JP. Sexual health issues in men with cancer. *Oncology (Williston Park)* 2006;20(3):294.

Thaler-DeMers D. Intimacy issues: sexuality, fertility, and relationships. *Semin Oncol Nurs* 2001;17(4):255.

Zippe CD, et al. Management of erectile dysfunction following radical prostatectomy. *Curr Urol Rep* 2001;2:495.

Web Sites

Fertile Hope: Fertility resources for cancer patients. www.fertilehope.org
Lance Armstrong Foundation. www.laf.org

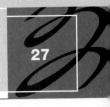

I. HYPERCALCEMIA

A. Mechanisms. Cancer is the most common cause of hypercalcemia in hospitalized patients. Hypercalcemia usually results from excessive bone resorption relative to bone formation.

1. **Bone metastases.** Most tumors capable of bone metastasis (see Chapter 33, section I) can also produce hypercalcemia. Local production of various substances by tumor cells may stimulate osteoclastic bone resorption.

2. **Ectopic parathyroid hormone** (PTH) secretion appears to be rare.

3. **Humoral hypercalcemia of malignancy** is caused by production of a PTH-like substance called PTH-related peptide (PTH-RP) by a variety of carcinomas (squamous tumors of many organs, hypernephroma, parotid gland tumors). PTH-RP has bone-resorbing activity and interacts with the renal PTH receptor to stimulate renal calcium resorption. PTH-RP is not measured in serum PTH assays.

4. **Vitamin D metabolites** (e.g., 1,25-dihydroxyvitamin D) may be produced by some lymphomas; these metabolites promote intestinal calcium absorption.

5. **Prostaglandins and interleukin-1** produced by various tumors may occasionally cause hypercalcemia, perhaps by enhancing bone resorption.

6. **Tumors** rarely or never associated with hypercalcemia despite high frequencies of bone metastases:
   a. Small cell lung cancer
   b. Prostate cancer
   c. Colorectal cancer

B. Diagnosis

1. **Symptoms of hypercalcemia** depend both on the serum level of ionized calcium and on how fast the level rises. Rapidly rising serum calcium levels tend to produce obtundation and coma with only moderately elevated serum calcium levels (e.g., 13 mg/dL). Slowly rising serum calcium levels may produce only mild symptoms, even with serum levels exceeding 15 mg/dL.
   a. **Early symptoms**
      (1) Polyuria, nocturia, polydipsia
      (2) Anorexia
      (3) Easy fatigability
      (4) Weakness
   b. **Late symptoms**
      (1) Apathy, irritability, depression, decreased ability to concentrate, mental obtundation, coma
      (2) Profound muscle weakness
      (3) Nausea, vomiting, vague abdominal pain, constipation, obstipation
      (4) Pruritus
      (5) Abnormalities of vision

2. **Differential diagnosis of hypercalcemia.** Idiopathic hypercalcemia is not a tenable diagnosis in adult patients. More and more often, benign causes of hypercalcemia are recognized to occur in patients with cancer. The possible etiologies of hypercalcemia include the following:

a. Malignancy
  (1) Metastases to bone
  (2) Secretion of PTH-like or other humoral factors
  (3) Production of vitamin D metabolites
b. Primary hyperparathyroidism
c. Thiazide diuretic therapy
d. Vitamin D or vitamin A intoxication
e. Milk–alkali syndrome
f. Familial benign hypocalciuric hypercalcemia
g. Others
  (1) Immobilization of patients with accelerated bone turnover (e.g., Paget disease or myeloma)
  (2) Sarcoidosis, tuberculosis, and other granulomatous diseases
  (3) Hyperthyroidism
  (4) Lithium administration
  (5) Adrenal insufficiency
  (6) Diuretic phase of acute renal failure
  (7) Severe liver disease
  (8) Theophylline intoxication
3. Laboratory studies. All patients with cancer and polyuria, mental status changes, or gastrointestinal symptoms should be evaluated for hypercalcemia.
  a. Routine studies
    (1) Serum calcium, phosphate, and albumin levels
      (a) Ionized calcium constitutes about 47% of the serum calcium and is in equilibrium with calcium bound to proteins, especially to albumin. Roughly 0.8 mg of calcium is bound by 1 g of serum albumin. An alkaline pH (e.g., resulting from repeated vomiting because of hypercalcemia) tends to decrease the fraction of ionized calcium. When serum albumin is low, the measured serum calcium can be corrected (to a normal albumin concentration of 4 g/dL) using the following formula:

$$\text{Corrected serum calcium (mg/dL)} = \text{measured calcium} + 0.8(4.0 - \text{measured albumin})$$

      (b) Long-standing hypercalcemia with hypophosphatemia suggests primary hyperparathyroidism.
    (2) Serum alkaline phosphatase. Elevated levels may be due to either hyperparathyroidism or metastatic disease to the bone or liver. Normal levels are typical in cases of hypercalcemia produced by myeloma.
    (3) Serum electrolytes. Serum chloride concentrations are frequently elevated in primary hyperparathyroidism. Renal tubular acidosis may complicate chronic hypercalcemia.
    (4) Blood urea nitrogen (BUN) and serum creatinine. The direct effect of hypercalcemia on the kidneys can result in azotemia and defective renal tubular water conservation (i.e., symptoms of polyuria) leading to dehydration.
    (5) Electrocardiogram (ECG). Hypercalcemia results in relative shortening of the Q-T interval and prolongation of the P-R interval. The T wave widens at blood levels above 16 mg/dL, paradoxically lengthening the Q-T interval.
    (6) Radiographs of the abdomen and bones
      (a) Nephrolithiasis is rare in hypercalcemia caused by malignancy and suggests hyperparathyroidism.
      (b) Nephrocalcinosis and other ectopic calcifications are common in long-standing hypercalcemia.
      (c) Subperiosteal reabsorption is pathognomonic of hyperparathyroidism, but osteopenia is the most common radiologic finding.
  b. Further studies. Results from preliminary evaluation may indicate the need for measuring serum PTH levels or for performing other tests.

(1) Evidence for concomitant primary hyperparathyroidism

(a) Documented long history of hypercalcemia or renal stones

(b) Radiographic evidence of hyperparathyroid bone disease (subperiosteal reabsorption, osteitis fibrosa cystica, or salt-and-pepper skull)

(c) Hyperchloremic acidosis, particularly with a serum chloride-to-phosphate ratio ≥ 34

(d) Elevated serum PTH level in the presence of hypercalcemia

(e) Absence of hypocalciuria; if the ratio of calcium clearance to creatinine clearance in a 24-hour urine specimen is < 0.01, the patient probably has familial hypocalciuric hypercalcemia, which can otherwise mimic primary hyperparathyroidism.

(2) Evidence for humoral hypercalcemia of malignancy

(a) Low or low-normal serum PTH levels in the presence of hypercalcemia

(b) Elevated level of PTH-RP

(c) Metabolic alkalosis

(d) Low serum level of 1,25-dihydroxyvitamin D

4. When should neck surgery for primary hyperparathyroidism be considered? Both primary hyperparathyroidism and humoral hypercalcemia of malignancy are characterized by hypercalcemia and, with many cancers, elevated urinary excretion of cyclic adenosine monophosphate. *Parathyroid surgery is justified if all of the following apply:*

a. Clinical and laboratory findings (see earlier) suggest hyperparathyroidism.

b. The malignancy is under control and the patient's expected survival is reasonably long.

c. The general condition of the patient makes the surgical risk acceptable.

d. The hypercalcemia is severe enough to warrant treatment. Mild hypercalcemia (e.g., ≤ 11.5 mg/dL) caused by primary hyperparathyroidism may remain stable and asymptomatic for many years and may never produce clinically significant complications during the patient's remaining life span.

e. Parathyroid scanning with technetium-99m sestamibi or neck sonography demonstrates a probable parathyroid adenoma. Neck exploration may also be undertaken in patients with negative radiologic studies but convincing biochemical findings of primary hyperparathyroidism; however, in such cases one must carefully weigh the possible benefits of surgery against the possibility of greater surgical morbidity and resultant chronic hypocalcemia.

C. Management

1. Acute, symptomatic hypercalcemia should be treated as an emergency.

a. Hydration and saline diuresis. Achieving and maintaining normal intravascular volume and hydration are the cornerstones of promoting calcium excretion. Normal saline containing potassium chloride (KCl; 10 mEq/L) is given at a dosage of 2 to 3 L per day IV. Calciuresis may be enhanced by administering furosemide, 40 to 80 mg IV given twice daily, but only after fluid and volume deficits have been corrected.

(1) Fluid intake and output and body weight are carefully monitored. Patients are evaluated for evidence of congestive heart failure 2 or 3 times daily. Patients with a history of congestive heart failure or renal insufficiency should be monitored with central venous pressure (CVP) measurements.

(2) Blood levels of calcium, potassium, and magnesium are measured every 8 to 12 hours, and concentrations of cations in the IV solutions are adjusted.

(3) Treatment is continued until the blood calcium concentration is below 12 mg/dL. Central nervous system manifestations in elderly or comatose patients may not improve until normal blood calcium levels are maintained for several days.

(4) More vigorous administration of fluids (e.g., 12 to 14 L over 24 hours) and diuretics (e.g., every 1 to 2 hours) requires excellent cardiac and renal function and necessitates close monitoring in an intensive care unit. Treatment at this intensity is rarely necessary for patients with malignancies.

b. Bisphosphonates are potent inhibitors of osteoclast activity and are effective in the treatment of hypercalcemia of malignancy. These drugs are relatively free of significant adverse effects. Zoledronate (Zometa) is the most effective of the available drugs; it is given as a single IV infusion of 4 mg in 100 mL of normal saline over 15 minutes. Pamidronate (Aredia) is slightly less effective; it is given as a single IV infusion of 60 to 90 mg in 250 to 500 mL of normal saline over 2 to 4 hours. With either drug, significant reductions in serum calcium occur in 1 to 2 days and generally persist for several weeks. Common side effects of both drugs include fever, nausea, and constipation; both drugs may also cause hypocalcemia, hypophosphatemia, and increased serum creatinine. Patients should be well hydrated both before and after administration of IV bisphosphonates. Doses may be repeated every 7 to 30 days.

A recently recognized adverse effect of bisphosphonates is osteonecrosis of the jaw. In this condition, patients typically develop a painful area of exposed, necrotic bone, usually on the medial aspect of the mandible. The majority of cases have occurred after repeated IV administration of potent bisphosphonates for malignancy, and may be precipitated by dental surgery; poor oral hygiene may also play a role. Although prospective data are lacking, some authorities have recommended that patients about to begin IV bisphosphonate therapy have routine dental care performed before treatment starts and biannually thereafter; patients who have already received >3 months of drug therapy have been cautioned to avoid or postpone extensive dental surgery, if possible. Treatment of osteonecrosis of the jaw usually consists of antibiotics and oral rinses; it is not yet clear if discontinuation of bisphosphonates is beneficial.

c. Gallium nitrate (Ganite), a potent inhibitor of bone resorption, is given intravenously in a dose of 200 mg/m^2 daily for 5 days. Serum calcium levels fall within a few days and remain normal for about 1 week. Renal function may worsen during gallium nitrate therapy, and the drug should not be given if the serum creatinine level is higher than 2.5 mg/dL.

d. Mithramycin (plicamycin). Patients who have congestive heart failure, fluid overload, or unresponding calcium levels during saline diuresis can be treated with mithramycin. The drug inhibits bone resorption by reversibly poisoning osteoclasts. Mithramycin, 25 mcg/kg, is given by rapid infusion into a well-established IV line; serum calcium levels are lowered in 24 to 48 hours. The dose may be repeated every 3 to 4 days. Hypocalcemia is averted by measuring blood calcium levels every 1 or 2 days or when mental status changes or tetany develops. Other important toxicities of mithramycin are discussed in Chapter 4, section III.I. The drug is contraindicated in the presence of severe thrombocytopenia or severe hepatocellular dysfunction. In patients with renal failure, mithramycin may be given in lower doses (10 mcg/kg), but calcitonin is preferred in these cases.

e. Calcitonin is useful for rapid reduction of blood calcium levels. Calcitonin can be given when bisphosphonates, mithramycin, or saline diuresis are contraindicated or ineffective (e.g., in severe thrombocytopenia, renal failure, congestive heart failure). The drug inhibits bone resorption and increases renal calcium clearance. Blood calcium levels are decreased within 2 to 3 hours of administration. The effect is transient but may be prolonged to 4 or more days by concurrent administration of prednisone, 10 to 20 mg given 3 times daily. Allergy is the only important complication of therapy. Synthetic salmon calcitonin is given in a dose of 3 U/kg (Medical Research Council Units) as a 24-hour infusion, or 100 to 400 units given SC every 8 to 12 hours.

f. Dialysis. Peritoneal dialysis and hemodialysis rapidly lower blood calcium levels but are rarely used.

g. **Dangerous therapies** that have little clinical usefulness and are not recommended:

(1) Intravenous phosphates (extraosseous calcification)

(2) Intravenous sodium sulfate (hypernatremia, heart failure)

(3) Calcium chelating agents (severe renal damage)

2. **Chronic hypercalcemia.** Ambulation is encouraged to minimize bone resorption that accompanies immobilization. Liberal fluid intake (2 to 3 L/day) is prescribed. Foods containing large amounts of calcium, such as milk products, are avoided. Thiazide diuretics aggravate hypercalcemia and should not be taken.

a. **Glucocorticoids.** Prednisone, 20 to 40 mg PO daily, or hydrocortisone, 100 to 150 mg IV every 12 hours, may be used for patients with tumors that are sensitive to glucocorticoids (e.g., lymphoma, multiple myeloma).

b. **Bisphosphonates.** Zoledronate (4 mg IV) or pamidronate (60 to 90 mg IV) may be given every 7 to 30 days as needed to control hypercalcemia (see section I.C.1).

c. **Phosphates** given orally lower blood levels by binding calcium in the gut. Because this may compromise renal function, effects of therapy should be monitored. Diarrhea nearly always accompanies phosphate therapy and is treated with diphenoxylate (Lomotil), 2 to 5 mg PO, with each dose of phosphate. Diarrhea may also be reduced by diluting the liquid or powder forms. The daily dose is 1 to 6 g of phosphate. *One gram of inorganic phosphate* is supplied by the following preparations:

(1) Fleet Phospho-soda, liquid, 6.7 mL

(2) Neutra-Phos, four capsules or 1 teaspoon of powder (Neutra-Phos-K contains no sodium)

(3) K-Phos Original Formula, six tablets (contains no sodium)

d. **Prostaglandin inhibitors,** such as aspirin and indomethacin, produce variable and inconsistent lowering of calcium levels but may be tried in patients with refractory hypercalcemia.

II. HYPOCALCEMIA

A. Mechanisms

1. **Paraneoplasia.** Hypocalcemia is an extremely rare paraneoplastic syndrome.

a. **Rapid uptake of calcium.** Patients with osteoblastic bone metastases may occasionally develop hypocalcemia due to uptake of calcium in the bone lesions. In addition, patients with bone metastases from prostate or breast cancer who are treated with hormonal agents may develop hypocalcemia, supposedly because of rapid bone healing. Calcifying chondrosarcoma is a rare tumor that has been associated with hypocalcemia.

b. **Calcitonin** production by medullary carcinoma of the thyroid rarely causes hypocalcemia.

2. **Magnesium deficiency.** Magnesium is necessary both for the release of PTH and for its peripheral action. Hypomagnesemia results in hypocalcemia that does not respond to calcium replacement therapy. Magnesium deficiency occurs in the following circumstances:

a. Patients who have prolonged nasogastric drainage

b. Patients who receive parenteral hyperalimentation without magnesium replacement

c. Cisplatin therapy–induced renal tubular dysfunction with urinary magnesium loss

d. Chronic diuretic therapy or diuresis due to glycosuria

e. Chronic alcoholism (alcohol interferes with renal conservation of magnesium)

f. Chronic diarrhea

3. **Other causes of hypocalcemia**

a. Therapy for hypercalcemia, especially if using mithramycin or IV bisphosphonates

    b. Hypoalbuminemia
    c. Hyperphosphatemia (see section III)
    d. Pancreatitis
    e. Renal disease
    f. Hypoparathyroidism
    g. Pseudohypoparathyroidism
    h. Rickets and osteomalacia
    i. Sepsis

B. Diagnosis

  1. Symptoms and signs are aggravated by hyperventilation or other causes of alkalosis.

    a. Tetany is the most prominent symptom of hypocalcemia and is manifested by paresthesias (especially numbness and tingling of the face, hands, and feet), muscle cramps, laryngospasm, or seizures. Other problems include diarrhea, headache, lethargy, irritability, and loss of recent memory. Chronic hypocalcemia may be well tolerated, however, with few symptoms.

    b. Dry skin, abnormal nails, cataracts, and papilledema may develop in long-standing cases.

    c. Chvostek's sign: twitching of muscles around the mouth, nose, or eyes after tapping the facial nerve.

    d. Trousseau's sign: spasm of the hand during 3 to 4 minutes of exercise while a blood pressure cuff on the arm is inflated midway between systolic and diastolic pressures.

  2. Routine laboratory studies. Serum levels of calcium, phosphate, magnesium, electrolytes, BUN, creatinine, and albumin should be obtained. The ECG may show a prolonged Q-T interval; the ECG is monitored during therapy.

  3. Differential diagnosis of hypocalcemia

    a. Severe alkalosis resulting from prolonged nasogastric suction, vomiting, or hyperventilation

    b. Severe muscle cramps resulting from vincristine or procarbazine therapy

C. Management

  1. Severe, acute, symptomatic hypocalcemia (blood calcium $\leq$6 mg/dL) is generally managed in an intensive care setting.

    a. Calcium gluconate or calcium chloride, 1 g by rapid IV injection is given every 15 to 20 minutes as long as tetany persists.

    b. Magnesium sulfate, 1 g IV or IM every 8 to 12 hours is also administered if the blood magnesium level is unknown or <1.5 mg/dL until the calcium or magnesium blood levels have normalized.

    c. Hyperventilating patients should breathe into a paper bag to decrease respiratory alkalosis.

    d. Serum calcium levels are obtained every 1 to 2 hours until the serum calcium level exceeds 7 mg/dL.

  2. Moderate hypocalcemia (blood calcium between 7 and 8 mg/dL)

    a. Calcium may be given either PO or, if the patient is severely symptomatic, IV.

      (1) Calcium carbonate, 2.5 g/day, or calcium citrate, 4 to 5 g/day PO; either form will provide about 1,000 mg of elemental calcium daily.

      (2) Calcium gluconate, 2 g IV in 500 mL of 5% dextrose in water, is given every 8 hours.

    b. Hypomagnesemia (<1.5 mg/dL) is treated with magnesium sulfate, 1 g IM or IV once or twice daily, until the blood level is normal.

    c. Patients recovering from hypercalcemia who were treated with IV bisphosphonates or mithramycin are in jeopardy of recurrent life-threatening hypocalcemia for as long as 4 days after treatment is stopped.

    d. Patients with postthyroidectomy hypoparathyroidism are discussed in Chapter 15, section III.F.1.a.

III. HYPERPHOSPHATEMIA

A. Mechanisms. Hyperphosphatemia (>4.5 mg/dL) is a rare complication of treatment of certain tumors, notably leukemia and lymphoma (especially Burkitt lymphoma). Rapid tumor lysis releases large amounts of potassium, phosphate, and nucleic acids (which are metabolized to uric acid). Elevated blood phosphate levels may not be observed until 2 days after beginning tumor therapy; elevations may persist for 4 to 5 days and can exceed 20 mg/dL.

B. Diagnosis. The serum phosphate level itself does not cause symptoms. Renal damage or acute renal failure results from precipitation of calcium phosphate in the kidneys. Tetany and seizures may develop if the ionized calcium concentration becomes inordinately reduced (e.g., with alkalosis from bicarbonate administration or vomiting).

1. Laboratory studies. Serum phosphate, calcium, and other electrolyte levels should be measured regularly in susceptible patients during the initial course of antitumor therapy.

2. Differential diagnosis
   a. Hypoparathyroidism
   b. Renal failure
   c. Rapid tissue breakdown after muscle trauma or burn
   d. Tumor lysis syndrome (see section XIII)
   e. Large oral or rectal doses of phosphates

C. Management. High phosphate levels must be lowered rapidly to avoid or reverse renal damage. Serum chemistries are monitored every 4 to 6 hours. The following methods are used *simultaneously* until the phosphate concentration reaches 5 mg/dL:

1. An IV infusion of 20% dextrose containing 10 U/L of regular insulin is administered at a rate of 50 to 100 mL/hour until the blood phosphate level falls below 7 mg/dL. The extracellular volume is expanded by infusing half-normal saline at 100 to 200 mL/hour. Potassium is added to the solution if the serum level is <4 mEq/L.

2. An aluminum hydroxide gel preparation (e.g., Amphojel), 30 to 60 mL PO, every 2 to 6 hours, is given to bind phosphate in the intestine.

3. Oral fluids are given at a rate of 2 to 4 L every 24 hours.

4. Dialysis may be necessary for patients with renal failure.

IV. HYPOPHOSPHATEMIA

A. Mechanism. Hypophosphatemia (<3 mg/dL) is occasionally associated with rapidly growing tumors (such as acute leukemia), presumably because tumor cells consume phosphate. Severe hypophosphatemia (<1 mg/dL) may result in rhabdomyolysis or hemolysis. Hypokalemia may be associated with hypophosphatemia, the reasons for which are unclear. In patients with cancer, hypophosphatemia more commonly accompanies marked nutritional deprivation or cachexia.

B. Diagnosis

1. Laboratory studies. Hypophosphatemia is usually recognized by routine serum electrolyte studies in patients with nutritional disturbances.

2. Differential diagnosis of hypophosphatemia
   a. Renal phosphate wasting accompanies certain syndromes associated with malignancies, including myeloma (Fanconi syndrome), multiple endocrine neoplasia (hyperparathyroidism), and oncogenic osteomalacia (see later discussion)
   b. Therapy with phosphate-binding antacids or other phosphate binders
   c. Starvation or malabsorption (decreased phosphate intake)
   d. Cachexia
   e. Alcoholism
   f. Nutritional recovery (e.g., during hyperalimentation) without adequate phosphate supplementation
   g. Massive, rapid tumor growth
   h. Alkalosis

i. Treatment of diabetic ketoacidosis

j. Use of IV bisphosphonates

k. Use of imatinib mesylate

l. Oncogenic osteomalacia appears to be caused by tumor products that interfere with the production of 1,25-dihydroxycholecalciferol and promote phosphaturia. This entity has been associated with mesenchymal neoplasms (usually benign) and prostate cancer. Oncogenic osteomalacia is characterized by hypophosphatemia, usually normocalcemia, elevated serum alkaline phosphatase, and decreased serum 1,25-dihydroxycholecalciferol.

C. Management

1. Patients with phosphate levels <1 mg/dL are given 30 to 40 mmol/L of neutral sodium phosphate or sodium potassium phosphate administered IV at a rate of 50 to 150 mL/hour. Doses and precautions are about the same as for IV potassium preparations.

2. Patients with blood phosphorus levels of 1 to 2 mg/dL may be given oral inorganic phosphate supplements (see section I.C.2.c). One bottle of Neutra-Phos (64 g of phosphorus) is dissolved in 4 L of water, and 2 to 3 ounces of the solution is given 4 times daily PO.

3. Patients with *simultaneous hypokalemia* are treated with 20 mEq of KCl in 10% solution 3 times daily, or with potassium-containing phosphate preparations. Neutra-Phos-K and Phos-Tabs both contain 50 to 57 mEq of potassium per gram of phosphate.

4. Oncogenic osteomalacia is treated by completely resecting the responsible tumor. If this is not possible, patients may be treated with a combination of 1,25-dihydroxycholecalciferol (calcitriol) 1.5 to 3.0 mcg/day and phosphorus supplementation of 2 to 4 g/day.

V. HYPERNATREMIA

A. Mechanisms.
Hypernatremia nearly always is due to a loss of water from the body fluids. Any hypotonic fluid loss (e.g., sweating, hyperventilation, fever, vomiting, nasogastric suction) causes mild hypernatremia if not treated. *Extreme elevations* of plasma sodium concentrations (>160 mEq/L) are usually encountered in only three clinical situations:

1. **Decreased or absent fluid intake** is the most common cause of hypernatremia, especially in patients who have disabilities that impair normal fluid intake.

2. **Diabetes insipidus** (insufficient production of antidiuretic hormone [ADH]) is usually caused by head trauma (accidental or neurosurgical) or pituitary or hypothalamic neoplasms (primary or metastatic). Breast and lung cancers appear to have a special propensity for metastasizing to the hypothalamus. Although there are other rare causes of diabetes insipidus, nearly half of the cases are idiopathic. Diabetes insipidus is an exceptionally rare paraneoplastic syndrome. Nephrogenic diabetes insipidus occurs when the kidney is unable to respond to normal circulating levels of ADH, and may be the result of hypercalcemia, hypokalemia, or medications.

3. **Osmotic diuresis** and often osmotic diarrhea are encountered in obtunded patients who receive a massive urea load from high-protein nasogastric tube feedings. Progressive dehydration develops, and the osmotic diuresis produces an apparently normal urine output. Daily weighing and twice-weekly measuring of serum electrolytes and urea nitrogen are necessary to detect or prevent this problem.

B. Diagnosis

1. **Signs and symptoms.** Most patients with severe hypernatremia are already seriously ill. The specific contribution of hypertonicity is frequently difficult to distinguish from the underlying disease. Polyuria draws attention to the problem in most cases. If the solute intake is low, however, urine output may not exceed 2 to 3 L/day.

2. **Laboratory studies.** To make a diagnosis of diabetes insipidus, a water-deprivation test is performed. Baseline body weight, serum sodium concentration,

serum osmolality, urine specific gravity, and urine osmolality are measured. Water intake is completely restricted; however, these patients should *never* be deprived of water without continuous observation. Beginning in the morning, urine volume and the baseline studies are determined hourly. The test must be *terminated* if the patient's weight decreases by >3% or serum osmolality exceeds 310 mOsm/kg. Pending results of direct measurement, the serum osmolality can be rapidly and accurately estimated from serum concentrations of sodium, urea nitrogen, and glucose by the following formula:

$$\text{Serum osmolality} = 2(\text{sodium}) + \text{BUN}/2.8 + \text{glucose}/18$$

a. **Criteria for diagnosing diabetes insipidus**
   (1) Urine osmolality never exceeds 200 mOsm/kg unless there is severe dehydration.
   (2) The initial serum osmolality determination exceeds 280 mOsm/kg.
   (3) Serum osmolality rises above the initial determination.
   (4) The urine flow rate consistently exceeds 1 mL/minute.

b. **Differentiating pituitary diabetes insipidus.** Significant diabetes insipidus is excluded if the urine osmolality is >600 mOsm/kg after water deprivation in the absence of glycosuria or recently injected contrast media. Urine osmolality between 200 and 600 mOsm/kg suggests partial diabetes insipidus. It is necessary to distinguish pituitary (central) diabetes insipidus from nephrogenic diabetes insipidus. To do this, the kidney's response to ADH is assessed. Desmopressin, 0.5 mcg, is given SC at the conclusion of the water-deprivation test, and hourly urine specimens are collected for an additional 3 hours. After desmopressin injection, urine osmolality exceeds 400 mOsm/kg in patients with ADH deficiency and 800 mOsm/kg in normal persons; values are lower in patients with nephrogenic diabetes insipidus.

C. **Management**
   1. **Severe hypernatremia** is life-threatening and must be carefully managed. Correcting the water deficit too rapidly may precipitate fatal cerebral edema. Therapy should not lower the serum sodium level by >2 to 4 mEq/hour. Emergency therapy for patients in shock consists of plasma volume expansion with normal saline solution (200 to 250 mL boluses IV over 10 minutes until the systolic blood pressure exceeds 90 mm Hg); volume expansion itself induces a saluresis and initiates reduction of the serum sodium level. When the patient is hemodynamically stable, **the total volume (in liters) of 5% dextrose in water** is given according to the following formula:

$$\frac{(\text{serum sodium concentration} - 140) \times (0.6 \times \text{body weight in kg})}{140}$$

   2. **Therapy for chronic ADH deficiency**
      a. **Desmopressin** (desamino-D-arginine vasopressin [DDAVP]), 5 to 10 mcg intranasally or 0.5 to 1.0 mcg by SC injection, produces 6 to 18 hours of antidiuresis. To avoid water intoxication, the next dose is not given until thirst and polyuria redevelop. Oral desmopressin is also available for chronic therapy; doses of 0.05 to 1.2 mg/day are given.
      b. **Chlorpropamide,** 250 to 500 mg PO each morning, appears to be effective only in patients with incomplete pituitary diabetes insipidus. The drug is not approved for this purpose by the U.S. Food and Drug Administration. Serious and prolonged hypoglycemia or hyponatremia may complicate therapy with chlorpropamide.

VI. **HYPONATREMIA: SYNDROME OF INAPPROPRIATE ANTIDIURETIC HORMONE (SIADH)**
A. **Mechanisms**
   1. **ADH** is normally released from the posterior pituitary gland in response to increased osmolality or decreased plasma volume. The release of ADH is normally

inhibited by decreased plasma osmolality and increased plasma volume. The hormone acts by increasing water resorption from the renal collecting tubules.

2. **SIADH.** Unregulated production of ADH results in increased water retention by the kidney, increased total-body water, and moderate expansion of plasma volume. Plasma hypotonicity fails to suppress the secretion of ADH. Hyponatremia, plasma hypo-osmolality, and inability to excrete maximally diluted urine are the consequences of SIADH.

3. **Associated tumors.** Ectopic production of ADH may occur with any malignancy but is most frequently associated with bronchogenic carcinoma, especially the small cell type, and mesothelioma.

    a. About half of the patients with small cell lung cancer are unable to excrete an exogenous free water load normally; however, only a small portion of these develop severe hyponatremia (<120 mEq/L).

    b. Abnormalities of serum electrolytes, other than hyponatremia and (occasionally) hypouricemia, do not occur in SIADH. Some tumors, however, produce multiple ectopic hormones. Concomitant hypokalemia suggests a complicating ectopic adrenocorticotropic hormone (ACTH) syndrome. Concomitant hypercalcemia suggests the presence of a paraneoplastic disorder of calcium metabolism.

4. **Central nervous system disease** (e.g., mass lesions, hemorrhage, infection) and pulmonary infection (e.g., pneumonia, tuberculosis, abscess) may result in excessive ADH release from the posterior pituitary.

5. **Drugs associated with hyponatremia**

    a. **Diuretics** commonly produce hyponatremia, particularly in patients with unrestricted fluid intake.

    b. **Vincristine and vinblastine** may produce SIADH and profound hyponatremia. Manifestations develop 1 to 2 weeks after treatment.

    c. **Cyclophosphamide,** when given intravenously, may produce SIADH. Mild hyponatremia develops 4 to 12 hours after a dose, persists for about 20 hours, and is usually asymptomatic.

    d. **Cisplatin, high-dose melphalan and thiotepa** have been associated with SIADH.

    e. **Chlorpropamide** occasionally causes SIADH; other oral hypoglycemics rarely do so.

    f. **Carbamazepine** induces ADH secretion.

    g. **Intravenous narcotics** have been associated with SIADH.

    h. **Antidepressants and antipsychotics** have occasionally been associated with SIADH.

B. **Diagnosis**

1. **Symptoms and signs.** Lethargy, nausea, anorexia, and generalized weakness are common symptoms in patients with hyponatremia; however, the symptoms may be related more to comorbid conditions than to the serum sodium concentration. Confusion, convulsions, coma, and death may ensue if the hyponatremia is severe or rapid in onset.

2. **Laboratory studies.** Laboratory results in conditions associated with hyponatremia are shown in Table 27.1. Measurements that should be obtained in patients with hyponatremia are as follows:

    a. **In all patients with hyponatremia**

       (1) Serum electrolytes, creatinine, urea nitrogen, calcium, phosphate, glucose, total protein, and triglycerides

       (2) Urine sodium

    b. **In patients with hyponatremia and without an elevated BUN**

       (1) Blood and urine osmolality

       (2) Chest radiograph to look for evidence of lung cancer

       (3) Patients who meet the diagnostic criteria for SIADH but in whom there is no obvious cause should have a bone marrow biopsy performed to look for metastases from small cell lung cancer (some patients have normal chest radiographs).

TABLE 27.1   **Hyponatremia: Differential Diagnosis and Laboratory Results**

Condition	BUN	Osmolality S	Osmolality U	Urine sodium concentration
SIADH	D,(N)	D	I	N,I
Edematous states	D,N,I	D	I	D
Myxedema	N	D	N,I	(D),N,I
Salt-wasting states				
Mineralocorticoid deficiency	I	D	I	I
Glucocorticoid deficiency	N	D	(N),I	N,I
Diuretics	N, I	D	I	(D),N,I
Chronic renal failure	I	D	D,N,I	D,N,I
GI loss with hypotonic replacement	N,I	D	D	D
Compulsive water drinking	N,D	D	D	N
Hypothalamic osmoregulatory defect	N	D	N	D,N,I
Pseudohyponatremia				
Hyperglycemia	N,I	I	D,N,I	N
Mannitol	N,I	N	D,N	D,N
Marked hyperlipidemia or paraproteinemia	N	N	N	N

BUN, blood urea nitrogen; S, serum; U, urine; SIADH, syndrome of inappropriate antidiuretic hormone; D, decreased; N, normal; I, increased; GI, gastrointestinal. Parentheses indicate slight or occasional amount.

   c. In patients with evidence of endocrine hypofunction
     (1) Thyroid function tests
     (2) Adrenal function tests
     (3) Pituitary gland function tests, as necessary
  3. Diagnostic criteria for SIADH include *all five* of the following:
   a. Hyponatremia with a disproportionately low BUN (often <10 mg/dL)
   b. Absence of intravascular volume contraction
     (1) Volume contraction is a potent stimulus for ADH secretion and overrides the suppressive effect of hypotonicity.
     (2) Persistent urinary excretion of sodium constitutes indirect evidence of volume expansion (urine sodium concentration >30 mEq/L; fractional excretion of sodium >1).
   c. Absence of abnormal fluid retention, such as peripheral edema or ascites
   d. Normal renal, thyroid and adrenal function
   e. Serum hypotonicity along with urine that is not maximally dilute. A normal adult should be able to dilute urine to an osmolality of 50 to 75 mOsm/kg in the presence of decreased plasma osmolality; higher values are presumptive evidence for ADH activity at the renal tubules. Urine must be less than maximally dilute but need not be hypertonic relative to serum. Urine osmolality >75 to 100 mOsm/kg (or urine specific gravity >1.003) with plasma osmolality <260 mOsm/kg is usually diagnostic of SIADH.
 C. Management. Control of the responsible cancer usually corrects the problems associated with ectopic SIADH.
  1. Severe hyponatremia (serum sodium <110 mEq/L). Comatose or seizing patients with severe hyponatremia must receive aggressive management. The development of mental status changes or seizures in patients with severe hyponatremia is *prima facie* evidence of cerebral herniation; dexamethasone, 10 to 20 mg IV, and mannitol, 50 g IV, are given immediately. Lowering the plasma volume is essential to promote proximal tubular reabsorption of sodium.

Administering saline solutions without diuresis to patients with SIADH does not correct the problem; saline increases plasma volume and results in further loss of sodium in the urine.

a. An IV infusion of 3% NaCl at a rate of 1 L every 6 to 8 hours is started.

b. Furosemide, 40 to 80 mg IV every 6 to 8 hours, is administered simultaneously.

c. The CVP is monitored every 15 to 30 minutes; serum sodium and potassium concentrations are obtained hourly. Give additional doses of furosemide, 20 to 40 mg IV, or decrease the saline infusion rate if the CVP exceeds 18 cm of water or if congestive heart failure becomes evident on physical examination.

d. Furosemide and saline are discontinued when the serum sodium concentration exceeds 110 mEq/L. More rapid treatment increases the risk for osmotic cerebral myelinolysis. The hyponatremia should then be further corrected more slowly as described in section VI.C.2; serum sodium should rise no >12 mEq/L in the first 24 hours to avoid myelinolysis. Correction to serum sodium values of 125 to 130 mEq/L is usually sufficient.

2. Moderately severe hyponatremia (serum sodium >110 mEq/L)

a. Fluid restriction is of paramount importance in treatment of all patients with SIADH and should result in correction of hyponatremia within 3 to 5 days. Patients with serum sodium levels <125 mEq/L should be restricted to 500 to 700 mL/day. Patients with higher serum sodium levels can be restricted to 1,000 mL/day.

b. Demeclocycline (Declomycin), 150 to 300 mg PO given 4 times daily, induces renal resistance to ADH and facilitates free water excretion. The drug is useful in patients who cannot tolerate chronic fluid restriction or who have insufficient improvement of hyponatremia with fluid restriction. The only significant toxicity of the drug is azotemia, which may be a problem in patients who receive the higher doses or simultaneous nephrotoxic agents.

c. Lithium salts are less reliable than demeclocycline.

VII. HYPERKALEMIA

A. Mechanisms

1. Hyperkalemia in patients with or without cancer usually develops as a consequence of renal failure.

2. Hyperkalemia may result from rapid tumor lysis after therapy, especially in patients with Burkitt lymphoma or acute leukemia.

3. Adrenal metastases are common in patients with many types of cancer, but clinical adrenal insufficiency from metastases is unusual.

4. Pseudohyperkalemia occurs in patients with persistent leukocytosis or thrombocytosis, especially in the myeloproliferative disorders (see Chapter 24, section II.G.3 in "Comparable Aspects").

B. Diagnosis

1. Symptoms mostly consist of weakness and other neuromuscular complaints.

2. Laboratory studies

a. Serum potassium concentration

b. The severity of the ECG abnormalities corresponds to the severity of hyperkalemia; as hyperkalemia gets worse, the ECG shows increased T-wave amplitude, decreased R-wave amplitude, and increased S-wave depth; prolongation of P-R intervals and widening of the QRS complex; and then a sine wave pattern, eventuating in asystole or ventricular tachyarrhythmias.

3. Differential diagnosis

a. Renal insufficiency

b. Excessive potassium intake, especially with renal insufficiency

c. Potassium-sparing diuretics

d. Adrenal insufficiency

e. Acidosis

f. Cell destruction (e.g., tumor lysis, rhabdomyolysis)

g. Angiotensin-converting enzyme inhibitors

h. Angiotensin receptor blockers

C. Management
1. In patients with significant ECG abnormalities, IVIV calcium gluconate (10 mL of 10% solution) may be given to antagonize the effect of hyperkalemia on cardiac cell membranes.
2. Immediate lowering of the potassium is achieved by IV administration of 10 units of regular insulin plus 50 to 100 mL of 50% dextrose solution. If the patient is acidotic, 150 to 300 mEq (one to two ampules) of sodium bicarbonate is given IV. Note that bicarbonate cannot be simultaneously given via the same IV line as calcium because of the precipitation of calcium carbonate.
3. Removal of potassium from the body can be achieved with cation exchange resins like Kayexalate, 15 to 30 g every 6 hours. Sorbitol, 20 mL of 70% solution PO 4 times daily, or 100 g in a water-retention enema, is given to expel the resin from the bowel.
4. Hemodialysis is necessary for management of chronic or refractory hyperkalemia.
5. Hyperkalemia due to adrenal insufficiency may be corrected with the synthetic mineralocorticoid, fludrocortisone, 0.05 to 0.20 mg/day.

VIII. HYPOKALEMIA: ECTOPIC SECRETION OF ACTH

A. Mechanism. A variety of tumors may ectopically synthesize ACTH and produce Cushing syndrome. Biologically active ACTH is secreted in varying proportions with biologically inactive prohormone and preprohormone. All of these substances possess antigenic activity for ACTH. Thus, assays based on ACTH antigenic activity do not prove the presence of Cushing syndrome.
1. **Tumors commonly producing ectopic ACTH syndrome**
   a. Small cell lung cancer
   b. Malignant thymoma
   c. Pancreatic cancer, especially islet cell tumors
   d. Bronchial carcinoids
2. **Tumors uncommonly or rarely producing ectopic ACTH syndrome**
   a. Ovarian cancer
   b. Thyroid cancer (except medullary)
   c. Colon cancer
   d. Prostate cancer
   e. Renal cancer
   f. Sarcomas
   g. Hematologic malignancies

B. Diagnosis
1. **Symptoms and signs.** The most common malignant causes of ectopic ACTH syndrome are rapidly fatal. The typical features of adrenal or pituitary Cushing syndrome are often absent. Presenting signs usually are cachexia, weakness, and hypertension. Slower-growing cancers and benign tumors give rise to the characteristic rounded facies, truncal obesity, purple striae in skin stretch areas, and overt diabetes mellitus.
2. **Laboratory studies**
   a. Cancer patients who complain of weakness should have serum electrolytes measured. Hypokalemia and metabolic alkalosis may be severe (serum potassium as low as 1 mEq/L, bicarbonate >30 mEq/L) in patients with ectopic ACTH syndrome.
   b. The diagnosis of ectopic ACTH syndrome may be quickly made by demonstrating the failure of dexamethasone to suppress ACTH levels in most cases (see Chapter 15, section V.C.2).
3. **Differential diagnosis**
   a. Gastrointestinal losses associated with alkalosis (vomiting, prolonged nasogastric suctioning, colonic neoplasms [villous adenoma], chronic laxative abuse)
   b. Gastrointestinal losses associated with acidosis (chronic diarrhea, ureterosigmoidostomy, Zollinger-Ellison syndrome)
   c. Potassium-wasting drugs (e.g., diuretics, cisplatin, corticosteroids)

    d. Hyperaldosteronism
    e. Hypercortisolism
    f. Licorice ingestion
    g. Renal tubular acidosis
    h. Hypercalcemia, hypomagnesemia
    i. Hypophosphatemia in anabolic states (e.g., rapid tumor growth)
    j. Respiratory therapy in patients with chronic carbon dioxide retention
    k. Correction of nutritional anemias

C. Management. Control of the underlying tumor is the most effective method. Hypokalemia is often difficult to correct. Potassium replacement consists of PO or IV doses of 80 to 150 mEq/day. Severe symptoms may occasionally improve with the use of adrenal suppressant medications, such as various combinations of mitotane, metyrapone, ketoconazole, and aminoglutethimide. The toxicity of these drugs may be worse than the symptoms from the underlying disease. Spironolactone, 100 to 400 mg daily, may be useful. Adrenalectomy is a consideration in the rare patient with an indolent, unresectable tumor that causes the ectopic ACTH syndrome.

IX. HYPERURICEMIA

A. Mechanisms. Hyperuricemia and hyperuricosuria pose a major problem for patients with myeloproliferative disorders, lymphomas, myeloma, or leukemias but usually not for patients with solid tumors.

    1. Hyperuricosuria. Urinary uric acid excretion is increased in untreated patients who have myeloproliferative disorders, acute or chronic myelocytic leukemia, or acute lymphoblastic leukemia. Patients with lymphoma have normal or slightly increased uric acid excretion. During treatment with either cytotoxic agents or radiation, massive tumor lysis releases nucleic acids and results in excess production of uric acid, especially in patients with lymphoma or leukemia.

    2. Uric acid nephropathy results from the precipitation of uric acid crystals in the concentrated, acidic urine of the renal medulla, distal tubules, and collecting ducts. The resultant sludge leads to intrarenal obstructive nephropathy and distinct inflammatory interstitial changes. Four types of renal disease comprise hyperuricemic nephropathy.

        a. Acute hyperuricemic nephropathy is seen in patients treated for hematologic malignancies. It is characterized by acute renal failure with a rapidly rising serum creatinine concentration. Blood uric acid levels of >20 mg/dL are consistently associated with acute renal functional impairment or failure. Lower levels may acutely compromise renal function if the patient is dehydrated or acidotic.

        b. Gouty nephropathy is usually mild to moderate and is characterized by the deposition of uric acid crystals (tophi) in the medulla or pyramids and a surrounding giant cell reaction.

        c. Uric acid nephrolithiasis develops in gouty and nongouty patients with or without hyperuricemia. Symptomatic uric acid calculi are usually manifested by renal colic. Acute or chronic renal failure may develop secondary to obstructive uropathy.

        d. Interstitial nephritis of hyperuricemia may lead to chronic renal failure after 20 to 30 years. This condition is almost always associated with hypertension and is questioned as an isolated cause of renal failure.

    3. Xanthine stones, resulting from the inhibition of xanthine oxidase by allopurinol in the setting of purine hypermetabolism, rarely complicates malignancies.

    4. Oxypurinol stones have rarely developed after therapy with massive doses of allopurinol.

B. Diagnosis is established by measurement of serum and urine uric acid concentrations. The normal excretory rate for uric acid is 300 to 500 mg/day.

C. Management

    1. Prevention is the cornerstone of management.

        a. Vigorous hydration is essential for increasing uric acid clearance and diluting the concentration of uric acid in the renal tubules. Urinary flow should be at least 100 mL/hour.

    b. Alkalinization of the urine. Traditionally, the urine pH is maintained between 7.0 and 7.5 (checked by dipstick). Sodium bicarbonate is given (one to three tablets PO every 4 hours) while the patient is awake. Acetazolamide (Diamox), 250 to 500 mg PO, is given at bedtime to maintain urine alkalinization. Other preparations that contain sodium or potassium citrate are also available. Recently, routine alkalinization of the urine has been questioned because it increases the risk of forming crystals of calcium phosphate and xanthine within the renal tubules, since these are both less soluble in an alkaline urine.

    c. Allopurinol should be given continuously to patients with myeloproliferative disorders and at least 12 hours before starting antitumor therapy to patients with the other hematologic malignancies. The usual dose is 300 to 600 mg/day PO; larger doses may be required. Intravenous allopurinol is also available but expensive. Allopurinol can be discontinued when the tumor burden has been sufficiently reduced.

  2. Treatment. Rapid lowering of established hyperuricemia may be accomplished with IV rasburicase, a recombinant form of urate oxidase. Rasburicase is currently approved only for pediatric use and is very expensive; doses of 0.15 to 0.2 mg/kg IV are given daily for several days.

  3. Renal failure because of uric acid nephropathy

    a. Ureteral lavage through nephrostomies and **surgical removal of stones** may be necessary to relieve acute renal pelvis and ureteral obstructions.

    b. Hemodialysis should be used if the previously discussed measures fail to improve renal function because uric acid nephropathy is usually a complication of effective antitumor therapy. Hemodialysis is superior to peritoneal dialysis for clearing uric acid.

X. HYPOURICEMIA

  A. Mechanisms. Hypouricemia is usually caused by defects in proximal renal tubular reabsorption of uric acid. Hypouricemia has also been reported to be associated with a variety of tumors, especially Hodgkin lymphoma and myeloma.

  B. Diagnosis

    1. Symptoms. Patients do not have symptoms.

    2. Laboratory studies. Blood uric acid levels identify the abnormality.

    3. Differential diagnosis

      a. Proximal renal tubular disease

        (1) Fanconi syndrome (myeloma is a common cause in adults)

        (2) Wilson disease

        (3) Isolated defect in otherwise healthy patients

      b. Uricosuric agents

        (1) Aspirin

        (2) Radiographic contrast agents

        (3) Glyceryl guaiacolate

      c. Treatment with xanthine oxidase inhibitors (allopurinol) or urate oxidase (rasburicase)

      d. Hereditary xanthinuria

      e. Neoplastic diseases, especially Hodgkin lymphoma

      f. Liver disease

      g. SIADH

  C. Management. Treatment of hypouricemia is not necessary.

XI. HYPERGLYCEMIA

  A. Mechanisms

    1. Diabetic glucose tolerance curves with relative insulin deficiency are present in many patients with cancer. Paradoxical hypersecretion of growth hormone from the pituitary gland occurs in most of these patients. Nutritional replenishment appears to improve the abnormal glucose tolerance, hyperinsulinemia, and paradoxical growth hormone secretion.

    2. Hyperglycemia occurs in patients with glucagonoma, somatostatinoma, pheochromocytoma, and hypercortisolism. Use of dexamethasone or other glucocorticoids as an antiemetic or as part of a chemotherapy regimen may cause hyperglycemia. Pancreatic destruction by carcinoma may also cause diabetes.

   3. Nonketotic hyperosmolar coma can be a complication of treatment with cyclophosphamide, vincristine, L-asparaginase, or prednisone in patients with even mild diabetes mellitus. Hyperosmolar coma also occurs as a result of hyperalimentation therapy.

B. Diagnosis. Random or 2-hour postprandial blood glucose determinations disclose the abnormality in most patients.

C. Management

   1. Nutritional status should be improved in cancer patients with glucose intolerance, if feasible. Management of substantial hyperglycemia on account of tumor is effected by control of the neoplasm and by administration of insulin or oral hypoglycemics as needed.

   2. Hyperosmolar coma must be vigorously treated with fluid replacement of volume losses with IV saline until the blood pressure is stable. Insulin infusion (1 to 4 U/hour) usually controls the hyperglycemia.

   3. Avoidance of glucocorticoids will prevent steroid-induced hyperglycemia.

XII. HYPOGLYCEMIA

A. Mechanisms. Insulinlike substances (probably insulinlike growth factor-2) may be produced by some tumors, especially large retroperitoneal sarcomas and occasionally other cancers. Hepatocellular carcinomas and extensive liver metastases from a variety of primary sites may deplete glycogen stores and impair gluconeogenesis. Insulinoma is discussed in Chapter 15, section VI.C.

   1. Etiologies of hypoglycemia

   a. Malignant tumors

      (1) Insulinoma
      (2) Large retroperitoneal tumor
      (3) Hepatocellular carcinoma
      (4) Extensive hepatic metastasis

   b. Drugs

      (1) Surreptitious or therapeutic insulin administration
      (2) Oral hypoglycemic agents
      (3) Alcohol
      (4) Salicylates
      (5) Gatifloxacin
      (6) Pentamidine
      (7) Jamaican vomiting sickness (akee fruit)
      (8) Quinine (in antimalarial doses)

   c. Metabolic disorders

      (1) Starvation
      (2) Chronic liver disease
      (3) Hypoadrenalism
      (4) Hypopituitarism
      (5) Myxedema
      (6) Glycogen storage diseases
      (7) Reactive hypoglycemias (e.g., prediabetes, postgastrectomy)

   2. Pseudohypoglycemia. Falsely low glucose levels may occur in patients with marked granulocytosis, especially patients with myeloproliferative disorders, because of *in vitro* consumption of glucose.

B. Diagnosis

   1. Symptoms and signs. Tumor-associated hypoglycemia produces mental status change, fatigue, convulsions, or coma. Some patients show features of fasting hypoglycemia, such as an altered morning personality that improves after breakfast. Tremors, sweating, tachycardia, and hunger pangs are suggestive of an acute decrease in blood sugar level.

2. **Laboratory studies.** A blood glucose concentration of <40 mg/dL establishes the presence of hypoglycemia. Further evaluation of fasting hypoglycemia is discussed in Chapter 15, section VI.C.1.b. Patients who surreptitiously abuse insulin should have C-peptide and insulin serum levels measured. Absent C-peptide with elevated insulin level suggests the diagnosis of exogenous insulin administration.

C. **Management**
1. **Intravenous glucose.** Any patient with suggestive signs, symptoms, or unexplained coma should have a blood sample drawn for glucose and insulin determination, followed immediately by rapid IV infusion of 50 mL of 50% dextrose solution. Serum glucose can remain low even while concentrated glucose solutions are being administered. All patients with glucose levels of <40 mg/dL and symptomatic patients with glucose levels of <60 mg/dL should be treated by continuous infusion of 20% glucose at 50 to 150 mL/hour; rates are adjusted to maintain glucose levels higher than 60 mg/dL. Blood glucose levels are measured every 3 to 4 hours until stabilization occurs.
2. **Glucagon,** 1 mg IM, also raises blood glucose by promoting glycogenolysis and gluconeogenesis.
3. **Octreotide,** a somatostatin analog, can decrease insulin hypersecretion.
4. **Other measures.** If the blood glucose cannot be increased to safe levels with infusions, prednisone or diazoxide should be administered (see Chapter 15, section VI.C.2.d).

XIII. TUMOR LYSIS SYNDROME
A. **Mechanisms.** Effective chemotherapy of several malignancies may result in the massive release into the blood of potassium, phosphate, uric acid, and other breakdown products of dying tumor cells. Hypocalcemia may occur with severe hyperphosphatemia. Tumor lysis syndrome develops within hours to a few days of treatment for the underlying neoplasm.
1. **Associated tumors** most commonly are acute leukemia, Burkitt lymphoma, and occasionally other lymphoreticular malignancies. The syndrome rarely occurs after the treatment of solid tumors. A high tumor burden and elevated serum lactate dehydrogenase levels increase the risk of tumor lysis syndrome.
2. **Life-threatening complications** include renal failure from precipitation of uric acid or calcium phosphate crystals in the kidney, seizures from hypocalcemia, and cardiac arrhythmias from hyperkalemia or hypocalcemia.
B. **Diagnosis**
1. **Physical examination.** Oliguria may call attention to the metabolic disorders. Tetany may be a presenting feature. Cardiac arrhythmias or cardiopulmonary arrest develop if the process is not controlled.
2. **Laboratory studies.** Patients treated for acute leukemia or Burkitt lymphoma should have measurements of serum levels of potassium, calcium, phosphate, uric acid, and creatinine performed daily for 1 week and every few hours if the syndrome develops.
C. **Management.** Vigorous IV hydration with half-normal saline is initiated. Severe metabolic problems are treated as follows:
1. Hypocalcemia, see section II.C.
2. Hyperphosphatemia, see section III.C.
3. Hyperkalemia, see section VII.C.
4. Hyperuricemia, see section IX.C.
5. Hemodialysis may be necessary on an emergency basis for patients who do not respond to treatment or who develop renal insufficiency.

Suggested Reading
Cairo MS, Bishop M. Tumour lysis syndrome: new therapeutic strategies and classification. *Br J Haematol* 2004;127:3.
Crowley RK, Thompson CJ. Syndrome of inappropriate antidiuresis. *Expert Rev Endocrinol Metab* 2006;1:537.

Gaasbeck A, Meinders AE. Hypophosphatemia: an update on its etiology and treatment. *Am J Med* 2005;118:1094.

Schaefer TJ, Wolford RW. Disorders of potassium. *Emerg Med Clin North Am* 2005;23:723.

Spinazze S, Schrijvers D. Metabolic emergencies. *Crit Rev Oncol Hematol* 2006;58:79.

Stewart AF. Hypercalcemia associated with cancer. *N Engl J Med* 2005;352:373.

Tanvetyanon T, Stiff PJ. Management of the adverse effects associated with intravenous bisphosphonates. *Ann Oncol* 2006;17:897.

Tisdall M, Crocker M, Watkiss J, et al. Disturbances of sodium in critically ill adult neurologic patients. *J Neurosurg Anesthesiol* 2006;18:57.

Woo S-B, Hellstein JW, Kalmar JR. Systematic review: bisphosphonates and osteonecrosis of the jaws. *Ann Intern Med* 2006;144:753.

CUTANEOUS COMPLICATIONS

Bartosz Chmielowski, Dennis A. Casciato, and Richard F. Wagner, Jr.

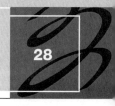

28

I. METASTASES TO THE SKIN

A. Incidence and pathology. Skin is not an uncommon metastatic site of solid tumors. Of patients with metastatic disease, 2% to 10% develop skin metastases. In men, the most common internal malignancies leading to cutaneous metastases are lung cancer (24%), colon cancer (19%), melanoma (13%), squamous cell carcinoma of the oral cavity (12%), and renal cell carcinoma (6%). In women, these are breast cancer (69%), colon cancer (9%), melanoma (5%), lung cancer (4%), and ovarian cancer (4%). Cutaneous involvement by cancer can occur both as a metastatic process and as a direct extension of the tumor to the skin.

B. Natural history. Metastases to the skin may be delayed 10 to 15 years after the initial surgical treatment of primary melanoma, breast carcinoma, and renal cancer or may be the first indication of an internal malignancy.

1. **Breast cancer** represents almost 75% of female patients with cutaneous metastases. It shows eight distinct clinicopathologic types of cutaneous involvement:

   a. Inflammatory (erysipelas-resembling erythematous patch or plaque with active border, usually affecting the breast, but other skin sites can also be involved)

   b. En cuirasse (a diffuse morphealike induration)

   c. Telangiectatic (papules with violaceous hue caused by accumulation of blood in vascular channels)

   d. Nodular (usually multiple firm papulonodules, sometimes ulcerated)

   e. Alopecia neoplastica (painless, well-demarcated, pinkish oval plaques of alopecia cause hematogeonous spread of breast carcinoma), which can occur with other neoplasms as well

   f. Paget's disease (a sharply demarcated, scaling plaque on the nipple or areola representing cutaneous infiltration of cancer)

   g. Breast carcinoma of the inframammary crease (a cutaneous nodule that may resemble basal cell carcinoma)

   h. Histiocytoid nodule of the eyelid (presents as a painless eyelid swelling with induration)

2. **Lung cancer.** Cutaneous metastases from lung cancer may appear on any surface, but they are most common on the chest wall and the posterior abdomen; small-cell lung cancer metastasizes most frequently to the skin of the back. Between 1.5% and 16% of patients with lung cancer develop skin metastases; in half of these patients, it is a presenting sign of the disease. Lung cancer also has a rare but peculiar tendency to metastasize to the anal area, fingertips, or toes.

3. **Gastrointestinal (GI) tract cancers.** Skin metastases from colon cancer and rectal cancer usually develop after malignancy has been recognized. Abdominal wall and the perineal area are the most common sites. They may appear as sessile or pedunculated nodules, vascular nodules, scalp cysts, inflammatory carcinoma, or persistent fistulation after appendectomy. Cutaneous metastasis of gastric cancer is rare, and most cutaneous metastases are typically solitary, nodular, have a firm consistency, and are red or hyperpigmented, but may present as dermatitis. Anal cancer metastases to skin involve unusual sites, such as the scalp, eyelid, nose, or legs.

4. **Melanoma.** Both cutaneous and extracuatneous melanoma can produce skin metastasis. They usually present as multiple pigmented nodules, but they can also be erythematous or apigmented.

5. **Urologic malignancies.** Of all urologic malignancies, renal cell carcinoma metastasizes to the skin most frequently, but skin metastasis from bladder, prostate, and testicular cancer have also been reported. These metastates are frequently the first sign of renal cell carcinoma, and they can appear very late—up to 10 years after diagnosis. Both clinically and histologically, they may resemble common dermatologic disorders, which leads occasionally to incorrect diagnosis.

6. **Subungual metastases.** Malignant lesions in the nail unit can be classified into three groups: metastatic lesions from a distant primary, cutaneous involvement of a hematopoetic or lymphoproliferative malignancy, and primary cancer at this location. Lung cancer is the most common type of malignancy that can metastasize to the nail bed, followed by genitourinary, breast, head and neck cancers, and sarcomas. Subungual metastases typically present as erythematous enlargement, swelling of the distal digit, or a violacious nodule. They are frequently painful, but they can also bleed, or be hot, pulsatile, and fluctuant. These lesions can be mistaken for infection or trauma; in almost half of affected persons, they are a presenting sign of malignancy.

7. **Umbilical metastasis** (Sister Mary Joseph's nodule) is encountered in 1% to 3% of patients with abdominopelvic malignancy. The term Sister Mary Joseph's nodule was assigned to the Mayo brothers' surgical nurse who recognized that umbilical metastasis-denoted incurable disease when the patient underwent laparotomy. The most common origins are GI (52%), gynecologic (28%), stomach (23%),and ovarian (16%) cancer. Survival in these patients, which depends on the type of tumor and treatment modalities, can range from 2 to 18 months.

C. **Prognosis.** Skin metastases usually indicate advanced disease and carry a poor prognosis. The average survival time from the recognition of skin metastases is 3 months, but it can be years for lymphomas, melanoma, and breast cancer.

D. **Diagnosis** is based on biopsy results, especially in patients who have not previously been diagnosed with malignancy.

E. **Management.** Most skin metastases are treated symptomatically, and they tend to regress when the primary tumor responds to systemic therapy. Occasionally, these lesions require treatment with local radiation therapy, surgery, cryotherapy, or photodynamic therapy. Intralesional injections of thiotepa (30 mg), bleomycin, or cisplatin, or electrochemotherapy (in which the effect of intralesional chemotherapy is enhanced by electroporation) have also been utilized.

II. CUTANEOUS PARANEOPLASTIC SYNDROMES

Cutaneous paraneoplastic syndromes comprise a heterogenous group of dermatologic syndromes describing skin lesions that do not contain malignant cells, but they appear in the presence of underlying malignancy.

A. **Acanthosis nigricans** is characterized by hyperpigmented, velvety plaques on the neck, in the axilla, groin, and antecubital fossa. In most cases, it reflects metabolic disturbances seen in patients with obesity, metabolic syndrome, or diabetes. If the lesions appear abruptly and progress rapidly, or they are associated with tripe palms or mucous membrane involvement, they can reflect underlying malignancy, mainly adenocarcinoma of the GI tract (in >50% of cases - gastric cancer). **Benign causes** of acanthosis nigricans include:

1. Acromegaly, gigantism
2. Adrenal insufficiency
3. Hyperthyroidism, hypothyroidism
4. Lipodystrophy
5. Diabetes mellitus
6. Syndrome with hirsutism, obesity, and amenorrhea
7. Inherited abnormality in humans (and Swedish dachshunds)

B. **Amyloidosis** secondary to nonmalignant disease rarely involves skin. Patients with multiple myeloma or, less commonly, Waldenstrom's macroglobulinemia may develop "pinch purpura" (ecchymoses or purpuric patches occurring spontaneously or with minor trauma). The lesions are primarily in flexural areas, paranasal skin, anogenital regions, the neck, and around the eyes.

C. **Bazex syndrome** (acrokeratosis paraneoplastica) consists of psoriasiform lesions in the acral areas (ears, nose, nails, hands, feet, elbows, knees). In 18% of cases, lesions can be pruritic. This syndrome is universally associated with malignancy, mainly carcinoma of the upper aerodigestive tract, but also prostate carcinoma, hepatocellular carcinoma, lymphoma, and bladder carcinoma. In nearly two-thirds of cases, cutaneous lesions precede the diagnosis of malignancy.

D. **Dermatomyosistis** and polymyositis belong to a group of idiopathic inflammatory myopathies. Between 15% and 25% of cases of dermatomysositis and about 10% of polymysositis are associated with malignancy. Almost any type of malignancy has been reported in patients with dermatomyosistis, but ovarian carcinoma and lung and breast cancer are the most common. Dermatomyositis may precede development of the neoplasm for up to 5 years. Treatment of the malignancy results in symptom improvement, and worsening of symptoms may herald tumor recurrence.

These myopathies are typified by proximal muscle weakness with or without tenderness. Patients typically report that they are not able to brush their hair. Flat-topped erythematous papules over the phalangeal joints (Gottron's papules) and pinkish-purple discoloration around the eyes (a heliotrope rash) are pathognomic signs of dermatomyositis. Other signs include periungual telangiectasias; patchy discoloration of the skin; red, scaly scalp rash; and photosensitivity. Laboratory work commonly reveals elevated creatinine kinase level, although the cases with normal level of creatinine kinase have been reported, and possibly they are more frequently associated with malignancy.

E. **Ectopic Cushing's syndrome** is caused by the secretion of an adrenocorticotrophic hormone (ACTH) prohormone or ACTH, most commonly by small-cell lung carcinoma and bronchial carcinoids, and occasionally by thymoma, islet cell tumor, non–small-cell lung carcinoma, and pheochromocytoma. It presents as proximal muscle wasting, hypertension, hypokalemia, usually weight loss (not a weight gain), and, because an ACTH prohormone contains pro-opiomelanocortin, frequently with hyperpigmentation.

F. **Erythema gyratum repens** is characterized by an extensive eruption of erythematous, scaly, rapidly progressing, ring-forming, wood-grain resembling lesions over most of the body, sparing the hands, feet, face. It is frequently accompanied by severe pruritus. It is almost always a representation of underlying malignancy, and it precedes the detection of malignancy by 1 to 24 months. Lung cancer is most commonly reported, followed by esophageal and breast cancer. The treatment consists of surgical removal of the primary tumor, but some improvement can sometimes be observed after therapy with systemic steroids, radiotherapy, and azathioprine.

G. **Exfoliative erythroderma syndrome** is a generalized erythema of the skin accompanied by a variable degree of scaling. It is frequently accompanied by severe pruritus and generalized lymphadenopathy. Malignancy accounts for 5% to 12% of cases, and it is most frequently associated with cutaneous T-cell lymphoma, rarely with solid tumors or acute myelogenous leukemia.

H. **Hypertrichosis lanuginosa acquisita** ("malignant down") refers to the development of fine, unpigmented hair predominantly localized to the head and neck. It has been associated with lung and colon cancer, but it can also occur in conjunction with shock, thyrotoxicosis, porphyria, and cyclosporine, minoxidil, phenytoin, and penicillin ingestion. Treatment should be directed toward the removal of malignancy.

I. **Ichthyosis.** Acquired ichthyosis is manifested by symmetric scaling ranging in severity from minor roughness and dryness to dramatic desquamation of white-to-brown scales. The diameter of the scales can range from <1 mm to >1 cm. It primarily affects the trunk and limbs. The lesions are usually more accentuated on extensor surfaces. It should be differentiated from the late-onset ichthyosis vulgaris, xerosis, and Refsum's disease. Hodgkin lymphoma is the most common malignancy associated with acquired ichthyosis, but it can also occur in patients with a cutaneous T-cell lymphoma or carcinomas of the breast, lung, or bladder. It may be also a result of nonmalignant disease (e.g., autoimmune syndromes, endocrinologic disorders, nutritional abnormalities, infectious diseases, and finally a drug reaction).

J. Multicentric reticulohistiocytosis is characterized by pink, brown, gray papules appearing initially on the hands and then spreading to the face. The lesions can be also present on the knees, elbows, ankles, shoulders, feet, or hips, and they may have pathognomic coral-bead appearance. Approximately 20% to 25% of multicentric reticulohistiocytosis cases are associated with malignancy, including hematologic, breast, ovarian, gastric, and cervical neoplasms.

K. Necrolytic migratory erythema (NME) is an uncommon inflammatory dermatosis usually associated with *glucagonoma*, and rarely with non-neoplastic conditions, such as liver disease, inflammatory bowel disease, pancreatitis, and malabsorption disorders. The postulated mechanism for NME involves a combination of zinc, amino acid, and fatty acid deficiencies. The clinical features of NME include transient eruptions of irregular erythematous lesions in which a central bulla develops, subsequently erodes, and heals with hyperpigmentation. The lesions follow a periorificial distribution or they are located in the areas subject to greater pressure and friction (i.e., the perineum, buttocks, groin, lower abdomen, and lower extremities).

L. Necrotizing leucocytoclastic vasculitis is a rare representation of malignancy. It appears as a palpable purpura, typically in dependent areas. This vasculitis is more common with hematologic malignancies than with solid tumors. Occasionally, it can also be a complication of antineoplastic therapy.

M. Pachydermoperiostosis exhibits thickening of skin and creation of new skin folds (leonine facies). The scalp, forehead, lids, ears, and lips are the typical sites. The tongue, thenar and hypothenar eminences, elbows, and knees may be enlarged. The fingers are clubbed. Biopsy shows thickening of the horny layer and hypertrophy of the sweat and sebaceous glands.

The familial form of pachydermoperiostosis is not usually associated with malignant tumors. The acquired variety occurs almost exclusively in patients with undifferentiated lung cancer. Clubbing and hypertrophic osteoarthropathy are also associated with a variety of nonmalignant disorders.

N. Paget's disease. *Extramammary* Paget's disease is a nonhealing neoplasm occurring in the apocrine gland-bearing areas, mainly axilla and the perineum. It can be associated with either contiguous or a distant cancer. Surgical excision is the primary treatment for the skin lesions. It can also respond to topical 5-fluorouracil or imiquimod.

O. Palmoplantar hyperkeratosis is characterized by yellowish, symmetric thickening of palms and soles. It occurs in hereditary and nonhereditary forms. Acquired form can be associated with Hodgkin lymphoma, leukemia, breast cancer, and gastric cancer. Familial forms are strongly associated with squamous cell carcinoma of the esophagus, breast, and ovarian carcinoma. In familial forms, the development of malignancy is delayed >30 years after the appearance of hyperkeratosis. Arsenic exposure can predispose to punctuate palmar hyperkeratosis and higher cancer risk.

P. Papillomatosis. Florid cutaneous papillomatosis describes the sudden appearance of multiple acuminate *keratotic papules* that morphologically resemble viral warts. They initially develop on hands and wrists, and later spread on the entire body and the face. This syndrome always reflects underlying malignancy, most commonly gastric adenocarcinoma.

Q. Pemphigus. Paraneoplastic pemphigus is a rare autoimmune bullous mucocutaneous disorder that presents typically with painful mucosal erosive lesions and pruritic papulosquamous eruptions that often progress to blisters. Immunofluorescence testing reveals IgG autoantibodies and C3 deposited intercellularly in the epidermis and in a linear fashion along the dermal–epidermal junction. The most common underlying neoplasms include non-Hodgkin lymphoma, chronic lymphocytic leukemia, and Castleman's disease.

R. Pityriasis rotunda manifests as round, scaly hyperpigmented lesions on the trunk, buttocks, and thighs. It is very rarely diagnosed in whites. In 6% of cases, it develops in patients with malignancies, mainly hepatocellular carcinoma and gastric carcinoma.

S. Pruritus. Refractory pruritus, in patients without liver disease, can be associated with iron deficiency, thyroid disorders, renal insufficiency and also with malignancy, most commonly lymphoma, myeloproliferative disorders, multiple myeloma, leukemia, and carcinoids.

T. Pyoderma gangrenosum is an idiopathic *neutrophilic dermatosis*. It presents classically as tender, fluctuant pustules or nodules, which expand peripherally to form ulcers with sharp, raised edges. Of cases, 50% to 70% are associated with underlying systemic disease, including ulcerative colitis, Crohn's disease, diverticulitis, hematologic and rheumatologic conditions, hepatopathies, visceral carcinomata, and immunodeficient states. The associated hematologic disorders include acute lymphoid and myeloid leukemia, myeloproliferative diseases, myeloma, Waldenström's macroglobulinemia, and Hodgkin and non-Hodgkin lymphomas. It has been also reported in patients with colon, bladder, prostate, breast, bronchus, ovary, and adrenocortical carcinoma.

U. Sweet's syndrome (acute febrile neutrophilic dermatosis) presents as an acute eruption of tender, erythematous plaques or nodules with irregular surfaces. The lesions can occur anywhere on the body, but are most common on the face and the trunk. Histologic examination reveals dense neutrophilic infiltration. The rash is usually accompanied by fever, peripheral blood neutrophilia, arthritis, and conjunctivitis. Approximately 10% of patients have underlying malignancy, and acute mylogenous leukemia has been reported most frequently. Therapy with prednisone appears to be most effective.

V. The sign of Leser-Trélat is ominous of internal malignancy and it describes the sudden eruption on multiple pruritic seborrheic keratoses. These lesions have frequently an inflammatory base. The sign of Leser-Trélat has to be differentiated from the presence of multiple benign seborrheic keratoses. The predominant types of malignancy are GI adenocarcinomas, lymphoproliferative disorders, and cancers of the lung or breast.

W. Urticaria pigmentosa is a presenting feature in 55% to 100% of patients with systemic mastocytosis. The primary lesion is a hyperpigmented macule or papule that transforms into a wheal when irritated mechanically (Darier's sign). In some cases, lesions can be pigmentless, telangiectatic, and nodular.

X. Vitiligo is the hypopigmentation of skin caused by the loss of melanocytes and it frequently occurs in individuals with malignant melanoma. It is thought that vitiligo is the consequence of the immune-mediated response against antigens shared by normal melanocytes and melanoma cells. The appearance of vitiligo in patients with melanoma is associated with better prognosis.

Y. Miscellaneous cutaneous paraneoplastic disorders

   1. Alopecia mucinosa can develop during the course of lymphoreticular neoplasms as a consequence of mucinous degeneration of collagen around hair follicles and sebaceous glands. The resultant alopecia is unrelated to therapy.

   2. Circinate erythemas. Erythema figuratum perstans is a circular elevation of the skin that remains stable for weeks to months. Erythema annulare centrifugum initially is a small erythematous area that slowly enlarges, leaving a central circle of normal-appearing skin. Lesions may be pruritic.

   Circinate erythemas are associated most commonly with nonmalignant diseases (especially collagen vascular syndromes, angiitides, and infections). Many cases are idiopathic. Less commonly, they are associated tumors that include lymphoma and, occasionally, visceral cancer.

   3. Erythromelalgia presents as painful, warm extremities (particularly, the digits) that appear erythematous. Myeloproliferative diseases are the most common associated malignancies. Aspirin provides relief.

   4. Pigmentation of the skin

   a. Gray discoloration of the skin because melanosis may develop in patients with extensive malignant melanoma

   b. Periorbital purplish discoloration can develop in patients who have amyloid deposition in the eyelids from infiltration and purpura. The syndrome of postproctoscopic palpebral purpura is well described in these patients.

5. **Porphyria cutanea tarda** (PCT) is a blistering disease that appears in skin exposed to sunlight. Hepatocellular carcinoma and metastatic liver tumors are occasionally associated with paraneoplastic PCT.

6. **Tripe palms** resemble bovine foregut and appear as thickened palmar skin with exaggerated dermatoglyphics. More than 90% of patients with tripe palms have associated malignancy, most frequently of the lung, stomach, and genitourinary tract.

III. INHERITED MALIGNANCY-ASSOCIATED SYNDROMES

Several genetic syndromes involving the skin predispose to internal malignancy without having a paraneoplastic association.

A. **Ataxia telangiectasia** is an autosomal-recessive disorder caused by mutations in the *ATM* gene, which has a crucial role in the cellular response to DNA damage. The syndrome is characterized by progressive neurodegeneration, ocular and cutaneous telangiectasias, immunodeficiency, and premature aging. These individuals are at high risk for development of hematologic malignancies, including Hodgkin and non-Hodgkin lymphoma, and leukemia.

B. **Basal cell nevus syndrome** (Gorlin's syndrome) (see Chapter 16).

C. **Cowden's disease** (multiple hamartoma-neoplasia syndrome) is an autosomal-dominant genodermatosis with incomplete penetrance characterized by multiple trichilemmomas (adnexal tumors), mucocutaneous papules, and high risk for malignancy. It is caused by an inactivation of PTEN (phosphatase and tensin homolog deleted on chromosome 10), a dual-phosphatase tumor suppressor gene. Patients with loss of wild-type PTEN expression from one allele carry an increased risk of malignant breast, thyroid, endometrial, and brain tumors.

D. **Cronkhite-Canada syndrome** is a rare, acquired, nonfamilial GI polyposis syndrome associated with protein-losing gastroenteropathy, alopecia, nail dystrophy, and hyperpigmentation. Patients are at high risk for the development of gastric, colon, and rectal carcinomas.

E. **Gardner's syndrome** is a variant of familial adenomatous polyposis (FAP) with extracolonic symptoms; it is caused by mutations in the tumor suppressor gene adenomatous polyposis coli (APC). It is an autosomal-dominant disease characterized by the presence of colonic polyposis, osteomas, and mesenchymal tumors of the skin and soft tissues. In most patients, cutaneous and bone abnormalities develop approximately 10 years before polyposis. The most common skin manifestations of Gardner's syndrome are epidermoid or sebaceous cysts (66%), which are found on the face, scalp, and extremities. Other skin manifestations are fibromas, neurofibromas, lipomas, leiomyomas, and pigmented skin lesions. The patients are at high risk for development of colon cancer and desmoid tumors.

F. **Howel-Evans syndrome** is a rare familial syndrome that links focal nonepidermolytic palmoplantar keratoderma (tylosis) with the early onset of esophageal squamous cell carcinoma. The locus has been located on chromosome 17q25 (*TOC* gene).

G. **Muir-Torre syndrome** is a rare genodermatosis associated with mutations in mismatch repair proteins, hMSH-2 and hMLH-1. It is most often diagnosed by the synchronous or metachronous occurrence of at least one sebaceous gland neoplasm and at least one internal malignancy. The syndrome is characterized by an autosomal-dominant inheritance pattern with variable penetrance and expression. The visceral malignancies include colorectal carcinoma or carcinoma of the urogenital system.

H. **Peutz-Jeghers syndrome** is an autosomal dominant disorder caused by germline mutations or epigenetic silencing of the serine/threonine kinase LKB1 (also known as STK11). It is characterized by skin and mucosal hyperpigmentation (perioral blue-black freckling), and development of multiple intestinal polyps that can transform into GI adenocarcinoma.

I. **Von Recklinghausen's disease (neurofibromatosis type 1)** is inherited as an autosomal-dominant condition caused by mutations in the tumor suppressor gene NF1. About one-half of affected individuals inherit the gene from an affected parent with the remainder of cases caused by spontaneous mutation. Hyperpigmented, oval-shaped macules with smooth borders (café au lait spots) are seen in the early childhood. Other skin lesions include freckling in non–sun-exposed areas, iris hamartomas, and cutaneous neurofibromas. Individuals with von Recklinghausen's disease have an increased risk of malignancy compared with the general population. A 10% lifetime risk exists of malignant peripheral nerve sheath tumors. Other malignancies (pheochromocytoma, urogenital rhabdomyosarcoma, astrocytoma, brainstem glioma, and juvenile chronic myelogenous leukemia) are seen less frequently.

J. Werner's syndrome is an autosomal recessive disorder caused by mutations in the WRN gene, which is involved in abnormal telomere maintenance. It is characterized by premature aging and by early onset of age-related pathologies (alopecia, ischemic heart disease, osteoporosis, cataracts diabetes mellitus, hypogonadism) and cancer (especially sarcomas).

K. Wiskott-Aldrich syndrome is an X-linked immunodeficiency disease caused by mutations in the WAS gene, which has a key role in actin polymerization. Its clinical phenotype includes thrombocytopenia with small platelets, typical in appearance and distribution eczema, recurrent infections caused by immunodeficiency, and an increased incidence of autoimmune manifestations and malignancies. The most frequent malignancy reported is B-cell lymphoma, often positive for Epstein-Barr virus.

IV. ADVERSE CUTANEOUS EFFECTS OF RADIATION THERAPY (RT)

Despite continuous improvement in methods of delivery of RT, >90% of patients experience a different degree of skin reactions. The severity of skin reactions is influenced by both treatment-related and patient-related factors. Treatment-related factors include a larger treatment volume per field, a larger total dose, a large fraction size, longer duration of treatment, and type of energy used. Patient risk factors include radiation to skin areas of increased moisture and friction (axilla, breast, perineum), poor skin hygiene, concurrent chemotherapy, older age, comorbid conditions, compromised nutritional status, smoking, and chronic sun exposure.

A. Early effects are usually defined as side effects occurring within 90 days from the initiation of therapy. Erythema, dryness, epilation, and pigmentation changes occur between the second and the fourth week. Dry desquamation can develop between weeks 3 and 6 of treatment. It can also be followed by moist desquamation, which usually occurs after week 5. Finally, skin damage may progress to dermal necrosis and secondary ulceration.

B. Late effects are associated with injury to the dermis. The list includes dermal atrophy, telangiectasias, and invasive fibrosis. There may be permanent loss of nails and skin appendages, alopecia, and decreased or absent sweating. Patients treated with RT are at higher risk for development of secondary cutaneous malignancy, especially squamous cell carcinoma.

C. Prophylaxis of skin damage. To decrease the risk of skin damage, patients should wash the skin gently with lukewarm water and mild soap to keep the irradiated area clean and to decrease the risk of superimposed bacterial infection. Moreover, they should avoid rubbing the skin, should not use skin irritants or metallic-based topical agents (zinc oxide-based creams, aluminum-containing deodorants), should wear loose cotton clothing, and avoid extreme temperatures.

D. Management of skin reactions. Patients with erythema and dry desquamation benefit from use of nonscented, lanolin-free hydrophilic or moisturizing creams. These creams should not be applied to skin breakdowns. Low-dose steroids (1% hydrocortisone, mometasone furoate) decrease the degree of inflammation and pruritus. Other products (e.g., aloe vera gels, biafine, hyaluronic acid) are of no proven benefit.

No standard recommendations on treatment of moist desquamation exist, but the general principle that wounds heal more rapidly in moist environment is usually applied. Hydrocolloid dressings and hydrogels in a form of sheets or amorphous gel are frequently utilized, but no compelling evidence suggests they are better than gentian violet (often not accepted esthetically) or dry dressings.

Atrophic skin has a high predisposition for ulcers and skin breakdowns; it is mainly treated with use of ointments and avoidance of trauma. The goal of treatment of chronic ulcers is to control the amount of secretions and prevent superimposed bacterial infections. These patients may require surgical intervention. Chronic fibrosis is the most difficult complication to treat, but some responses were seen with use of pentoxifylline and liposomal superoxide dismutase.

V. ADVERSE CUTANEOUS EFFECTS OF CHEMOTHERAPY

A. **Alopecia** induced by chemotherapy usually begins 1 to 2 weeks after the initial treatment, and it becomes most prominent in 1 to 2 months. In most cases, it is reversible and hair frequently regrows with a change of color and structure. The use of cranial prostheses (wigs) and scarves should be encouraged. Chemotherapy drugs associated with alopecia are shown in Appendix B-1.

B. **Hypersensitivity reactions** have been documented with almost all chemotherapeutic agents. The types of reaction can range from urticaria, pruritus, angioedema, through erythema multiforme, up to toxic epidermal necrolysis. Cutaneous vasculitis, contact dermatitis, and exanthematous drug rashes are also not uncommon.

Asparaginase can cause reactions ranging from uticaria to anaphylactic shock in 25% of patients, and an intradermal skin testing with two units of the drug before the initial administration is generally recommended. Taxanes (paclitaxel and docetaxel) are routinely administered together with steroids, H1 and H2 blockers. In the case of paclitaxel, the reaction may be owing to polyoxyethylated castor oil that is used to solubilize the drug. Chimeric and humanized monoclonal antibodies, such as rituximab, cetuximab, alemtuzumab, gemtuzumab, and trastuzumab, are given together with diphenhydramine and acetaminophen to reduce the incidence of infusion-related reactions. Panitumumab, a fully human antibody, has been reported to cause hypersensitivity reactions in 1% of patients.

C. **Hyperpigmentation** can occur locally in the infusion site, or diffusely throughout the skin; it can also affect nails and mucous membranes. Busulfan is known to cause "busulfan tan," a dusky diffuse hyperpigmentation that may resemble Addison disease. Bleomycin is a cause of flagellate hyperpigmentation, linear, bandlike streaks of discoloration in areas of trauma predominantly on the trunk and the proximal extremities. Repetitive administration of fluorouracil results in serpentine supravenous hyperpigmentation of the skin overlying veins. Methotrexate given weekly can cause the "flag sign," the hyperpigmented bands alternating with the normal color of the patient's hair. Other drugs that can result in hyperpigmentation include cisplatin, cyclophosphamide, dactinomycin, daunorubicin, doxorubicin, etoposide, hydroxyurea, ifosfamide, nitrosoureas, paclitaxel, plicamycin, procarbazine, thiotepa, and vinca alkaloids.

D. **Hand-foot syndrome** (acral erythema, palmar-plantar erythrodysesthesia) presents initially with tingling and burning of the palms and soles that progress to severe pain, tenderness, edema, and development of well-demarcated, symmetric erythematous plaques. The lesions can spread to the dorsum of the hands and feet. Areas of pallor progress into formation of vesicles and bullae that desquamate. This syndrome is traditionally associated with use of high-dose cytarabine, fluorouracil, and liposomal doxorubicin. Currently, newer agents, such as capecitabine, which causes hand-foot syndrome of various degree in >50% of patients, and multikinase inhibitors, such as sorafenib and sunitinib, are the main causes.

Hand-foot syndrome is generally treated by cessation of the chemotherapeutic agent or a decrease in the dose. Patients are recommended to wear cotton socks or gel inserts and to avoid pressure points, to soak the affected skin in lukewarm water mixed with Epsom salts, to use urea-containing creams to remove callus build-up (prophylactic callus removal may decrease the risk of the development of hand-foot syndrome), and to apply moisturizing creams to prevent skin hardening.

Pyridoxine in doses >200 mg/day has been shown to provide symptomatic relief. Application of cold during infusion of chemotherapy may prevent acral erythema. Celecoxib at a dose of 200 mg orally twice a day may attenuate the incidence and the intensity of hand-foot syndrome in patients treated with capecitabine.

E. **Extravasation of chemotherapeutic agents** describes the process of leakage or direct infiltration of a chemotherapeutic drug into tissue. The agents are divided into three groups, based on their potential to cause local tissue injury: **vesicant drugs** (they induce the formation of blisters and ulcers and cause tissue destruction);

irritant drugs (they cause pain at the extravasation site or along the vein, with or without inflammatory response; if a large amount is extravasated they can cause ulcers, too); and **nonvesicant drugs** (they rarely produce reactions). The group of vesicant agents includes drugs with a high vesicant potential (actinomycin D, amsacrine, daunorubicin, doxorubicin, epirubicin, idarubicin, mechlorethamine, mitomycin C, vinblastine, vincristine, vindesine, vinorelbine) and with a low vesicant potential (cisplatin, dacarbazine, docetaxel, etoposide, fluorouracil, liposomal doxorubicin, mitoxantrone, oxaliplatin, paclitaxel). Irritant drugs include bleomycin, carboplatin, cyclophosphamide, carmustine, gemcitabine, ifosfamide, irinotecan, melphalan, pentostatin, plicamycin, streptozocin, and topotecan.

1. **Prevention.** All vesicant chemotherapeutics should be administered through the central line whenever possible. Central lines significantly reduce, but do not eliminate, the chance of drug extravasation. If peripheral lines have to be used, they should be used only for short infusions under direct monitoring of nursing staff. The dorsum of the hand and the areas near joints should be avoided, because extravasation can cause significant functional damage. When an IV line is placed, the vein should be accessed using a single approach and the entry site should not be covered by tape. Line patency is checked by gently withdrawing blood and administering IV fluids before a cytotoxic agent is started. Patients are asked to report any discomfort promptly.

2. **Clinical presentation.** Extravasation usually causes immediate pain, which is followed by erythema and edema within a few hours and increasing induration over a period of several days. Skin ulceration and necrosis can occur within the next 1 to 3 weeks. Necrosis can involve underlying tendon, fascia, and periostium. Occasionally, extravasation is painless, and it may be detected late, resulting in worsening of tissue damage.

3. **Management.** As soon as extravastion is noted, the drug infusion must be stopped and the affected extremity elevated. The IV catheter should not be removed immediately; it should be used for aspiration of the fluid from the site and administration of a possible antidote. If no antidote is available, the catheter can be removed.

   Never flush the line and avoid applying pressure to the area. Intermittent cooling for 24 to 48 hours with ice or cold packs is recommended in all cases of extravasation, except the vinca alkaloids and epidophyllotoxins (etoposide). Warm compresses are used for drugs from these two groups. Most clinicians also use cold compresses for paclitaxel and docetaxel extravasation, but some recommend treatment with heat.

   Patients who develop nonhealing ulcers and tissue necrosis are treated surgically. A limited number of specific antidotes is available.

   a. **Sodium thiosulfate** is used as antidote for mechlorethamine, cisplatin, and dacarbazine: 4 mL of 10% sodium thiosulfate solution is mixed with 6 mL sterile water and 2 mL for each milligram of mechlorethamine or 100 mg of cisplatin is injected through the existing IV line, followed by SC injection of 1 mL around the area of extravasation.

   b. **Hyaluronidase** (150 to 900 U through the IV line and around the site) is used for treatment of extravasation of vinca alkaloids, paclitaxel, ifosfamide, and epidophyllotoxins.

   c. **Dimethyl sulfoxide (DMSO):** 1 to 2 mL of 50% DMSO is applied topically and allowed to air-dry in patients with extravasation of anthracyclines, or mitomycin C.

   d. **Dexrazoxane** has been reported as a part of successful treatment of anthracycline extravasation.

   e. **Corticosteroids.** Despite the common use of corticosteroids, they are most probably ineffective. Hydrocortisone is recommended for the treatment of doxorubicin-induced venous flare reactions, which are more common than extravasation, and it may be helpful in cases of oxaliplatin extravasation.

F. **Acneiform rash.** Both small molecules (erlotinib) and monoclonal antibodies (cetuximab, panitumumab) that target epidermal growth factor receptor (EGFR) are associated with the development of a unique acneiform rash in up to 90% of patients. Typical lesions consist of pruritic maculopapullar eruptions that may evolve into pustules. The rash has predilection to the seborrheic areas (upper trunk, face, scalp, neck).

No standard management guidelines have been developed. Avoidance of sun exposure and use of moisturizing or colloidal oatmeal lotions are recommended. Topical clindamycin or erythromycin might be helpful, and corticosteroid use is usually discouraged. Similar rash can also be seen with imatinib.

G. Radiation reactions

1. **Photosensitivity** can be observed in patients receiving dacarbazine, dactinomycin, fluorouracil, hydroxyurea, methotrexate, mitomycin, procarbazine, and vinblastine.

2. **Enhancement of skin toxicity caused by RT** has been associated with bleomycin, dactinomycin, doxorubicin, fluorouracil, gemcitabine, hydroxyurea, methotrexate, and paclitaxel.

3. **Radiation recall** (i.e., inflammatory reaction of a previously radiated area after exposure to a chemotherapeutic agent) has been described with bleomycin, capecitabine, cyclophosphamide, cytarabine, dactinomycin, daunorubicin, docetaxel, doxorubicin, etoposide, fluorouracil, gemcitabine, hydroxyurea, lomustine, methotrexate, melphalan, paclitaxel, tamoxifen, and vinblastine.

4. **Reactivation of UV light-induced erythema** has been associated with methotrexate, gemcitabine, and taxanes.

H. Nail dystrophies. Nails are commonly affected by chemotherapy. Bleomycin, cyclophosphamide, and doxorubicin can be responsible for development of Beau lines, transverse ridgings that move distally and disappear in the treatment-free intervals. Mees lines, multiple white lines whose number correlates with the number of cycles of chemotherapy, are associated with daunorubicin. Onycholysis can result from therapy with docetaxel, doxorubicin, fluorouracil, and mitoxantrone.

I. Neutrophilic eccrine hidradenitis has a distinct histopathology consisting of neutrophilic infiltrates in eccrine glands with areas of necrosis. It appears as an erythematous eruption of hemorrhagic nodules, pustules, and plaques typically confined to the head, neck, trunk, or extremities. The rash usually presents 2 to 3 weeks after chemotherapy, and it was most frequently described with use of cytarabine, but also bleomycin, chlorambucil, daunorubicin, doxorubicin, and mitoxantrone. The eruption clears spontaneously without scar formation.

J. Eccrine squamous syringometaplasia is a rare chemotherapy-related skin eruption characterized by squamous metaplasia of the eccrine ducts, which presents as well-circumscribed erythematous macules or papules that can coalesce. It is usually located in the intertriginous areas.

Suggested Reading

Hymes SR, Strom EA, Fife C. Radiation dermatitis: clinical presentation, pathophysiology, and treatment 2006. *J Am Acad Dermatol* 2006;54:28.

Sabir S, James WD, Schuchter LM. Cutaneous manifestations of cancer. *Curr Opin Oncol* 1999;11:139.

Schwartz RA. Cutaneous metastatic disease. *J Am Acad Dermatol* 1995;33:161.

Susser WS, Whitaker-Worth DL, Grant-Kels JM. Mucocutaneous reactions to chemotherapy. *J Am Acad Dermatol* 1999;40:367.

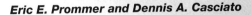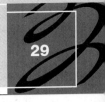

THORACIC COMPLICATIONS
Eric E. Prommer and Dennis A. Casciato

29

I. SUPERIOR VENA CAVA (SVC) OBSTRUCTION

A. Epidemiology and etiology

1. **Malignant etiologies** (85% to 95% of cases)

    a. **Lung cancer** (mainly with *small cell* histology) accounts for 80% of cases of SVC obstruction. SVC syndrome develops in about 5% of patients with lung cancer.

    b. **Malignant lymphoma** accounts for 15% of cases of SVC obstruction. Nearly all cases have high-grade histology. Hodgkin lymphoma or low-grade nodular lymphomas rarely cause SVC obstruction.

    c. **Other etiologies.** Metastatic disease (most commonly the result of breast adenocarcinoma or testicular seminoma), sarcomas, and other malignancies, such as gastrointestinal tumors, transitional-cell carcinomas, and melanomas, account for the small remainder of cases.

2. **Benign etiologies** (<15% of cases)

    a. **Mediastinal fibrosis**

        (1) Idiopathic fibrosing mediastinitis

        (2) Histoplasmosis (in endemic regions), actinomycosis

        (3) Tuberculosis and pyogenic infections

        (4) Associated with Riedel thyroiditis, retroperitoneal fibrosis, sclerosing cholangitis, and Peyronie disease

        (5) After radiation therapy (RT) to the mediastinum

    b. **Thrombosis of vena cava**

        (1) Long-term central venous catheterization, transvenous pacemakers, balloon-tipped pulmonary artery catheters, peritoneal venous shunting

        (2) Polycythemia vera, paroxysmal nocturnal hemoglobinuria

        (3) Behçet syndrome

        (4) Idiopathic

    c. **Benign mediastinal tumors**

        (1) Aneurysm of aorta or right subclavian artery

        (2) Dermoid tumors, teratomas, thymoma

        (3) Goiter, sarcoidosis

B. Pathogenesis

1. **Obstruction and thrombosis.** Tumors growing in the mediastinum compress the thin-walled vena cava, leading to its collapse. Venous thrombosis because of stasis or vascular tumor invasion often appears to be responsible for acute-onset SVC syndrome.

2. **Collateral circulation.** Vena cava obstruction caused by malignancy often progresses too rapidly to develop sufficient collateral circulation, which might alleviate the syndrome. If the obstruction occurs above the azygos vein, the obstructed SVC could then drain into the azygos system. The azygos vein, however, is frequently obstructed by malignancy below its origin.

3. **Incompetent internal jugular vein valves,** a rare occurrence, cause a dire emergency that is manifested by the filling of these veins. Approximately 10% of patients can experience a rapid demise due to cerebral edema.

C. Diagnosis. The diagnosis is usually based on the clinical findings and the presence of a mediastinal mass. CT scan evidence of collateral flow due to a mass is also supportive evidence for the presence of SVC. *SVC syndrome rarely has to be treated before a histological diagnosis is made.*

1. **Symptoms** of SVC syndrome are present for <2 weeks before diagnosis in 20% of patients and for >8 weeks in 20%.
   a. The most common presenting symptoms are shortness of breath (50% of patients), neck and facial swelling (40%), and swelling of trunk and upper extremities (40%). Sensations of choking, fullness in the head, and headache are also frequent symptoms. Chest pain, cough, lacrimation, dysphagia, mental status changes, and convulsions are less frequent.
   b. SVC obstruction may occasionally be accompanied by spinal cord compression, usually involving the lower cervical and upper thoracic vertebrae. The SVC syndrome consistently precedes spinal cord compression in these cases. The coexistence of these two complications should be seriously suspected in patients with upper back pain.
2. **Physical findings.** The most common physical findings are thoracic vein distention (65%), neck vein distention and edema of face (55%), tachypnea (40%), plethora of the face and cyanosis (15%), edema of upper extremities (10%), and paralysis of vocal cords and Horner syndrome (3%). Veins in the antecubital fossae are distended and do not collapse when elevated above the level of the heart. Retinal veins may be dilated on funduscopic examination. Dullness to percussion over the sternum may be present. Laryngeal stridor and coma are grave signs.
3. **Radiographs**
   a. **Chest radiograph** demonstrates a mass in >90% of patients. The mass is located in the right superior mediastinum in 75% of cases and is combined with a pulmonary lesion or hilar adenopathy in 50%. Pleural effusions are present in 25% of cases, nearly always on the right side.
   b. **Chest CT scan.** Contrast-enhanced CT can pinpoint the area of obstruction, the degree of occlusion, and the presence of collateral veins. CT scans show absence of contrast in central venous structures with opacification of collateral routes. It can guide fine-needle aspiration.
   c. **Superior venocavogram.** Digital subtraction angiography demonstrates the exact site of obstruction and is the procedure of choice in planning stenting procedures. This information is rarely needed for localization of RT ports.
   d. **MRI scans** of the cervical and upper thoracic vertebrae should be planned in patients with SVC syndrome and back pain, particularly in the presence of Horner syndrome or vertebral destruction on plain films.
4. **Histological diagnosis** is important for identifying malignancies that must be treated with cytotoxic agents to improve survival (e.g., lymphoma, small-cell lung cancer). After RT is started, tissue diagnosis is difficult to interpret due to nondescript necrosis from radiation. Likewise, steroids can affect histology if the underlying diagnosis is lymphoma.
   a. **Cytology** of sputum is positive in 67% of patients and of pleural effusion fluid in nearly all patients with SVC syndrome.
   b. **Bronchoscopy** and bronchial brushings are positive in 60% of patients. Bronchoscopy and bronchial biopsy are rarely associated with serious complications when performed by experienced endoscopists.
   c. **Lymph node biopsy** of palpable nodes can be helpful. Biopsy of *palpable* scalene nodes in patients with SVC syndrome reveals tumor in 85% of cases; biopsy of nonpalpable scalene nodes reveals tumors in only 30% to 40% of cases.
   d. **Transthoracic fine-needle aspiration** can be attempted for peripheral lesions that cannot easily be approached by bronchoscopy or in whom bronchoscopy results are nondiagnostic. The risk for pneumothorax is small but real.
   e. **Minithoracotomy or video-assisted thoracoscopic surgery** (VATS) nearly always results in a definitive histological diagnosis. Bleeding points are usually visualized and can be controlled.

    f. Mediastinoscopy with biopsy risks hemorrhage and other complications. However, when mediastinoscopy is performed on a highly selected group of patients, positive results are obtained in 80% of cases.

    g. Bone marrow biopsy is helpful in patients suspected of having small-cell lung cancer or lymphoma, especially in patients with cytopenia or leukoerythroblastic blood smear. It is especially useful in the young patient with a mediastinal mass.

D. Management. There is little clinical or experimental evidence that unrelieved SVC syndrome is life-threatening. Emergency treatment is indicated only in the presence of cerebral dysfunction, decreased cardiac output, or upper airway obstruction.

  1. Supportive therapy. Airway obstruction should be corrected and hypoxia treated by oxygen administration. Corticosteroids reduce brain edema and improve the obstruction by decreasing the inflammatory reaction associated with the tumor and early RT. Diuretics may be helpful.

  2. Stenting. Percutaneous placement of self-expanding metal endoprostheses gives rapid symptomatic relief in 90% to 100% of patients. When available, stenting is the procedure of choice, especially in the setting of recurrent SVC obstruction after RT. Complications are infrequent, but interventional radiologists experienced in stent placement are not universally available.

  3. RT. The total dose of RT varies between 3,000 and 5,000 cGy, depending on the general condition of the patient, severity of the symptoms, anatomic site, and histological type of underlying malignant tumor. Symptoms may resolve dramatically even without establishment of patency of the SVC.

    a. Response. Improvement is evident within 3 to 7 days for most patients. Complete response is observed in about 75% of patients with lymphoma and in 25% with lung cancer. Virtually all patients with lymphoma have at least a partial response, whereas about 15% of patients with lung cancer experience no real benefit from treatment.

    b. Median survival is about 10 months for small-cell lung cancer and 3 to 5 months for other types of lung cancer.

    c. Local relapse and recurrent SVC syndrome occur in 15% to 20% of patients but rarely after RT for lymphoma.

  4. Chemotherapy is indicated in patients with malignant lymphoma or with small-cell lung cancer. Chemotherapy is used in combination with RT in these conditions.

  5. Anticoagulants and antifibrinolytic agents may be helpful if the underlying cause of the SVC thrombosis is an indwelling catheter. These agents rarely result in disappearance of caval thrombosis but may be used in conjunction with stent placement.

  6. Surgical decompression of acute SVC obstruction and incompetence of jugulosubclavian valves consists of reconstructing or bypassing the SVC using a spiral saphenous vein graft or left saphenoaxillary vein bypass, which can be done under local anesthesia. The experience with this procedure has been mainly in SVC associated with nonmalignant causes.

II. PULMONARY METASTASES

A. Epidemiology and etiology

  1. Incidence. The lungs are the most frequent site of distant metastases for nearly all malignant tumors except those arising in the gastrointestinal tract.

  2. Dissemination. Malignant melanoma, bone and soft-tissue sarcomas, trophoblastic tumors, and renal cell, colonic, and thyroid carcinomas tend to spread to vascular routes and usually produce discrete metastatic lung nodules. Malignant tumors of the breast, pancreas, stomach, and liver may spread directly through lymphatic channels, involve mediastinal lymph nodes, and produce diffuse interstitial or lymphangitic infiltration, focal or segmental atelectasis, and pleural metastasis or effusion. Germ-cell tumors and sarcomas may also involve the mediastinum.

3. Metastatic sites
   a. Endobronchial metastasis is not uncommon in Hodgkin lymphoma, hypernephroma, and breast adenocarcinoma.
   b. Solitary pulmonary metastasis is relatively uncommon but can occur in patients with malignant melanoma or carcinoma of the breast, uterus, testis, kidney, or urinary bladder.
   c. Isolated pulmonary metastasis. Osteogenic sarcoma, soft-tissue sarcoma, and testicular carcinoma are the tumors that are most likely to have lung metastases without involvement of other organs. Renal and uterine carcinomas may also produce isolated lung metastases. Colonic adenocarcinoma and malignant melanoma rarely have pulmonary metastases without other organ involvement as well.

B. Natural history and prognostic factors
   1. Nodular lung metastases have a highly variable course ranging from slow-growing cystic adenoid carcinoma to rapidly growing teratocarcinoma and osteogenic sarcoma.
      a. Symptoms. Most patients with solitary or multiple pulmonary metastases do not have symptoms; the presence of symptoms portends a poor prognosis.
      b. Histology. Well-differentiated tumors have a better prognosis than undifferentiated tumors. Melanoma has a worse prognosis than breast, colonic, or renal cell carcinoma.
      c. Hilar lymphadenopathy worsens the prognosis.
      d. Tumor doubling time (TDT) is calculated by plotting tumor volumes against time on semilogarithmic graph paper. Pulmonary metastases with a TDT of <40 days are associated with a distinctly poorer prognosis than those with a TDT of >60 days.
      e. Disease-free interval (DFI) is the time that elapses from resection of the primary tumor to detection of metastases. Patients with long DFIs have a better prognosis than patients with short DFIs.
      f. Multiple metastases. Multiple or bilateral pulmonary nodules usually, but not invariably, have a worse prognosis than single or unilateral metastases.
      g. Amenability to chemotherapy. Responsive tumors (e.g., trophoblastic and testicular tumors) obviously have a better prognosis.
   2. Lymphangitic pulmonary metastases are rapidly lethal. Median survival <2 to 3 months for patients without effective treatment.
   3. Central pulmonary metastases. Malignant tumors that invade hilar or mediastinal structures may result in SVC obstruction, major airways obstruction, postobstructive pneumonia, and invasion of the pericardium, myocardium, or esophagus. Consequently, this type of pulmonary metastases is associated with a poorer prognosis than nodular metastases.

C. Diagnosis
   1. Symptoms and signs. Most patients with solitary pulmonary metastasis do not have symptoms. Patients with multiple pulmonary metastases; central, hilar, or mediastinal metastatic involvement; or lymphangitic metastasis are more often symptomatic with cough, chest pain, hemoptysis, or progressive dyspnea. Dyspnea out of proportion to the radiographic findings in the absence of radiological findings should raise suspicion of lymphangitic spread. Paraneoplastic syndromes such as hypertrophic pulmonary osteoarthropathy can occur with sarcoma or lung cancer. Physical examination may also be absolutely negative.
   2. Radiographic studies. No current imaging modality can distinguish a benign tumor from a malignant tumor or a primary tumor from a metastasis. Plain films do not detect lesions smaller than 1 cm in diameter. CT scans can detect nodules as small as 0.5 mm in diameter, however. About half of patients with lymphangitic lung metastases have normal chest radiographs; the remainder of patients have interstitial changes that are indistinguishable from radiation fibrosis, chemotherapy-induced lung disease, or a variety of infectious processes.
   3. Sputum cytologies are positive in only 5% to 20% of patients with nodular metastases.

4. **Pulmonary function studies.** Lymphangitic pulmonary metastases characteristically produce a restrictive defect with hypocapnia but without hypoxemia. Restrictive lung disease can be confirmed by finding impaired diffusion capacity of the lung for carbon monoxide DLco and low residual and total-lung volumes.

5. **Bronchoscopy.** Bronchoscopy with biopsy or brushings of the lesion identified on chest radiograph may be necessary to establish the diagnosis in patients with a history of malignancy (especially with tumors that do not typically metastasize to the lung), pulmonary lesions appearing 4 to 5 years after the original tumor was resected, or lesions that are likely to be a new primary lung carcinoma.

D. Management

1. **Nodular lung metastases**

   a. **Surgery.** The type of histology, number of lesions, and whether they are bilateral do not appear to contraindicate resection or adversely influence the survival if the selection criteria discussed here are adhered to. The 5-year survival rate of patients who undergo successful resection is as high as 30%. Prognosis is best for patients with a long disease-free interval (>36 months) and a solitary metastasis.

      Resection (preferably wedge resection) is the recommended treatment of pulmonary metastases in patients who meet all of the following criteria:

      (1) The patient's general medical condition and pulmonary function status are suitable for surgery.

      (2) The primary tumor is under control (no evidence of local recurrence) or controllable.

      (3) Metastases are limited to the lung (no extrapulmonary tumor exists).

      (4) Metastases appear more than 1 year after definitive treatment of the primary lesion.

      (5) TDT is prolonged (>41 to 60 days).

      (6) Complete resection is possible as suggested by CT scan.

      (7) No better method of treatment exists.

   b. **Surgical resection of metastases with specific primary cancers.** Resection of a solitary metastasis is appropriate in patients with colon, renal, and head and neck cancer, especially if they fulfill the criteria listed above for resection.

      (1) Head and neck cancers. Patients with a history of head and neck carcinoma (especially laryngeal carcinoma) and who develop a lung nodule should be approached as if they have developed a new primary lung cancer. There is no way to differentiate a solitary metastasis from a second primary cancer in these patients.

      (2) Testicular carcinoma. Solitary lung nodules in the treated patient may develop into malignant teratomas or be lesions harboring active cancer. These have to be considered for resection.

      (3) Sarcomas. Osteogenic sarcomas are best treated with preoperative chemotherapy if the tumors are multiple. Patients with sarcomas are routinely followed with CT scans of the chest, monitoring for the development of pulmonary metastases amenable to resection, because the lungs are frequently the only site of metastasis.

      (4) Breast cancer. Resection of pulmonary metastasis that are solitary in patients with a previous history of breast cancer is appropriate as 50% of these patients may have a benign lesion or a new primary lung cancer.

      (5) Melanoma. Resection of lung metastases does not appear to benefit patients with malignant melanoma.

   c. **RT** is useful for palliation of local complications of metastatic tumors, such as bronchial obstruction, vena cava obstruction, hemoptysis, or pain caused by tumor invasion of the chest wall.

   d. **Chemotherapy or hormonal therapy** can be applied in responsive tumors. Germ-cell and trophoblastic tumors can be cured despite the presence of pulmonary metastasis.

2. **Lymphangitic lung metastases** represent an emergent problem in diagnosis and management. Symptomatic relief of dyspnea can often be rapidly achieved with prednisone, 60 mg PO daily. Chemotherapy is effective in responsive tumors. Hormonal manipulation is usually ineffective or achieves a response too slowly to be helpful. Symptoms from refractory lymphangitic lung metastases may be palliated by low-dose lung irradiation.

3. **Terminal problems in patients with lung cancer** such as hemoptysis and air hunger are discussed in Chapter 5, section VI.C.

III. MALIGNANT PLEURAL EFFUSIONS

A. Pathogenesis

1. **Etiology.** Malignant tumors causing pleural effusions are as follows (in order of decreasing frequency): lung cancer (especially adenocarcinoma), breast carcinoma, lymphoma, unknown primary, gastric carcinoma, ovarian carcinoma, melanoma, and sarcoma.

2. **Types of malignant effusions.** Pleural effusions are usually caused by direct involvement of the pleura by tumor or by lymphatic or venous obstruction or both. Central effusions, particularly those caused by lymphoma or nerve-tissue tumors, may be chylous, and have high-triglyceride and low-cholesterol concentrations. Atelectasis, pneumonia, and severe hypoalbuminemia that complicates malignancy may also cause pleural effusion.

B. Natural history.
Malignant pleural effusion is a sign of advanced disease. The pleural space is progressively obliterated by fibrosis and serosal tumor. Patients with carcinomatous pleural effusions have a mean survival of 3 months from the time of diagnosis, but this varies with the underlying tumor type.

C. Differential diagnosis.
The differentiation of pleural fluid from pleural fibrosis or pulmonary consolidation may not be possible by physical examination or chest radiographs. Aspiration of fluid may be difficult because of loculation. Ultrasonography is helpful for identifying and sampling small pockets of effusion.

1. **Symptoms and signs.** Cough and dyspnea are the most common symptoms of pleural effusion. Dullness to percussion, decreased breath and voice sounds, decreased vocal fremitus, and egophony are the classic physical findings. The trachea may be shifted to the side opposite the effusion. Thickened pleura from fibrosis or neoplastic involvement also produce dullness and decreased vibration.

2. **Thoracentesis** should be performed in any patient with a suspected malignant, infectious, or empyemic pleural effusion. Pleural fluid should be assayed for protein, lactate dehydrogenase (LDH) level, specific gravity, pH, glucose, cell count, and cytology and stained and cultured for bacteria (especially mycobacteria) and fungi. If the effusion appears chylous, triglyceride and cholesterol concentrations should be measured. Malignant effusions are usually exudative but may be transudative. Results of fluid examination frequently are nonspecific.

   a. **Discrimination between transudates and exudates** is facilitated by calculating the ratios of pleural fluid/serum values. **Ratios for transudates** are <0.5 for protein, <0.6 for LDH, and >1.2 for albumin. **Ratios for exudates** are >0.5 for protein, >0.6 for LDH, and/or <1.2 for albumin.

   b. **Cytology** is positive in half of the malignant pleural effusions. Repeated cytologic analysis increases the yield if the first thoracentesis is negative.

   c. **Leukocyte counts** in malignant pleural fluid may be low or high; the predominant cells may be either neutrophils or lymphocytes. Eosinophilia is nonspecific in pleural effusions and can be associated with cancer, infection, trauma, pulmonary embolism, and even prior thoracentesis.

   d. **pH.** In patients with bronchopneumonia, a pH <7.2 at the initial thoracentesis may be predictive for the development of an empyema that has to be drained by tube. Values of <7.2, however, may also be found in patients with malignancy or collagen vascular disease.

   e. **Tumor markers** or a combination of markers have not been definitive in proving malignancy.

3. Pleural biopsy
  a. Pleural needle (Cope) biopsy is a blind procedure and is less sensitive than cytology. Among patients with a cytology-negative malignant effusion, the yield of this procedure is only about 7%.
  b. VATS is more commonly used in the United States and is usually performed by thoracic surgeons. The entire costal pleura and a good portion of the diaphragmatic and mediastinal pleura can be visualized, thus allowing direct biopsy of any pleural lesion. Although VATS is well tolerated, it does have some risks and carries with it a significant expense due to the requirement for general anesthesia and expensive instruments. On occasion, it requires conversion to an open procedure if there are significant adhesions or if there are undue risks noted with the insertion of a thoracoscope.

D. Management. Respiratory insufficiency caused by malignant effusion may be relieved by removing up to 1,500 mL of fluid by needle aspiration. The effusion should be later tapped dry if possible. Removal of excessive amounts of pleural fluid can be associated with reactive pulmonary edema. In a small percentage of patients, no recurrence of the effusion develops after a single evacuation. In most cases, the effusion recurs, and more definitive methods of therapy are required.

  1. Chemotherapy. Pleural effusion secondary to metastatic tumors that are sensitive to chemotherapy (lymphoma, breast, ovarian, or testicular carcinoma) should be treated with appropriate combinations of agents. The results may be dramatic if the effusion presents early in the disease before resistance to the chemotherapeutic drugs develops. Pleural effusions that occur in the late or terminal stage are usually resistant to chemotherapy.

  2. RT. Pleural effusions caused by mediastinal lymphadenopathy are best treated with RT.

  3. Pleurodesis (visceroparietal pleural symphysis) is accomplished with tube thoracostomy.
    a. Patient selection. Pleurodesis should be performed in patients who meet the following conditions:
      (1) The patient's symptoms (shortness of breath) are caused by the pleural effusion and not by lymphangitic or intrapulmonary metastasis (i.e., symptoms improve after aspiration of fluid).
      (2) The pleural effusion recurs after repeated needle aspirations (two times) or rapidly reaccumulates (within a few days).
      (3) The patient's life expectancy is estimated to be longer than 1 month.
    b. Drainage procedure
      (1) The chest tube is inserted in the most dependent location, preferably at the anterior axillary line. The pleural fluid is first allowed to drain through a water-seal gravity drainage system. Negative suction may be later applied to ensure completeness of drainage.
      (2) When <100 mL drains in 24 hours, a chest radiograph is obtained to assess the amount of residual fluid and the extent of re-expansion of the underlying lung.
      (3) The evacuation of pleural fluid may take 1 to 3 days. The expansion of the underlying lung is necessary to bring the visceral and parietal pleural surfaces in close proximity in preparation for symphysis. Injecting sclerosing agents without apposition of the pleural surfaces is ineffective and may result in loculation.
    c. Instilling sclerosing agents
      (1) The chest tube is first cross-clamped and is cleaned with antiseptic solution. A narcotic is given to prevent pain.
      (2) The sclerosing agent in 30 mL of normal saline is injected into the chest tube, which is then flushed with 50 mL of saline. Changing the patient's position to distribute the agent throughout the pleural space usually is not necessary.

TABLE 29.1 Drugs Used for Pleural and Pericardial Instillation	
Drug	**Dosage**
Bleomycin	1 U/kg (40 U maximum in the elderly)
Cisplatin	100 mg/m^2 (pleural)
Cytarabine	1,200 mg (pleural)
Doxorubicin	30 mg
Doxycycline	500 mg (may be repeated)
5-Fluorouracil	750–1,000 mg
Thiotepa	30–45 mg
Talc, dry powder or 50-mL suspensions	1–2 g (pericardial), 2–6 g (pleural)

(3) The chest tube should remain clamped for 6 hours for all other drugs. The pleural fluid is then allowed to drain, preferably with negative suction, until <100 mL drains in 24 hours.

(4) After a drug has been instilled, there may be a great deal of drainage because of pleural weeping from drug irritation. A nonfunctioning or blocked tube may produce complications (pain, atelectasis, and infection) and should be removed.

d. Choice of sclerosing agents. Drugs and doses used for the treatment of malignant effusions are shown in Table 29.1. These agents are successful in 70% to 85% of cases.

(1) Talc. Asbestos-free, sterilized talc may be used as a powder at thoracotomy (poudrage) or thoracoscopy (insufflation) or as a slurry through a chest tube. The last example is associated with efficacy rates of 90% to 100% in control of malignant pleural effusions.

(2) Doxycycline. Replacement of parenteral tetracycline (no longer available) for pleurodesis with doxycycline has been suggested. Studies reveal that doxycycline may require repeat installations to achieve response rates of 60% to 85% with a relatively low cost.

(3) Antineoplastic agents. Bleomycin is the most commonly used of the antineoplastic agents for control of malignant pleural effusion. It is associated with 60% to 85% response rates. This agent is nearly 50% systemically absorbed but rarely causes systemic effects. The antineoplastic agents are generally more costly than the alternatives.

e. Complications of pleural sclerosis

(1) Pneumothorax. Suction may be applied to the chest bottles to re-expand the lung if the chest tube is not blocked. If the chest tube is obliterated (no fluid oscillation), insertion of a new chest tube is indicated.

(2) Cough may result from re-expansion of an atelectatic lung after the compressing pleural fluid is removed. This symptom is self-limited and may be advantageous because it further clears atelectasis.

(3) Chest pain may be secondary to the chest tube insertion or the instillation of drugs. Pain usually dissipates within 5 days but may require opioids.

(4) Fever may be caused by atelectasis or pneumonitis or by the sclerosing agent.

(5) Loculation of fluid may be caused by inadequate drainage or the instillation of sclerosing agents before the lung has completely re-expanded. Injection of radiopaque material (Hypaque) into the pleural space followed by upright and lateral decubitus chest radiographs may confirm this problem. Trying to break the loculation by tube manipulation is not recommended.

(6) Empyema and pleurocutaneous draining sinus may occur when tumor seeds the chest tube site. Empyema may be the result of either contamination or bronchopleural communication.

4. Pleurectomy carries high morbidity and mortality and is indicated only for otherwise healthy patients in whom all of the more conservative measures have failed.

IV. OTHER PULMONARY COMPLICATIONS

A. Chemotherapy lung

1. Etiology

a. Associated drugs. Bleomycin, carmustine (BCNU), busulfan, cytarabine, mitomycin C, and methotrexate have been associated with pulmonary toxicity with significant frequency (Table 29.2. Many drugs, in a growing list of offending agents, have been associated with pulmonary toxicity rarely (see legend to Table 29.2). Most alkylating agents have been associated with the development of pulmonary fibrosis on rare occasions. The pathogenesis of these reactions is unknown.

b. Association with RT. Cytotoxic drugs and thoracic RT, administered concomitantly or sequentially, may produce pulmonary toxicity. The interaction of RT with bleomycin has been particularly well documented in patients with testicular carcinoma. Severe pulmonary irradiation reactions have been associated with concurrent doxorubicin or gemcitabine therapy, prior busulfan therapy, and concurrent or prior actinomycin D therapy; doxorubicin and actinomycin D have not been associated with pulmonary disease in the absence of RT.

2. Differential diagnosis.
Chemotherapy lung has no characteristic radiographic pattern and may be associated with a normal chest radiograph or diffuse infiltrates. Hilar or mediastinal lymphadenopathy or a purely segmental or lobar pattern should make other diagnostic possibilities more likely. Establishing the diagnosis of drug pulmonary toxicity is often difficult because cancer patients may also have pulmonary abnormalities caused by the following:

a. Chronic lung disease

b. Opportunistic pulmonary infection

c. Lymphangitic lung metastases

d. RT of the thorax

e. Pulmonary hemorrhage, collagen disease, vasculitis, or granulomatous angiitis

f. Pulmonary toxicity from oxygen therapy

g. Pulmonary toxicity from blood component therapy

h. Graft-versus-host disease

3. Diagnosis.
Drug-induced pulmonary toxicity may be insidious or acute in onset, and it rarely develops after the drugs have been discontinued. Clinical features are similar regardless of the specific drug involved.

a. Symptoms. Dry cough and dyspnea are prominent.

b. Signs. Fever, tachypnea, and rales are common. Incomplete or asymmetric chest expansion (respiratory lag) may be an early finding. Skin eruptions are common with methotrexate pulmonary toxicity.

c. Eosinophilia is often an associated finding, especially if methotrexate, procarbazine, or tretinoin have been used.

d. Chest radiographs may be normal. The most typical abnormalities are bibasilar linear densities. Nodular, interstitial, alveolar, and mixed patterns also occur. Pleural effusions are distinctly uncommon.

e. Pulmonary function tests usually show hypoxemia, a decreased D_{LCO}, and a restrictive ventilatory defect (decreased vital and total-lung capacities).

f. Lung biopsy may be necessary. Histology reveals acute and organizing interstitial pneumonia with hyaline membranes, atypical epithelial desquamation, and nodular inflammation or fibrosis. Busulfan lung toxicity may result in atypical, malignant-appearing cells on sputum cytology.

4. Management
includes careful patient selection before administering potentially pulmonary toxic drugs or using drugs that potentiate the effect of radiation. Drugs should be discontinued in patients who get symptoms and signs of toxicity, or who get significant changes in their pulmonary function tests, as in the case of bleomycin. Corticosteroids are advocated to minimize lung injury in the symptomatic patient who does not improve with drug withdrawal.

TABLE 29.2 Chemotherapy Lung

Drug[a]	Incidence (%)	Dose dependent	Onset after therapy	Reaction type[b]	Reversibility (steroids)	Risk factors[c]
Bleomycin	1–10	Yes, >450 U[d]	Immediate to months	A, B, F, H	Possible	Age >70, RT, CT, O_2, renal insufficiency
Busulfan	1–10	Yes	At least 1 yr (usually 4 yr)	F	Occasional	RT, CT
Carmustine (BCNU)	2–30	Yes, >1,500 mg[d]	2 mo to 17 yr	A, F	Rare	Pre-existing lung disease, younger age, RT, CT
Cytarabine	20	Yes	2 to 21 days (usually <6 days)	E	Uncertain	Total dose
Mitomycin C[e]	3–10	Possible	2 to 6 wk	A, F	50% recover	RT, CT, FA, O_2
Methotrexate	8	No	10 days to 5 yr	E, F, H, P	Common	CT, FA, steroid tapering, previous adrenalectomy
Chlorambucil	Rare	Yes	6 to 9 mo	A, F	Occasional	CT
Cyclophosphamide	Rare	Possible	3 wk to 3 yr	E, F, H	Common	CT, possibly RT
Procarbazine	Rare	No	2 to 6 mo	H	Possible	

[a]Cases of chemotherapy lung have also been **rarely** associated with azathioprine (A), bortezomib (A), cetuximab (A), erlotinib (A), fludarabine (A), gefitinib (A), gemcitabine (A), hydroxyurea (E), lomustine (A,F), melphalan (F), mercaptopurine (A), mitoxantrone (A), nitrogen mustard (F), teniposide, tretinoin (H), vinblastine (A), and vindesine (A).

[b]A, acute pneumonitis; B, bronchiolitis obliterans; E, pulmonary edema; F, pulmonary fibrosis; H, hypersensitivity pneumonitis; P, pleuritis.

[c]CT, combination chemotherapy regimens; RT, radiation therapy; FA, frequency of administration; O_2, oxygen administration.

[d]Pulmonary toxicity is related to the total cumulative dose.

[e]This complication occurs more frequently when vinblastine or vindesine is given with mitomycin C.

B. Radiation pneumonitis
1. **Acute radiation pneumonitis.** An acute alveolar infiltrate can develop 3 to 10 weeks after the completion of RT. Withdrawal of corticosteroids while the lungs are being irradiated or soon thereafter may precipitate this process. Pneumonitis is more frequent the higher the radiation dose and the greater the portal size.
   a. **Manifestations.** The patient usually does not have symptoms, although a dry cough, dyspnea, fever, and leukocytosis may be present. Symptoms usually subside within 2 weeks. On radiograph, the infiltrate is the shape of the RT portal, which is usually sharply outlined. Pneumonitis may progress to interstitial fibrosis.
   b. **Management.** Corticosteroids are useful in relief of symptoms of pneumonitis caused by drugs and radiation. The usual dose is 30 to 60 mg of prednisone (1 mg/kg) per day for 2 to 3 weeks with a slow taper for 3 to 4 weeks or more. Higher doses at longer periods may be needed. Antibiotics are generally not helpful unless infection is present. Opioids are reliable medications for the treatment of dyspnea and cough.
2. **Pulmonary interstitial fibrosis** may appear as early as 4 months after RT. Patients may develop restrictive lung disease, alveolar-capillary block, or cor pulmonale. Corticosteroids have an uncertain role in preventing progression of fibrosis.
C. Pulmonary tumor thrombotic microangiopathy with pulmonary hypertension is characterized by fibrocellular intimal proliferation of small pulmonary arteries and arterioles in patients with metastatic carcinoma, particularly adenocarcinoma. This condition develops when microscopic tumor cell embolism induces both local activation of coagulation and fibrocellular proliferation of intima but does not occlude the affected vessels. The increased vascular resistance results in pulmonary hypertension. This complication should be considered in the differential diagnosis in patients with known carcinoma who develop acute or subacute cor pulmonale.
D. Pulmonary infections are discussed in Chapter 35.

V. PERICARDIAL AND MYOCARDIAL METASTASES
A. Epidemiology and etiology
1. Malignant pericardial effusion is usually a preterminal event. About 10% to 20% of patients who die from carcinoma have metastases in the heart or pericardium at autopsy. The epicardium is involved in 75% of metastatic lesions, and pericardial effusions are associated with 35% of epicardial metastases.
2. Carcinomas of the lung and breast constitute about 75% of all cases of malignant pericardial effusion. Melanoma, leukemia, and lymphoma also commonly affect the heart. Pericardial effusion, which is usually insignificant, occurs in 20% of patients with non-Hodgkin lymphoma at the time of presentation.
B. Natural history
1. Most myocardial and pericardial metastases are clinically silent; about two-thirds are not diagnosed antemortem. Prognosis appears to be related to tumor type.
2. Pericardial metastases produce symptoms by causing pericardial effusion with tamponade, constrictive pericarditis, or arrhythmias.
3. Myocardial metastases produce symptoms by causing conduction blocks and arrhythmias. Metastases infrequently cause myocardial rupture, valvular disease, or emboli to other organs.
C. Diagnosis of pericardial effusion. Clinical manifestations arise from decreased cardiac output and venous congestion.
1. **Symptoms.** Frequently, pericardial tamponade develops slowly, and symptoms resemble those of congestive heart failure.
2. **Signs of pericardial tamponade**
   a. Neck vein distention that increases on inspiration (Kussmaul sign)
   b. A fall in systolic pressure of >10 mm Hg at the end of inspiration (pulsus paradoxus)
   c. Distant heart sounds with decreased cardiac impulse; possible pericardial friction rub
   d. Pulmonary rales, hepatosplenomegaly, or ascites may be seen.

3. **Differential diagnosis.** The differential diagnosis of malignant pericardial effusion includes SVC syndrome, radiation pericarditis, and a variety of nonmalignant causes of pericarditis, including myocardial infarction, connective tissue disorders, acute and chronic infections, uremia, myxedema, trauma, and drugs (hydralazine, procainamide).
4. **Diagnostic studies**
   a. **Chest radiographs** may show enlargement of the cardiac silhouette or a "water bottle" configuration.
   b. **Electrocardiogram (ECG) abnormalities** are generally not specific. Total electrical alternans involving both the P wave and QRS complex is almost pathognomonic of pericardial tamponade. Alternans of only the QRS complex is suggestive of but not specific for cardiac tamponade.
   c. **Echocardiography.** Echocardiography can detect as little as 15 mL of fluid. The findings on echocardiogram of right atrial and ventricular collapse in diastole strongly suggest tamponade.
   d. **Cardiac catheterization** is the gold standard for diagnosis and monitoring. Equalization of pressures across the chambers defines tamponade.
   e. **Pericardiocentesis.** A small catheter should be introduced through the needle into the pericardial sac and attached to water-seal gravity drainage to prevent the recurrence of effusion until the final diagnosis is made.
   f. **Fluid analysis.** Malignant pericardial fluids are usually exudative and often hemorrhagic. Fluid analysis and interpretation are the same as for pleural effusions (see section III.C.2). Cytological findings may be difficult to interpret in patients who have received RT. Negative cytological results do not exclude the diagnosis of malignant effusion.
D. **Management**
   1. **Pericardiocentesis and catheter drainage.** Conservative treatment of malignant pericardial effusion using pericardiocentesis or short-term catheter drainage as needed (with or without instillation of intrapericardial chemotherapeutic drugs) may be effective treatment for some patients. Serious complications of pericardial aspiration through a left parasternal or xiphosternal approach are rare, but they include laceration of the heart or coronary arteries, other vessels, liver, or stomach and (very rarely) a dramatic shocklike reaction. Pneumothorax and arrhythmia occur rarely. Emergency subxiphoid pericardial decompression under local anesthesia, however, is reported to be associated with no operative mortality. The drainage catheter can be left in place for several days if necessary without increased risk of infection. The catheter can be removed when drainage is <75 to 100 cc/hour. Systemic therapy should always be considered and used whenever possible.
   2. **RT** may be used in radiosensitive tumor types. Overall response rates are reported to be 60% with a dose of 3,500 cGy given for 3 to 4 weeks.
   3. **Sclerosing agents.** Chemotherapeutic drugs or doxycycline may be instilled intrapericardially to induce pericardial sclerosis and obliterate the pericardial space. Pericardial sclerosis results in decreased pericardial fluid reaccumulation in 50% to 75% of patients. The dose and method of administration of intrapericardial drugs are similar to those for malignant pleural effusion (Table 29.1). Drug instillation should be performed with ECG monitoring and an intravenous line in place in case arrhythmia develops. The development of constrictive pericarditis and refractory heart failure has been reported. There have been no trials comparing pericardial drug instillation to the creation of a pericardial window.
   4. **Pericardiectomy.** The length of hospital stay for any surgical procedure represents a major portion of the life expectancy of these patients. Surgery should be reserved for patients with (a) rapidly accumulating pericardial effusions that cannot be controlled conservatively, (b) radiation-induced constrictive pericarditis, and (c) a life expectancy of 6 months or more.
      a. **Subtotal pericardiectomy** (resection of entire pericardium anterior to the phrenic nerves) is the surgical procedure of choice in patients whose expected survival is reasonably long. Subtotal pericardiectomy is superior to the

pericardiopleural window, which may seal off shortly after surgery. Surgery may be performed by means of thoracotomy or with video-assisted thoracostomy. Success rates range from 90% to 95%.

b. Alternative surgical interventions for pericardial tamponade
- **(1)** **Percutaneous balloon pericardiotomy** proved successful in relieving the cardiac tamponade in >90% of cases with few complications.
- **(2)** **Subxiphoid pericardiotomy** was safe and efficacious in 85% of patients at 6 months.
- **(3)** **VATS** offers a minimally invasive technique for treatment of pericardial effusions but still requires general anesthesia and the ability to tolerate single-lung ventilation. VATS offers little advantage over subxiphoid pericardiostomy and should be applied in situations for which the subxiphoid approach failed.

5. Myocardial metastases. Patients with disseminated malignancy and new, unexplained cardiac arrhythmias that are refractory to treatment should be considered for cardiac irradiation, particularly if there is known mediastinal or pericardial involvement.

VI. OTHER CARDIAC COMPLICATIONS

A. Nonbacterial thrombotic endocarditis is most common in patients with mucinous adenocarcinoma of the lung, stomach, or ovary, but it can complicate any systemic cancer. Fibrin vegetations appear on heart valves that are otherwise normal. Heart murmurs and other stigmata of bacterial endocarditis usually are not present. Endocarditis is manifested by embolic peripheral or cerebral vascular occlusions that may become clinically apparent as acute peripheral arterial insufficiency, progressive encephalopathy, acute focal neurological defects suggesting a stroke, or acute multifocal neurological disease. Treatment with anticoagulants or antiplatelet drugs may be reasonable in some cases, but the results of such treatment are not encouraging.

B. Bacterial endocarditis is not more frequent in cancer patients than in the general population.

C. Radiation pericarditis and pancarditis
1. **Acute pancarditis or pericarditis** is dependent on the volume of heart irradiated and the radiation dose. This complication develops in about 3% of patients who have received >4,000 cGy to the internal mammary chain for breast carcinoma or to the mantle for Hodgkin lymphoma. Pancarditis or pericarditis can occur weeks, or even years, after treatment is completed.
   - **a. Manifestations.** Symptoms and signs resemble acute or chronic pericarditis of other etiologies: pleuritic chest pain, pericardial friction rub, ECG abnormalities, and enlargement of the cardiac silhouette on radiographs. Most patients, however, do not have symptoms. Cytological findings from irradiated mesothelium may suggest malignancy and obfuscate the cause of the effusion.
   - **b. Management.** Treatment in the acute phase includes giving corticosteroids and antipyretics and doing pericardiocentesis. The disease is usually self-limiting but may become chronic. In the chronic phase, a pericardial window for symptomatic effusions or pericardiectomy for constrictive pericarditis may become necessary.
2. **Myocardiopathy** is a rare sequela of large doses of irradiation to the heart, particularly with concomitant or prior use of doxorubicin. Refractory heart failure may result.

D. Anthracycline-induced cardiomyopathy. A major dose-limiting toxicity of the anthracyclines (doxorubicin, liposomal doxorubicin, daunorubicin, epirubicin, and idarubicin) is cardiomyopathy. Mitoxantrone appears to be less cardiotoxic and is discussed below. Proposed mechanisms of cardiac toxicity involve the generation of free radicals, which damages cell membranes through peroxidation of membrane lipids; the binding of drug to a variety of membrane sites (including cardiolipin and spectrum), which can cause alterations in membrane structure and ion transport; and the selective inhibition of cardiac muscle gene expression.

1. Types of cardiac toxicity

   a. Acute myocardiopathy is not related to total dose. Manifestations include the following:

   (1) Arrhythmias, especially sinus tachycardia, which do not correlate with subsequent development of chronic cardiomyopathy

   (2) Nonspecific ST-T–wave changes

   (3) Pericardial and pleural effusions (after 1 to 2 days)

   (4) Clinically inapparent decrease in left ventricular ejection fraction. Reversible congestive heart failure may develop after the first dose.

   (5) *Myocarditis–pericarditis syndrome:* Decreased myocardial function can be persistent in these patients.

   (6) Rarely, sudden death or myocardial infarction

   b. Chronic myocardiopathy is related to the total dose and method of administration. The overall incidence of congestive heart failure related to doxorubicin use is about 3% to 4%. The incidence is 1% to 2% for total doses of 300 mg/m^2, 3% to 5% for 400 mg/m^2, 5% to 8% for 450 mg/m^2, and 6% to 20% for 500 mg/m^2. The heart becomes dilated and may contain mural thrombi. Microscopy is nonspecific and reveals interstitial edema, cytoplasmic vacuolization, muscle fiber degeneration, and deformed mitochondria. Manifestations include the following:

   (1) Subclinical left ventricular dysfunction

   (2) Overt congestive heart failure, which usually develops within 2 months of the last dose but can occur 6 months to many years later

2. Evaluation of cardiac injury. Symptoms, physical findings, and ECG abnormalities (reduction of QRS voltage by 30%) occur too late to be helpful.

   a. Endomyocardial biopsy is the most specific method for determining anthracycline cardiotoxicity (short of waiting for overt heart failure). Semiquantitative scoring systems reveal a linear correlation of abnormalities with cumulative dose. This technique can be safely performed in an outpatient setting. Only specially trained personnel, however, can perform the biopsies and interpret the results.

   b. Echocardiogram and multigated radionuclide angiography are noninvasive methods for determining left ventricular ejection fraction (LVEF); they should be obtained at baseline, especially in patients with risk factors. Suggested intervals to repeat echocardiography are at 300 mg/m^2, 450 mg/m^2, and each 100 mg/m^2 thereafter.

3. Prevention

   a. Infusion rates. The development of cardiac toxicity is related to peak serum levels of doxorubicin. Weekly administration (20 mg/m^2) is associated with a lower incidence of cardiotoxicity when compared with monthly administration (60 mg/m^2). Continuous infusion over 24 to 96 hours through a central venous catheter also is less cardiotoxic than bolus administration; cumulative dosages much greater than 500 mg/m^2 have been administered by this technique without significant cardiac toxicity.

   b. Liposomal anthracyclines have efficacy in various malignancies (such as ovarian cancer, breast cancer, and Kaposi sarcoma) and may be used trying to decrease cardiac toxicity. One trial showed lower endomyocardial biopsy scores for those getting liposomal anthracycline as opposed to free anthracycline.

   c. Dexrazoxane (Zinecard) is a cardioprotectant that can decrease the incidence and severity of cardiomyopathy associated with doxorubicin when >300 mg/m^2 is given. It is indicated for women with metastatic breast cancer to whom >300 mg/m^2 of doxorubicin has been given and who are believed will benefit from further doxorubicin.

4. Recommendations

   a. Recognize patients who are at high risk for developing cardiac toxicity; risk factors are the following:

(1) Age >70 years

(2) Pre-existing heart disease or hypertension

(3) Prior chest or mediastinal RT (especially if >4,000 cGy)

(4) Concurrent treatment with cyclophosphamide or mitomycin C

b. Limit the total cumulative dose of doxorubicin to 450 to 500 mg/m^2.

c. Consider altering the schedule of administration (weekly or infusion).

d. If one or more risk factors (see section VI.D.4.a) are present, measure LVEF before starting treatment and after every 100 mg of doxorubicin. Discontinue the drug if the LVEF is <45% of predicted value or if the LVEF decreases by 10% on subsequent measurements.

e. If expertise in endomyocardial biopsy and interpretation are available, interpret abnormal LVEFs in the light of biopsy results.

f. Discontinue the drug at the first sign of an unexplained tachycardia, cough, dyspnea, or S3 gallop. Manifestations of congestive heart failure often do respond to therapy, but there are still a large number of patients with refractory symptoms.

E. Other chemotherapy-induced cardiotoxicity

1. Arrhythmias can be associated with the use of anagrelide, cetuximab (including cardiac arrest, particularly during the first infusion), cisplatin, interleukin-2, procarbazine, and rituximab.

2. Ischemic cardiotoxicity

a. 5-Fluorouracil can cause cardiac ischemia with angina, hypotension, or congestive heart failure. The incidence of such toxicity is uncertain but has been reported to occur in 2% to 8% of patients, particularly when the drug is given by continuous intravenous infusion in patients with a prior history of cardiac disease. These manifestations are reversible when the drug is stopped; patients respond well to conventional cardiac treatments.

b. Capecitabine therapy has been associated with observations similar to those with 5-fluorouracil.

c. Other agents associated with ischemic cardiotoxicity on rare occasions are sofafenib, paclitaxel, and vinblastine.

3. Alkylating agents

a. Cyclophosphamide can potentiate doxorubicin-induced cardiotoxicity. When given in high doses, cyclophosphamide can cause myocardial necrosis and hemorrhagic myocarditis.

b. Cisplatin has occasionally caused bradycardia, bundle branch block, and congestive heart failure.

c. Busulfan can cause endocardial fibrosis.

4. Mitoxantrone can cause a decrease in ejection fraction in 3% to 6% of patients and overt congestive heart failure in 1% to 3% of patients. This toxicity is related to cumulative dose and occurs in >10% of patients who receive >120 mg/m^2 and who have received prior doxorubicin.

5. Taxanes

a. Paclitaxel (Taxol) commonly results in asymptomatic bradycardia but can also occasionally cause conduction defects, cardiac ischemia, and ventricular tachycardia.

b. Docetaxel (Taxotere) occasionally causes pericardial effusion, but other cardiac events are rare.

6. Trastuzumab (Herceptin), which is a monoclonal antibody to the *Her2/neu* receptor, can cause decreased left ventricular ejection fraction, particularly when used with anthracyclines.

7. Tretinoin (ATRA) can cause pericardial effusions, myocarditis, pericarditis, and, rarely, cardiac ischemia.

8. Miscellaneous

a. Cytarabine has caused pericarditis and cardiomegaly rarely.

b. Interferon-α has been associated with reversible cardiac dysfunction.

Suggested Reading

Abelhoff MD, Armitage JO, Lichter AS, et al., eds. *Clinical Oncology.* 2nd ed. New York: Churchill Livingstone; 2004.

Keefe DL. Cardiovascular emergencies in the cancer patient. *Semin Oncol* 2000;27:244.

Light RW, et al. Pleural effusions: the diagnostic separation of transudates and exudates. *Ann Intern Med* 1972;77:507.

Movas B, et al. Pulmonary radiation injury. *Chest* 1997;111:1061.

Pass HI. Surgical management of pulmonary metastases. *Curr Opin Oncol* 1998;10:146.

Rashmi A, Milite F, Vander Els NJ. Respiratory emergencies. *Semin Oncol* 2000;27:256.

Shan K, Lincoff AM, Young JB. Anthracycline-induced cardiotoxicity. *Ann Intern Med* 1996;125:47.

ABDOMINAL COMPLICATIONS
Eric E. Prommer and Dennis A. Casciato

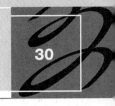

30

I. GASTROINTESTINAL (GI) BLEEDING
A. Etiology
1. **Benign causes.** GI bleeding in patients with active cancer is usually caused by erosive gastritis, peptic ulcer disease, esophageal or gastric varices, or other benign diseases; only 10% to 15% is caused by direct tumor bleeding. Hemorrhage is often related to the use of aspirin or glucocorticoids.
2. **Malignant causes.** Most primary GI cancers produce slow blood loss; massive hemorrhage is not common. Melanomas and leiomyosarcomas involving the GI tract, on the other hand, are likely to result in bleeding. Blood or clots from ostomies or mucous fistulas usually signify recurrent cancer.

B. Management
1. **Benign conditions causing GI bleeding** in patients with advanced cancer should be managed in the same way as in patients without cancer, with the following exceptions:
   a. Surgery should not be undertaken in patients who have a life expectancy of <2 months even if the bleeding is correctable.
   b. Nonsurgical therapy to control benign causes of bleeding is preferred for patients who have advanced cancer and a prognosis of >2 months, even if surgery is usually indicated. Surgery should generally be considered, however, for large gastric peptic ulcers or recurrent peptic ulcer bleeding.
2. **Patients with persistent GI bleeding from unresectable tumors** may be managed with RT. Resection of local tumor recurrence may be used if permitted by the patient's general condition.

II. BOWEL OBSTRUCTION
A. Etiology.
Bowel obstruction in patients with a history of cancer is due to the original tumor or its metastases in 60% to 70% of cases. About 20% to 30% of patients have a benign cause of obstruction, and 10% to 20% have a new, and often resectable, primary lesion. Bowel obstruction caused by malignancy occurs most often as a complication of ovarian carcinoma or GI tumors.
1. **Mechanisms** of bowel obstruction in malignancy
   a. External pressure on the intestine
   b. Obstructing masses in the bowel lumen
   c. Invasion of the intestine's neural plexus, causing localized or diffuse ileus clinically indistinguishable from mechanical obstruction
   d. Intussusception with certain tumors, notably melanoma
   e. Pseudo-obstruction as a paraneoplastic syndrome (see section IX)
2. **Differential diagnosis.** Diagnostic considerations in cancer patients include the following:
   a. **Vinca alkaloid neurotoxicity** may produce constipation. Particularly in elderly patients, paralytic ileus or decreased bowel tone may lead to high fecal impaction with bowel obstruction. Impaction is better prevented than treated.
   b. **Radiation injury of small bowel** (see section VI.C) may be seen on small bowel radiographs or CT scan as mucosal effacement, ulcers, rigidity, narrowing, adhesions, bowel wall thickening, and bowel dilation.

    c. Diverticulitis may produce tightly narrowed areas in the distal colon that are often radiologically indistinguishable from constricting carcinoma. In the absence of metastatic disease elsewhere, these lesions must be resected regardless of coexistent tumor.

    d. Other nonmalignant causes of ileus and obstruction include adhesions, hernia, inflammatory bowel disease, volvulus, spontaneous intussusception, acute pancreatitis, and bowel infarction.

B. Management of bowel obstruction caused by cancer

  1. Decompression. Patients with evidence of intestinal obstruction should have decompression by placement of a nasogastric (NG) tube and intermittent suction. Complications of prolonged NG tube use include nasal erosion and sinusitis. The goal is to use decompression with other modalities listed later to minimize time with the NG tube. In refractory cases, venting gastrostomy/ percutaneous endoscopic gastrostomy tube decompression is often the only palliative modality available when other measures fail.

  2. Stents. Expandable metallic stents have been used to treat obstruction in nearly all portions of the GI tract, including the esophagus, gastric outlet, duodenum, proximal jejunum, terminal ileum, colon, and rectum. Although stent placement requires a trained endoscopist or interventional radiologist, this procedure palliates obstruction in >80% of patients and may obviate the need for surgery in patients who cannot be cured. Complication rates are low but include bleeding, stent migration, and tumor growth into stent. Stents can be used as a "bridge" to improve symptoms while awaiting definitive treatments for obstruction.

  3. Operative intervention

    a. A history of cancer or even the presence of active tumor is not necessarily a contraindication to surgery. About 75% of patients with a bowel obstruction resume normal bowel function after surgery. Function is maintained until death in 45% of patients. About 25% of these patients do not experience improvement of symptoms with surgery.

    b. Surgical intervention should be considered if the obstruction does not improve after 4 to 5 days of decompression and if the following conditions are met:

      (1) The patient's medical condition makes the operative risk low.

      (2) The patient does not have malignant ascites.

      (3) The patient's life expectancy would be >2 months if the bowel obstruction were relieved.

      (4) The patient underwent no more than one surgical intervention for obstruction during the previous year and was significantly palliated by that operation for >4 months.

      (5) The most recent operative intervention did not disclose multiple or widespread tumor sites causing obstruction.

  4. Other modalities of management

    a. Chemotherapy may be tried in patients with obstruction caused by carcinomatosis. Specific regimens depend on the type of primary tumor.

    b. RT to relieve bowel obstruction may be beneficial in patients who have peritoneal carcinomatosis from ovarian carcinoma or extensive abdominal lymphoma that is resistant to chemotherapy. Abdominal irradiation produces severe side effects and is not recommended for other types of malignant bowel obstruction.

    c. Treatment of preterminal patients with refractory obstruction caused by cancer

      (1) NG suction is used to alleviate abdominal pain. Intravenous fluids are given to maintain hydration.

      (2) Opioids are given SC or IV for pain control.

      (3) Anticholinergic agents, such as hyoscine butylbromide, 60 to 380 mg/ day, may alleviate pain and can also reduce nausea and vomiting. Nausea and vomiting can be treated with various drugs.

(4) Metoclopramide probably should be used cautiously, if at all, in the setting of bowel obstruction because of its prokinetic effects.

(5) Haloperidol, 1 to 5 mg SC 3 times daily, is useful because of its effect on the chemoreceptor trigger zone.

(6) Dexamethasone, 8 mg/day, can help decrease edema and possibly help decrease obstructive symptoms.

(7) Octreotide, 0.2 to 0.9 mg/day SC, is an effective drug that decreases GI secretions, decreases distention, and in many cases allows the NG tube to be taken out.

III. METASTASES TO THE LIVER AND BILIARY TRACT
A. Incidence and pathology

1. Liver. The liver is a common site of metastases. Liver metastases account for more than half of the deaths in certain malignancies, such as colorectal cancer.

   a. The relative risks of tumor metastasizing to the liver during the course of advanced disease are as follows:

      (1) Liver commonly involved: GI tract cancers (including carcinoids, pancreatic adenocarcinoma, and islet cell tumors), lung cancer (especially small cell), breast cancer, choriocarcinoma, melanoma, lymphomas, and leukemias

      (2) Liver occasionally involved: carcinoma of the distal esophagus, kidney, prostate, endometrium, adrenal gland, and thyroid; testicular cancers, thymoma; angiosarcoma

      (3) Liver rarely involved: carcinoma of the proximal esophagus, ovary, and skin; plasma cell myeloma; most sarcomas

   b. Types of metastases

      (1) Nodular metastases are the most common type and occur with all tumors capable of metastasizing to the liver, including lymphoma.

      (2) Diffuse metastases most frequently occur with lymphomas. Breast cancer, small cell lung cancer, poorly differentiated GI tumors, and, rarely, other types of tumors can also produce diffuse metastases.

2. Extrahepatic biliary obstruction can occur from lymph node metastases in the porta hepatis, particularly from GI cancers and lung cancers (especially the small cell type).

B. Natural history.
The clinical course of liver metastases depends on the tumor's behavior and responsiveness to chemotherapy. In patients with solid tumors, death commonly occurs within 6 months with nodular metastases and more rapidly with diffuse metastases. A liver that appreciably increases in size in <8 weeks is typical in small cell lung cancer and high-grade lymphoma; both of these tumors respond well to treatment. Rapid liver enlargement in patients with other tumor types is less common.

C. Diagnosis

1. Symptoms and signs. Any combination of pain or discomfort in the right upper quadrant, weight loss, fatigue, anorexia, jaundice, or fever should raise the possibility of liver metastases, particularly in patients with a history of cancer. Symptoms are present in 65% of patients and hepatomegaly in 50% when liver metastases are discovered.

2. Laboratory studies

   a. LFTs should be obtained in all patients suspected of having liver metastases. An elevation of the alkaline phosphatase level that is out of proportion to that of the transaminases suggests either a mass lesion or a biliary obstruction.

   b. Liver imaging is obtained in all patients with history, physical findings, or laboratory values suggestive of hepatic metastases. Hepatic CT or MRI scans are the most sensitive techniques. Ultrasonography and ^{99m}Tc colloid liver scans have lower diagnostic accuracy. Ultrasound may be useful in determining whether a lesion is solid or fluid. The evaluation of a single focal lesion in the liver is discussed in Chapter 9.

3. **Selective hepatic angiography** is the most predictive diagnostic test to assess the presence, number, and distribution of hepatic metastases but is usually unnecessary unless an embolization procedure is planned.

4. **Liver biopsy** should be performed to confirm the presence and type of tumor in the following circumstances:

   a. There is no *primary history of cancer,* and the liver is the only obvious site of disease.

   b. There has been a *long disease-free interval* (>2 years) since the removal of the primary tumor.

   c. The liver abnormality is *not typical* of the natural history of the primary cancer. Suggestive evidence for hepatic metastases in patients with primary tumor type that does not usually metastasize to the liver indicates biopsy *if the results are likely to affect therapeutic decisions.*

   d. **Relative contraindications** for liver biopsy include the following:

      (1) Coagulation protein or platelet abnormalities

      (2) Evidence of a vascular tumor (e.g., angiosarcoma)

5. **Extrahepatic biliary obstruction.** These patients must have special studies to exclude benign causes of obstruction, such as gallstones or bile duct strictures.

   a. **CT scan** or DISIDA (diisopropyl iminodiacetic acid) scan of the liver is performed to look for parenchymal or porta hepatis masses and obstruction of the biliary tree.

   b. **Percutaneous transhepatic cholangiogram** or retrograde contrast study of the biliary tree is performed, depending on the availability of experienced radiologists and gastroenterologists.

   c. **Laparotomy** is indicated for both definitive diagnosis and treatment if the other studies suggest extrahepatic obstruction and if other sites of tumor are well controlled or not evident.

D. **Management**

1. **Surgery**

   a. **Resection of hepatic metastases** has been used in highly selected patients and should be considered, especially in patients with colon cancer and metastasis only to the liver. Modern anatomic techniques have decreased surgical mortality to <6%. Overall, in properly selected patients (those with four or fewer metastases, absence of disease outside the liver, and good performance status), 20% to 40% of patients survive 5 years. Success is greater in patients with slow-growing tumors and with a disease-free interval of >1 year. Experience with hepatic resection is greatest in patients with colon cancer.

   b. **Extrahepatic biliary tract obstruction** may be decompressed surgically if pruritus is severe. Jaundice per se is generally not an indication for surgery unless the patient must have a laparotomy for diagnosis. Biliary cirrhosis occurs only after 6 to 8 months of total obstruction, a period that exceeds the life expectancy of most patients with malignant obstructive jaundice.

      (1) Percutaneous drainage through internal or external catheter placement offers reasonable palliation. Drainage is achieved in 60% to 85% of cases. This procedure has a 25% to 40% morbidity rate and a 2.5% to 5% mortality rate. The most frequent complication is cholangitis, which appears to relate to multiple sites of obstruction or inadequate drainage. Further intervention with tube manipulation, tube replacement, or surgery is required in 20% to 75% of patients. The success rate for palliation is about 80%, similar to that achieved with cholecystojejunostomy.

      (2) Endoscopic placement of prostheses is another option that is successful in about 80% of patients. The difficulties of cholangitis from inadequate drainage result in a 2% to 5% mortality rate. Morbidity rates are similar to those associated with percutaneous procedures. Drainage is internal and more convenient for patients.

   c. **Hepatic artery ligation or hepatic dearterialization** alone or in combination with perfusion produces no significant benefit.

2. RT in low doses (<2,400 cGy) is useful to palliate refractory pain from liver metastases. RT to portal masses may relieve biliary tract obstruction. External-beam therapy is best suited for patients with a good performance status, bilirubin <1.5 mg/dL, and no extrahepatic metastasis.

3. Chemotherapy

    a. Oral and IV chemotherapy is useful for treating responsive tumors such as lymphomas, breast cancer, and small cell lung cancer. The primary tumor determines the selection of drugs. Dexamethasone (4 mg PO, IV, or SC twice daily) can reduce pain due to distention and inflammation of the hepatic capsule.

    b. Direct perfusion of chemotherapy into the liver through hepatic artery cannulation is used by some physicians to treat isolated liver metastases when no other organs are involved. The most extensively used drugs are fluorouracil, floxuridine, and doxorubicin (Adriamycin). Compared with systemic chemotherapy (including continuous peripheral venous infusion), hepatic artery infusion is associated with more responses, less systemic drug toxicity, significantly greater development of extrahepatic metastases, and no difference in survival. Complications of hepatic artery infusion include hospitalization for catheter placement and perfusion (if a portable pump is not used), hemorrhage, thrombosis of the perfused vessels, embolization, catheter displacement or breakage, catheter sepsis, GI bleeding, chemical hepatitis, acalculous cholecystitis, and biliary sclerosis.

4. Other options under investigation for hepatic metastases include selective chemoembolization, alcohol instillation, cryoablation, and radiofrequency ablation. Large randomized studies have not yet been conducted to determine whether these modalities affect survival.

IV. MALIGNANT ASCITES

A. Pathogenesis

1. Peritoneal carcinomatosis with malignant ascites is most often caused by ovarian, unknown primary, colon, gastric, and biliary tract carcinomas. The most common extra-abdominal malignancies to produce peritoneal carcinomatosis include breast and lung carcinomas. Mesothelioma is a rare cause.

2. Hepatic venous obstruction from hepatocellular carcinoma or extensive hepatic metastases from other tumors may result in ascites. Hyperviscosity states, particularly polycythemia vera, may result in the Budd-Chiari syndrome. Patients with hepatic venous obstruction have large, tender livers and rapidly evolving ascites.

3. Chylous ascites may result from obstruction or rupture of the major abdominal lymphatic passages. More than 80% of cases in adults are caused by abdominal neoplasms, usually lymphoma.

4. Peritonitis caused by *Streptococcus bovis* may be a presenting feature for right-sided colon carcinoma. Ascites from any cause may become infected.

B. Diagnosis

1. Differential diagnosis of ascites. Neoplastic diseases that cause ascites include liver metastases, peritoneal metastases, pseudomyxoma peritonei, and primary mesothelioma. The etiologies of ascites can be best classified by the serum–ascites albumin gradient, which is the difference between serum and ascitic fluid albumin concentration (Table 30.1). This gradient predicts the presence or absence of portal hypertension and, in parallel, the responsiveness to treatment with diuretics.

2. Paracentesis should be done in all patients with presumed malignant ascites for diagnosis and to rule out complicating infections. Ascites from carcinomatosis is usually exudative and often bloody. Ascitic fluid should be studied for the following:

    a. Culture for bacteria (including acid-fast bacilli) and fungi

    b. Albumin should be measured to calculate the gradient.

TABLE 30.1	Serum–Ascites Albumin Gradient

High albumin gradient (≥ 1.1 g/dL; portal hypertension likely)	Low albumin gradient (<1.1 g/dL; portal hypertension unlikely)
Massive hepatic metastases	Peritoneal carcinoma
Chronic liver disease	Peritoneal inflammation (fungal, tuberculous, vasculitic)
Hepatic vein obstruction (Budd-Chiari syndrome)	Oncotic ascites (hypoalbuminemia): nephritic syndrome, protein-losing enteropathy, chronic disease
Hepatic veno-occlusive disease	Hollow organ leak: pancreatic, biliary, ureteric, chylous
Cardiac failure	
Hemodialysis with fluid overload	
Myxedema (possibly)	Idiopathic

    c. Exudates are associated with total protein values >2.5 g/dL, white blood cell count >250/μL (lymphocytosis suggests tuberculous peritonitis), and a lactate dehydrogenase level >50% of serum values.

    d. Values in ascitic fluid significantly greater than in serum of **amylase or triglyceride** indicate a pancreatic etiology or chylous content, respectively.

    e. Glucose level is often <60 mg/dL in carcinomatosis.

    f. Fibronectin levels >75 mcg/mL in the absence of infection or pancreatic disease or carcinoembryonic antigen levels >12 ng/mL are rarely caused by benign disease.

    g. Cytology is positive in more than half of the cases of peritoneal carcinomatosis.

C. Management. With the exception of ovarian cancer–associated malignant ascites, which is treated with cytoreductive surgery and chemotherapy, management of malignant ascites is principally directed toward the palliation of symptoms.

    1. Diuretics, such as furosemide and spironolactone, may be tried but are unlikely to be effective for ascites from peritoneal carcinomatosis. Diuretics may be beneficial for patients with a high albumin gradient.

    2. Large-volume paracentesis is reserved for patients with symptoms of shortness of breath, anorexia, early satiety, nausea, vomiting, or pain. A 14- to 16-gauge plastic catheter or a peritoneal dialysis catheter can be used; the latter is preferred for removing a large volume of fluid. A single suture should hold the catheter in place.

        a. Removal of large volumes of peritoneal fluid should not be done if a hepatic cause, such as cirrhosis or Budd-Chiari syndrome, is suspected.

        b. If cancer is suspected, as much fluid as possible should be removed; nonpalpable abdominal masses may later become evident. Removal of large volumes of ascites fluid that is a result of peritoneal carcinomatosis does not usually cause dangerous fluid shifts.

    3. Systemic chemotherapy is the treatment of choice for responsive tumors.

    4. Intraperitoneal chemotherapy. Instillation of chemotherapy directly into the abdomen may control some malignant effusions. The abdomen is drained to be as dry as possible, preferably using a peritoneal dialysis catheter. The chosen drug is dissolved in 100 mL of normal saline, injected into the catheter, and followed by another 100 mL of normal saline for flushing. The patient's position is shifted every few minutes for an hour to disperse the drug. If treatment is effective, the dose may be repeated at intervals. Fever or abdominal pain or tenderness may develop after the procedure, may persist for up to 1 week, and may require paracentesis to confirm that the peritonitis is sterile.

        a. Effective agents include bleomycin (15 units), 5-fluorouracil (1,000 mg), thiotepa (45 mg), doxorubicin (30 mg), cisplatin (various doses), and mitoxantrone (10 mg).

    b. Radioactive phosphorus may be tried, but leakage of the radioisotope through the needle tract is a major problem. Radioactive gold and vesicant drugs, such as nitrogen mustard, are extremely hazardous and can cause bowel necrosis, especially if the fluid is loculated.

  5. Peritoneovenous shunts (LeVeen and Denver) may be used to treat refractory cases if the patient has a life expectancy of >1 month and does not have significant cardiac or renal disease or disseminated intravascular coagulation (DIC). The ascitic fluid should not be hemorrhagic, infected, or loculated, and it should not contain large numbers of malignant cells. Complications of these shunts include primary fibrinolysis or clinically silent DIC (virtually 100%), sepsis (20%), pulmonary edema (15%), pulmonary emboli (10%), upper GI bleeding, fever without sepsis, superior vena cava thrombosis, pneumonia, shunt displacement, seromas around the catheter (10%), and neoplastic seeding to the superior vena cava on adjacent subcutaneous tissues. Thrombocytopenia is caused by both DIC and hemodilution. There is no evidence that shunts improve quality of life.

  6. Pseudomyxoma peritonei. Mucinous adenocarcinomas, benign mucin-producing tumors, and appendiceal mucoceles can produce abundant gelatinous material that is impossible to remove by paracentesis. Recurrent bowel obstruction and progressive ascites develop. Laparotomy with removal of as much of the jelly-like substance as possible is indicated. The procedure may be repeated if there is recurrence, depending on the changing anatomy and formation of adhesions.

V. PANCREATITIS AND METASTASES TO THE PANCREAS

  A. Etiology. Pancreatitis rarely complicates primary or metastatic cancer of the pancreas. When abdominal carcinomatosis with secondary pancreatic involvement is excluded, metastases to the pancreas is rare. Small cell lung cancer metastasizes to the pancreas most commonly, but lymphoma and carcinomas of the breast, colon, and kidney do also.

  B. Diagnosis of pancreatitis depends on signs and laboratory findings. CT scan of the abdomen is the best technique to demonstrate a mass in the pancreas. Differential diagnosis includes the following:

    1. Pancreatitis associated with hypercalcemia

    2. Drug-induced pancreatitis from the following:

      a. Alcohol

      b. Glucocorticoids, indomethacin, salicylates

      c. L-Asparaginase, mercaptopurine, azathioprine

      d. Isoniazid, thiazides, oral contraceptives, certain antibiotics

  C. Management. Pancreatitis complicating metastatic cancer should be treated with analgesics. Intravenous fluids should be administered to replace losses.

VI. ADVERSE EFFECTS OF RADIATION TO THE LIVER AND ALIMENTARY CANAL

  A. Radiation hepatitis. Clinical hepatitis is uncommon at doses of <2,500 cGy to the liver. This dose is usually not exceeded except in the treatment of Wilms' tumor. Acute hepatitis from radiation can be mild to severe and may result in cirrhosis.

  1. Manifestations. Signs and symptoms become evident 2 to 6 weeks after irradiation. Hepatomegaly and ascites develop. Enzyme abnormalities are indistinguishable from those in viral hepatitis. Decreased uptake of ^{99m}Tc in the treatment portal is observed on liver scan. Liver biopsy demonstrates endophlebitis with thickening and obstruction of central veins and mild cellular necrosis or atrophy, findings similar to those seen with veno-occlusive disease (VOD) induced by chemotherapy.

  2. Management is symptomatic. Corticosteroids may help.

  B. Radiation esophagitis

  1. Acute esophagitis. Transient esophageal dysphagia and odynophagia may occur toward the end of a course of RT to the mediastinum. Analgesics or viscous lidocaine solution may be helpful. Occasionally, nutritional supplementation may be required through a gastrostomy tube.

2. **Esophageal stricture** is a rare late complication that is more common when chemotherapy, particularly doxorubicin or methotrexate, is given concomitantly. Endoscopy may be needed to distinguish stricture from cancer recurrence. Dilation is performed in patients with symptoms.

C. **Radiation enteritis**

1. **Acute radiation enteritis**

   a. **Manifestations** are usually related to the volume of the bowel irradiated and to the daily dose. Most injuries involve the terminal ileum.

      (1) Nausea, vomiting, and anorexia usually do not persist >3 days after RT is stopped.

      (2) Diarrhea is more severe in patients who have had laparotomies and have developed adhesions. Symptoms can occur after the second week of RT and usually disappear within 2 weeks after its completion.

   b. **Management**

      (1) **Antiemetics** are given regularly throughout the day for patients with persistent vomiting. If symptoms are severe, parenteral hyperalimentation and reduction of the daily dose of radiation may be necessary. The serotonin antagonists are excellent agents for the treatment of radiation-induced nausea and vomiting.

      (2) **Diarrhea** is managed by eliminating alcoholic beverages, roughage, and milk products from the diet. Paregoric (tincture of opium), cholestyramine, or diphenoxylate–atropine (Lomotil) may be useful.

2. **Chronic radiation enteritis.** Abdominal pain syndromes, malabsorption, bowel strictures, hemorrhage, perforations, and fistulas usually occur with doses to the abdomen of >4,500 cGy and are more frequent in the presence of postsurgical adhesions. Symptoms may develop months to many years after completion of therapy. Parenteral hyperalimentation may be necessary while the bowel abnormality is being corrected.

   a. **Abdominal pain syndromes** are treated with analgesics, bulk laxatives, and dietary modifications.

   b. **Perforations and fistulas** indicate a poorer prognosis than strictures and hemorrhage; malignancy recurs in 70% of these patients.

   c. **Bowel obstruction.** Tube decompression may lead to resolution. Laparotomy should be avoided if possible. If the obstruction progresses, intestinal bypass (10% mortality rate) rather than bowel resection should be performed in the absence of gangrenous bowel (75% mortality rate).

   d. **Chronic diarrhea** with malabsorption is rare and is treated symptomatically. Anorexia, nausea, and vomiting may occur. Medium-chain triglycerides may be of help to decrease stool fat loss and to relieve radiation-induced intestinal lymphangiectasia with protein loss. Steatorrhea may result from bacterial overgrowth; tetracycline, 250 mg given 4 times daily, may be tried for 10 to 14 days on an empiric basis. Prednisone and sulfasalazine may also be used.

D. **Radiation proctitis**

1. **Acute transient proctitis**

   a. **Manifestations.** Tenesmus, diarrhea, and, occasionally, minor bleeding develop. Symptoms usually resolve soon after RT is completed.

   b. **Management** is usually not indicated. If symptoms are prolonged or severe, steroid enemas and suppositories, stool softeners, mineral oil, low-residue diet, or paregoric or diphenoxylate–atropine may be helpful.

2. **Late radiation proctitis** occurs 6 months to 2 years after RT.

   a. **Manifestations.** Symptoms include tenesmus, diarrhea, and hematochezia. Proctoscopic examination reveals hemorrhagic, edematous mucosa with decreased pliability, and, occasionally, ulcers.

   b. **Management**

      (1) **For severe inflammation,** treat as described for acute proctitis.

      (2) **For rectal ulcers** refractory to conservative management, surgery is advised.

      (3) **For late rectal narrowing,** treat with dilation and stool softeners.

VII. HEPATIC VENO-OCCLUSIVE DISEASE (VOD). Hepatic VOD is a nonthrombotic obliterative process of the central or sublobular hepatic veins characterized by rapid onset of hyperbilirubinemia, ascites, and painful hepatomegaly, and by varied clinical outcome.

A. Causes

1. The hepatotoxic pyrrolizidine alkaloids that occur naturally in plants (other implicated dietary contaminants include aflatoxin and nitrosamines) are the most common cause worldwide. Chemotherapy and irradiation, especially in patients who have had bone marrow or kidney transplantation and graft-versus-host disease, are important causes in the Western world.

2. Virtually any high-dose chemotherapeutic regimen can cause hepatic VOD. Azathioprine, 6-mercaptopurine (a metabolite of azathioprine), 6-thioguanine (a compound related to 6-mercaptopurine), and dacarbazine have been implicated as causes of hepatic vascular damage.

3. Other causes include postnecrotic cirrhosis, metastatic or primary hepatic malignancy, myeloproliferative disorders (particularly polycythemia vera), and a variety of other hypercoagulable states.

B. Diagnosis. The diagnosis of hepatic VOD is suggested by reversal of flow in the portal vein by Doppler ultrasound. The diagnosis is established by liver biopsy, which should be done early when hepatic dysfunction is evident because alteration of therapy may improve subsequent clinical outcome. The transvenous approach is useful for patients with thrombocytopenia.

C. Management

1. **Supportive care** is indicated because most patients recover (70%). Management of fluid balance and diuretics are useful. In those with severe VOD, modalities such as dialysis and mechanical ventilation have little impact on outcome and the continued use of these modalities will have to be discussed based on the overall prognosis of the patient.

2. **Thrombolytic therapy with tissue plasminogen activator (** tPA) has efficacy, even in severe VOD. The use of tPA/heparin must be balanced against the risk of bleeding. The dose of tPA is 20 mg on 4 consecutive days along with heparin at 150 U/kg/day.

3. **Liver transplant** for severe VOD has been tried in patients where the underlying disease has a good chance of being cured with cytoreductive therapy.

4. **Other surgical procedures,** such as peritoneovenous or intrahepatic shunts, have had variable outcomes with VOD.

VIII. CHEMOTHERAPY DOSE MODIFICATION FOR LIVER DYSFUNCTION is shown in Appendix B-1.

IX. PARANEOPLASTIC GI TRACT SYNDROMES. The cause of paraneoplastic gastrointestinal tract syndromes is not known.

A. Esophageal achalasia may accompany gastric cancer and is reversible when the cancer is resected. Patients present with dysphagia for all foods and liquids.

1. **Diagnosis.** The barium esophagogram reveals a large, aperistaltic esophagus. Esophageal manometry shows weak contractions with a hypertensive lower esophageal sphincter.

2. **Therapy.** Patients with achalasia and unresectable cancer must have gastrostomy, an esophageal tube (e.g., Celestin tube), or forced pneumatic dilation.

B. Intestinal pseudo-obstruction occurs in patients with peritoneal carcinomatosis in the absence of mechanical obstruction. Signs of obstruction are crampy abdominal pain, absence of stools, nausea, vomiting, hyperactive bowel sounds, and nonlocalized air–fluid levels on abdominal plain films.

1. **Diagnosis.** Pseudo-obstruction and mechanical obstruction are clinically indistinguishable. Pseudo-obstruction, however, often remits spontaneously. Hypokalemia, hypomagnesemia, fecal impaction, history of vincristine use, and other causes of ileus should be sought.

2. **Therapy** is the same as for suspected bowel obstruction (see section II).

X. SYMPTOM CARE FOR ALIMENTARY CANAL PROBLEMS is discussed in Chapter 5.

   A. Oral problems, including stomatitis, xerostomia, abnormal taste, halitosis, caked material in the mouth, and dysphagia: see Chapter 5, section II.

   B. Nausea and vomiting: see Chapter 5, section III.

   C. Colorectal symptoms, including constipation and rectal discharge: see Chapter 5, section IV.

   D. Anorexia, including hyperalimentation: see Chapter 5, section XII.

Suggested Reading

Ensimnger WD. Intrahepatic arterial infusion of chemotherapy: pharmacologic principles. *Semin Oncol* 2002;29:119.

Geoghegan JG, Scheele J. Treatment of colorectal liver metastases. *Br J Surg* 1999;86:158.

Hinson FL, Ambrose NS. Pseudomyxoma peritonei. *Br J Surg* 1998;85:1332.

King PD, Perry MC. Hepatotoxicity of chemotherapy. *Oncologist* 2001;6:162.

Malik U, Mohiuddin M. External-beam radiotherapy in the management of liver metastasis. *Semin Oncol* 2002;29:196.

Nevitt AW, et al. Expandable metallic prostheses for malignant obstructions of gastric outlet and proximal small bowel. *Gastrointest Endosc* 1998;47:271.

Parikh AA, et al. Radiofrequency ablation of hepatic metastasis. *Semin Oncol* 2002;29:168.

Prat F, et al. A randomized trial of endoscopic drainage methods for inoperable malignant strictures of the common bile duct. *Gastrointest Endosc* 1998;47:1.

Richardson P, Bearman SI. Prevention and treatment of hepatic veno-occlusive disease after high-dose cytoreductive therapy. *Leuk Lymphoma* 1998;31:267.

Sasson AR, Sigurdson ER. Surgical treatment of metastasis. *Semin Oncol* 2002;29:107.

Sussman-Schnoll F, Kurtz RC. Gastrointestinal emergencies in the critically ill cancer patient. *Semin Oncol* 2000;27:270.

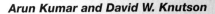

RENAL COMPLICATIONS
Arun Kumar and David W. Knutson

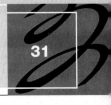

$\mathcal{C}$ ancer patients are prone to developing renal failure (especially acute renal failure; ARF). The renal failure may be due to direct or indirect consequences of the tumor, anticancer therapy, infectious complications, or complications of drugs other than chemotherapeutics. Many patients with ARF will have more than one possible cause. All three major categories of renal failure are increased: **prenal failure, obstructive uropathy,** and **intrinsic renal disease** (acute tubular necrosis, tubular interstitial disorders, and glomerulonephritis).

I. PRERENAL FAILURE
A. Pathogenesis. In all patients with prerenal failure, a decrease in effective circulating volume (ECV) leads to a decrease in renal blood flow with a consequent reversible decrease in glomerular filtration rate (GFR). Decreased ECV provides a baroreceptor-mediated stimulus for the secretion of antidiuretic hormone (ADH). The simultaneous decrease in renal blood flow stimulates the production of renin with consequent increases in circulating levels of angiotensin II (AII) and aldosterone. The combined effects of decreased renal blood flow and increased levels of ADH, AII, and aldosterone result in excretion of urine that is low in volume, is highly concentrated, and contains little sodium but relatively large amounts of potassium. Table 31.1 shows laboratory values that distinguish prerenal failure from renal failure in oliguric patients.

   1. Decreased GFR leads to a retention of urea (along with sodium) and creatinine. Reabsorption of filtered urea is increased in the proximal nephron as well as in the distal nephron due to slow tubular flow, a high concentration of urea in tubular fluid, and elevated ADH. Thus, more urea than creatinine is retained, leading to a characteristic elevated blood urea nitrogen (BUN) to serum creatinine ratio.

   2. Creatinine production is proportional to muscle mass, and urea production is dependent on protein intake, among other things. Thus, these values may be lower than normal in the wasted cancer patient who often has poor nutritional intake. In such patients, normal or borderline high values of BUN and serum creatinine may suggest significant impairment of renal function.

B. Causes of prerenal failure. Table 31.2 shows general causes of prerenal failure with specific factors that may predispose patients with malignancies to prerenal failure.

C. Diagnosis and management. The history often reveals likely causes of increased fluid loss (e.g., diarrhea, vomiting) or sequestration [e.g., congestive heart failure (CHF), ascites, and edema]. Decreased intake may be more difficult to elicit. The physical examination is of paramount importance in assessing volume status and finding clues to the pathogenesis of aberrations, as follows.

   1. Supine systolic blood pressure of <90 mm Hg, orthostatic decreases of >10 mm Hg diastolic, or orthostatic increases in pulse rate of >10 beats/minute suggest intravascular volume depletion.

   2. Flat neck veins in the supine position (in patients whose neck veins can be demonstrated by gentle occlusion) suggest volume depletion.

   3. In patients without the finding of volume depletion, careful palpation and percussion of the bladder, rectal examination of the prostate of male patients, and pelvic examination in female patients may divert attention to an obstructive cause.

621

TABLE 31.1 Distinguishing Prerenal from Renal Causes of Azotemia

Characteristic	Prerenal	Renal
Fractional excretion of sodium: $FE_{Na} = [(U_{Na} \times S_{creat}) \div (S_{Na} \times U_{creat})] \times 100$	$\leq 1\%$	$\geq 2\%$
U_{Na}	<15 mEq/L	>30 mEq/L
$U_{creat} : S_{creat}$ ratio	>40	<20
BUN : S_{creat} ratio	>20	<20
Response to fluid or loop diuretics	Positive	Negative

FE, Fractional excretion; U, concentration in urine; S, concentration in serum; Na, sodium; creat, creatinine; BUN, blood urea nitrogen.

TABLE 31.2 Cause of Decreased Effective Circulating Volume and Prerenal Failure in Patients With Malignancies

General cause	Predisposing factors in patients with malignancies
Hypovolemia	
Decreased intake	Anorexia from malignancy or chemotherapy, intercurrent illness, obtundation, neglect
Increased loss	
Vomiting	Intestinal obstruction, chemotherapy
Diarrhea	Enteral hyperalimentation, carcinoid, VIPoma, chomotherapy, antibiotic-associated
Blood loss	Tumor- or chemotherapy-related
Renal	
Diabetes insipidus (DI)	Primary pineal tumor, craniopharyngioma, metastasis (breast cancer)
Nephrogenic DI	Chronic renal insufficiency, myeloma kidney, lithium, demeclocycline, nephrocalcinosis
Osmotic diuresis	Hypercalcemia, hyperglycemia
Hypoalbuminemia	Poor nutrition, severe liver disease, nephrotic syndrome
Intra- & extravascular shifts	
Congestive heart failure, low cardiac output	Malignant pericardial effusion, radiation-induced pericarditis or myocarditis
Sepsis, shock	Lymphoma, leukemia, myeloma, neutropenia due to chemotherapy
Decreased renal blood flow per se	
Renal artery obstruction	
Intrinsic	Renal artery stenosis, atheroemboli
Extrinsic	Tumor (rare)
Hepatorenal syndrome	Hepatic metastases
Drugs	Angiotensin-converting enzyme inhibitors, cyclosporine, tacrolimus, nonsteroidal anti-inflammatory drugs (NSAIDs), angiotensin receptor blockers

4. **Occult prerenal failure** may be present that escapes detection by any of the above measures. Thus, many clinical scenarios require the careful administration of a fluid challenge. In the absence of clear physical findings of fluid overload, 1 L of normal saline can be safely administered to most normal-sized adults without untoward effect. Often, a gratifying increase in urinary output results, and BUN and serum creatinine values subsequently return to normal.

5. **Loop diuretics** given as an intravenous challenge are often used in acutely oliguric patients. An increased urinary output suggests that obstruction is not present and that the renal tubules are functioning. Such response, however, does not clarify or correct the underlying abnormality causing the initial decrease in urine production, and except for overload states such as CHF, the diuretic may make the prerenal failure worse.

6. **Overall management** of prerenal failure is to correct the underlying cause and, when possible, to restore ECV to normal. In hypovolemic patients, this usually requires large volumes of salt-containing solutions. Although albumin solutions specifically increase intravascular volume, they are expensive and the effect is often transient. Obstruction to urinary outflow should be considered in all patients who do not respond to a fluid challenge. In such patients (especially men), insertion of a Foley catheter should be performed. If the problem is still not corrected, all such patients should undergo an imaging procedure to visualize the kidneys and collecting system. Ultrasonography is often the safest and most convenient choice although computed tomography (CT) scan of the pelvis may also be useful.

II. OBSTRUCTIVE UROPATHY CAUSING RENAL FAILURE
A. Pathogenesis
1. **Ureteral obstruction.** Uremia may be caused by bilateral obstruction (or unilateral obstruction in the case of a single functioning kidney) as a result of the following:
   a. Bladder tumors and tumors of the collecting systems
   b. Uterine tumors, especially carcinoma of the cervix
   c. Retroperitoneal tumors (rare), including lymphoma, sarcomas, and metastatic tumors
   d. Intrinsic renal tumors (rare)
   e. Retroperitoneal fibrosis, including that induced by irradiation, drugs (busulfan), carcinoid tumors (especially rectal), Gardner's syndrome (intestinal polyposis), or desmoplastic reactions to metastases
   f. Nephrolithiasis
   g. Blood clots
2. **Outlet obstruction of the urethra.** Causes include primary cancer of the prostate, urethra, cervix, ovary, bladder, or endometrium. Metastases from the lung, gastrointestinal tract, breast, and melanoma to the pelvic organs, prostate, or urethra are rare causes of this complication.

B. Diagnosis
1. **Symptoms** are often absent or insidious in onset. Anuria is highly suggestive, but partial high-grade obstruction of ureters can occasionally cause renal failure with a normal urine volume. A variable urine output or overflow incontinence causing dribbling (and the strong smell of urine during physical examination) suggests bladder outlet obstruction.
2. **Physical findings** are those of the underlying disease. Dullness to percussion in the suprapubic region suggests a mass or distended bladder.
3. **Postvoid residual urine** determination is often useful in evaluating for outlet obstruction.
4. **Ultrasonography** may show hydronephrosis. However, acute obstruction or chronic obstruction wherein the collecting system is encased in tumor may show minimal abnormalities. A normal-appearing but full collecting system in an oliguric patient suggests obstruction.
5. **Cystoscopy** demonstrates bladder outlet obstruction, shows the extent of bladder tumors, and permits retrograde ureterography.

C. Management

1. **Obstruction of the urinary tract** accompanied by infection **above** the obstruction is a medical emergency requiring immediate drainage and intravenous antimicrobials.

2. **Stones** may pass spontaneously or can be removed by shock lithotripsy or by one of several available urologic procedures.

3. **Blood clots** in the collecting system will lyse spontaneously; larger clots in the bladder should be removed by continuous bladder irrigation and/or cystoscopy.

4. **Retroperitoneal fibrosis** may be treated by percutaneous nephrostomies or by surgical release of the involved ureters.

5. **Obstructing lymphomas** are usually successfully managed with chemotherapy, with or without focal radiation therapy.

6. **Solid tumors** usually require percutaneous catheter placement under combined ultrasound and fluoroscopic guidance. Stents placed from below are less commonly used. Systemic chemotherapy may be considered for responsive tumors. High-dose pelvic irradiation may be considered as an alternative, as may diverting ureteral surgery. Most patients with pelvic tumors causing obstruction, however, are at an advanced stage of disease; therapy, including percutaneous drainage of the renal pelvis, must be carefully considered in light of the potential for palliation, the extent of disease, and the overall prognosis.

III. INTRINSIC RENAL DISEASE CAUSING RENAL FAILURE

A. **Acute renal failure** may have an abrupt onset immediately after renal insult (e.g., radiocontrast administration). Acute renal failure may also arise more insidiously over days to weeks as an indirect consequence of malignancy (e.g., hypercalcemia, myeloma kidney resulting from deposits of Bence Jones proteins) or therapy (e.g., hyperuricemia after tumor lysis, nephrotoxicity, interstitial nephritis after administration of certain therapeutic agents).

Oliguria is often present in more dramatic episodes of acute renal failure; in this case, laboratory parameters in Table 31.1 may be useful in distinguishing it from prerenal failure. Most causes of acute renal failure and many patients with acute renal failure, however, present with normal or nearly normal urine volumes.

Although acute renal failure is often transient and reversible, certain causes can result in permanent renal failure (e.g., cisplatin toxicity, mitomycin-induced hemolytic–uremic syndrome). Drugs may cause injury to the kidney by a variety of mechanisms (Table 31.3).

B. **Acute tubular necrosis (ATN)** usually has an abrupt onset and is often oliguric. Urine specific gravity is usually near isosthenuria, and mild proteinuria is typical. ATN can often be suspected by the presence of many "dirty brown" granular casts in the urine. Usually only small numbers of white and red blood cells and tubular epithelial cells are present. Early on, the sediment may be remarkably bland. Red blood cell casts are rare.

1. **Several pathogenetic mechanisms** are recognized, and multiple mechanisms may be responsible in a given patient. Direct tubular toxicity is likely the mechanism for ATN as a result of aminoglycosides and many chemotherapeutic agents (see Table 31.3). Intratubular obstruction with cellular debris, protein casts, or crystal deposition (uric acid, acyclovir, methotrexate, and sulfa drugs) may play a role. Ischemic injury due to sepsis or shock is probably the most common cause.

2. **The major histological findings** are death and sloughing of tubular epithelial cells with preservation of tubular basement membranes and evidence of epithelial regeneration (mitotic figures). Proteinaceous casts and inflammatory cells may be present. Glomeruli are generally preserved. The lesion may be spotty with some nephrons appearing nearly normal. Disruption of tubular basement membranes (tubulorrhexis) and disrupted glomeruli suggest cortical necrosis, which carries a poor renal prognosis. Management includes avoidance of fluid imbalance and other supportive measures until function returns. Dialysis may be needed in some cases.

TABLE 31.3	**Drugs That Affect the Kidneys of Cancer Patients**

Acute tubular necrosis	
Antibiotics	Aminoglycosides, amphotericin, pentamidine, cephalosporin (rare), vancomycin (rare, but especially with aminoglycosides)
Chemotherapeutics	Methotrexate, cisplatin (often irreversible damage), carboplatin (especially in high doses), streptozocin and other nitrosoureas, cyclosporine (acute: hemodynamic changes; chronic: interstitial fibrosis), tacrolimus, ifosfamide (especially when combined with cyclophosphamide), interferon-α, (mainly by intravascular volume depletion), suramin, and pentostatin
Tubular obstruction	Acyclovir, methotrexate, and sulfa drugs (crystal-induced acute renal failure)
Acute interstitial nephritis	Penicillins, cephalosporins, ciprofloxacin (possibly with other fluoroquinolones as well), sulfa drugs, thiazide, furosemide, bumetanide (but not ethacrynic acid), antituberculous drugs, nonsteroidal anti-inflammatory drugs (NSAIDs, usually after 3 to 6 months of use), and allopurinol
Chronic irreversible renal failure (mild to severe)	
Acute hemolytic–uremic syndrome	Mitomycin (most often reported cytotoxic agent; potentiated by tamoxifen), cisplatin, cyclosporine, gemcitabine, streptozocin, deoxycoformycin, and interferon-α (rare)
Tubular interstitial fibrosis	Cisplatin, cyclosporine, tacrolimus, ifosfamide, carmustine, streptozocin, semustine
Fanconi's syndrome (partial or complete)	Ifosfamide, azactidine, diaziquone

3. **Radiocontrast** is a particularly important cause of acute renal failure in patients with malignancies because of the frequency with which these patients undergo radiocontrast studies. Predisposing factors include age older than 60 years, diabetes mellitus, volume depletion, other recent radiocontrast studies, high dose of contrast, concomitant nephrotoxic drug therapy, and, possibly, hyperuricemia.

4. **Prevention of ATN** is often difficult in complicated patients who may be septic or hypotensive and who may have received or require nephrotoxic drugs and/or participated in studies using radiocontrast materials. The following measures are reasonable:

   a. Avoid nephrotoxics when possible and monitor drug levels when such drugs are needed.

   b. Keep patients optimally hydrated with attention to intravascular volume, blood pressure, and cardiac output.

   c. Maintain high urine flow rates in patients at risk of crystal deposition in tubules, with fluids and, when necessary, loop diuretics; and alkalinize the urine for patients with rhabdomyolysis, hyperuricemia, or high-dose methotrexate therapy.

   d. Prevention of radiocontrast-induced ATN is best managed by hydrating patients and avoiding serial studies in a short period of time. Most patients can tolerate 1 L of normal saline administered intravenously over 2 to 6 hours before the procedure. Data also support the use of *N*-acetylcysteine (Mucomyst) 600 mg PO twice daily on the day preceding and the day of the procedure.

Small series suggest benefit from the selective dopamine (D1) receptor agonist fenoldopam (Corlopam) given at a dose of 1 mcg/kg/minute 1 hour prior to procedure. Animal data suggest a benefit from intravenous mannitol; however, data in humans are not compelling. The use of loop diuretics is not supported by current data. The use of low-ionic contrast has been somewhat disappointing. However, recent data with nonionic, iso-osmolar, dimeric contrast agents are more promising.

C. Tubulointerstitial nephritis occurs acutely after the administration of a growing list of drugs but can occur more insidiously after 6 to 12 months of therapy with nonsteroidal anti-inflammatory drugs (NSAIDs; see Table 31.3). The acute presentation is that of nonoliguric acute renal failure with variable systemic findings of allergic skin rash, fever, or arthralgias. Leukocytosis with eosinophilia may be seen, but pyuria with eosinophiluria is probably more common. Microscopic hematuria is a remarkably frequent finding in acute allergic tubulointerstitial nephritis.

1. **Histologically,** there is a diffuse inflammatory reaction in the interstitium, sometimes with invasion of tubules by white blood cells. Eosinophils may dominate or may be only minimally present.

2. **The renal prognosis** is good if the offending agent is discontinued. Anecdotal evidence favors the use of a short course of corticosteroids (40 to 60 mg/day of prednisone) if renal failure is severe or persists. Dialysis is only rarely required.

D. Tumor invasion

1. **Primary renal tumors** commonly invade renal parenchyma, of course, but renal failure requires extensive bilateral renal involvement and is a rare event. The more common cause of renal failure in patients with primary renal tumors is surgical ablation of renal tissue, the consequence of attempts to extirpate the tumor. Because renal cell carcinomas occur bilaterally in at least 5% of patients, preservation of renal tissue by segmental or heminephrectomy is an option to consider; it is a necessity in the patient with only one kidney if dialysis is to be avoided. Such selective ablative surgery may be impossible if tumor has invaded the renal vein (as it tends to do). Patients with renal vein involvement extending into the inferior vena cava often have degrees of renal vein thrombosis and occasionally consequent renal failure.

2. **Solid tumor metastasis** to kidneys occurs frequently late in the course of many tumors but is a rare cause of renal failure or death.

3. **Lymphoproliferative tumors.** Renal involvement is common in acute lymphoblastic leukemia (about half of the cases) and lymphoma. Renal failure is less common but does occur. Urinary findings include mild proteinuria, hematuria, and often tumor cells that, when present, are highly suggestive of renal invasion. Imaging studies show large, poorly functioning kidneys without hydronephrosis. Treatment with local irradiation or chemotherapy is associated with resolution of renal failure and diminution of renal size to or toward normal; both abnormalities may recur with recurrence of the tumor.

4. **Retinoic acid syndrome.** Leukocytes may infiltrate the kidney and cause ARF as part of the retinoic acid syndrome, which is caused by the treatment of acute promyelocytic leukemia with all-*trans*-retinoic acid (see Chapter 25, section VII.D). The syndrome responds to corticosteroids.

E. Acute glomerulonephritis causing renal failure is as rare in patients with underlying malignancies as it is in the general population. Certain lymphoproliferative disorders may result in mixed cryoglobulinemia that can cause rapidly progressive (crescentic) glomerulonephritis. Occasionally, tumor antigen interferon-α can cause membranoproliferative glomerulonephritis, both presumably by immune complex–mediated processes that can result in renal failure (see section IV).

F. Radiation nephritis can occur 6 to 12 months after doses to the kidneys exceeding 2,000 cGy as a function of dose and proportion of kidney tissue irradiated. Cases with earlier onset may manifest as severe or malignant hypertension, proteinuria of

<2 g/day, and an active urinary sediment with microscopic hematuria and granular casts. Cases occurring later mimic chronic interstitial nephritis with a bland urinary sediment, possible salt wasting, or hyporeninemic hypoaldosteronism. Treatment of either presentation involves controlling the blood pressure when elevated.

IV. **THE NEPHROTIC SYNDROME** is an unusual but recognized complication of neoplasms. The syndrome may be caused by glomerular deposits of amyloid, by the deposition of immune complexes, or by less well-defined immunologic mechanisms.

   A. **Incidence.** The incidence of nephrotic syndrome as a consequence of malignancies is unknown. From 6% to 10% of patients with nephrotic syndrome eventually manifest a malignancy, but the duration before clinical onset of the malignancy, the large number of patients with a wide variety of malignancies, and the number of isolated (single) case reports make some associations questionable.

      Accordingly, the clinical maxim that "patients older than 50 years of age with nephrotic syndrome should have a diligent search for cancer" probably overstates the case. Thus, we apply the age-appropriate cancer screening tests in nephrotic patients as would be done in the normal population. This includes a careful history and physical examination with attention to the lymphatic system, coupled with a complete blood count, chest radiograph, and stool for occult blood unless symptoms or findings suggest the need for further workup. Colonoscopy should be done in patients over age 50 years or with a family history of colon cancer. Women should undergo mammography and pelvic examination with Papanicolaou's smear as part of their routine examination.

   B. **Associations of nephrotic syndrome** exist with many malignancies, including: Hodgkin lymphoma (most common); many other lymphoproliferative disorders (including cutaneous T-cell lymphoma); thymoma; plasma cell myeloma; squamous cell carcinoma; adenocarcinomas of the lung, breast, kidney, thyroid, cervix, prostate, and gastrointestinal tract (including esophagus, stomach, pancreas, and colon); mesothelioma; and multiple melanoma. Membranous nephropathy has been frequently reported in patients undergoing graft-versus-host disease following bone marrow transplantation. The nephrotic syndrome may occur simultaneously with the clinical manifestation of malignancy. More often, what appear to be true associations of nephrotic syndrome occur months before or after the tumor manifestations, and such associations may occasionally exceed a year. Recurrence of previously treated tumor may be heralded by the return of the nephrotic syndrome by weeks or months.

   C. **Pathology** is correlated with the most common tumors (Table 31.4).

   D. **Pathogenesis.** Because of the similarity between the minimal change lesion seen in lipoid nephrosis and the lesion sometimes seen with Hodgkin lymphoma, a defect in T-lymphocyte function causing the generation of an aberrant T-cell factor (yet to be defined) has been postulated for both of these lesions. Glomerular deposition of immune complexes containing specific tumor antigens, viral antigens, and normal autoantigens has been described in single case reports regarding a number of tumors.

   E. **Management.** Remission of nephrotic syndrome may occur with partial or complete elimination of the tumor, especially in Hodgkin lymphoma. Corticosteroid therapy for tumor-associated nephrotic syndrome is usually ineffective if the tumor cannot be controlled.

TABLE 31.4   **Renal Pathology in the Nephrotic Syndrome Associated With Malignancy**

Renal pathology	Minimal change (%)	Membranous nephropathy (%)	Membranoproliferative glomerulonephritis (%)
Carcinoma	4–6	80	4–6
Hodgkin lymphoma	50–67	8–12	—
Non-Hodgkin lymphoma	33	33	33

Suggested Reading

Aspelin P, et al. Nephrotoxic effects in high-risk patients undergoing angiography. *N Engl J Med* 2003;348:491.

Kapoor M, Chan G. Malignancy and renal disease. *Crit Care Clin* 2001;17:571.

Kini A, et al. A protocol for prevention of radiographic contrast nephropathy during percutaneous coronary intervention: effect of selective dopamine receptor agonist fenoldopam. *Catheter Cardiovasc Interv* 2002;169.

Kintzel PE. Anticancer drug-induced kidney disorders. *Drug Saf* 2001;24:19.

Kintzel PE, et al. Anti-cancer drug renal toxicity and elimination: dosing guidelines for altered renal function. *Cancer Treat Rev* 1995;21:33.

Tepel M, et al. Prevention of radiographic-contrast-agent-induced reductions in renal function by acetylcysteine. *N Engl J Med* 2000;343:180.

Trish AB, et al. Presentation and survival of patients with severe renal failure and myeloma. *Q J Med* 1997;90:773.

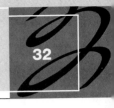

NEUROMUSCULAR COMPLICATIONS
Lisa M. DeAngelis

32

I. METASTASES TO THE BRAIN
A. Pathogenesis

1. **Incidence.** Autopsy series show that 25% of patients who die of cancer have intracranial metastases; 15% have brain metastases and 10% have dural and leptomeningeal metastases.

2. **Tumor of origin.** The tumor that most commonly metastasizes to the brain is lung cancer, which is responsible for 30% of brain metastases. Brain metastases from pulmonary tumors can occur early in the course of malignancy, and their diagnosis is synchronous (i.e., before or at the same time as the primary tumor) in about one-third of cases. Other types of tumors that commonly metastasize to the brain include renal cancer, breast cancer, and melanoma (each comprising 10% of cases), along with metastases from tumors of unknown primary sites (15%). Carcinomas of the ovary, uterus, and prostate rarely produce intracerebral metastases.

3. **Mechanism.** Tumor dissemination to the central nervous system (CNS) is usually by the hematogenous route, and the distribution of lesions parallels the distribution of arterial blood flow. Of brain metastases, 80% are supratentorial, 15% are cerebellar, and 5% are in the brainstem. However, metastases from certain primaries have a predilection for particular regions in the brain. For example, colon cancer and pelvic primaries have a propensity to metastasize to the posterior fossa, whereas lung cancer tends to metastasize to the supratentorial compartment. About one-half of the metastases are solitary, especially those from lung, renal, and colon cancers; metastases from melanoma and breast cancer are more likely to be multiple. Metastases can be solid, cystic, or hemorrhagic (especially choriocarcinoma, melanoma, and thyroid carcinoma).

B. Natural history.
Left untreated, metastatic brain tumors cause progressive neurologic deterioration leading to coma and death; the median survival time is only 1 month. About one-half of patients with brain metastases die of their neurologic disease, and the remainder die of systemic causes. Among treated patients, the overall median survival is 3 to 8 months; however, patients with limited systemic disease and one to three brain metastases can have vigorous focal treatment and survive longer, sometimes years.

C. Clinical presentation.
Metastases can cause focal or global cerebral dysfunction at presentation. Symptoms usually develop insidiously and progress over a few weeks. Occasionally, the onset is sudden when there is an acute hemorrhage into a metastatic lesion.

1. **Global signs and symptoms.** Headache and mental status changes are each seen in 50% of patients. Other nonlocalizing findings include symptoms of increased intracranial pressure, such as papilledema, nausea, and vomiting.

2. **Focal signs and symptoms,** including hemiparesis, visual field defect, and aphasia, depend on the site of metastasis.

3. **Seizures** are the presenting manifestation in about 20% of patients.

4. **Differential diagnosis.** Conditions that should be considered in the differential diagnosis of brain metastasis include the following:
   a. **Metabolic encephalopathy,** including hyponatremia, hypercalcemia, hypoxemia, uremia, hepatic encephalopathy, and hypothyroidism

629

b. **Drug-induced encephalopathy** from analgesics, sedatives, steroids, chemotherapeutic agents, and other drugs

c. **CNS infections,** including bacterial and fungal meningitis, herpes encephalitis, progressive multifocal leukoencephalopathy, cerebral abscess (see Chapter 35, section III.B).

d. **Nutritional deficiency,** such as Wernicke's encephalopathy

e. **Cerebrovascular disease (CVD),** including stroke, hemorrhage, and venous obstruction owing to thrombotic disorders and disseminated intravascular coagulation (DIC)

f. **Paraneoplastic disorders,** especially subacute paraneoplastic cerebellar degeneration (see section V.A)

D. Evaluation. An MRI is the optimal test to detect brain metastases. A CT scan should only be used in those patients unable to undergo MRI (e.g., pacemaker). Most metastatic tumors enhance after administration of contrast material and both a noncontrast and contrast study should be performed in every patient. Lesions detectable by CT or MRI that may resemble brain metastases include cerebral abscesses, parasitic disease, and occasionally stroke. Lumbar puncture is not useful in diagnosing brain metastases and is often contraindicated.

E. Management. The aims of therapy for patients with brain metastases are to relieve neurologic symptoms and prolong survival. Exact treatment recommendations depend on the histology of the tumor, the degree of systemic dissemination of the tumor, and the patient's clinical condition.

1. **Dexamethasone,** usually 16 mg IV followed by 4 mg PO or IV every 6 hours, results in a dramatic reversal of neurologic deficits and alleviates headaches. The effect is short-lived (weeks), however, but further improvement is possible with dose escalation and definitive treatment. Dexamethasone is unnecessary for asymptomatic patients whose brain metastases were identified on a screening MRI. In most patients, steroids can be tapered off once definitive therapy has been administered.

2. **Anticonvulsant therapy** should be administered only to patients with seizures. No role is seen for prophylactic anticonvulsants in patients with brain metastases. They do not protect against future seizures, are associated with frequent side effects, and can enhance the metabolism and thus reduce the efficacy of many chemotherapeutic agents.

3. **Radiation therapy** is the standard treatment of brain metastases. The field usually encompasses the whole brain, and doses range from 2,000 to 4,000 cGy, administered by larger fractions in the lower dose regimen.

4. **Surgery** provides a significant survival advantage for patients with single brain metastasis. Median survival for surgically treated patients is 10 to 12 months, and 12% of patients live 5 years or longer. Candidates for surgical resection should have single or possibly two brain metastases and limited or controlled systemic disease. Surgical resection is considered in other cases on an individual basis and may be influenced by the need for a tissue diagnosis. Whole-brain RT after surgical resection improves control of CNS disease but does not prolong survival.

5. **Radiosurgery** delivers a single large dose of radiation to a well-defined target; the steep dose curve of this technique ensures that little radiation is delivered to surrounding tissues. Radiosurgery can be delivered with equal efficacy by a gamma knife or linear accelerator. It is an effective, minimally invasive outpatient procedure that is a treatment option for patients with one to three intracranial metastases. Radiosurgery may be used in place of surgical resection or whole-brain radiation therapy or as an adjunct to either treatment. Local control rates appear to be equal for surgery and radiosurgery. Radiosurgery offers an advantage for metastases that are not surgically accessible, for multiple metastases, or for tumor types that are resistant to standard radiation therapy (e.g., renal cell carcinoma, melanoma) where control by radiosurgery appears to be superior. Radiosurgery must be limited to lesions ≤3 cm in diameter and can occasionally produce symptomatic radionecrosis or a prolonged dependence on corticosteroids.

6. **Chemotherapy.** Cytotoxic agents are primarily used to treat brain metastases at relapse or occasionally asymptomatic lesions found on screening MRI. Responses have been documented in patients with metastatic breast cancer, small-cell lung cancer, and lymphoma. Effective regimens are selected on the basis of the underlying primary and the patient's prior therapies. Temozolomide is effective for some patients with brain metastases from non–small-cell lung cancer and melanoma.

II. METASTASES TO THE MENINGES

A. Pathogenesis

1. **Incidence.** Leptomeningeal metastases have been demonstrated at autopsy in 8% of patients with systemic malignancy.

2. **Associated tumors.** Although any systemic tumor can metastasize to the leptomeninges, those that do so most commonly are lymphoma, leukemia (especially acute), lung carcinoma (especially small cell), breast carcinoma, and melanoma.

3. **Mechanism.** Metastasis to the leptomeninges occurs by hematogenous spread through arachnoid vessels or the choroid plexus, by infiltration along nerve roots, and by extension from brain or dural metastases. The sites of heaviest infiltration are usually at the base of the brain, the major brain fissures, and the cauda equina.

B. Natural history.
Leptomeningeal metastasis can involve any area of the CNS in direct contact with the cerebrospinal fluid (CSF). Tumor can grow as a sheet along the surface of the brain, spinal cord, cranial nerves, or nerve roots, and can also invade these structures, causing focal dysfunction. Tumor cells can obstruct the arachnoid villi and impair CSF reabsorption, causing hydrocephalus.

C. Clinical presentation.
The hallmarks of leptomeningeal metastasis are evidence of multilevel, noncontiguous neurologic signs and more neurologic findings identified on examination than the patient has symptoms. There are four basic clinical presentations that may be seen alone or in combination; meningismus is rarely present.

1. **Spinal.** At least 50% of patients with leptomeningeal metastasis have spinal symptoms. Signs and symptoms include back pain, radicular pain, weakness, and numbness (leg more often than arm) and loss of bowel and bladder control.

2. **Cerebral.** About one-half of the patients present with cerebral signs and symptoms, including headache, lethargy, change in mental status, ataxia, and seizures (partial and generalized).

3. **Cranial nerve.** Signs and symptoms include visual loss, diplopia, facial numbness, facial weakness, dysphagia, and hearing loss.

4. **Hydrocephalus.** Signs and symptoms of increased intracranial pressure include headache, decreased level of consciousness, gait apraxia, and urinary incontinence.

D. Evaluation.
The diagnosis of leptomeningeal metastasis is often strongly suspected on clinical grounds, but it can sometimes be difficult to make a definitive diagnosis. The diagnosis may be confirmed by characteristic findings on MRI or by the demonstration of tumor cells in the CSF.

1. **Imaging studies.** Contrast-enhanced MRI of the brain and complete spine should be obtained in all patients to evaluate the full extent of disease. If the patient cannot have an MRI, CT scan of the head and CT myelography of the spine can be performed. Definitive neuroimaging findings include nodules on the cauda equina, enhancement of the cranial nerves, enhancement within sulci or the cisterns, or enhancement along the surface of the spinal cord. These findings suffice to establish the diagnosis and do not require CSF confirmation of tumor cells in patients known to have cancer. Radiographic evidence of communicating hydrocephalus or brain metastases adjacent to a ventricular surface or deep within sulci are suggestive of leptomeningeal disease but require the demonstration of tumor cells in the CSF to confirm the diagnosis.

2. **CSF examination.** CSF is examined for protein and glucose concentrations, cell count, and cytology. Routine cultures should be performed because the

differential diagnosis includes chronic infectious meningitis. CSF may be obtained by lumbar puncture or, in cases of suspected spinal block, by cervical puncture under radiographic guidance. The opening pressure should always be measured to assess the intracranial pressure.

a. Routine studies. Elevated protein and pleocytosis (usually lymphocytic) are nonspecific findings that occur in about 75% of patients with leptomeningeal metastases. A low glucose concentration occurs in <25%.

b. Cytologic examination confirms the diagnosis in about one-half of patients on the first lumbar puncture. The diagnostic yield increases to about 90% by the third tap, but 10% of patients remain undiagnosed. The use of molecular diagnostic techniques, particularly for hematopoietic neoplasms, may be useful. Immunohistochemical staining and fluorescence *in situ* hybridization (FISH) to detect aneusomy of chromosome 1 may enhance the diagnostic yield. Flow cytometry studies, which evaluate DNA abnormalities and estimate the degree of aneuploidy, may also be useful in cases of suspected leptomeningeal metastasis (especially from leukemia or lymphoma) with a nondiagnostic CSF cytology.

c. Tumor markers may serve as additional diagnostic tests and are useful in following response to therapy. Tumor-specific biochemical markers include β_2-microglobulin (leukemia and lymphoma), carcinoembryonic antigen (solid tumors such as lung, colon, and breast cancer), cancer antigen 15-3 (breast cancer), human chorionic gonadotropin and α-fetoprotein (germ cell tumors), and lymphocyte markers (especially B-cell markers) to differentiate leukemic or lymphomatous cells from normal reactive T-lymphocytes. Nonspecific markers that may be elevated in a variety of tumor types include β-glucuronidase and lactate dehydrogenase isoenzyme 5; newer markers also include telomerase and vascular endothelial growth factor (VEGF).

E. Management. The optimal therapy for neoplastic meningitis has not been established. The basic premise is to treat clinically active or bulky disease with RT and to treat the remainder of the neuraxis with intrathecal chemotherapy. Systemic chemotherapy appears, however, to have an important role and may be associated with improved outcome. A response can be achieved in about one-half of patients, but the median survival is <6 months. Patients with breast cancer and lymphoma have the best prognosis.

1. Dexamethasone is of limited benefit in patients with leptomeningeal disease, except in patients with lymphoma where it acts as a chemotherapeutic agent. It should be avoided unless the patient has elevated intracranial pressure.

2. RT is limited to areas of clinical involvement and areas of bulky disease defined radiographically. The typical dose is 3,000 cGy delivered in 10 fractions. This frequently relieves pain and may stabilize the patient neurologically. Fixed neurologic deficits do not usually improve. Complete neuraxis RT is avoided because it is associated with a high morbidity, causes myelosuppression, and does not improve outcome.

3. Intrathecal chemotherapy may be used to treat the entire subarachnoid space, although intrathecal drug does not penetrate into nodules of subarachnoid disease. The drug can be administered by lumbar puncture or preferably by intraventricular reservoir (an Ommaya reservoir). The drug is usually given twice weekly until abnormal cells are no longer found in the CSF, and it is then given at progressively longer intervals. Preservative-free agents should be used. The dose is fixed and not calculated on a meter-squared basis because the volume of CSF is identical in all adults regardless of size. There must be normal CSF flow dynamics for intrathecal chemotherapy to be effective. Patients with large bulky lesions or hydrocephalus always have impaired CSF flow, and intrathecal drug should not be administered to these patients until normal CSF flow is documented by an intrathecal indium radionuclide study. Intrathecal chemotherapy can be complicated by an acute chemical meningitis or arachnoiditis. This can cause headache, nausea, fever, and neck stiffness, mimicking an infectious meningitis. Arachnoiditis may be seen with any agent but is pronounced with liposomal cytarabine (DepoCyt), and patients must be treated with corticosteroids for several days before and after each DepoCyt injection to minimize this toxicity.

    a. Methotrexate, 12 mg twice weekly followed by leucovorin rescue

    b. Cytarabine, 30 to 60 mg twice weekly

    c. Thiotepa, 10 mg twice weekly

    d. DepoCyt (liposomal cytarabine), 50 mg every other week

  4. Systemic chemotherapy has the advantage of reaching all areas of disease, penetrating into bulky lesions that intrathecal drug cannot reach, and being independent of CSF flow to reach the whole subarachnoid space. The choice of drug is based on its ability to penetrate into the CSF and on the chemosensitivity spectrum of the underlying primary. The most widely used agents are high-dose methotrexate (≥ 3 g/m^2), high-dose cytarabine (3 g/m^2), and thiotepa. A wide variety of other drugs, however, have been used effectively, such as capecitabine (Xeloda) for breast cancer.

III. EPIDURAL SPINAL CORD COMPRESSION

Epidural spinal cord compression is a neuro-oncologic emergency. Any cancer patient with back pain should receive a prompt and thorough evaluation, and those with neurologic dysfunction localizing to the spinal cord or cauda equina require emergency evaluation and treatment.

A. Pathogenesis

  1. Incidence. About 5% of patients with cancer develop clinical evidence of spinal cord compression.

  2. Distribution. About 10% of epidural metastases occur in the cervical spine, 70% in the thoracic spine, and 20% in the lumbosacral spine. About 10% to 40% of patients have multifocal epidural tumor.

  3. Responsible tumors. Any tumor can cause spinal cord compression, but lung cancer accounts for 15% of cases; breast, prostate, carcinoma of unknown primary site, lymphoma, and myeloma each account for about 10% of cases.

  4. Mechanisms. A tumor reaches the epidural space by several mechanisms. The most common is direct extension from a metastasis to the vertebral body growing into the epidural space, resulting in cord compression. Other tumors, particularly neuroblastoma and lymphoma, can grow into the spinal canal through the intervertebral foramina without destroying bone. Secondary vascular compromise can also occur, resulting in venous infarction that can cause the sudden, irreversible deterioration seen in some patients. Direct metastasis to the spinal cord parenchyma is a rare cause of spinal cord dysfunction in cancer patients.

B. Diagnosis

  1. Natural history. The progression of disease from the spinal column to the epidural space with neural encroachment is manifested clinically as local back pain followed by radicular symptoms and eventually myelopathy.

    a. The initial stage of localized pain can last for several weeks or, in tumors such as breast or prostate cancer and lymphoma, for several months.

    b. Radicular symptoms, such as pain radiating in a root distribution, usually herald further progression of the metastatic tumor but are still a relatively early symptom.

    c. Once paraparesis or ascending numbness of the legs occurs, the progression may be extremely rapid and a complete myelopathy may develop within hours. Rapid progression is especially common with lung cancer, renal cancer, and multiple myeloma.

  2. Clinical presentation depends on the level of spinal involvement.

    a. Back pain is the initial symptom in >95% of patients with spinal cord compression caused by malignancy. The pain is dull, aching, and often localized to the upper back; it typically worsens with recumbency, unlike back pain from spinal degenerative disease. Tenderness over the appropriate spinal level may be readily elicited.

    b. Radiculopathy is usually manifested by pain in a dermatomal distribution, but can also include sensory or motor loss in the distribution of the involved roots. Cervical and lumbar disease usually cause unilateral radiculopathy, whereas thoracic disease causes bilateral radiculopathy, resulting in a band-like distribution of pain. The pain from thoracic radiculopathies can sometimes be similar to pain from pleurisy, cholecystitis, or pancreatitis. The pain from cervical or lumbar radiculopathies can simulate disk herniation.

  c. **Myelopathy** can rapidly result from further disease progression. Depending on the level of spinal involvement, the signs of myelopathy include bilateral weakness and numbness in the legs and loss of bowel and bladder function. Associated neurologic findings include hyperactive deep tendon reflexes, Babinski responses, and decreased anal sphincter tone. Disease at the level of the cauda equina usually causes urinary retention and saddle anesthesia. Unusual presentations of spinal cord compression include ataxia without motor, sensory, or autonomic dysfunction. Metastasis to the spinal cord parenchyma can cause a myelopathy without back pain.

3. **Evaluation.** Because the prognosis worsens when myelopathy develops, the diagnosis of epidural metastasis should be established before the onset of spinal cord injury. The extent of workup depends on the clinician's suspicion for metastatic disease and the degree and rate of neurologic progression of the patient.

  a. **MRI** is the procedure of choice for evaluating patients with suspected cord compression. MRI defines the degree of neural impingement and the extent of bone involvement; it is noninvasive, and accurately detects other entities in the differential diagnosis of myelopathy. In addition, the entire spine can be imaged, which is essential in any patient with an epidural metastasis. Images should be obtained without gadolinium; a negative, nonenhanced spine MRI excludes epidural tumor. If leptomeningeal metastasis is a diagnostic consideration, the scan can be obtained without and with contrast, but this is not required in the emergency setting and postcontrast images can always be obtained at a later date.

  b. **CT myelography** can be used if the patient cannot undergo an MRI. If myelography shows a complete block, contrast material needs to be administered at both the lumbar and the high cervical levels to establish the extent of disease. If myelography is performed, CSF should always be sent for routine studies and cytologic examination. Myelography is contraindicated in patients with coagulopathy and may worsen a neurologic deficit below the level of a complete spinal block.

  c. **Bone scan** can identify metastatic disease to the spinal column and may suggest the level of tumor involvement. It cannot, however, visualize the epidural space and should never be done in a patient suspected of cord compression.

  d. **Plain radiographs** have no role in the assessment of epidural metastasis.

4. **Differential diagnosis**

  a. **Structural lesions.** Epidural hematoma (may occur spontaneously or after invasive procedures, especially in patients with a coagulopathy), epidural abscess, herniated disk, osteoporotic vertebral collapse

  b. **Nonstructural lesions.** Paraneoplastic syndromes (see section V), radiation myelopathy (see section VI.B.3), Guillain-Barré syndrome

  c. **Back pain** in the absence of neurologic findings in patients with normal imaging studies of the spine may be caused by leptomeningeal, lumbosacral, or brachial plexus or retroperitoneal metastases, which can be diagnosed by enhanced MRI, CSF studies, or body MRI or CT scans.

C. **Prognosis.** The outcome is greatly improved if treatment is initiated before spinal cord symptoms appear. In general, if the patient is walking at diagnosis, he or she will remain ambulatory after treatment, but if the patient is not walking at diagnosis, restoration of ambulation is less likely. Other prognostic factors include the level of spinal cord involvement and the rate of neurologic progression. Patients with breast cancer and lymphoma tend to do better because their tumors respond to therapy. Patients with lung or prostate cancer that is refractory to treatment, and who have cord compression that has progressed rapidly, tend to do poorly.

D. Management. Once the diagnosis of epidural tumor has been established, rapid therapeutic intervention is essential.

1. **Dexamethasone** is useful for alleviating neurologic symptoms and helps to control pain associated with epidural cord compression. Treatment should begin immediately, even before diagnostic studies are performed, unless the patient has lymphoma in which case corticosteroids can cause tumor regression and a false–negative finding on MRI. Dosing depends on the degree of neurologic involvement. For radiculopathy only, doses are usually 16 mg IV followed by 4 to 6 mg IV or PO every 6 hours. For rapidly evolving disease, or with evidence of myelopathy, treat with 100 mg IV followed by 24 mg IV every 6 hours. A rapid taper is essential for these high-dose regimens and should start within 48 hours.

2. **RT** has been the primary treatment for spinal cord compression. It not only retards tumor growth but also alleviates pain. RT is especially useful for tumors that are sensitive to radiation (e.g., lymphoma, breast), early and slowly progressive lesions, and metastases below the conus medullaris. The usual dose is 3,000 to 4,000 cGy over 2 to 4 weeks.

3. **Surgery** is used in the treatment of some patients with tumor metastatic to the spine. A recent randomized, prospective trial suggests that surgery followed by RT is superior to RT alone, giving significantly longer survival and better neurologic outcome, including restoration of ambulation in paraplegic patients. These operations usually involve resection of the vertebral body through an anterior surgical approach; the body is reconstructed and the spine stabilized with hardware. Patients must be in reasonable condition with controlled systemic disease to qualify for this approach. RT is performed after surgery. Laminectomy has limited value in the management of metastatic spinal disease because the tumor usually originates anteriorly and posterior decompression does not relieve pressure on the spinal cord. Other specific indications for surgery include the following:
   a. Need for a pathologic diagnosis
   b. Progression of neurologic abnormalities during RT; surgery rarely restores lost neurologic function in this situation
   c. Recurrent spinal cord compression in a previously irradiated area
   d. Spinal instability

4. **Chemotherapy** is rarely used for treatment of malignant spinal cord compression. It is occasionally used in highly responsive tumors, such as lymphoma, if neurologic involvement is limited.

IV. METASTASES TO THE PERIPHERAL NERVOUS SYSTEM

A. Brachial plexus

1. **Anatomy.** The brachial plexus is composed of the C5 through T1 nerve roots. The upper portion of the plexus (C5 and C6) innervates the proximal arm musculature and sensation to the forearm and thumb. The lower portion (C8 and T1) innervates the hand musculature and sensation to the fifth digit. In the axillary region, the lower portion of the plexus is in close proximity to the lymphatic system.

2. **Mechanism.** Tumor is most likely to involve the brachial plexus by contiguous growth from the upper lobe of the lung or the axillary or paraspinal lymph nodes. Lung cancer, breast cancer, and lymphoma are the most common tumors to cause a metastatic brachial plexopathy.

3. **Clinical presentation.** The most common presenting symptom is pain, which tends to radiate from the shoulder to the digits in a radicular fashion and is exacerbated by shoulder movement. Paresthesias and weakness, with loss of deep-tendon reflexes and evidence of muscle atrophy, occur in relation to the extent of involvement of the brachial plexus. Associated findings may include a palpable axillary or supraclavicular mass, or Horner syndrome.

4. **Differential diagnosis.** The primary differential diagnosis is radiation plexopathy in patients who have been irradiated as treatment for their primary disease

(e.g., breast cancer). Metastatic tumors tend to involve the lower trunk of the plexus because of its close proximity to lymphatic vessels, whereas RT plexopathy is more likely to involve the upper trunk. Features of both upper and lower plexus involvement are usually found, however, so this distinction is not diagnostic. Other causes of plexopathy include surgical trauma, trauma secondary to poor limb placement during anesthesia, brachial neuritis, and radiation-induced tumors of the plexus.

 a. Metastatic plexopathy is suggested by early severe pain, hand weakness, and Horner syndrome.

 b. Radiation plexopathy is suggested by absent or mild pain, weakness of the shoulder girdle, and progressive lymphedema. Often cutaneous radiation changes, such as telangiectasias, can be identified within the previous RT port.

 5. Evaluation. Imaging with CT or MRI will demonstrate a tumor mass in the plexus in most patients with metastatic plexopathy. Surgical exploration and biopsy are rarely required to confirm the diagnosis but are necessary in patients who have diffusely infiltrative disease that does not form a discrete mass. Epidural disease of the cervical or upper thoracic spine may accompany metastatic plexopathy in some patients, particularly those with Horner syndrome; therefore, additional imaging of the spine may be required.

 6. Management. The tumor is usually treated with RT if not previously administered; otherwise, chemotherapy may be helpful. The primary management problem is often pain control; neurologic function may not return even with effective treatment of the metastatic lesion. No treatment exists for radiation plexopathy. Physical therapy can help maintain residual arm and hand function after both types of plexus injury.

B. Lumbosacral plexus

 1. Mechanism. Malignant lumbosacral plexopathy is caused primarily from direct extension of intra-abdominal tumors, but 25% of cases are from metastases of extra-abdominal tumors. Nearly one-half of the patients with metastatic plexopathy also have spinal epidural disease. Radiation plexopathy can result from pelvic irradiation and present in a similar fashion.

 2. Clinical presentation. The most common presenting symptom is pain; severe, unremitting low back or pelvic pain usually radiates into one leg. Pain is later followed by paresthesias, weakness, and loss of deep tendon reflexes. Bladder function is usually preserved. Lymphedema, painless weakness, and paresthesias are more commonly seen with radiation plexopathy.

 3. Evaluation. CT or MRI scans will detect tumor involving the plexus, presacral areas, or sacral erosion. MRI of the spine may also be required.

 4. Management. RT and chemotherapy are used to treat the malignancy as indicated. Pain control and physical therapy are often required.

C. Peripheral nerves. Spread of systemic tumors to peripheral nerves is an unusual neurologic complication of malignancy. It occurs primarily in two settings.

 1. Infiltrative polyneuropathy can result from invasion of the endoneurium by lymphoma or leukemia. This syndrome is rare, even at autopsy, but produces a recognizable clinical picture. Over weeks to months, it causes a widespread, asymmetric, multifocal neuropathy, which may be fulminant in some cases and lead to death. Secondary seeding of the CSF may develop with subsequent leptomeningeal metastasis. The diagnosis is made by biopsy of an involved sensory nerve or demonstration of tumor cells in the CSF.

 2. Perineural spread of tumors is seen with cutaneous and primary cancers of the head and neck (i.e., cancers of the larynx, pharynx, and tongue). Tumors invade the perineural space, spread proximally along the nerve, and may enter the intracranial cavity and extend into the brainstem. The trigeminal and facial nerves are most commonly involved, often together, probably because of their rich co-innervation of the face. Orbital nerves may also be involved. The tumors most likely to disseminate along nerves are spindle cell variant and atypical squamous cell carcinomas. The diagnosis is based on clinical suspicion and is confirmed by biopsy of a cutaneous nerve. MRI rarely shows thickened, enhancing cranial nerves.

V. PARANEOPLASTIC SYNDROMES

Rare neuromuscular complications of cancer, paraneoplastic syndromes frequently present before the cancer is diagnosed and can be associated with neoplastic disease that is not yet radiographically detectable but is potentially curable. Patients with paraneoplastic syndromes tend to present with less extensive tumor and have a prolonged survival time compared with the standard population with the same cancer. An autoimmune pathogenesis has been demonstrated for some of these disorders, and specific antibodies are associated with many of the paraneoplastic disorders. These antibodies are generated as an antitumor response and are directed against the patient's tumor; they are thought to cross-react with specific neuronal subgroups, producing neurologic dysfunction and the clinical syndrome. It is important to realize that clinically identical disorders can occur in patients without cancer, but such patients do not demonstrate these autoantibodies.

A. **Paraneoplastic cerebellar degeneration (PCD)** is a syndrome of pancerebellar dysfunction of subacute onset. Manifestations include truncal and appendicular ataxia, dysarthria, and nystagmus; patients are usually so severely affected that they are bedridden, have unintelligible speech, and are unable to care for themselves. Associated neurologic symptoms, such as dementia or neuropathy, may be present, but they tend to be much less severe.

1. **Pathogenesis.** This disorder is associated with circulating antibodies that bind to both tumor and Purkinje cells in the cerebellum. The tumors in patients with PCD express antigens normally present only in the cerebellum, and the paraneoplastic syndrome is believed to result as a consequence of an immune response against the tumor. About one-half of the affected patients have antitumor antibodies, the most common of which is anti-Yo. Anti-Yo is seen in women with breast and gynecologic malignancies. Other antibodies that may be associated with this syndrome include anti-Hu (mostly with small-cell lung cancer), anti-Ri (breast cancer), and anti-Tr (mostly in men with Hodgkin lymphoma).

2. **Diagnosis.** The diagnosis should be suggested on the basis of the neurologic presentation. A definitive diagnosis is possible when anti-Yo, anti-Hu, or anti-Ri antibodies are detected in the patient's serum or CSF. Other diagnostic features include inflammatory cells in the CSF, normal brain scans except for cerebellar atrophy, and the absence of other causes of cerebellar dysfunction. If there is no known malignancy, a thorough search for cancer must be undertaken. Body positron emission tomography (PET) is the most sensitive test to detect these small cancers. The diagnosis is sometimes not made until autopsy, when an occult malignancy is discovered, and examination of the brain shows loss of Purkinje cells of the cerebellum.

3. **Therapy is ineffective.** Patients with PCD do not respond to plasmapheresis, immunosuppressive treatment with steroids or cytotoxic agents, or treatment of the underlying malignancy. The patient's condition usually stabilizes at a level of severe disability.

B. **Paraneoplastic sensory neuronopathy** (PSN), also referred to as *dorsal root ganglionitis*, is a syndrome of subacute progressive loss of proprioception and vibratory sense. Pain, temperature, and touch modalities of sensation are also affected but to a lesser degree. Painful dysesthesias and paresthesias are usually present. The result is a severe sensory ataxia that leaves patients unable to walk. The neuropathy may affect the autonomic system, causing urinary retention, hypotension, pupillary changes, impotence, and hyperhidrosis. Sparing of the motor system is a hallmark of the syndrome, although patients are usually so impaired that they may have mild weakness from disuse atrophy. In patients with more widespread neurologic disease, such as dementia, myelopathy, or cerebellar dysfunction, the disorder is referred to as *paraneoplastic encephalomyelitis* (PEM).

1. **Pathogenesis.** A circulating antibody, called anti-Hu (also called ANNA-1 for antineuronal nuclear antibody type 1), has been demonstrated in patients with

PSN or PEM; it is primarily associated with small-cell lung cancer. This antibody reacts with all small-cell carcinomas as well as with neurons throughout the nervous system. Clinically, the antibody mainly targets the dorsal root ganglia, causing inflammation and loss of neurons. Despite the presence of antigen in all small-cell cancers, only about 15% of patients develop the antibody and few of these patients develop the neurologic syndrome that is associated with very high titers of anti-Hu. Anti-Hu antibody is also associated with PCD and PEM, again primarily in patients with small-cell carcinoma (see parts A, E, F, and G of section V); sites of antibody binding in the nervous system roughly correlate with a patient's neurologic symptoms and signs.

  2. Diagnosis. The diagnosis is often suspected clinically because the neurologic syndrome is highly specific. Electromyographic (EMG) studies in patients with PSN usually show a total absence of sensory action potentials and normal or nearly normal compound muscle action potentials. A definitive diagnosis can be made by detecting the anti-Hu antibody in serum and CSF. CSF studies show increased protein, a mild pleocytosis, and oligoclonal bands. A thorough attempt to diagnose an underlying malignancy must be made in patients who present without known cancer.

  3. Therapy is ineffective. Plasmapheresis, immunosuppressive therapy, or treatment of the underlying malignancy does not reverse neurologic deficits, although treatment may arrest progression of the disorder.

C. Opsoclonus–myoclonus. Opsoclonus is an ocular motility disorder consisting of irregular, involuntary, multidirectional eye movements that persist with eye closure and sleep. It may be associated with myoclonus (brief, jerking contractions of flexor muscles). Opsoclonus–myoclonus is classically associated with neuroblastoma in children, in whom it heralds a good prognosis. Less commonly, it is associated with ataxia and encephalopathy in adults with breast cancer. In the latter disorder, opsoclonus–myoclonus is associated with the anti-Ri antibody (or ANNA-2). Unlike PCD and PSN, opsoclonus–myoclonus can be relapsing and remitting and may resolve spontaneously.

D. Cancer-associated retinopathy is a syndrome of visual loss that begins with obscurations and night blindness and proceeds to total blindness. It is most commonly associated with small-cell lung carcinoma and melanoma. This disorder is associated with an antibody that recognizes the protein *recoverin* in the photoreceptor cells of the retina. It can be diagnosed by detection of this antibody in serum and by electroretinography.

E. Limbic encephalitis. Early manifestations of this disorder include personality changes (depression and anxiety), which are followed by a profound loss of short-term memory. Seizures, hallucinations, and hypersomnia may also be present. Limbic encephalitis is most commonly associated with small-cell lung cancer and, in some cases, is attributable to the anti-Hu antibody.

F. Brainstem encephalitis causes vertigo, nystagmus, facial numbness, oculomotor disorders, dysphagia, dysarthria, deafness, and long-tract signs. It is most commonly seen in small-cell lung carcinoma and may be associated with the anti-Hu antibody.

G. Motor neuronopathy, or motor neuron disease, is a spectrum of disorders involving the motor system for which the association with malignancy is still poorly characterized. Unlike most other paraneoplastic disorders, this syndrome can arise late in the course of the malignancy, even during remission. It is most commonly seen in lymphoma (both non-Hodgkin and Hodgkin lymphoma), where it is frequently associated with a paraproteinemia. A similar condition can be seen as part of the spectrum of disease associated with the anti-Hu antibody and small-cell lung carcinoma.

  These disorders are characterized by a progressive loss of motor function that may resolve spontaneously; the sensory system is spared. Loss of anterior horn cells is seen pathologically. EMG studies can help establish the diagnosis.

H. Neuropathies associated with plasma cell dyscrasias. A symmetric, distal sensorimotor polyneuropathy may be associated with plasma cell dyscrasias, including monoclonal gammopathy of undetermined significance (MGUS), multiple myeloma with or without systemic amyloidosis, osteosclerotic myeloma, and Waldenström's macroglobulinemia. The polyneuropathy can occur as part of the POEMS (**p**olyneuropathy, **o**rganomegaly, **e**ndocrinopathy, **m**onoclonal gammopathy, and **s**kin changes) syndrome. It is often associated with a monoclonal paraprotein (often immunoglobulin M-κ), which reacts with a myelin-associated glycoprotein, resulting in a demyelinating neuropathy. The neuropathy is progressive, but usually no pain or autonomic involvement occurs. Treatment of the underlying disease or with plasmapheresis is beneficial in some patients.

I. Polymyositis and dermatomyositis. These disorders cause painful symmetric, proximal muscle weakness manifested as difficulty rising from a chair or combing hair. Only a small minority of patients with polymyositis or dermatomyositis have an associated malignancy. These disorders are discussed further in Chapter 28, section II.D.

J. Myasthenia gravis causes progressive fatigue with exercise. It occurs in 30% of patients with a thymoma, and 10% of patients with myasthenia gravis have a thymoma. The syndrome is caused by antiacetylcholine receptor antibodies that block function at the postsynaptic membrane of the neuromuscular junction. The diagnosis is made by detecting the antibody in the serum, by the response to edrophonium chloride (the Tensilon test), and by the characteristic EMG response to repetitive stimulation. Treatments include pyridostigmine bromide (Mestinon), steroids, plasmapheresis, resection of an associated thymoma, and often resection of the thymus. Myasthenia gravis may be difficult to treat, especially during the postoperative period after tumor resection. Treatment should be undertaken only by those familiar with the disorder.

K. Lambert-Eaton myasthenic syndrome (LEMS) is characterized by proximal muscle weakness, especially of the pelvic girdle. In contrast to myasthenia gravis, the weakness improves with exercise, and this can be demonstrated on physical examination. Hyporeflexia, muscle tenderness, and autonomic dysfunction (orthostatic hypotension, impotence, dry mouth) may be associated with the condition. LEMS results from an autoantibody that reacts with voltage-gated calcium channels (VGCC) of peripheral cholinergic nerve terminals.

  1. Associated tumors. Mostly small-cell lung cancers are found; LEMS may also be seen in association with lymphoma and thymoma. One-third of patients have no malignancy.

  2. Diagnosis. The diagnosis of LEMS is established by detection of the antibody against P/Q-type VGCC and by EMG, which demonstrates small compound muscle action potentials that increase after brief exercise or repetitive stimulation at high frequencies (20 to 50 Hz).

  3. Therapy. Effective therapies include treatment of the underlying malignancy, guanidine hydrochloride (125 to 500 mg PO three or four times daily), 3-4-diamino-pyridine (5 to 25 mg PO three or four times daily), steroids, IV immune globulin, and plasmapheresis.

VI. ADVERSE EFFECTS OF RADIATION TO THE NERVOUS SYSTEM

A. Mechanism. The CNS is highly susceptible to damage from radiation. The degree of neural dysfunction depends on the total radiation dose and fraction size, the volume of irradiated brain or spinal cord, and the time elapsed since RT. Reactions are classified as acute, early delayed, and late delayed. Acute reactions during RT are believed to be caused by a transient breakdown in the blood–brain barrier, leading to increased intracranial pressure. The risk for acute reactions increases with fraction sizes >200 cGy. Early delayed reactions, occurring weeks to months after irradiation, are usually self-resolving and are thought to be caused by demyelination. Late delayed reactions, usually occurring months to years after irradiation, result in permanent CNS damage. Tissue destruction with coagulative necrosis of the involved white matter is seen pathologically. Hyalinization of blood vessels leading to vascular thrombosis is a specific feature of radionecrosis.

B. Radiation syndromes. Specific neurologic syndromes occur in response to RT, depending on the site of irradiation. The skin, hair, subcutaneous tissues, and bone are at risk as well. Hair loss occurs when the dose to the brain is >2,000 cGy over 2 weeks; incomplete regrowth is common after higher doses.

1. **Radiation encephalopathy.** Acute radiation encephalopathy manifests as headache, nausea, and vomiting. Early delayed encephalopathy often mimics tumor recurrence, both clinically and radiographically, and consists of headache, lethargy, and worsening or reappearance of neurologic symptoms. Children undergoing prophylactic whole-brain RT for acute lymphoblastic leukemia may develop the radiation somnolence syndrome that causes profound lethargy and sleep for 18 or more hours per day; this resolves spontaneously over several weeks. Chronic radiation encephalopathy is associated with atrophy of the brain and is more likely to occur after whole-brain RT than after focal RT. Clinical findings include memory loss, cognitive dysfunction (learning disabilities in children), gait abnormalities, and urinary incontinence. This chronic disorder sometimes responds to CSF shunting.

2. **Radiation necrosis** is a late delayed reaction to RT that mimics tumor recurrence. It causes worsening focal neurologic deficits and progressive enhancing lesions on imaging studies. PET or MRI spectroscopy may be useful in differentiating radiation necrosis from tumor recurrence. Because the necrotic lesion has mass effect, surgical extirpation is often useful.

3. **Radiation myelopathy.** No acute reactions to irradiation of the spine occur. Early delayed reactions occur as electric shock-like sensations in the arms or legs that last for several seconds and are precipitated by flexion of the neck (Lhermitte sign). The condition is usually self-limited. Late delayed damage to the spinal cord results in a progressive myelopathy that may be asymmetric in onset; typically, numbness and weakness ascend and progress to symmetric paraplegia. This disorder is secondary to necrosis of the white matter and usually occurs with doses ≥5,000 cGy given over 5 weeks by conventional fractionation.

4. **Radiation plexopathy.** Brachial and lumbosacral plexopathy, a late delayed reaction to RT, are discussed in section IV.A.4.

5. **Loss of special senses.** Loss of vision and hearing are relatively common sequelae of cranial irradiation. Visual loss can result from radiation-induced optic neuropathy, retinopathy, glaucoma, cataract formation, and dry-eye syndrome. Hearing loss is caused by otitis media (acute or early delayed effect) or by sensorineural damage (late delayed effect).

6. **Hormonal deficiencies** occur as a result of hypothalamic and pituitary dysfunction after cranial irradiation. The most common deficiency involves growth hormone, but thyroid, adrenal, and gonadal dysfunctions also occur.

C. **Management.** Acute and early delayed reactions are self-limited, but often respond to treatment with steroids. Acute reactions and some early delayed reactions, such as the somnolence syndrome, may be prevented by premedicating patients with steroids before the start of cranial RT. Patients with large CNS tumor(s) and surrounding edema should always receive steroids for at least 48 hours before RT is started. Late delayed reactions, which are usually caused by neuronal and glial injury, do not recover with treatment; however, steroids can reduce swelling and symptoms in patients with radionecrosis. If small, the radionecrosis will eventually resolve on its own, but if the involved region is large, resection of the dead tissue may be necessary.

D. **Radiation-induced tumors** tend to occur decades after irradiation and include meningiomas, nerve sheath tumors, astrocytomas, and sarcomas.

E. **Radiation-induced CVD disease** is caused by accelerated atherosclerosis that becomes manifest years after irradiation. It is thought to result from occlusion of the vasa vasorum. Patients are at high risk for transient ischemic attacks and strokes.

VII. NEUROLOGIC COMPLICATIONS OF CHEMOTHERAPY

Neurologic complications of chemotherapy are common and depend on the dose of the chemotherapeutic agent, whether the drug is given as part of a multidrug regimen, and whether it is given in conjunction with radiation therapy. Chemotherapeutic agents may be toxic to the entire nervous system or cause more limited neurotoxicity, affecting only the central or peripheral nervous system. A variety of clinical syndromes are seen, many of which are drug-specific.

A. **Encephalopathy** (insomnia, agitation, drowsiness, depression, confusion, headache) usually develops acutely after administration of the offending agent. Responsible agents include methotrexate, cytarabine, procarbazine, mitotane, L-asparaginase, ifosfamide, cisplatin, vincristine, 5-fluorouracil, tamoxifen, nitrosoureas, etoposide, interferon-α, pentostatin, tegafur, levamisole, and, rarely, hexamethylmelamine, fludarabine, and 5-azacitidine.

B. **Cerebellar syndrome** (ataxia, nausea and vomiting, nystagmus) can be seen after the use of cytarabine, procarbazine, fluorouracil, and the nitrosoureas.

C. **Seizures** may occur after cisplatin, hydroxyurea, L-asparaginase, ifosfamide, procarbazine, and rarely vincristine.

D. **Peripheral neuropathy** (paresthesias, loss of deep tendon reflexes, distal extremity weakness) is a common neurologic complication of chemotherapy. Vincristine, paclitaxel (Taxol), and cisplatin cause some degree of peripheral neuropathy in almost all patients. The neuropathy is cumulative and is at least partially (if not completely) reversible with discontinuation of the offending agent. Other drugs that can cause neuropathy include bortezimab (Velcade), docetaxel (Taxotere), paclitaxel (Taxol), thalidomide, vindesine, vinblastine, procarbazine, suramin, hexamethylmelamine, etoposide, and teniposide.

E. **Cranial neuropathy** (loss of hearing, vision, taste) may develop from the use of cisplatin, vincristine, and the nitrosoureas.

F. **Myelopathy** (quadriparesis, paraparesis, bowel and bladder dysfunction) is a rare complication of intrathecal chemotherapy, including methotrexate and cytarabine.

G. **Combined radiation and chemotherapy induced neurotoxicity.** The combination of cranial irradiation and chemotherapy, particularly with methotrexate, nitrosoureas, or cytarabine, can have a synergistic toxic effect on normal brain structures. This can lead to permanent damage, often affecting the white matter and causing a leukoencephalopathy that produces a progressive dementing process. No known treatment exists, but some patients temporarily benefit from a ventriculoperitoneal shunt. Other drugs can have this effect but are less well studied than those mentioned.

VIII. OTHER COMPLICATIONS OF CANCER

A. **Cerebrovascular disease.** Strokes and hemorrhages are the second most common cause of CNS lesions in cancer patients. (Metastases are the most common.) Autopsy series show that 15% of cancer patients have CVD, of whom one-half have symptoms during their lifetime. In addition to standard risk factors that apply to the general population, patients with cancer have additional conditions that predispose to CVD.

1. **Cerebral embolism** can result from the following:

   a. Nonbacterial thrombotic endocarditis, seen especially with adenocarcinoma of the lung and gastrointestinal tract, is probably the most common cause of cerebral infarction in patients with carcinoma, although it is difficult to diagnose. Diagnosis of the valvular lesions is best established by transesophageal echocardiogram.

   b. Septic emboli from systemic fungal infections, most commonly *Aspergillus* species

   c. Tumor emboli (uncommon)

2. **Thrombosis** can cause strokes (arterial) as well as occlusion of the superior sagittal sinus (venous). The latter syndrome presents with headache, obtundation, and sometimes bilateral venous infarcts that may be hemorrhagic. Thrombotic disorders in cancer are caused by the following:

   a. DIC

   b. Hyperviscosity syndromes

      c. Chemotherapy, especially with L-asparaginase, which causes venous sinus thrombosis

      d. Vasculitis, usually as a complication of herpes zoster infection or seen in patients with Hodgkin disease

  3. Hemorrhages are more common in patients with leukemia, but can occur in those with solid tumors as well. Specific causes include the following:

      a. Thrombocytopenia

      b. DIC

      c. Hyperleukocytosis (acute myelogenous leukemia)

      d. Tumor invasion of blood vessels

      e. Bleeding diatheses (e.g., in hepatic failure)

      f. Brain metastasis

  4. Subdural hematomas can result from the following:

      a. Metastases

      b. Lumbar puncture producing intracranial hypotension

      c. Thrombocytopenia

B. CNS infections are discussed in Chapter 35, section III.B.

C. Ocular complications in cancer

  1. Metastases to the eye and orbit

    a. Etiology. Ocular and orbital metastases occur most frequently in breast cancer. Hematogenous dissemination to the eye also complicates acute leukemia, melanoma, sarcoma, and carcinomas of the lung, bladder, and prostate. Lymphoma can also invade the globe or orbit. Several head and neck cancers can erode directly into the orbit.

    b. Diagnosis

      (1) Signs. Patients develop eye pain, diplopia, loss of vision, and exophthalmos. Fundal hemorrhages, leukemic infiltrates, or masses may be evident on ophthalmoscopy.

      (2) MRI or CT scans of the orbits, brain, and surrounding tissues must be obtained in patients with symptoms of ocular or orbital metastases.

      (3) Biopsy is performed if the retro-orbital mass is the sole site of disease.

    c. Management. Prednisone, 40 mg/m^2 PO daily, should be given to decrease pain. RT to the orbit is the treatment of choice for metastatic disease and can improve vision. Emergency treatment of the eye with small doses of RT may prevent blindness in patients with ocular involvement from acute leukemia. Ocular or orbital RT can produce subsequent cataracts, but rarely causes permanent visual loss.

  2. Central retinal vein thrombosis

    a. Etiology. Central retinal vein thrombosis occurs in hyperviscosity syndromes associated with Waldenström's macroglobulinemia and occasionally with plasma cell myeloma. Marked erythrocytosis from polycythemia vera may also cause the problem.

    b. Diagnosis. Patients develop a sudden, painless loss of vision. "Sausage-link" widening of conjunctival and fundal veins may be present. The fundus may also have hemorrhages, hard and soft exudates, and microaneurysms.

    c. Management. Plasmapheresis is used for malignant paraproteinemias (see Chapter 22, section IX.A.1), and phlebotomy for polycythemia vera (see "Polycythemia Vera" in Chapter 24).

  3. Retinal artery occlusion

    a. Etiology. Embolic retinal artery occlusion is most commonly caused by atherosclerosis but may rarely be seen with atrial myxoma, nonbacterial thrombotic endocarditis, and cryoglobulinemia.

    b. Diagnosis. Patients develop sudden, painless loss of vision and a pale fundus with a bright red spot over the fovea.

    c. Management. Ophthalmologic consultation should be obtained immediately in all cases. Emergency measures include vigorous massage of the eye, administration of tolazoline (Priscoline, 75 mg IV) as a vasodilator, and aspiration of aqueous humor.

4. Amaurosis fugax can occur in patients with marked thrombocytosis (platelet count >800,000/μL) caused by myeloproliferative diseases, especially essential thrombocythemia or polycythemia vera. Treatment consists of antiplatelet drugs (e.g., aspirin, 81 to 325 mg/day) and chemotherapy. Plateletpheresis may also be used in severe cases.

Suggested Reading

Kesari S, Batchelor TT. Leptomeningeal metastases. *Neurol Clin* 2003;21:25.

Nguyen TD, Abrey LE. Brain metastases: old problem, new strategies. *Hematol Oncol Clin North Am* 2007;21(2):369.

Nguyen T, DeAngelis LM. Stroke in cancer patients. *Curr Neurol Neurosci Rep* 2006;6(3): 187.

Patchell RA, Tibbs PA, Regine WF, et al. Direct decompressive surgical resection in the treatment of spinal cord compression caused by metastatic cancer: a randomized trial. *Lancet* 2005;366(9486):643.

Peak S, Abrey LE. Chemotherapy and the treatment of brain metastases. *Hematol Oncol Clin North Am* 2006;20(6):1287.

Schiff D, Wen P. Central nervous system toxicity from cancer therapies. *Hematol Oncol Clin North Am* 2006;20(6):1399.

Sul JK, DeAngelis LM. Neurologic complications of cancer chemotherapy. *Semin Oncol* 2006;33(3):324.

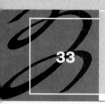

BONE AND JOINT COMPLICATIONS

33

Howard A. Chansky, Dennis A. Casciato, and James R. Berenson

I. **METASTASES TO CORTICAL BONE.** Metastases to bone marrow are discussed in Chapter 34, section I.A in "Cytopenias."

A. **Pathogenesis.** The bones most frequently involved with metastases are the femur, pelvis, spine, and ribs. Tumor cells may metastasize to vertebral bodies or the skull without entering the systemic circulation by seeding through Batson's vertebral venous plexus (a valveless system of veins along the entire vertebral column that communicates with other venous systems, from the pelvis to the brain).

1. **Mechanisms.** Osteoclast-mediated destruction and direct tumor cell–mediated destruction are the two mechanisms by which skeletal metastases destroy bone. Stimulation or inhibition of osteoblastic activity also occurs. The relative balance of osteoclastic and osteoblastic activity determines whether a lesion is lytic or blastic. Malignant cells secrete many factors known to both stimulate the proliferation and activity of osteoclasts and produce osteolysis, possibly indirectly through the osteoblasts. These factors include the following:

   a. Transforming and fibroblastic growth factors; tumor necrosis factors
   b. Prostaglandins; interleukin-1 (IL-1), IL-6, and IL-11
   c. Parathyroid hormone–related protein
   d. Bone morphogenic proteins
   e. Matrix-degrading proteins, such as specific metalloproteinases
   f. Receptor activator of nuclear factor-kappa B ligand (RANKL), the essential osteoclast differentiation factor (discussed in Chapter 22, section II.D.3.a)
   g. Chemokines and chemokine receptors

2. **Frequency.** A relatively small number of malignancies account for most tumors that spread to bone.

   a. **Tumors that commonly metastasize to bone.** Carcinomas of unknown primary site, lung, breast, kidney, prostate, and thyroid; plasmacytoma; melanoma; and occasionally Ewing sarcoma
   b. **Tumors that rarely metastasize to bone.** Ovarian carcinoma and most soft-tissue sarcomas

B. **Natural history.** Bone metastases are usually confined within the bony substance and generally do not cross joint spaces. They lead to pain, pathological fracture, neurological compromise, and progressive immobility. Crippling bone disease can make bedridden patients susceptible to decubitus ulcers, hypercalcemia, and infections.

1. Cervical spine metastases compressing the cord may result in myelopathy and weakness of the muscles of respiration, resulting in paralysis, pneumonia, and possibly death. Thoracic spine metastases compressing the cord can result in paraplegia.

2. Dense osteoblastic metastases (e.g., with prostate cancer) or extensive involvement of bone marrow spaces can result in refractory pancytopenia. Pathological fracture is less likely in the osteoblastic variant of metastatic prostate cancer.

C. **Prognosis.** The expected survival of patients with skeletal metastasis varies. Patients with lung cancer survive only a few months. The median survival of patients with breast cancer and only skeletal metastases, however, is 2 years. The median survival time of patients with stage IV renal cancer is 11 months, but 20% to 30% of those with a solitary metastasis survive 5 years after the lesion is surgically resected. About 20% of patients with skeletal metastases from prostate cancer survive 5 years.

D. Diagnosis

1. **Symptoms and signs**

   a. **Dull, aching, or boring pain** that is worse at night than with physical activity is characteristic of pain from bone metastases. This pain pattern also occurs with malignant invasion of retroperitoneal structures without bony involvement. These characteristics are directly opposite to the typical pain of degenerative diseases, in which pain related to activity is worse than pain at rest.

   b. **Bone pain intensified by activity** is often the first symptom of imminent fracture. On the other hand, pathological fractures can also be painless. Patients often report falling down, but it is often not clear whether the fracture was the cause or the effect of the fall.

   c. **Spinal instability secondary to bone loss** can cause excruciating pain, which is mechanical in origin. The patient is comfortable only when lying absolutely still.

   d. **C-7 to T-1 vertebral pain** is usually referred to the interscapular region; radiography of both cervical and thoracic spines is essential in these patients.

   e. **T-12 to L-1 vertebral pain** is usually referred to the iliac crest or sacroiliac joint.

   f. **Sacral pain** is usually referred to the buttocks, perineum, and posterior thighs. The pain typically is exacerbated by sitting or lying down and relieved by standing.

2. **Serum alkaline phosphatase levels** are usually elevated in patients with bone metastases. Elevations appear to reflect an osteoblastic (or healing) response to tumor destruction. In pure osteolytic tumors, such as plasma cell myeloma, the serum alkaline phosphatase level is normal.

   a. **Nonneoplastic causes** of increased bone alkaline phosphatase include primary hyperparathyroidism, thyrotoxicosis, acromegaly, renal disease, Paget disease, osteomalacia, and healing fractures.

   b. **Physiological increases** occur in the pediatric age group (before bony epiphyseal closure) and pregnancy (placental source).

3. **Radionuclide bone scan,** using ^{99m}Tc-methylene bisphosphonate, is the most effective screening test for skeletal metastases. The scan often detects metastases several months before radiological changes are evident. Radionuclide bone scans reflect osteoblastic activity; thus, purely lytic lesions with a preponderance of osteoclastic activity may not be apparent on a bone scan.

   a. **Specificity.** Patients with a known cancer and bone pain have positive bone scans in 60% to 70% of cases; patients without bone pain have positive scans in 10% to 15% of cases. Multiple "hot spots" are more specific than one or two.

      (1) Retroperitoneal tumors often cause a bony response, characterized by diffuse isotope uptake over the anterior aspect of the spine.

      (2) Patients with metastases from breast or prostate cancer, when clinically responding to endocrine therapy, may develop new abnormal areas on scans because of bone healing and increased osteoblastic activity.

      (3) Multiple myeloma is the most frequent cause of false-negative bone scans. These patients rarely have positive bone scans except in fractured areas.

      (4) Decreased uptake of radioisotope is seen in irradiated bone that never did contain metastases and thus cannot be interpreted as a sign of absence of metastases or of reduced tumor burden.

   b. **Benign conditions that can cause a positive bone scan**

      (1) Bone healing after fracture

      (2) Radiation osteitis

      (3) Arthritis and spondylitis

      (4) Osteomyelitis

      (5) Osteonecrosis

      (6) Regional osteoporosis

      (7) Paget disease of bone

      (8) Hyperostosis frontalis interna

TABLE 33.1 Radiological Characteristics of Bone Metastases

Predominantly lytic tumors	Mixed lytic and blastic tumors	Predominantly blastic tumors	Other causes of blastic bone lesions
Non–small-cell lung cancer	Breast cancer	Small-cell lung cancer	Tuberculosis
Renal cancer	Squamous cell cancers (most	Prostate cancer	Fluorosis
Multiple myeloma	primary sites)	Carcinoids	Osteoarthritis
Melanoma	Gastrointestinal	Gastrinoma	Osteopetrosis
	cancers (most)	Gastric cancers (some)	Paget disease
	Thyroid cancer	Hodgkin lymphoma	Tuberous sclerosis
		Lymphomas	
		Mastocytosis	

    (9) Osteopetrosis (Albers-Schönberg disease)
    (10) Osteogenesis imperfecta

4. Plain radiographs remain essential for the diagnosis and characterization of bone metastases. Metastatic lesions must involve 30% to 50% of bone matrix to be visualized on plain radiographs. Some tumors typically produce osteolytic or osteoblastic metastases, but both processes are accelerated in affected bone, and most tumors produce mixed lesions (Table 33.1). *Diffuse osteoporosis* may be the only radiological abnormality in some patients with extensive bony involvement (e.g., multiple myeloma). *Skeletal infections* with many pyogenic bacteria are frequently associated with sclerotic reactions; chronic granulomatous infections, however, may result in purely lytic lesions.

    a. Indications. Radiographs should be obtained and compared with previous films of the involved areas in patients with bone pain, abnormalities on physical examination suggestive of fracture, or asymptomatic abnormalities in bone scans.

    b. Routine skeletal surveys are not indicated except in patients with plasma cell myeloma, which may be associated with painless osteolytic lesions in crucial bone sites, such as the femora or cervical spine.

    c. Vertebral involvement from metastatic cancer is manifested by loss of the pedicles or lateral spinous processes and vertebral collapse with sparing of the intervertebral space. Infections that involve the intervertebral disk space destroy it. Some chronic infections (e.g., tuberculosis or brucellosis), however, may involve the vertebrae and not the intervertebral spaces, result in vertebral collapse, and thereby mimic malignancy.

    d. Postirradiation osteitis produces irregular, diffuse (rather than localized) lytic or mixed lesions confined to the radiation portal.

5. CT scan is useful to diagnose early metastases of bone, particularly the spine, when hot spots are detected on the radionuclide scan but corresponding plain radiographs are normal. CT scans elucidate cortical erosion, subtle fractures, and matrix calcification or ossification. In addition, they are useful to evaluate epidural compression, the extent of metastases (e.g., in the femur), and areas difficult to image by conventional radiographs (e.g., costovertebral junction, sternum, and sacrum).

6. MRI scanning is best at delineating the extraosseous extension of a soft-tissue mass through the bone cortex (e.g., epidural compression). This technique is also ideal for demonstrating the intraosseous extension of tumor into the cancellous bone.

7. Biopsy. If a fracture has already occurred, care must be taken to sample the tumorous area adequately rather than the healing area of fibrous tissue and osteoid formation. Specific expertise in bone histopathology must be available. If only a single bone is involved, the biopsy must be approached as if the lesion were resectable for cure. Potentially curable lesions include a solitary renal cell metastasis and sarcoma.

    a. Indications. If other sites associated with a lower risk for morbidity are not available, bone biopsy for the differential diagnosis of cancer is indicated in patients with the following conditions:

        (1) An isolated bone lesion that the radiologist interprets as being compatible with a primary bone tumor

        (2) An osteolytic bone lesion in a crucial area (e.g., cervical spine or femoral neck) and no history of cancer

        (3) A history of a cancer that metastasizes to bone, localized bone pain, normal radiographs of the area, equivocal bone scan and alkaline phosphatase results, and no evidence of disease elsewhere

        (4) Isolated bone pain in a region that was previously irradiated and radiographic findings that are not typical of postirradiation osteitis

    b. Contraindications. Bone biopsy should not be done in asymptomatic patients known to have cancer but with isolated, osteolytic lesions in noncrucial areas that are suspected to be benign lesions or metastatic disease. Biopsy in these patients often results in chronic pain at the biopsy site. If a cancer is discovered, it is a metastasis for which treatment could have awaited the development of symptomatic disease.

  8. Bone markers. The availability of markers for bone resorption (N-telopeptide) and formation (bone alkaline phosphatase) has allowed more accurate assessment of the risk of patients with metastatic bone disease to develop skeletal complications including fractures, spinal cord compression, or the need for radiotherapy or surgery to the affected bone. These tests have also been used to assess the efficacy of anti–bone-resorptive therapies such as IV bisphosphonates. However, their usefulness in the clinic to follow individual patients with metastatic bone disease has still not been demonstrated.

E. Management

  1. Medical management is necessary in patients with multiple painful metastatic sites.

    a. Chemotherapy and endocrine therapy are useful for treating metastatic tumors known to respond to these modalities. Chemotherapy doses may need to be attenuated because of compromised marrow function from neoplastic invasion or irradiation.

    b. Bisphosphonates. Pyrophosphonates are natural compounds that are potent inhibitors of osteoclast-mediated bone resorption and contain two phosphonate groups bound to a common oxygen. Bisphosphonates (such as pamidronate or clodronate) are analogs of the endogenous pyrophosphonate with a carbon replacing the oxygen atom. The wide variety of alternative carbon substitutions results in marked differences in antiresorptive properties and side effects. Bisphosphonates have become the standard treatment for tumor-induced hypercalcemia (see Chapter 27, section I), have been successfully used in the treatment of conditions characterized by increased osteoclast-mediated bone resorption (such as Paget disease of bone or osteoporosis), and are a valuable form of therapy for bone metastases.

        (1) These drugs are poorly absorbed and often poorly tolerated when administered orally. They are highly concentrated in bone and become biologically inactive once the drug becomes a part of bone that is not remodeling. As a result, continued administration of bisphosphonates is required to achieve the desired lasting inhibition of bone resorption.

        (2) Intravenous zoledronic acid (Zometa, 4 mg IV over 15 minutes) **or pamidronate** (Aredia, 90 mg IV over 2 hours) every 3 to 4 weeks as a supplement to antitumor therapy substantially reduces morbidity and subsequent skeletal events for patients with myeloma and metastatic bone disease. Although both pamidronate and zoledronic acid have shown efficacy for patients with osteolytic bone disease caused by breast cancer or myeloma, only zoledronic acid has reduced skeletal events among patients with other cancers, regardless of whether the disease results from osteolytic, osteoblastic, or mixed metastatic bone lesions. Pain is improved in about half of the patients given pamidronate even without anticancer treatments. Oral clodronate is also helpful but appears to be less effective than the intravenous forms.

Several recent studies have shown the ability of these drugs administered less frequently to prevent bone loss and actually increase bone density and, in some cases, reduce fracture risk among cancer patients receiving therapies that induce bone loss. However, more studies are needed to establish the long-term safety and efficacy of this approach for this at-risk cancer population.

(3) Side effects of bisphosphonates. It is important to recognize that these agents occasionally are associated with side effects, including renal dysfunction and osteonecrosis of the jaw (ONJ).

(a) Renal dysfunction. The type of renal lesion is different between the two bisphosphonates. Pamidronate more often will cause a glomerular lesion initially associated with proteinuria, which may be at nephrotic levels. By contrast, zoledronic acid more often causes tubular dysfunction and thus is not often associated with albuminuria.

(b) Osteonecrosis of the jaw. Reports suggest that bisphosphonates are associated with an increased risk of ONJ. This complication occurs more frequently among patients who have had recent dental surgery or trauma, poor dental hygiene, or abuse alcohol or use tobacco. Before initiating bisphosphonate treatment, patients should have a complete dental exam, and any dental extractions or removal of jawbone(s) should be completed several months before initiating these drugs to reduce the risk of ONJ.

The course of ONJ is quite variable, and many patients do not show worsening of the condition, although this can occur. There are no studies evaluating whether discontinuing these drugs among patients with this complication affects the course of ONJ. It is clear that surgical intervention to treat this problem should be minimized and only undertaken by dental professionals experienced with this problem.

(4) Bisphosphonates may also have an antitumor effect; some randomized trials have shown a reduction in both skeletal and visceral metastases in patients with myeloma or breast cancer.

c. Criteria for response of bone metastases to therapy. The appearance of new osteoblastic lesions on radiographs or bone scans or increasing size of sclerotic lesions does not necessarily indicate progression of metastases. Indeed, these findings may represent clinical improvement. Although the response of bone metastases to treatment is difficult to quantitate, it may be evaluated by assessing the following:

(1) Pain relief and quality of life

(2) Serum tumor markers

(3) Biochemical markers of bone resorption (e.g., urinary hydroxyproline excretion)

(4) CT scans

(5) Positron emission tomography (PET) is a promising but not yet validated technique to assess response of metastases to therapy.

d. Bracing of the vertebral column helps relieve pain and protect neurovascular structures while the lesions are resolving with radiation therapy (RT) or chemotherapy. Bony strength to resist gravitational forces must be adequate. Bracing of the lower extremities is seldom helpful.

2. RT ameliorates pain and may produce bone union and prevent fracture. The optimal dose of RT has not been defined. Smaller doses (e.g., 800 cGy given once) may be as effective as 2,500 to 4,000 cGy given over 2 to 4 weeks. This undoubtedly convenient, single or very short dose schedule, however, may not be adequate for patients with a relatively good prognosis.

a. **Pathological fractures.** The administration of RT after orthopedic fixation of pathological fractures is considered standard therapy. After orthopedic fixation, the bone encompassing the entire prosthesis is typically included in the radiation portal. RT may begin as soon as the patient can be moved if the incision can be spared; otherwise, treatment is delayed until the skin has healed.

b. **Isolated sites of bone pain.** RT controls local pain from bony metastases in more than 80% of patients within 2 weeks to 3 months. Irradiating a few severely painful sites may reduce the analgesic dose needed to manage patients with multiple sites of pain.

c. **Asymptomatic osteolytic lesions** of the cervical spine and long bones are irradiated to prevent complications.

d. **Hemibody irradiation** is used by some centers for control of pain caused by bone metastases. The treatment is effective in about 60% of patients, but it is associated with gastrointestinal upset and hematosuppression, particularly transfusion-dependent anemia.

3. **Radiopharmaceuticals,** especially ^{89}Sr (Metastron), can decrease pain for several months in about 75% of patients with skeletal metastases from breast or prostate cancer. Such agents are useful when endocrine therapy fails to control the disease (see Chapter 2, section IV.B).

a. ^{89}Sr is preferentially taken up and retained at sites of increased bone mineral turnover; uptake in bone adjacent to metastases is up to five times greater than for normal bone. This agent appears to provide effective adjuvant therapy to local-field RT with decreased new sites of pain, decreased need for further RT, decreased analgesic requirement, and improved quality of life.

b. Hematologic toxicity is the major precaution but is usually transient. Other agents (including ^{32}P, ^{153}Sm, and ^{186}Re) generally are associated with more hematologic toxicity or have undergone fewer clinical trials than ^{89}Sr.

c. Unfortunately, substantial numbers of patients achieve incomplete pain resolution, and some patients get no pain relief at all. None of the radiopharmaceuticals affects survival. Relatively few patients exhibit antitumor activity when treated with radiopharmaceuticals.

4. **Surgery** plays a crucial role in managing bony metastases that endanger neurological function or ambulation. Surgery can usually be avoided when RT or chemotherapy is effective and adequate stability of the bone permits natural repair.

Orthopedic consultation should be obtained in all patients with metastatic lesions of the femoral neck or shaft or with pathological limb fracture. When considering operative treatment, the major factors include the patient's general medical condition, functional goals, and comfort and quality of life; the anticipated responsiveness of the tumor to RT alone; the ease of delivering nursing care; and the morbidity of the contemplated procedure.

a. **Methyl methacrylate,** an acrylic bone cement, replaces deficient bone and greatly enhances the ability to use metal implants. It increases compressive strength and torque capacity, promotes hemostasis, and should be used with fixation devices whenever bone stock is inadequate to permit rigid fixation or implantation. The use of methyl methacrylate entails considerable potential for local complications, and the circulating monomer may be associated with intraoperative cardiac complications.

b. **Complications.** Surgical treatment for pathological fractures is associated with an operative mortality rate of about 8% and an infection rate of about 4%. The risk for infection increases in previously irradiated sites and in immunocompromised patients. Common reasons for failure of internal fixation include poor initial fixation, improper implant selection, and progression of disease within the operative field.

c. **Embolization.** Blood loss during surgical stabilization or biopsy of a metastatic lesion may be life-threatening. Metastatic breast cancer, myeloma, and particularly renal cell cancers are notoriously hypervascular. Preoperative angiography and occlusion of feeding vessels, particularly for lesions of the acetabulum or spine, may be indicated. The embolization of vertebral lesions, however, is associated with a risk for spinal cord injury.

    d. Rehabilitation. Patients treated surgically for pathological fractures caused by metastases are good candidates for intensive rehabilitation programs unless they have hypercalcemia or require parenteral narcotics, which are associated with very short survival times.

F. Surgical management of the appendicular skeleton. The threshold to treat lower extremity lesions is lower than that for upper extremity disease as a result of the weight-bearing function of the legs. However, lifting and pulling with the arms generate high distractive forces. In addition, patients with metastases to the lower extremities often require crutches or a walker, which generate high compressive loads in the bones of the arms. These issues must be factored into the decision of how to best treat an upper extremity (usually humeral) lesion.

    1. Surgical methods for metastases to long bones of the limbs include the following:

        a. Reinforcement of the involved bone with internal splints (bone plates, compression hip screws and side plates, intramedullary rods). Whenever possible, intramedullary fixation (nails or endoprostheses) is preferred over extramedullary fixation (plates) because the former results in smaller dissections, more durable fixation, and more rapid return to weight bearing.

        b. Removal of the metastatic tumor from the bone (either by surgical resection or by curettage), insertion of an internal fixation device or prosthesis, and supplemental fixation with bone cement

        c. Reconstruction of the articular surfaces of the proximal humerus, hip, or knee after *en bloc* excision of involved segments of periarticular bone with either total joint arthroplasty or hemiarthroplasty. Prosthetic arthroplasty is useful in the following circumstances:

            (1) Reconstruction of large destructive areas that are not amenable to internal fixation

            (2) Salvage of failed internal fixation devices

            (3) Salvage of lesions in which there are no RT options to prevent disease progression

        d. Amputation of dysfunctional extremities riddled with tumor in patients with intractable pain, reasonable life expectancy, and an absence of limb-sparing treatment options

    2. Upper extremities. Small lesions involving the humerus that are unlikely to fracture and that are sensitive to RT may be treated successfully with nonoperative measures, including RT. Lesions that are larger and in patients using walkers or crutches may be best treated with prophylactic fixation or endoprosthetic replacement followed by RT.

        Pathological fracture of the humerus usually occurs at the junction of its proximal and middle thirds and in the past was often treated by stabilizing the extremity in a cast or sling. Internal fixation or prosthetic replacement is now the treatment of choice for these patients because the risk for nonunion and infection increases when surgery is performed on an irradiated limb, and pain relief is predictable with modern orthopedic techniques and radiotherapy.

    3. Lower extremities: prophylactic orthopedic surgery. Prophylactic internal fixation, followed by RT to inhibit further tumor growth, is always considered in patients with lytic lesions in the femoral neck or shaft that are at risk for pathological fracture. Prophylactic surgery should be considered in the following circumstances:

        a. The patient is in good general medical condition, and

        b. The lytic lesion of the femur or tibia is >2.5 cm in diameter or involves more than half of the total cortical width (implies a 50% likelihood of fracture if untreated), or

        c. Spontaneous avulsion of the lesser trochanter has occurred, or

        d. Pain from lytic lesions persists despite RT.

    4. Lower extremities: pathological fractures. Untreated pathological fractures rarely heal, and although RT may achieve local control, bony union remains unlikely. Internal fixation is indicated for pathological fractures of the femur or tibia to decrease pain and to permit early ambulation.

   a. Femoral head and neck fractures. Internal fixation may be considered but is usually inadequate. A long-stem cemented femoral hemiarthroplasty is safe, provides long-lasting relief from pain, permits early ambulation without the need for postoperative RT, and is preferred. Prosthetic replacement is particularly required if extensive cortical destruction would not allow a stable construction even with bone cement augmentation. If the articular cartilage and subchondral bone of the acetabulum are intact, an endoprosthesis is used. The complication rate is 20%. Insertion of long femoral stems with bone cement can create dangerous embolic loads, and some surgeons routinely vent the distal femur to minimize pressure within the medullary canal. Biological porous ingrowth fixation is rarely indicated as protected weight bearing is difficult in debilitated patients and life expectancy may be short. In addition, RT interferes with ingrowth.

   b. Intertrochanteric fractures. Nail-plate devices are used when sufficient residual bone is present to allow stable bony fixation and to support body weight, but intramedullary devices are frequently required. Prosthetic replacement is considered if there is extensive bony loss; if pathological fracture has developed slowly, resulting in extensive destruction; or if there is no possibility of obtaining structural stability. The complication rate, however, is substantial.

   c. Subtrochanteric fractures are more difficult to repair because the fracture often extends into the intertrochanteric area or femoral shaft. The fractures are usually stabilized with a reconstruction nail. Nail-plate devices are associated with a high frequency of implant failure, but intramedullary devices are helpful, especially with the use of methyl methacrylate. Extensive destruction may require the use of a modular oncological or calcar-replacing prosthesis, but local morbidity is significant, and the ideal device to attach the abductor muscles to the prosthesis has yet to be devised.

   d. Femoral shaft fractures require intramedullary fixation supplemented with interlocking screws and bone cement if there has been extensive cortical loss.

   e. Lesions of the acetabulum may respond to chemotherapy, but they still leave the patient with a painful hip if subchondral collapse and deformity have already begun. Reconstructive surgery with total-hip replacement is often beneficial in patients with reasonable life expectancy (e.g., those with breast cancer). This procedure is demanding because acetabular support and fixation may require the use of flexible Steinmann pins and bone cement in the superior ilium and across the sacroiliac joints to transmit the weight-bearing stresses to intact bone. A protrusio acetabulum ring is often needed to provide additional structural support.

G. Management of the axial skeleton. Most cancer patients with mild mechanical instability of the spine and neck or back pain can be successfully treated with bracing and RT. Surgery is associated with a significant rate of complications (about 20%) but can be very important when the spine becomes unstable. Segmental spinal fixation systems use pedicle screws to attach rods to the posterior spine at multiple vertebral levels. Newer techniques use combinations of bone cement, allograft bone, and metallic implants (cages) to replace or supplement diseased vertebral bodies. Patients may get out of bed on the first postoperative day and typically require a custom-fitted, low-profile plastic orthosis.

   Patients in whom spinal instability is likely to develop should undergo surgical stabilization before RT. Whenever possible, adjuvant RT should be delayed 3 to 6 weeks after surgery to minimize wound complications.

   1. Surgery for spinal metastases may be indicated in the following circumstances:

      a. The diagnosis of metastatic cancer has escaped diagnosis at other sites. Percutaneous trocar biopsy may be necessary when needle biopsy fails to provide a diagnosis.

      b. Mechanical instability from fracture causes pain and progressive deformity.

    c. Pathological fracture or tumor extension causes compression of the spinal cord or nerve roots.

    d. A symptomatic tumor is known to be resistant to RT (e.g., renal cell carcinoma).

    e. A spinal tumor continues to progress despite adequate RT.

2. Restabilization of the spine may not be indicated in the following circumstances:

    a. Multiple osseous and soft-tissue metastases exist.

    b. More than two or three vertebrae are destroyed and need replacement.

    c. The patient has poor nutritional, immunologic, or pulmonary status or severe disease not related to the malignancy.

    d. Life expectancy is very limited.

3. Cervical spinal metastases must be irradiated regardless of symptoms and often require immobilization of the head and neck. A soft cervical collar is the least uncomfortable method but should be used only in patients with minimal disease. A rigid collarlike brace is adequate support if there is some intrinsic stability.

    As in the thoracic and lumbar spine, metal implants to replace vertebral bodies anteriorly, and screws into the pedicles or lateral masses posteriorly, can restore spine and spinal cord integrity. In patients with severely limited life expectancy, in lieu of major surgery, the head can be immobilized with a special halo device and placement of screws into the skull. These prosthetic devices are often used until the patient succumbs.

4. Thoracolumbar spinal metastases

    a. Painful lesions should be irradiated. MRI should be done first to search for potential sites of epidural compression and to map out radiation fields. Many patients have a soft-tissue mass extending around the involved vertebra. These masses compress nerves, contribute to pain, and should be included in the radiation port. Fiberglass braces and corsets may reduce back pain and help stabilize the spine.

    b. Rapidly progressive metastases that are refractory to RT may be manifested by increasing pain, worsening destruction on radiographs, or the development of neurological deficits. Open decompression of the spinal cord and internal fixation to permit early mobility (1 to 3 weeks) should be considered, but the outlook for these patients is poor.

5. Spinal decompression

    a. Laminectomy provides direct access to posterior and posterolateral tumors but compromises the stability of the spine. Spinal cord compression is usually a result of tumors of the vertebral body (i.e., anterior to the spinal cord); thus, laminectomy does not reliably relieve symptoms. Below the level of the third cervical vertebra, laminectomy should only be used for lesions in the dorsal elements, laminae, and pedicles.

    b. Anterior surgical decompression of the spinal cord is performed using thoracotomy or laparotomy, especially for RT-resistant tumors (e.g., renal cell carcinoma). Anterior decompression involves the removal of the vertebral body and all tumor anterior to the spinal cord (vertebrectomy). The spinal column is reconstructed with a graft or cage, and posterior stabilization with rods and pedicle screws is also usually needed. Custom-shaped methyl methacrylate in combination with plates can be used to supplement fixation; bone grafts are preferred in patients when life expectancy exceeds 6 months because any purely mechanical construct will eventually fail if there is no bony healing. The anterior route provides immediate mechanical stability and the best chance for neurological improvement. The associated success rate is reported to be 75% to 90%, with less blood loss and fewer complications than with laminectomy.

    c. Posterolateral surgical decompression is an alternative for the technically difficult lesions above the sixth thoracic vertebra and is useful in more debilitated patients. Patients are able to sit in a chair on the night of surgery and to begin walking the next day.

(1) Posterolateral decompression removes a part of the rib and lamina to gain access to the vertebral body and decompress the anterior aspect of the spinal cord from the side. After completing vertebrectomy and removing the disks, the surgeon inserts a vertical strut (graft or cage) between the end plates of the healthy vertebrae above and below the tumor site. Posterior fixation rods, which can be placed through the same incisions, provide immediate stability.

(2) The advantage of this approach is that it does not require thoracotomy. Posterior spinal instrumentation can be carried out at the same time as tumor removal, often with video-assisted endoscopic techniques. This procedure may reduce patient morbidity, days in intensive care, and days of hospitalization while providing the same quality of neurological recovery and maintenance of function as anterior resection. Access to the tumor, however, is usually limited because the surgeon is working around the spinal cord. Neurological recovery has been less reliable than with a formal anterior approach.

d. Vertebroplasty and kyphoplasty are evolving new procedures consisting of the percutaneous injection, under fluoroscopic guidance, of methyl methacrylate into a diseased vertebral body. These procedures have been most commonly used to treat osteoporotic compression fractures, but experience in treating myeloma and metastatic carcinoma has been accumulating. Unlike vertebroplasty, the kyphoplasty procedure uses a balloon to restore vertebral height and compress both cancellous bone and tumor before injecting the cement. Both procedures can be done quickly, have been shown to lead to very rapid and sustained reduction in back pain for patients with vertebral compression fractures, and are associated with low surgical risk and minimal morbidity.

II. OCCURRENCE OF CANCER IN CONNECTIVE TISSUE DISORDERS.
The associations of rheumatic conditions with the development of malignancies probably reflect immune dysregulation, chronic immune stimulation, and the use of immunosuppressive drugs in their treatment.

A. Sjögren syndrome is associated with a 44-fold increased risk for non-Hodgkin lymphoma (NHL), particularly of the monocytoid B-cell type. An intermediate stage of "pseudolymphoma" may persist for years.

B. Dermatomyositis and polymyositis. Various kinds of malignancy develop in about 25% of patients with these disorders, particularly dermatomyositis. The cancer may present at the time of diagnosis or at a significantly later time. Thus, an extensive radiographic or invasive search for malignancy at the time of diagnosis is not recommended.

C. Rheumatoid arthritis is associated with a fourfold increased incidence of malignancies (which are usually hematopoietic) in the United States and an increased risk for oropharyngeal carcinomas in Japan. Felty syndrome, which has been extended to include the presence of increased numbers of circulating CD16-positive large granular lymphocytes, is associated with a 13-fold increased occurrence of NHL. The use of cytotoxic agents is believed to be involved in the pathogenesis of malignancies in rheumatoid arthritis, but patients have developed cancer without such exposure.

D. Scleroderma with pulmonary fibrosis has previously been reported to be associated with bronchoalveolar cell carcinoma, but this association has not been observed in more recent series. Fibrosing disorders that resemble scleroderma and are associated with a significant risk of malignancy include the following:

1. Palmar fasciitis with inflammatory polyarthritis. This syndrome is accompanied by thickening of the palmar fascia, which can progress to Dupuytren contracture. The syndrome can precede recognition of the malignancy by several months and is most often associated with ovarian carcinoma.

2. Reflex sympathetic dystrophy syndrome shows several clinical features of the palmar fasciitis syndrome and is associated with Pancoast's tumor when it affects the upper extremities and with gynecologic tumors when it affects the lower extremities.

E. Vasculitis

1. **Cutaneous leukocytoclastic vasculitis** is the form of vasculitis that is most strongly associated with coexistent malignancy, including both hematopoietic neoplasms and solid tumors. This association is strongest for hairy cell leukemia, which is also associated with a high occurrence of polyarteritis nodosum.

2. **Sweet syndrome** (acute febrile neutrophilic dermatitis) is associated with malignancy in 15% of cases, usually acute leukemia. Fever, leukocytosis, and a characteristic eruption of painful, erythematous papules on the head, neck, and upper extremities compose the syndrome.

3. **Erythema nodosum,** a variety of panniculitis, is associated with Hodgkin lymphoma and leukemia.

4. **Mixed cryoglobulinemia** is associated with hepatocellular carcinoma, NHL, and hepatitis C virus infection.

F. Other connective tissue diseases

1. **Systemic lupus erythematosus.** About 5% of patients develop malignancies, usually hematopoietic and probably related to the use of immunosuppressive drugs.

2. **Lymphatoid granulomatosis** affects the lungs and may result in NHL.

3. **Gout.** Two-thirds of patients with myeloproliferative disorders have hyperuricemia and hyperuricosuria. The occurrence of acute gouty arthritis in these patients has been markedly reduced with the routine prescription of allopurinol.

III. PARANEOPLASTIC AND INFILTRATIVE BONE AND JOINT CONDITIONS

A. Hypertrophic osteoarthropathy is manifested by clubbing of the fingers, pain and effusion in large joints, and periosteitis. The ankles, knees, elbows, and wrists are the most frequently involved joints. The extremely painful periosteal reaction usually involves the extensor surfaces of the legs and forearms. The change in the overlying skin resembles cellulitis with induration, erythema, and *peau d'orange.*

1. **Associated tumors.** Hypertrophic osteoarthropathy develops most frequently with lung adenocarcinomas, less frequently with other lung carcinomas, and occasionally with gastrointestinal adenocarcinomas and intrathoracic sarcomas.

2. **Benign causes of clubbing** include hereditary clubbing, lung abscess, bronchiectasis, tuberculosis, endocarditis, biliary cirrhosis, Crohn disease, and cyanotic congenital heart disease.

3. **Diagnosis.** Clubbing should be self-evident; patients should be questioned about the duration of the abnormality. Sponginess, by palpation, of the proximal nail beds may indicate early clubbing. Radiographs of painful joints or long bones often show periosteal reactions.

4. **Therapy.** Control of the associated tumor usually alleviates symptoms of hypertrophic osteoarthropathy. The pain can be relieved by a variety of nonsteroidal anti-inflammatory drugs (NSAIDs). Patients with severe pain require narcotic analgesics.

B. Rheumatic manifestations that suggest an occult malignancy. No distinguishing features of rheumatic syndromes define the coexistence of cancer. Manifestations may improve or disappear with therapy directed at the malignancy. The following syndromes should strongly suggest a thoughtful search for malignancy, *particularly if they first occur at ≥50 years of age.*

1. Explosive seronegative polyarthritis presenting with swollen and tender joints, with a predilection for the lower extremities sparing the small joints and wrists, and with mild nonspecific synovitis identified by synovial biopsy

2. Monoclonal gammopathy in a patient with typical rheumatoid arthritis

3. Palmar fasciitis and polyarthritis

4. Eosinophilic fasciitis unresponsive to steroidal therapy

5. Raynaud phenomenon (often with asymmetric involvement of the fingers and progression to necrosis)

6. Cutaneous leukocytoclastic vasculitis

C. Pachydermoperiostosis associated with lung cancer consists of a dense overgrowth of periosteum resulting in clubbing and leonine facies (see Chapter 28, section II.M).

D. Joint pain, subcutaneous fat necrosis (panniculitis), and eosinophilia occasionally constitute the presenting features of pancreatic cancer.

E. Hypercalcemia and hypocalcemia; see Chapter 27, sections I.A and II.A.

F. Direct infiltration of malignancy into articular tissues

  1. Sarcomas can present as primary malignancies of any joint.

  2. Metastases can affect any joint and mimic inflammatory arthritis.

  3. Acute leukemic arthritis is caused by leukemic infiltration of synovium. It is usually symmetric and may resemble rheumatic fever or juvenile rheumatoid arthritis. Effusions may occur. In 25% of cases, adjacent bone may develop lytic lesions, osteoporosis, or osteoblastic changes. Brief symptomatic responses can be obtained with ibuprofen or aspirin. Treatment of the underlying leukemia resolves with arthritis.

  4. Chronic leukemic arthritis is uncommon; it is usually symmetric but is otherwise similar to the acute type both in radiographic patterns and in response to therapy.

  5. Myeloma-induced amyloidosis produces carpal tunnel syndrome and, rarely, a rheumatoid arthritis–like syndrome. Synovial tissues may be densely infiltrated with myeloma cells.

IV. ADVERSE EFFECTS OF RADIATION TO BONE

A. Radio-osteonecrosis of the mandible may complicate RT of head and neck cancers. The problem occurs more often in patients with large tumors, bone invasion, history of large alcohol intake and heavy smoking, poor dentition, poor oral hygiene, and poor nutritional status. The mandible becomes brittle and superinfected, resulting in pain, fractures, and draining fistulas.

  1. Diagnostic criteria

    a. Localized pain and tenderness

    b. Mucosal ulceration or necrosis (occasionally, a fistula) with exposure of bone and, occasionally, cutaneous fistulas

    c. Loose teeth in the suspected area

    d. Radiographs showing a lytic lesion of the mandible, sometimes with a radiodense sequestrum or involucrum

    e. Manifestations should not be clinically evident for at least 4 months after completion of treatment.

  2. Prevention of radio-osteonecrosis involves proper dental extractions before RT and oral hygiene and fluoride treatment regimen during and after RT. If possible, the patient should not have any dental extractions for 2 years after RT. Even with these precautions, osteonecrosis develops in 5% to 10% of patients when a high-dose RT portal overlies the mandible.

  3. Treatment

    a. Conservative management

      (1) Frequent mouthwashes with dilute hydrogen peroxide or a baking soda and salt solution

      (2) Systemic antibiotics, usually penicillin; topical nystatin or bacitracin ointment

      (3) Gentle débridement

    b. Aggressive management

      (1) Hyperbaric oxygen treatments

      (2) Surgical resection of the nonviable portion of the mandible

      (3) A combination of hyperbaric oxygen and surgical resection

B. Radiation osteitis may mimic bony metastases. Differentiation of these disorders is discussed in section I.D. Postirradiation pathological fractures of the femoral neck may rarely complicate pelvic irradiation.

C. Radiation-induced bone sarcomas have been reported after high-dose irradiation of both benign and malignant lesions. The incidence is <0.1% of all 5-year survivors; the latent period is >5 years.

D. Premature closure of bone epiphyses and apophyses can result in shortening, kyphosis, and asymmetry of osseous structures in children who have received RT.

V. ADVERSE EFFECTS OF CHEMOTHERAPY ON BONE

A. Aseptic necrosis of the hip is a complication of high doses of glucocorticoids. The risk is proportional to the dose of drug and not to the duration of therapy. Increased pressure in the intramedullary space causes the sudden onset of hip pain. Capsular irritability is demonstrated by flexing the hip and medially rotating the thigh. Early diagnosis is best established by MRI. Radionuclide bone scan is the diagnostic test of second choice. Removal of bony cores from the necrotic areas predictably, if incompletely, relieves pain and may favorably alter the natural history of osteonecrosis if done before the occurrence of secondary changes, such as collapse of subchondral bone and articular cartilage.

B. Postchemotherapy rheumatism is a syndrome of myalgias and arthralgias that develops within 1 to 3 months after completing adjuvant chemotherapy for breast cancer using cyclophosphamide and 5-fluorouracil. Mild periarticular swelling occurs in some cases. NSAIDs are not effective. Symptoms are self-limiting and generally resolve over several months. Extensive workups for breast cancer recurrence or for inflammatory rheumatologic disease are not needed in this setting.

   1. Arthralgias associated with paclitaxel therapy usually begin 2 to 3 days after treatment and resolve within 5 days.

   2. Arthralgias associated with hormonal therapy occur frequently in patients being treated with aryl aromatase inhibitors (anastrozole, letrozole, exemestane) for breast cancer. The problem often is not solved by changing agents within that class of drugs and may lead to discontinuation of such therapy. Arthralgias have also been reported in patients treated with tamoxifen, but to a lesser extent and severity. The relative incidence of these phenomena are difficult to determine by published studies, but the significance of their occurrences remains important because long-term treatment is affected by their development.

C. Raynaud's phenomenon is a common toxicity of treatment with cisplatin, oxaliplatin, vinblastine, or bleomycin.

D. Osteoporosis. Many therapeutic regimens in cancer treatment carry the risk of promoting osteoporosis. Therapies involving corticosteroids or causing hypogonadism are the most common causes. Cytotoxic drugs that have been implicated in the development of osteoporosis include methotrexate and ifosfamide. The risk of osteoporosis should be assessed with osteodensitometry when indicated. Treatment with hormone replacement and/or bisphosphonates can be considered when appropriate.

Suggested Reading

Bauer HCF. Controversies in the surgical management of skeletal metastases. *J Bone Joint Surg Br* 2005;87:608.

Berenson J, et al. Long-term pamidronate treatment of advanced multiple myeloma patients reduces skeletal events. *J Clin Oncol* 1998;16:593.

Carsons S. The association of malignancy with rheumatic and connective tissue diseases. *Semin Oncol* 1997;24:360.

Coleman RE, ed. Treatment of skeletal complications of cancer with zoledronic acid (Zometa). *Semin Oncol* 2002;29(Suppl 21):1.

Coleman RE, et al. Predictive value of bone resorption and formation markers in cancer patients with bone metastases receiving the biphosphonate zoledronic acid. *J Clin Oncol* 2005;23:4925.

Dougall WC, Chaisson M. The RANK/RANKL/OPG triad in cancer-induced bone diseases. *Cancer Metastasis Rev* 2006;25:541.

Giehl JP, Kluba T. Metastatic spine disease in renal cell carcinoma: indication and results of surgery. *Anticancer Res* 1999;19:1619.

Lipton A. Treatment of bone metastases and bone pain with bisphosphonates. *Supportive Cancer Therapy* 2007;4:92.

Loprinzi CL, Duffy J, Ingle JN. Postchemotherapy rheumatism. *J Clin Oncol* 1993;11:768.

Muller A, et al. Involvement of chemokine receptors in breast cancer metastasis. *Nature* 2001;410:50.

Naschitz JE, Yeshurun D, Rosner I. Rheumatic manifestations of occult cancer. *Cancer* 1995;75:2954.

Pfeilschifter J, Diel IJ. Osteoporosis due to cancer treatment: pathogenesis and management. *J Clin Oncol* 2000;18:1570.

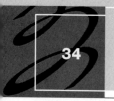

34 HEMATOLOGIC COMPLICATIONS
Dennis A. Casciato

INCREASED BLOOD CELL COUNTS

I. ERYTHROCYTOSIS (POLYCYTHEMIA). Erythrocytosis is defined as an elevation of the hematocrit and red blood cell (RBC) count above the *upper limits of normal.* Normal limits in adults are as follows:

	Men	**Women**
Hematocrit	52%	47%
Red blood cell count	$5.9 \times 10^6/\mu L$	$5.2 \times 10^6/\mu L$
Red blood cell mass	36 mL/kg	32 mL/kg (or >25% above mean normal predicted value)

A. Relative erythrocytosis is characterized by normal RBC mass and decreased plasma volume. Causes of relative erythrocytosis include dehydration, diuretics, burns, capillary leak, decreased oncotic pressure ("third-spacing"), hypertension, and stress ("Gaisböck syndrome"). The majority of patients with Gaisböck syndrome have an RBC mass that is at the upper limits of normal and a plasma volume that is toward the lower limits.

B. Primary erythrocytosis is caused by intrinsic defects of erythroid progenitors.

  1. Acquired primary erythrocytosis (polycythemia vera [PV]) is a clonal disorder. The majority of patients with PV have a somatic mutation in a gene on chromosome 9p (the *JAK2* gene). Erythrocytosis develops independently of serum erythropoietin (EPO) concentration. Uncontrolled proliferation of marrow elements results in an increased RBC mass. PV, including diagnostic criteria, is discussed in Chapter 24, "Polycythemia Vera."

  2. Primary familial and congenital polycythemias result from germ line rather than somatic mutations.

  a. Chuvash polycythemia is the most common congenital polycythemia in the world and the only known endemic polycythemia. The condition is named after the Chuvash population in the mid-Volga River region of Russia. The condition results from an abnormality in the oxygen-sensing pathway. Inheritance is as an autosomal recessive involving mutation of the von Hippel Lindau (*VHL*) gene. Marked erythrocytosis occurs in the presence of normal to increased levels of EPO.

  b. Primary erythrocytosis due to mutations of the EPO receptor (usually truncation) can be congenital or familial. Inheritance is as an autosomal dominant. An increased proliferation of erythrocytes, elevated RBC mass, hypersensitivity of erythroid progenitors to EPO, low serum EPO levels, and normal hemoglobin oxygen dissociation characterize this rare disorder.

C. Secondary erythrocytosis is associated with increased RBC mass due to extrinsic stimulation of progenitors by circulating substances such as EPO.

  1. Appropriate erythrocytosis

  a. Chronic hypoxemia is a potent stimulus for EPO production. Causes of hypoxemia include pulmonary diseases, right-to-left intracardiac shunts, low atmospheric pressure (high altitudes), alveolar hypoventilation (brain disease or pickwickian syndrome), and portal hypertension. Intermittent arterial desaturation and erythrocytosis may be caused by sleep apnea or by supine posture, particularly in obese patients with pulmonary disease.

   b. Heavy smoking. Excessive and sustained exposure to carbon monoxide from cigarettes or cigars, which produces an increased affinity between the remaining oxygen and the hemoglobin molecule, is a common cause of erythrocytosis.

   c. Congenital disorders include hemoglobinopathies with high oxygen affinity (abnormal oxyhemoglobin dissociation), overproduction of EPO, and familial deficiency of 2,3-biphosphoglycerate (rare).

   d. Androgen therapy stimulates erythropoiesis.

   e. Cobalt chloride induces tissue hypoxia and consequent EPO production.

   f. Chuvash polycythemia has elements of both primary and secondary erythrocytosis.

  2. Inappropriate erythrocytosis occurs with elevated EPO levels in the absence of generalized tissue hypoxia and is seen in a variety of diseases.

   a. Renal diseases account for about 60% of all cases of inappropriate erythrocytosis, and renal adenocarcinomas account for half of those cases. Cysts, other tumors, hydronephrosis, and transplantation make up the remaining renal causes of erythrocytosis.

    (1) Renal cell carcinomas synthesize EPO in association with erythrocytosis in 1% to 5% of cases.

    (2) Renal transplantation is associated with erythrocytosis in 10% of patients. The erythrocytosis has been ascribed to transplanted artery stenosis, graft rejection, hypertension, hydronephrosis, diuretic use, and EPO overproduction from residual renal tissue, especially in polycystic disease.

   b. Hepatocellular carcinoma and cerebellar hemangioblastoma each account for 10% to 20% of the cases of inappropriate erythrocytosis in the literature.

   c. Other causes of inappropriate erythrocytosis are rare. Huge uterine leiomyomas and ovarian carcinoma can cause renal hypoxia or ectopic EPO production. Pheochromocytomas and aldosteronomas cause erythrocytosis through multiple mechanisms.

D. Evaluation of patients with erythrocytosis

  1. Initial evaluation. The following studies are obtained in all patients with persistent erythrocytosis:

   a. Perform a complete history and physical examination to search for known causes of elevated hematocrits. Search for treatments that are associated with absolute or relative erythrocytosis (androgen therapy, diuretics) and for splenomegaly, which would suggest PV. If intravascular volume depletion is suspected, replete the volume and then reassess.

   b. Analyze the hemogram. The presence of granulocytosis, eosinophilia, basophilia, or thrombocytosis suggests PV.

   c. Measure arterial oxygen saturation. The RBC mass is roughly proportional to the degree of arterial desaturation. Arterial oxygen saturation <90% and a PaO_2 of <60 to 65 mm Hg may result in erythrocytosis.

   d. If the patient smokes tobacco, measure the carboxyhemoglobin concentration; values of >5% are associated with erythrocytosis. Smoking may also cause granulocytosis.

   e. Serum EPO level is decreased in PV and abnormalities of the EPO receptor. The concentration is normal or increased in the other disorders associated with erythrocytosis.

  2. Special diagnostic studies

   a. RBC mass determination previously was paramount for distinguishing absolute erythrocytosis from relative erythrocytosis. RBC mass is measured with ^{51}Cr-labeled erythrocytes and plasma volume is measured concomitantly with ^{125}I-labeled albumin to assess for intravascular volume reduction. However, this useful test is becoming increasingly unavailable.

   b. Abdominal radiography (ultrasonography or CT scanning) is indicated in all patients with absolute erythrocytosis that is not explained by either PV or hypoxemia because the frequency of renal causes is high.

   c. *JAK2* gene mutation should be sought if PV is suspected.

   d. Oxyhemoglobin dissociation curve is indicated in patients with a family history of unexplained erythrocytosis.

   e. Other diagnostic studies for inappropriate erythrocytosis are obtained *only if* the screening evaluation exposes abnormalities that could indicate pathology of a specific organ.

   f. Bone marrow examination is not diagnostic of any disorder associated with erythrocytosis.

II. GRANULOCYTOSIS

A. Definitions

1. **Granulocytosis.** The upper limit of normal for neutrophils is 8,000/µL.

2. **Leukemoid reactions.** The term *leukemoid reaction* should be restricted to granulocytosis with circulating promyelocytes and myeloblasts.

3. **Leukoerythroblastic reactions** are characterized by immature granulocytes in association with nucleated erythrocytes in the peripheral blood. Platelet counts may be normal, increased, or decreased. *Differential diagnosis* includes the following:

   a. Metastatic tumor in the marrow

   b. Marrow fibrosis with extramedullary hematopoiesis

   c. Marrow recovery after severe hematosuppression

   d. Shock, hemorrhage

   e. Brisk hemolysis, hereditary anemias

B. Causes of granulocytosis

1. **Increased proliferation in the marrow** is seen in the myeloproliferative disorders (MPDs), marrow rebound after suppression by drug or virus, and as a chronic response to infection, inflammation, or tumor. The mechanism of tumor-induced granulocytosis most often involves increased production of granulocyte and granulocyte-macrophage colony-stimulating factors (G-CSF, GM-CSF), interleukin (IL)-1, and IL-3.

2. **Increased marrow proliferation and increased granulocyte survival** are seen in chronic myelogenous leukemia (CML).

3. **Shift from the marrow storage pool into the circulation** is seen in response to stress, endotoxin, corticosteroids, and etiocholanolone.

4. **Demargination** (resulting in granulocytosis involving only mature neutrophils) is seen in stress, including emotional upset, epinephrine administration, exercise, infection, hypoxia, and intoxication.

5. **Decreased egress into the tissues** is seen after chronic treatment with corticosteroids.

C. Differentiation of leukemoid reactions from MPDs and CML involves complete clinical evaluation, especially for the history and presence of splenomegaly. The leukocyte differential count, neutrophil alkaline phosphatase score, and cytogenetics may be helpful (see Table 24.1). Bone marrow biopsies are frequently not discriminatory.

1. **Neutrophil alkaline phosphatase** scores are normal or increased in MPDs and reactive granulocytosis and decreased in CML.

2. **Vitamin B$_{12}$.** Transcobalamins I and III are synthesized by granulocytes. The total-body granulocyte mass, when increased, is reflected by increased serum levels of vitamin B$_{12}$ and unsaturated B$_{12}$-binding capacity. These levels are usually elevated in patients with MPD and CML and normal in patients with erythrocytosis or granulocytosis of other causes. Transcobalamin I is increased in CML, and transcobalamin III is increased in PV.

III. THROMBOCYTOSIS

- **A. Thrombocytosis in cancer patients.** Persistent thrombocytosis may indicate cancer. Thrombocytosis in neoplastic disease may be idiopathic or the result of bleeding or bone marrow metastases. Generally, thrombocytosis associated with solid tumors is mild, but values may exceed $1,000,000/\mu L$.
- **B. Common causes of transient thrombocytosis**
  1. Acute hemorrhage or phlebotomy
  2. Acute infection
  3. Recovery from myelosuppression (viruses, ethanol, cytotoxic agents)
  4. After surgery (persists for about 1 week)
  5. Response to therapy for folic acid or vitamin B_{12} deficiency
  6. Certain drugs (epinephrine, vinca alkaloids, and perhaps miconazole)
- **C. Causes of chronic thrombocytosis**
  1. Iron deficiency (the most common cause of thrombocytosis)
  2. MPDs
  3. Neoplasms (idiopathic or bone marrow metastases)
  4. Chronic inflammatory diseases
  5. Hyposplenism (postsplenectomy states, hemolytic anemias, regional enteritis, sprue, and splenic atrophy from repeated infarctions)
- **D. Differentiation of causes of chronic thrombocytosis.** After history and physical examination, helpful screening tests for the evaluation of chronic thrombocytosis include the following:
  1. **Peripheral blood.** Megathrombocytes and fragments of megakaryocytes are rarely seen in disorders other than the MPDs and CML. A normal mean platelet volume suggests reactive thrombocytosis. The granulocyte differential is helpful for recognizing MPDs and CML. The presence of hypochromia and microcytosis supports iron deficiency.
  2. **Serum iron, iron-binding capacity, and serum ferritin** to evaluate for iron deficiency
  3. **Bone marrow** aspirate examination demonstrates panmyelosis in MPDs and CML. Bone marrow biopsy may detect tumor involvement. Iron staining is unreliable in patients with cancer or chronic inflammatory diseases if the results show low or absent iron stores.

IV. EOSINOPHILIA

- **A. Definition.** The upper limit of normal in absolute cell count is $550/\mu L$.
- **B. Nonneoplastic causes of eosinophilia**
  1. Allergies and drug hypersensitivities
  2. Skin diseases (many types)
  3. Infection with fungus, protozoan, or metazoan; convalescence after a febrile illness
  4. Eosinophilic gastroenteritis, inflammatory bowel disease
  5. Eosinophilic pulmonary syndromes (e.g., Löffler syndrome)
  6. Collagen vascular diseases, especially rheumatoid arthritis, polyarteritis nodosa, and Churg-Strauss syndrome
  7. Contaminated tryptophan eosinophilia–myalgia syndrome
  8. Chronic active hepatitis, pernicious anemia, immunodeficiency syndromes
  9. Hyposplenism (see section III.C.5)
  10. Hypereosinophilic syndrome/chronic eosinophilic leukemia
- **C. Eosinophilia associated with neoplasia**
  1. Hodgkin lymphoma (up to 20% of cases)
  2. MPDs and CML (common)
  3. Acute lymphocytic leukemia and lymphoma (especially T-cell types)
  4. Acute monocytic leukemia with *inv(16)*
  5. Angiolymphoid hyperplasia with eosinophilia (Kimura disease)
  6. Pancreatic acinar cell carcinoma (syndrome of polyarthritis, subcutaneous panniculitis, and peripheral eosinophilia)
  7. Tumors undergoing central necrosis or metastasizing to serosa

8. Malignant histiocytosis
9. Eosinophilia related to treatment: RT to the abdomen, hypersensitivity to cyto-toxic agents

V. BASOPHILIA
A. Definition. The upper limit of normal is $50/\mu L$.
B. Causes of basophilia
1. Hypersensitivity reactions
2. MPDs
3. CML
4. Mastocytosis
5. Hyposplenism (see section III.C.5)
6. Infections: tuberculosis, influenza, hookworm
7. Endocrine: diabetes mellitus, myxedema, menses onset
8. Miscellaneous: hemolytic anemia, ulcerative colitis, carcinoma

VI. MONOCYTOSIS
A. Definition. The upper limit of normal is 500 to $800/\mu L$.
B. Causes of monocytosis
1. Hematologic neoplasms (leukemias, lymphomas, myeloma), myelodysplastic syndromes, immune hemolytic anemias, immune thrombocytopenia, and other hematologic disorders
2. Solid tumors with and without metastases
3. Inflammatory bowel disease, sprue, and alcoholic liver disease
4. Collagen vascular disease (including rheumatoid arthritis, systemic lupus erythematosus, polyarteritis nodosa, and temporal arteritis)
5. Sarcoidosis
6. Mycobacterial infections, subacute bacterial endocarditis, syphilis, and resolution from acute infection
7. Infections with varicella-zoster virus or cytomegalovirus (CMV)
8. Hyposplenism (see section III.C.5)
9. Factitious monocytosis may occur when blood samples are taken from fingertips affected by peripheral vascular disease

VII. LYMPHOCYTOSIS. The differential diagnosis of lymphocytosis is discussed in Chapter 23, section III.D in "Chronic Lymphocytic Leukemia."

 CYTOPENIA

Decreased formed elements in the circulating blood can result from decreased or ineffective production within the bone marrow, increased destruction of cells, or sequestration in the spleen. Patients with cancer often have a combination of these abnormalities. The type and duration of cytopenia depend on several factors (Table 34.1).

I. PANCYTOPENIA BECAUSE OF BONE MARROW FAILURE
A. Metastases to the marrow
1. **Occurrence.** Carcinomas of the breast, prostate, and lung are the solid tumors most likely to be associated with extensive marrow metastases. Melanoma, neuroblastoma, and carcinomas of the kidney, adrenal gland, and thyroid also frequently have marrow metastases.
2. **Findings.** Tumor volume in the marrow does not correlate directly with the degree of hematosuppression. Marrow metastases are often found in patients without any hematologic abnormality. Patients may have bone pain, bone tenderness, radiographic evidence of cortical bone involvement, or elevated serum alkaline phosphatase levels.
   a. **Bone marrow paraneoplastic alterations** can result in qualitative and quantitative abnormalities in hematopoiesis. In the absence of marrow

TABLE 34.1	Hematopoiesis, Cell Kinetics, and Bone Marrow Injury			

Characteristic	Erythrocytes	Platelets	Neutrophils	Lymphocytes
Bone marrow				
Storage cell	Reticulocyte	Megakaryocyte ($32n$ ploidy); platelets	Metamyelocyte	Lymphocyte
From blast to storage cell	3 days	5 days	5 days	Unknown
Storage time	2 days	<1 day	3–4 days	Unknown
Circulation				
Cells replaced daily	1%	10%	300%–400%	25%–40%
Half-life	60 days	5 days	7 hr	Days to years
Onset of cytopenia[a]	5 days[b]	3–30 days	5 days	2–3 weeks

[a]The type, severity, and duration of cytopenia depends on the etiology of the injury, its dose and exposure time, and other factors.
[b]Reticulocytopenia; anemia requires prolonged and repeated arrests of erythropoiesis.

metastases, changes can develop that are comparable to those seen in the primary myelodysplastic syndromes, including myelodysplasia in all cell lines, marked reactive changes, stromal modifications, and bone marrow remodeling.

  b. Desmoplastic reactions to metastases can result in myelofibrosis.

  c. Bone marrow biopsy is superior to aspiration (with examination of the clot specimen) for detection of metastases; both techniques are complementary. Cytologic preparations of bone marrow aspirates must be inspected at the edges of the smears for clumps of tumor cells. Immunohistochemical staining for epithelial markers may be helpful in identifying carcinomas.

  d. Peripheral blood abnormalities. Nearly all patients with solid tumors and leukoerythroblastosis have demonstrable marrow metastases. Thrombocytopenia (in the absence of RT or chemotherapy) is the next best indicator. Leukocytosis, eosinophilia, monocytosis, and thrombocytosis each is associated with positive marrow biopsies in about 20% of cases.

B. Marrow fibrosis

  1. Occurrence. Extensive primary marrow fibrosis is characteristic of myelofibrosis with agnogenic myeloid metaplasia and late-stage polycythemia vera. Marrow fibrosis may also be secondary to neoplastic infiltration with leukemia or metastatic carcinoma or as a distant effect of some tumors without demonstrable tumor cells in the marrow. *Secondary fibrosis* in the marrow may also be seen in reaction to the following:

    a. Collagen vascular disorders (particularly systemic lupus erythematosus, in which the fibrosis can reverse after treatment with high-dose corticosteroids)

    b. Toxic agents (benzene, radiation, cytotoxic agents)

    c. Infectious agents (especially tuberculosis and syphilis)

    d. Hematologic diseases (myelodysplasia, pernicious anemia, hemolytic anemia)

    e. Miscellaneous disorders (osteopetrosis, mastocytosis, renal osteodystrophy, Gaucher disease, giant lymph node hyperplasia, angioimmunoblastic lymphadenopathy)

  2. Findings. Splenomegaly and a leukoerythroblastic blood smear are characteristic of marrow fibrosis of any cause.

C. Marrow necrosis

  1. Occurrence. When diagnosed antemortem, marrow necrosis nearly always is due to either sickle cell disease or a malignancy, particularly a hematologic neoplasm. Systemic embolization of fat and marrow frequently occurs. The median survival of patients with marrow necrosis from a malignancy is <1 month. Patients with severe weight loss may develop *gelatinous transformation* of the marrow with marrow hypoplasia and fat atrophy; this condition is reversible.

   2. Findings. Patients have severe bone pain in the back, pelvis, or extremities (75%), fever (70%), cytopenias, and a leukoerythroblastic blood smear.

   a. Serum levels of alkaline phosphatase and lactate dehydrogenase (LDH) are usually elevated.

   b. Radiographs are normal.

   c. Bone marrow aspiration demonstrates characteristic findings: Individual hematopoietic cells are not recognizable, and cells with indistinct margins and intensely basophilic nuclei are usually surrounded by amorphous acidophilic material.

D. Bone marrow failure secondary to treatment. Ionizing radiation and most chemotherapeutic agents cause suppression of bone marrow function. Although recovery is usual after chemotherapy, recovery after irradiation is inversely proportional to dose and volume treated and may never be complete. Indeed, after doses in excess of 3,000 cGy, the bone marrow may be replaced by fatty and fibrous tissue. The distribution of marrow in the human skeleton is shown in Figure 34.1.

   The occurrence of **therapy-related myelodysplasia and acute myelogenous leukemia (AML)** is even more worrisome for the development of treatment strategies. To develop this complication, the patient must have been treated long enough and then live long enough to manifest this long-term toxicity.

   1. Occurrence. Nearly half of the patients have a primary hematologic malignancy. The risk for AML is increased 10- to 50-fold in patients treated for multiple myeloma, Hodgkin lymphoma, non-Hodgkin lymphoma, ovarian cancer, germ cell tumors, small cell lung cancer, and childhood acute lymphoblastic leukemia (ALL). For children with ALL who achieve complete remission, the risk for therapy-related AML is greater than the risk for developing relapsed ALL. Adjuvant chemotherapy for breast cancer is not associated with an increased risk for AML.

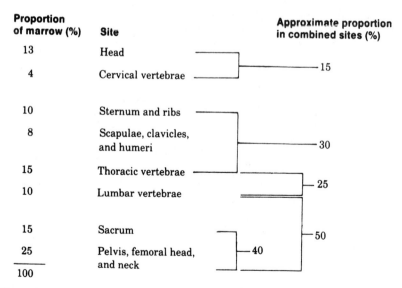

Figure 34.1. Distribution of bone marrow in healthy 40-year-old persons. Marrow cellularity is relatively decreased and amounts of fat increased in elderly subjects. (Data from Ellis RE. The distribution of active bone marrow in the adult. *Phys Med Biol* 1961;5:255.)

2. **Leukemogenic agents.** The risk of inducing AML is directly related to the total cumulative dose and probably to dose intensity. The risk may also depend on the schedule of administration; for example, the risk in children with ALL is greatest in those undergoing weekly or biweekly therapy with epipodophyllotoxins.

   a. **Alkylating agents** are the drugs with the most clearly demonstrated leukemogenic potential. Melphalan and chlorambucil are most often associated with AML in this class of drugs.

   b. **Other drugs.** Epipodophyllotoxins (etoposide, teniposide), nitrosoureas, and procarbazine are also leukemogenic. Cisplatin is not a classic alkylating agent and is possibly leukemogenic; however, it is nearly always given in combination with other drugs, some of which are leukemogenic. Hydroxyurea has been implicated as being possibly leukemogenic in the treatment of MPDs, but the risk has been found to be low.

   c. **RT** is associated with a minimally increased risk for AML when given alone but with a synergistically increased risk when combined with leukemogenic drugs.

3. **Chromosome abnormalities,** particularly involving chromosomes 5q or 7q, are found in 70% of therapy-linked AML associated with alkylating agents. These same aberrations are seen in patients developing AML after exposure to leukemogenic solvents and pesticides. In contrast, certain balanced translocations involving 11q23 appear to be characteristic of myelodysplasia and AML occurring after treatment with cytostatic agents acting on DNA topoisomerase II, such as etoposide.

4. **Natural history.** AML usually develops 3 to 5 years after initiation of therapy but can arise after 10 years or longer; the syndrome rarely develops within 1 year. Therapy-induced AML is usually preceded by months to years of myelodysplasia. After AML develops, the course is rapid and usually refractory to treatment. Death usually occurs within 2 to 4 months of diagnosis. An important predictive factor for favorable response to intensive antileukemic therapy is the absence of a preceding myelodysplastic phase.

II. PANCYTOPENIA BECAUSE OF HYPERSPLENISM

A. **Pathogenesis.** Splenic enlargement from any cause (including carcinomatous metastases) may result in phagocytosis of the circulating blood cells and the development of cytopenias. Hypersplenism with severity sufficient to beg the question of splenectomy develops most often in lymphoproliferative disorders and myelofibrosis.

B. **Diagnosis.** The diagnosis of hypersplenism is based on clinical judgment. The only true diagnostic test for hypersplenism is improvement in the cytopenias after splenectomy.

C. **Treatment**

1. **Indications for splenectomy** for hypersplenism are all of the following:

   a. The patient has palpable splenomegaly.

   b. The cytopenia is severe (e.g., anemia requiring frequent transfusions; severe neutropenia associated with recurrent, serious bacterial infections; or thrombocytopenia with hemorrhagic manifestations).

   c. Other causes of cytopenia have been ruled out (e.g., disseminated intravascular coagulation [DIC]).

   d. A reasonable survival time after splenectomy is expected.

   e. The patient's general medical condition is satisfactory enough to make the operative mortality risk acceptable.

   f. Surgeons experienced in performing splenectomy under adverse conditions are available.

2. **Consequences of splenectomy**

   a. **Postsplenectomy blood picture** is characterized by Howell-Jolly bodies, neutrophilia, eosinophilia, basophilia, lymphocytosis, monocytosis, and thrombocytosis.

   b. Postsplenectomy sepsis is a potentially fatal complication, especially in children younger than 6 years of age. The most common infecting organisms are *Streptococcus pneumoniae* and *Haemophilus influenzae*. The incidence of sepsis in patients with Hodgkin lymphoma who undergo splenectomy has been reported to be 1% to 3%. Immunization may be helpful. Febrile episodes must be treated immediately and aggressively.

III. PANCYTOPENIA DUE TO HISTIOCYTOSIS

A. **Hemophagocytic histiocytosis** is an acquired syndrome of exaggerated histiocytic proliferation and activation. It is usually associated with systemic viral infection (particularly with Epstein-Barr virus [EBV]), although other micro-organisms have also occasionally been implicated. These syndromes often develop on the background of another primary disease, such as autoimmunity or cancer (especially lymphomas).

1. **Pathogenesis.** EBV enters T cells, and proliferation of these cells leads to disruption of immune regulation and cytokine storm, which may cause major organ failure of the liver, kidneys, or lung. The severity of the syndrome varies from mild to lethal.

2. **Clinical findings** include fever, severe malaise, myalgias, and often hepatosplenomegaly (which is less prevalent in adults than in children). At least two cytopenias are seen in nearly all cases.

   a. **Bone marrow biopsy** is often hypocellular with an increase in marrow macrophages. The macrophages are vacuolated and contain ingested RBCs and erythroblasts (and perhaps other hematopoietic elements).

   b. **Lymph node biopsy** shows normal nodal architecture with hemophagocytic histiocytes.

   c. **Blood studies**

   (1) Acute phase reactants and proinflammatory cytokines are elevated.

   (2) Triglycerides, ferritin, and LDH are frequently elevated.

   (3) Parameters indicating DIC are frequently present.

3. **Treatment**

   a. Patients with mild to moderately severe disease may recover in weeks if the infectious agent is treatable or the disease may resolve naturally if the patient's immune system is intact.

   b. Patients receiving immunosuppressive therapy may require drug dosage reduction.

   c. Patients with the severe EBV-induced syndrome may require 2 months of treatment with dexamethasone, etoposide, and cyclosporine A to suppress the cytokine release and reverse proliferation of T cells. Etoposide alone, antithymocyte globulin, and γ-globulin have been used for less severe manifestations.

B. **Sinus histiocytosis with massive lymphadenopathy** (Rosai-Dorfman syndrome) is a polyclonal disorder manifested by massive lymphadenopathy (particularly cervical) and is usually self-limited. It usually occurs in the first 2 decades of life.

1. **Pathogenesis.** The etiology is unknown.

2. **Clinical findings.** Lymphadenopathy may be isolated or generalized. Extranodal involvement, especially in the head and neck region, is common. Virtually any organ may be involved. Fever is common and weight loss may occur. Blood studies are nonspecific and consistent with chronic inflammation.

   a. **Bone marrow biopsy** is nondiagnostic.

   b. **Lymph node biopsy.** Lymphophagocytosis and erythrophagocytosis by histiocytes in the lymph node sinus are characteristic. Marked fibrosis in the capsular areas and distention and engorgement of medullary and subcapsular sinusoids by phagocytic histiocytes are usually diagnostic. The polyclonal histopathologic appearance of extranodal biopsies is very similar to that of lymph nodes.

3. **Treatment.** Lymph node enlargement progresses for weeks to months, then gradually recedes so that most patients have no evidence of disease after 12 to

18 months. Surgical excision of problematic masses is often successful. Other forms of therapy have had no consistent effect.

C. Other disorders of macrophages that are relevant to the differential diagnosis of hemophagocytic histiocytosis include:

1. Langerhans cell histiocytosis

2. Familial hemophagocytic lymphohistiocytosis

3. Malignant histiocytosis

IV. ANEMIA IN PATIENTS WITH CANCER

A. Anemia because of blood loss or iron deficiency

1. Pathogenesis includes ulcerating tumors, extensive surgery, benign gastrointestinal (GI) tract diseases, gastrectomy (unable to use heme iron but able to use ferrous salts), and hemosiderinuria from chronic intravascular hemolysis.

2. Diagnosis. Patients with known GI tract malignancies must not be presumed to be bleeding from an ulcerating tumor (see Chapter 30, section I). Stools should be tested for occult blood.

a. Blood studies may demonstrate microcytosis and hypochromia. Important clues that may signify a recent hemorrhage are polychromasia (often prominent 5 to 10 days after acute hemorrhage) or thrombocytosis (as a reaction to bleeding). Hypoferremia and hypertransferrinemia are often obfuscated in cancer patients by the presence of concomitant anemia of chronic disease; serum ferritin levels are usually more helpful. Assays of soluble transferrin receptor (which is elevated in iron deficiency but not in anemia of chronic diseases) may be helpful.

b. Bone marrow examination demonstrating the absence of stainable iron is unreliable in patients with cancer. The presence of stainable iron eliminates iron deficiency.

c. Therapeutic trials. Ferrous sulfate, 325 mg PO given 3 times daily for 30 days, should elevate the hemoglobin concentration in patients with iron deficiency and otherwise intact hematopoiesis.

B. Anemia because of nutritional deficiencies results in megaloblastic anemia, macro-ovalocytosis, neutrophil hypersegmentation, and in severe cases, pancytopenia.

1. Folic acid deficiency is the most common cause of megaloblastic anemia in cancer patients. Decreased intake of folate is common with any advanced cancer. Increased requirements for folate develop with autoimmune hemolytic anemia, the postoperative state, prolonged IV therapy, and competition for use of folate by rapidly proliferating tumor cells. Folate deficiency may also develop after the use of folate antagonist drugs (e.g., methotrexate).

2. Vitamin B$_{12}$ deficiency is usually seen in cancer patients who have undergone gastrectomy (the site of intrinsic factor production) or who have malabsorption secondary to lymphoma that involves the ileum (the site of vitamin B$_{12}$ absorption).

C. Anemia of chronic diseases (ACD)

1. Pathogenesis. ACD is caused by immune activation in reaction to foreign antigens with the production of cytokines that directly inhibit both the action and production of EPO. ACD is more severe with widespread metastases but may be observed in patients with localized tumors.

The increased levels of tumor necrosis factor (TNF) and IL-1 seen in malignancies and inflammatory conditions result in anemia indirectly by means of interferons (IFNs). TNF stimulates marrow stromal cells to produce IFN-β, and IL-1 acts on T lymphocytes to produce IFN-γ. Both IFN-β and IFN-γ inhibit erythropoiesis directly.

Neopterin levels, which indicate the activation of macrophages by IFN-γ, are also increased in malignancies. The hemoglobin concentrations are inversely proportional to the blood concentrations of neopterin and IFN-γ. IFN-γ also inhibits granulocytopoiesis, but neutropenia is not a manifestation of ACD.

IL-1 also stimulates the release of G-CSF and GM-CSF, which can overcome the inhibitory effects of IFN-γ.

2. Diagnosis

a. Hemogram. The erythrocytes in ACD are usually normocytic and normochromic. Some patients have microcytosis and hypochromia. The reticulocyte count is normal or slightly increased.

b. Serum iron studies. The diagnosis of ACD involves the demonstration of decreased levels of both serum iron and transferrin (total iron-binding capacity). Serum ferritin values are normal or increased. The levels of soluble transferrin receptor are normal.

c. Bone marrow studies demonstrate ineffective erythropoiesis that is manifested by decreased polychromasia of nonnucleated marrow RBCs, shortened RBC life spans, and decreased numbers of sideroblasts. Reticuloendothelial iron may be normal, increased, or decreased.

3. Treatment. ACD is rarely severe enough to necessitate RBC transfusions. However, recombinant human EPO can correct ACD in most situations in which it is encountered.

D. Anemia caused by parvovirus B19. Parvovirus B19 is the etiologic agent of transient acute aplastic crises in patients with underlying hemolytic anemias. This complication is also seen in patients receiving chemotherapy, particularly as treatment of leukemia. An acute infection is manifested by worsening anemia, exanthem, and polyarthralgia.

In immunocompromised hosts who are unable to produce neutralizing antibodies against the virus, an infection can persist and cause chronic bone marrow failure, usually manifested by anemia. The viral target is an erythroid progenitor cell. The bone marrow shows erythroid hypoplasia. Treatment with commercial hyperimmune γ-globulins may be helpful.

E. Pure red cell aplasia (PRCA) is the isolated severe hypoplasia of erythroid elements in the marrow.

1. Pathogenesis. Although previously reported to be associated with thymoma in more than half of the cases of PRCA, modern series show this association to be approximately 10%. Lymphoproliferative disorders and various carcinomas have also been associated with PRCA. Rare cases of thymoma have been associated with pure neutropenia.

2. Diagnosis. A normocytic, normochromic anemia and reticulocytopenia are present. Bone marrow biopsy demonstrates markedly decreased-to-absent erythroid precursors and normal megakaryocytes and myeloid elements. Chest radiographs demonstrate a mediastinal mass if associated with thymoma.

3. Treatment. Removal of a thymoma results in remission of PRCA in about 20% of these cases. Patients with and without thymoma have responded to therapy with cyclophosphamide, cyclosporine, or antithymocyte globulin.

F. Warm antibody (IgG) immune hemolysis

1. Pathogenesis. Autoimmune hemolysis because of IgG antibodies most commonly occurs in patients with lymphoproliferative neoplasms. More than half of the patients in some series have an associated malignancy, but only 2% of cases are associated with solid tumors. This complication has also been reported after treatment with various cytostatic drugs (e.g., fludarabine). The IgG-coated erythrocytes are removed from the circulation by the reticuloendothelial system, predominantly by the spleen (extravascular hemolysis).

2. Diagnosis. Patients with warm antibody autoimmune hemolysis usually have an insidious onset of severe anemia, mild jaundice, and splenomegaly. The blood smear shows polychromasia, a significant degree of spherocytosis, and, often, nucleated RBCs. Reticulocytes are typically increased but may be normal if any other cause of anemia is also present. The direct antiglobulin test (DAT, or Coombs' test) is positive with anti-IgG or anticomplement antisera, usually with specificity for the Rh blood group system.

3. Treatment. Prednisone and successful treatment of the tumor are necessary. Patients with solid tumors associated with immune hemolysis respond to prednisone infrequently. Patients who have an unsatisfactory response or need chronic corticosteroid therapy require splenectomy if their general condition permits. Treatment with rituximab may be considered.

G. Cold antibody (IgM) immune hemolysis

1. **Pathogenesis.** Cold agglutinins are IgM molecules that attach to RBC membranes at cold temperatures and fix complement. At $37°C$, the IgM molecules dissociate from the cell, but the complement remains fixed. Cold agglutinins are most common in lymphoma and are rare in other malignancies. Overt hemolysis (often intravascular) is unusual except in patients with very high titers ($>1:10,000$) of cold agglutinins.

2. **Diagnosis.** Patients with high titers of cold agglutinins may have acrocyanosis or Raynaud phenomenon. RBC agglutination may be observed on blood smears, but spherocytes are not prominent. The DAT is strongly positive when performed at $4°C$ but is positive only with anticomplement antisera at $37°C$.

3. **Treatment.** Rituximab, 375 mg/m² weekly for 4 weeks is often effective. Chlorambucil or cyclophosphamide may be helpful for patients with symptomatic chronic cold agglutinin disease.

H. Microangiopathic hemolytic anemia hemolysis (MAHA) with erythrocyte fragmentation has been described in patients with adenocarcinoma (particularly gastric cancer) and hemangioendothelioma. The pathophysiology of MAHA involves fibrin strands of DIC, pulmonary intraluminal tumor emboli, narrowing of pulmonary arterioles by intimal proliferations, or a side effect of chemotherapy. Most patients with MAHA, however, probably have DIC or chemotherapy-associated thrombotic thrombocytopenia (see section V.C).

V. THROMBOCYTOPENIA BECAUSE OF INCREASED PLATELET DESTRUCTION. Decreased production is by far the most common cause of thrombocytopenia in patients with cancer. Splenic sequestration may cause thrombocytopenia, almost always in association with anemia. Increased destruction of platelets is usually associated with normal megakaryocytes in the bone marrow and decreased platelet life spans.

A. DIC is the most common cause of increased destruction of platelets in cancer patients (see "Coagulopathy," section II).

B. Idiopathic thrombocytopenic purpura (ITP) complicates lymphoproliferative diseases, especially malignant lymphoma and chronic lymphocytic leukemia, and is rarely associated with carcinoma. Thrombocytopenia in ITP is due to reticuloendothelial system destruction of IgG-coated platelets.

1. **Diagnosis** of ITP is made presumptively in the absence of evidence of DIC or of drug-induced thrombocytopenia with the finding of a nondiagnostic bone marrow containing normal or increased numbers of megakaryocytes.

2. **Treatment.** Control of the underlying disease is essential for satisfactory control of ITP.

   a. Patients are treated with prednisone, 60 to 80 mg/day PO. Single alkylating agents or vinca alkaloids successfully achieve remission in some patients. Splenectomy is indicated in patients who fail these measures and have symptomatic thrombocytopenia or require relatively high doses of prednisone chronically.

   b. Many cases of ITP are chronic; platelet counts are 50,000 to 80,000/μL. In the absence of symptoms, it is best to observe these patients without giving long-term immunosuppressive therapy.

C. Chemotherapy-induced thrombotic thrombocytopenic purpura (TTP) or hemolytic–uremic syndrome (HUS). TTP/HUS can develop during the treatment of patients with cancer, particularly when using mitomycin C for adenocarcinoma. More than 90% of cases have been associated with mitomycin C. About 10% of patients treated with mitomycin C develop TTP/HUS, especially when the cumulative dose is >60 mg. Manifestations are often precipitated or exacerbated by transfusion of blood products. Therapy with cisplatin, bleomycin, cyclosporine, or gemcitabine has also been associated with this complication. TTP has also occurred with clopidogrel (Plavix), ticlopidine (Ticlid), and tacrolimus (used for transplant rejection prophylaxis).

Chemotherapy-induced TTP/HUS usually occurs 2 to 9 months after cessation of treatment, even when the cancer is in remission (about one-third of patients). Noncardiogenic pulmonary edema develops in 65% of patients with this syndrome, which is rapidly lethal if not successfully treated.

1. **Diagnosis.** TTP/HUS is characterized by the extensive deposition of hyalin-like material in arterioles and capillaries. Diagnostic hallmarks of TTP/HUS are microangiopathic hemolysis and severe thrombocytopenia; other features often include markedly elevated serum LDH levels, rapidly changing neurologic abnormalities, fever, and renal dysfunction. Coagulation abnormalities associated with DIC are absent.

2. **Treatment.** Transfusion of plasma and intensive plasmapheresis have been successful in achieving remissions in classic TTP/HUS. Treatment of chemotherapy-induced TTP/HUS with staphylococcal protein A extracorporeal immunoabsorption of circulating IgG immune complexes also achieves significant responses in half of the patients. Normalization of platelet counts and LDH values is seen 7 to 14 days after starting treatment.

VI. GRANULOCYTOPENIA
Granulocytopenia in cancer patients is usually the result of chemotherapy, radiotherapy, other drugs, severe infection, or myelophthisis. An immune or cytokine basis is involved in the granulocytopenia associated with T-γ-lymphoproliferative disease (syndrome of large granular T lymphocytes) and rare cases of thymoma. Experimental evidence also supports the existence of paraneoplastic suppression of granulopoiesis. These entities are discussed elsewhere in this book.

VII. MONOCYTOPENIA
Monocytopenia as an isolated finding has no clinical significance. Monocytopenia is seen in all causes of aplastic anemia and is a constant finding in hairy cell leukemia, for which it can represent an important diagnostic clue.

VIII. BLOOD COMPONENT THERAPY
A. Transfusion of erythrocytes
1. **Indications** for transfusion of packed RBCs (PRBCs) are for increasing blood volume (with saline or colloid solutions when acute blood loss threatens the integrity of the cardiovascular system) and for increasing oxygen-carrying capacity (when anemia causes or threatens tissue hypoxia). Most patients tolerate chronic, moderately severe anemia well. No specific hemoglobin value mandates transfusion. PRBCs are given to increase the oxygen-carrying capacity of blood for actual or incipient congestive heart failure or to reverse cardiac or central nervous system ischemic symptoms. When the hemoglobin level that precipitated symptoms is determined, patients with chronic anemia are transfused prophylactically to exceed that level.

2. **Transfusion reactions**
   a. **Fever and chills.** Most febrile reactions are caused by antibodies in the recipient directed against granulocytic antigens and specific human leukocyte antigens (HLAs) on leukocytes in the donor blood. Febrile reactions occur in up to 80% of patients who receive multiple transfusions. The reaction usually starts shortly into the transfusion, continues for 2 to 6 hours, and may persist for 12 hours.

   b. **Allergic reactions** involving urticaria develop in 5% of transfused patients. Some of these reactions are due to antibodies in the recipient directed against immunoglobulin components and other proteins in the plasma of the donor. These reactions are usually mild and respond to antihistamines.

   These kinds of reactions or anaphylaxis are particularly likely to occur in patients with congenital IgA deficiency who have formed anti-IgA antibody (1 per 800 people). Reactions can be prevented by using washed or frozen

RBCs because these components are prepared by procedures that remove donor plasma.

c. **Major acute intravascular hemolytic transfusion reactions** are most likely to occur as a result of human error during blood preparation or administration. Fever and chills usually develop within the first 30 minutes into the transfusion and are often accompanied by back pain, sensations of chest compression, tachycardia, hypotension, tachypnea, nausea, vomiting, oliguria, hemoglobinuria, and DIC. The risk for a fatal hemolytic transfusion reaction is about 1:100,000. Plasma is examined for confirmatory findings and compared with the pretransfusion specimen: increased free plasma hemoglobin (pink plasma) and methemalbumin (brown plasma). Detailed evaluation of antibodies evaluated in the cross-matching process follows.

d. **Delayed hemolytic transfusion reactions** occur 5 to 14 days after transfusion, particularly in association with alloantibodies to antigens of the Kidd, Duffy, Kell, or Rh blood group systems. Hemolysis is extravascular and is manifested by jaundice and the absence of an improvement of hemoglobin levels after transfusion. In these cases, patients have become alloimmunized by a previous transfusion or pregnancy, but the antibody concentration was too low to be detected at the time of transfusion; an anamnestic antibody response was generated by the subsequent transfusion.

e. **Posttransfusion purpura** is manifested by severe thrombocytopenia developing 5 to 8 days after transfusion and occurs in the 2% of patients who lack the platelet antigen Pl^{A1}.

f. **Bacterial contamination** occurs rarely in packed RBC units (usually with cryopathic gram-negative bacteria) but is more likely with platelet packs that are stored (at room temperature) for >4 days.

g. **Viral contamination.** Predonation screening interviews and postdonation serologic testing have significantly reduced the incidence of some transfusion-transmitted viral infections (hepatitis B, hepatitis C, and human immunodeficiency virus [HIV]). The risks (per unit for blood units that are negative in laboratory testing) of transmitting viruses through transfusion are as follows:

Hepatitis B virus, 1:150,000
Hepatitis C virus, 1:1,200,000 to 1,900,000
HIV, 1:1,400,000 to 2,100,000
Human T-cell lymphotrophic virus types 1 and 2, 1:640,000

h. **Graft-versus-host disease** (GVHD; see Chapter 37) can occur after blood cell transfusion in patients who have undergone a conditioning regimen for bone marrow transplantation (BMT) or who have acute lymphoblastic leukemia or congenital immunodeficiency. GVHD can also occur in patients who are not immunocompromised if the blood donor is homozygous for one of the HLA haplotypes of the recipient, and particularly if the donor is a first-degree relative. GVHD is preventable by irradiation of blood prior to transfusion.

i. **Other complications** include those associated with massive transfusion (blood volume overload, hypocalcemia, hyperkalemia, hypothermia), iron overload with chronic transfusions, and alloimmunization.

3. **Uses for erythrocyte preparations**
   a. **Fresh whole blood.** None
   b. **PRBCs.** The mainstay of erythrocyte transfusion therapy
   c. **Saline-washed PRBCs** are indicated in patients who have IgA deficiency (particularly those with high anti-IgA titers), prior urticarial reactions with transfusions, the need to avoid transfusion of complement, or the rare patient who is hypersensitive to plasma.
   d. **Leukocyte-reduced PRBCs** are used for patients requiring chronic transfusion therapy and those with prior febrile nonhemolytic transfusion reactions; also, immunocompromised patients in whom reducing the risk for transfusion-transmitted CMV is sought (particularly when seronegative units

for CMV are not available). Leukocytes can be removed by centrifugation, washing, or filtration (the latter technique is most frequently used). These products yield less than 5×10^8 leukocytes per unit of blood.

  e. Frozen RBCs. Source for rare blood types, a backup supply for the common blood types, a substitute for saline-washed or leukocyte-filtered PRBCs when those methods fail to prevent febrile or allergic transfusion reactions, and an additional method of autologous donation. The extensive washing required to remove the cryopreservatives in frozen RBCs renders the suspension totally free of all leukocytes, platelets, and plasma constituents. The major limitations are the cost and the time required to prepare and store cells.

  f. Gamma-irradiated PRBCs are given to prevent viable T lymphocytes from causing transfusion-induced GVHD in the recipient. A dose of 1,500 cGy is usually administered.

  g. Directed or designated donors from among family members or friends, contrary to expectation, are no safer for viral transmission than volunteer blood donors (probably because of the sometimes unreliability of the history taken from these candidates in the screening process prior to donation). Furthermore, these units are associated with an increased risk for GVHD when provided by first-degree relatives to immunocompromised patients.

B. Transfusion of granulocytes. Granulocytes collected by apheresis are rarely helpful in treating patients with granulocytopenia. The paramount factor in determining the outcome of sepsis is the recovery of marrow function. Transfusion of leukocytes often results in GVHD and transmission of CMV. Prophylactic transfusions are useless. If granulocyte transfusion is used, the transfused cells should be irradiated for severely immunocompromised patients, and donors who are seronegative for CMV should be used for seronegative recipients.

Granulocyte harvesting from the donor is promoted by the use of G-CSF and/or glucocorticoids. The donor and recipient must be compatible for Rh and ABO erythrocyte antigens. Daily granulocyte transfusions may be occasionally helpful *only if all of the following criteria are met:*

  1. Recovery of bone marrow function is a reasonable expectation but is not expected to occur for 1 week.

  2. The absolute granulocyte count is $<200/\mu L$.

  3. A serious bacterial or fungal infection is proved by culture.

  4. The infection is not responding to the appropriate antibiotics.

C. Transfusion of platelets

  1. Factors influencing the decision to transfuse platelets

  a. Platelet count. Spontaneous hemorrhage rarely occurs with platelet counts above $20,000/\mu L$. Platelet counts of $<10,000/\mu L$ are associated with an increased risk for spontaneous hemorrhage, especially when the thrombocytopenia results from decreased production rather than from increased platelet destruction. Progressively worsening thrombocytopenia is more likely to be associated with active hemorrhage than with stable or increasing platelet counts.

  b. Platelet age. Young platelets (i.e., produced after peripheral destruction) are larger and better able to provide hemostasis than old platelets. Usually, patients with immune or postinfectious severe thrombocytopenia have no serious hemorrhagic sequelae.

  c. Active bleeding, uncontrollable by local measures, or bleeding into vital or inaccessible organs, is an absolute indication for platelet transfusion in patients with thrombocytopenia of nearly any severity.

  d. Fever, infection, and corticosteroid therapy increase the risk for serious hemorrhage in patients with very low platelet counts.

  e. Drugs and diseases adversely affecting platelet function may necessitate platelet transfusions in times of hemorrhage or surgery despite adequate platelet counts (see section VIII.C.6).

  f. Immune thrombocytopenia usually makes platelet transfusions useless.

g. **Patients with thrombocytopenia that is refractory to platelet transfusion** may be alloimmunized, but they also may have DIC, TTP/HUS, or ITP.

2. **Problems associated with platelet transfusion.** The majority of platelets are now produced by plateletpheresis, wherein the platelet concentrate contains less than 5×10^6 white blood cells (WBCs); these products can be considered "leukocyte-depleted."

   a. **Alloimmunization.** Compatibility between donor and recipient for both ABO and HLAs is important for achieving a successful platelet count increment after transfusion. Alloimmunization requires the presence of class I and class II HLAs. Platelets alone do not result in the development of antibodies because they carry only class I HLAs and platelet-specific antigens; the class II antigens necessary for the development of alloimmunization are provided by transfused monocytes, lymphocytes, and dendritic cells. Rh antigens play a minor role in alloimmunization after platelet transfusions.

   b. **Reactions to platelet transfusion.** Infectious contamination occurs rarely, but more commonly than with PRBCs because platelets are stored at room temperature for 5 days. Hemolysis of the small numbers of contaminating donor RBCs in donor platelet concentrates is of minor consequence. **Febrile reactions,** however, occur often in ABO-compatible platelet transfusions because:

      (1) **Recipient antibodies to WBCs** attack donor WBCs contained in transfused platelet packs. This reaction is prevented by effective leukodepletion of platelet packs.

      (2) **Cytokines released by leukocytes during storage,** particularly TNF-α and IL-1β (which are exceptional pyrogens), are passively transfused. This reaction is prevented by performing leukodepletion before storage of the platelet packs.

      (3) **Recipient antibodies to cells and proteins** in the donor unit form immune complexes that trigger the release of cytokines. This reaction involving incompatible platelets is unaffected by leukodepletion and justifies further testing for HLA antibodies or platelet-specific antibodies, if available.

   c. **Leukodepletion filters** remove donor leukocytes by barrier retention of the filters' microfibers, by adherence to the filter material, and by platelet-leukocyte–mediated interactions.

3. **Selection of which platelet preparation to transfuse** depends on expected future transfusions and the presence of alloimmunization.

   a. **Random (ABO-compatible) units** are obtained from multiple donors of whole blood. Platelet concentrates (without regard to ABO compatibility) may be used in patients with transient thrombocytopenia that is not expected to recur and when platelets are needed immediately.

   b. **Single-donor platelets** (plateletpheresis packs) are obtained by density centrifugation. About 6 to 8 units may be obtained from one donor 2 or 3 times weekly. Single-donor platelet packs are the preferred blood product in conditions that require recurrent platelet transfusions because alloimmunization is delayed. Chemotherapy tends to reduce the risk of alloimmunization to platelets.

   c. **Platelets cross-matched for ABO compatibility** are available for potential use in alloimmunized patients.

   d. **HLA-compatible platelets.** HLA-matched platelets are required in alloimmunized patients but are not always available. The likelihood of an identical HLA match is 1 in 4 among siblings and 1 in 1,000 in the general population.

   e. **Platelets from family members should be avoided** in patients who are possible candidates for BMT. The marrow donor may be used as the source of HLA-identical platelets, however, after the transplantation conditioning program has begun.

4. Prophylactic transfusions

   a. **Acute leukemia.** Prophylactic transfusion of these patients with platelets is recommended to maintain the count above 10,000/μL if they are afebrile and above 20,000/μL if they are febrile.

   b. **In aplastic anemia,** prophylactic transfusions are avoided if possible.

   c. **Pregnancy.** Platelet packs are administered to patients with a platelet count of <100,000/μL just before delivery. After delivery, platelet counts should be maintained above 50,000/μL for 1 week. The possibility of DIC should be evaluated in patients with continued or massive postpartum bleeding associated with thrombocytopenia. Pregnant patients with thrombocytopenia induced by myelosuppressive therapy or leukemia are given platelet transfusions empirically.

5. Effectiveness of platelet transfusions

is determined by measuring platelet counts just before, 1 hour after, and 24 hours after transfusions. If the patient does not respond with an increase of about 25,000 in the platelet count after 1 hour, the transfusion should be considered a failure. The result at 24 hours can be further affected by concurrent hematologic complications.

6. Other measures

   a. **Diseases affecting platelet function.** Patients with uremia require dialysis, cryoprecipitate, or desmopressin acetate (DDAVP) with ε-aminocaproic acid (EACA; Amicar) to improve platelet function. In patients with platelet dysfunction secondary to paraproteins, it is necessary to control the underlying disease or to perform plasmapheresis.

   b. **DDAVP** may be useful in patients with aspirin-induced platelet dysfunction at a dose of 0.3 mcg/kg given over 20 minutes.

   c. **Alloimmunized patients who are refractory to transfused platelets.** High-dose intravenous γ-globulin (400 mg/kg per day for 5 days) occasionally permits better platelet increments in patients who are refractory to platelet transfusion. Cross-matched platelets may be helpful. Plasmapheresis may be tried empirically in difficult situations.

   d. **Menorrhagia in patients with thrombocytopenia** should be treated with medroxyprogesterone, 20 mg PO daily, to induce amenorrhea. Alternatively, leuprolide, 3.75 mg IM monthly, can be used if the platelet count is high enough to permit IM administration. Treatment is continued until the platelet count exceeds 60,000/μL.

D. Transfusion of plasma proteins

1. Preparations

   a. **Fresh-frozen plasma (FFP)** contains all coagulation factors and is useful in replacement of all acquired clotting factor deficiencies (e.g., DIC, massive transfusion, liver disease). The indications for FFP are as follows:

   (1) Replacement of isolated coagulation factor deficiencies

   (2) Reversal of documented coagulation factor deficiencies after massive blood transfusions

   (3) Reversal of warfarin effect in patients requiring immediate surgery or having active bleeding

   (4) Treatment of antithrombin (AT) deficiency or TTP

   b. **Cryoprecipitate** contains von Willebrand factor, fibrinogen (factor I), factor VIII, and factor XIII. Cryoprecipitate is useful in treating acquired deficiencies of fibrinogen and factor VIII (e.g., DIC) when volume overload from plasma treatment is to be avoided and in severe von Willebrand disease.

   c. **Plasma protein fractionation** has resulted in the following commercially available products, which are obtained by pooling plasma from thousands of donors:

   (1) Fibrinogen. This form is never indicated because of the 100% risk for hepatitis.

   (2) Prothrombin complexes (factors II, VII, IX, X, protein C, and protein S) are used in congenital factor deficiencies and in occasional cases of coumarin overdose with life-threatening hemorrhage. The risk for hepatitis with this blood product is 60%. This product carries the risk of inducing venous thrombosis and/or DIC, but the risk appears to have been reduced with modern preparations.

(3) Albumin and purified protein fraction have the same concentration of albumin and the same cost. They are useful for blood volume expansion, but their use in chronic hypoalbuminemia of malabsorption, nephrosis, or cirrhosis or as a nutritional supplement is futile.

(4) Gamma globulin is useful for passive immunization.

d. Hyperimmune IV γ-globulin must be infused at a rate slower than 1 mL/minute to avoid complications. This very expensive product is of definite therapeutic importance in only a few clinical circumstances:

(1) Congenital humoral immunodeficiency states

(2) Acquired humoral immunodeficiency states (e.g., chronic lymphocytic leukemia, lymphoma, myeloma) when complicated by recurrent bacterial infections that do not respond to prophylactic antibiotics

(3) Platelet alloimmunization in conjunction with platelet transfusion

(4) ITP when severe or life-threatening hemorrhage occurs, when severe thrombocytopenia refractory to steroids occurs during pregnancy, or when splenectomy is performed and hemostasis is a problem

2. Hazards

a. Allergy. All plasma preparations are associated with a small incidence of serum sickness reactions. Fever, urticaria, or erythema may also occur in reaction to residual leukocyte antigens.

b. Volume overload is an important consideration when administering FFP. Citrate toxicity may occur with very rapid transfusion rates (100 mL/minute).

c. Infection with hepatitis B, hepatitis C, delta agent hepatitis, HIV, CMV, and EBV is a potential risk for all plasma products.

(1) Very high risk: fibrinogen, prothrombin complex, repeated use of cryoprecipitate

(2) Intermediate risk: single-donor units screened for hepatitis B surface antigen of plasma

(3) Very low risk: γ-globulin, albumin, purified protein fraction (nil for HIV)

COAGULOPATHY

I. THROMBOSIS IN PATIENTS WITH CANCER. Multiple or migratory venous thromboembolism (VTE) in cancer patients has been repeatedly documented since Trousseau's description in 1865. An accelerated course of intermittent claudication and of ischemic heart disease has also been described in cancer patients and probably represents additional variants of Trousseau syndrome. Thus, the presence of cancer is recognized to be a "hypercoagulable" or "thrombophilic" state.

Fibrin-platelet vegetations may form on mitral or aortic valves, resulting in noninfectious ("marantic") endocarditis with paradoxical emboli to peripheral organs. Fewer than one-third of affected afebrile patients have heart murmurs. Most vegetations, which are smaller than 2 mm, are not detected by echocardiography.

A. Incidence. The overall incidence of thrombotic episodes in cancer patients is 10% to 15%, especially during postoperative periods. The postoperative risk of VTE in cancer patients is about double that in patients without cancer (37% vs. 20%) and the risk of fatal pulmonary embolism is about fourfold higher in cancer patients.

About 5% to 10% of patients with idiopathic VTE (see section I.E.) ultimately are proved to have a malignancy, particularly during the first 6 months after diagnosis. Pulmonary emboli have been found at necropsy in about half of the patients with disseminated cancer and have antedated the diagnosis of cancer in 1% to 15% of patients. The malignancies most commonly associated with thrombosis are MPDs and carcinomas of the GI tract, lung, or ovary. Only 7% of patients with pancreatic cancer develop classic Trousseau syndrome.

B. Mechanisms for hypercoagulability
  1. **Cancer is associated with the following thrombophilic factors:**
     a. The tumor's **disruption of blood vessels** exposes collagen and endothelial basement membrane, which may trigger clotting. Tumor neovascularization activates both factor XII and platelet reactions.
     b. Cancers can directly produce various procoagulants. The best characterized is **tissue factor–like procoagulant (TF).** TF forms a complex with factor VIIa to activate factors IX and X, initiating the activation cascade of clotting protease complexes.
        (1) TF is normally expressed only on fibroblasts of the vascular adventitia and other stromal cells. TF is produced by many solid tumor cells and leukemic blasts.
        (2) TF also appears to be an important promoter of tumor growth and of angiogenesis. TF expression directly correlates with the malignant phenotype of various tumors. TF up-regulates expression of vascular endothelial growth factor (VEGF) by tumor cells. VEGF in turn up-regulates TF. The induction of angiogenesis by TF also involves its interaction with the protease-activated receptors (PARs).
     c. **Inflammatory cytokines** (CKs), particularly TNF and IL-1, can be released by tumor cells and immune regulatory cells under pathologic conditions. These CKs can induce TF expression on tumor-associated macrophages and endothelial cells. The endothelial cells become procoagulant under the influence of these CKs.
        (1) The CKs also up-regulate adhesion molecules, platelet-activating factor, and plasminogen activator inhibitor type-1 (PAI-1).
        (2) The CKs down-regulate the expression of thrombomodulin and endothelial cell protein C receptor.
     d. Thus, a **hypercoagulable state** is established in cancer patients through activation of the clotting cascade, activation of platelets, enhancement of endothelial cell adhesion, suppression of fibrinolysis, and inhibition of the anticoagulant protein C pathway.
  2. **Comorbid factors,** such as advanced age, surgery, catheterization, infection, and concomitant chemotherapy, play contributory roles for blood hypercoagulability to become manifest clinically. Venous stasis as a result of bed rest or extrinsic vessel compression from tumor masses also contributes.
  3. **Cancer therapies** associated with enhanced risk for thrombosis are high-dose chemotherapy with BMT, bevacizumab (Avastin), 5-fluorouracil, thalidomide and its derivatives, and high doses of estrogen. Several cytotoxic agents (asparaginase, bleomycin, carmustine, cisplatin, mitomycin C, vinca alkaloids) have been reported to cause VTE but the true incidence and mechanisms are not clear.
     a. Tamoxifen increases the risk for venous thrombosis slightly (1.5-fold to twofold) when given alone and significantly increases the risk for venous and arterial thrombosis when given concomitantly with chemotherapy, particularly in premenopausal women. The aryl aromatase inhibitors used in the treatment of postmenopausal women with breast cancer also increase the risk for thrombosis.
     b. The presence of the prothrombin G20210A gene mutation or of activated protein C resistance as a result of the inheritance of factor V^{Leiden} may increase the risk further for hormonal therapies. However, these mutations have been shown not to be contributing factors for the development of VTE in patients receiving cytotoxic chemotherapy.
C. Management of recurrent thrombosis in cancer patients is difficult because it is often resistant to therapy and because patients often have worrisome sites for potential hemorrhage.
  1. **Anticoagulant therapy.** Standard-dose intravenous unfractionated heparin (UH), low-dose UH (LDUH), adjusted-dose SC UH (while monitoring the partial thromboplastin time), and weight-adjusted low-molecular-weight heparin

(LMWH) are options for initiating therapy, depending on the clinical and social circumstances.

   a. The attractiveness of LMWH is the ability to treat venous thrombosis outside the hospital setting without the need for monitoring clotting tests; the switch to oral warfarin is made after 8 to 12 days.

   b. Treatment with LMWH may be extended well beyond the usual transition period to oral therapy with warfarin. For secondary prophylaxis of VTE in cancer patients, studies indicate more favorable efficacy for LMWH with treatment extended for 3 to 6 months compared to warfarin.

   c. If there are concerns about potential bleeding, low-dose warfarin may be used with an international normalized ratio (INR) target of 1.4 to 1.9. The dose of warfarin can be increased to maintain a higher INR for recurrent thrombosis. The necessary duration of warfarin therapy in cancer patients is unclear.

  2. Contraindications to anticoagulant therapy include the following:

   a. Pre-existing clotting defect or bleeding source

   b. Inaccessible ulceration (e.g., GI tract)

   c. Recent hemorrhage or surgery in the eye or central nervous system

   d. Severe hypertension or bacterial endocarditis

   e. Regional or lumbar anesthesia; T-tube drainage

   f. Pregnancy (if anticoagulation is mandatory, UH or LMWH is used because it crosses the placenta less readily than warfarin)

  3. Vena caval interruption, usually with a Greenfield filter, is performed if anticoagulants are contraindicated. The filter is effective for preventing pulmonary embolism, but the risk for recurrent VTE increases.

  4. Graduated compression stockings should be used, if practical, particularly in postoperative patients.

  5. Removal of the tumor may control thrombotic episodes but is often impossible.

  6. Special considerations for anticoagulation in cancer patients. The objective in treating VTE (prevention of death due to and other complications of pulmonary embolism) is not necessarily applicable in the preterminal patient with cancer. The goal of anticoagulation in these patients is more likely to prevent pain in the extremities or chest. Therapy with warfarin in cancer patients is often chaotic and associated with unpredictable changes in dose response because of the presence of poor nutrition, impaired liver function, infection, and concomitant medications (especially antibiotics). Furthermore, temporary cessation of anticoagulation may be necessary because of thrombocytopenia induced by chemotherapy.

D. Prophylaxis against venous thrombosis in cancer patients

  1. Cancer surgery is associated with a 35% risk of venous thrombosis without prophylaxis. The use of either LMWH or LDUH decreases the rate to 13%. The addition of mechanical prophylaxis to either anticoagulant program reduces the risk to 5%. There appears to be no difference between the anticoagulation agents, but higher doses are more effective than lower doses (e.g., 1.5 mg/kg rather than 1.0 mg/kg daily for enoxaparin or 5,000 units SQ 3 times daily rather than twice daily for LDUH). Some authorities have advised prophylaxis to continue for at least 1 month, which is very effective and does not increase the risk of hemorrhage. Published rates of major bleeding complications are low, particularly in those patients without significant risk factors for bleeding.

   a. Issues with anesthesia. Patients receiving thienopyridine platelet inhibitors (clopidogrel, ticlopidine) should discontinue those drugs 2 weeks prior to surgery. The timing of spinal anesthesia should coincide with the trough blood levels of heparin.

   b. Heparin-induced thrombocytopenia occurs in 1% to 5% of patients treated with LDUH and in <1% of patients receiving LMWH under these circumstances.

  2. Central venous catheters. Low doses of warfarin or LMWH seem to have no effect on reducing catheter-related thrombotic complications. Increased risk for thrombosis is seen in those patients with a poorly positioned catheter tip, insertion of the catheter in left-sided veins, age >60 years, or metastatic disease.

3. **Chemotherapy.** The risk of VTE in cancer patients undergoing chemotherapy is particularly high. Current evidence, however, does not support the use of generalized prophylaxis in these patients.

E. **Diagnostic tests in patients with idiopathic VTE**

1. **The clinical diagnosis of venous thrombosis** is made by physical examination and venous ultrasonography or venography. Venography and the fibrinogen uptake test have higher rates of detection than ultrasonography. The presence of venous thrombosis, a heart murmur, and arterial embolism suggests an underlying mucin-producing carcinoma.

2. **An occult malignancy should be sought** in patients who present with any of the following:

   a. Idiopathic deep vein thrombosis or pulmonary emboli
   b. Idiopathic deep vein thrombosis combined with arterial thrombosis
   c. Idiopathic thrombosis that is recurrent or at multiple sites
   d. Thrombosis that is resistant to anticoagulation therapy
   e. Associated paraneoplastic syndromes and thrombosis

3. **A reasonable screening evaluation for occult cancer** in patients with thrombotic disease includes a thorough history and physical examination (including rectal or pelvic examination), CBC, LFTs, LDH, prostate-specific antigen in men older than 50 years, urinalysis, stool for occult blood, and chest radiograph. An abdominopelvic CT scan and carcinoembryonic antigen assay may be considered for patients who are suspected to have cancer.

   Routine screening for cancer in patients with unprovoked VTE using extensive studies evaluating systems not suggested by basic screening is not justified. Detecting cancers in this way has not been shown to provide a survival advantage.

4. **Laboratory tests of coagulation** can be obtained during the first idiopathic thromboembolic event in an otherwise healthy person to seek a possible biological defect predisposing to thrombosis. Such assays would include the following:

   a. Assays for lupus anticoagulant and serologic tests for antiphospholipid antibodies
   b. Functional assays for protein C and AT
   c. Functional assays for protein S (immunologic assays of total and free protein S)
   d. Clotting assay for resistance to activated protein C (genetic test for factor V^{Leiden} if clotting assay is positive)
   e. Screening for dysfibrinogenemia (thrombin time, immunologic and functional assays of fibrinogen)
   f. Total plasma homocysteine
   g. Genetic test for prothrombin gene mutation (prothrombin 20210A)
   h. Various laboratory findings that are *not predictive* of thromboembolic disease in cancer patients include increased levels of platelets, markers of platelet activation, markers of thrombin generation, fibrinogen, and factors V, VIII, IX, and XI; decreased plasma levels of AT; suppression of fibrinolytic activity.

II. **DIC** is provoked by numerous disorders. If series of cases with disproportionate numbers of obstetrics and trauma cases are excluded, the vast majority of cases result from infectious diseases or cancer. DIC is a frequent complication for patients with metastatic cancer, either as a consequence of the metastases themselves or complicating infections. Local or diffuse thrombosis or hemorrhage can occur in all combinations. The incidence depends on the definition of DIC and assays used. Severe DIC is common in only two malignancies: metastatic carcinoma of the prostate and acute hypergranular promyelocytic leukemia (type M3).

A. **Factors in pathogenesis of DIC.** With all inciting conditions, procoagulants are produced or introduced into the blood and overcome the anticoagulant mechanisms, leading to the generation of thrombin and DIC. The endothelium of the capillary bed in conjunction with mononuclear inflammatory cells are the mainstays of host defense against organ and tissue injury. Compromising the endothelium with injury or infection can trigger the sequential "systemic inflammatory response syndrome," which can lead to microvascular thrombosis and ensuing multiorgan dysfunction. The following is an overview of the extraordinarily complex interactions that result in the clinical syndrome of DIC.

1. **Tissue factor** and the cascade of cytokines leading to thrombosis are discussed in section I.B. Once TF is expressed on the membrane of monocytes and endothelial cells, thrombin is generated and fibrin and platelets are deposited.

2. **Thrombin** generation amplifies both clotting and inflammation by activating:
   a. Factors VIII, V, and XI, yielding further thrombin generation
   b. Platelets, giving rise to platelet aggregation and activation
   c. Proinflammatory factors via PARs
   d. Factor XIII, which makes fibrin insoluble by covalent cross-linking
   e. Thrombin-activatable fibrinolysis inhibitor, making clots resistant to fibrinolysis
   f. Inflammatory effects of leukocytes

3. **Activation of complement** (C'5 and C'5–9) by injury or inflammation accelerates the rate of coagulation reactions. C'4b binding protein can become a procoagulant and proinflammatory by binding protein S, thereby decreasing free protein S levels and slowing the quenching of inflammation via the endothelial protein C receptor pathway.

4. **Up-regulation of inflammation** is induced by the coagulation proteases (e.g., thrombin, Xa, VIIa-TF) via PARs, which are located on endothelial cells, platelets, and leukocytes.

5. **Activated protein C,** which has an anti-inflammatory effect, decelerates thrombin generation by inactivating factors Va and VIIIa in the presence of protein S. Protein C is activated by thrombin-thrombomodulin complexes on endothelial cells. Thrombomodulin is most ubiquitous in the capillary beds of the microcirculation where the disruptions and inflammations are occurring.

6. **AT** is an important circulating serine protease inhibitor that neutralizes thrombin, factor Xa, and the other coagulation serine proteases. AT is consumed in DIC.

7. **Fibrinolysis** often becomes impaired in DIC, resulting in persistent microthrombosis. In patients with DIC and multiorgan failure tissue plasminogen activator antigen and PAI-1 are often elevated and α-antiplasmin is reduced.

8. **Superoxides and hydroxyl radicals** generated during sepsis and other organ injury states are proinflammatory agents that induce endothelial apoptosis, which would exacerbate capillary leak.

9. **Elastase** released by damaged endothelium interacting with activated neutrophils promotes DIC by inhibiting thrombomodulin function, causing detachment of endothelial cells and inhibiting fibrinolysis.

B. **Diagnosis.** The widespread generation of thrombin in DIC induces the deposition of fibrin, which results in the consumption of platelets, fibrinogen, factors V and VIII, protein C, AT, and components of the fibrinolytic system. The severity of DIC manifestations depends on the underlying diagnosis, the acuteness of the DIC, the integrity of the reticuloendothelial system, and the intensity of secondary fibrinolysis. Some patients hemorrhage profusely and have marked abnormalities of all of the tests for DIC. On the other hand, DIC may be subclinical and manifested only by a positive paracoagulation test and mild thrombocytopenia.

1. **Clinical features**
   a. **Type of bleeding.** Patients with severe DIC bleed from multiple sites simultaneously. Petechiae, ecchymoses, mucosal bleeding, and oozing from venipunctures, lines, and catheters are common. Patients with chronic DIC (the usual DIC seen with malignancies) may have minimal bleeding.
   b. **End-organ damage.** Microangiopathic hemolysis, hypotension, oliguria, and renal failure are frequent complications of serious DIC. Renal cortical ischemia induced by microthrombosis of afferent glomerular arterioles and acute tubular necrosis due to hypotension are the major causes of renal dysfunction in DIC. Both the diseases underlying DIC and DIC itself can cause shock.

Microvascular thrombi and thromboembolism can result in dysfunction of any organ (e.g., acral necrosis, neurologic manifestations, and pulmonary dysfunction).

2. **Laboratory tests.** No single test is diagnostic for DIC.

   a. **Blood smear.** The numbers of circulating platelets are decreased and fragmented erythrocytes or microspherocytes may be seen.

   b. **Platelet count.** Thrombocytopenia occurs nearly always, but DIC alone rarely causes platelet counts of <50,000/μL. Concomitant causes of thrombocytopenia should be sought for severe thrombocytopenia in the presence of DIC.

   c. **Clotting tests.** Prothrombin time (PT) and activated partial thromboplastin time (aPTT) may be slightly shortened, normal, or prolonged. Thrombin time (TT) prolongation occurs with severe hypofibrinogenemia (<50 mg/dL) or clinically significant elevation of fibrin degradation products; the TT can also be prolonged with heparin therapy, dysfibrinogenemia, or malignant paraproteinemia.

   d. **Fibrinogen level** is usually decreased. Fibrinogen concentrations >50 mg/dL (normal range is 200 to 400 mg/dL) should not result in abnormalities of the TT. It is important to remember that fibrinogen is a phase reactant protein and is normally elevated in pregnancy and inflammatory states; thus, a normal result may actually be abnormal.

   e. **Paracoagulation tests for fibrin monomers** (protamine sulfate or D-dimers) are positive in >95% of patients with DIC.

3. **DIC versus primary fibrinolysis.** Although primary fibrinolysis is rare and DIC is common, differentiation between these disorders is important to plan treatment. These disorders are compared in Table 34.2. The platelet count, paracoagulation test, and euglobulin lysis separate the disorders.

C. **Management.** Few patients with DIC are helped if the underlying problem is not corrected. Treatment is not necessary for laboratory manifestations alone. The following sequence is recommended:

1. **Treat the underlying disease.** This may be futile for patients with disseminated cancer alone, but the possible advantages of antimicrobial therapy, further surgery, RT, or chemotherapy should be considered. Hypotension, tissue perfusion, acidosis, hypoxemia, and the triggering event (e.g., sepsis) must be addressed vigorously.

2. **Administration of blood components.** Platelet packs are given in the presence of thrombocytopenia and serious bleeding. DIC microangiopathy can induce organ failure long before the bleeding risk from DIC becomes relevant; thus, the threshold platelet count to prompt transfusion is dependent on the patient and the diseases that are evident.

   FFP or cryoprecipitate (for fibrinogen and factor VIII) usually improve factor deficiencies unless the clotting process is severe. Replacement therapy may need to be repeated every 8 hours, with adjustment of doses according to platelet count,

 TABLE 34.2 **Comparison of Acute Disseminated Intravascular Coagulation (DIC) and Primary Fibrinolysis**

Feature	Acute DIC	Primary fibrinolysis
Incidence	Common	Very rare
Platelets[a]	Decreased	Usually normal
Paracoagulation test (fibrin monomers)[a]	Positive	Negative
Clot lysis or euglobulin lysis time[a]	Normal or long	Rapid
Fibrinogen	Decreased	Decreased
Fibrin degradation products	Increased	Large amounts

[a]Discriminatory assays.

PT, aPTT, fibrinogen level, and volume status. Cryoprecipitate is useful in patients with borderline cardiac reserve who cannot tolerate large volumes of FFP.

3. The use of heparin remains controversial. At best, heparin has improved the levels of hemostatic factors in treated patients, but has not reduced mortality. However, heparin can seriously aggravate bleeding. Heparin appears to have most benefit in patients with chronic DIC and can be considered if DIC is causing end-organ damage.

4. Fibrinolysis is inhibited only if necessary, that is, if the patient has documented primary fibrinolysis or DIC with life-threatening bleeding and evidence of extensive secondary fibrinolysis (i.e., shortened euglobulin lysis time). Use of these agents in patients with active DIC has been complicated by severe thrombosis. Fibrinolysis may be inhibited by EACA (Amicar) or tranexamic acid; renal failure is a relative contraindication for EACA use. A loading dose of 5 g is followed by 0.5 to 1 g/hour IV or 2 g every 2 hours PO. If the episode of DIC has abated, EACA may be given alone. If the status of DIC is uncertain or ongoing, heparin should be given with EACA.

5. Antiplatelet drugs (aspirin and dipyridamole) may be useful in patients with chronic DIC who are not bleeding.

6. Other measures. Activated protein C infusion can reduce mortality in septicemia, particularly if DIC is demonstrable. Infusion of AT also has been tested but has not be shown to be beneficial.

7. Patient surveillance. The platelet count, fibrinogen level, and clinical evaluation are the most useful factors to follow. Following paracoagulation tests is not useful for monitoring therapy because their clearance can be delayed. The *reptilase time* (performed like the TT) is sensitive to the presence of fibrin degradation products; unlike the TT, the reptilase test is not affected by heparin.

III. PRIMARY FIBRINOLYSIS. Primary fibrinolysis occurs essentially only in metastatic prostatic carcinoma, advanced cirrhosis of the liver, heat stroke, or amniotic fluid embolism.

A. Malignancies may promote fibrinolysis by releasing plasminogen activators, such as urokinase or other proteolytic enzymes. Extensive metastatic liver disease may result in decreased clearance of plasminogen and its activators. Prostatic carcinoma and, to a lesser extent, benign prostatic conditions are capable of triggering both thrombosis and fibrinolysis. Other cancers that have been reported to activate fibrinolysis are sarcoma and carcinomas of the breast, thyroid, colon, and stomach.

B. Diagnosis of primary fibrinolysis: see section II.B.3.

C. Management of primary fibrinolysis: see section II.C.4.

IV. OTHER HEMOSTATIC DEFECTS ASSOCIATED WITH CANCER

A. Platelet function abnormalities are common in malignancies.

1. Mechanisms

a. Coating of platelet surfaces by fibrin degradation products with DIC

b. Coating of platelets by paraproteins with myeloma

c. Concomitant azotemia

d. Inherent platelet dysfunction associated with myelodysplastic disorders or MPDs

e. Patients may be taking drugs with antiplatelet activity, such as aspirin, other nonsteroidal anti-inflammatory drugs, clopidogrel, or ticlodipine.

2. Diagnosis

a. Signs of platelet dysfunction include easy bruisability, gingival bleeding with toothbrushing, and other minor mucosal bleeding.

b. Laboratory studies. A variety of *in vitro* platelet function tests have uncertain clinical validity. Thrombocytopenia, DIC, and azotemia should be ruled out by appropriate tests.

3. Treatment. Patients with bleeding and platelet dysfunction require treatment of the underlying disorder and may require platelet transfusions. DDAVP, 0.3 mcg/kg IV over 20 minutes, may also be helpful temporarily.

B. **Paraproteinemia.** Hemostatic abnormalities associated with plasma cell myeloma were discussed in Chapter 22, section IX.A.1.a.(1).

C. **Liver metastases,** when extensive, can result in the inability to synthesize clotting factors. Treatment with vitamin K is ineffective. Bleeding may be controlled by the administration of FFP, which also may be impractical.

D. **Dysfibrinogenemia.** Dysfibrinogens are abnormal fibrinogen molecules, which may be inherited or acquired in association with hepatocellular carcinoma or liver metastases. The PT, aPTT, and TT are all markedly abnormal. Fibrinogen concentrations are low when measured by clotting methods but are normal when measured by immunologic or physical precipitation methods. Hemorrhage is not common with dysfibrinogenemia but may occur.

E. **Acquired circulating inhibitors of coagulation** occur in a wide variety of tumors (e.g., a heparinlike inhibitor has been described in mastocytosis). It is doubtful that these inhibitors are responsible for hemorrhage in the absence of other causes, such as uremia or thrombocytopenia.

F. **Specific factor deficiencies**
   1. **Factor XIII deficiency or dysfunction** is common in patients with cancer but usually does not cause clinical problems. The PT, PTT, and TT are normal, but the assay for factor XIII is abnormal. Hemorrhagic episodes are treated with FFP, 5 mL/kg weekly.
   2. **Factor X deficiency** may occasionally be an isolated coagulation abnormality in patients with amyloidosis, which can also be associated with systemic fibrinolysis. Hemorrhagic episodes are treated with FFP or prothrombin complexes.
   3. **Factor XII and Fletcher factor (prekallikrein) deficiencies** have been described in patients with cancer but have little clinical significance.
   4. **Acquired von Willebrand disease** has been reported in cancer patients, particularly in the MPDs in association with marked thrombocytosis. (See Chapter 24, section II.C.2 in "Comparable Aspects.")

G. **Hemostatic abnormalities associated with cytotoxic agents**
   1. **Hypofibrinogenemia** or dysfibrinogenemia is an almost universal complication of treatment with L-asparaginase.
   2. **Vitamin K antagonism** occurs with actinomycin D therapy.
   3. **DIC** is a common complication of administration of mithramycin.
   4. **Primary fibrinolysis** has been reported to be activated by the anthracyclines.
   5. **Platelet dysfunction** (of questionable significance) has been reported with cytarabine, daunorubicin, melphalan, vincristine, mitomycin C, L-asparaginase, and high-dose chemotherapy in preparation for BMT.
   6. **Budd-Chiari syndrome** is associated with dacarbazine therapy.

Suggested Reading

Thrombosis and Cancer

Bergqvist D, et al. Duration of prophylaxis against thromboembolism with enoxaparin after surgery for cancer. *N Engl J Med* 2002;346:974.

Bergqvist D. Risk of venous thromboembolism in patients undergoing cancer surgery and options for thromboprophylaxis. *J Surg Oncol* 2007;95:167.

Falciani M, Imberti D, Prisco D. Prophylaxis and treatment of venous thromboembolism in patients with cancer: an update. *Intern Emerg Med* 2006;1:273.

Leonardi MJ, McGory ML, Ko CY. A systematic review of deep venous thrombosis prophylaxis in cancer patients: Implications for improving quality. *Ann Surg Oncol* 2007;14:929.

Nash, GF, Walsh DC, Kakkar AK. The role of the coagulation system in tumor angiogenesis. *Lancet Oncol* 2001;2:608.

Prandoni P, et al. Recurrent venous thromboembolism and bleeding complications during anticoagulant treatment in patients with cancer and venous thrombosis. *Blood* 2002;100:3484.

Rickles FR. Relationship of blood clotting and tumor angiogenesis. *Haemostasis* 2001; 31(suppl 1):16.

Sallah S, et al. Disseminated intravascular coagulation in solid tumors: clinical and pathologic study. *Thromb Haemost* 2001;86:828.

Sørenson HT, et al. The risk of a diagnosis of cancer after primary deep vein thrombosis or pulmonary embolism. *N Engl J Med* 1998;338:1169.

Thompson CA, Steensma DP. Pure red cell aplasia associated with thymoma: clinical insights from a 50-year single-institution experience. *Br J Haematol* 2006;135:405.

Trousseau A. Phlegmasia alba dolens. *Clin Med Hotel Dieu Paris* 1865;3:94.

Other Topics

Castello A, Coci A, Magrini U. Paraneoplastic marrow alterations in patients with cancer. *Haematologica* 1992;77:392.

Chapman JF, et al. Guidelines on the clinical use of leucocyte-depleted blood components. *Transfus Med* 1998;8:59.

Dodd RY, Notari IV, Stamer SL. Current prevalence and incidence of infectious disease markers and estimated window-period risk in the American Red Cross blood donor population. *Transfusion* 2002;42:975.

Jannssens AM, Offner FC, Van Hove WZ. Bone marrow necrosis. *Cancer* 2000;88:1769.

Kuderer NM, et al. Impact of primary prophylaxis with granulocyte colony-stimulating factor on febrile neutropenia and mortality in adult cancer patients receiving chemotherapy: a systematic review. *J Clin Oncol* 2007;25:3158.

Kuter DJ. New thrombopoietic growth factors. *Blood* 2007;109:4607.

Tas F, et al. Anemia in oncology practice: relation to diseases and their therapies. *Am J Clin Oncol* 2002;25:371.

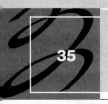

INFECTIOUS COMPLICATIONS
W. Lance George

I. BACKGROUND

The development of infection in patients undergoing treatment for malignancies is a complex interplay of a number of factors. These include alterations in the host's natural mechanical barriers to infection, reduction in the number and function of "professional" phagocytes (particularly, neutrophils), and alterations in both humoral and cell-mediated immunity. These various alterations may be a consequence of the malignancy itself or of the treatment (chemotherapy and radiation therapy).

Certain patterns of infection have been recognized and form the basis for empirical management. For example, neutropenia is a major predisposition to bacterial infection, yet it is clear that chemotherapy-induced neutropenia can occur in association with alterations in the host's mechanical barriers to infection, and alterations in both humoral and cell-mediated immunity. These interactions likely account both for the different infectious complications that occur during therapy of malignancies and for the types of infections that may be seen with different malignancies.

II. NEUTROPENIA AND FEVER

A. Principles. Development of fever in neutropenic patients should always be regarded as a medical emergency caused by infection. The patient who has signs or symptoms of infection, in the absence of fever, should still be treated in a manner similar to that of the febrile patient.

Early in the period of neutropenia, bacterial infections predominate; hence, management of suspected infection is usually directed initially toward bacterial processes. Diagnosis of a specific infectious process is not possible, however, in a significant proportion of febrile neutropenic patients; much of the clinical uncertainty in treating patients with neutropenia is related to the lack of a specific diagnosis. This should not, however, deter the physician from performing a thorough evaluation and continuing to reassess the patient. Management of infection in the neutropenic patient continues to evolve as new diagnostic tests and antimicrobial therapies (particularly, antifungal) are developed.

1. Definitions

   a. Fever. A single oral temperature measurement of $\geq 101°F$ ($38.3°C$), or a temperature of $\geq 100.4°F$ ($38.0°C$) for >1 hour constitutes fever.

   b. Neutropenia. A neutrophil count of $\leq 1,000$ cells/μL represents neutropenia and is associated with an increased risk of infection. The risk of infection is substantially increased, however, when the absolute neutrophil count (ANC) is ≤ 500 cells/μL, and it is quite high when the count is ≤ 100 cells/μL.

2. Prevention of infection in neutropenic patients

   a. General measures

   (1) Handwashing by the staff before touching patients is the most important preventive technique.

   (2) Skin care may be important in preventing infections with *Staphylococcus aureus* and other pathogens. Occlusive antiperspirants should be avoided. Electric shavers are preferred; not shaving at all may be best.

   (3) Avoidance of fresh flowers and foods with high bacterial contents (e.g., fruits, uncooked foods, and tap water) is commonly practiced, but has no established value.

(4) Teeth should be brushed daily. Procedures involving the use of tubes, tapes, and instruments should be minimized because they may be sources of infection.

b. Isolation methods

(1) Reverse or neutropenic isolation (caps, masks, gloves, and gowns) has no established benefit. In addition, it deters good patient care by limiting patient contact with the hospital staff and family.

(2) High-efficiency particulate air filters and laminar airflow rooms, which are expensive, are of questionable benefit.

c. Prophylactic antibiotics. Using absorbable, orally administered antibiotics in neutropenic patients alters the endogenous flora, particularly in the gastrointestinal (GI) tract. Many have advocated this as a form of prophylaxis in the neutropenic patient. The disadvantage of routine oral prophylaxis is the risk of inducing significant resistance of the bacterial and fungal flora to the agents being used for prophylaxis; this, in turn, would limit the availability of effective agents to treat infection.

(1) Prophylaxis with fluoroquinolones (e.g., levofloxacin, 500 mg PO daily) reduces the incidence of fever, "probable" infection, and hospitalization, but does not reduce overall mortality. Subsequent infections are more likely to be the result of resistant organisms. Significant concern exists regarding the rising incidence of resistance to quinolones and the relationship of this resistance to *Clostridium difficile* diarrhea and colitis. If routine prophylactic antimicrobial therapy is adopted at a cancer center, it should be done in association with rigorous infection control practices and monitoring for emergence of resistant microorganisms.

(2) The routine use of sulfamethoxazole-trimethoprim (Bactrim or Septra) for bacterial prophylaxis in neutropenic patients is of limited benefit and possesses some of the same risks associated with quinolone prophylaxis. Patients at risk for *Pneumocystis carinii* (renamed *P. jiroveci*) infection, such as those with leukemia, certain solid tumors, and acquired immunodeficiency syndrome (AIDS), should, however, receive prophylaxis in the form of one double strength tablet (800 mg of sulfamethoxazole plus 160 mg of trimethoprim) once daily during the period of neutropenia. Sulfamethoxazole-trimethoprim *is not recommended*, however, for bacterial prophylaxis.

(3) Intravenous vancomycin prophylaxis has been used to prevent catheter-associated gram-positive infections or as combination prophylaxis with quinolones. This practice is *strongly discouraged.*

(4) Linezolid, daptomycin, and quinupristin-dalfopristin (Zyvox, Cubicin, and Synercid, respectively) are newer agents with activity against some resistant gram-positive organisms; they *should not be used* as prophylactic agents.

(5) Antifungal agents. Posaconazole prophylaxis was recently shown to improve survival when compared with fluconazole and itraconazole in patients with certain types of immunosuppression. Patients studied were those who received chemotherapy for acute myelogenous leukemia or myelodysplastic syndrome, and those undergoing allogeneic hematopoietic stem-cell transplantation recipients with graft-versus-host disease (GVHD). Serious side effects of prophylaxis were noted. Although there is debate regarding the overall benefit of antifungal prophylaxis in severely immunosuppressed patients, *antifungal prophylaxis in patients with lesser degrees of immunosuppression is not recommended.*

3. Predisposition to infection

a. The degree and the duration of neutropenia are the most important and easily measured risk factors that predispose to the development of infection. Neutropenia of relatively brief duration (5 to 7 days) is most likely to be associated with bacterial infection, reflecting the important role of granulocytes in the prevention or control of bacterial infection. Defects in granulocyte function, humoral immunity, and cell-mediated immunity are likely contributing factors, particularly when neutropenia is of longer duration, but these defects are difficult to assess clinically.

b. Defects in the normal mechanical barriers of the host to infection are important predispositions to infection.

(1) Defects in mechanical barriers related to treatment of malignancy are major predisposing factors. The most common sites of such breaches are the skin, the paranasal sinuses, and the alimentary tract; breaches of these barriers allow for local and disseminated infection by the indigenous (normal) and colonizing (environmental) flora of the skin and alimentary tract. Placement of vascular access devices creates a portal for infection of the surrounding soft tissues and bloodstream by micro-organisms. Other invasive procedures pose risks for infection that relate to the site of the procedure.

(2) Other types of impairment of the host's normal barriers to infection include tumor invasion of mucosal surfaces and of the integument; loss of protective reflexes, such as cough; and obstruction to drainage of hollow organs, such as the urinary bladder and the gall bladder.

c. Hospitalization, per se, does not increase the risk of infection, but it does influence the types of infecting organisms and their antimicrobial susceptibility.

4. Infecting organisms

a. Early in the course of neutropenia, bacteria predominate as the microbiologically documented pathogens. Gram-positive bacteria now account for approximately two-thirds of isolates, gram-negative bacilli account for approximately one-fourth, and *Candida* species and other fungi are occasional pathogens, although fungi are usually not of major concern early in neutropenia. Gram-negative bacilli that are encountered frequently include *Escherichia coli, Klebsiella pneumoniae,* and *Pseudomonas aeruginosa.*

Increasing antimicrobial resistance among gram-positive bacteria has made management difficult. *S. aureus* and *Streptococcus pneumoniae* may be resistant to traditional antimicrobial agents (penicillins and cephalosporins) and produce rapidly fatal infections. Other gram-positive organisms may also display significant antimicrobial resistance, but typically have a more indolent course; these include coagulase-negative staphylococci, vancomycin-resistant enterococci, and *Corynebacterium jeikeium.*

b. Later in the course of neutropenia, fungi, particularly *Candida* species and *Aspergillus* species, must be considered as potential pathogens. In addition, multiply drug-resistant bacteria must be considered.

c. *Clostridium difficile*-associated diarrhea or colitis is now frequently hospital acquired; it is often associated with fever and almost invariably follows antimicrobial therapy. Of note, onset of symptoms may occur during antimicrobial treatment or as many as 6 weeks after cessation of antimicrobial therapy.

B. Diagnosis

1. History and physical examination. A careful history should be taken, with a focus on new symptoms and on sites that are most commonly infected. Classic signs of inflammation may not be present because of the absence of neutrophilic exudates in infected tissues, although the presence of localized pain may be an important clue. Perform a detailed examination of the ocular fundus; oropharynx, including teeth and supporting structures; lungs; perineum and perianal areas; and the skin, including vascular access catheter sites and other breaks in the integument related to diagnostic procedures. Digital rectal examination and pelvic examination are usually not performed because trauma to the mucosa during the examination may cause bacteremia.

2. Laboratory evaluation. At least two samples of blood for bacterial and fungal culture should be obtained promptly by percutaneous collection. The practice of obtaining blood cultures via a central venous catheter (CVC) is not necessary; if micro-organisms are present in blood, they will be detected by percutaneously collected cultures. Recovery of organisms from cultures collected from a CVC may reflect true infection, but frequently reflects contamination of the external port or connection hardware of the CVC; this often leads to much confusion, unnecessary use of antimicrobial agents, with the attendant risks of adverse side effects and colonization of the patient by increasingly resistant micro-organisms.

If a CVC is present, the skin exit site should be carefully inspected. If there is drainage from the CVC exit site, the exudate should be submitted to the laboratory for Gram stain, bacterial culture, and fungal culture and microscopic examination.

Cutaneous lesions should be either aspirated or biopsied for bacterial and fungal cultures. Sputum for bacterial culture should be obtained if pulmonary symptoms are present or radiographic abnormalities are seen. Urine culture is indicated if there are symptoms, a bladder catheter is present, or the urinalysis is abnormal. If diarrhea is present, then samples should be submitted for *Clostridium difficile* toxin test and routine bacterial cultures; if diarrhea has been present for >7 days, tests for *Giardia, Cryptosporidium, Cyclospora,* and *Isospora* should be submitted.

3. **Surveillance cultures.** No clinical value is seen in obtaining *surveillance* cultures from sites such as the anterior nares, pharynx, urine, and rectum or perianal area.

4. **Imaging studies.** A baseline chest radiograph (posteroanterior and lateral views) should always be done as part of the initial evaluation. CT, MRI, ^{67}Ga scanning, and other isotopic scans and imaging studies may occasionally be of diagnostic value, depending on the particular clinical circumstances. Generally, CT and MRI scans are the imaging studies most likely to yield useful information.

C. **Empiric therapy. Initial antimicrobial therapy.** Treatment of febrile neutropenic patients has traditionally been with IV antimicrobial agents in an inpatient setting. Studies have demonstrated that selected low-risk patients can be safely treated with oral antimicrobial therapy as outpatients. Useful antibacterial and antifungal agents for the treatment of neutropenic fever are shown in Table 35.1.

1. **Intravenous antimicrobial therapy.** Most patients will fall into this category. Several different themes for treatment have been found to be effective. Each of these, however, requires knowledge of the antimicrobial susceptibility patterns of bacteria isolated at the facility where the patient has been receiving care and consideration of the particular infection, if a diagnosis is known. Information regarding antimicrobial susceptibility, often termed the hospital "antibiogram," can usually be obtained from the microbiology laboratory. The goal of empiric therapy is to provide coverage against likely pathogens pending receipt of culture results. Information from the antibiogram can be used to tailor empiric treatment based on local resistance patterns.

The three themes are (*a*) administration of a single broad-spectrum agent; (*b*) two-drug therapy that does not include vancomycin; and (*c*) two- to three-drug therapy that includes vancomycin. Any treatment regimen should contain a nonaminoglycoside antipseudomonal agent, because single-drug coverage of *Pseudomonas* with an aminoglycoside is not reliably effective in the presence of neutropenia.

A reasonable clinical approach is first to select one of the agents listed under monotherapy and then to determine whether vancomycin therapy is also warranted. Finally, determine whether an aminoglycoside is needed because of the risk of a multiply drug-resistant gram bacillus.

a. **Agents appropriate for monotherapy** are a broad-spectrum carbapenem (imipenem-cilastatin or meropenem), a combination of a broad spectrum β-lactam with a β-lactamase inhibitor (e.g., piperacillin-tazobactam), or cefepime (a fourth-generation cephalosporin). Other cephalosporins and carbapenems are not appropriate for initial therapy because of limitations in their spectrum of activity.

TABLE 35.1 Useful Antibiotics for Neutropenic Fever

Antibiotic (brand name)[a]	Standard dose in NF	Comments
Carbapenems		
Imipenem-cilastatin (Primaxin)[b]	0.5 g IV q6h	1.0 g q6 to 8h may be given in certain situations, but these higher doses predispose to seizures
Meropenem (Merrem)	1.0 g IV q8h	Less likely than imipenem-cilastatin to induce seizures when given in standard doses. Up to 2 g q8h have been given in instances of CNS infection or infection caused by relatively resistant bacteria
Extended spectrum penicillins		
Piperacillin-tazobactam (Zosyn)	3.375 g IV q6h	3.375 g IV q4h or 4.5 g q6h for life-threatening infection or nosocomial pneumonia
Ticarcillin-clavulanate (Timentin)	3.1 g IV q6h	Dosing interval for serious infection is q4h; however, piperacillin-tazobactam may be preferred in such situations because of a broader spectrum of activity
Cephalosporins		
Cefepime (Maxipime)	2.0 g IV q8h	
Ceftazidime (multiple)	2.0 g IV q8h	Poor activity vs. gram-positive organisms
Aminoglycosides[c]		
Gentamicin (Garamycin)[c]	1.7 to 2.0 mg/kg IV q8h, or 5 to 7 mg/kg q24h	Dosing is based on ideal body weight
Tobramycin (Nebcin)[c]	1.5 to 2 mg/kg IV q8h, or 5 to 7 mg/kg q24h	Dosing is based on ideal body weight
Amikacin (Amikin)[c]	7.5 mg/kg IV q12h, or 15 mg/kg q24h	Dosing is based on ideal body weight
ANTIFUNGAL AGENTS		
Echinocandins		
Caspofungin (Cancidas)[d]	70 mg IV × 1, followed by 50 mg IV q24h	Offers good activity vs. essentially all *Candida* species and *Aspergillus*; considered by many to be the antifungal of choice for NF. FDA-approved for treatment of NF
Anidulafungin (Eraxis)[d]	200 mg IV × 1, followed by 100 mg IV q24h	Efficacy and dosing for treatment of NF have not been well-studied
Micafungin (Mycamine)[d]	150 mg q24h	Efficacy and dosing for treatment of NF have not been well-studied

Triazoles

Drug	Dose	Comments
Fluconazole (Diflucan)	400 mg IV or PO q24h	Generally not preferred for NF because of increasing incidence of resistant *Candida* and lack of activity vs. *Aspergillus*
Itraconazole (Sporanox)	200 mg IV q12 hr × 4, then 200 mg q24h	Generally not preferred because of limited experience
Voriconazole (VFEND)	6 mg/kg q12h × 2, followed by 4 mg/kg q12h	Good activity vs. *Candida* and *Aspergillus*; many drug–drug interactions; reasonable choice if echinocandins are not tolerated
Posaconazole (Noxafil)	200 mg PO t.i.d. (IV preparation not available)	Limited experience; existing data are for prophylaxis of fungal infection, rather than treatment of NF or of documented systemic infection

Amphotericin preparations

Drug	Dose	Comments
Amphotericin B deoxycholate (Fungizone, AmBD)[e]	0.5 to 0.7 mg/kg IV q24h	Certain fungal infections (e.g., aspergillosis) require higher doses than is used for empiric treatment of NF; utility limited by nephrotoxicity
Liposomal amphotericin B (AmBisome, LAmB)[e]	3 mg/kg IV q24h	Higher doses may be required for certain documented fungal infections
Amphotericin B colloidal dispersion (Amphotec, ABCD)[e]	3 to 6 mg/kg IV q24h	Higher doses may be required for certain documented fungal infections
Amphotericin B lipid complex (Abelcet, ABLC)[e]	3 to 5 mg/kg IV q24h	Higher doses may be required for certain documented fungal infections

NF, neutropenic fever; CNS, central nervous system; FDA, U.S. Food and Drug Administration.

[a] All of the agents listed require dose adjustment for impairment of renal function. Many of these agents are available as generic products.

[b] 1.0 g q8h to q6h may be given in life-threatening situations or for infections by organisms that are only *moderately* susceptible to imipenem-cilastatin (primarily some strains of *P. aeruginosa*) and resistant to most other agents.

[c] Monitoring of blood levels (peak and trough) and adjustment of dosing of aminoglycosides are indicated to ensure efficacy and to minimize oto- and nephrotoxicity. Once-daily aminoglycoside dosing should not be done unless a β-lactam or carbapenem is also being administered; dose adjustments are needed in the case of renal dysfunction and obesity, regardless of the dosing regimen.

[d] Of the three echinocandins, only caspofungin has an FDA indication for treatment of NF. Many hospitals will maintain a supply of only one echinocandin. Based on available data, it is reasonable to use one of the other echinocandins for treatment of NF, if caspofungin is not available.

[e] Of the three lipid preparations of amphotericin, only LAmB has an FDA indication for treatment of NF. Because most hospitals will only maintain a supply of AmBD and one of the three lipid formulations, it is reasonable to use the available lipid formulation if AmBD cannot be used. All amphotericin-containing products possess multiple toxicities, including nephrotoxicity.

Combinations of extended spectrum penicillins and β-lactamase inhibitors (e.g., ticarcillin-clavulanate or piperacillin-tazobactam) have spectra of activity that resemble the broad-spectrum carbapenems. Piperacillin-tazobactam is generally considered to have greater activity than other β-lactam or β-lactamase inhibitors, however. Piperacillin-tazobactam (but not piperacillin alone) has a spectrum of activity similar to that of imipenem-cilastatin, meropenem, and cefepime against both gram-positive cocci and gram-negative bacilli and has been effective as monotherapy. Generally, these agents would be appropriate when the patient has not been exposed repeatedly to antimicrobial therapy, and the microbiology laboratory at the facility providing treatment has not recorded appreciable resistance to these agents.

Extended spectrum β-lactamase (ESBL) production by certain gram-negative bacilli, particularly *Escherichia coli* and *Klebsiella* sp., renders most cephalosporins inactive. Evidence suggests that cefepime and piperacillin-tazobactam are less effective against ESBL-producing organisms. If the microbiology laboratory reports an appreciable incidence of ESBL-producing organisms, it may be prudent to use a carbapenem as the β-lactam of first choice.

(1) Ceftazidime, because of activity against *Pseudomonas*, has been used as monotherapy in the past, but it is susceptible to degradation by ESBL-producing organisms and is less active against gram-positive organisms than the carbapenems, β-lactam–β-lactamase inhibitor combinations, and cefepime. Ceftazidime should not be used for empiric monotherapy.

(2) The use of quinolones, such as ciprofloxacin and levofloxacin, and of aminoglycosides for monotherapy has major limitations and should be avoided.

(3) The most significant limitation of monotherapy with imipenem-cilastatin, meropenem, piperacillin-tazobactam, or cefepime is that methicillin-resistant *S. aureus* are not susceptible to these three agents.

b. Two-drug therapy without vancomycin usually involves an aminoglycoside (gentamicin, tobramycin, or amikacin) plus an extended-spectrum penicillin (piperacillin-tazobactam), an aminoglycoside plus an antipseudomonal cephalosporin (ceftazidime or cefepime), or an aminoglycoside plus a carbapenem (imipenem-cilastatin or meropenem). The major advantage of these types of regimens is their potential benefit in situations in which antimicrobial-resistant gram-negative bacilli are of concern.

(1) The combination of ceftazidime and aminoglycoside has inferior gram-positive activity to the other drug regimens.

(2) The spectrum of activity, per se, of these two drug regimens is not necessarily greater than that of the monotherapy regimens, and the potential ototoxicity and nephrotoxicity of the aminoglycoside are major disadvantages. The selection of the aminoglycoside should be based on the microbial-resistance patterns (antibiogram) of the hospital at which the patient is receiving care.

(3) Extensive analysis of the literature has led to the conclusion that the efficacy of the two-drug regimen (without vancomycin) is not superior to monotherapy as outlined above. Such analyses, however, cannot account for local factors, such as the likelihood of a drug-resistant organism in patients receiving care at a particular health care facility. A key concept is that a two-drug regimen, in some instances, provides broader coverage for potential pathogens, rather than so-called "double coverage." Thus, it is incumbent on the physician to communicate with the microbiology laboratory and to be aware of any local trends.

c. Therapy with vancomycin plus one or two other drugs is not recommended as routine empiric therapy because of the emergence of vancomycin-resistant organisms. When used, the preferred other agents in this two- or three-drug regimen are those listed above for monotherapy or two-drug therapy without vancomycin. Adoption of a regimen that includes vancomycin is appropriate in the following types of patients:

(1) Have a suspected CVC-related infection

(2) Have been previously infected by, or are known to be colonized by, methicillin-resistant *S. aureus,* or penicillin- and cephalosporin-resistant *S. pneumoniae*

(3) A gram-positive organism has been recovered from the patient's blood (but before susceptibility data are available)

(4) Demonstrate clinical deterioration that is reasonably attributed to infection

2. Oral antimicrobial therapy. Oral antimicrobial therapy with ciprofloxacin (Cipro), 750 mg q12h, **plus** amoxicillin/clavulanate (Augmentin) 875 mg/125 mg q12h has been shown to be safe and appropriate, when limited to adult patients who are at low risk for complications of neutropenia. Such patients do not have an identifiable focus of infection and lack clinical findings of systemic infection other than fever.

A number of factors that favor a low risk for severe infection have been identified and a scoring index has been developed to identify low-risk subjects who would be suitable for oral therapy (Hughes, et al. 2002 in *Suggested Reading*). These patients, however, still require careful observation and immediate access to medical care. Outpatient oral antibiotic therapy may not be suitable for many patients and health care facilities, but likely greater use will be seen in the future as additional experience is gained with this form of management.

D. Empiric therapy. Management of antimicrobial therapy during the first 7 days. Response to initiation of antimicrobial therapy, if it is to occur, often requires 3 to 5 days. After initiation of antimicrobial therapy, several possible outcomes exist: deterioration during the ensuing 1 to 3 days, resolution of fever during the first 3 to 5 days, and persistence of fever during the first 3 to 5 days. In the event of rapid deterioration, immediate reassessment of the patient and the treatment regimen is essential.

In most studies, the median time to defervescence after initiation of therapy is approximately 5 days. Therefore, in a patient who is clinically stable, except for persistent fever, the physician should consider waiting approximately 5 days before entertaining changes in the antimicrobial regimen, unless initial cultures yield an organism resistant to the treatment regimen. Changes in antimicrobial therapy should generally be made for specific reasons; an unintended consequence of aggressive, unjustifiably escalating antimicrobial therapy is the promotion of infection by more highly resistant microorganisms.

1. In patients who become afebrile within 3 days, broad-spectrum therapy should be maintained for at least 7 days, with appropriate modifications to the regimen based on results of cultures and other diagnostic tests. After 7 days of treatment, cessation of therapy is appropriate when cultures and clinical assessment indicate eradication of infection and the ANC is ≥ 500 cells/μL. Discontinuation of therapy after 7 days in carefully selected patients with prolonged neutropenia (ANC ≤ 500 cells/μL) has been recommended by some experts.

2. In patients whose fever persists during the first 3 to 5 days of empiric therapy and in whom a specific infectious process has not been identified, a number of possibilities exist. In the event of persistent fever of unknown cause for 5 days, the most appropriate actions are (*a*) continue treatment with the initial regimen, (*b*) change or add antibacterial agents to the original regimen, or (*c*) add an antifungal agent to the regimen (with or without making changes to the antibacterial regimen).

a. Causes of persistent fever include:

(1) Slow response to the treatment regimen

(2) Bacterial infection resistant to the treatment regimen

(3) Development of a second infection

(4) Inadequate antibiotic levels owing to suboptimal dosing

(5) Inadequate penetration of drugs into an infected site, such as infected necrotic tissue, an abscess, or a CVC site

(6) A nonbacterial infection

(7) Drug fever

b. **Reevaluation.** In reevaluating the patient's status after 3 to 4 days of therapy, the physician should repeat the initial diagnostic evaluation, review results of culture, obtain additional cultures, and consider obtaining radiographic imaging studies, if new localizing symptoms or signs are present. Any changes in therapy should be dictated by findings on reevaluation.

c. **If the patient has remained clinically stable** and the reevaluation was unrevealing, continuation of the initial regimen is reasonable. If neutropenia is expected to resolve within 5 days, this approach is quite appropriate.

d. **With evidence of progressive disease,** consideration should be given to changes in the antimicrobial regimen. The nature of these changes should be dictated by findings made during clinical reassessment and the components of the initial antimicrobial regimen. Examples of new findings include development of abdominal pain (suggesting cecitis, enterocolitis, or other intra-abdominal processes), development of diarrhea (suggesting *C. difficile* disease), detection of pulmonary infiltrates, drainage or inflammation at catheter entry sites, worsening stomatitis, and so forth.

e. **Addition of antifungal therapy** to the treatment regimens of patients who are febrile after initial antimicrobial therapy has been controversial, particularly with regard to the timing of such therapy and the particular antifungal agent to be used. Most experts believe that a patient with persistent fever and profound neutropenia after 5 days of empiric antimicrobial therapy should be considered for antifungal therapy. A thorough evaluation to detect systemic fungal infection should be done; this should include consideration of biopsy of suspicious lesions, chest radiographs, sinus radiographs or CT, and chest and abdomen CT. If a focus of infection is not found, consider fungal infection; fungi most likely to cause fever relatively early in the course of neutropenia are *Candida* species.

Detailed discussion of treatment of fungal infections is provided in section VII. The use of antifungal agents in patients with prolonged neutropenic fever is discussed in section VII.B.

E. Empiric therapy: duration of therapy

1. Antibacterial therapy

a. **The most important indicator in deciding to discontinue antibacterial therapy is the neutrophil count.** If the ANC is ≥ 500 cell/μL and the patient is afebrile for 2 consecutive days, therapy may be stopped unless more prolonged therapy is needed to provide adequate treatment of a specific, documented infection (e.g., pneumonia or bacteremia).

b. **For the patient who becomes afebrile but remains neutropenic,** no consensus exists regarding management. Some experts would change to oral therapy in the low-risk patient. In the completely healthy-appearing patient, some would discontinue antimicrobial therapy and engage in close monitoring, particularly with early evidence of bone marrow recovery.

c. **For the patient who remains profoundly neutropenic** (ANC ≤ 100 cells/μL), IV antimicrobial treatment should be continued.

2. Antifungal therapy

a. **If a specific fungal infection has been documented,** then the duration of antifungal therapy will be determined by the pathogen and the nature of the infection. Because of the differing activities of the three main groups of antifungal agents (echinocandins, triazoles, and amphotericin preparations), a greater need now exists for establishing an etiologic diagnosis. Knowledge of the infecting fungus should allow for selection of the most effective therapeutic agent and facilitate limitation of toxicity.

b. **If a fungal infection is not documented,** then it is less clear how long antifungal therapy should be given. Antifungal therapy can be discontinued if neutropenia and fever have resolved, the patient appears well, and CT of the abdomen and chest do not reveal lesions suspicious for fungal infection. If the patient is clinically well but has prolonged neutropenia, antifungal therapy can be discontinued after 2 weeks of treatment if CT scans of the thorax and abdomen are benign.

3. **Persistent fever after resolution of neutropenia.** The persistence of fever after broad-spectrum antimicrobial therapy and recovery of bone marrow function (ANC ≥ 500 cells/μL) suggests infection with a mycobacterium or fungus (e.g., aspergillosis or systemic candidiasis).

F. **Further issues involving neutropenic fever**
   1. **Antiviral therapy.** Empiric use of antiviral agents is not recommended. Localized lesions caused by herpes simplex or varicella zoster virus may provide a portal of entry for other pathogens and can be treated with oral acyclovir, valacyclovir, or famciclovir. Disseminated cytomegalovirus (CMV) infection is rare in the absence of profound immunosuppression that occurs in patients with AIDS or stem cell transplant.
   2. **Granulocyte transfusion.** The routine use of granulocyte transfusions is not recommended. Some investigators believe that patients with severe bacterial of fungal infections may benefit from granulocyte transfusion. This procedure should still be considered investigational (see Chapter 34, section V.B in "Cytopenia").
   3. **Use of colony-stimulating factors (CSF).** The hematopoietic growth factors G (granulocyte)-CSF (filgrastim) and GM (granulocyte-macrophage)-CSF (sargramostim) have long been used for the treatment of patients with febrile neutropenia. Although they may reduce the period of neutropenia, they do not reliably reduce the duration of fever, the need for antimicrobial therapy, the duration of hospitalization, or other measures of febrile morbidity. The American Society of Clinical Oncology, through an update of its clinical practice guidelines (see Smith, et al. in *Suggested Reading*) has recommended the routine use of CSF when the risk of febrile neutropenia is approximately 20%, based on the conclusion that reduction of febrile neutropenia was, per se, an important clinical outcome.

III. SPECIFIC INFECTIONS IN THE COMPROMISED HOST
A. **Pulmonary infections**
   1. **Differential diagnosis**
      a. **Noninfectious causes.** About 25% to 30% of cases of fever with pulmonary infiltrates in cancer patients are owing to noninfectious causes, which include radiation pneumonitis, drug-induced pneumonitis, pulmonary emboli and hemorrhage, and leukoagglutinin transfusion reaction.
      b. **Predicting the infecting agent.** Acute, severe symptoms that progress in 1 to 2 days suggest a common bacterial pathogen, a virus, or a noninfectious process (pulmonary emboli, pulmonary hemorrhage). A subacute course (5 to 14 days) suggests pneumocystis, or, occasionally, aspergillosis or nocardiosis. A chronic course (over several weeks) is more typical of mycobacterial or fungal infections, radiation fibrosis, or drug-induced pneumonitis.
         (1) **Infection acquired outside the hospital.** Despite the susceptibility of cancer patients to opportunistic pathogens, *S. pneumoniae* and influenza virus are the most likely pulmonary infections in the outpatient setting.
         (2) **Infection acquired inside the hospital.** *E. coli, K. pneumoniae, Serratia marcescens, P. aeruginosa, Acinetobacter* sp., and *S. aureus* are the most frequently acquired nosocomial bacterial pathogens. *Aspergillus* sp., *Legionella pneumophila*, and *P. carinii* are also hospital acquired.
         (3) **The association between lung carcinoma and pulmonary tuberculosis** is related to the increased susceptibility to opportunistic infections and tuberculosis in cancer patients. Erosion of tumor into a quiescent tuberculous focus likely accounts for some cases. Diagnosis of tuberculosis requires pathologic evidence from biopsies or bacteriology samples.

Surgical treatment of early stage bronchopulmonary carcinoma may have to be postponed and may even be contraindicated in the presence of active tuberculosis. Chemotherapy and radiotherapy may result in extension of the tuberculosis.

2. **Diagnostic approach**

   a. **Sputum examination.** If the sputum contains neutrophils or macrophages and <10 epithelial cells per low-power field, the sputum culture results are probably valid. Problems with interpretation include the following:

      (1) Neutropenic patients usually have no neutrophils in the sputum.

      (2) Aspiration pneumonia is usually caused by mouth flora, which renders routine culture meaningless in this condition.

      (3) *S. pneumoniae* is a fastidious organism that is difficult to recover from sputum, although approximately 25% of pneumococcal pneumonias are associated with concomitant bacteremia.

      (4) Many opportunistic organisms that produce pneumonia are infrequently retrieved from sputum (e.g., *Nocardia asteroides* and *Aspergillus* species).

      (5) Sputum cultures of hospitalized patients, particularly those receiving antibiotics, often yield *Candida* on culture. Although candidemia and disseminated candidiasis are frequent complications of immunosuppression, pneumonia because of *Candida* is remarkably uncommon. Therefore recovery of *Candida* from sputum should not be considered to be diagnostic of infection.

   b. **Serology** may be useful for identifying infection caused by *Coccidioides immitis*. Serology is less useful for diagnosis of infections caused by *Aspergillus* species, *L. pneumophila*, *Mycoplasma pneumoniae*, *Toxoplasma gondii*, and CMV. There is a delay associated with most serologic tests and some are not highly sensitive or specific.

   c. **Antigen tests.** Blood antigen tests are useful for diagnosis of infections caused by *C. neoformans*. Urinary antigen tests are valuable tools for diagnosis of infections caused by *S. pneumoniae*; *L. pneumophila*, serogroup 1; and *Histoplasma capsulatum*. The detection of cryptococcal antigen in any body fluid is considered diagnostic of infection.

   The use of nonculture tests for diagnosis of other fungal infections has been disappointing. Detection of *Candida* species depends primarily on culture.

   The serum galactomannan test for aspergillosis is not particularly helpful. A meta-analysis found the test sensitivity ranged from 61% to 71% and specificity from 89% to 93%; the positive values ranged from 26% to 53%, whereas the negative predicative values ranged from 95% to 98%. These findings indicate that the main value of the galactomannan assay is that a negative test finding helps to exclude the disease.

   d. **Blood cultures** should be obtained in all patients.

   e. **CT and high-resolution CT (HRCT).** A neutropenic patient with a normal chest radiograph and CT scan is at low risk for the development of subsequent pneumonia. HRCT scans may be even more reliable as a screening tool. Neutropenic patients with fever of unknown origin and normal chest radiographs should undergo CT scanning (and perhaps HRCT) to detect occult inflammatory pulmonary disease. CT is of particular value for diagnosis of invasive pulmonary mycoses, such as aspergillosis.

   f. **Thoracentesis** should be performed in patients with pleural effusion.

   g. **Lung biopsy procedures.** Diagnosis is paramount in the immunocompromised host. The highest yield and best control of bleeding is by direct visualization with open-lung biopsy. This procedure may be mandatory when the patient is rapidly deteriorating. If the pneumonic process is less rapid, then bronchoscopy with lavage appears to be the best approach. When a mass or consolidation is present, fine-needle biopsy is more frequently performed because of less chance of complications.

Invasive techniques are often not justified late in the course of malignancy because they often add morbidity with little hope of benefit. Empiric antibiotic therapy directed at the most likely pathogen(s) may be justified in these cases.

3. Therapy for acute pneumonia should be initiated immediately after cultures are obtained. Patients with acid-fast bacilli, *Nocardia asteroides, Cryptococcus,* or *Aspergillus* species in sputum should not be regarded as colonized and should be treated.

B. Central nervous system infections. Infections of the CNS can present either with simple changes to mentation or motor skills or with seizures and coma. Meningismus is a hallmark of disease, but this condition may be absent. MRI is indicated when cerebral edema, abscess, or demyelinating encephalitis is suspected. This scan is particularly useful in defining viral encephalitis and areas where enhanced foci are seen, such as in toxoplasmosis.

Special considerations in cancer patients suspected or proved to have CNS infections are as follows:

1. Meningitis. Cancer patients have an increased incidence of atypical pathogens. These can occur as a direct result of immune suppression, CNS involvement by the malignancy, or opportunistic infections after craniofacial surgery.

   a. Neutropenic patients rarely develop gram-negative meningitis despite a relatively high incidence of gram-negative bacteremia. When meningitis does develop, the pathogens usually are members of the family *Enterobacteriaceae* (e.g., *E. coli, Klebsiella*), *P. aeruginosa, Listeria monocytogenes,* or *Bacillus subtilis.* Meningitis caused by aspergillosis or zygomycosis has also been described.

   b. Patients with defects in cell-mediated immunity. *L. monocytogenes* and *C. neoformans* are the most likely pathogens. Meningitis and meningoencephalitis from varicella zoster virus (VZV), herpes simplex virus (HSV), JC virus (progressive multifocal leukoencephalopathy), human immunodeficiency virus (HIV), CMV, *T. gondii,* and *Strongyloides stercoralis* also occur.

2. Brain abscesses are most likely caused by mixed aerobic and anaerobic bacteria. In the immunocompromised patient, brain abscesses are often caused by *Aspergillus* species, the agents of mucormycosis, *N. asteroides,* or *T. gondii. Toxoplasma* can produce meningitis, necrotizing encephalitis, or abscess. In atypical cases, brain biopsy should be performed at the time of surgical drainage.

3. Lumbar puncture (LP)

   a. Papilledema. An emergency CT scan of the brain must be performed first. Patients with space-occupying lesions seen on CT scan should have LP or cisternal puncture performed by a qualified neurologist or neuroradiologist.

   b. Thrombocytopenia. Spinal subdural hematoma occasionally complicates LP in patients with severe thrombocytopenia. Clinical evidence of CNS infection, however, supersedes consideration of risks. The following guidelines are recommended:

      (1) If the platelet count is <50,000/mm^3, transfuse platelets just before performing LP. Transfuse additional platelets, if back pain or neurologic signs develop.

      (2) A highly skilled physician should perform the LP using a 22-gauge needle and the patient should be observed closely afterward. The role of needle aspiration and surgical intervention in patients with spinal subdural hematomas induced by LP is not known.

   c. Cerebrospinal fluid should be evaluated for the following:

      (1) Glucose and protein concentrations, cell counts, routine bacterial culture and sensitivity, Gram stain, and cytology. The WBC count in the cerebrospinal fluid is >100/μL in about 90% of patients with bacterial meningitis and >1,000/μL in 15% to 20%. Neutrophils constitute >80% of the WBC count in 80% to 90% of patients; occasionally, lymphocytes predominate in the cerebrospinal fluid, especially in neutropenic patients and in about 25% of patients with meningitis caused by *L. monocyto-genes*.

(2) Acid-fast culture and stain; fungal stains of smears and fungal cultures; India ink preparation; cryptococcal antigen; and "screening" and complement fixation serology for *Coccidioides immitis* (depending on geography and predominant soil fungus) should be done.

(3) Polymerase chain reaction (PCR) assays for HIV, JC virus, herpesviruses, *Toxoplasma, Mycobacterium tuberculosis, Listeria,* and other pathogens should be performed only if clinical or laboratory findings suggest the likelihood of that specific infection.

C. Skin infections

1. **Neoplasms invading the skin** (e.g., mycosis fungoides) are associated with infections involving common pathogens such as *S. aureus*.

2. **Cell-mediated immunity deficiencies** are typically associated with skin infection by VZV or HSV.

3. **Neutropenic patients** may have skin infections with atypical or few physical findings. *S. aureus* and *Streptococcus pyogenes* are common. More serious manifestations represent systemic infections; these include bullae formation, raised ecchymotic plaques or nodules, black necrotic ulcers, or ecthyma gangrenosum. These more pronounced manifestations of systemic infection are typically caused by gram-negative bacilli, such as *P. aeruginosa, Aeromonas hydrophila,* and members of the family *Enterobacteriaceae* and fungi, including *Candida* species, *Aspergillus* species, and members of the class *Zygomycetes* (the latter infections are often referred to as mucormycosis or zygomycosis).

D. Alimentary tract and intra-abdominal infections

1. **Esophagitis** may be caused by *Candida* or HSV.

2. **Colitis** with ulceration is occasionally produced by CMV. Aspergillus and zygomycosis may also involve the GI tract.

3. **Cecitis and ileocolitis** are processes that probably develop as a consequence of several factors that include mucosal injury, neutropenia, and the resident bowel flora. They can usually be appreciated on CT scan of the abdomen and may be confused with *Clostridium difficile*-induced colitis when colonic wall thickening is present.

4. **Intra-abdominal abscesses** develop when the bowel or genital tract becomes obstructed, necrotic, or perforated because of tumor. Mixed infections derived from colonic flora involve gram-negative enteric bacilli; various species of streptococci and members of the *Bacteroides fragilis* family are common. *Streptococcus bovis* abscess and sepsis may occur with colonic, pancreatic, or oropharyngeal carcinoma.

5. **Perirectal abscesses** frequently develop in neutropenic patients, especially those with acute leukemia; usually, they are caused by mixtures of aerobic and anaerobic bacteria. The hallmark of perirectal abscess in neutropenic patients is pain.

6. **Liver infections.** Multiple abscesses secondary to systemic bacterial or fungal infection also occur. Hepatosplenic candidosis can be an extremely difficult infection to diagnose and treat, and it is often found at autopsy to involve other organs; it may not become clinically evident until there is recovery from neutropenia. Even herpesviruses, such as VZV, HSV, HHV-8 (human herpesvirus 8), CMV, or Epstein-Barr virus (EBV), can present as mass or necrotic lesions in the liver of immunocompromised patients.

E. Urinary tract infections

E. Urinary tract infections are frequent in cancer patients because of obstructive uropathies, the use of urinary catheters, and prolonged and repeated hospitalizations. These infections are often caused by resistant gram-negative bacteria or *Candida* species.

F. Infection of bone marrow usually reflects systemic or disseminated disease, particularly with *M. tuberculosis, Mycobacterium avium* complex, fungi, *Salmonella,* and *Listeria*. Bone marrow biopsy for culture can be a useful diagnostic tool. **Bone**

marrow suppression mimicking aplastic anemia occurs with parvovirus B19, mycobacterial infection, histoplasmosis, and brucellosis.

G. **Central line infections.** The incidence of infection of IV catheters, including nontunneled central lines, tunneled silicone catheters (e.g., Hickman, Broviac, or Groshong), or implantable devices (e.g., Portacath), is significant and often poses a major challenge for the clinician.

1. Most central-line infections are caused by *S. aureus* (coagulase-positive *Staphylococcus*) or coagulase-negative *Staphylococcus* species (often incorrectly referred to as "Staph epi" or "Staph epidermidis"). The neutropenic patient is also at risk for infection of venous catheters by a variety of gram-negative bacilli, including *P. aeruginosa*, and by a variety of *Candida* species and other fungi.

2. In almost all instances, infected peripheral vascular catheters and nontunneled CVC should be removed and appropriate antimicrobial therapy administered. In addition, CVC in which there is a tunnel (pocket) infection or a periport abscess should always be removed. Attempts at salvage of the CVC can sometimes be made, if the organism is of low virulence (e.g., coagulase-negative staphylococci), by the use of appropriate IV antibiotics. Clinical guidelines have been developed to assist clinicians with this vexing problem (see Mermel LA, et al. in *Suggested Reading*).

3. Vancomycin, with dosage adjustment for renal dysfunction, should be used for initial therapy of gram-positive organisms; if the organism is susceptible, high-dose oxacillin should be used.

4. "Antibiotic lock therapy," in which the catheter is filled with a high concentration of an appropriate antibiotic and then capped for varying periods of time, has been advocated by some, but controlled clinical studies are insufficient to permit conclusions to the utility of this method in the setting of neutropenia.

5. **All venous catheters must be removed** in the following circumstances:
   a. All nontunneled peripheral and central catheters (the latter are often referred to colloquially as "PICC lines") if bacteremia has been documented or there is evidence of insertion site infection.
   b. All tunnel infections or periport abscesses
   c. All catheter infections caused by fungi
   d. Persistence of infection after 48 to 72 hours of treatment, regardless of the pathogen
   e. Bacteremia caused by *S. aureus*, vancomycin-resistant *Enterococcus*, *Bacillus* species, *Corynebacterium jeikeium*, or gram-negative bacilli
   f. Infections associated with thrombophlebitis, septic emboli, or hypotension
   g. Nonpatent (i.e., plugged) catheter

IV. VACCINATION OF IMMUNOSUPPRESSED PATIENTS

A. **Vaccines contraindicated in immunosuppressed patients** are those that contain living organisms. These include the viral vaccines for rubeola (measles), varicella, rubella, mumps, oral poliovirus, smallpox, yellow fever, and live-attenuated, intranasally administered influenza vaccine (FluMist).

B. **Permissible vaccines.** Immunosuppressed patients often do not attain an effective response to active immunization. Permissible vaccines, however, are those for diphtheria, tetanus, pertussis, typhoid, cholera, plague, influenza, hepatitis A and B, and *S. pneumoniae*. Influenza immunization should be done on an annual basis because immunity is short lived, and antigenic drift of the "epidemic" strain(s) occurs each year. Pneumococcal vaccination is strongly indicated for all cancer patients. Although the efficacy is diminished in severely immunosuppressed patients, a potential benefit still exists. Reimmunization every 5 years is recommended for patients with AIDS and is reasonable in non-AIDS subjects who have cancer.

V. VIRAL INFECTIONS

A. **Cytomegalovirus** often presents as EBV-negative mononucleosis. Fever, interstitial pneumonia, and alimentary canal ulcerative disease are the most common manifestations of CMV in adults with neoplasms. CMV, which is tropic for endothelial cells, also causes retinitis, encephalitis, and peripheral neuropathy. CMV can suppress cell-mediated immunity, reticuloendothelial cell function, and granulocyte reserves.

1. **Infection, latency, and recurrence.** Primary CMV infection can occur perinatally or later in life and inevitably results in latent infection. Infection is especially likely after transfusions of blood that contains granulocytes. Latent CMV burden and risk for recurrence are related to the extent of virus multiplication during primary infection. The risk for CMV recurrence is relatively high in immunocompromised patients.

2. **CMV infection of the GI tract** can cause serious inflammatory or ulcerative disease in immunocompromised patients. Manifestations include pain, ulceration, bleeding, diarrhea, and perforation. All levels of the GI tract, particularly the stomach and colon, may be involved. Pathologic examination reveals diffuse ulcerations and necrosis with scattered CMV inclusions.

3. **Diagnosis**
   a. **Culture.** CMV is slow growing (up to 6 weeks) and culture is generally not practical. Early antibody detected by application of enzyme-linked immunosorbent assay (ELISA) in cultures may accelerate identification.
   b. **Histocytology** shows the characteristic enlarged cells with dense nuclear inclusions and wide peri-inclusion halos. Cytoplasmic inclusions are frequent, but multinucleation is absent.
   c. **Serologic assays**
      (1) Seropositivity for antibodies against CMV is indicative of latent infection, but is insufficient as a predictor for the risk for recurrence.
      (2) Elevated IgM antibody showing fourfold titer increases is highly suggestive of acute disease.
      (3) Anticomplementary immunofluorescent assay, ELISA, and indirect fluorescent antibody (FA) assays are sensitive indicators of infection. IgG antibody occurs during the acute phase of the illness and persists for life, whereas IgM antibodies occur early and often disappear after 4 to 8 weeks. Recurrent IgM spikes occur in certain patients, indicating either partial immunity to CMV or exposure to new variants of the virus.
   d. **PCR assay,** both *in situ* and in DNA extracted from gross specimens, is the most useful tool to isolate and identify the presence and location of CMV in clinical disease. Interpretation of the PCR results is sometimes difficult, given that shedding of low levels of CMV does not necessarily indicate clinical infection.

4. **Management**
   a. **Ganciclovir**
      (1) The efficacy of this drug for CMV retinitis and colitis is well documented, but it is less effective with CMV pneumonia or meningoencephalitis. After stem cell transplantation, the prophylactic administration of ganciclovir abrogates CMV pneumonitis and considerably reduces the incidence of CMV infection.
      (2) Ganciclovir is given for 14 days at a dose of 5 mg/kg IV q12h. Patients with AIDS often require maintenance treatment (5 mg/kg/day). Dosage is modified according to the predicted creatinine clearance and ANC.
      (3) Valganciclovir, a derivative of ganciclovir, is effective when given orally. The usual treatment is 900 mg b.i.d. for 21 days, followed by 900 mg daily for suppression.
   b. **Foscarnet** and cidofovir are other agents that may be useful for treatment of CMV infection.

B. **Varicella-Zoster virus (VZV).** Chickenpox is often associated with extensive visceral dissemination and appreciable mortality in immunocompromised patients, particularly stem cell transplant recipients. Shingles is characterized by the development of vesicles in clusters on erythematous bases, usually distributed along one to three dermatomes. Although disseminated VZV infection does occur, the presence of several lesions outside a dermatomal distribution does not necessarily indicate dissemination. Disseminated VZV infections may be manifested by encephalopathy, Guillain-Barré syndrome, transverse myelitis, myositis, pneumonia, thrombocytopenia, hepatitis, and arthritis.

1. **Diagnosis.** VZV can usually be diagnosed on physical examination.
    a. **Histocytology.** Multinucleated cells with intranuclear inclusions is suggestive.
    b. **Culture.** Inoculate early vesicular fluid.
2. **Management.** VZV is transmissible; patients should be isolated.
    a. **IV acyclovir** is the treatment of choice for ophthalmic zoster and disseminated VZV infection in immunocompromised patients (10 mg/kg IV every 8 hours for 7 to 10 days; renal function should be monitored for evidence of nephrotoxicity). "Localized" or nondisseminated zoster can be treated with IV acyclovir initially, and then with oral agents to complete 7–10 days of treatment: acyclovir (800 mg five times daily), vancyclovir (1,000 mg t.i.d. or q.i.d.), or famciclovir (500 mg t.i.d.).
    b. **Ganciclovir** has considerable activity for VZV as well as for CMV.
    c. **VZV live vaccine** is available for primary immunization against chicken pox but has no role in the immunocompromised patient.
    d. **VZV immuno globulin or plasma** may prevent or ameliorate the severity of infection in non-immunocompromised subjects if given soon after exposure, but are only sporadically available.
C. **Herpes simplex virus.** Patients with reticuloendothelial neoplasms, T-lymphocyte defects, or cytotoxic chemotherapy treatment may develop HSV viremia. The viremia often produces alimentary tract ulceration and hemorrhage, hepatitis (occasionally manifested by abscesslike lesions), and respiratory tract infections. Patients with Sézary's syndrome or atopic dermatitis can develop progressive fulminant mucocutaneous disease (eczema herpeticum), which can recur and disseminate to visceral organs.

1. **Diagnosis**
    a. **Histocytology** demonstrates the characteristic intranuclear mass surrounded by marginated chromatosis and often a peri-inclusion halo. Cytoplasmic inclusions are absent. Electron microscopy analysis of vesicular fluid, which can be performed in <30 minutes, strongly suggests the diagnosis. Immunofluorescence for HSV antigen is also rapid and specific.
    b. **Culture.** HSV grows rapidly in tissue cultures (24 to 72 hours) and produces a unique cytopathologic picture.
    c. **Assays.** Hemagglutination and indirect FA titers are useful if fourfold increases are demonstrated. Differentiation of IgG from IgM antibody assists in clarifying recent infection. An HSV IgG-capture ELISA has demonstrated intrathecal synthesis of antibodies to the virus. Furthermore, a PCR assay has demonstrated amplification of HSV DNA in cerebrospinal fluid. Both ELISA and PCR are rapid, noninvasive means of diagnosing HSV encephalitis in a very early stage of the disease.

2. **Management**
    a. **Topical idoxuridine,** especially using dimethyl sulfoxide as a carrier, is effective for HSV keratitis.
    b. **Acyclovir** is safe, effective treatment for HSV infections in normal and immunocompromised patients. The dose is 200 mg PO five times daily for 7 to 10 days. As an ointment, acyclovir is useful for primary local infections but does not appear to prevent recurrent disease. **Famciclovir** and **valacyclovir** are now superseding acyclovir because they have easier dosing regimens of 500 mg PO t.i.d. and have evidence of better penetration into tissue.

    Serious infections requiring IV therapy should be treated with acyclovir, 10 mg/kg IV q8h for 7 to 10 days.
    c. **Ganciclovir** has excellent activity against HSV, although its primary usefulness has been directed at CMV.
    d. **Vidarabine** is effective topically for keratitis.

VI. BACTERIAL INFECTIONS

A. Mycobacteria. Active tuberculosis (TB) develops in 0.5% to 1% of patients with malignancies. Infection is predominantly pulmonary in 70%, is widely disseminated in 20%, and involves lymph nodes or other nonpulmonary sites in 10% of cases.

1. **The incidence** of atypical *Mycobacterium* infection (particularly with *M. kansasii* and *M. avium* complex [MAC]) is significantly higher in patients with cancer, HIV, or AIDS than in the general population. *M. kansasii* infection has been associated with hairy cell leukemia. *M. malmoense* is an opportunistic pathogen mainly isolated in northern Europe, most often in patients with pulmonary infections. All of these organisms are commonly resistant to isoniazid or rifampin. A variety of other atypical mycobacteria is occasionally isolated from patients with malignancy.

2. **Pathogenesis.** Cutaneous anergy and treatment with corticosteroids, cytotoxic agents, or irradiation predispose to reactivation of quiescent *M. tuberculosis*. It is now appreciated, however, that some cases of tuberculosis in adults represent new acquisition of infection, rather than reactivation.

3. **Resistant TB.** Immigration from high-prevalence countries, coinfection with HIV, and outbreaks in congregate facilities are primarily responsible for the increased incidence of TB cases during the past decade. Coincident with the increase in TB, outbreaks of multidrug-resistant (MDR) TB have occurred. MDR TB occurs late in the course of HIV infection and is refractory to treatment. A history of antituberculous therapy is the strongest predictor of the presence of resistance.

4. **Diagnosis**

   a. **Chest radiographic** evidence of infiltrates in apical or posterior segments of the upper lobe or superior segment of the lower lobe are the most frequent manifestations of postprimary TB. Radiographic features may be confusing in immunosuppressed patients, however, in whom intrathoracic adenopathy, pleural effusions, miliary infiltrates, or cavities are important clues to the presence of TB. Chest radiographs are normal in 10% to 15% of immunosuppressed patients with TB.

   b. **Smears and cultures.** The tuberculin skin test is often negative in immunocompromised patients with TB and is not helpful in evaluating patients thought to have active TB. The diagnosis of TB can be established by visualizing the organism in stained sputum smears or culturing *M. tuberculosis* from sputum or from extrapulmonary sites; blood cultures may be occasionally be positive when blood is sampled utilizing specialized media or techniques. Three sputum cultures from separate days are necessary for routine culturing; more samples do not increase the yield. Expectorated sputum may be adequate for smears and culture. Aerosol-induced sputum is superior to expectorated sputum or gastric juice aspiration in patients who produce little sputum, however, and it is the preferred means for sputum collection. Bronchoalveolar lavage or transbronchial biopsy may be required when other material is not diagnostic.

   c. **Effusions.** Pleural fluid samples may yield the organism in up to 30% of cases, and percutaneous needle pleural biopsies (three biopsies in three locations) provide up to a 75% yield. Culture of pericardial fluid may be positive in up to 50% of cases, and pericardial biopsy yields 80% positive results on either histology or culture. Analysis of ascitic fluid findings is not helpful unless the fluid is concentrated; peritoneal biopsy is preferred. PCR and detection of elevated adenosine deaminase levels in fluids is occasionally useful, but neither is highly sensitive.

   d. **TB meningitis.** Spinal fluid analysis is variable, although mononuclear cell pleocytosis and low glucose concentrations are common. Concentrated spinal fluid reveals TB bacillus on smear in 30% to 50% of cases in some reports and on culture in about 50%. Most often, however, the diagnosis is made on clinical grounds and treatment is empiric. PCR has been disappointing for diagnosing tuberculous meningitis.

5. **Management**
   a. **TB prophylaxis in cancer patients.** Any patient who is to receive immuno-suppressive therapy should be skin tested for TB and anergy. Prophylaxis with isoniazid (INH), 300 mg/day for 9 months, should be given to any cancer patient who has a positive tuberculin skin test.
   b. **Active TB.** Because of increasing drug resistance, the U.S. Public Health Service has issued new guidelines for the initial treatment of TB. Until drug susceptibility data are available, patients with active TB should be treated with daily administration of isoniazid, rifampin, pyrazinamide, and ethambutol. After 2 months of therapy, the regimen for patients with drug-sensitive organisms should be changed to isoniazid and rifampin administered daily for an additional 4 months or until sputum cultures are negative for 3 months. Alternative regimens are recommended for patients who require directly observed therapy to ensure compliance.
   c. **MDR TB,** defined as resistance to at least isoniazid and rifampin, is readily transmitted among hospitalized patients with AIDS. The management of MDR TB is exceedingly difficult, and early diagnosis with individualized therapy is crucial. To interrupt the transmission of MDR TB, stringent isolation procedures and aggressive chemotherapy with a combination of drugs are essential. The choice of agents depends on susceptibility testing, but until such results are available, the drugs most likely to be effective include pyrazinamide, streptomycin, ciprofloxacin, ofloxacin, cycloserine, and ethambutol.

   The treatment of patients exposed to MDR TB is also difficult. Such patients should be evaluated for the closeness of their contact with infected patients and their immune status. People at high risk are candidates for chemoprophylaxis.
   d. **MAC.** Treatment for dissemination should include either azithromycin or clarithromycin and ethambutol. When resistance to a two-drug regimen or multisystem disease develops, one or two additional drugs should be selected from the following: rifabutin, a fluoroquinolone, or in some instances, amikacin.
B. ***Nocardia asteroides* infection (nocardiosis).** Several types of cell-mediated immune defects have been described in association with nocardiosis. About 20% of cases occur in patients receiving corticosteroids. In immunocompromised subjects, 75% of nocardiosis involves the lung.

   Nocardiosis can be asymptomatic, heal spontaneously, or produce a lower lobe bronchopneumonia with cavities, abscesses, or empyema. Disseminated nocardiosis typically involves subcutaneous tissue, muscle, and brain.
   1. **Diagnosis.** Gram stain of sputum reveals gram-positive, beaded, branching filaments. Sputum should also be examined with modified Ziehl-Neelsen stain, because the organism is typically weakly acid-fast.
   2. **Management.** Sulfa drugs have been the mainstay of therapy for *Nocardia;* in recent years, the convenience, safety, and efficacy of the combination of sulfamethoxazole and trimethoprim (Bactrim or Septra) have led most experts to consider this combination as the first line of therapy. High initial daily doses (15 mg/kg of trimethoprim and 75 mg/kg of sulfamethoxazole per day) are used for severe infection, such as disseminated infection or cerebral abscess. Several different species are found in the *Nocardia asteroides* complex. Poor response to therapy in some patients in the past may have been because of differing antimicrobial susceptibilities of these organisms. In addition, a number of other conventional antibacterial agents are active against many *Nocardia* isolates and their use may be beneficial, depending on the nature of the specific infection.
C. ***Listeria monocytogenes*** may be confused with gram-positive cocci, *H. influenzae,* or diphtheroids on Gram stain of specimens. Infections are more common in patients with defects in cell-mediated immunity.

   Listeria monocytogenes is the most common cause of bacterial meningitis in patients with carcinoma and in patients receiving corticosteroids or other immunosuppressive therapy, especially for lymphoma. CNS infection with cerebritis or brain abscess accounts for 80% of cases. The mortality rate for CNS infections is 15% to 45%. Bacteremia or sepsis accounts for 20% of cases in adults. Pulmonary involvement is always in the form of an empyema.

1. Diagnosis

   a. Culture. After *L. monocytogenes* is isolated, the organisms have a unique tumbling motion when viewed in a hanging drop, thereby allowing for rapid tentative identification.

   b. Spinal fluid. Either lymphocytes or polymorphonuclear neutrophils are predominant. Spinal fluid protein concentration ranges from normal to 1 g/dL. Glucose levels are low in only half of the cases.

2. Management

   a. Sepsis. Ampicillin, 200 mg/kg/day, is given IV in six divided doses. Most experts recommend adding gentamicin to ampicillin for synergy. In patients who cannot tolerate ampicillin, the best alternative appears to be high-dose sulfamethoxazole-trimethoprim.

   b. Meningoencephalitis is treated in the same manner as sepsis. Intrathecal gentamicin, 3 to 5 mg every 24 hours, may be synergistic with IV antibiotics.

D. *Legionella pneumophila*. Legionnaires' disease can affect normal and immunosuppressed hosts, especially patients receiving glucocorticoids. The disease typically produces lobar pulmonic consolidation evolving from patchy infiltrates. Features that suggest Legionnaires' disease include nonproductive cough, pulmonary consolidation, diarrhea, hyponatremia, and confusion.

1. Diagnosis

   a. Cultures on specialized media developed specifically for recovery of *Legionella* should be requested.

   b. Legionella urine antigen should be obtained. This test only detects Legionella pneumophila serogroup 1; however, serogroup 1 organisms cause the most severe forms of disease in humans.

   c. Tissue examination. Dieterle staining can be used to detect bacteria in tissue. Positive direct FA examination of tissue strongly suggests Legionnaires' disease.

   d. Serology. Antibody titers do not help early in the disease course.

2. Management

   a. Newer macrolides, such as clarithromycin and azithromycin, and the so-called respiratory fluoroquinolones (e.g., levofloxacin) have efficacy. Azithromycin, 500 mg/day, is an effective and well-tolerated agent. High-dose levofloxacin or can be used if azithromycin therapy is not possible.

   b. Rifampin 300 to 600 mg/day PO may be effective as adjunctive therapy and can be added if the patient does not respond to initial therapy.

E. *Clostridium difficile*. This toxin-mediated diarrheal disease of the colon is almost invariably associated with recent or concurrent use of antimicrobial therapy. Horizontal spread of *C. difficile* within health care facilities has become extremely common.

An epidemic clonal strain (NAP1) of *C. difficile* was found to be associated with increased morbidity and mortality. The spread of this strain may be owing to resistance to newer fluoroquinolones, whereas the apparent increase in virulence may result from dysregulation of toxin production. Preliminary data suggest this strain has spread globally.

Clinical correlates of infection with the NAP1 strain appear to be more severe disease as manifested by high fever (>102.5°F), marked leukocytosis (>25,000 cells/μL), protein-losing enteropathy, extensive colitis on CT scanning, and more frequent need for emergent colectomy because of loss of colonic wall integrity or toxic dilation of the colon.

1. Diagnosis. Of the number of tests for *C. difficile* toxins in feces, the most rapidly available is an enzyme immunoassay (EIA) for toxins A and B. The sensitivity of this and other EIA for *C. difficile* toxins is often relatively poor (ranges are from ~65% to 90%), however. Tissues culture cytotoxin assay for toxin B is appreciably more sensitive, but is not a rapid test, is expensive and is not widely available. Stool culture alone for *C. difficile* is not clinically useful. The presence of colonic pseudomembranes or characteristic plaques is considered diagnostic, but these findings are present in no more than 50% of patients and require lower GI endoscopy for detection.

2. **Management.** Nosocomial diarrhea that is not attributable to hyperosmolar nutritional supplements or tube feeding preparations suggests the presence of symptomatic *C. difficile* disease. Such patients should be placed in contact isolation, a test for *C. difficile* toxin ordered, and empiric treatment considered.

   a. If the diarrhea is trivial and the offending antimicrobial agent can be stopped, resolution of diarrhea occurs in approximately 90% of patients without significant risk of relapse or recurrence.

   b. If the illness is mild to moderate (high fever, marked leukocytosis, and abdominal pain or tenderness are absent), then treatment with metronidazole is appropriate. Standard doses of metronidazole for *C. difficile*-associated diarrhea are 250 mg q.i.d. or 500 mg t.i.d. daily orally for 10 to 14 days, although higher doses (2 to 2.25 g/day) are recommended for treatment of other anaerobic infections. Intravenously administered metronidazole penetrates the colonic lumen poorly and has not been established as reliably effective therapy for *C. difficile* diarrhea.

   c. If the illness is severe, then oral vancomycin, 125 or 250 mg q.i.d. for 10 to 14 days, may be prudent.

   d. Surgical consultation for consideration for colectomy is indicated with clinical evidence of progressive toxicity, radiographic evidence of progressive colonic dilation, or concern regarding loss of bowel wall integrity.

   e. Approximately 25% of patients treated for *C. difficile* diarrhea with oral metronidazole or vancomycin have a relapse or recurrence of diarrhea. Generally, retreatment is effective, although multiple relapses are not uncommon and may require a tapering schedule of drug.

VII. FUNGAL INFECTIONS

The profoundly immunosuppressed host, particularly if there is prolonged neutropenia, is at risk for infection by a variety of fungi, many of which rarely cause infection in healthy hosts. Some organisms cause infection so rarely that identification of genus and species by a clinical microbiology laboratory may not be possible, and, if identified by the laboratory, they may not be familiar even to many clinically astute infectious diseases clinicians.

In this section are reviewed the more common fungal pathogens, rather than an encyclopedic review of the literature. Recovery of "nonpathogenic" fungi (or members of other classes of "nonpathogenic" micro-organisms) from normally sterile body fluids, such as spinal fluid or blood, or from biopsy samples should prompt the clinician to consider whether that "nonpathogenic" organism could be a pathogen.

A. **Antifungal agents.** The three major classes of antifungal agents that may be useful in the patient with neutropenia and persistent fever are echinocandins, triazoles, and amphotericin B (AmB) preparations. Detailed information is available via the package inserts, including dosing instructions and warnings regarding potential adverse reactions. Dosages are shown in Table 35.1.

   1. **Echinocandins.** The echinocandins are the newest group of antifungal agents; those currently marketed are caspofungin (Cancidas), anidulafungin (Eraxis), and micafungin (Mycamine). Although the greatest clinical experience is with caspofungin, many experts believe these three agents have similar antifungal activities and toxicities. The echinocandins have excellent activity against most species of *Candida* (including fluconazole-resistant *C. glabrata*) and *Aspergillus*.

   2. **Triazoles** are clinically useful antifungal agents that have substantially differing spectra of activity, adverse effects, and potential for drug–drug interactions. All are effective for treatment of infections caused by *Candida albicans*. The four agents with potential clinical utility in cancer patients are

      a. **Fluconazole** (Diflucan). Although highly effective against *C. albicans*, fluconazole has much less activity against non-*albicans Candida* than do the newer triazoles. In the past, fluconazole had been considered an acceptable alternative to AmB at institutions in which infections with certain *Candida* species (*C. krusei* and some isolates of *C. glabrata*) and molds (e.g., *Aspergillus* species) were relatively uncommon.

b. Itraconazole (Sporanox) has a broader spectrum of activity than fluconazole. Its main clinical utility is against the agents of histoplasmosis and blastomycosis. It also has modest activity against *Aspergillus*.

c. Voriconazole (VFEND) has a broader spectrum of activity than fluconazole or itraconazole and is active against most species of *Candida*, *Aspergillus*, and several less common fungi. The potential for drug–drug interactions can be a problem with the use of voriconazole.

   (1) Adverse reactions. The most common adverse reactions are several different types of visual disturbances that usually do not require discontinuation of therapy and skin reactions. IV voriconazole is solubilized in sulfobutylether-β-cyclodextrin (SBECD), which accumulates with moderate real dysfunction; it is recommended that the IV preparation not be used if the creatinine clearance is <50 mL/minute.

   (2) Bioavailability of oral voriconazole is excellent and the oral preparation does not contain SBECD. In selected patients with appreciably impaired renal function, a change to oral therapy with voriconazole may be feasible.

d. Posaconazole (Noxafil), available only in an oral formulation, appears promising as an agent for prophylaxis of infection in severely immunosuppressed patients, such as those with GVHD. Additional study of this agent is needed to define its role in treatment of fungal infections in cancer patients.

e. Drug–drug interactions. Of importance, a number of important drug–drug interactions involve voriconazole and the other triazoles. Most of these interactions involve cytochrome P450 isoforms and may result in significantly increased or decreased concentrations of voriconazole or of the interacting drug, resulting in either potential toxicity or lack of efficacy, respectively.

3. AmB preparations

   a. Amphotericin B deoxycholate (AmBD, Fungizone) had been the gold standard for treatment of fungal infections, but there is reluctance to use it in *non-neutropenic* patients because of nephrotoxicity. In neutropenic patients, this concern is heightened by the frequent concomitant use of nephrotoxic chemotherapeutic agents and antimicrobial agents.

   b. Lipid formulations of AmB have not been shown to be more effective than AmBD for treatment of fungal infections, but they are much less likely to cause nephrotoxicity. Their major drawbacks have been other potential side effects and their much greater cost. These lipid preparations include

   (1) Amphotericin B lipid complex (ABLC, Abelcet)

   (2) Amphotericin B colloidal dispersion (ABCD, Amphotec)

   (3) Liposomal amphotericin B (LAmB, AmBisome), which currently is the only U.S. Food and Drug Administration (FDA)-approved lipid formulation for empiric therapy for presumed fungal infections in febrile neutropenic patients.

B. Antifungal agents in patients with neutropenic fever. Reasonably clear guidelines can be developed for antifungal therapy early in the course of neutropenia. With prolonged broad-spectrum antibacterial therapy and empiric antifungal therapy, increasing opportunity and selective pressure tend to result in unusual infections. The availability of the newer triazoles and echinocandins has provided greater therapeutic options with reduced toxicity; it has also created more opportunity for administration of an antifungal agent that is not active against the patient's present fungal pathogen. This makes microbiologic diagnosis of infection imperative, and may require invasive procedures to procure biopsy material for culture and fungal staining.

The strategy for providing empiric antifungal therapy in cancer patients with neutropenia is based on the following principles:

1. During the first 3 to 5 days of neutropenic fever, the major concern is infection by *Candida* spp., followed by *Aspergillus* spp. The echinocandins and newer triazoles have excellent activity against *Candida* and most *Aspergillus* spp. and possess limited toxicity.

2. AmBD and the lipid formulations of AmB possess the broadest spectrum of antifungal activity of all groups of antifungal agents. The echinocandins may lack the broader activity of AmB preparations and of the newer triazoles against genera of clinically important fungi that may be cause infection later in neutropenia.

3. Among the echinocandins, the greatest clinical experience is with caspofungin; however, many experts believe that micafungin and anidulafungin are likely to have similar clinical efficacies, based on *in vitro* and limited *in vivo* data. It is important to note that echinocandins are inactive against *Cryptococcus neoformans*, the endemic mycoses (e.g., *Coccidioides* spp., *Histoplasma capsulatum*), and many molds (e.g., *Fusarium* spp., *Scedosporium apiospermum*, *Zygomyces*). Drug–drug interactions are generally less than those seen with triazoles.

4. Among the triazoles, voriconazole may be a reasonable alternative to an echinocandin or AmB preparation. With voriconazole, attention must be paid to potential side effects and drug–drug interactions; also, it is recommended that the drug not be given intravenously, if at all possible, when the creatinine clearance is <50 mL/minute to avoid accumulation of the diluent used to solubilize the drug. Of the other azoles, fluconazole and itraconazole are thought not to have a sufficiently broad spectrum of activity against *Candida* spp. Clinical experience with posaconazole is quite limited and this drug is not currently available in an IV formulation.

5. If an AmB preparation were to be used for empiric antifungal coverage of the febrile neutropenic patient, most clinicians would use one of the more expensive lipid preparations to avoid the potentially more severe nephrotoxicity of AmBD.

6. Substantial variation exists in the costs of all of the all antifungal agents. Cost plus an institution's clinical experience with fungal infections may determine the choice of an initial antifungal agent.

7. **Summary.** With concerns regarding renal function (pre-existing impairment of renal function, concomitant use of nephrotoxic agents, or development of renal dysfunction during AmB administration), use of an echinocandin (preferably caspofungin) is reasonable and appropriate. Voriconazole would be a reasonable alternative. With substantial clinical deterioration that might be caused by fungal infection, the initiation of antifungal therapy with an AmB lipid preparation would be prudent.

C. **Cryptococcus.** Patients receiving corticosteroids and those with AIDS or Hodgkin lymphoma have the highest incidence of infection with *C. neoformans*.

1. **Clinical presentation.** Pulmonary infection can be asymptomatic. Chest radiographs reveal local bronchopneumonia, lobar involvement, or discrete nodules that may cavitate. CNS infection usually presents as insidious meningoencephalitis without evidence of infection outside the meninges. A variety of skin findings, ranging from maculopapular or nodular lesions to cellulitis, can be seen in disseminated infection.

2. **Diagnosis**

   a. **Culture.** *C. neoformans*, an encapsulated yeast that replicates by budding, can easily be grown from blood, respiratory secretions, spinal fluid, and skin biopsies on common laboratory media.

   b. **Cerebrospinal fluid** typically reveals an elevated opening pressure and lymphocytic pleocytosis in cryptococcal meningoencephalitis. A low glucose concentration is found in half of the cases. The India ink preparation is positive in approximately 40% of cases.

   c. **Serology.** The presence of cryptococcal polysaccharide antigen in spinal fluid is diagnostic and is detected in cerebrospinal fluid in >90% of meningitis cases. The presence of cryptococcal antigen in serum documents infection and can be used as a rapid screen. Antibody assays are not useful.

3. **Management.** The major difficulty the clinician faces with management of cryptococcal infection is determining whether meningeal infection exists. The greatest clinical experience with treatment of cryptococcal infection is that from HIV-infected patients; this experience heavily influences management algorithms. All echinocandins lack activity against *Cryptococcus*.

   a. **Meningitis or disseminated disease** is treated with AmBD, 0.7 mg/kg/day, with adjunctive flucytosine for 2 weeks. Amphotericin lipid preparations are sometimes substituted. This 2-week induction is followed by fluconazole given at a dose of 400 mg/day (after a 400-mg loading dose) either PO or IV. In patients with intracranial hypertension, depressed sensorium, or other ominous CNS findings, AmB should be given in a dose of 1.0 mg/kg/day. Intracranial hypertension in the absence of intracranial mass lesions may require repeated lumbar puncture to reduce intracranial pressure and ensure adequate perfusion of the brain.

   b. **Extrameningeal infection.** Most patients with extrameningeal infection can be treated with fluconazole (400 to 800 mg/day), if meningeal infection has been excluded.

D. **Candidiasis.** The major risk factors for systemic candidiasis include treatment with immunosuppressive agents, antibiotics, glucocorticoids, or parenteral hyperalimentation. Indwelling central venous catheters, IV drug abuse, and underlying diseases that produce defects in polymorphonuclear neutrophil function or cell-mediated immunity (e.g., leukemia, lymphoma, diabetes mellitus) also are associated with this infection.

1. **Clinical presentation.** Localized candidiasis can involve the skin, mouth, esophagus, rectum, or vagina. Disseminated candidiasis can present with fever alone, sepsis, endophthalmitis, skin nodules, renal disease, arthritis, or myositis. With dissemination, *C. albicans* and occasionally other *Candida* species may produce discrete, yellow–white retinal lesions of *Candida* endophthalmitis. Visceral involvement (hepatosplenic candidosis) is another sequel of dissemination and typically becomes evident following resolution of neutropenia.

2. **Diagnosis**

   a. **Cultures.** Although studies have shown that blood cultures were positive in only 50% of patients with disseminated candidiasis at autopsy, the yield using modern culture media is undoubtedly higher. Recovery of *Candida* in the laboratory allows for speciation; this may have implications for selection of therapeutic agents. Documentation of disseminated candidiasis may also avoid a continued search for causes of fever.

   b. **Serology.** A useful test for diagnosis of candidiasis has yet to be developed.

   c. **Esophagogram** shows a typical shaggy, moth-eaten appearance in cases of esophageal candidiasis; the diagnosis can also be made by esophagoscopy.

3. **Management.** Infected foreign bodies, such as CVC, should be promptly removed.

   a. **Local therapy.** Nystatin liquid suspension (100,000 U/mL) is used to treat oropharyngeal candidiasis; the usual regimen is 500,000 to 2,000,000 U every 4 to 6 hours ("swish and swallow"). If this fails, clotrimazole (Mycelex troches) five times daily or fluconazole, 50 to 100 mg once daily, should be used.

   b. **Prophylaxis.** Topical agents such as nystatin or clotrimazole may be used for prophylaxis, although no good data support a clear-cut benefit. The prophylactic use of fluconazole (or other triazole antifungals) is not recommended because of the risk of selecting resistant organisms that would preclude fluconazole and possibly other triazoles as therapeutic agents for subsequent treatment of suspected or documented infections.

   c. **Systemic therapy.** If a *Candida* species is isolated from the patient, then treatment with an echinocandin would be appropriate. When the isolate has been speciated or susceptibility testing has been done, changing to a triazole might be appropriate, depending on the species of *Candida* recovered, whether the patient is tolerating the echinocandin, and whether there has been resolution of neutropenia.

E. Aspergillosis. Infection usually occurs via inhalation of spores leading to infection of lung parenchyma or, occasionally, of the paranasal sinuses; dissemination usually occurs from the lung. Approximately 70% to 80% of isolates are *Aspergillus fumigatus*.

The typical presentation for aspergillosis in immunosuppressed patients is fever and pulmonary nodules or infiltrates; as disease progresses, there may be infarction, hemoptysis, and gangrene from vascular invasion. Nearly one-third of patients have no radiologic abnormalities early in the disease.

Dissemination complicates pulmonary disease in 25% to 50% of cases. Various skin lesions, multiple abscesses, brain infarction, or GI ulceration with hemorrhage can result. Aspergillosis is the second most frequent fungal infection that affects the face and mouth of patients receiving chemotherapy. In these patients, bone marrow recovery may lead to the liquefaction of pulmonary foci. Potentially lethal erosion and bleeding may then occur because of the vasculotropic nature of the infection.

1. Diagnosis. The "gold standard" for diagnosis is recovery of the organism by the laboratory from an appropriate clinical sample; this invariably involves culture of a biopsy specimen. *Aspergillus* species are infrequently recovered from tracheobronchial secretions and essentially never from blood cultures. The galactomannan assay, which detects a cell wall polysaccharide of *Aspergillus* species, has poor sensitivity, poor specificity, and poor positive-predictive value.

The diagnosis of aspergillosis is often based on demonstration of septate, acutely branching hyphae in tissue. Other fungi (e.g., *Scedosporium apiospermum*, *Fusarium* species, *Penicillium* species), however, may not be distinguishable from *Aspergillus* in tissue section and other fungi (e.g., the Zygomycetes) may require an experienced microscopist to recognize their distinct morphology. Chest radiographic studies may reveal nodules, with or without cavitation, or pleural-based infiltrates. The presence of a "halo sign" (low attenuation surrounding a nodular lesion) on high-resolution CT may be seen in early pulmonary aspergillosis. Later an "air-crescent" sign indicative of cavitation may be noted. Similar radiographic findings may, however, be present with other vasculotropic organisms. Hence, the emphasis should be on biopsy and culture, whenever possible.

2. Management

   a. Optimal antifungal treatment of invasive aspergillosis is unclear at this time. The main difficulty is that no single antifungal agent is active against all species and isolates of *Aspergillus* and reliable, reproducible means of susceptibility testing of agents against *Aspergillus* do not exist. The greatest experience is with AmBD, given in a dose of 1.0 to 1.5 mg/kg/day; this dose regimen almost invariably results in significant renal dysfunction. The lipid preparations of AmB (ABLC and LAmB) are better tolerated and are usually given in a daily dose of at least 5 mg/kg/day; some patients with refractory disease have been treated with doses as high as 15 mg/kg/day.

   b. Voriconazole has FDA approval for treatment of invasive aspergillosis, and is rapidly becoming a mainstay of treatment of invasive aspergillosis. Recent reports of *in vitro* resistance of *Aspergillus* to voriconazole are of concern, although the clinical impact of these findings is unclear. Therapy should be initiated with two doses of 6 mg/kg given IV 12 hours apart, followed by 4 mg/kg every 12 hours. Patients who respond to this treatment can be switched to oral drugs at 7 days. (See section VII.A.2 for adverse reactions, bioavailability, and drug interactions.)

   c. The other triazoles (fluconazole, itraconazole, and posaconazole) are either not active against *Aspergillus* or offer no advantage over voriconazole.

   d. Caspofungin has FDA approval for treatment of aspergillosis in patients who cannot tolerate or who have failed other forms of therapy. The other echinocandins, anidulafungin and micafungin, possess *in vitro* activity against *Aspergillus*, but clinical data are exceedingly limited.

e. Data to support the use of **combination therapy** for aspergillosis are extremely limited. Triazoles have been shown to be antagonistic when given in conjunction with AmB preparations. Although the combined use of caspofungin and voriconazole has biologic plausibility, insufficient clinical data exist regarding efficacy and toxicity to support their use.

f. Surgical resection of localized invasive pulmonary aspergillosis with a cavitating lesion may prevent hemoptysis and recurrence in selected patients. In leukemic patients, the achievement of complete remission combined with aggressive antifungal therapy has led to markedly increased cure rates for aspergillosis.

F. Zygomycosis. Members of the taxonomic class *Zygomycetes* are a complicated group of organisms. Infection has been recognized with increasing frequency in patients who have leukemia or lymphoma, immunoincompetence, glucocorticoid therapy, diabetes mellitus, malnutrition, burns, stem cell transplantation, or solid-organ transplantation.

1. Manifestations. The genera *Rhizopus, Absidia,* and *Mucor* produce similar pathologic and clinical manifestations because of neutrophil exudation, tissue necrosis, and vascular invasion that results in thrombosis and infarction.

a. Pneumonia can be associated with a dry cough or hemoptysis. Radiographs may show interstitial infiltrates, lobar consolidation, or cavitation.

b. Cerebral disease is usually secondary to pulmonary involvement and presents as brain infarcts or abscesses. Spinal fluid studies are not usually helpful. In contrast, rhinocerebral mucormycosis occurs most frequently in uncontrolled diabetes mellitus.

c. Disseminated disease can result in gastroenteritis, bowel perforation or hemorrhage, peritonitis, or abscess in any organ.

2. Diagnosis. *Zygomycetes* organisms have broad, nonseptate hyphae, often with right-angle branching in tissue specimens. The agents of zygomycosis may be difficult to recover by culture. Diagnosis is made by demonstrating the organism by culture or, more commonly, by special stains of tissue sections.

3. Management. A high dose of either AmBD or one of the AmB lipid formulations is recommended, although these drugs are largely adjunctive. Reversal of the predisposing condition and resection of infected tissue, if feasible, are the mainstays of therapy. Posaconazole appears to provide some benefit following treatment with an AmB preparation, but experience is quite limited. Mortality is high.

G. Other systemic mycoses

1. *Histoplasma capsulatum, Coccidioides immitis, and Blastomyces dermatitidis* can readily be recovered from tissues and display typical (pathognomonic) histopathologies. These common human pathogens can present as opportunistic infections in patients who are immunocompromised. Dissemination is often associated with cutaneous anergy.

2. *Trichosporon beigelii* refers to a group of fungi that cannot readily be distinguished without the use of molecular techniques. *Trichosporon beigelii* causes white piedra, an infection of hair shafts, is an emerging opportunistic mycosis that is can be difficult to diagnose, and has a high attributable mortality rate. Systemic infection has been most frequently described in neutropenic patients receiving chemotherapy.

a. Cutaneous involvement occurs in about 30% of patients and frequently presents as purpuric papules and nodules with central necrosis or ulceration. Biopsy specimens of these lesions reveal dermal invasion by fungal elements. Culture is positive in >90% of cases.

b. Resolution of disseminated infection appears to require resolution of neutropenia. The antifungal triazoles are most active. AmBD, liposomal AmB, and the echinocandins appear not to be very effective.

3. **Scedosporiasis** is caused by the asexual form *Scedosporium apiospermum* (*Pseudallescheria boydii*); it is an increasingly common cause of opportunistic infection and may cause CNS disease and fungemia in patients with leukemia. Although infections are usually resistant to AmB, the triazoles may be effective, with voriconazole being preferred.

4. **Fusariosis.** Members of the genus *Fusarium* are ubiquitous fungi uncommonly associated with infection. Disseminated fusariosis typically occurs in neutropenic patients, carries a high mortality rate, and presents with fever and diffuse cutaneous macules, papules, and nodules. *Fusarium* species can be isolated from biopsy of skin lesions (hyphae are often observed on direct microscopy) or bronchial aspirates of lung lesions. AmBD and AmB lipid formulations may eradicate this infection; voriconazole is indicated for those with fusariosis who are intolerant of, or refractory to, other therapy. Some clinicians prefer a lipid preparation of AmB plus voriconazole.

5. **Fungemic shock.** As the use of empiric antibiotics for bacteria has increased, the likelihood has increased that fungi, particularly *Candida* species, can cause a septic shock-type picture.

VIII. PARASITIC INFECTIONS

A. **Toxoplasmosis.** The incidence of asymptomatic disease based on serology ranges from 10% to 40% in the United States to 96% in western Europe. Of those patients with AIDS who are seropositive for *T. gondii*, about 25% to 50% originally developed *Toxoplasma* encephalitis. This has decreased dramatically because of the use of trimethoprim-sulfamethoxazole for *Pneumocystis* prophylaxis in severely CD4 lymphopenic patients and the availability of highly active antiretroviral therapy.

Patients with symptomatic disease present with a low-grade febrile illness characterized by localized or generalized lymphadenopathy, hepatosplenomegaly, malaise, and fatigue. Any organ may become involved. Infection in patients with abnormal cellular immunity may mimic brain tumor or lymphoproliferative disorder.

1. **Diagnosis**
   a. **Histology.** Identification of trophozoites rather than cysts is important because cysts can persist for decades. Lymph node pathology is characteristic of toxoplasmosis.
   b. **Culture** is rarely used.
   c. **Serology** suggests the disease. IgM antibody is suggestive of recent infection. Many patients, however, develop symptomatic disease as a result of reactivation of a quiescent infection. In the latter instance, only IgG antibody will likely be detectable.

2. **Management.** Pyrimethamine (a folic acid antagonist) and a sulfa derivative are given in divided doses for 3 to 6 weeks. The development of hematologic toxicity often interrupts treatment. Leucovorin is also given to minimize marrow suppressive effects.
   a. **Pyrimethamine** is given as a loading dose of 200 mg PO followed by maintenance of 50 to 75 mg/day in association with leucovorin, 10 to 20 mg/day orally.
   b. **Sulfadiazine,** 1.0 to 1.5 g q.i.d. is given in conjunction with pyrimethamine.
   c. **Another combination** for acute disease is pyrimethamine (100 mg/day PO) and leucovorin plus clindamycin (1.2 g/day IV in divided doses).

B. **Pneumocystis.** *P. carinii* (which has been reclassified as a fungus and renamed *P. jiroveci*) causes pneumonia in immunodeficient patients, including those with AIDS. Children with acute lymphoblastic leukemia in remission and patients in whom corticosteroid therapy is being tapered are particularly susceptible to infection. Manifestations include dyspnea, fever, nonproductive cough, pulmonary rales, hypoxemia, and hypocapnia. Chest radiographs early in the disease may appear benign, whereas blood gases often demonstrate hypoxemia. Chest radiographs most often show diffuse symmetric, bilateral, perihilar infiltrates that progress at variable rates.

1. **Diagnosis.** In patients infected with HIV, the organism is usually easily visualized because of the large numbers often present; in patients with other forms of immunosuppression, detection of cysts is much more difficult. The most commonly used diagnostic techniques are direct fluorescent antibody (DFA) stain or methenamine silver stain of pulmonary secretions or lung biopsy material. Giemsa stain detects sporozoites within the cyst wall but not the wall. Sputum specimens are diagnostic in 10% to 15% of cases, bronchoscopic brushings in 65% to 75%, and open-lung biopsy in 90%.

   In patients who are critically ill or severely thrombocytopenic, lung biopsy should be deferred. Less invasive procedures or possibly an empiric trial of therapy may be considered because the biopsy procedure has high morbidity and mortality rates.

2. **Management.** In patients with significant respiratory difficulties (arterial oxygen pressure <70 mm Hg or an alveolar–arterial oxygen gradient >35 mm Hg), corticosteroids (prednisone 40 mg b.i.d., tapering over a 21-day course) should be added to the antimicrobial treatment for pneumocystis. Treatment is normally given for 21 days and options include the following:

   a. Sulfamethoxazole-trimethoprim (Bactrim or Septra), two double-strength tablets PO or two ampules IV every 6 to 8 hours; this schedule is considered to be the therapy of choice.

   b. Pentamidine, 4 mg/kg IM daily, can be used in patients intolerant to sulfa drugs.

   c. Trimetrexate in combination with leucovorin may be effective when other regimens have failed. Trimetrexate is relatively toxic and does not offer any advantages over sulfamethoxazole-trimethoprim or pentamidine.

   d. Atovaquone or the combination of clindamycin-primaquine is sometimes used for mild cases in patients infected with HIV, but these are definitely second-line therapies and less likely to produce a good outcome in the severely ill patient.

C. **Strongyloidiasis.** Humans are infected by both filariform larvae and adult forms, resulting in self-perpetuating autoinfection. Defective cell-mediated immunity, high-dose corticosteroid therapy, and decreased bowel motility enhance the chance of massive GI tract, pulmonary, or CNS infection. The characteristics of *Strongyloides stercoralis* allow it to be harbored within a host for prolonged periods, only to disseminate after cell-mediated immunity is suppressed.

   1. **Diagnosis.** A diagnosis of strongyloidiasis should be considered in an immunocompromised patient with a petechial rash. Larvae can be recovered from the stool in 25% to 60% of patients and from duodenal aspirates in 40% to 90%. Peripheral eosinophilia is typical but may be absent in the hyperinfected state.

   2. **Management.** Prompt diagnosis and initiation of thiabendazole therapy, 1.5 g PO twice daily for 2 to 4 days, provides the greatest opportunity for patient survival. Secondary bacterial infections should be aggressively sought. The mortality rate from disseminated strongyloidiasis approaches 80%.

D. **Other parasites**

   1. *Giardia lamblia* infection is associated with hypogammaglobulinemia, small bowel lymphoma, and pancreatic carcinoma. Manifestations include diarrhea, nausea, flatulence, and cramps.

   2. **Malaria and babesiosis** may infect immunosuppressed hosts, especially after splenectomy. Infection results in high fever and hemolysis.

Suggested Reading

Hubel K, et al. Suppressed neutrophil function as a risk factor for severe infection after cytotoxic chemotherapy in patients with acute nonlymphocytic leukemia. *Ann Hematol* 1999;78:73.

Hughes WT, et al. 1997 guidelines for the use of antimicrobial agents in neutropenic patients with unexplained fever. Infectious Diseases Society of America. *Clin Infect Dis* 1997;25:551.

Hughes WT, et al. 2002 guidelines for the use of antimicrobial agents in neutropenic patients with cancer. *Clin Infect Dis* 2002;34:730.

Marr KA, et al. Combination antifungal therapy for invasive aspergillosis. *Clin Infect Dis* 2004;39:797.

Mermel LA, et al. Guidelines for the management of intravascular catheter–related infections. *Clin Infect Dis* 2001;32:1249.

Ostrosky-Zeichner L, et al. Amphotericin B: time for a new "gold standard." *Clin Infect Dis* 2003;37:415.

Ozer H, et al. 2000 update of recommendations for the use of hematopoietic colony-stimulating factors: evidence-based, clinical practice guidelines. *J Clin Oncol* 2000;18:3558.

Pappas PG, et al. Guidelines for treatment of candidiasis. *Clin Infect Dis* 2004;38:161.

Pfeiffer CD, et al. Diagnosis of invasive aspergillosis using a galactomannan assay: a meta-analysis. *Clin Infect Dis* 2006;42:1417.

Pizzo PA. Fever in immunocompromised patients. *N Engl J Med* 1999;341:893.

Rex JH. Practice guidelines for the treatment of Candidiasis. *Clin Infect Dis* 2000;30:662.

Smith TJ, et al. 2006 update of recommendations for use of white blood cell growth factors: an evidence-based clinical practice guideline. *J Clin Oncol* 2006;24:3187.

Spellberg BJ, et al. Current treatment strategies for disseminated candidiasis. *Clin Infect Dis* 2006;42:244.

Note: The Infectious Diseases Society of America publishes clinical practice guidelines; publication of the guidelines on the following subjects can be expected in the next 6 to 18 months: Candidiasis; Aspergillus; management of neutropenic patients with cancer; and management of vascular catheter-related infections. These guidelines can be found at the Infectious Diseases Society of America website: http://www.idsociety.org/Content/NavigationMenu/Practice_Guidelines/Standards_Practice_Guidelines_Statements/Standards,_Practice_Guidelines,_and_Statements.htm,
http://www.idsociety.org/Content.aspx?id-9088, or
http://www.idsociety.org/default.aspx (under the heading "Practice Guidelines")

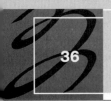

AIDS-RELATED MALIGNANCIES
Alexandra M. Levine

36

I. INTRODUCTION
Highly active antiretroviral therapy (HAART) consists of the use of multiple antiretroviral agents comprising different classes of agents used in combination. With the first advent of protease inhibitors, used in combination with reverse transcriptase inhibitors, such HAART therapy became widely available in the United States and other resource-rich areas of the world between 1996 and 1997. In that short period, a stunning change in the outcome of infection by human immunodeficiency virus (HIV) among HAART users was observed. The death rate in patients with full-blown acquired immunodeficiency syndrome (AIDS) decreased by approximately 80%, and the development of an AIDS-defining condition among HIV-infected patients declined by approximately 75%. These changes have persisted over the past decade and have resulted in dramatic changes in the course of HIV infection and in the malignant diseases that may occur as a consequence of AIDS.

The cancers that are considered AIDS defining include Kaposi sarcoma (KS), non-Hodgkin lymphoma, and invasive cervical carcinoma. Each of these malignancies is associated with infection by an etiologic organism, including human herpesvirus type 8 (HHV-8) in KS, Epstein-Barr virus (EBV) and others in lymphoma, and human papillomavirus (HPV) in cases of cervical (and anal) carcinoma. With the widespread use of HAART, the incidence of these tumors has changed as dramatically as the natural history and disease outcome of AIDS.

II. AIDS-RELATED LYMPHOMA
A. Incidence
1. Lymphoma is now one of the most common of the initial AIDS-defining conditions, occurring in approximately 16% of all new cases of AIDS. All age groups and all groups at risk for acquisition of HIV infection are equally likely to develop lymphoma.
2. Lymphoma is a late manifestation of HIV disease. As the immune system weakens with progressive loss of CD4 lymphocytes, the risk of lymphoma increases significantly. With widespread use of HAART in various areas of the world, resulting in populationwide increases in CD4 cells, the incidence of lymphoma has decreased dramatically. In this setting, the risk for lymphoma depends on the latest CD4 cell count, and not the nadir count, before the time that HAART was used.
3. Although the risk of lymphoma has decreased significantly in patients or populations treated effectively with HAART, this decrease in lymphoma has been far less substantial than that seen in KS or the various opportunistic infections, resulting in a relative increase in the occurrence of lymphoma as an initial AIDS-defining illness.

B. Pathology.
Most AIDS-related lymphomas are B-cell tumors of high-grade pathological type. About 70% of patients are diagnosed with immunoblastic lymphoma or small noncleaved lymphoma; the latter may be Burkitt or non-Burkitt subtype. In contrast, only 10% to 15% of patients with *de novo* lymphoma are diagnosed with one of these rather unusual forms of lymphoma. Intermediate-grade, diffuse, large B-cell lymphomas have been reported in 30%.

With the advent of HAART, a change in the spectrum of AIDS lymphoma has occurred, with a greater percentage of patients now diagnosed with Burkitt or atypical Burkitt lymphomas and relatively fewer numbers of individuals diagnosed with diffuse large B-cell lymphoma.

Aggressive B-cell lymphomas are expected, but HIV-infected patients have also been shown to have an increased incidence of low-grade B-cell lymphoma and of various T-cell lymphomas, as well.

A newly recognized entity, termed *primary effusion lymphoma* (PEL), has been identified among HIV-infected patients who are also infected with HHV-8. PEL is a B-cell neoplasm with the morphological appearance of an anaplastic or immunoblastic lymphoma. Patients present with malignant serous effusions, usually in the absence of specific mass lesions. Median survival time is in the range of 6 months, despite therapy.

C. Clinical features

1. About 80% to 90% of patients with newly diagnosed AIDS-related lymphoma present with systemic B symptoms, consisting of fever, drenching night sweats, and/or weight loss.

2. About 60% to 90% of patients have far-advanced disease presenting in extranodal sites. This occurrence is in sharp distinction to patients with *de novo* lymphoma, of whom approximately 40% present with extranodal disease.

   a. The more common sites of initial extranodal disease include the central nervous system (CNS; about 30% prevalence at diagnosis), gastrointestinal (GI) tract (25%), bone marrow (20% to 33%), and liver (10%).

   b. Any anatomic site may be involved, with lymphoma reported in the myocardium, earlobe, gallbladder, rectum, gingiva, and elsewhere.

D. Diagnosis and staging evaluation

1. **Biopsy.** Immunophenotypic or genotypic studies are often helpful to confirm the monoclonal (and thus the malignant) nature of the process.

2. **Computed axial tomography (CAT) scans.** Staging evaluation should begin with a CAT scan of the chest, abdomen, and pelvis. Nearly two-thirds of patients with AIDS-related lymphoma have evidence of intra-abdominal lymphomatous disease, which most commonly involves the lymph nodes, GI tract, liver, kidney, and/or adrenal gland. Isolated hepatic or splenic enlargement is not usually seen in the absence of other intra-abdominal findings.

3. **Positron-emission tomography (PET) scanning** is now used quite commonly in conjunction with CAT scans and can detect more minimal disease activity that may not be evident on a CAT scan. This staging tool is helpful in evaluating residual stable masses after completion of chemotherapy and may be used to differentiate residual active lymphomatous disease from scar and fibrosis. Caution should be taken in the interpretation of PET scans, however, as sites of infection or inflammation, common in the setting of HIV infection, may also yield positive PET scan findings.

4. **Bone marrow** aspiration and biopsy should be performed, usually from two sites.

5. **Lumbar puncture (LP).** Although not required in most patients with *de novo* lymphoma, LP should be performed routinely as part of the staging evaluation of patients with AIDS-related lymphoma. About 20% of HIV-infected patients are found to have leptomeningeal involvement even when they have no CNS symptoms. Because prophylactic intrathecal chemotherapy has become an integral part of initial therapy, it is now common practice to inject the first dose of methotrexate or cytosine arabinoside at the time of this initial staging LP in an attempt to prevent isolated CNS relapse. In the presence of active cerebrospinal fluid (CSF) involvement by lymphoma, abnormalities may be relatively minor, with median white cell count of approximately 10 cells/cc. Nonetheless, elevated protein and decreased CSF glucose levels are expected in the majority; abnormal lymphoma cells are clearly recognizable upon cytologic evaluation.

E. Prognostic factors

1. **Decreased survival** in AIDS-related lymphoma is associated with the following factors:

   a. CD4 cells $<100/\mu L$

   b. Karnofsky performance status $<70\%$

    c. Age >35 years

    d. Stage III or IV

    e. Elevated lactate dehydrogenase in serum

  2. Primary CNS lymphoma (PCNSL). In the era of HAART, a stunning decline in PCNSL (see section II.G.1) has occurred, and affected patients are only rarely seen at this time. Before the availability of HAART, patients with PCNSL fared significantly worse than patients with AIDS-related systemic lymphoma, with a median survival of only 2 to 3 months despite therapy, probably because of the far-advanced degree of HIV disease. Use of HAART, along with chemotherapy and/or radiation, has resulted in a significant prolongation of survival in these patients.

  3. Leptomeningeal involvement in patients with AIDS-related systemic lymphoma is a poor prognostic indicator.

F. Management

  1. Low-dose regimens. Before the availability of HAART, use of low-dose modifications of standard regimens (such as m-BACOD or CHOP) was advocated because prospective clinical trials indicated that standard dose regimens provided no benefit over lower doses but were clearly associated with significantly increased toxicity. In the era of HAART, *these recommendations are no longer valid.*

    A phase III randomized trial was completed within the AIDS Malignancy Consortium (AMC). Patients were randomized to receive either standard CHOP for six cycles or standard dose CHOP with rituximab given on day 1 of each cycle, with an additional 3 doses at the conclusion of all therapy. Results of this trial indicated better complete remission rates and decreased risk of relapse in patients treated with rituximab, but these differences were not significantly different. This study comprised only 150 patients and was not powered to detect such statistically significant differences, which were of the same magnitude as those reported by Coiffier and his colleagues, who studied the use of CHOP with or without rituximab in 400 HIV-negative patients. Of importance, HIV-infected patients on the AMC trial who received rituximab were at increased risk of developing fatal infections, although the risk of neutropenia, neutropenic fever, and hypogammaglobulinemia was equivalent in the two groups. Patients who died of infection were more likely to have entered study with CD4 cell counts <50/μL, indicating severe immunocompromise. It is now recommended that patients with CD4 cells <100/μL receive prophylactic antibiotics along with combined rituximab and chemotherapy.

  2. Antiretroviral therapy may be used simultaneously with multiagent chemotherapy or may be discontinued until chemotherapy has been completed and then restarted immediately. If used simultaneously with chemotherapy, *zidovudine (AZT) should not be incorporated into the antiretroviral regimen because this drug is myelosuppressive.* With this exception, however, pharmacokinetic studies have indicated no clinically significant interactions between HAART (including protease inhibitors) and multiagent anti-lymphoma chemotherapy. *Accepted practice now includes the combined use of chemotherapy with HAART.*

  3. Infusional chemotherapy: EPOCH. A dose-adjusted EPOCH regimen has been used in a limited number of patients studied at the National Cancer Institute (NCI) with excellent preliminary results. Three of the five drugs are given by continuous IV infusion (CIV). Cycles are repeated every 21 days for a total of six cycles. The specific dose-adjusted regimen for patients with AIDS is as follows:

Etoposide, 50 mg/m^2/day on Days 1 through 4 by CIV

Hydroxydaunomycin (doxorubicin, Adriamycin), 10 mg/m^2/day on Days 1 through 4 by CIV

Oncovin (vincristine), 0.4 mg/m^2/day on Days 1 through 4 by CIV (with no maximum dose)

Prednisone, 60 mg/m^2/day PO on Days 1 through 5

Cyclophosphamide IV on Day 5; 375 mg/m^2 if CD4 $\geq$100; 187 mg/m^2 if CD4 <100

a. On subsequent cycles, the dose of cyclophosphamide was adjusted in increments of 187 mg/m^2 to a maximum dose of 750 mg/m^2 IV. If the nadir absolute neutrophil count (ANC) was >500 cells/μL, the subsequent dose was increased by 187 mg/m^2. If the nadir ANC was <500 cells/μL, the dose was decreased by 187 mg/m^2.

b. Granulocyte colony–stimulating factor was given at a dose of 5 mcg/kg/day subcutaneously from Day 6 until the ANC was >5,000 cells/μL after the nadir.

c. Intrathecal methotrexate was given at a dose of 12 mg on Days 1 and 5 of cycles 3 through 6.

d. Prophylaxis for *Pneumocystis pneumonia* was mandated, and prophylaxis against *Mycobacterium avium* was given to patients with CD4 cells <100/μL. Antifungal prophylaxis was not given.

e. Antiretroviral therapy was suspended for the duration of EPOCH chemotherapy and was reinstituted immediately at its conclusion.

f. Results of EPOCH in AIDS-related lymphoma

(1) The overall complete remission rate was 74%, including 56% of patients with CD4 cells <100/μL and 87% of patients with CD4 cells >100/μL. With a median follow-up of 56 months, there have only been two relapses, and the disease-free survival is 92%. Several patients with Burkitt lymphoma experienced CNS relapse, necessitating a change in protocol to include CNS prophylaxis (intrathecal methotrexate) in all subsequent patients. Overall survival at 56 months is 60%, whereas the overall survival of patients with CD4 cells >100/μL at entry is 87%.

(2) Neutropenia (<500 cells/μL) was evident in 30% of cycles, febrile neutropenia was seen in 13% of cycles, and 21% of cycles were associated with a platelet count <50,000/μL.

(3) In the absence of concomitant HAART, the HIV viral load increased by 0.83 log over the first month of chemotherapy, but fell promptly to pre-EPOCH levels very quickly after reinstitution of HAART at the conclusion of chemotherapy. Likewise, although the CD4 cells fell by a median of 189 cells/μL by the completion of cycle 6, they had returned to baseline levels by 12 to 18 months following completion of chemotherapy.

g. Rituximab plus EPOCH. Further study on larger numbers of patients has recently been accomplished within the multi-institutional AMC, sponsored by the NCI. In this randomized phase II study, patients received either EPOCH with concomitant rituximab (375 mg/m^2 on Day 1 of each cycle) or EPOCH followed sequentially by weekly rituximab for 6 weeks. The group receiving concomitant rituximab fared better than those who received rituximab at the conclusion of chemotherapy, with a statistically superior rate of complete remission and with no increase in infectious death or any non-lymphoma cause of death.

h. Role of HAART. HAART therapy may be delayed until completion of combination chemotherapy. However, opportunistic infections did occur within 3 months of completion of EPOCH. It is possible that concomitant HAART with chemotherapy might have prevented these complications.

G. Primary CNS lymphoma (PCNSL; see also Chapter 21, section VIII.C in "Non-Hodgkin lymphoma")

1. Clinical features. Patients with PCNSL present with far-advanced HIV disease, with median CD4 cells of <50/μL and history of AIDS before the lymphoma in about 75% of cases. Initial symptoms and signs are variable and include seizures, headache, or focal neurological dysfunction. Isolated subtle changes in personality or behavior may also be seen.

2. Diagnosis. Radiographic scanning reveals mass lesions in the brain, occurring at any site. These masses are likely to be relatively large (2 to 4 cm) and relatively few in number (one to three). Ring enhancement may be seen. No specific radiographic findings on CT scans are characteristic of PCNSL. PET scans or thallium single-photon emission computed tomography (SPECT) scans may provide more specific information in terms of the differentiation of PCNSL from other space-occupying lesions within the brain of HIV-infected patients. Further, because AIDS-related PCNSL is essentially always associated with infection by EBV, determination of latent EBV proteins within the CSF may also be used to diagnose PCNSL. In the case of equivocal results, definitive diagnosis requires brain biopsy.

3. **Management.** Radiation therapy (RT) is associated with complete remission in 20% to 50% of cases, but the median survival time has been only 2 to 3 months, with death often due to opportunistic infection. Although RT may not improve the duration of survival, the quality of life does improve, often dramatically, in about 75% of patients. Use of HAART with antineoplastic therapy has been shown to improve survival substantially. Combined use of chemotherapy and radiation improves survival in PCNSL unrelated to AIDS, but such information is lacking in AIDS-related disease. High-dose methotrexate is recommended for the treatment of patients with PCNSL without AIDS but has not been tested in patients with PCNSL and AIDS.

III. HODGKIN LYMPHOMA

A. **Incidence.** Hodgkin lymphoma (HL) is not considered an AIDS-defining condition, although the incidence of HL has increased significantly in HIV-infected patients. All groups at risk for HIV infection appear equally at risk for HL.

   The incidence of HL has increased substantially in the era of HAART when compared when the pre-HAART time period. This finding is likely a result of the fact that the Reed-Sternberg cell (RS), the malignant cell of HL, requires a certain milieu in which to grow and survive. This milieu requires the presence of CD4+ lymphocytes, which provide proliferation and survival signals to the malignant RS cells. With the use of HAART and its associated increased CD4+ lymphocyte counts, this milieu is more advantageous to the RS cells, and clinically diagnosable HL is now seen with increasing frequency.

B. **Biology.** An association of HL with EBV has been suggested for years based on epidemiological data in HIV-negative patients; approximately half of these patients have presence of clonally integrated EBV within the diagnostic Reed-Sternberg cells. In the setting of HIV infection, EBV is almost universally present within the malignant RS cells.

C. **Clinical features.** Patients with underlying HIV infection have different clinical and pathological manifestations of HL than those expected in patients without HIV disease.

   1. **Sites of disease.** Most HIV-infected patients with HL have widespread extranodal disease at diagnosis, with about 80% to 90% presenting with stage III or IV disease. Systemic B symptoms (e.g., fever, drenching night sweats, weight loss) are seen in about 80% to 90% of patients.

      Unusual extranodal sites of disease may be seen, including the anus and rectum and CNS. Bone marrow is involved in approximately 50% to 60% at diagnosis and may be the only site of disease in patients with B symptoms, usually in the setting of peripheral cytopenias.

   2. **Pathology.** Mixed cellularity and lymphocyte depletion subtypes of HL are prominent. Nodular sclerosis and lymphocyte predominant subtypes are relatively decreased in prevalence in the setting of HIV infection when compared with HIV negative patients with *de novo* HL.

D. **Management.** The ABVD regimen (see Appendix D-1) is used most frequently, along with hematopoietic growth factors. The Stanford V regimen (Appendix D-1), when used with concomitant HAART, has been associated with marked improvements in response rate and overall survival. Whether this improvement is due to the addition of HAART or to that specific regimen is not known, though HAART is probably the most important factor. The median survival after definitive therapy is about 1 to 2 years in the absence of HAART, as opposed to the median survival of HIV-uninfected patients with HL, of whom approximately 80% to 90% may be cured. Further work will be required to ascertain the outcome of patients with HIV-HL treated with ABVD and concomitant HAART.

IV. KAPOSI SARCOMA

A. Incidence and epidemiology. AIDS-related KS is seen primarily in homosexual or bisexual men, for reasons that are not understood. With the advent of effective antiretroviral therapy (HAART), the incidence of KS has fallen dramatically in the United States and other resource-rich areas. This dramatic change in the incidence of disease, coincident with the marked decrease in HIV viral load and improvement in immune function associated with HAART, serves to emphasize the crucial role of immunity in the development of KS.

B. Pathogenesis: HHV-8

   1. HHV-8 is associated with all types of KS, including that associated with HIV, with organ transplantation, and with the classic KS seen in elderly men of Mediterranean descent. HHV-8 infection occurs before the development of KS and is associated with a history of greater numbers of sexual partners.

   2. The specific mechanisms of HHV-8 transmission are not yet thoroughly understood, although the virus is found at highest titer and greatest frequency in saliva. The salivary transmission of HHV-8 infection would be consistent with the primary mode of transmission of other human herpesviruses, such as EBV.

   3. HHV-8 infection is clearly required for development of KS, although the virus itself may not be sufficient for KS outcome. About 2% to 10% of normal, healthy people in the United States have evidence of antibody to HHV-8, without clinical illness.

   4. HHV-8 infection of vascular endothelial cells results in a change to spindle-cell morphology, with most cells latently infected. A few lytically infected cells within the endothelium express certain genes (e.g., G-coupled protein, vGCP) that have transforming potential, leading to a proliferating angiogenic KS lesion.

C. Pathogenesis: inflammatory cytokines and angiogenic factors. HIV infection induces an inflammatory cytokine response, with secretion of interleukin-6 (IL-6), IL-1, tumor necrosis factor-α, and others. These cytokines serve as growth factors for endothelial cells infected with HHV-8 and may also be operative in changing the morphology of these cells to the typical spindle cell, which characterizes the KS lesion. Further, secretion of angiogenic factors, such as basic fibroblast growth factor, vascular-endothelial growth factor, and others, by HIV-1–infected mononuclear cells serves to induce the prominent proliferation of vascular tissue that characterizes the KS lesion. HHV-8 itself has genes that encode a viral IL-6 and other proteins that further contribute to the growth and dissemination of the tumor.

D. Clinical features

   1. Natural history of disease. Some patients experience slowly progressive disease over many years, whereas others have fulminant, rapidly advancing KS that quickly leads to death.

   2. Sites of involvement. The patient with KS usually presents with disease on the skin that may consist of nodular or irregular hyperpigmented lesions. The lesions are often remarkably symmetric. Lymphedema may be profound, occasionally in the absence of visible skin lesions. Lymphadenopathy, sometimes in the absence of KS lesions on the skin, is often seen.

   Another common site of involvement is the oral cavity, which is associated with the presence of KS in the lower in the GI tract about 50% of the time. Literally any visceral organ may be involved, although CNS involvement is rare. KS in the lung is associated with a poor prognosis and mandates immediate chemotherapy.

E. Diagnosis and staging evaluation. An initial biopsy with pathological confirmation should be obtained. Routine staging is not necessary in the patient with KS. Assessment of visible disease on the skin and oral cavity, a baseline chest radiograph, and determination of the number of CD4 cells in blood should be performed. If the patient has symptoms suggestive of GI involvement (e.g., abdominal pain, weight loss, or diarrhea), endoscopy should be performed. With unexplained abnormalities on chest radiograph, bronchoscopy should be performed; the diagnosis of KS is usually made by visualization and not by biopsy, which may be associated with significant hemorrhage.

F. Prognostic factors. Factors associated with poor prognosis include (a) history or presence of opportunistic infection; (b) presence of systemic B symptoms, consisting of fever, drenching night sweats, or weight loss in excess of 10% of the normal body weight; and (c) CD4 cells <300/μL. In the absence of all such factors, the median survival is about 3 years. A history of opportunistic infection is the most significant poor prognostic factor, with a median survival time of only 7 months.

G. Management

1. **HAART.** Multiple case reports have documented significant regression of KS after HAART therapy alone. The initial treatment of patients with KS should be an effective antiretroviral regimen alone. In patients who have never taken HAART before, the overall response rate of KS to HAART alone is approximately 60% after 6 months of use (with complete remission in 11%) and increases to a 75% response rate at 24 months, with complete remissions seen in approximately 60%. If the KS does not regress despite a reduction in HIV viral load and an increase in CD4 cells, alternative treatment for KS may be considered.

2. **Antiherpetic therapy.** *In vitro*, HHV-8 may be suppressed by ganciclovir, cidofovir, and foscarnet; acyclovir is ineffective. A prospective trial in patients with cytomegalovirus retinitis suggested that KS could be prevented by the use of systemic ganciclovir. However, prospective studies of cidofovir, used in patients with known KS, revealed no efficacy to this anti–HHV-8 approach. Such lack of efficacy may be due to the fact that the majority of KS cells are only latently infected with HHV-8, making this viral target less useful in terms of anti-HHV8 treatment approaches.

3. **Local therapy.** KS is a disseminated disease at the time of diagnosis in patients with AIDS, even though only localized disease may be clinically evident. Thus, the role of local therapy often includes considerations of cosmesis as opposed to "cure."

   Topical 9-*cis*-retinoic acid (Panretin) is associated with a 30% to 50% response rate and has been licensed for use in cutaneous KS. Individual lesions may be injected with vincristine (0.1 mg) or vinblastine (0.1 mg), or with interferon-α (1 million U), although these modalities are painful and associated with the possibility of secondary infection. Such local injections are rarely advocated at this time.

   Local lesions may also be treated effectively with cryotherapy, laser, or surgical excision. Local radiation may be helpful; however, great care must be taken to avoid undue toxicity, as has been reported in HIV-infected patients after receipt of standard doses and dose schedules of radiation.

4. **Immune response modifiers.** Oral 9-*cis*-retinoic acid may be useful in the therapy of KS, working by means of its ability to down-regulate IL-6, which is a growth factor for KS. Interferon-α (1 million to 2 million U/day) is also effective, especially when combined with antiretroviral agents. Of great interest, interferon-α in low doses is known to function as an antiangiogenic factor, which may explain its efficacy in AIDS-related KS. Recently, additional biological agents that aim to decrease either inflammatory cytokines or angiogenic factors have been studied, with preliminary evidence of efficacy. These agents include imatinib (Gleevec), thalidomide, IL-12, and others. The spectrum of available biologic or targeted therapies for KS is expected to change considerably over the next several years.

5. **Chemotherapy** is indicated for rapidly progressive disease, severe lymphedema, pulmonary involvement, and symptomatic visceral disease. Low doses of doxorubicin (10 mg/m^2 IV), bleomycin (10 mg/m^2 IV), and vincristine (2 mg IV), given every 2 weeks, may result in response rates of 25% to 50%. Liposomal preparations of anthracyclines (Doxil and DaunoXome) have shown greater efficacy with lesser degrees of toxicity and have been licensed for use in KS. Taxol (100 mg/m^2 or 135 mg/m^2 given IV every 2 to 3 weeks) is also highly effective and has been licensed for this purpose.

V. CERVICAL CANCER

A. Incidence. Cervical cancer is now an AIDS-defining diagnosis. Women constitute the fastest rising group of new AIDS cases in the United States. The primary risk factor for HIV infection in these patients is heterosexual transmission, usually from a partner who was not known to be infected by the woman in question.

The precise incidence of cervical carcinoma, while increased statistically when compared with that in HIV-negative women, is still very low in the United States and other countries in which routine Papanicolaou (Pap) screening is common. The incidence of the precursor lesions (cervical intraepithelial neoplasia [CIN] on biopsy or squamous intraepithelial lesions [SIL] on Pap smear) is unknown, although various large cohort studies of HIV-infected women have indicated a high prevalence. HAART has been associated with spontaneous clearing of these precursor lesions. Although the incidence of invasive cervical carcinoma has not changed in the era of HAART, it remains quite low in Pap smear–screened populations.

B. Biological factors

    1. Role of human papillomavirus (HPV). Cervical cancer is associated with prior infection by HPV, usually involving serotypes 16, 18, 31, 33, or 35. Immunosuppression may allow more rapid development of *in situ* or invasive disease in the setting of such HPV infection. Preliminary data indicate that infection by more than one serotype may increase the risk for cervical cancer or CIN. Furthermore, lower CD4+ lymphocyte counts have been associated with greater prevalence of HPV infection among HIV-infected women.

    2. Role of HPV vaccine. Recently, an HPV vaccine against serotypes 6, 11, 16, and 18 has been licensed in the United States and is suggested for use in girls from the age of 9 to 26 years for prevention of primary HPV infection. The vaccine has been remarkably effective in inducing immunity against HPV and in decreasing the risk of incident CIN/SIL. The vaccine is composed of viral-like particles (VLPs) and is thus not a "live" viral vaccine in any sense. Although it should theoretically be safe in HIV-infected women, neither safety nor efficacy of the vaccine in the setting of HIV infection has yet been demonstrated. Such studies are currently under way. Nonetheless, because most HIV-infected women have already been infected by multiple types of HPV, the actual effectiveness of this approach in preventing CIN or invasive cervical cancer remains questionable.

C. Clinical features of cervical cancer in the HIV-infected woman are not different from those in uninfected women. Preliminary evidence suggests that HIV-infected women are more likely to have advanced-stage disease, high-grade pathological type, and relapse after definitive therapy.

D. Management. Because of the aggressive nature of cervical carcinoma in HIV-infected women, it becomes extremely important to diagnose such patients early, at the time of precancerous abnormalities on the Pap smear. It is recommended that HIV-infected women undergo routine Pap testing every 12 months with evaluation of HPV status as well. Colposcopy and biopsy should be performed in the presence of positive HPV status or any abnormal Pap smear results, including atypia. After definitive therapy for CIN II or III, about half of patients relapse within 1 to 2 years. Topical 5-fluorouracil may reduce the short-term recurrence rate of CIN II or III. Invasive cervical cancer is treated in the usual manner.

VI. ANAL CARCINOMA. Although not diagnostic of AIDS, the incidence of HPV-related anal carcinoma is known to be increased in homosexual men, even independent of HIV infection. Large cohort studies are being conducted to determine the natural history of anal cancer in HIV-infected patients and its response to therapy. Anal HPV infection is quite common in HIV-infected women and also in HIV-infected men without history of homosexual activity.

Suggested Reading

Biggar RJ, Jaffe ES, Goedert JJ, et al. Hodgkin lymphoma and immunodeficiency in persons with HIV/AIDS. *Blood* 2006;108:3786.

Harris TG, Burk RD, Palefsky JM, et al. Incidence of cervical squamous intraepithelial lesions associated with HIV serostatus, CD4 cell counts and human papillomavirus test results. *JAMA* 2005;293:1471.

Kaplan LD, Lee JY, Ambinder RF, et al. Rituximab does not improve clinical outcome in a randomized phase 3 trial of CHOP with or without rituximab in patients with HIV-associated non-Hodgkin lymphoma: AIDS Malignancies Consortium Trial 010. *Blood* 2005;106:1538.

Levine AM. Evaluation and management of the HIV-infected woman: review. *Ann Intern Med* 2002;136:228.

Levine AM, Tulpule A. Clinical aspects and management of AIDS related Kaposi's sarcoma. *Eur J Cancer* 2001;37:88.

Lim ST, Karim R, Nathwani BN, et al. AIDS related Burkitt's lymphoma versus diffuse large cell lymphoma in the pre-HAART and HAART eras: significant differences in survival with standard chemotherapy. *J Clin Oncol* 2005;23:4430.

Lim ST, Levine AM. AIDS related Hodgkin's disease. *Abstr Hematol Oncol* 2005;8:24.

Lim ST, Levine AM. Recent advances in AIDS related lymphoma. *CA Cancer J Clin* 2005;55:229.

Little RF, et al. Highly effective treatment of acquired immunodeficiency syndrome–related lymphoma with dose adjusted EPOCH: impact of antiretroviral therapy suppression and tumor biology. *Blood* 2003;101:4653.

Little RF, Yarchoan R. Treatment of gammaherpesvirus-related neoplastic disorders in the immunosuppressed host. *Semin Hematol* 2003;40:163.

Massad LS, Fazzari MJ, Anastos K, et al. Outcomes after treatment of cervical intraepithelial neoplasia among women with HIV. *Journal of Lower Genital Tract Disease* 2007;11:90.

Yarchoan R. Key role for a viral lytic gene in Kaposi's sarcoma. *N Engl J Med* 2006;355:1383.

HEMATOPOIETIC STEM CELL TRANSPLANTATION

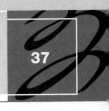

37

Mary C. Territo

I. PRINCIPLES

A. Hematopoietic stem cell transplantation (HSCT) is an important treatment option for an increasing number of malignant and nonmalignant disorders that are listed in Table 37.1. HSCT has been used in malignant diseases for the following situations:

  1. To restore marrow function for the patient following the administration of very high doses (myeloablative/immunoablative) of chemotherapy with or without radiotherapy (CT/RT) to kill off tumor cells. The following requirements apply when using this approach to treat tumors:

    a. The tumor must have a steep dose-response curve so that escalating doses of drug results in increased tumor killing.

    b. The drugs that give that steep dose-response curve must have the bone marrow as their main dose-limiting toxicity (since HSCT will not protect any of the other organ toxicity).

    c. The types of tumors that are usually treated in this manner include primarily the hematologic malignancies (leukemias, lymphomas, myelomas), but also germ cell tumors, neuroblastoma, and selected other solid tumors.

  2. To replace deficient or defective hematopoietic cells for diseases such as aplastic anemia, and congenital hematologic, immunologic, and metabolic disorders.

  3. To effectively administer adoptive immunotherapy against tumor cells (the graft vs. tumor effect of allogeneic transplants).

B. The choice of the type of transplant that is performed and the type of conditioning therapy used will depend on the disease being treated, the clinical status of the patient, and the donor cells that are available.

C. Outcomes of transplantation will depend on multiple factors including age of the patient, stage of disease, disease risk factors, prior therapies, comorbid conditions, and the type of conditioning therapy used. For allogeneic transplants, donor relationship, HLA matching and donor cell dose (for cord blood) are also important variables impacting on outcome.

II. STEM CELL SOURCES

Hematopoietic stem cells (HSCs) normally reside in the bone marrow with only rare HSCs circulating in the blood. HSCs can be found in increased numbers in the blood during recovery from chemotherapy-induced cytopenias, and can also be mobilized from the bone marrow into the blood with granulocyte colony-stimulating factor (GCSF). Umbilical cord blood is a very rich source of HSCs that can also be used for transplantation.

A. Bone marrow (BM) is collected in the operating room under general or spinal anesthesia. Multiple aspirations (of 5 to 10 mL each) are obtained to a desired target dose of about 3×10^8 nucleated cells per kilogram of recipient weight (about 1 to 1.5 liters for an adult). The collection is then filtered to remove any bone particles, can be processed to deplete red blood cells (RBCs) or plasma if needed for ABO-incompatible transplants, and can then be cryopreserved for later use, or directly infused intravenously into the patient. This was the original product used for HSCT.

B. Peripheral blood stem cells (PBSCs). Donors are first given GCSF to mobilize the HSC into the blood (for autologous donors chemotherapy is frequently given prior

TABLE 37.1 Uses for Hematopoietic Stem Cell Transplantation	
Allogeneic transplants	**Autologous transplants**
Acute leukemias	Acute leukemias
Chronic leukemias	Hodgkin lymphoma
Myelodysplasia	Non-Hodgkin lymphomas
Aplastic anemia	Myelomas
Hodgkin lymphomas	Neuroblastoma
Non-Hodgkin lymphomas	Breast carcinoma
Myelomas	Testicular/germ cell neoplasms
Congenital metabolic disorders	Selected other malignancies
Congenital immunologic disorders	
Hemoglobinopathies/thalassemias	

to the GCSF). PBSCs are then obtained in the nucleated cell fraction of the blood by apheresis. Multiple collections may be required to reach the target dose (1 to 5×10^6 CD34-positive cells per kilogram of patient weight). The cells can then be cryopreserved for later use, or directly infused intravenously into the patient. This product engrafts a little faster than BM, has a similar incidence of acute graft-versus-host disease (GVHD) as BM, but has a greater occurrence of chronic GVHD.

C. Umbilical cord blood (UCB) cells are obtained from the umbilical vein in the placenta after the umbilical cord has been severed from the newborn. This blood is rich in HSC and the lymphocytes are naive. This product has less GVHD than either BM or PBSC but is slower to engraft.

D. Manipulation. Stem cell sources can be manipulated in a variety of ways depending on the intent of the transplant. Some of the manipulations used include depletion of T cells, enrichment of CD34-positive cells, and stem cell expansion.

III. TYPES OF HSCT

A. Autologous transplant. The patient's own cells are used as the HSC source. This is primarily used to permit the administration of very high doses (myeloablative) of CT/RT to kill tumor cells. The advantage of this approach is that you do not have to search for an allogeneic donor and there is no GVHD. The disadvantage is that you may have residual tumor cells in the graft and you achieve no graft-versus-tumor effect from the graft.

B. Allogeneic transplant. The HSCs are obtained from someone other than the patient. The donor of the HSCs must be matched by HLA tissue typing with the patient. Genes for the HLA antigen system are found on chromosome 6. HLA typing is performed for the class I antigens (A, B, and C) and the class II antigens (DR and DQ) to identify properly matched donors. The advantage of this approach is that the product has normal stem cells, which are free of tumor or abnormal cells In addition to allowing recovery after myeloablative CT/RT, allogeneic HSCs can be used to replace deficient or defective stem cells. It also is a way of providing adoptive immunotherapy against tumor cells (graft-vs.-tumor effect). The disadvantages are that you need to find an appropriately matched donor and that the patient is at risk for GVHD.

  1. Related donors. The best donor is usually a sibling with the same two HLA haplotypes as the recipient (matched on both chromosomes for HLA A, B, C, DR, and DQ; a "10 of 10 HLA match"). Only about 30% of patients will have an identifiable sibling donor. Identical twin (syngeneic) donors are the best donors immunologically, but have a higher risk of relapse (less graft-vs.-tumor effect) after transplant. Rarely, HLA identical family members other than siblings can be identified.

  2. Unrelated donors. There are large registries of individuals around the world who have volunteered to donate HSCs for unrelated patients in need of a transplant.

With sensitive DNA-based typing, HLA-matched unrelated donors can be found for many patients. The chances of finding an appropriate unrelated donor for an individual patient depends on the specific HLA typing of the patient and varies with different ethnic groups. Transplants using unrelated donor HSCs have some increased risk of GVHD but are an appropriate treatment option if no matched related donors are available. The use of unrelated UCB requires less stringent HLA compatibility but may be limited by cell dose.

IV. CONDITIONING THERAPY

Patients are given high doses of CT/RT prior to the transplant. For autologous transplants, the therapy is aimed at getting the greatest tumor killing while ignoring the myeloablative toxicity of the agents, but is limited by toxicity to other organs. Immune ablation (to allow for engraftment of the foreign HSCs) is necessary for allogeneic transplants, in addition to tumor killing. Many different "conditioning protocols" have been used with similar outcomes depending on the clinical situation of the patient. Examples of some standard conditioning regimens follow.

A. Total body irradiation and cyclophosphamide (Cy)

1. Total body irradiation: Patients receive 12 Gy given in 8 fractions (1.5 Gy each) on Days minus 7 to minus 4.
2. Cy, 60 mg/kg/day in normal saline solution, is given IV over 1 hour for 2 days (on Days minus 3 and minus 2). Patients also receive mesna, 60 mg/kg/day by constant IV infusion beginning with the start of Cy and continuing until 24 hours following completion of Cy.
3. Rest on Day minus 1.
4. HSCT on Day 0

B. High-dose busulfan and Cy

1. Busulfan (Busulfex) at a dose of 0.8 mg/kg of ideal body weight or actual body weight (whichever is lower) is administered IV over 2 hours every 6 hours for 4 days for a total of 16 doses on Days minus 7 to minus 4. Phenytoin (300 mg/day and adjusted for therapeutic blood levels) should be given prophylactically to prevent seizures beginning on the day prior to starting the busulfan and continued until 2 days after busulfan is completed.
2. Cy (to start after busulfan finishes) at a dose of 60 mg/kg/day is given in normal saline solution IV over 1 hour daily for 2 days (on Days minus 3 and minus 2). Patients receive mesna, 60 mg/kg/day by constant IV infusion, beginning with the start of Cy and continuing until 24 hours following completion of Cy.
3. Rest on Day minus 1.
4. HSCT on Day 0

C. High-dose BEAM (BCNU/Etoposide/Cytarabine/Melphalan)

1. BCNU (carmustine), 300 mg/m^2 in 500 mL normal saline, is given IV over 2 hours on Day minus 7.
2. Etoposide, 100 mg/m^2 is given IV over 2 hours every 12 hours for 8 doses on Days minus 6, minus 5, minus 4, and minus 3.
3. Cytarabine, 200 mg/m^2, is given IV over 1 hour every 12 hours for 8 doses on Days minus 6, minus 5, minus 4, and minus 3.
4. Melphalan, 140 mg/m^2, is given IV over 1 hour on Day minus 2.
5. Rest on Day minus 1.
6. HSCT on Day 0.

D. On Day 0, donor BM, PBSC, or UCB is administered IV without a filter. Patients should be premedicated with acetaminophen (650 mg PO), diphenhydramine (Benadryl, 50 mg PO or IV), and hydrocortisone (50 mg IV) 30 minutes prior to HSC infusion. Benadryl (50 mg), epinephrine (1:10,000; 10 mL), and hydrocortisone (100 mg) should be at bedside for standby IV use. Oxygen with a nasal canula setup should also be on standby in the room during the stem cell infusion.

V. SUPPORTIVE CARE

A. All blood products (except the HSC) should be irradiated with 1.5 Gy (to prevent transfusional GVHD) as soon as the conditioning regimen is initiated.

1. **RBC transfusions:** Packed RBCs should be given to maintain the hematocrit at 27% (or higher, if clinically indicated).
2. **Platelet transfusions:** Platelets should be maintained at 10,000/μL or higher depending on clinical status and evidence of bleeding.
3. **For allogeneic transplants when there is an ABO mismatch** (of any type) between patient and donor, the patient should be transfused with type O blood for all RBC transfusions starting at the time of admission.

B. **Specific supportive care measures**
1. **Hydration.** Patients should receive adequate hydration throughout the preparative regimen, such as 5% dextrose in 0.5 normal saline with 20 mEq normal saline containing potassium chloride per liter at 100 mL/m²/hour.
2. **Antiemetics.** Patients will require intensive antiemetic therapy prior to and during the conditioning CT/RT. They should receive a 5-HT3 (serotonin) antagonist plus dexamethasone, prochlorperazine, and other agents as necessary.
3. **Allopurinol** (300 mg/day for adults) should be started on admission for transplant for all patients with bulky tumors. The allopurinol should be stopped on Day minus 1 or soon after the transplant depending on the original tumor burden and the patient's response.
4. **Menstruating females** should be started on nonovulatory agents prior to initiation of the conditioning regimen (norethindrone [Aygestin], 5 to 10 mg PO daily) and remain on it until the platelet count exceeds 50,000/μL.
5. **Vitamin K1** (AquaMEPHYTON), 10 mg SQ, is given weekly.
6. **Growth factors:** Depending on the clinical status and the underlying malignancy, GCSF or granulocyte-macrophage colony-stimulating factor can be given starting Day plus 2 following transplantation.

C. **Protective isolation and prophylaxis**
1. **Protective isolation** should begin when the absolute neutrophil count is ≤500/μL.
   a. Hospital rooms should be equipped with air-filtration units. Individuals entering the patient's room must perform good hand washing or gloving prior to entering the patient area. While in isolation, patients will wash daily with a microbicidal cleaning solution.
   b. A low-bacterial diet should be ordered.
   c. Antibacterial, antifungal, and antiviral prophylaxis can be initiated at the beginning of the conditioning regimen.
2. **Pneumocystis prophylaxis.** All allogeneic transplant patients and patients receiving autologous transplants who have had extensive corticosteroid exposure should receive *Pneumocystis* prophylaxis. Start trimethoprim-sulfamethoxazole (Bactrim DS, one tablet PO every 8 hours) at the onset of the conditioning therapy and stop at Day minus 1 before transplantation. Prophylaxis should be restarted after sustained neutrophil engraftment (Bactrim DS, one tablet PO t.i.d. twice a week along with folinic acid 5 mg twice a week) and continued until Day 100 after transplant, or longer if the patient is receiving immunosuppression (i.e., for GVHD prophylaxis). Dapsone, 50 to 100 mg PO daily; atovaquone (Mepron), 1,500 mg (10 mL) suspension once daily; or pentamidine (aerosolized 300 mg, or 4 mg/kg IV) monthly can be used as an alternative for patients with an allergy to sulfa.
3. **Cytomegalovirus (CMV) prophylaxis/prevention.** Patients who are CMV seronegative prior to transplant should receive only blood products that are CMV seronegative or leukoreduced. CMV seropositive patients undergoing an allogeneic transplant should receive ganciclovir (6 mg/kg IV piggyback [IVPB]/day) starting at the onset of conditioning therapy and stopping at Day minus 1 prior to the transplant. After allogeneic transplantation, the ganciclovir (6 mg/kg IVPB/day, 5 days/week) can be restarted after sustained neutrophil engraftment and continued to Day 100 for prophylaxis. Alternatively, after engraftment, patients can be monitored for viremia weekly with evaluation of blood CMV-DNA for antigenemia to determine when treatment is needed.

D. Prevention and suppression of GVHD. Patients undergoing an allogeneic HSC transplant require immunosuppression treatment to prevent or suppress GVHD.

1. **Calcineurin inhibitors.** *Cyclosporine or tacrolimus* should be given to all allogeneic transplant recipients starting on Day minus 2. Cyclosporine is initially given at a dose of 3. 0 mg/kg IV infusion over 12 hours, followed by 3 mg/kg/day continuous infusion (or 1.5 mg/kg every 12 hours). Doses are adjusted to maintain therapeutic serum cyclosporine levels (between 150 and 350 by Syva's EMIT [enzyme multiplied immunoassay technique]). Tacrolimus is given at a dose of 0.03 mg/kg/day continuous IV infusion (or 0.12 mg/kg/day PO in two divided doses). Doses are adjusted to maintain therapeutic whole-blood tacrolimus levels (between 5 and 20 by microparticle enzyme immunoassay). Doses are adjusted for renal failure.

2. **Other agents** can also be used depending on the GVHD risk of the transplant. These include corticosteroids (i.e., methylprednisolone 1 mg/kg/day IV), antithymocyte globulin (ATG-equine [20 to 30 mg/kg/day] or rabbit-Thymoglobulin [3 mg/kg/day] for 3 to 5 days), mycophenolate (1 g b.i.d.), rapamycin (2 mg/day), or methotrexate (15 mg/m^2 IV Day plus 1, and 10 mg/m^2 on Days plus 3 and plus 6).

3. **T-cell depletion.** GVHD is a T-cell–mediated process. Extensive depletion of T cells from the HSC graft can markedly reduce the incidence and severity of GVHD. Extensive T-cell depletion, however, is accompanied by an increased risk of graft failure, posttransplant lymphoproliferative disease, and an increased risk of tumor relapse so that disease-free survival is not improved. Programs using partial T-depletion or adding back of T-cell subpopulations at various times posttransplant are used in some centers.

VI. COMPLICATIONS OF HSCT

A. GVHD is a syndrome resulting from the reaction of immunocompetent donor cells against the tissues of an immunocompromised recipient. The immunologic reaction is traditionally divided in an "afferent phase" (antigen presentation) and an "efferent phase," and is favored by the release of proinflammatory cytokines during immune activation and tissue damage associated with the conditioning therapy. Recipient antigen presentation results in activation and proliferation of donor T-lymphocytes. Thus, host-specific cytotoxic lymphocytes are generated that mediate tissue damage. During this process, cytokines are secreted and enhance tissue damage by recruiting nonspecific cytotoxic mechanisms (e.g., by direct cytokine damage, natural killer cells, macrophages). Manipulations that include T-cell depletion of the graft, anti–T-lymphocyte agents, and antibodies to certain cytokines have been used to reduce GVHD.

GVHD can be subclassified as acute GVHD (AGVHD), which occurs 2 to 8 weeks following allogeneic HSCT, and chronic GVHD (CGVHD), which usually occurs beyond the eighth week. The distinction is not always clear by timing because AGVHD often evolves into CGVHD, and findings characteristic of CGVHD can sometimes occur early. Manifestations of GVHD are shown in Table 37.2.

1. **Incidence.** The incidence of GVHD is influenced by a number of factors including the degree of histoincompatibility, patient age, intensity of conditioning regimen, type of GVHD prophylaxis, and stem cell source.

   a. The probability of grade II-IV AGVHD is <30% in HLA-matched siblings but is 60% to 90% with mismatched unrelated transplants. The incidence of grade III-IV AGVHD is about 35% for 9 of 10 mismatched adult donor transplants, but only about 10% for mismatched UCB donor transplants.

   b. CGVHD occurs in 25% to 60% of patients surviving >4 months after allogeneic transplant. About two-thirds of the patients who develop CGVHD had preceding AGVHD.

2. **Diagnosis**

   a. **AGVHD** is manifested primarily by the involvement of the skin, liver, and gastrointestinal (GI) tract. Table 37.3 shows the grading system for AGVHD depending on the severity of organ involvement.

TABLE 37.2 Clinical Manifestations of Graft-Versus-Host Disease (GVHD)

Organ	Acute GVHD	Chronic GVHD
Skin, mucous membranes	Maculopapular rash; bullous lesions; mucositis, conjunctivitis	Scleroderma, lichenoid lesions, dyspigmentation, mucositis, conjunctivitis
Liver	Elevation of serum bilirubin and/or alkaline phosphatase; liver failure	Cholestatic hepatitis
Gut	Diarrhea, abdominal pain, ileus; anorexia, dyspepsia, nausea, vomiting	Malabsorption, hypomotility, dysphagia
Immunodeficiency	Hypogammaglobulinemia, anergy, infections	Infections
Lung	—	Bronchiolitis obliterans
Autoimmune syndromes	—	Arthritis, sicca syndrome, polymyositis, immune cytopenias

 TABLE 37.3 Staging and Grading of Acute Graft-Versus-Host Disease (GVHD)

Organ	Extent of involvement	Stage
Skin	Maculopapular rash <25%	1
	Maculopapular rash 25%–50%	2
	Maculopapular rash >50%	3
	Rash >50% with desquamation, with or without bullae	4
Liver	Bilirubin 2–3 mg/dL	1
	Bilirubin 3.1–6 mg/dL	2
	Bilirubin 6.1–15 mg/dL	3
	Bilirubin >15 mg/dL	4
Gastrointestinal	Diarrhea >500 mL/day (>500 mL/m^2 for pediatrics)	1
	Diarrhea >1,000 mL/day (500–1,000 mL/m^2 for pediatrics)	2
	Diarrhea >1,500 mL/day (1,000–1,500 mL/m^2 for pediatrics)	3
	Diarrhea >1,500 mL/day and pain/ileus/blood (>1,500 mL/m^2, blood or ileus for pediatrics)	4

Overall GRADING of acute GVHD

Grade I	Rash involving <50% of body surface (skin stage 1–2); bilirubin levels <2 mg/dL; diarrhea <500 mL/day
Grade II	Rash up to entire body surface (skin stage 1–3); bilirubin <3 mg/dL (liver stage 1); diarrhea <1,000 mL/day (intestine stage 1)
Grade III	Skin stage 1–3; bilirubin <15 mg/dL (liver stage 2–3); diarrhea >1,500 mL/day (intestine stage 2–3)
Grade IV	Any organ with stage IV involvement

Adapted from Glicksberg H, Stoub R, Fefer A, et al. Clinical manifestations of graft-versus-host disease in human recipients of marrow from HLA-matched sibling donors. *Transplantation* 1974;18:295.

(1) Usually the onset of AGVHD is marked by a maculopapular rash on the face, palms, and soles that can subsequently spread and involve the entire body. Bullae or desquamation may follow.

(2) Initially, bilirubin levels are elevated with a subsequent rise in alkaline phosphatase; transaminase elevations may occur later.

(3) The presence of secretory watery diarrhea, which can be quite severe, is characteristic of the GI involvement; paralytic ileus can occur. Persistent nausea and vomiting can be seen with upper GI involvement. Radiographically, bowel wall edema, sometimes with a "thumb-printing" appearance, can be demonstrated.

(4) The clinical diagnosis of AGVHD is occasionally confounded by the presence of chemotherapy-related toxicity, infection, allergic reactions, or veno-occlusive disease, which can mimic some of the findings of AGVHD. Biopsy of the involved organ affected by AGVHD typically shows epithelial cell destruction and apoptosis, but does not show significant lymphocytic infiltration (suggesting a major role for cytokine destruction in the process).

b. CGVHD is characterized by immune dysregulation and the presence of autoreactive lymphocytes that stimulate a chronic inflammatory process leading to fibrosis and collagen vascular disease–like syndromes. CGVHD can involve the skin, eyes, mouth, lungs, GI tract, liver, genitourinary tract, and musculoskeletal, immune, and hematopoietic systems. Disorders mimicking autoimmune processes such as arthritis, immune cytopenias, polymyositis, and sclerodermatous skin, GI, and lung changes can also be seen.

3. Treatment. All patients undergoing allogeneic HSCT receive prophylaxis (see section V.D) to help prevent significant complications from GVHD. Despite this, most patients will develop some degree of GVHD posttransplant. Development of GVHD posttransplant also correlates with a graft-versus-tumor effect so that in some cases GVHD may be beneficial.

a. Patients with grade I AGVHD do not necessarily need to have additional treatment unless they become symptomatic.

b. Patients with grade II-IV AGVHD are usually taking a calcineurin inhibitor when diagnosed. Dose adjustment can be undertaken if serum levels are subtherapeutic. Further T-cell suppression with agents such as corticosteroids, mycophenolate, or rapamycin can be instituted. Treatment with ATG or daclizumab (an anti-interleukin-2R antibody) has also been used. Treatments aimed at specific organ problems, such as topical skin treatments, antiperistalsis (loperamide), antisecretory (octreotide), and bile acid (ursodiol) agents can also be instituted.

c. Treatment of CGVHD includes calcineurin inhibitors, corticosteroids, mycophenolate, rapamycin, and thalidomide (200 to 1600 mg/day). Extracorporeal photochemotherapy (photopheresis with exposure of blood mononuclear cells to the photosensitizing compound PUVA [psoralen plus ultraviolet A] prior to reinfusion) and rituximab (Rituxan; anti-CD20 antibody; 375 mg/m^2 weekly) have also been used with success in some patients.

(1) CGVHD patients are at increased risk of infections and thus need prophylaxis and early treatment of infections, monitoring of immunoglobulin G (IgG) levels and infusion of intravenous IgG (IVIG) for patients with significant hypoglobulinemia.

(2) Supportive care measures include topical steroids, skin lubricants, eye drops, artificial saliva, and nystatin or acyclovir when indicated for oral infections.

(3) Patients with sclerodermatous GVHD and restricted range of motion can benefit from physical therapy.

(4) Patients should use sun screen and avoid sun exposure.

B. Infections. Although many advances in antimicrobial therapies have improved the overall posttransplant survival, infectious complications remain among the most common causes of morbidity and mortality following allogeneic or autologous HSCT. Treatments of specific micro-organisms are discussed in Chapter 35.

1. **Conditioning therapy** results in severe neutropenia for prolonged periods (2 to 4 weeks and more) and patients are at high risk for infections. Gram-positive and gram-negative bacteria, as well as *Candida, Aspergillus*, and other fungal infections are common. Patients should receive treatment with broad-spectrum antibiotics and antimycotic agents either prophylactically after the transplant, or therapeutically at the earliest signs of fever or infection.

2. **Reactivation of herpes viral infections** is common. CMV infection is particularly problematic after allogeneic transplantation. Infections usually occur after patients have engrafted. Treatment doses of ganciclovir (5 mg/kg IV every 12 hours for 3 weeks) should be used. Patients with CMV pneumonia should additionally receive IVIG (500 mg/kg every other day for 10 doses).

   Infections with adenovirus, respiratory syncytial virus, influenza, and other viruses posttransplant can be quite severe and are associated with a high rate of mortality. Treatment with ribavirin, vidarabine, IVIG, or other agents should be instituted early.

3. ***Pneumocystis jirovecil*** infections can be problematic posttransplant and patients should receive prophylactic treatment with trimethoprim-sulfamethoxazole as discussed in section V.C.2. Patients who develop *Pneumocystis* infections should be treated with therapeutic doses of trimethoprim-sulfamethoxazole (15 to 20 mg/kg/day [trimethoprim component] IV administered in three to four divided doses every 6 to 8 hours).

4. **Infections with encapsulated bacteria** (*Pneumococcus, Meningococcus, Haemophilus*) can be seen late in the course (sometimes a year or more) after engraftment has been complete. This complication is related to poor opsonization of the organisms. Patients should receive vaccination for these agents (as well as other primary and booster vaccinations) once their prophylactic GVHD immunosuppressive drugs have been discontinued. Rapid treatment of symptomatic patients is important.

C. **Delayed immune reconstitution.** HSCT results in profound and protracted immune dysfunction. The type of transplantation (autologous vs. allogeneic, UCB vs. adult source), the conditioning regimen, and the presence of GVHD affect both the severity and the duration of immunodeficiency. After transplant, the entire immune system of the patient will be reconstituted with the donor cells. The development of this new immune system, however, can be a slow process. In addition to quantitative impairment of lymphocytes, loss of skin test reactivity, impaired proliferative responses, and reduced cytokine production by lymphocytes and macrophages can be seen and predispose the patient to infections and posttransplant lymphoproliferative syndromes. Antibody response can also be impaired and may result in poor response to vaccinations as well as susceptibility to bacterial pathogens. Replacement doses of IVIG should be given to patients who fail to normalize their IgG level. The presence of GVHD further delays immunologic recovery as do the therapeutic interventions aimed at treating GVHD.

D. **Bleeding.** Patients are at risk of bleeding from thrombocytopenia until platelet engraftment occurs. Platelet engraftment usually lags behind neutrophil engraftment but spontaneous platelet counts of $>20,000/\mu L$ are attained by most patients by Day 21 following autologous transplants, and by Day 28 following allogeneic transplants (but may require >40 days for UCB transplants). Prophylactic platelet transfusions are usually used to keep platelets above $10,000/\mu L$, but higher levels are needed if patients are febrile or having bleeding symptoms.

E. **Nonmarrow organ toxicity.** The use of high doses of CT/RT for conditioning patients prior to transplant ignores the marrow toxicity of the agents used, but we must be mindful of the nonmarrow toxicity of these agents.

1. Infections, sepsis, tumor lysis, and other drug exposures can also add to the insult experienced by the nonmarrow organs after transplantation.

2. Toxicity to the lungs, kidneys, heart, liver, GI tract, endocrine glands, and central nervous system can be seen posttransplant.

3. GVHD can also result in toxicity to target organs following allogeneic transplants.

4. Veno-occlusive disease of the liver (VOD) probably results from injury to the sinusoidal endothelial cells and hepatocytes from the high-dose conditioning therapy. Patients with hepatitis, extensive prior chemotherapy, or certain drug exposures (i.e., gemtuzumab) are at higher risk for development of VOD. VOD is usually seen within the first 1 to 2 months posttransplant and is characterized by hepatomegaly with right upper quadrant pain, unexplained fluid retention, and jaundice. Mild VOD may occur in up to 60% of patients and usually is reversible without treatment. When severe, however, VOD is frequently fatal. Symptomatic treatments should be used but attempts at treatment with various anticoagulants and antioxidants have been unimpressive. Initial studies using defibrotide have been encouraging.

Suggested Reading

Afessa B, Peters SG. Major complications following hematopoietic stem cell transplantation. *Semin Respir Crit Care Med* 2006;27:297.

Chaidos A, Kanfer E, Apperley JF. Risk assessment in haemotopoietic stem cell transplantation: disease and disease stage. *Best Pract Res Clin Haematol* 2007;20:125.

Copelan EA. Hematopoietic stem-cell transplantation. *N Engl J Med* 2006;354:1813.

Komanduri KV, Couriel D, Champlin RE. Graft-versus-host disease after allogeneic stem cell transplantation: evolving concepts and novel therapies including photopheresis. *Biol Blood Marrow Transplant* 2006;12(1 suppl 2):1.

Laughlin MJ, et al. Outcomes after transplantation of cord blood or bone marrow from unrelated donors in adults with leukemia. *N Engl J Med* 2004;351:2265.

Petersdorf EW. Risk assessment in haematopoietic stem cell transplantation: histocompatibility. *Best Pract Res Clin Haematol* 2007;20:155.

Schmitz N, et al. International Bone Marrow Transplant Registry; European Group for Blood and Marrow Transplantation. Long-term outcome of patients given transplants of mobilized blood or bone marrow: a report from the International Bone Marrow Transplant Registry and the European Group for Blood and Marrow Transplantation. *Blood* 2006;108:4288.

Villanueva ML, Vose JM. The role of hematopoietic stem cell transplantation in non-Hodgkin lymphoma. *Clin Adv Hematol Oncol* 2006;4:521.

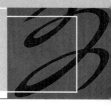

Appendixes

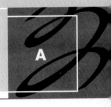

Symbol	Definition	Example
p	**Short arm** of a chromosome (arm above centromere); a prefix number gives the number of the chromosome and a suffix number refers to a particular band on the chromosome	22p5 is the 5th band from the centromere on the short arm of chromosome 22.
q	**Long arm** of a chromosome (arm below centromere); numbering is the same as for **p**	22q5 is the 5th band from the centromere on the long arm of chromosome 22
t	**Translocation** of part of one chromosome to another. The first set of parentheses indicates the chromosomes involved and the second set indicates the bands affected by the breakpoints on the respective chromosomes.	t(3;21)(q26;q22) is the translocation of material between the long arms of chromosomes 3 and 21 with breakpoints at band q26 for chromosome 3 and band q22 for chromosome 21
	Insertion of extra material (e.g., portions of a chromosome) within a chromosome	ins(3;3)(q26;q21q26) is the insertion of band 26 to a position between bands 21 and 26 in the long arms of chromosome 3 (for different chromosomes being involved, the conventions for **t** are followed)
	·sion (or turn in the opposite ·on) of a portion of the ·some	inv(3)(q21q26) is inversion of bands of 21 through 26 on the long arm of chromosome 3
	·hromosome: Addition ·(−) of a whole	+8 or −7 is an extra chromosome 8 or a missing chromosome 7 (see **del**)
	·dditional material ·erial (−) in the the specified	7q⁻ is missing material in the long arm of chromosome 7 (see **del**)
	·f a	del (7q) or del (7)(q22) is deletion of the long arm or of band 22 in the long arm of chromosome 7, respectively (see "+ or −")

(continued)

Symbol	Definition	Example
der	**Derivative chromosome:** an abnormal chromosome resulting from structural rearrangement, generally of a balanced nature, involving two or more chromosomes	der(1;7)(q10;p10) (see **t, ins, inv**)
i	**Isochromosome:** a symmetric chromosome composed of duplicated long or short arm with associated centromere	i(17q) is chromosome 17 with duplicated long arms
idic	**Isocentric:** symmetrical abnormal chromosome composed of the duplication of a total arm and its centromere with part of the adjacent other arm	Idic(X)(q13)
dic	**Dicentric:** chromosome with two centromeres	

TOXICITY OF CHEMOTHERAPY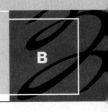

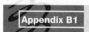

| Appendix B1 | Major Toxicities and Dose Modifications for Chemotherapeutic Agents | | | |

Drug	Cyto-penias	Nausea and vomiting	Hair loss	Other major toxicities [dose modifications]
CYTOTOXIC AGENTS				
Actinomycin D[V]	3	2	2	M, Skin [L*, R*]
Aminoglutethimide	0	1	0	Adrenal, skin, fever [R#]
Anagrelide	1	1	0	C [L*]
Asparaginase	0	2	0	N, allergy [R*]
Azacytidine (Vidaza)	3	2	3	M, N, L [L# N*]
Bexarotene (Targretin)	0	0	0	Oc, skin, metabolic, thyroid
Bleomycin	0	1	2	P, Skin, allergy [R*]
Bortezomib (Velcade)	2	2	0	N*, C [L#, R#]
Busulfan	3	1	1	P [R#]
Carboplatin	2	2	0	[R*]
Capecitabine	1	1	0	D, Skin [R*]
Carmustine (BCNU)[V]	3	3	1	P, R, [R#]
Chlorambucil	2	0	0	
Cisplatin[I]	2	3	2	R, N [N#, R*]
Cladribine	2	1	0	
Cyclophosphamide	3	2	2	Urothelium [L#, R*]
Cytarabine	3	2	1	M, Cho, fever [L#, R#]
Cytarabine, high dose	3	3	1	M, N, Cho, Oc [L*, R#]
Dacarbazine (DTIC)[V]	2	3	1	Flulike symptoms [L*, R*]
Dasatinib (Sprycel)	3	2	0	Skin, edema, bleeding
Daunorubicin[V]	3	2	3	C [L*]
Decitabine (Dacogen)	3	1	0	D, Hypoglycemia [L# R*]
Denileukin diftitox (Ontak)	0	1	0	D, Skin, hypersensitivity, vascular leak syndrome
Docetaxel (Taxotere)	2	1	3	Edema, Skin [L*]
Doxorubicin[V] (Adriamycin)	3	2	3	C [L*]
Doxorubicin, liposomal[I] (Doxil)	2	2	3	C, IRCRS, skin [L*]
Epirubicin	3	2	3	C [L#]
Erlotinib (Tarceva)	0	1	0	D, Skin, Oc, [L#]
Estramustine (Emcyt)	0	2	0	Thrombosis
Etoposide[I] (VePesid)	2	1	2	N [L*, R*]
Fludarabine (Fludara)	2	1	1	Immunosuppression, N [R#]
Fluorouracil[I] (5-FU)	1	1	0	D, M, Oc, C

(continued)

Appendix B1 **Major Toxicities and Dose Modifications for Chemotherapeutic Agents (*Continued*)**

Drug	Cyto-penias	Nausea and vomiting	Hair loss	Other major toxicities [dose modifications]
Gefitinib (Iressa)	0	2	0	D, Skin, Oc, edema [L#]
Gemcitabine (Gemzar)	2	2	1	P [L#, R#]
Hexamethylmelamine	1	3	0	N [L#]
Hydroxyurea	2	1	0	Skin [L#, R*]
Idarubicin^V	3	2	3	C [L*, R#]
Ifosfamide^I	3	1	3	N, Urothelium [R#]
Imatinib (Gleevec)	2	1	0	Edema [L*]
Interferon	1	1	0	Flulike symptoms, depression
Irinotecan	2	1	2	D [L#]
Ixabepilone (Ixempra)	2	1	3	L*, N*
Lapatinib (Tykerb)	2	2	0	D, Skin [L#]
Lenalidomide (Revimid)	2	1	0	D, Thrombosis [R*]
Lomustine (CCNU)	3	2	1	P, R [R#]
Mechlorethamine^V	2	3	1	
Melphalan	2	1	0	[R#]
Mercaptopurine	2	1	0	Cho [L#, R#]
Methotrexate	2	1	0	M, N [L#, R*]
Mithramycin^I	2	1	0	Hypocalcemia
Mitoguazone^V	2	1	0	M, N
Mitomycin^V	3	1	1	P, R, TTP [L*]
Mitotane	0	2	1	Adrenal insufficiency [L#]
Mitoxantrone^V	2	1	1	C, Cho [L*]
Nilotinib (Tasigna)	2	2	0	C*, L*, Sk, Mg
Oxaliplatin^I	1	2	0	N [N*]
Paclitaxel^V (Taxol)	2	1	3	N, Weak vesicant [L*, N#]
Pemetrexed (Alimta)	2	1	0	M, Skin [R*]
Pentostatin	1	1	0	R [R*]
Procarbazine	2	1	0	Drug interactions [L#, R*]
Raltitrexed (Tomudex)	2	1	0	Fatigue [R*]
Sorafenib (Nexavar)	2	1	2	D, Skin, HT, bleeding
Streptozocin$^{V, I}$	1	3	0	L, R, Hypoglycemia [R*]
Sunitinib (Sutent)	2	2	1	D, HT, bleeding
Suramin	2	1	1	N
Temozolomide (Temodar)	2	2	0	[L#, R*]

(continued)

Major Toxicities and Dose Modifications for Chemotherapeutic Agents (*Continued*)

Drug	Cyto-penias	Nausea and vomiting	Hair loss	Other major toxicities [dose modifications]
Temsirolimus (Toricel)	1	0	0	L, R, P
Teniposide[I]	2	1	1	N [L#, R#, N#]
Thalidomide	0	1	0	N, Skin, thrombosis
Thioguanine	2	1	0	Cho [L*]
Thiotepa	2	1	0	[L#, R#]
Topotecan	3	2	2	[R*]
Trimetrexate	2	1	2	M, Skin [L#, R#]
Uracil/Tegafur	1	1	0	D, Skin
Vinblastine[V]	2	1	1	Cramps [L*, N#]
Vincristine[V]	0	1	1	N [L*, N#]
Vindesine[V]	1	1	2	N [L*, N#]
Vinorelbine[V, I]	2	1	1	[L*]
MONOCLONAL ANTIBODIES				
Alemtuzumab (Campath)	2	0	0	IRCRS, Immunosuppression
Bevacizumab (Avastin)	0	0	0	IRCRS, HT, Thrombosis, hemorrhage, proteinuria
Cetuximab (Erbitux)	0	2	0	Severe IRCRS, Skin, D, Mg++
Gemtuzumab (Mylotarg)	2	0	0	IRCRS, L
Panitumumab (Vectibix)	0	2	0	IRCRS, Skin, Oc, Mg++
Rituximab (Rituxan)	1	0	0	IRCRS, C
Trastuzumab (Herceptin)	0	0	0	IRCRS, C

C, cardiac; Cho, cholestasis; D, diarrhea; HT, hypertension; I, irritant; IRCRS, infusion-related cytokine release syndrome; L, liver function tests; M, mucositis; Mg++, hypomagnesemia; N, neurologic; Oc, ocular; P, pulmonary; R, renal; TTP, thrombotic thrombocytopenia-like syndrome; V, vesicant.
[L*, N*, R*] = Reduce dose for liver, neurologic, or renal dysfunction, respectively.
[L#, N#, R#] = Use with caution for liver, neurologic, or renal dysfunction, respectively.
Scale: 0 = none or rare; 1 = mild; 2 = moderate; 3 = marked or severe.

| Appendix B2 | Abridged Common Toxicity Criteria |

Toxicity	Grade 1	Grade 2	Grade 3	Grade 4
Hematologic				
Hemoglobin	10.0–LLN	8.0–10.0	6.5–7.9	<6.5 g/dL
Platelets	75,000–LLN	50,000–74,000	25,000–49,000	<25,000/μL
White blood cells	3,000–LLN	2,000–3,000	1,000–2,000	<1,000/μL
Neutrophils	1,500–LLN	1,000–1,500	500–1,000	<500/μL
Lymphocytes	1,500–2,000	1,000–1,500	500–1,000	<500/μL
INR or PTT	>1.0–1.5 × ULN	1.6–2 × ULN	>2 × ULN	—
Fibrinogen	0.99–0.75 × ULN	0.74–0.50 × ULN	0.49–0.25 × ULN	≤0.24 × ULN
Clinical hemorrhage	Mild, no transfusion	Gross, 1–2 units transfused per episode	Gross, 3–4 units transfused per episode	Massive, >4 units transfused per episode
Thrombotic microangiopathy	Schizocytes without clinical consequences	—	With clinical consequences	Life-threatening or disabling consequences
Constitutional				
Weight gain/loss	5.0%–9.9%	10.0%–19.9%	>20% of baseline	—
Fatigue	Mild fatigue over baseline	Moderate; or causing some difficulty with ADL	Severe fatigue IWADL	Disabling
Allergic reaction	Transient rash or flushing; drug fever ≤100.4°F	Urticaria, rash; drug fever ≥100.4°F, dyspnea	Serum sickness or bronchospasm; requires parenteral medication	Anaphylaxis
Fever without infection	38.0–39.0°C (100.4–102.2°F)	39.1–40.0°C (102.3–104.0°F)	>40.0°C (>104.0°F) for ≤24 h	>40.0°C (>104.0°F) for >24 h

(continued)

Appendix B2 Abridged Common Toxicity Criteria (*Continued*)

Toxicity	Grade 1	Grade 2	Grade 3	Grade 4
Febrile neutropenia	—	—	Present	Life-threatening consequences
Chills/rigors	Mild	Moderate; narcotics indicated	Severe or prolonged; not responsive to narcotics	—
Dermatologic				
Local injection site reaction	Pain; itching; erythema	Pain or swelling with inflammation or phlebitis	Ulceration or necrosis requiring surgery	—
Rash	Asymptomatic macular or papular eruption or erythema	Eruption or erythema with pruritus or other symptoms; desquamation <50% BSA	Severe generalized symptomatic macular, papular, or vesicular eruption; desquamation ≥50% BSA	Exfoliative or ulcerating dermatitis
Alopecia	Thinning or patchy	Complete	—	—
Hand-foot syndrome	Minimal skin changes or dermatitis without pain	More severe skin changes or pain not IWF	Ulceration or pain IWF	—
Alimentary				
Taste alteration (dysgeusia)	Altered taste but no change in diet	Altered taste with change in diet; unpleasant or loss of taste	—	—
Stomatitis	Minimal symptoms; normal diet	Can eat and swallow modified diet	Cannot aliment or hydrate PO; symptoms IWADL	Life-threatening consequences
Nausea	Reduced but reasonable intake	Intake significantly decreased but still can eat	IVF or alimentation ≥24 h	Life-threatening consequences
Vomiting	One episode in 24 h	Two to five episodes in 24 h; IVF <24 h	Six or more episodes in 24 h; IVF ≥24 h	Life-threatening consequences

Diarrhea	Increase of <4 stools/day over baseline	Increase of 4–6 stools/day; IVF <24 h; not IWADL	Increase of ≥7 stools/day, or incontinence; hospitalization; IWADL	Life-threatening consequences
Constipation	Occasional or intermittent	Persistent with regular use of laxatives	Symptoms IWADL; manual evacuation indicated	Life-threatening consequences (e.g., obstruction)
Liver function				
Liver failure (clinical)	—	Jaundice	Asterixis	Hepatic coma
Amylase	ULN–1.5 × ULN	1.6–2.0 × ULN	2.1–5.0 × ULN	>5.0 × ULN
Bilirubin	ULN–1.5 × ULN	1.6–3.0 × ULN	3.1–10 × ULN	>10 × ULN
Transaminase	ULN–2.5 × ULN	2.6–5.0 × ULN	5.1–20.0 × ULN	>20.0 × ULN
Alkaline phosphatase	≤2.5 × ULN	2.6–5.0 × ULN	5.1–20.0 × ULN	>20.0 × ULN
Urinary/Metabolic				
Renal failure	—	—	Chronic dialysis not indicated	Chronic dialysis indicated
Creatinine	ULN–1.5 × ULN	1.6–3.0 × ULN	3.1–6.0 × ULN	>6.0 × ULN
Proteinuria	1+ or 0.15–1.0 g/24 h	2+ to 3+ or 1.1–3.5 g/24 h	4+ or >3.5 g/24 h	Nephrotic syndrome
Hypercalcemia	ULN–11.5	11.6–12.5	12.6–13.5	>13.5 mg/dL
Hypocalcemia	LLN–8.0	7.9–7.0	6.9–6.0	<6.0 mg/dL
Hypomagnesemia	LLN–1.2	1.1–0.9	0.8–0.7	<0.7 mg/dL
Hyperglycemia	ULN–160	161–250	251–500	>500 mg/dL
Hyperkalemia	>ULN–5.5	5.6–6.0	6.1–7.0	>7.0 mmol/L
Hypokalemia	<LLN–3.0	—	2.9–2.5	<2.5 mmol/L

(continued)

| Appendix B2 | Abridged Common Toxicity Criteria *(Continued)* | | | |

Toxicity	Grade 1	Grade 2	Grade 3	Grade 4
Cardiovascular				
Hypertension (increase by >20 mm Hg diastolic or to >150/100 if previously WNL)	No treatment required; asymptomatic transient diastolic increase	Monotherapy may be required; recurrent or persistent diastolic increase	Requires more than one drug or more intensive therapy than previously	Hypertensive crisis
Hypotension	Changes requiring no therapy	Brief (<24 h) fluid replacement or other therapy	Requires sustained (≥24 h) therapy	Shock (e.g., impairment of vital organ function)
Arrhythmias	Asymptomatic; no therapy indicated	Nonurgent medical intervention indicated	Symptomatic and incompletely controlled medically or requires a device	Life-threatening
Left ventricle function	Asymptomatic; LVEF 50%–59%	Asymptomatic; LVEF 40%–49%	Mild CHF responsive to therapy; LVEF 20%–39%	Severe or refractory CHF; LVEF <20%
Cardiac ischemia	Nonspecific T-wave flattening	Asymptomatic; testing suggests ischemia	Unstable angina without evidence of infarction	Acute myocardial infarction
Pericarditis or pericardial effusion	Asymptomatic effusion or pericarditis	Symptomatic pericarditis	With physiological consequences	Life-threatening; emergency intervention required
Pulmonary				
Respiratory distress (ARDS)	—	—	Present, intubation not indicated	Present, intubation indicated
Bronchospasm	Asymptomatic	Symptomatic; not IWF	Symptomatic; IWF	Life-threatening consequences
Diffusing capacity (D_LCO)	90%–75%	74%–50%	49%–25%	<25% of predicted value
Neurologic				
Syncope	—	—	Present	Life-threatening consequences

Seizures	—	Well-controlled seizures; or infrequent focal seizures not IWADL	Seizures with altered consciousness; poorly controlled seizure disorder	Seizures of any type that are prolonged, repetitive, or difficult to control (status epilepticus)
Mood alteration	Mild, not IWF	Moderate, IWF but not IWADL	Severe, IWADL	Suicide ideation; danger to others or self
Confusion	Transient confusion, disorientation, or attention deficit	Confusion, disorientation, or attention deficit IWF but not IWADL	Confusion or delirium IWADL	Harmful to others or self; hospitalization indicated
Somnolence	—	Somnolence IWF but not IWADL	Obtundation or stupor IWADL	Coma
Ataxia	Asymptomatic	Symptomatic, not IWADL	Symptomatic; IWADL; mechanical assistance needed	Disabling
Involuntary movements	Mild, not IWF	Moderate, IWF but not IWADL	Severe, IWADL	Disabling
Motor neuropathy, muscle weakness	Asymptomatic; weakness on exam	Symptomatic, IWF; not IWADL	Weakness IWADL; brace, cane, or walker indicated	Life-threatening, disabling
Sensory neuropathy	Tingling; loss of deep tendon reflexes but not IWF	Sensory loss or paresthesias IWF but not IWADL	Sensory alteration or paresthesias IWADL	Disabling
Vision	—	Blurred vision or diplopia	Symptomatic subtotal loss of vision	Blindness (20/200)
Hearing (without monitoring program)	—	Hearing loss not requiring hearing aid	Requires hearing aid	Profound bilateral hearing loss (>90 dB)

Note: Grade 5, death.
ADL, Average daily living; ARDS, acute respiratory distress syndrome; BSA, body surface area; CHF, congestive heart failure; INR, international normalized ratio (for prothrombin time); IVF, intravenous fluids indicated for; IWADL, interfering with average daily living; IWF, interfering with function; LLN, lower limit of normal; LVEF, left ventricular ejection fraction; PTT, partial thromboplastin time; ULN, upper limit of normal; WNL, within normal limits.
Extracted from the National Cancer Institute. Common Terminology Criteria for Adverse Events, v. 3.0. Published: June 10, 2003. The entire 71-page document defining Adverse Events can be downloaded from www.nci.nih.gov/

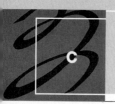

TUMOR IDENTIFIERS

Russell K. Brynes, Nancy Klipfel, and Dennis A. Casciato

Appendix C1 **Microscopic Clues of Tumor Origin**

Potentially helpful findings	Primary site or tumor type
HISTOPATHOLOGY	
Signet ring cells	Gastrointestinal tract, pancreas, ovary, breast (lobular)
Psammoma bodies	Ovary (papillary serous), thyroid, breast, meningioma
Papillary	Thyroid, ovary, breast, pancreas, mesothelioma, renal, lung (sometimes)
Single file tumor cells	Breast (lobular), small cell carcinoma
Nonacinar cell nests	Carcinoid, melanoma, paraganglioma, pancreatic islet cell tumor
Intranuclear inclusions	Papillary thyroid, melanoma, meningioma, bronchoalveolar carcinoma, hepatocellular carcinoma
Rosettes	Neuroblastoma, retinoblastoma, neuroendocrine carcinoma, PNET/Ewing sarcoma, ependymoma
Clear cell neoplasms	See Chapter 20, section **II.C.4.**
Very poorly differentiated small cell neoplasms	See Chapter 20, section **II.C.5.**
HISTOCHEMISTRY	
Mucin stains (e.g., mucicarmine)	Adenocarcinoma (absent in renal cell and hepatocellular carcinoma)
Glycogen stains (PAS-positive, removed by diastase)	Abundant in renal cell carcinoma; seminoma, Ewing sarcoma
Silver impregnation (e.g., Fontana-Masson, Grimelius, Sevier-Munger)	Polypeptide-forming endocrine cells, melanoma
PAS, periodic acid-Schiff; PNET, primitive neuroectodermal tumor.	

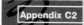 **Appendix C2**   Selected Immunohistochemical Tumor Markers

Detectable antigen	Tumor type
Alpha-fetoprotein (AFP)	Germ cell tumors, hepatocellular carcinoma
Calretinin	Mesothelioma, sex cord/stromal tumors, adrenal cortex, synovial sarcoma
Carcinoembryonic antigen, monoclonal (mCEA)	Gut, pancreas, cervix uteri, lung, ovary, breast, urinary tract
CD34	SFT/HPC, pleomorphic lipoma, GIST, DFSP
CD99	Ewing sarcoma/PNET, SFT/HPC, synovial sarcoma, lymphoma/leukemia, sex cord/stromal tumors
CD117	GIST, mastocytosis, seminoma
Chromogranin	NET
Cytokeratin	Broad range of carcinomas, some sarcomas
Desmin	Sarcomas (smooth or skeletal muscle, endometrial stromal sarcoma)
Epithelial membrane antigen (EMA)	Broad range of carcinomas, meningioma, some sarcomas
Factor VIII; CD31, CD34, FL1	Sarcomas (vascular)
Glial fibrillary acid protein (GFAP)	Gliomas (astrocytoma, ependymoma)
Gross cystic disease fluid protein (GCDFP-15)	Breast, ovary, salivary gland
Hormones, specific	Endocrine glands, gut, or pancreatic tumors
HMB-45	Melanoma, PEComas (e.g., angiomyolipoma), clear cell sarcoma, adrenal cortex
Human chorionic gonadotropin (hCG)	Trophoblastic and germ cell tumors, carcinomas
Immunoglobulin molecules	Lymphomas/leukemias
Inhibin	Sex cord/stromal tumors, adrenal cortex, hemangioblastoma
Keratin (various types)	Carcinomas, some sarcomas
Leucocyte common antigen (LCA, CD45)	Lymphomas/leukemias, histiocytic tumors
Lymphoid cell epitopes and activation markers	Lymphomas/leukemias
MART-1 / Melan A	Melanoma, steroid (adrenal and gonadal) tumors
Myo D1	Muscle: rhabdomyosarcoma, PSBRCT
Muscle-specific actin (MSA)	Sarcomas (leiomyosarcoma, rhabdomyosarcoma)
Neurofilaments	NET; Lung (small cell carcinoma)
Neuron-specific enolase (NSE)	NET; Lung (small cell carcinoma); breast (some)
Placental alkaline phosphatase (PLAP)	Seminoma/dysgerminoma, embryonal carcinoma
Prostate-specific antigen (PSA)	Prostate

(continued)

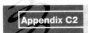

Appendix C2   **Selected Immunohistochemical Tumor Markers (*Continued*)**

Detectable antigen	Tumor type
S100 protein	Melanoma; sarcomas (neural, lipomatous, chondroid); astrocytoma, GIST, salivary gland, some adenocarcinomas, histiocytic (dendritic cell and macrophage) tumors
Smooth muscle actin (SMA)	GIST, leiomyosarcoma, PEComas,
Synaptophysin	NET
Thyroglobulin	Thyroid (except medullary)
TTF-1 (Thyroid transcription factor-1)	Thyroid (all types), lung
Vimentin	Sarcomas; renal cell, endometrial, lung and other carcinomas; lymphomas/leukemias; melanoma

DFSP, dermatofibrosarcoma protuberans; GIST, gastrointestinal stromal tumor; NET, neuroendocrine tumors (neuroblastic, Merkel cell, and carcinoid tumors; paragangliomas; pheochromocytoma; small cell carcinoma); PEComas, perivascular epithelioid cell tumors; PNET, primitive neuroectodermal tumor; PSBRCT, pediatric small blue round cell tumors; SFT/HPC, solitary fibrous tumor/hemangiopericytoma.

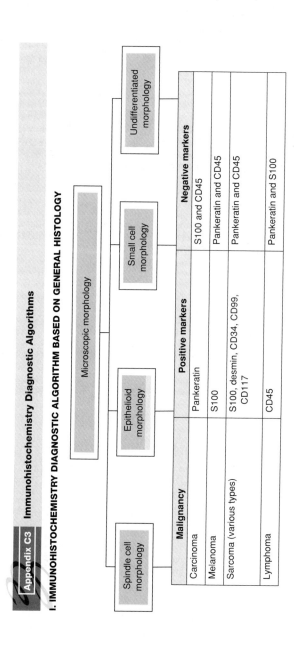

Appendix C3 Immunohistochemistry Diagnostic Algorithms

I. IMMUNOHISTOCHEMISTRY DIAGNOSTIC ALGORITHM BASED ON GENERAL HISTOLOGY

Microscopic morphology

- Epithelioid morphology
- Small cell morphology
- Undifferentiated morphology
- Spindle cell morphology

Malignancy	Positive markers	Negative markers
Carcinoma	Pankeratin	S100 and CD45
Melanoma	S100	Pankeratin and CD45
Sarcoma (various types)	S100, desmin, CD34, CD99, CD117	Pankeratin and CD45
Lymphoma	CD45	Pankeratin and S100

II. IMMUNOHISTOCHEMISTRY DIAGNOSTIC ALGORITHM FOR CARCINOMA OF UNKNOWN ORIGIN

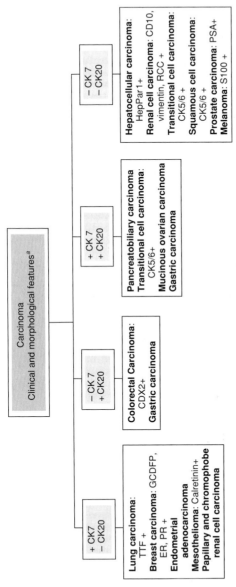

Carcinoma
Clinical and morphological features[a]

+ CK7
– CK20

Lung carcinoma:
TTF +
Breast carcinoma: GCDFP,
ER, PR +
Endometrial
adenocarcinoma
Mesothelioma: Calretinin+
Papillary and chromophobe
renal cell carcinoma

– CK7
+ CK20

Colorectal Carcinoma:
CDX2+
Gastric carcinoma

+ CK7
+ CK20

Pancreatobiliary carcinoma
Transitional cell carcinoma:
CK5/6+
Mucinous ovarian carcinoma
Gastric carcinoma

– CK7
– CK20

Hepatocellular carcinoma:
HepPar1+
Renal cell carcinoma: CD10,
vimentin, RCC +
Transitional cell carcinoma:
CK5/6 +
Squamous cell carcinoma:
CK5/6 +
Prostate carcinoma: PSA+
Melanoma: S100 +

+, positive; –, negative. CD, clusters of differentiation; CK, cytokeratin; ER, estrogen receptor; HepPar-1, hepatocyte paraffin-1; GCDFP, gross cystic disease fluid protein-15; PR, progesterone receptor; PSA, prostate-specific antigen; RCC, renal cell carcinoma; TTF, thyroid transcription factor; See Appendix C4.IX for expanded evaluations of carcinoma of unknown origin.

[a]Glandular, squamoid, epithelioid, small cell, large cell, spindle cell

Modified from Voigt JJ, Mathieu MC, Bibeau F. The advent of Immunohistochemistry in carcinoma of unknown primary site: a major progress. In: Fizazi K, ed. *Carcinoma of an Unknown Primary Site.* New York: Taylor & Francis; 2006:25–35.

Appendix C4   Expected Immunophenotypes of Tumors

I. EXPECTED IMMUNOPHENOTYPES FOR SPECIFIC MALIGNANT CELL TYPES

Cell Type	CK	Vim	CEA	S100	NET	CD45	EMA	Other
Adenocarcinoma	+	0	+	±	0	0	+	+: CD15, B72.3, BerEP4 ±: Mucin
Islet cell, carcinoids	±	±	±	±	+	0	±	+ Hormones
Lymphoma	0	+	0	0	0	+	0	See Appendix C5
Melanoma	0	+	0	+	0	0	0	+ MEL See II.A, III.A, VII, VIII
Mesothelioma	+	+	0	0	0	0	+	0: CD15, B72.3, BerEP4 +: Calretinin, CK5/6
Neuroendocrine tumors	±	±	±	±	+	0	+	Carcinomas: Punctate keratin
Sarcoma	0	+	0	±	0	0	0	See III
Small cell carcinoma	+	0	±	0	+	0	+	
Squamous cell carcinoma	+	0	±	0	0	0	0	+: CK5/6
Transitional cell carcinoma	+	0	±	0	0	0	+	

II. SMALL BLUE CELL TUMUORS

A. Small blue cell tumors in adults

Tumor	CK	EMA	CD99	S100	NET	Inh	Des	CD45
Carcinoma	+	+	0	0	0	0	0	0
Carcinoma, small cell	±	±	±	0	±	0	0	0
Desmoplastic small round cell tumor	+	+	±	0	±	0	±	0
Granulosa cell tumor[a]	±	0	±	±	0	+	0	0
Lymphoma	0	±	0	0	0	0	0	+
Melanoma[b]	0	0	0	+	0	0	0	0

[a]Calretinin, Vim, Melan-A/Mart-1 +.
[b]Vim +, MEL +.

B. Small blue cell tumors in children

Tumor	CK	EMA	CD99	S100	NET	Vim	Musc
Neuroblastoma	0	0	0	±	+	+	0
PNET/Ewing sarcoma	0	0	+	±	±	+	0
Rhabdomyosarcoma	0	0	0	0	0	+	+
Synovial cell sarcoma	+	+	+	±	0	+	0

See footnote to all parts of Appendix C4 at end of C4.IX.

Appendix C4 | **Expected Immunophenotypes of Tumors (*Continued*)**

III. SARCOMAS
A. Soft-tissue tumors

Tumor	CK	Vim	Des	SMA	MyoD1	CD34	S100	Other
Alveolar soft parts	0	+	±	+	±	0	0	TFE3 +
Angiosarcoma	0	+	0	±	0	+	0	CD31 +, vWF +, FL1 +
Epithelioid	+	±	0	±	0	+	0	mCEA ±
Fibrosarcoma	0	+	0	± 0	± 0	0	0	
Gastrointestinal stromal tumor (GIST)	±	+	±	±	0	+	0	MSA +, CD117+ (c-*kit*)
Granular cell tumor	0	+	0	0	0	0	+	Inh +, CD68 +
Kaposi sarcoma	0	+	0	0	0	+	0	HHV8 +
Leiomyosarcoma	0	+	+	+	0	0	0	
Liposarcoma, myxoid	0	+	0	0	0	0	+	
Malignant peripheral nerve sheath tumor	0	0	0	0	0	0	±	Focal S100 +
Pleomorphic high grade sarcoma[a]	0	+	0	0	0	0	0	
Rhabdomyosarcoma	0	+	+	+	+	0	0	
Synovial	+	+	0	0	0	0	±	CD99 + *BCL2*+
Melanoma	0	+	0	0	0	0	+	MEL +

[a]Pleomorphic high-grade sarcoma was previously designated malignant fibrous histiocytoma.

B. Osseous and chondroid tumors

Tumor	CK	Vim	Des	SMA	MyoD1	CD34 CD31	S100	Other
Chondroblastoma	0	+	0	0	0	0	+	CD57 −
Chondrosarcoma	0	+	0	0	0	0	+	CD57 +
Chordoma	+	+	0	0	0	0	+	CD57 ±
Osteosarcoma	0	+	0	±	0	0	0	CD57 ± EMA ±
PNET/Ewing sarcoma	0	+	0	0	0	0	0	+: NET, CD99, FL1

IV. LIVER, PANCREAS, AND BILIARY TRACT

Carcinoma	CK 7/20	CK CAM5.2	mCEA	pCEA	CA19-9 BerEP4	AFP	HepPar-1	AAT
Cholangiocarcinoma	+/±	0	+	+	+	0	0	0
Hepatocellular	0/0	+	±	+[a]	0	+	+	±
Pancreas adenocarcinoma	+/±	+	+	0	+	0	0	0

[a]Canalicular pattern.

See footnote to all parts of Appendix C4 at end of C4.IX.

Appendix C4 Expected Immunophenotypes of Tumors (*Continued*)

V. NEURAL TUMORS

Tumor	CK	Vim	mCEA	S100	NSE	Syn	GFAP	EMA
Astrocytoma	0	±	+	+	0	0	+	0
Chordoma	+	+	±	+	0	0	0	+
Choroid plexus papilloma	+	0	0	0	0	+	0	0
Craniopharyngioma	+	0	0	0	0	0	±	0
Ependymoma	Rare	0	+	+	0	0	±	±
Ganglioneuroma	0	0	0	+	+	0	0	0
Medulloblastoma	0	+	±	±	+	+	±	0
Meningioma	0	+	±[a]	Rare	0	0	0	+
Neuroblastoma	0	+	+	±	+	+	0	±
Neurofibroma	0	+	0	+	0	0	±	+
Oligodendroglioma	0	0	±	+	0	0	±	0
Paraganglioma	0	0	0	±[b]	0	+	0	0
Schwannoma	0	+	0	+	0	0	0	0

[a]Secretory type of meningioma.
[b]Sustentacular cells surrounding the zellballen are S100 +.

VI. GERM CELL TUMORS

Tumor	CK	CD30	PLAP	OCT4	CD117	HCG	AFP	EMA
Choriocarcinoma	I	0	+	0	0	+	0	±
Embryonal carcinoma[a]	+	+	+	+	0	0[a]	±	0
Seminoma	±	0	+	+	+	0[a]	0	0
Sertoli-Leydig[b]	Weak	0	0	0	0	0	0	+
Teratoma	+	0	0	0	±	0	±	0
Yolk sac tumor	+	0	+	0	±	0	+	0

[a]Positive in syncytiocytotrophoblasts.
[b]Sertoli-Leydig: Inh +, Vim +, Des +, S100 +.

VII. SKIN TUMORS

Tumor	CK 7/20	CAM 5.2[a]	CK 903[b]	EMA	BerEP4	S100	MEL	NET
Melanoma	0/0	0	0	0	0	+	+	0
Basal cell carcinoma	0/0	0	0	0	+	0	0	0
Squamous cell carcinoma	0/0	0	+	0	+	0	0	0
Merkel cell carcinoma	0/+	0	0	0	+	0	0	±
Paget disease	+/0	+	0	+	+	±	0	0

[a]Low-molecular-weight keratin.
[b]High-molecular-weight keratin.

See footnote to all parts of Appendix C4 at end of C4.IX.

Appendix C4 **Expected Immunophenotypes of Tumors (*Continued*)**

VIII. SPINDLE CELL TUMORS OF SKIN

Tumor	CK	Vim	Des	S100	CD34	SMA
Dermatofibrosarcoma protuberans	0	+	0	0	+	0
Leiomyosarcoma	0	+	+	0	0	+
Melanoma, spindle cell	0	+	0	+	0	0
Small cell carcinoma, spindle cell	+	0	0	0	0	0

IX. TUMORS OF UNKNOWN ORIGIN

CK7	CK20	Carcinoma	Additional markers
+	+	Ovarian mucinous Gastric (30%) Pancreatic Transitional cell	CA 125 –, mCEA + mCEA + CA 19-9 +, BerEP4 +, mCEA +; see IV CK5/6 +
0	+	Gastric (40%) Colorectal Merkel cell	mCEA + CEA +, CDX2 + NET +
+	0	GYN serous GYN endometrioid Breast, ductal Breast, lobular Gastric (20%) Bile ducts Lung adenocarcinoma Mesothelioma Thyroid, follicular/papillary Thyroid, medullary Renal cell (chromophobe)	CA 125 +, p53 +, mCEA – CA 125 +, Vim +, Inh – mCEA +, GCDFP +; E-cadherin + mCEA +, GCDFP +; E-cadherin – mCEA + CA 19-9 +, CA 125 +, BerEP4 +, mCEA +; See IV TTF-1 +, mCEA +; CDX2 – Calretinin +, CK5/6 +; mCEA –, TTF1 – TTF-1 +, Thyg +, Calc – TTF-1 +, Thyg –, Calc +, NET +, mCEA + mCEA –, Vim –, CD10 –, RCC –, HCl +
0	0	Ovarian Granulosa cell Hepatocellular Prostate Small cell Squamous cell Renal cell (clear cell) Renal (oncocytoma) Renal cell (chromophobe)	Cam 5.2 (punctate), GCDFP –; Inh + HepPar1 +, AFP +; CA 19-9 –, BerEP4 –; See IV PSA +, PAP +, AMACR + NET +, mCEA ±, pankeratin (punctate) ± CK5/6 + mCEA –, Vim +, CD10 +, RCC + mCEA –, Vim –, CD10 ±, RCC–, HCl – mCEA –, Vim –, CD10 –, RCC ±, HCl +

Key to all parts of Appendix C4: +, Positive; – or 0, negative; AFP, α-fetoprotein; AMACR, P504S α-methylacyl-CoA racemase; CA, cancer antigen; Calc, calcitonin; CD, clusters of differentiation; CD45, leukocyte common antigen (LCA); CEA, carcinoembryonic antigen; CK, cytokeratins; Des, desmin; EMA, epithelial membrane antigen; GCDFP, gross cystic disease fluid protein-15; GFAP, glial fibrillary acid protein; GYN, gynecologic cancers; HCG, human chorionic gonadotropin; HCl, Hales colloidal iron; HepPar-1, hepatocyte paraffin-1; Inh, inhibin; LCA, leukocyte common antigen (CD45); mCEA, monoclonal CEA; MEL, melanocyte markers, which include HMB-45 and Mart-1 (Melan-A); Musc, muscle markers (Des, MSA, MyoD1); MyoD1, striated muscle specific; MSA, muscle-specific actin (especially smooth muscle); NET, neuroendocrine tumor markers, which include neuron-specific enolase (NSE), chromogranin, and synaptophysin (Syn), CD56, and CD57; Oct4, octamer transcription factor 4; PAP, prostatic acid phosphatase; pCEA, polyclonal CEA; PLAP, placental alkaline phosphatase; PNET, primitive neuroectodermal tumor; PSA, prostate-specific antigen; RCC, renal cell carcinoma; S100, S100 protein; SMA, smooth muscle actin; Thyg, thyroglobulin; TTF-1, thyroid transcription factor-1; TFE3, thyroid transcription factor-E3; Vim, vimentin; vWF, von Willebrand factor (factor VIII-related antigen).

Appendix C5 Discriminatory Immunophenotypes for Lymphocytic Neoplasms

Cells or neoplasm	Positive	Negative
B Cells	CD10, 19, 20*, 22, 23, 45RA, 79a; Pax-5 *Generally absent following anti-CD20 (rituximab) therapy	
Precursor B-lymphoblastic leukemia/lymphoma	CD10, 19, 79a, [CD20, 22, 34]; HLA-DR, Pax-5, Tdt	
CLL/SLL, B-cell prolymphocytic leukemia	CD5, 19, 20, 23, 38**, 43, [CD11c]; BCL-2, Zap-70** **Defines a group with more aggressive disease	CD10; FMC7
Lymphoplasmacytic lymphoma	CD19, 20, 22	CD5, 10
Follicular lymphomas (FL)	CD10, 19, 20, 22; BCL-2, BCL-6	CD5, 11c, 23, 43
Marginal zone lymphomas (MALT)	CD19, 20, 22, [CD11c, 43]	CD5, 10, 23, 103
Hairy cell leukemia (HCL)	CD11c, 19, 20, 25, 103; FMC7; TRAP	CD5, 10, 23
Mantle cell lymphoma (MCL)	CD5, 19, 20, 43; FMC7; Cyclin D1, BCL-2	CD11c, 23, 25
Diffuse large B-cell lymphoma (DLBCL)	CD19, 20, 22, [CD10, BCL-2, BCL-6, Mum-1]	CD5
Mediastinal large B-cell lymphoma	CD19, 20, 23, 30 (weak), 79a	Igs, CD5, 10
Intravascular large B-cell lymphoma	CD5 (many cases), 19, 20, 22, 79a,	
Burkitt lymphoma	CD10, 19, 20, 22 [21]; BCL-6, Ki67 (100%), c-Myc rearrangement	CD5, 23, Tdt, BCL-2, Mum-1
Primary effusion lymphoma	CD30, 45, 138; EBER, HHV8, EMA	CD19, 20, 22, 79a
Plasma cell myeloma	CD10, 38, 43, 56, 138 (syndecan-1) [Cyclin D1] Cytoplasmic light/heavy chain	[CD45, 79a]
T Cells	CD1, 2, 3, 4, 5, 7, 8, 43, 45RO	
Precursor T-lymphoblastic leukemia/lymphoma	CD2, 3, 5, 7, [CD1a, 4, 8]; Tdt	
Adult T-cell leukemia/lymphoma	CD2, 3, 4, 5, 25; HTLV-1	CD7, 8, 16, 56, 57
T-cell prolymphocytic leukemia	CD2, 3, 4, 5, 7, [CD8]	CD1a, Tdt, HLA-DR

Large granular lymphocyte
leukemia
   T-cell type
   NK-cell type
	
	CD2, 3, 5, 7, 8, 11c, 57; TIA-1
	CD2, 7, 11c, 16, 56, 57; TIA-1
		
		CD4
		CD3, 4, 5

(continued)

Appendix C5 | **Discriminatory Immunophenotypes for Lymphocytic Neoplasms (Continued)**

Cells or neoplasm	Positive	Negative
Peripheral T-cell lymphoma, unspecified	CD2, 3, 5, 7, [CD4 > CD8] loss of pan-T antigens common;	
Anaplastic large cell lymphoma (ALCL)	CD2, 4, 25, 30, 43, [CD3, 45]; ALK-1, TIA-1, EMA; loss of pan-T antigens common	CD5, 7
Angioimmunoblastic T-cell lymphoma	CD3, 10, [CD2, 3, 5, 7], CD4 > CD8, Bcl-6, EBER, loss of pan-T antigens common,	
Extranodal NK/T-cell lymphoma, nasal type	CD2, CD3-cytoplasmic, CD56, EBER, TIA-1	CD3 (surface), CD4, 5, 8
Hepatosplenic T-cell lymphoma	CD2, 3, 7, [56]; TIA-1, TCRγδ	CD4, 5, 8, TCRαβ
Enteropathy-type T-cell lymphoma	CD2, 3, 7,11c, 43, 30, 103, [CD8]	CD4, 5
Subcutaneous panniculitis–like T-cell lymphoma	CD3, 8; TIA-1	CD4
Mycosis fungoides and Sézary syndrome	CD2, 3, 4, 5, 25**, 45RO **Defines a group with more aggressive disease	CD7, 8, 25
Hodgkin Lymphoma (HL)		
L & H cell of "nodular lymphocyte-predominant" type	CD20, 45, 79a, [EMA], Pax-5, Oct2, BOB.1	CD15, 30
Reed-Sternberg cells of classical HL	CD15, 30, [20], Pax-5	CD45; EMA, ALK-1, Oct2, BOB.1

[X], occasionally positive.
ALK-1, anaplastic lymphoma kinase [upregulated by t(2;5) in ALCL]; BCL, breakpoint cluster location (BCL-2 is positive in MCL, most FL, CLL/SLL, and some DLBCL, BCL-6 is positive in FL and some DLBCL); BOB.1 positive in Reed-Sternberg cells of lymphocyte-predominant Hodgkin lymphoma; CD, clusters of differentiation; CD45, leukocyte common antigen (LCA); CLL/SLL, chronic lymphocytic leukemia/small lymphocytic lymphoma; Cyclin D1 (BCL-1) is positive in MCL, some HCL, and plasma cell malignancies; EBER, Epstein-Barr virus–encoded RNA; EMA, epithelial membrane antigen; FMC7, B-cell surface antigen found on mantle cell lymphoma, follicular lymphoma, and HCL; HHV8, human herpesvirus type 8; HLA-DR, Human leukocyte antigen-DR; HTLV-1, human T-cell lymphotropic virus type I; Igs, immunoglobulins; L & H, lymphocytic and histiocytic; Mum-1, multiple myeloma oncogene-1; NK, natural killer; OCT2 positive in Reed-Sternberg cells of lymphocyte predominant Hodgkin lymphoma; Pax-5, pan-B antigen positive in B-cell lymphomas and in lymphocyte-predominant and classical Hodgkin lymphomas; TCR, T-cell receptor protein (TCRαβ recognizes αβ chains of the TCR, TCRγδ recognizes the γδ chains of the TCR); Tdt, terminal deoxytransferase (positive in cortical thymic lymphoid cells and lymphoblastic neoplasms); TIA-1, T-cell intracellular antigen (found in cytotoxic T-cell and NK-cell cytoplasmic granules); TRAP, tartrate-resistant acid phosphatase.

Appendix C6 Classification of Lymphoproliferative Disorders

I. WORLD HEALTH ORGANIZATION CLASSIFICATION OF NEOPLASTIC DISEASES OF LYMPHOID TISSUES[a]

B-Cell neoplasms	%NHL	Variants [synonyms]
Precursor B-Cell Neoplasms		
Precursor B-cell lymphoblastic leukemia/lymphoma[H]		[B-cell ALL; lymphoblastic lymphoma]
Mature B-Cell Neoplasms		
Diffuse large B-cell lymphoma (LBCL)[M]	30.6	Centroblastic; anaplastic LBCL; immunoblastic; T-cell/histiocyte-rich; plasmablastic; lymphomatoid granulosis-type
Mediastinal (thymic) LBCL[M]	2.4	[Mediastinal large cell lymphoma]
Intravascular LBCL[M,H]	—	
Primary effusion lymphoma[H]	—	[Body cavity–based lymphoma]
Follicular lymphoma[L] (Grades 1, 2, and 3)	22.1	Diffuse follicular center cell lymphoma (FCC); cutaneous FCC
Marginal zone B-cell lymphoma (MZL)		
Extranodal MZL of mucosa-associated lymphoid tissue[L]	7.6	[MALToma]
Nodal MZL[L]	1.8	[Monocytoid B-cell lymphoma]
Splenic MZL[L]	—	Splenic lymphoma with/without villous lymphocytes
Mantle cell lymphoma[M]	6.0	Blastoid
Chronic lymphocytic leukemia (CLL)[L]/ small lymphocytic lymphoma[L] (SLL)	6.7	[CLL, SLL]
Lymphoplasmacytic lymphoma[L] [Waldenström macroglobulinemia]	1.2	
B-cell prolymphocytic leukemia[M]	—	
Hairy cell leukemia[L]	—	[Leukemic reticuloendotheliosis]
Burkitt lymphoma/leukemia[H] (Subtypes: Endemic, Sporadic, AIDS-associated)	2.5	Classical; atypical with plasmacytoid differentiation (AIDS-associated)
B-Cell Proliferations of Uncertain Malignant Potential		
Lymphomatoid granulomatosis (grades 1–3)		[Angiocentric immunoproliferative lesion]
Posttransplant lymphoproliferative disorder		
Plasma Cell Neoplasms		
Monoclonal gammopathy of undetermined significance (MGUS)		[Benign monoclonal gammopathy, MGUS]
Plasma cell myeloma (multiple myeloma)		Indolent, smoldering, nonsecretory; plasma cell leukemia
Osteosclerotic myeloma		[POEMS syndrome]
Plasmacytomas		Solitary plasmacytoma of bone; extraosseous plasmacytoma
Immunoglobulin deposition diseases		Primary amyloidosis; monoclonal light chain deposition disease
Heavy chain disease (HCD)		γ-HCD, α-HCD, μ-HCD

(*continued*)

Appendix C6 Classification of Lymphoproliferative Disorders (*Continued*)

B-Cell neoplasms	%NHL	Variants [synonyms]
Hodgkin Lymphoma (HL)		
Nodular lymphocyte predominant HL		[Nodular L & H]
Classical HL (CHL)		
Nodular sclerosis CHL		
Mixed cellularity CHL		
Lymphocyte-rich CHL		
Lymphocyte-depleted CHL		

T-Cell and NK-Cell neoplasms	%NHL	Variants [synonyms]
Precursor T-Cell Neoplasms		
Precursor T-cell lymphoblastic leukemia/lymphoma[H]	1.7	T-cell ALL; T-lymphoblastic lymphoma
Mature T-Cell and NK-Cell Neoplasms		
Adult T-cell leukemia/lymphoma (HTLV-1)	<1	Acute[H], lymphomatous[H], chronic[L], smoldering[L], Hodgkin-like
Aggressive NK cell leukemia[H]	—	
Blastic NK cell leukemia[H]	—	
T-cell prolymphocytic leukemia[H]	—	Small cell, "cerebriform" cell
T-cell large granular lymphocytic leukemia[M]	—	
Peripheral T-cell lymphoma, unspecified[H]	3.7	
Anaplastic large cell lymphoma (ALCL)[L,M]	2.4	Common; lymphohistiocytic; small cell; ALK-positive, ALK-negative,
Angioimmunoblastic T-cell lymphoma[M,H]	1.2	
Extranodal NK/T-cell lymphoma, nasal-type[M,H]	1.4	[Lethal midline granuloma]
Hepatosplenic T-cell lymphoma[M,H]	<1	
Enteropathy-type T-cell lymphoma[M]	<1	
Mycosis fungoides (MF)[L] and Sézary syndrome[M]	—	Pagetoid reticulosis; MF-associated follicular mucinosis; Granulomatous slack skin
Subcutaneous panniculitis–like T-cell lymphoma[M]	—	
Primary cutaneous CD30-positive T-cell lymphoproliferative disorders[M]	—	Lymphomatoid papulosis (LyP); Primary cutaneous ALCL; Borderline
Incidence of all nonspecified NHL types	7.4	

ALK, anaplastic lymphoma kinase; ALL, acute lymphoblastic leukemia; AIDS, acquired immunodeficiency syndrome; HTLV-1, human T-cell lymphotropic virus type I; L & H, lymphocytic and histiocytic; NHL, non-Hodgkin lymphoma; NK, natural killer; POEMS, polyneuropathy, organomegaly, endocrinopathy, monoclonal gammopathy, and skin changes.

[a]Lymphoma grades: [L], low; [M], intermediate/high; [H], high.

Extracted from Jaffe ES, Harris NL, Stein H, et al. World Health Organization classification of tumors. Pathology and genetics of tumors of hematopoietic and lymphoid tissue. Lyon, France: IARC Press; 2001.

Appendix C6   Classification of Lymphoproliferative Disorders (*Continued*)

II. WORLD HEALTH ORGANIZATION AND EUROPEAN ORGANIZATION OF RESEARCH AND TREATMENT OF CANCER CLASSIFICATION OF CUTANEOUS LYMPHOMAS WITH PRIMARY CUTANEOUS MANIFESTATIONS

Cutaneous T-cell and NK-cell lymphomas
Mycosis fungoides (MF)
MF variants and subtypes
Folliculotropic MF
  - Pagetoid reticulosis
  - Granulomatous slack skin
Sézary syndrome
Adult T-cell leukemia/lymphoma
Primary cutaneous CD30[+] lymphoproliferative
  disorders
  - Primary cutaneous anaplastic large cell lymphoma
  - Lymphomatoid papulosis
Subcutaneous panniculitis-like T-cell lymphoma
Extranodal NK/T-cell lymphoma, nasal type

Primary cutaneous peripheral T-cell lymphoma,
  unspecified
  - Primary cutaneous aggressive epidermotropic
    CD8[+] T-cell lymphoma (provisional)
  - Cutaneous γ/δ T-cell lymphoma (provisional)
  - Primary cutaneous CD4[+] small/medium-sized
    pleomorphic T-cell lymphoma (provisional)

Cutaneous B-cell lymphomas
Primary cutaneous marginal zone
  B-cell lymphoma
Primary cutaneous follicle center
  lymphoma
Primary cutaneous diffuse large B-cell
  lymphoma, leg type
Primary cutaneous diffuse large B-cell
  lymphoma
  - Intravascular large B-cell
    lymphoma

Precursor hematologic neoplasm
CD4[+]/CD56[+] hematodermic
  neoplasm (blastic NK-cell
  lymphoma)

NK, natural killer.
Abstracted from Willemze R, et al. WHO-EORTC classification for cutaneous lymphomas. *Blood*
2005;105:3768.

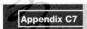

I. ACUTE LEUKEMIAS: CYTOLOGY AND THE WORLD HEALTH ORGANIZATION (WHO) CLASSIFICATION

WHO subtype of acute leukemia	Characteristics of immature cells		Recurrent cytogenetic abnormalities and comments
	Nuclei	Granules, AR	
Acute myeloid leukemia (AML) with t(8;21)	Round, indented	Present,; AR ++	Blasts and early promyelocytes predominate; secondary neutrophil granules present; thin, sharp ends in AR; splenomegaly; MS
Acute promyelocytic leukemia [APL; AML with t(15;17)]	Round, folded, twisted	Large; AR +++	t(15;17), t(11;17), and t(5;17) and variants; "Faggot cells" (bundles of AR); DIC common
APL variant with t(15;17)	Twisted, bilobed	Few; AR +	Submicroscopic size granules gives appearance of their paucity; MPO strongly +; easily mistaken for AMML
AML with 11q23 abnormalities	Round, reniform, folded	Rare, AR −/+	Large cells, monoblastic or myelomonocytic features MPO −, NSE +, associated with topoisomerase II inhibitor therapy, MS
AML with abnormal eosinophils and inv(16) or t(16;16)	Reniform, folded	Variable,	Myelomonocytic morphology, some eosinophil granules are darkly stained, MS
AML, minimally differentiated	Round	Absent; AR—	Confused with ALL and AMegL; requires CD13+, CD33+, or CD117+ to confirm
AML without maturation	Round to indented	Scarce; rare AR	Some cases confused with ALL
AML with maturation	Round to reniform, to PPH	Present; AR +	Cases with increased basophils are associated with t(6;9), and 12p abnormalities
Acute myelomono-cytic leukemia (AMML)	Round to reniform to folded	Present; AR +	Both granulocytic and monocytic differentiation; MS
Acute Monoblastic and Monocytic (AMoL)	Large, round to reniform; large nucleoli	Present; AR—	Monoblastic composed of >80% monoblasts; monocytic composed of >80% promonocytes, MS

(continued)

Appendix C7 Acute Leukemias (*Continued*)

WHO subtype of acute leukemia	Characteristics of immature cells		Recurrent cytogenetic abnormalities and comments
	Nuclei	Granules, AR	
Acute erythroid leukemias (AEL; erythroleukemia and pure erythroid leukemia)	Round	Few; AR +	Erythroleukemia (erythroid/myeloid): ≥50% erythroid precursors and ≥20% myeloblasts in nonerythroid population. Pure erythroid leukemia: >80% erythroid lineage; florid erythroid hyperplasia and dysplasia with bi- and multinucleated, vacuolated forms, and ringed sideroblasts; important to distinguish from megaloblastic anemias
Acute mega-karyoblastic leukemia (AMegL)	Round to indented	Scarce to numerous and fine; AR—	CD41+ & CD61+ (platelet glycoproteins); often with prominent marrow fibrosis
Acute panmyelosis with myelofibrosis	Round to indented	Scarce to numerous	Dry tap, distinguished from AMegL by panmyelosis. Blasts are MPO+, lysozyme+, CD34+, and CD68+
AML with multilineage dysplasia			Dysplasia in two or more myeloid cell lines
Bilineal acute leukemia			Dual populations of blasts, each expressing myeloid or lymphoid markers
Biphenotypic cute leukemia			Blasts express myeloid and B or T markers
AML, therapy-related: alkylating agent-related; topoisomerase II inhibitor-related			
Precursor B lymphoblastic leukemia/ lymphoma	Round, to convoluted	Absent; AR—	Homogeneous cell population (synonymous with ALL)

(*continued*)

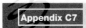

Acute Leukemias (*Continued*)

| WHO subtype of acute leukemia | Characteristics of immature cells | | Recurrent cytogenetic abnormalities and comments |
	Nuclei	Granules, AR	
Precursor T lymphoblastic leukemia/ lymphoma	Round to convoluted	Absent; AR—	Homogeneous cell population (synonymous with T-cell ALL)

+, positive or present;—, negative or absent.
ALL, acute lymphoblastic leukemia; AR, Auer rods; DIC, disseminated intravascular coagulation; MPO, myeloperoxidase; MS, myeloid sarcoma; NSE, nonspecific esterase; PPH, pseudo-Pelger-Huet anomaly.

Appendix C7 **Acute Leukemias (Continued)**

II. ACUTE LEUKEMIAS: CYTOCHEMISTRY AND FLOW CYTOMETRY

WHO subtype[a]	Cytochemistry (Degree of reaction)[b]						Flow cytometry[d]
	MPO	Lyso[c]	NSE	Panmy	HPC	Mono	Other
AML, min diff	A	A	A	+	+	−	CD15−, CD38+; TdT+ in one-third; CD10−, CD20−
AML w/o diff	M	A	A	+	+	−	CD15±; CD10−, CD20−
AML w/diff	S	A	A	+	+		CD15+; CD10−, CD20−
APL, APL variant	S	A	A	+	−	−	CD15− or dim; CD15 never coexpressed with CD34; frequent coexpression of CD2 & CD9; CD10−, CD20−
AMML w/abn BM Eos	M	M	M	+	−	+	Suspect this if CD2+ and coexpressed with myeloid markers; CD10−, CD20−
AMML	M	M	M-S	±	±	+	CD56+, CD64+; CD15+; CD10−, CD20−
AMoL	A	S	S	±	−	+	CD14−, CD4+, CD11b+, CD11c+, CD56+, CD64+, CD68+; CD10−, CD20−
AEL	A-M		A	+	±		Hemoglobin A+, Glycophorin ±, CD36+;CD71+; CD10−, CD20−
AMegL	A	M	M	+	−		CD41+ (GpIIb/IIIa), CD61+ (GpIIIa), CD36+; CD10−, CD20−
Precursor B ALL	A	A	A				See Appendix C5; CD10+, CD19, CD79a, TdT, HLA-DR, PAX-5+
Precursor T ALL	A		A				See Appendix C5; CD2, CD3, CD5, CD7, TdT+

AEL, acute erythroid leukemia; AMegL, acute megakaryoblastic leukemia; AML, acute myeloid leukemia; AMML, acute myelomonocytic leukemia; AMoL, acute monoblastic and monocytic leukemia; APL, acute promyelocytic leukemia; diff, differentiation; Gp, platelet glycoprotein; HPC, hematopoietic progenitor cell antigens CD34, HLA-DR; Lyso, lysozyme (muramidase); Mono, monocytic antigens CD11b, CD14 (also CD4, CD11c, CD56, CD64); MPO, myeloperoxidase and Sudan black B; NSE, nonspecific esterase; Panmy, panmyeloid antigens CD13, CD33, CD117; TdT, terminal deoxytransferase; w/, with; w/abn BM EOS, with abnormal bone marrow eosinophils; w/o, without; WHO, World Health Organization.

[a]Subtypes of AML are described in Appendix C7.I.

[b]A, absent or weak; M, moderate; S, strong.

[c]Increased lysozyme levels are measured in the serum and characterize mixed (AMML) or pure (AMoL) monocytic leukemias.

[d]+, usually positive; −, usually negative or weak; ±, variable.

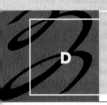

CHEMOTHERAPY REGIMENS FOR LYMPHOMAS

Appendix D1   Regimens for Hodgkin Lymphoma (HL)[a]

Regimen (cycle frequency)	Alkylating agent	Plant alkaloid	Anthracycline or antibiotic	Antimetabolite	Corticosteroid	Other
I. Traditional first-line regimens for HL						
MOPP (28 d)	Mechl 6 [d 1 + 8]	Vcr 1.4 [d 1 + 8]			Pred 40 PO [d 1 → 14]	Pcz 100 PO [d 1 → 14]
COPP (21 d)	Cyclo 400–650 [d 1 + 8]	Vcr 1.4[b] [d 1 + 8]			Pred 40 PO [d 1 → 14]	Pcz 100 PO [d 1 → 14]
ABVD (28 d)		Vbl 6 [d 1 + 15]	Doxo 25 [d 1 + 15] Bleo 10 [d 1 + 15]			DTIC 375 [d 1 + 15]
MOPP–ABVD (alternate cycles of MOPP & ABVD)						
MOPP–ABV Hybrid (28 d)	Mechl 6 [d 1]	Vcr 1.4[b] [d 1] Vbl 6 [d 8]	Doxo 35 [d 8] Bleo 10 [d 8]		Pred 40 PO [d 1 → 14]	Pcz 100 PO [d 1 → 7]
Chl-VPP (28 d)	Chl 6 [d 1 → 14] (Max 10 mg)	Vbl 6 [d 1 + 8] (Max 10 mg)			Pred 40 PO [d 1 → 14]	Pcz 100 PO [d 1 → 14] (Max 150 mg)

II. Dose-intense regimens for HL

Regimen					
Stanford V (28 d)	Mechl 6 [d 1 + 15]	Vbl 6 [d 1 + 15] Vcr 1.4[b] [d 8 + 22] Etop 60 [d 15]	Doxo 25 [d 1 + 15] Bleo 5 [d 8 + 22]	Pred 40 PO [every other day for three cycles]	
BEACOPP (21 d)	Cyclo 650 [d 1]	Etop 100 [d 1 → 3] Vcr 1.4[b] [d 8]	Doxo 25 [d 1] Bleo 10 [d 8]	Pred 40 PO [d 1 → 14]	Pcz 100 PO [d 1 → 7]
BEACOPP escalated (21 d)	Cyclo 1250 [d 1]	Etop 200 [d 1 → 3] Vcr 1.4[b] [d 8]	Doxo 35 [d 1] Bleo 10 [d 8]	Pred 40 PO [d 1 → 14]	Pcz 100 PO [d 1 → 7]

Bleo, bleomycin (dose in units/m^2); Chl, chlorambucil; Cyclo, cyclophosphamide; Doxo, doxorubicin (Adriamycin); DTIC, dacarbazine; Etop, etoposide; Max, maximum dose; Mechl, mechlorethamine (nitrogen mustard); Pcz, procarbazine; Pred, prednisone; Vbl, vinblastine; Vcr, vincristine.
[a]Drugs and dosage in mg/m^2 [days given in cycle]. All doses are given intravenously (IV) except when they are oral (PO), where indicated.
[b]Maximum, 2.0-mg dose.

Appendix D2   Regimens for Non-Hodgkin Lymphoma (NHL)[a]

Regimen (cycle frequency)	Alkylating agent	Plant alkaloid	Anthracycline or antibiotic	Antimetabolite	Corticosteroid	Other
I. Low-grade NHL						
Chl & P (14–28 d)	Chl 16 PO [d 1 or d 1 → 5]				Pred 40 PO [d 1 → 5]	
CVP (21 d)	Cyclo 1000 [d 1] or, Cyclo 400 PO [d 1 → 5]	Vcr 1.4[b] [d 1]			Pred 100[c] PO [d 1 → 5]	
FMD (28 d)			Mitox 10 [d 1]	Flud 25 [d 1 → 3]	Dexa 8–20[c] PO [d 1 → 4]	
II. Intermediate high-grade NHL						
CHOP (21 d)	Cyclo 750 [d 1]	Vcr 1.4[b] [d 1]	Doxo 50 [d 1]		Pred 100[c] PO [d 1 → 5]	
M-BACOD (21 d)	Cyclo 600 [d 1]	Vcr 1.0 [d 1]	Doxo 45 [d 1] Bleo 4 [d 1]	Mtx 3000 [d 14] (monitor Mtx levels)	Dexa 6 PO [d 1 → 5]	Leuc[d] 10 PO q6h × 12 doses
m-BACOD (21 d)	Cyclo 600 [d 1]	Vcr 1.0 [d 1]	Doxo 45 [d 1] Bleo 4 [d 1]	Mtx 200 [d 8 + 15]	Dexa 6 PO [d 1 → 5]	Leuc[d] 10 PO q6h × 8 doses
ProMACE/CytaBOM	Cyclo 650 [d 1]	Vcr 1.4 [d 8] Etop 120 [d 1]	Doxo 25 [d 1] Bleo 5 [d 8]	Mtx 120 [d 8] Cytar 300 [d 8]	Pred 60 PO [d 1 → 14]	Leuc[d] 25 PO q6h × 5 doses
MACOP-B (28 d for 3 cycles)	Cyclo 350 [d 1 + 15]	Vcr 1.4 [d 8 + 22]	Doxo 50 [d 1 + 15] Bleo 10 [d 22]	Mtx 400 [d 8]	Pred 75[c] PO [for 12 weeks, tapered over last 14 d]	Leuc[d] 15[c,d] PO q6h × 6 doses Antimicrobials[e]

III. High-grade NHL (e.g., Mantle cell lymphoma)

CODOX-M/IVAC						
Regimen A: **Codox-M** (2 cycles alternating with Regimen B)	Cyclo 800 [d 1]; Cyclo 200 [d 2 → 5]	Vcr 1.5 [d 1 + 8]	Doxo 40 [d 1]	Mtx 1200 over 1 h, then 240/h × 23 h [d 10]	IT Cytar 70^c [d 1 + 3]; IT Mtx 12^c [d 15]	Leuc^f; GCSF from d 13 until ANC >1,000
Regimen B: **IVAC** (2 cycles alternating with Regimen A)	Ifos 1500 over 1–2 h with Mesna 360 over 1 h q3h [d 1 → 5]	Etop 60 [d 1 → 5]		Cytar 2000 over 1–2 h q12h [d 1 & 2]	IT Mtx 12^c [d 5]	GCSF from d 7 until ANC >1,000
R-HyperCVAD Induction course 1	Cyclo 300 q12h [d 1 → 3]	Vcr 2^c [d 4 + 11]	Doxo 25/d CIV [d 4 + 5]		Dexa 40^c PO or IV [d 1 → 4 & d 11 → 14]	Ritux 375 [d 1 + 8]; GCSF from d 6 until WBC >4,500
R-HyperCVAD Induction course 2				Mtx 200 bolus, then 800 over 24 h [d 1]	Cytar 3000^g over 1 h q12h × 4 doses [d 2 & 3]	Leuc^h; Ritux 375 [d 1]

ANC, absolute neutrophil count per μL; Bleo, Bleomycin (dose in units/m^2); Chl, chlorambucil; Cyclo, cyclophosphamide; Cytar, cytarabine; Dexa, dexamethasone; Doxo, doxorubicin (Adriamycin); Etop, etoposide; Flud, fludarabine; GCSF, granulocyte colony stimulating factor (5 mcg/kg SQ or IV daily); Ifos, ifosfamide; Leuc, leucovorin; Mtx, methotrexate; Pred, prednisone; Ritux, rituximab (Rituxan); Vcr, vincristine; WBC, white blood cell count per μL.

^{a} Drugs and dosage in mg/m^2 [days given in cycle]. All doses are given intravenously (IV) except when they are oral (PO) or intrathecal (IT), where indicated. Rituximab, 375 mg/m^2 weekly for 4 weeks is frequently added to these regimens for CD20-positive NHLs.

^{b} Maximum, 2.0-mg dose.

^{c} Total dose (not per m^2).

^{d} Leucovorin begins at 24 h after Mtx is started.

^{e} Antimicrobials PO daily for 12 weeks: cotrimoxazole 2 b.i.d. and ketoconazole 200 mg qd.

^{f} Leucovorin 192 mg/m^2 given at 36 h after Mtx started, and then 12 mg/m^2 q6h until serum Mtx level $<10^{-8}$ M.

^{g} Reduce cytarabine dosage to 1,000 mg/m^2 per dose for patients older than 60 years or with serum creatinine levels higher than 1.5 mg/dL.

^{h} Leucovorin 50 mg PO given 24 h after Mtx is finished, then 15 mg q6h × 8 doses (adjusted according to serum Mtx level).

Appendix D3   Salvage Regimens for Hodgkin and Non-Hodgkin Lymphoma[a]

Regimen (cycle frequency)	Alkylating agent	Plant alkaloid	Anthracycline/ antibiotic	Other
EPOCH (21 d)	Cyclo 750 IV bolus [d5]	Etop 50/d CIV [d 1 → 4] Vcr 0.4/d CIV [d 1 → 4]	Doxo 10/d CIV [d 1 → 5]	Prednisone 60/d PO [d 1 → 5] GCSF daily d 6 until ANC ≥10,000 Cotrimoxazole 2 tablets b.i.d. × 3 consecutive days/wk Doses modified according to CD4 count in AIDS (see Chapter 36, Section II.F.3)
EVA (28 d)		Etop 100 [d 1 → 3] Vbl 6 [d 1]	Doxo 50 [d 1]	
CEPP-B (28 d)	Cyclo 600 [d 1 + 8]	Etop 70 [d 1 → 3]	Bleo 15 [d 1 → 15]	Prednisone 60 PO [d 1 → 10] Procarbazine 60 [d 1 → 10]
DHAP (21–28 d)	Cispl 100 CIV [d 1]			Cytarabine 2,000 over 2 h q12h [d 2 × 2 doses] Dexamethasone 40[b] [d 1 → 4]
ESHAP (21–28 d)	Cispl 25/d CIV [d 1 → 4]	Etop 40 [d 1 → 4]		Cytarabine 2,000 over 2 h [d 5 × 1 dose] Solu-Medrol 500[b] [d 1 → 4]
VAPEC-B (28 d for total of 3 cycles)	Cyclo 350 [d 1]	Vcr 1.4 [d 8 + 22] Etop 100 [d 15→19]	Doxo 35 [d 1 + 15] Bleo 10 [d 8]	Prednisone 50[b] PO daily × 6 wk, then 25[b] PO daily × 6 wk Cotrimoxazole 2 tablets b.i.d.
ICE (21–28 d)	Ifos 5,000 CIV [d 2]	Etop 100 [d 1 → 3]		Carboplatin AUC = 5 using Calvert's formula [d 2] Mesna 5,000 by 24 h CIV [d 2]
MINE (21–28 d)	Ifos 1,330 over 1 h [d 1 → 3]	Etop 65 [d 1 → 3]	Mitox 8 [d 1]	Mesna 1,330 IV over 1 h with Ifos [d 1 → 3] and 500 mg[b] PO 4 h after Ifos ends

AIDS, acquired immunodeficiency syndrome; ANC, absolute neutrophil count per μL; AUC, area under the curve; b.i.d., twice daily PO; Bleo, bleomycin (dose in units/m²); Cispl, cisplatin; CIV, by 24-h continuous intravenous infusion; Cyclo, cyclophosphamide; Doxo, doxorubicin; Etop, etoposide; GCSF, granulocyte colony-stimulating factor; Ifos, ifosfamide; Mitox, mitoxantrone; Vbl, vinblastine; Vcr, vincristine.

[a]Drugs and dosage in mg/m² [days given in cycle]. All doses are intravenous (IV) bolus except when they are oral (PO) or CIV, where indicated. Rituximab, 375 mg/m² IV is frequently added to these regimens.

[b]Total dose (not per m²).

Page numbers followed by t indicate table; those in *italics* indicate figure.